the calorie carb and fat bible

The UK's Most Comprehensive Calorie Counter

Juliette Kellow BSc RD, Lyndel Costain BSc RD & Rebecca Walton

The Calorie, Carb & Fat Bible

Published by:
Weight Loss Resources Ltd
2C Flag Business Exchange
Vicarage Farm Road
Peterborough
PE1 5TX.

Tel: 01733 345592
www.weightlossresources.co.uk

Companies and other organisations wishing to make bulk purchases of the Calorie, Carb and Fat Bible should contact their local bookstore or Weight Loss Resources direct.

Whilst every effort has been made to ensure accuracy, the publishers cannot be held responsible for any errors or omissions.

ISBN 978-1-904512-20-2

Authors: Lyndel Costain BSc RD
Juliette Kellow BSc RD
Rebecca Walton, Weight Loss Resources

Database Editor: Sam Holt
Design and Layout: Joanne Putney

Printed and bound in the UK

Contents

Losing weight – the easy way

Juliette Kellow BSc RD

PIZZA, curries, chocolate, chips and the odd glass of wine! Imagine being told the best diet to help you lose weight can include all these foods and more. It sounds too good to be true, doesn't it? But the truth is, these are exactly the types of foods you can still enjoy if you opt to lose weight by counting calories.

But you'd be forgiven for not knowing you can still eat all your favourite foods *and* lose weight. In recent years, endless trendy diets that cut carbs, or skip entire groups of foods, have helped to make dieting a complicated business. Added to this, an increasing number of celebrities and so-called nutrition experts have helped mislead us into thinking that dieting is all about restriction and denial. Is it any wonder then that most of us have been left feeling downright confused and miserable about what we should and shouldn't be eating to shift those pounds?

Dieting doesn't have to be complicated or an unhappy experience. In fact, there's really only one word you need to remember if you want to shift those pounds healthily and still eat all your favourite foods. And that's CALORIE!

It's calories that count

When it comes to losing weight, there's no getting away from the fact that it's calories that count. Ask any qualified nutrition expert or dietitian for advice on how to fight the flab and you'll receive the same reply: quite simply you need to create a calorie deficit or shortfall. In other words, you need to take in fewer calories than you use up so that your body has to draw on its fat stores to provide it with the energy it needs to function properly. The result: you start losing fat and the pounds start to drop off!

Fortunately, it couldn't be easier to create this calorie deficit. Regardless of your age, weight, sex, genetic make up, lifestyle or eating habits, losing weight is as simple as reducing your daily calorie intake slightly by modifying your diet and using up a few more calories by being slightly more active each day.

Better still, it's a complete myth that you need to change your eating and exercise habits dramatically. You'll notice I've said you need to reduce your calorie intake 'slightly' and be 'slightly' more active. It really is just LITTLE differences between the amount of calories we take in and the amount we use up that make BIG differences to our waistline over time. For example, you only need to consume one can of cola more than you need each day to gain a stone in a year. It's no wonder then that people say excess weight tends to 'creep up on them'.

10 simple food swaps you can make every day *(and won't even notice!)*

Make these simple swaps every day and in just 4 weeks you'll lose 7lb!

SWAP THIS...	FOR THIS...	SAVE...
300ml full-fat milk (195 calories)	300ml skimmed milk (100 calories)	95 calories
1tsp butter (35 calories)	1tsp low-fat spread (20 calories)	15 calories
1tbsp vegetable oil (100 calories)	10 sprays of a spray oil (10 calories)	90 calories
1tsp sugar (16 calories)	Artificial sweetener (2 calories)	14 calories
1tbsp mayonnaise (105 calories)	1tbsp fat-free dressing (10 calories)	95 calories
Regular sandwich (600 calories)	Low-fat sandwich (350 calories)	250 calories
Can of cola (135 calories)	Can of diet cola (1 calorie)	134 calories
Large (50g) packet of crisps (250 calories)	Small (25g) packet of crisps (125 calories)	125 calories
1 chocolate digestive (85 calories)	1 small chocolate chip cookie (55 calories)	30 calories
1 slice thick-cut wholemeal bread (95 calories)	1 slice medium-cut wholemeal bread (75 calories)	20 calories
	TOTAL CALORIE SAVING:	*868 calories*

The good news is the reverse is also true. You only need to swap that daily can of cola for the diet version or a glass of sparking water and you'll lose a stone in a year – it really is as easy as that!

Of course, most people don't want to wait a year to shift a stone. But there's more good news. To lose 1lb of fat each week you need to create a calorie deficit of just 500 calories a day. That might sound like a lot, but you can achieve this by simply swapping a croissant for a wholemeal fruit scone, a regular sandwich for a low-fat variety, a glass of dry white wine for a gin and slimline tonic and using low-fat spread on two slices of toast instead of butter. It is also important to become more active and increase your level of exercise. Losing 1lb a week, amounts to a stone in 14 weeks, or just under 4 stone in a year!

Taking control of calories

By now you've seen it really is calories that count when it comes to shifting those pounds. So it should be no surprise that a calorie-controlled diet is the only guaranteed way to help you shift those pounds – and that's a scientific fact! But better still, a calorie-controlled diet is one of the few that allows you to include anything, whether it's pizza, wine or chocolate. A healthy diet means including a wide range of foods *(see 'Healthy Eating Made Easy' page 32).*

And that's where this book can really help. Gone are the days when it was virtually impossible to obtain information about the calorie contents of foods. This book provides calorie information for more than 22,000 different branded and unbranded foods so that counting calories has never been easier.

The benefits of counting calories

- *It's guaranteed to help you lose weight providing you stick to your daily calorie allowance*

- *You can include favourite foods*

- *No foods are banned*

- *It's a great way to lose weight slowly and steadily*

- *Nutrition experts agree that it's a proven way to lose weight*

Calorie counting made easy

Forget weird and wacky science, complicated diet rules and endless lists of foods to fill up on or avoid every day! Counting calories to lose weight couldn't be easier. Quite simply, you set yourself a daily calorie allowance to help you lose between ½-2lb (¼-1kg) a week and then add up the calories of everything you eat and drink each day, making sure you don't go over your limit.

To prevent hunger from kicking in, it's best to spread your daily calorie allowance evenly throughout the day, allowing a certain amount of calories for breakfast, lunch, dinner and one or two snacks. For example, if you are allowed 1,500 calories a day, you could have 300 calories for breakfast, 400 calories for lunch, 500 calories for dinner and two snacks or treats of 150 calories each. You'll find more detailed information on p26-31 (Your step-by-step guide to using this book and shifting those pounds).

QUESTION
What affects the calorie content of a food?

ANSWER:
Fat, protein, carbohydrate and alcohol all provide the body with calories, but in varying amounts:

- *1g fat provides 9 calories*

- *1g alcohol provides 7 calories*

- *1g protein provides 4 calories*

- *1g carbohydrate provides 3.75 calories*

The calorie content of a food depends on the amount of fat, protein and carbohydrate it contains. Because fat provides more than twice as many calories as an equal quantity of protein or carbohydrate, in general, foods that are high in fat tend to contain more calories. This explains why 100g of chips (189 calories) contains more than twice as many calories as 100g of boiled potato (72 calories).

DIET MYTH:
Food eaten late at night stops you losing weight

DIET FACT:
It's not eating in the evening that stops you losing weight. It's consuming too many calories throughout the day that will be your dieting downfall! Providing you stick to your daily calorie allowance you'll lose weight, regardless of when you consume those calories. Nevertheless, it's a good idea to spread your calorie allowance throughout the day to prevent hunger from kicking in, which leaves you reaching for high-calorie snack foods.

Eat for good health

While calories might be the buzz word when it comes to shifting those pounds, it's nevertheless important to make sure your diet is healthy, balanced and contains all the nutrients you need for good health. Yes, you can still lose weight by eating nothing but, for example, chocolate, crisps and biscuits providing you stick to your calorie allowance. But you'll never find a nutrition expert or dietitian recommending this. And there are plenty of good reasons why.

To start with, an unbalanced diet is likely to be lacking in essential nutrients such as protein, vitamins, minerals and fibre, in the long term putting you at risk of nutritional deficiencies. Secondly, research proves that filling up on foods that are high in fat and/or salt and sugar can lead to many different health problems. But most importantly, when it comes to losing weight, it's almost impossible to stick to a daily calorie allowance if you're only eating high-calorie foods.

Filling up on lower-calorie foods also means you'll be able to eat far more with the result that you're not constantly left feeling unsatisfied. For example, six chocolates from a selection box contain around 300 calories, a lot of fat and sugar, few nutrients – and are eaten in just six mouthfuls! For 300 calories, you could have a grilled skinless chicken breast (packed with protein and zinc), a large salad with fat-free dressing (a great source of fibre, vitamins and minerals), a slice of wholemeal bread with low-fat spread (rich in fibre and B vitamins) and a satsuma (an excellent source of vitamin C). That's a lot more food that will take you a lot more time to eat! Not convinced? Then put six chocolates on one plate, and the chicken, salad, bread and fruit on another!

Bottom line: while slightly reducing your calorie intake is the key to losing weight, you'll be healthier and far more likely to keep those pounds off if you do it by eating a healthy diet *(see 'Healthy Eating Made Easy' page 32).*

Eight steps to a healthy diet

1 Base your meals on starchy foods.

2 Eat lots of fruit and vegetables.

3 Eat more fish.

4 Cut down on saturated fat and sugar.

5 Try to eat less salt - no more than 6g a day.

6 Get active and try to be a healthy weight.

7 Drink plenty of water.

8 Don't skip breakfast.

SOURCE: www.nhs.uk/Livewell/Goodfood/Pages/eatwell-plate.aspx

Fat facts

Generally speaking, opting for foods that are low in fat can help slash your calorie intake considerably, for example, swapping full-fat milk for skimmed, switching from butter to a low-fat spread, not frying food in oil and chopping the fat off meat and poultry. But don't be fooled into believing that all foods described as 'low-fat' or 'fat-free' are automatically low in calories or calorie-free. In fact, some low-fat products may actually be higher in calories than standard products, thanks to them containing extra sugars and thickeners to boost the flavour and texture. The solution: always check the calorie content of low-fat foods, especially for things like cakes, biscuits, crisps, ice creams and ready meals. You might be surprised to find there's little difference in the calorie content when compared to the standard product.

Uncovering fat claims on food labels

Many products may lure you into believing they're a great choice if you're trying to cut fat, but you need to read between the lines on the labels if you want to be sure you're making the best choice. Here's the lowdown on what to look for:

LOW FAT	by law the food must contain less than 3g of fat per 100g for solids. These foods are generally a good choice if you're trying to lose weight.
REDUCED FAT	by law the food must contain 25 percent less fat than a similar standard product. This doesn't mean the product is low-fat (or low-calorie) though! For example, reduced-fat cheese may still contain 14g fat per 100g.
FAT FREE	the food must contain no more than 0.5g of fat per 100g or 100ml. Foods labelled as Virtually Fat Free must contain less than 0.3g fat per 100g. These foods are generally a good choice if you're trying to lose weight.
LESS THAN 8% FAT	this means the product contains less than 8g fat per 100g. It's only foods labelled 'less than 3% fat' that are a true low-fat choice.
X% FAT FREE	claims expressed as X% Fat Free shall be prohibited.
LIGHT OR LITE	claims stating a product is 'light' or 'lite' follows the same conditions as those set for the term 'reduced'.

10 easy ways to slash fat (and calories)

1 Eat fewer fried foods – grill, boil, bake, poach, steam, roast without added fat or microwave instead.

2 Don't add butter, lard, margarine or oil to food during preparation or cooking.

3 Use spreads sparingly. Butter and margarine contain the same amount of calories and fat – only low fat spreads contain less.

4 Choose boiled or jacket potatoes instead of chips or roast potatoes.

5 Cut off all visible fat from meat and remove the skin from chicken before cooking.

6 Don't eat too many fatty meat products such as sausages, burgers, pies and pastry products.

7 Use semi-skimmed or skimmed milk instead of full-fat milk.

8 Try low-fat or reduced-fat varieties of cheese such as reduced-fat Cheddar, low-fat soft cheese or cottage cheese.

9 Eat fewer high-fat foods such as crisps, chocolates, cakes, pastries and biscuits.

10 Don't add cream to puddings, sauces or coffee.

Getting Ready for Weight Loss Success

Lyndel Costain BSc RD

THIS BOOK not only provides tools to help you understand more about what you eat and how active you are, but guidance on how to use this information to develop a weight loss plan to suit your needs. Getting in the right frame of mind will also be a key part of your weight control journey, especially if you've lost weight before, only to watch the pounds pile back on.

The fact is that most people who want to lose weight know what to do. But often there is something that keeps stopping them from keeping up healthier habits. The same may be true for you. So what's going on? For many it's a lack of readiness. When the next diet comes along with its tempting promises it's so easy to just jump on board. But if you have struggled with your weight for a while, will that diet actually help you to recognise and change the thoughts and actions that have stopped you shifting the pounds for good?

Check out your attitude to weight loss programmes

Before starting any new weight loss programme, including the Weight Loss Resources approach, ask yourself:

Am I starting out thinking that I like myself as a person right now?	(YES or NO)
OR I feel I can only like myself once I lose weight?	(YES or NO)
Do I want to stop overeating, but at the same time find myself justifying it – in other words I want to be able to eat what I want, but with no consequences?	(YES or NO)
Do I believe that I need to take long-term responsibility for my weight?	(YES or NO)
OR Am I relying on 'it' (the diet) to do it for me?	(YES or NO)

Keep these questions, and your replies, in mind as you read through this chapter.

Next Steps

You may have already assessed the healthiness of your weight using the BMI guide on page 37. If not, why not do it now, remembering that the tools are a guide only. The important thing is to consider a weight at which you are healthy and comfortable – and which is realistic for the life you lead *(see opposite - What is a healthy weight?).*

The next step is to have a long hard think about why you want to lose weight. Consider all the possible benefits, not just those related to how you look. Psychologists have found that if we focus only on appearance we are less likely to succeed in the long-term. This is because it so often reflects low self-esteem or self-worth – which can sabotage success – as it saps confidence and keeps us stuck in destructive thought patterns. Identifying key motivations other than simply how you look - such as health and other aspects of physical and emotional well being - is like saying that you're an OK person right now, and worth making changes for. Making healthy lifestyle choices also has the knock on effect of boosting self-esteem further.

Write down your reasons for wanting to lose weight in your Personal Plan *(see page 42)* – so you can refer back to them. This can be especially helpful when the going gets tough. It may help to think of it in terms of what your weight is stopping you from doing now. Here's some examples: to feel more confident; so I can play more comfortably with my kids; my healthier diet will give me more energy; to improve my fertility.

What is a Healthy Weight?

With all the 'thin is beautiful' messages in the media it can be easy to get a distorted view about whether your weight is healthy or not. However, as the BMI charts suggest, there is no single 'ideal' weight for anybody. Research also shows that modest amounts of weight loss can be very beneficial to health and are easier to keep off. Therefore, health professionals now encourage us to aim for a weight loss of 5-10%. The ideal rate of weight loss is no more than 1-2 pounds (0.5-1kg) per week – so averaging a pound a week is great, and realistic progress.

The health benefits of modest weight loss include:

- *Reduced risk of developing heart disease, stroke and certain cancers*

- *Reduced risk of developing diabetes and helping to manage diabetes*

- *Improvements in blood pressure*

- *Improvements in mobility, back pain and joint pain*

- *Improvements with fertility problems and polycystic ovarian syndrome*

- *Less breathlessness and sleep/snoring problems*

- *Increased self esteem and control over eating*

- *Feeling fitter and have more energy*

Are You Really Ready to Lose Weight?

When you think of losing weight, it's easy just to think of what weight you'd like to get to. But weight loss only happens as a result of making changes to your usual eating and activity patterns – which allow you to consume fewer calories than you burn *(see 'It's calories that count' page 5)*.

So here comes the next big question. Are you really ready to do it? Have you thought about the implications of your decision? If you have lost weight in the past, and put it all back on - have you thought about why that was? And how confident do you feel about being successful this time?

To help you answer these questions, try these short exercises.

Where would you place yourself on the following scales?

Importance

How important is it to you, to make the changes that will allow you to lose weight?

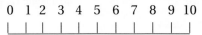

0 1 2 3 4 5 6 7 8 9 10

Not at all important   *Extremely important*

If you ranked yourself over half way along the scale then move on to the next question. If you were half way or less along the scale, you may not be mentally ready to make the required changes to lose weight. To further explore this, go to *'The Pros and Cons of Weight Loss' (page 17)*.

Confidence

How confident are you in your ability to make the changes that will allow you to lose weight?

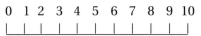

0 1 2 3 4 5 6 7 8 9 10

Not at all confident   *Extremely confident*

Now ask yourself (regarding your confidence ratings):

1. Why did I place myself here?

2. What is stopping me moving further up the scale (if anything)?

3. What things, information, support would help me move further up the scale? (if not near 10)

If you aren't sure about answers to question 3, then keep reading for some pointers.

The Pros and Cons of Weight Loss

Making lifestyle changes to lose weight is simpler if there are lots of clear benefits or pros, for example, clothes fit again, more energy, helps back pain - but there will also be associated downsides or cons. For example, some may feel it interferes with their social life, or don't have the time to plan meals or check food labels. Or overeating can help, if only temporarily, as a way of coping with unwanted feelings. Being overweight allows some people to feel strong and assertive, or to control their partner's jealousy. So in these cases there are downsides to losing weight, even if the person says they are desperate to do it.

If you are aware of the possible downsides, as well as the pros, you will be better prepared to deal with potential conflicts. Understanding what could be (or were with past weight loss efforts) barriers to success gives you the chance to address them. This boosts confidence in your ability to succeed this time, which in turn maintains your motivation.

Have a go at weighing up the pros and cons using the charts below and on page 18. Some examples are included. If you decide that the pros outweigh the cons, then great. You can also use the cons as potential barriers to plan strategies for *(see page 42)*. If you find it's the other way around, this may not be the best time to actively lose weight. Try the exercise again in a month or so.

Making Lifestyle Changes to Lose Weight Now

CONS *e.g. Must limit eating out, take aways*	PROS *e.g. Feel more energetic, slimmer*

Not Making Changes Now – how would I feel in 6 months time?

PROS *e.g. Haven't had to worry about failing;* *Still able to eat take aways a lot*	CONS *e.g. Probably gained more weight;* *Back pain may be worse*

To change your weight, first change your mind

To lose weight you may already have a list of things to change, such as eating more fruit and veg, calculating your daily calorie intake, going for a walk each morning or buying low fat options. Others could also give you tips to try. But knowing what to do isn't the same as feeling motivated or able to do it. To be effective, you have to believe the changes are relevant, do-able and worth it.

What you think, affects how you feel, and in turn the actions you take.

Self-efficacy

In fact, research is telling us that one of the most important factors that influences weight loss success are your feelings of 'self-efficacy'. Self-efficacy is a term used in psychology to describe a person's belief that any action they take will have an effect on the outcome. It reflects our inner expectation that what we do will lead to the results we want. Not surprisingly, high levels of self-efficacy can enhance motivation, and allow us to deal better with uncertainty and conflict, and recovery from setbacks. But low levels, can reduce our motivation. We fear that whatever we do will not bring about our desired goal. This can lead self-defeating thoughts or 'self-talk', which make it hard to deal with set-backs, meaning we are more likely to give up. Here's some examples.

Examples: Low self-efficacy

'*No matter how carefully I diet, I don't lose weight . . .*'

'*I have eaten that chocolate and as usual blown my diet, so I may as well give up now.*'

'*I had a rich dessert – I have no willpower to say no. I can't stand not being able to eat what I want.*'

If you have a strong sense of self-efficacy, your mindset and 'self-talk' will be more like:

Examples: High self-efficacy

'*I know from previous weight loss programmes, that if I stay focussed on what I am doing I do lose weight. I have always expected to lose too much too quickly which frustrates me. I know that I will lose weight if I keep making the right changes, and this time it is important to me.*'

'*The chocolate bar won't ruin my diet, but if I think it has and keep on eating, then my negative self-talk will. So I will get back on track.*'

'*I don't like having to eat differently from others, but losing weight is very important to me, so I **can** stand it. After all, the world won't stop if I say no to dessert, and I will feel great afterwards. If I think about it, I am not hungry so would just feel bloated and guilty if I ate it.*'

Willpower is a Skill

Many people feel that they just need plenty of willpower or a good telling off to lose weight. But willpower isn't something you have or you don't have. Willpower is a skill. Like the dessert example on page 19, it's a sign that you've made a conscious choice to do something, because you believe the benefits outweigh any downsides. In reality everything we do is preceded by a thought. This includes everything we eat. It just may not seem like it because our actions often feel automatic *(see 'Look out for trigger eating' page 21)*.

When it comes to weight loss, developing a range of skills – including choosing a lower calorie diet, coping with negative self-talk and managing things that don't go to plan - will boost your sense of self-efficacy to make the changes you want. This is especially important because we live in such a weight-promoting environment.

Our weight-promoting environment

We are constantly surrounded by tempting food, stresses that can trigger comfort eating and labour-saving devices that make it easy not to be physically active. In other words, the environment we live in makes it easy to gain weight, unless we stop and think about the food choices we make and how much exercise we do. In fact, to stay a healthy weight/maintain our weight, just about all of us need to make conscious lifestyle choices everyday. This isn't 'dieting' but just part of taking care of ourselves in the environment we live in.

It is also true that some people find it more of a challenge than others to manage their weight, thanks to genetic differences in factors such as appetite control, spontaneous activity level and emotional responses to food – rather than metabolic rate, as is often believed. The good news is that with a healthy diet and active lifestyle a healthier weight can still be achieved. But do talk to your doctor if you feel you need additional support.

Coping with Common Slimming Saboteurs

Lyndel Costain BSc RD

Look out for 'trigger' eating

Much of the overeating we do or cravings we have are actually down to unconscious, habitual, responses to a variety of triggers. These triggers can be external, such as the sight or smell of food, or internal and emotion-led, such as a response to stress, anger, boredom or emptiness. Your food diary (see page 43) helps you to recognise 'trigger' or 'non-hungry' eating which gives you the chance to think twice before you eat (see below).

Get some support

A big part of your success will be having someone to support you. It could be a friend, partner, health professional, health club or website. Let them know how they can help you most.

Make lapses your ally

Don't let a lapse throw you off course. You can't be, nor need to be perfect all the time. Doing well 80-90% of the time is great progress. Lapses are a normal part of change. Rather than feel you have failed and give up, look at what you can learn from a difficult day or week and use it to find helpful solutions for the future.

Understand why you eat

When I ask people what prompts them to eat, hunger usually comes down near the bottom of their list of reasons. Some people struggle to remember or appreciate what true hunger feels like. We are lucky that we have plenty of food to eat in our society. But its constant presence makes it harder to control what we eat, especially if it brings us comfort or joy.

If you ever find yourself in the fridge even though you've recently eaten, then you know hunger isn't the reason but some other trigger. The urge to eat can be so automatic that you feel you lack willpower or are out of control. But it is in fact a learned or conditioned response. A bit like Pavlov's dogs. He rang a bell every time he fed them, and from then on, whenever they heard the bell ring they were 'conditioned' to salivate in anticipation of food.

Because this 'non-hungry' eating is learned, you can reprogramme your response to the situations or feelings that trigger it. The first step is to identify when these urges strike. When you find yourself eating when you aren't hungry ask yourself 'why do I want to eat, what am I feeling?' If you aren't sure think back to what was happening before you ate. Then ask yourself if there is another way you can feel better without food. Or you could chat to your urge to eat in a friendly way, telling it that you don't want to give into it, you have a planned meal coming soon, and it's merely a learned response. Whatever strategy you choose, the more often you break into your urges to eat, the weaker their hold becomes.

Practise positive self-talk

Self-talk may be positive and constructive (like your guardian angel) or negative and irrational (like having a destructive devil on your shoulder).

If you've had on-off battles with your weight over the years, it's highly likely that the 'devil' is there more often. 'All or nothing' self-talk for example, 'I ate a "bad food" so have broken my diet', can make you feel like a failure which, can then trigger you into the action of overeating and/or totally giving up *(see 'Diet-binge cycle' page 23)*. One of the most powerful things about it is that the last thoughts we have are what stays in our mind. So if we think 'I still look fat' or 'I will never be slim', these feelings stay with us.

To change your self-talk for the better, the trick is to first recognise it's happening (keeping a diary really helps, *see Keep a Food Diary, page 29*). Then turn it around into a positive version of the same events *(see Self-efficacy, page 18)* where the resulting action was to feel good and stay on track. Reshaping negative self-talk helps you to boost your self-esteem and feelings of self-efficacy, and with it change your self-definition - from someone who can't 'lose weight' or 'do this or that', to someone 'who can'. And when you believe you can…

The Diet – Binge Cycle

If this cycle looks familiar, use positive self-talk, and a more flexible dietary approach, to help you break free.

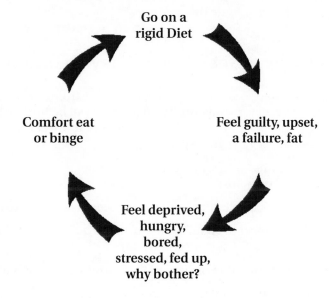

Go on a rigid Diet

Feel guilty, upset, a failure, fat

Feel deprived, hungry, bored, stressed, fed up, why bother?

Comfort eat or binge

Really choose what you want to eat

This skill is like your personal brake. It also helps you to manage 'trigger/non-hungry' eating and weaken its hold. It legalises food and stops you feeling deprived. It helps you to regularly remind yourself why you are making changes to your eating habits, which keeps motivation high. But it doesn't just happen. Like all skills it requires practise. Sometimes it will work well for you, other times it won't – but overall it will help. Basically, ask yourself if you really want to eat that food in front of you. This becomes the prompt for you to make a conscious choice, weighing up the pros and cons or consequences of making that choice, and feeling free to have it, reject it or just eat some. Remembering all the while that you can eat this food another time if you want to.

Action Planning

Successful people don't just wait for things to happen. They believe in themselves, plan ahead, take action and then refine their plan until it gets, and keeps on getting the results they want. Successful slimmers use a very similar approach. They don't rely on quick-fixes or magic formulas, but glean information from reliable sources to develop a plan or approach that suits their needs, tastes and lifestyle. Thinking of weight management as a lifelong project, which has a weight loss phase and a weight maintenance phase, is also a route to success.

When the Going Gets Tough - Staying on Track

If things start to go off track, don't panic. Learning new habits takes time. And life is never straightforward so there will be times when it all seems too much, or negative 'self- talk' creeps in to try and drag you back into old ways. So if the going gets tough:

- Value what you've achieved so far, rather than only focus on what you plan to do.

- Look back at your reasons to lose weight and refer to the list often.

- Don't expect to change too much, too quickly. Take things a step at a time.

- Accept difficulties as part of the learning and skill building process.

- Enjoy a non-food reward for achieving your goals (including maintaining your weight).

- Use recipes and meal ideas to keep things interesting.

- Talk to your supporters and get plenty of encouragement. This is really vital!

Strategies of Successful Slimmers

Thanks to research conducted by large studies such as the US National Weight Control Registry and the German Lean Habits Study, we now know more about what works best for people who have lost weight and successfully kept it off. So be inspired!

The key elements of success are to:

- Believe that you can control your weight and the changes involved are really worth it.
- Stay realistic and value what you have achieved rather than dwell on a weight you 'dream' of being.
- Be more active – plan ways to fit activity into your daily life – aim for 1 hour of walking daily.
- Plan ahead for regular meals and snacks, starting with breakfast.
- Choose a balanced, low-fat diet with plenty of fruit and vegetables *(see Healthy Eating Made Easy, page 32).*
- Watch portion size and limit fast food.
- Sit down to eat and take time over meals, paying attention to what you are eating.
- Have a flexible approach – plan in and enjoy some favourite foods without guilt.
- Recognise and address 'all or nothing' thinking and other negative 'self-talk'.
- Keep making conscious choices.
- Learn to confront problems rather than eat, drink, sleep or wish they would go away.
- Enlist ongoing help and support from family, friends, professionals or websites.
- Regularly (at least once a week but not more than once daily) check your weight.
- Take action before your weight increases by more than 4-5lb (2kg).
- Accept that your weight management skills need to be kept up long-term.
- Take heart from successful slimmers, who say that it gets easier over time.

Your step-by-step guide to using this book and shifting those pounds

Juliette Kellow BSc RD and Rebecca Walton

1. Find your healthy weight

Use the weight charts, body mass index table and information on pages 36-43 to determine the right weight for you. Then set yourself a weight to aim for. Research shows it really helps if you make losing 10% of your weight your first overall target. It also brings important health benefits too *(see 'What is a Healthy Weight?' page 15)*. You can break this down into smaller manageable steps, for example, 3kg/6.5lbs at a time. If 10% is too much, then go for a 5% loss – this has important health benefits too. In fact, just keeping your weight stable is a great achievement these days, because of our weight-promoting environment *(see page 20)*.

Waist Management

In addition to BMI, another important way to assess your weight is by measuring your waist just above belly button level. It is especially useful for men as they tend to carry more excess weight around their bellies, but women should test it out too. Having excess weight around your middle (known as being 'apple-shaped') increases your risk of heart disease and type 2 diabetes. A simple way to stay aware of your waist is according to how well, or otherwise, skirts and trousers fit. Talk to your doctor about any weight and health concerns.

WAIST MEASUREMENT

	Increased Health Risk	High Risk to Health
Women	32-35in (81-88cm)	more than 35in (88cm)
Men	37-40in (94-102cm)	more than 40in (102cm)

---

2. Set a realistic time scale

With today's hectic lifestyles, everything tends to happen at breakneck speed, so it's no wonder that when it comes to losing weight, most of us want to shift those pounds in an instant. But it's probably taken years to accumulate that extra weight, with the result that it's unrealistic to expect to lose the excess in just a few weeks! Instead, prepare yourself to lose weight slowly and steadily. It's far healthier to lose weight like this. But better still, research shows you'll be far more likely to maintain your new, lower weight.

If you only have a small amount of weight to lose, aim for a weight loss of around 1lb (½kg) a week. But if you have more than 2 stone (28kg) to lose, you may prefer to aim for 2lb (1kg) each week. Remember though, it's better to keep going at 1lb (½kg) a week than to give up because trying to lose 2lb (1kg) a week is making you miserable! The following words may help you to keep your goal in perspective:

'Never give up on a goal because of the time it will take to achieve it – the time will pass anyway.'

Weight Fluctuations

Weight typically fluctuates on a day to day basis. You know that shock/horror feeling when you weigh yourself in the morning then later in the day, or after a meal out, and it looks like youve gained pounds in hours! But this is due to fluid not fat changes. Real changes in body fat can only happen more gradually (remember, to gain 1lb you need to eat 3500 calories more than you usually do). Don't be confused either by seemingly very rapid weight loss in the first week or so.

When calorie intake is initially cut back, the body's carbohydrate stores in the liver and muscles (known as glycogen) are used up. Glycogen is stored with three times its weight in water, meaning that rapid losses of 4.5- 6.6lb (2 -3 kg) are possible. These stores can be just as rapidly refilled if normal eating is resumed. True weight loss happens more gradually and this book helps you to lose weight at the steady and healthy rate of no more than 1-2 lbs per week.

3. Calculate your calorie allowance

Use the calorie tables on pages 39-40 to find out how many calories you need each day to maintain your current weight. Then use the table below to discover the amount of calories you need to subtract from this amount every day to lose weight at your chosen rate. For example, a 35 year-old woman who is moderately active and weighs 12 stone (76kg) needs 2,188 calories a day to keep her weight steady. If she wants to lose ½lb (¼kg) a week, she needs 250 calories less each day, giving her a daily calorie allowance of 1,938 calories. If she wants to lose 1lb (½kg) a week, she needs 500 calories less each day, giving her a daily calorie allowance of 1,688 calories, and so on.

TO LOSE...	Cut your daily calorie intake by	In three months you could lose...	In six months you could lose...	In one year you could lose...
½lb a week	250	6.5lb	13lb	1st 12lb
1lb a week	500	13lb	1st 12lb	3st 10lb
1½lb a week	750	1st 5.5lb	2st 11lb	5st 8lb
2lb a week	1,000	1st 12lb	3st 10lb	7st 6lb

TO LOSE...	Cut your daily calorie intake by	In three months you could lose...	In six months you could lose...	In one year you could lose...
¼kg a week	250	3.25kg	6.5kg	13kg
½kg a week	500	6.5kg	13kg	26kg
¾kg a week	750	9.75kg	19.5kg	39kg
1kg a week	1,000	13kg	26kg	52kg

4. Keep a food diary

Writing down what you eat and drink and any thoughts linked to that eating helps you become more aware of your eating habits. Recognising what is going on helps you feel in control and is a powerful way to start planning change. Keeping a food diary before you start to change your eating habits will also help you identify opportunities for cutting calories by substituting one food for another, cutting portion sizes of high-calorie foods or eating certain foods less often. Simply write down every single item you eat or drink during the day and use this book to calculate the calories of each item. Then after a few days of eating normally, introduce some changes to your diet to achieve your daily calorie allowance. Remember to spread your daily calorie allowance fairly evenly throughout the day to prevent hunger. You'll find a template for a daily food and exercise diary on page 43. Try to use it as carefully as you can as research shows that people who do, do best.

Top Tip

If you only fill in your main food diary once a day, keep a pen and notepad with you to write down all those little extras you eat or drink during the day – that chocolate you ate in the office, the sliver of cheese you had while cooking dinner and the few chips you pinched from your husband's plate, for example! It's easy to forget the little things if they're not written down, but they can make the difference between success and failure.

QUESTION: Why are heavier people allowed more calories than those who have smaller amounts of weight to lose?

ANSWER: This confuses a lot of people but is easily explained. Someone who is 3 stone overweight, for example, is carrying the equivalent of 42 small packets of butter with them everywhere they go – up and down the stairs, to the local shops, into the kitchen. Obviously, it takes a lot more energy simply to move around when you're carrying that extra weight. As a consequence, the heavier you are, the more calories you need just to keep your weight steady. In turn, this means you'll lose weight on a higher calorie allowance. However, as you lose weight, you'll need to lower your calorie allowance slightly as you have less weight to carry around.

5. Control your portions

As well as making some smart food swaps to cut calories, it's likely you'll also need to reduce your serving sizes for some foods to help shift those pounds. Even 'healthy' foods such as brown rice, wholemeal bread, chicken, fish and low-fat dairy products contain calories so you may need to limit the amount you eat. When you first start out, weigh portions of foods like rice, pasta, cereal, cheese, butter, oil, meat, fish, and chicken rather than completing your food diary with a 'guesstimated' weight! That way you can calculate the calorie content accurately. Don't forget that drinks contain calories too, alcohol, milk, juices and sugary drinks all count.

6. Measure your success

Research has found that regular weight checks do help. Weighing yourself helps you assess how your eating and exercise habits affect your body weight. The important thing is to use the information in a positive way – to assess your progress - rather than as a stick to beat yourself up with. Remember that weight can fluctuate by a kilogram in a day, for example, due to fluid changes, premenstrually, after a big meal out, so weigh yourself at the same time of day and look at the trend over a week or two.

People who successfully lose weight and keep it off, also tend to continue weighing themselves at least once a week, and often daily (but not in an obsessive way), because they say it helps them stay 'on track'. Probably because they use it as an early warning system. People who weigh themselves regularly (or regularly try on a tight fitting item of clothing) will notice quickly if they have gained a couple of kilograms and can take action to stop gaining more. Checking your weight less often can mean that you might discover one day that you gained 6kg. That can be pretty discouraging, and it might trigger you to just give up.

Top Tip

Don't just focus on what the bathroom scales say either – keep a record of your vital statistics, too. Many people find it doubly encouraging to see the inches dropping off, as well as the pounds!

7. Stay motivated

Each time you lose half a stone, or reach your own small goal – celebrate! Treat yourself to a little luxury – something new to wear, a little pampering or some other (non-food) treat. It also helps replace the comfort you once got from food and allows you to take care of yourself in other ways. Trying on an item of clothing that used to be tight can also help to keep you feeling motivated. Make sure you keep in touch with your supporters, and if the going gets tough take another look at the *'Coping with Common Slimming Saboteurs' section on page 21*. Once you've reviewed how well you've done, use this book to set yourself a new daily calorie allowance based on your new weight to help you lose the next half stone *(see point 3 - page 28 - Calculate your calorie allowance)*.

8. Keep it off

What you do to stay slim is just as important as what you did to get slim. Quite simply, if you return to your old ways, you are likely to return to your old weight. The great thing about calorie counting is that you will learn so much about what you eat, and make so many important changes to your eating and drinking habits, that you'll probably find it difficult to go back to your old ways – and won't want to anyway. It's still a good idea to weigh yourself at least once a week to keep a check on your weight. The key is to deal with any extra pounds immediately, rather than waiting until you have a stone to lose *(see page 30)*. Simply go back to counting calories for as long as it takes to shift those pounds and enjoy the new slim you. Page 25 has more information about how successful slimmers keep it off.

QUESTION: Do I need to stick to exactly the same number of calories each day or is it OK to have a lower calorie intake during the week and slightly more at the weekend?

ANSWER: The key to losing weight is to take in fewer calories than you need for as long as it takes to reach your target, aiming for a loss of no more than 2lb (1kg) a week. In general, most nutrition experts recommend a daily calorie allowance. However, it's just as valid to use other periods of time such as weeks. If you prefer, simply multiply your daily allowance by seven to work out a weekly calorie allowance and then allocate more calories to some days than others. For example, a daily allowance of 1,500 calories is equivalent to 10,500 calories a week. This means you could have 1,300 calories a day during the week and 2,000 calories a day on Saturday and Sunday.

Healthy Eating Made Easy

Juliette Kellow BSc RD

GONE ARE THE DAYS when a healthy diet meant surviving on bird seed, rabbit food and carrot juice! The new approach to eating healthily means we're positively encouraged to eat a wide range of foods, including some of our favourites – it's just a question of making sure we don't eat high fat, high sugar or highly processed foods too often.

Eating a healthy diet, together with taking regular exercise and not smoking, has huge benefits to our health, both in the short and long term. As well as helping us to lose or maintain our weight, a healthy diet can boost energy levels, keep our immune system strong and give us healthy skin, nails and hair. Meanwhile, eating well throughout life also means we're far less likely to suffer from health problems such as constipation, anaemia and tooth decay or set ourselves up for serious conditions in later life such as obesity, heart disease, stroke, diabetes, cancer or osteoporosis.

Fortunately, it couldn't be easier to eat a balanced diet. To start with, no single food provides all the calories and nutrients we need to stay healthy, so it's important to eat a variety of foods. Meanwhile, most nutrition experts also agree that mealtimes should be a pleasure rather than a penance. This means it's fine to eat small amounts of our favourite treats from time to time.

To help people eat healthily, the Food Standards Agency recommends eating plenty of different foods from four main groups of foods and limiting the amount we eat from a smaller fifth group. Ultimately, we should eat more fruit, vegetables, starchy, fibre-rich foods and fresh products, and fewer fatty, sugary, salty and processed foods.

The following guidelines are all based on the healthy eating guidelines recommended by the Food Standards Agency.

Bread, other cereals and potatoes

Eat these foods at each meal. They also make good snacks.

Foods in this group include bread, breakfast cereals, potatoes, rice, pasta, noodles, yams, oats and grains. Go for high-fibre varieties where available, such as wholegrain cereals, wholemeal bread and brown rice. These foods should fill roughly a third of your plate at mealtimes.

TYPICAL SERVING SIZES

* *2 slices bread in a sandwich or with a meal*

* *a tennis ball sized serving of pasta, potato, rice, noodles or couscous*

* *a bowl of porridge*

* *around 40g of breakfast cereal*

Fruit and vegetables

Eat at least five portions every day.

Foods in this group include all fruits and vegetables, including fresh, frozen, canned and dried products, and unsweetened fruit juice. Choose canned fruit in juice rather than syrup and go for veg canned in water without added salt or sugar.

TYPICAL PORTION SIZES

* *a piece of fruit eg: apple, banana, pear*

* *2 small fruits eg: satsumas, plums, apricots*

* *a bowl of fruit salad, canned or stewed fruit*

* *a small glass of unsweetened fruit juice*

* *a cereal bowl of salad*

* *3tbsp vegetables*

Milk and dairy foods

Eat two or three servings a day.

Foods in this group include milk, cheese, yoghurt and fromage frais. Choose low-fat varieties where available such as skimmed milk, reduced-fat cheese and fat-free yoghurt.

TYPICAL SERVING SIZES

- *200ml milk*

- *a small pot of yoghurt or fromage frais*

- *a small matchbox-sized piece of cheese*

Meat, fish and alternatives

Eat two servings a day

Foods in this group include meat, poultry, fish, eggs, beans, nuts and seeds. Choose low-fat varieties where available such as extra-lean minced beef and skinless chicken and don't add extra fat or salt.

TYPICAL SERVING SIZES

- *a piece of meat, chicken or fish the size of a deck of cards*

- *1-2 eggs*

- *3 heaped tablespoons of beans*

- *a small handful of nuts or seeds*

Healthy Eating on a plate

A simple way to serve up both balance and healthy proportions is to fill one half of your plate with salad or vegetables and divide the other half between protein-rich meat, chicken, fish, eggs or beans, and healthy carbs (potatoes, rice, pasta, pulses, bread or noodles).

Fatty and sugary foods

Eat only small amounts of these foods

Foods in this group include oils, spreading fats, cream, mayonnaise, oily salad dressings, cakes, biscuits, puddings, crisps, savoury snacks, sugar, preserves, confectionery and sugary soft drinks.

TYPICAL SERVING SIZES:

- *a small packet of sweets or a small bar of chocolate*
- *a small slice of cake*
- *a couple of small biscuits*
- *1 level tbsp mayo, salad dressing or olive oil*
- *a small packet of crisps*

Useful Tools

Body Mass Index

The Body Mass Index (BMI) is the internationally accepted way of assessing how healthy our weight is. It is calculated using an individual's height and weight. Use the Body Mass Index Chart to look up your BMI, and use the table below to see what range you fall into.

BMI Under 18.5	*Underweight*
BMI 18.5-25	*Healthy*
BMI 25-30	*Overweight*
BMI 30-40	*Obese*
BMI Over 40	*Severely Obese*

This is what different BMI ranges mean.

- **Underweight:** you probably need to gain weight for your health's sake. Talk to your doctor if you have any concerns, or if you feel frightened about gaining weight.

- **Healthy weight:** you are a healthy weight, so aim to stay in this range (note that most people in this range tend to have a BMI between 20-25).

- **Overweight:** aim to lose some weight for your health's sake, or at least prevent further weight gain.

- **Obese:** your health is at risk and losing weight will benefit your health.

- **Severely obese:** your health is definitely at risk. You should visit your doctor for a health check. Losing weight will improve your health.

Please note that BMI is not as accurate for athletes or very muscular people (muscle weighs more than fat), as it can push them into a higher BMI category despite having a healthy level of body fat. It is also not accurate for women who are pregnant or breastfeeding, or people who are frail.

Body Mass Index Table

HEIGHT IN FEET / INCHES

WEIGHT IN STONES / LBS	4'6	4'8	4'10	5'0	5'2	5'4	5'6	5'8	5'10	6'0	6'2	6'4	6'6	6'8	6'10
6st 7	22.0	20.5	19.1	17.8	16.7	15.7	14.7	13.9	13.1	12.4	11.7	11.1	10.6	10.0	9.5
7st 0	23.7	22.1	20.6	19.2	18.0	16.9	15.9	15.0	14.1	13.3	12.6	12.0	11.4	10.8	10.3
7st 7	25.4	23.6	22.0	20.6	19.3	18.1	17.0	16.0	15.1	14.3	13.5	12.8	12.2	11.6	11.0
8st 0	27.1	25.2	23.5	22.0	20.6	19.3	18.1	17.1	16.1	15.2	14.4	13.7	13.0	12.3	11.8
8st 7	28.8	26.8	25.0	23.3	21.8	20.5	19.3	18.2	17.1	16.2	15.3	14.5	13.8	13.1	12.5
9st 0	30.5	28.4	26.4	24.7	23.1	21.7	20.4	19.2	18.1	17.2	16.2	15.4	14.6	13.9	13.2
9st 7	32.2	29.9	27.9	26.1	24.4	22.9	21.5	20.3	19.2	18.1	17.1	16.2	15.4	14.7	14.0
10st 0	33.9	31.5	29.4	27.4	25.7	24.1	22.7	21.4	20.2	19.1	18.0	17.1	16.2	15.4	14.7
10st 7	35.6	33.1	30.8	28.8	27.0	25.3	23.8	22.4	21.2	20.0	18.9	18.0	17.0	16.2	15.4
11st 0	37.3	34.7	32.3	30.2	28.3	26.5	24.9	23.5	22.2	21.0	19.8	18.8	17.9	17.0	16.2
11st 7	39.0	36.2	33.8	31.6	29.6	27.7	26.1	24.6	23.2	21.9	20.7	19.7	18.7	17.8	16.9
12st 0	40.7	37.8	35.2	32.9	30.8	28.9	27.2	25.6	24.2	22.9	21.6	20.5	19.5	18.5	17.6
12st 7	42.3	39.4	36.7	34.3	32.1	30.1	28.3	26.7	25.2	23.8	22.5	21.4	20.3	19.3	18.4
13st 0	44.0	41.0	38.2	35.7	33.4	31.4	29.5	27.8	26.2	24.8	23.5	22.2	21.1	20.1	19.1
13st 7	45.7	42.5	39.6	37.0	34.7	32.6	30.6	28.8	27.2	25.7	24.4	23.1	21.9	20.8	19.8
14st 0	47.4	44.1	41.1	38.4	36.0	33.8	31.7	29.9	28.2	26.7	25.3	23.9	22.7	21.6	20.6
14st 7	49.1	45.7	42.6	39.8	37.3	35.0	32.9	31.0	29.2	27.6	26.2	24.8	23.5	22.4	21.3
15st 0	50.8	47.3	44.0	41.2	38.5	36.2	34.0	32.0	30.2	28.6	27.1	25.7	24.4	23.2	22.0
15st 7	52.5	48.8	45.5	42.5	39.8	37.4	35.2	33.1	31.2	29.5	28.0	26.5	25.2	23.9	22.8
16st 0	54.2	50.4	47.0	43.9	41.1	38.6	36.3	34.2	32.3	30.5	28.9	27.4	26.0	24.7	23.5
16st 7	55.9	52.0	48.5	45.3	42.4	39.8	37.4	35.2	33.3	31.4	29.8	28.2	26.8	25.5	24.2
17st 0	57.6	53.6	49.9	46.6	43.7	41.0	38.6	36.3	34.3	32.4	30.7	29.1	27.6	26.2	25.0
17st 7	59.3	55.1	51.4	48.0	45.0	42.2	39.7	37.4	35.3	33.3	31.6	29.9	28.4	27.0	25.7
18st 0	61.0	56.7	52.9	49.4	46.3	43.4	40.8	38.5	36.3	34.3	32.5	30.8	29.2	27.8	26.4
18st 7	62.7	58.3	54.3	50.8	47.5	44.6	42.0	39.5	37.3	35.3	33.4	31.6	30.0	28.6	27.2
19st 0	64.4	59.9	55.8	52.1	48.8	45.8	43.1	40.6	38.3	36.2	34.3	32.5	30.8	29.3	27.9
19st 7	66.1	61.4	57.3	53.5	50.1	47.0	44.2	41.7	39.3	37.2	35.2	33.3	31.7	30.1	28.6
20st 0	67.8	63.0	58.7	54.9	51.4	48.2	45.4	42.7	40.3	38.1	36.1	34.2	32.5	30.9	29.4
20st 7	69.4	64.6	60.2	56.3	52.7	49.4	46.5	43.8	41.3	39.1	37.0	35.1	33.3	31.6	30.1
21st 0	71.1	66.2	61.7	57.6	54.0	50.6	47.6	44.9	42.3	40.0	37.9	35.9	34.1	32.4	30.9
21st 7	72.8	67.7	63.1	59.0	55.3	51.9	48.8	45.9	43.3	41.0	38.8	36.8	34.9	33.2	31.6
22st 0	74.5	69.3	64.6	60.4	56.5	53.1	49.9	47.0	44.4	41.9	39.7	37.6	35.7	34.0	32.3
22st 7	76.2	70.9	66.1	61.7	57.8	54.3	51.0	48.1	45.4	42.9	40.6	38.5	36.5	34.7	33.1
23st 0	77.9	72.5	67.5	63.1	59.1	55.5	52.2	49.1	46.4	43.8	41.5	39.3	37.3	35.5	33.8
23st 7	79.6	74.0	69.0	64.5	60.4	56.7	53.3	50.2	47.4	44.8	42.4	40.2	38.2	36.3	34.5
24st 0	81.3	75.6	70.5	65.9	61.7	57.9	54.4	51.3	48.4	45.7	43.3	41.0	39.0	37.0	35.3
24st 7	83.0	77.2	71.9	67.2	63.0	59.1	55.6	52.3	49.4	46.7	44.2	41.9	39.8	37.8	36.0
25st 0	84.7	78.8	73.4	68.6	64.2	60.3	56.7	53.4	50.4	47.6	45.1	42.8	40.6	38.6	36.7
25st 7	86.4	80.3	74.9	70.0	65.5	61.5	57.8	54.5	51.4	48.6	46.0	43.6	41.4	39.4	37.5
26st 0	88.1	81.9	76.3	71.3	66.8	62.7	59.0	55.5	52.4	49.5	46.9	44.5	42.2	40.1	38.2
26st 7	89.8	83.5	77.8	72.7	68.1	63.9	60.1	56.6	53.4	50.5	47.8	45.3	43.0	40.9	38.9
27st 0	91.5	85.1	79.3	74.1	69.4	65.1	61.2	57.7	54.4	51.5	48.7	46.2	43.8	41.7	39.7
27st 7	93.2	86.6	80.8	75.5	70.7	66.3	62.4	58.7	55.4	52.4	49.6	47.0	44.7	42.4	40.4
28st 0	94.9	88.2	82.2	76.8	72.0	67.5	63.5	59.8	56.4	53.4	50.5	47.9	45.5	43.2	41.1
28st 7	96.5	89.8	83.7	78.2	73.2	68.7	64.6	60.9	57.5	54.3	51.4	48.7	46.3	44.0	41.9
29st 0	98.2	91.4	85.2	79.6	74.5	69.9	65.8	62.0	58.5	55.3	52.3	49.6	47.1	44.8	42.6
29st 7	99.9	92.9	86.6	80.9	75.8	71.1	66.9	63.0	59.5	56.2	53.2	50.5	47.9	45.5	43.3

Weight Chart

BMI

Underweight
BMI less than 18.5

HEALTHY
WEIGHT
BMI 18.5-25

Overweight
BMI 25-30

Obese
BMI 30-40

Severely
Obese
BMI 40 or more

BMI: 10 11 12 13 14 15 16 17 18 19 20 21 22 23 24 25 26 27 28 29 30 31 32 33 34 35 36 37 38

Heights:
6ft 6" / 197.5cm
6ft 5" / 195cm
6ft 4" / 192.5cm
6ft 3" / 190cm
6ft 2" / 187.5cm
6ft 1" / 185cm
6ft 0" / 182.5cm
5ft 11" / 180cm
5ft 10" / 177.5cm
5ft 9" / 175cm
5ft 8" / 172.5cm
5ft 7" / 170cm
5ft 6" / 167.5cm
5ft 5" / 165cm
5ft 4" / 162.5cm
5ft 3" / 160cm
5ft 2" / 157.5cm
5ft 1" / 155cm
5ft 0" / 152.5cm
4ft 11" / 150cm
4ft 10" / 147.5cm
4ft 9" / 145cm
4ft 8" / 142.5cm
4ft 7" / 140cm
4ft 6" / 137.5cm

Weights:
23st 7lb / 149kg
23st 0lb / 146kg
22st 7lb / 143kg
22st 0lb / 140kg
21st 7lb / 137kg
21st 0lb / 133kg
20st 7lb / 130kg
20st 0lb / 127kg
19st 7lb / 124kg
19st 0lb / 121kg
18st 7lb / 118kg
18st 0lb / 114kg
17st 7lb / 111kg
17st 0lb / 108kg
16st 7lb / 105kg
16st 0lb / 102kg
15st 7lb / 98kg
15st 0lb / 95kg
14st 7lb / 92kg
14st 0lb / 89kg
13st 7lb / 86kg
13st 0lb / 83kg
12st 7lb / 79kg
12st 0lb / 76kg
11st 7lb / 73kg
11st 0lb / 70kg
10st 7lb / 67kg
10st 0lb / 64kg
9st 7lb / 60kg
9st 0lb / 57kg
8st 7lb / 54kg
8st 0lb / 51kg
7st 7lb / 48kg
7st 0lb / 45kg
6st 7lb / 41kg
6st 0lb / 38kg
5st 7lb / 35kg
5st 0lb / 32kg
4st 7lb / 29kg

Calories Required to Maintain Weight
Adult Females

ACTIVITY LEVEL / AGE

WEIGHT IN STONES / LBS	VERY SEDENTARY			MODERATELY SEDENTARY			MODERATELY ACTIVE			VERY ACTIVE		
	<30	30-60	60+	<30	30-60	60+	<30	30-60	60+	<30	30-60	60+
7st 7	1425	1473	1304	1544	1596	1412	1781	1841	1630	2138	2210	1956
8st 0	1481	1504	1338	1605	1629	1450	1852	1880	1673	2222	2256	2008
8st 7	1537	1535	1373	1666	1663	1487	1922	1919	1716	2306	2302	2059
9st 0	1594	1566	1407	1726	1696	1524	1992	1957	1759	2391	2349	2111
9st 7	1650	1596	1442	1787	1729	1562	2062	1996	1802	2475	2395	2163
10st 0	1706	1627	1476	1848	1763	1599	2133	2034	1845	2559	2441	2214
10st 7	1762	1658	1511	1909	1796	1637	2203	2073	1888	2644	2487	2266
11st 0	1819	1689	1545	1970	1830	1674	2273	2111	1931	2728	2534	2318
11st 7	1875	1720	1580	2031	1863	1711	2344	2150	1975	2813	2580	2370
12st 0	1931	1751	1614	2092	1897	1749	2414	2188	2018	2897	2626	2421
12st 7	1987	1781	1648	2153	1930	1786	2484	2227	2061	2981	2672	2473
13st 0	2044	1812	1683	2214	1963	1823	2555	2266	2104	3066	2719	2525
13st 7	2100	1843	1717	2275	1997	1861	2625	2304	2147	3150	2765	2576
14st 0	2156	1874	1752	2336	2030	1898	2695	2343	2190	3234	2811	2628
14st 7	2212	1905	1786	2397	2064	1935	2766	2381	2233	3319	2858	2680
15st 0	2269	1936	1821	2458	2097	1973	2836	2420	2276	3403	2904	2732
15st 7	2325	1967	1855	2519	2130	2010	2906	2458	2319	3488	2950	2783
16st 0	2381	1997	1890	2580	2164	2047	2976	2497	2362	3572	2996	2835
16st 7	2437	2028	1924	2640	2197	2085	3047	2535	2405	3656	3043	2887
17st 0	2494	2059	1959	2701	2231	2122	3117	2574	2449	3741	3089	2938
17st 7	2550	2090	1993	2762	2264	2159	3187	2613	2492	3825	3135	2990
18st 0	2606	2121	2028	2823	2298	2197	3258	2651	2535	3909	3181	3042
18st 7	2662	2152	2062	2884	2331	2234	3328	2690	2578	3994	3228	3093
19st 0	2719	2182	2097	2945	2364	2271	3398	2728	2621	4078	3274	3145
19st 7	2775	2213	2131	3006	2398	2309	3469	2767	2664	4162	3320	3197
20st 0	2831	2244	2166	3067	2431	2346	3539	2805	2707	4247	3366	3249
20st 7	2887	2275	2200	3128	2465	2383	3609	2844	2750	4331	3413	3300
21st 0	2944	2306	2235	3189	2498	2421	3680	2882	2793	4416	3459	3352
21st 7	3000	2337	2269	3250	2531	2458	3750	2921	2836	4500	3505	3404
22st 0	3056	2368	2303	3311	2565	2495	3820	2960	2879	4584	3552	3455
22st 7	3112	2398	2338	3372	2598	2533	3890	2998	2923	4669	3598	3507
23st 0	3169	2429	2372	3433	2632	2570	3961	3037	2966	4753	3644	3559
23st 7	3225	2460	2407	3494	2665	2608	4031	3075	3009	4837	3690	3611
24st 0	3281	2491	2441	3554	2699	2645	4101	3114	3052	4922	3737	3662
24st 7	3337	2522	2476	3615	2732	2682	4172	3152	3095	5006	3783	3714
25st 0	3394	2553	2510	3676	2765	2720	4242	3191	3138	5091	3829	3766
25st 7	3450	2583	2545	3737	2799	2757	4312	3229	3181	5175	3875	3817
26st 0	3506	2614	2579	3798	2832	2794	4383	3268	3224	5259	3922	3869
26st 7	3562	2645	2614	3859	2866	2832	4453	3307	3267	5344	3968	3921
27st 0	3618	2676	2648	3920	2899	2869	4523	3345	3310	5428	4014	3973
27st 7	3675	2707	2683	3981	2932	2906	4594	3384	3353	5512	4060	4024
28st 0	3731	2738	2717	4042	2966	2944	4664	3422	3397	5597	4107	4076
28st 7	3787	2768	2752	4103	2999	2981	4734	3461	3440	5681	4153	4128

Calories Required to Maintain Weight
Adult Males

ACTIVITY LEVEL / AGE

WEIGHT IN STONES / LBS	VERY SEDENTARY			MODERATELY SEDENTARY			MODERATELY ACTIVE			VERY ACTIVE		
	<30	30-60	60+	<30	30-60	60+	<30	30-60	60+	<30	30-60	60+
9st 0	1856	1827	1502	2010	1979	1627	2320	2284	1878	2784	2741	2254
9st 7	1913	1871	1547	2072	2026	1676	2391	2338	1933	2870	2806	2320
10st 0	1970	1914	1591	2134	2074	1724	2463	2393	1989	2955	2871	2387
10st 7	2027	1958	1636	2196	2121	1772	2534	2447	2045	3041	2937	2454
11st 0	2084	2001	1680	2258	2168	1820	2605	2502	2100	3127	3002	2520
11st 7	2141	2045	1724	2320	2215	1868	2677	2556	2156	3212	3067	2587
12st 0	2199	2088	1769	2382	2262	1916	2748	2611	2211	3298	3133	2654
12st 7	2256	2132	1813	2444	2310	1965	2820	2665	2267	3384	3198	2720
13st 0	2313	2175	1858	2506	2357	2013	2891	2719	2322	3470	3263	2787
13st 7	2370	2219	1902	2568	2404	2061	2963	2774	2378	3555	3329	2854
14st 0	2427	2262	1947	2630	2451	2109	3034	2828	2434	3641	3394	2920
14st 7	2484	2306	1991	2691	2498	2157	3106	2883	2489	3727	3459	2987
15st 0	2542	2350	2036	2753	2545	2205	3177	2937	2545	3813	3525	3054
15st 7	2599	2393	2080	2815	2593	2253	3248	2992	2600	3898	3590	3120
16st 0	2656	2437	2125	2877	2640	2302	3320	3046	2656	3984	3655	3187
16st 7	2713	2480	2169	2939	2687	2350	3391	3100	2711	4070	3721	3254
17st 0	2770	2524	2213	3001	2734	2398	3463	3155	2767	4155	3786	3320
17st 7	2827	2567	2258	3063	2781	2446	3534	3209	2823	4241	3851	3387
18st 0	2884	2611	2302	3125	2828	2494	3606	3264	2878	4327	3917	3454
18st 7	2942	2654	2347	3187	2876	2542	3677	3318	2934	4413	3982	3520
19st 0	2999	2698	2391	3249	2923	2591	3749	3373	2989	4498	4047	3587
19st 7	3056	2741	2436	3311	2970	2639	3820	3427	3045	4584	4112	3654
20st 0	3113	2785	2480	3373	3017	2687	3891	3481	3100	4670	4178	3721
20st 7	3170	2829	2525	3434	3064	2735	3963	3536	3156	4756	4243	3787
21st 0	3227	2872	2569	3496	3112	2783	4034	3590	3211	4841	4308	3854
21st 7	3285	2916	2614	3558	3159	2831	4106	3645	3267	4927	4374	3921
22st 0	3342	2959	2658	3620	3206	2880	4177	3699	3323	5013	4439	3987
22st 7	3399	3003	2702	3682	3253	2928	4249	3754	3378	5098	4504	4054
23st 0	3456	3046	2747	3744	3300	2976	4320	3808	3434	5184	4570	4121
23st 7	3513	3090	2791	3806	3347	3024	4392	3862	3489	5270	4635	4187
24st 0	3570	3133	2836	3868	3395	3072	4463	3917	3545	5356	4700	4254
24st 7	3627	3177	2880	3930	3442	3120	4534	3971	3600	5441	4766	4321
25st 0	3685	3220	2925	3992	3489	3168	4606	4026	3656	5527	4831	4387
25st 7	3742	3264	2969	4054	3536	3217	4677	4080	3712	5613	4896	4454
26st 0	3799	3308	3014	4116	3583	3265	4749	4135	3767	5699	4962	4521
26st 7	3856	3351	3058	4177	3630	3313	4820	4189	3823	5784	5027	4587
27st 0	3913	3395	3103	4239	3678	3361	4892	4243	3878	5870	5092	4654
27st 7	3970	3438	3147	4301	3725	3409	4963	4298	3934	5956	5158	4721
28st 0	4028	3482	3191	4363	3772	3457	5035	4352	3989	6042	5223	4787
28st 7	4085	3525	3236	4425	3819	3506	5106	4407	4045	6127	5288	4854
29st 0	4142	3569	3280	4487	3866	3554	5177	4461	4101	6213	5354	4921
29st 7	4199	3612	3325	4549	3913	3602	5249	4516	4156	6299	5419	4987
30st 0	4256	3656	3369	4611	3961	3650	5320	4570	4212	6384	5484	5054

Calories Burned in Exercise

This table shows the approximate number of extra* calories that would be burned in a five minute period of exercise activity.

ACTIVITY	CALORIES BURNED IN 5 MINUTES	ACTIVITY	CALORIES BURNED IN 5 MINUTES
Aerobics, Low Impact	25	Situps, Continuous	17
Badminton, Recreational	17	Skiing, Moderate	30
Cross Trainer	30	Skipping, Moderate	30
Cycling, Recreational, 5mph	17	Squash Playing	39
Dancing, Modern, Moderate	13	Tennis Playing, Recreational	26
Fencing	24	Toning Exercises	17
Gardening, Weeding	19	Trampolining	17
Hill Walking, Up and Down, Recreational	22	Volleyball, Recreational	10
Jogging	30	Walking, Uphill, 15% Gradient, Moderate	43
Kick Boxing	30	Walking Up and Down Stairs, Moderate	34
Netball Playing	23	Walking, 4mph	24
Rebounding	18	Weight Training, Moderate	12
Roller Skating	30	Yoga	13
Rowing Machine, Moderate	30		
Running, 7.5mph	48		

*Extra calories are those in addition to your normal daily calorie needs.

My Personal Plan

Date: _____

Body Mass Index: _____

Weight: _____

Waist Measurement: _____

Height: _____

Body Fat % (if known) _____

10% Weight Loss Goal: _____

Current weight	16stone (224lb)	100kg
- 10% weight	1stone 8½lb (22½lb)	10kg
= 10% loss goal	14stone 5½lb (201½lb)	90kg

My smaller weight targets on the way to achieving my 10% goal will be:

_____ _____ _____ _____

Reasons why I want to lose weight:

_____

Changes I will make to help me lose weight:

Diet:

_____

_____

_____

Activity:

_____

_____

_____

Potential saboteurs or barriers will be:

_____

_____

_____

Ways I will overcome these:

_____

_____

_____

My supporters will be:

_____

I will monitor my progress by:

_____

_____

_____

_____

I will reward my progress with:

In the short term:

_____

_____

In the long term:

_____

_____

Food and Exercise Diary

Date:

| / / |

Daily Calorie Allowance: [ ] **A**

Food/Drink Consumed	Serving Size	Calories

Total calories consumed [ ] **B**

Exercise/Activity	No. mins	Calories

Calories used in exercise [ ] **C**

Calorie balance [ ] **D**

You are aiming for your Calorie Balance (Box D) to be as close to zero as possible - ie. you consume the number of calories you need.

Your Daily Calorie Allowance (Box A) should be set to lose ½-2lb (¼-1kg) a week, or maintain weight, depending on your goals.

Daily Calorie Allowance (A) *plus* Extra Calories used in Exercise (C) *minus* Total Calories Consumed (B) *equals* Calorie Balance (D)

$A + C - B = D$

You can also write down any comments or thoughts related to your eating if you want to.

Food Information

Nutritional Information

CALORIE AND FAT values are given per serving, plus calorie and nutrition values per 100g of product. This makes it easy to compare the proportions of fat, protein, carbohydrate and fibre in each food.

The values given are for uncooked, unprepared foods unless otherwise stated. Values are also for only the edible portion of the food unless otherwise stated. ie - weighed with bone.

Finding Foods

The Calorie, Carb & Fat Bible has an Eating Out section which is arranged alphabetically by brand. In the General Foods and Drinks A-Z most foods are grouped together by type, and then put in to alphabetical order. This makes it easy to compare different brands, and will help you to find lower calorie and/or fat alternatives where they are available.

This format also makes it easier to locate foods. Foods are categorised by their main characteristics so, for example, if it is bread, ciabatta or white sliced, you'll find it under "Bread".

Basic ingredients are highlighted to make them easier to find at a glance. You'll find all unbranded foods in bold - making the index easier to use, whether it's just an apple or all the components of a home cooked stew.

There are, however, some foods which are not so easy to categorise, especially combination foods like ready meals. The following pointers will help you to find your way around the book until you get to know it a little better.

FILLED ROLLS AND SANDWICHES - Bagels, baguettes, etc which are filled are listed as "Bagels (filled)" etc. Sandwiches are under "Sandwiches".

CURRIES - Popular types of curry, like Balti or Jalfrezi, are listed under their individual types. Unspecified or lesser known types are listed under their main ingredient.

BURGERS - All burgers, including chicken-type sandwiches from fast-food outlets, are listed under "Burgers". CHIPS & FRIES - Are listed separately, depending on the name of the particular brand. All other types of potato are listed under "Potatoes".

SWEETS & CHOCOLATES - Well-known brands, eg. Aero, Mars Bar, are listed under their brand names. Others are listed under "Chocolate" (for bars) and "Chocolates" (for individual sweets).

READY MEALS - Popular types of dishes are listed under their type, eg. "Chow Mein", "Casserole", "Hot Pot", etc. Others are listed by their main ingredient, eg. "Chicken With", "Chicken In", etc.

EATING OUT & FAST FOODS - By popular demand this edition has the major eating out and fast food brands listed separately, at the back of the book. They are alphabetised first by brand, then follow using the same format as the rest of the book, with calories provided per serving.

Serving Sizes

Many ready-meal type foods are given with calories for the full pack size, so that an individual serving can be worked out by estimating the proportion of the pack that has been consumed. For example, if you have eaten a quarter of a packaged pasta dish, divide the calorie value given for the whole pack by 4 to determine the number of calories you have consumed. Where serving sizes are not appropriate, or unknown, values are given per 1oz/28g. Serving sizes vary greatly from person to person and, if you are trying to lose weight, it's very important to be accurate – especially with foods that are very high in calories such as those that contain a fair amount of fat, sugar, cream, cheese, alcohol etc.

Food Data

Nutrition information for basic average foods has been compiled by the Weight Loss Resources food data team using many sources of information to calculate the most accurate values possible. Some nutrition information for non-branded food records is from The Composition of Foods 6th Edition (2002). Reproduced under licence from The Controller of Her Majesty's Stationary Office. Where basic data is present for ordinary foodstuffs such as 'raw carrots'; branded records are not included.

Nutrition information for branded goods is from details supplied by retailers and manufacturers, and researched by Weight Loss Resources staff. The Calorie Carb & Fat Bible contains data for over 1400 UK brands, including major supermarkets and fast food outlets.

The publishers gratefully acknowledge all the manufacturers and retailers who have provided information on their products. All product names, trademarks or registered trademarks belong to their respective owners and are used only for the purpose of identifying products.

Calorie & nutrition data for all food and drink items are typical values.

Caution

The information in The Calorie, Carb and Fat Bible is intended as an aid to weight loss and weight maintenance, and is not medical advice. If you suffer from, or think you may suffer from a medical condition you should consult your doctor before starting a weight loss and/or exercise regime. If you start exercising after a period of relative inactivity, you should start slowly and consult your doctor if you experience pain, distress or other symptoms.

Weights, Measures & Abbreviations

ABBREVIATIONS

kcal	kilocalories / calories
prot	protein
carb	carbohydrate
sm	small
med	medium
av	average
reg	regular
lge	large
tsp	teaspoon
tbsp	tablespoon
dtsp	dessertspoon
gf	gluten free

BRAND ABBREVIATIONS USED

ASDA

Good for You	GFY
Chosen by You	CBY
Good & Counted	G&C

MARKS & SPENCER — M & S

Count on Us	COU
Balanced For You	BFY

MORRISONS

Better For You	BFY

SAINSBURY'S

Be Good to Yourself	BGTY
Way to Five	WTF
Taste the Difference	TTD

TESCO

Healthy Eating	HE
Healthy Living	HL
Light Choices	LC

WAITROSE

Perfectly Balanced	PB

Cambridge Weight Plan	CWP

	Measure INFO/WEIGHT	per Measure KCAL	FAT	Nutrition Values per 100g / 100ml KCAL	PROT	CARB	FAT	FIBRE
ABSINTHE								
Average	*1 Pub Shot/35ml*	*127*	*0*	*363*	*0*	*38.8*	*0*	*0*
ACKEE								
Canned, Drained, Average	*1oz/28g*	*43*	*4.3*	*151*	*2.9*	*0.8*	*15.2*	*0*
ADVOCAAT								
Average	*1 Pub Shot/35ml*	*91*	*2.2*	*260*	*4.7*	*28.4*	*6.3*	*0*
AERO								
Creamy White Centre, Nestle*	1 Bar/46g	244	13.8	530	7.6	57.4	30	0
Honeycomb, Nestle*	1 Serving/40g	199	10	497	5.9	62.2	25	0
Milk Chocolate, Bubbles, Sharing Bag, Aero, Nestle*	1 Bag/113g	610	34.7	540	6.5	57.8	30.7	0
Milk, Giant, Bar, Nestle*	1 Bar/125g	674	38.6	539	6.6	57.7	30.9	2.2
Milk, Medium, Bar, Nestle*	1 Bar/43g	232	13.3	539	6.6	57.7	30.9	2.2
Milk, Snacksize, Bar, Nestle*	1 Bar/20.5g	110	6.5	537	6.6	55.9	31.9	2.2
Milk, Standard, Bar, Nestle*	1 Bar/31g	165	9.6	531	6.3	56.9	30.9	0.8
Minis, Nestle*	1 Bar/11g	57	3.2	518	6.8	58.1	28.7	0.8
Mint, Bubbles, Aero, Nestle*	1 Bubble/3g	16	0.9	538	5.4	60.5	30.1	1.4
Mint, Nestle*	1 Bar/41g	221	12.3	538	5.1	61.5	29.9	0.9
Mint, Snack Size, Nestle*	1 Bar/20.5g	112	6.7	548	7.7	55.3	32.8	0.9
Mint, Standard, Aero, Nestle*	1 Bar/43g	233	13.2	542	5.2	60.5	30.8	0.9
Orange Chocolate, Limited Edition, Aero, Nestle*	1 Bar/41g	221	12.3	539	5.1	61.4	29.9	0.9
Orange, Bubbles, Aero, Nestle*	1 Bubble/3g	16	0.9	538	5.4	60.5	30	1.4
Orange, Nestle*	6 Squares/22g	119	6.8	542	5.1	60.7	30.7	0.9
ALCOPOPS								
Smirnoff Apple Bite, Frozen, Smirnoff*	1 Pint/568ml	523	0	92	0	15	0	0
Smirnoff Ice, Frozen, Smirnoff*	1 Pint/568ml	511	0	90	0	15	0	0
Smirnoff Ice, Smirnoff*	1 Bottle/275ml	188	0	68	1.8	12	0	0
Smirnoff Lemon Sorbet, Frozen, Smirnoff*	1 Pint/568ml	517	0	91	0	15	0	0
Smirnoff Mango Sorbet, Frozen, Smirnoff*	1 Pint/568ml	511	0	90	0	15	0	0
Smirnoff Raspberry Sorbet, Frozen, Smirnoff*	1 Pint/568ml	517	0	91	0	15	0	0
ALFALFA SPROUTS								
Raw, Average	*1 Serving/33g*	*8*	*0.3*	*24*	*3*	*3*	*0.9*	*3*
ALLSPICE								
Ground, Schwartz*	1 Tsp/3g	11	0.1	358	6.1	74.3	4	0
ALMONDS								
& Edamame, Honey Wasabi	*1 Pack/140g*	*191*	*10.7*	*478*	*13.5*	*48.2*	*26.8*	*6*
Aasani, Tesco*	1 Serving/25g	160	14.1	640	23.6	5.8	56.4	7.2
Blanched, Average	*1 Serving/100g*	*617*	*54.3*	*617*	*25.1*	*6.9*	*54.3*	*8.1*
Candied, Sugared	*1 Serving/100g*	*458*	*16.3*	*458*	*8.4*	*69.2*	*16.3*	*2.2*
Flaked, Average	*1oz/28g*	*172*	*15.2*	*613*	*24.9*	*6.5*	*54.3*	*7.6*
Flaked, Toasted, Average	*1oz/28g*	*176*	*15.8*	*629*	*24.6*	*5.8*	*56.4*	*7.5*
Ground, Average	*1 Serving/10g*	*62*	*5.6*	*625*	*24*	*6.6*	*55.8*	*7.4*
Marcona, Average	*1 Serving/100g*	*608*	*53.7*	*608*	*22.1*	*13*	*53.7*	*9.7*
Moroccan Spiced, Mr Filbert's*	1 Pack/110g	684	54.1	622	22.4	17.1	49.2	10.4
Spicy BBQ, Krunchies, Blue Diamond*	1 Serving/30g	161	10.5	537	12.9	39.5	34.9	6.6
Toasted, Average	*1oz/28g*	*178*	*15.8*	*634*	*25*	*6.6*	*56.4*	*6.6*
Wasabi, Roasted, Deluxe, Lidl*	1 Serving/25g	160	13.6	639	19.2	14.3	54.6	6.6
Whole, Average	*1 Serving/20g*	*122*	*11*	*612*	*23.4*	*6.9*	*54.8*	*8.4*
Yoghurt Coated, Holland & Barrett*	1 Pack/100g	536	37	536	10.9	45.3	37	2.8
ALOO								
Bombay, M&S*	½ Pack/114g	108	5.2	95	1.8	10.3	4.6	2.3
Gobi Saag, Indian Cuisine, Microwaved, Aldi*	½ Pack/145g	106	5.5	73	1.8	6	3.8	3.6
Saag, Canned, Tesco*	½ Can/200g	124	3.8	62	1.8	9.3	1.9	2
Saag, Fresh, Sainsbury's*	1 Pack/400g	388	13.2	97	2	14.7	3.3	4.8
Saag, Gobi, Indian Takeaway, Sainsbury's*	1 Pack/334g	164	3.7	49	1.7	8	1.1	1.5

A

Measure INFO/WEIGHT		per Measure KCAL	FAT	Nutrition Values per 100g / 100ml KCAL	PROT	CARB	FAT	FIBRE
ALOO								
Saag, Gobi, Indian, Tesco*	1 Pack/225g	225	16.4	100	2.1	6.5	7.3	1.8
Saag, Gobi, M Kitchen, Morrisons*	1 Pack/225g	130	6.1	58	2	4.6	2.7	3.8
Saag, Gobi, M&S*	1 Pack/225g	270	19.1	120	1.9	9.3	8.5	2.4
Saag, Gobi, Retail	*1 Serving/330g*	*314*	*22.8*	*95*	*2.2*	*7.1*	*6.9*	*1.4*
Saag, Gobi, Takeaway, Microwaved, Morrisons*	½ Pack/105g	88	3.6	84	2	9.5	3.4	3.9
Saag, Gobi, Tesco*	1 Serving/175g	166	8.9	95	2.1	9.5	5.1	1.9
Saag, Gobi, Waitrose*	½ Pack/150g	140	8.4	93	2	6.6	5.6	4.1
Saag, North Indian, Sainsbury's*	1 Pack/300g	354	24	118	2.4	9	8	1.6
Saag, Sainsbury's*	1 Pack/300g	441	31.8	147	2.1	10.7	10.6	3.5
Saag, Tesco*	1 Serving/200g	144	7	72	2.1	8	3.5	2
Tikki, Average	*1 Serving/25g*	*48*	*2*	*191*	*4.5*	*25.2*	*8*	*3.5*
ALPACA								
Fillet, Average*	1 Serving/100g	169	3	169	34.8	0.6	3	0
AMARANTH								
Grain, Cooked	*1 Serving/100g*	*102*	*2*	*102*	*4*	*19*	*2*	*2*
ANCHOVIES								
Drained, Finest, Tesco*	1 Fillets/3g	7	0.4	220	21.3	0.8	14.6	0.5
Fillets, Flat, John West*	1 Can/50g	113	7	226	25	0.1	14	0
Fillets, Tesco*	1 Serving/15g	34	2.1	226	25	0	14	0
in Oil, Canned, Drained	*1 Anchovy/4g*	*8*	*0.5*	*195*	*23.4*	*0*	*11.3*	*0*
Marinated, Sainsbury's*	¼ Pot/44g	78	4	177	22	2	9	0.1
Paste, Lusso Vita*	1 Tsp/5g	9	0.6	185	17.7	3.9	11	0
Paste, with Olive Oil, Admiral*	1 Tsp/5g	11	0.8	215	15.7	0	16.7	0
Salted, Finest, Tesco*	1 Serving/10g	9	0.2	93	18.2	0	2.2	0
ANGEL DELIGHT								
Banana, Kraft*	1 Sachet/59g	280	12.3	474	2.3	69.3	20.9	0.3
Butterscotch, no Added Sugar, Kraft*	1 Sachet/47g	224	11.3	477	4.2	60.9	24.1	0
Butterscotch, no Added Sugar, with Semi Skimmed, Kraft*	1 Portion/89g	93	4.1	104	3.4	12.4	4.6	0
Chocolate Flavour, Kraft*	1 Sachet/67g	305	12.1	455	3.7	69.5	18	0.4
Raspberry Flavour, no Added Sugar, Kraft*	1 Sachet/59g	292	15.3	495	4.8	59.5	26	0
Strawberry Flavour, Kraft*	1 Sachet/59g	286	12.4	485	2.5	71	21	0
Strawberry Flavour, no Added Sugar, Kraft*	1 Sachet/47g	230	12.5	490	4.8	59	26.5	0
Toffee Flavour, Kraft*	1 Sachet/59g	283	12.4	480	2.6	70	21	0
Vanilla Ice Cream Flavour, Kraft*	1 Sachet/59g	289	12.7	490	2.5	71.5	21.5	0
ANGEL HAIR								
Konjac, Slim Pasta*	1 Serving/100g	8	0	8	0.6	0.6	0	5.6
Pasta, Dry	*1 Serving/50g*	*181*	*1.1*	*362*	*12.4*	*73.6*	*2.2*	*4.4*
ANTIPASTO								
Artichoke, Sainsbury's*	1 Serving/50g	68	6.2	135	2	3.6	12.5	2.3
Coppa, from Selection Platter, TTD, Sainsbury's*	1 Serving/100g	255	17.1	255	25.2	0.1	17.1	0
Felino, from Selection Platter, TTD, Sainsbury's*	1 Serving/100g	349	24.9	349	31.1	0.1	24.9	0
Italian, Specially Selected, Aldi*	¼ Pack/30g	97	6.9	323	28	0	23	0
Mixed Mushroom, Sainsbury's*	¼ Jar/72g	70	6.5	97	2.7	1.4	9	3.7
Mixed Pepper, Sainsbury's*	½ Jar/140g	48	1.8	34	1.3	4.2	1.3	3.5
Mixed, Misto Cotto, Arrosto Erbe, Waitrose*	1 Slice/9g	11	0.4	129	22.2	0	4.4	0
Parma Ham, from Selection Platter, TTD, Sainsbury's*	1 Serving/100g	236	12.9	236	29.9	0.1	12.9	0
Parma, Salami Milano, Bresaola, Finest, Tesco*	¼ Pack/30g	104	7.9	345	26.4	0.5	26.3	0
Roasted Pepper, Drained, Tesco*	1 Jar /170g	128	9.4	75	0.9	5.5	5.5	4.1
Seafood, Drained, Sainsbury's*	½ Jar/84g	150	9.7	178	14.3	4.1	11.6	1.4
Sun Dried Tomato, Sainsbury's*	¼ Jar/70g	275	25	393	4.5	13.4	35.7	6.2
APPLES								
& Grapes, Ready to Eat, Garden Gang, Asda*	1 Bag/80g	46	0.1	58	0.4	12.4	0.1	2.4
Bites, Average	*1 Pack/118g*	*58*	*0.1*	*49*	*0.3*	*11.6*	*0.1*	*2.2*

	Measure INFO/WEIGHT	per Measure KCAL	FAT	Nutrition Values per 100g / 100ml KCAL	PROT	CARB	FAT	FIBRE
APPLES								
Braeburn, Average	*1 Apple/123g*	*52*	*0.1*	*42*	*0.3*	*10.2*	*0.1*	*1.8*
Cape, Tesco*	1 Apple/100g	50	0.1	50	0.4	11.8	0.1	1.8
Cooking, Baked with Sugar, Flesh Only, Average	*1 Serving/140g*	*104*	*0.1*	*74*	*0.5*	*19.2*	*0.1*	*1.7*
Cooking, Raw, Peeled, Average	*1oz/28g*	*10*	*0*	*35*	*0.3*	*8.9*	*0.1*	*1.6*
Cooking, Stewed with Sugar, Average	*1 Serving/140g*	*104*	*0.1*	*74*	*0.3*	*19.1*	*0.1*	*1.2*
Cooking, Stewed without Sugar, Average	*1 Serving/140g*	*46*	*0.1*	*33*	*0.3*	*8.1*	*0.1*	*1.5*
Cox, English, Average	*1 Apple/123g*	*53*	*0.1*	*43*	*0.4*	*10.2*	*0.1*	*1.8*
Discovery, Average	*1 Apple/182g*	*82*	*0.9*	*45*	*0.4*	*10.6*	*0.5*	*1*
Dried, Average	*1 Pack/250g*	*537*	*0.7*	*215*	*0.8*	*52.8*	*0.3*	*5.9*
Empire, Average	*1 Apple/120g*	*52*	*0.1*	*44*	*0.4*	*10.7*	*0.1*	*1.8*
Fuji	*1 Apple/132g*	*64*	*0.1*	*48*	*0.4*	*11.8*	*0.1*	*1.8*
Gala, Average	*1 Apple/152g*	*66*	*0.2*	*43*	*0.3*	*10.4*	*0.1*	*1.4*
Golden Delicious, Average	*1 Med/102g*	*44*	*0.1*	*43*	*0.3*	*10.1*	*0.1*	*1.6*
Granny Smith, Average	*1 Sm/125g*	*56*	*0.1*	*45*	*0.3*	*10.7*	*0.1*	*1.8*
Green, Raw, Average	*1 Med/182g*	*86*	*0.2*	*48*	*0.4*	*11.3*	*0.1*	*1.8*
Kanzi, Tesco*	1 Apple/134g	71	0.1	53	0.4	11.8	0.1	1.8
Mackintosh, Red, Average	*1 Apple/165g*	*81*	*0.5*	*49*	*0.2*	*12.8*	*0.3*	*1.8*
Pink Lady, Average	*1 Apple/125g*	*56*	*0.1*	*45*	*0.4*	*10.6*	*0.1*	*1.9*
Puree, Biona Organic*	1 Serving/100g	48	0.1	48	0.2	10.5	0.1	1.5
Red, Average	*1 Med/149g*	*71*	*0.2*	*48*	*0.3*	*11.8*	*0.1*	*2*
Sliced, Average	*1oz/28g*	*14*	*0*	*49*	*0.4*	*11.6*	*0.1*	*1.8*
Stewed, & Rice, Wiltshire Farm Foods*	1 Serving/155g	144	3.3	93	2	16.1	2.1	0.6
Sticks, with Crispy Rice, Little, Fruit Bowl*	1 Portion/15g	47	0.1	316	2	70	1	7.5
APPLETISER*								
Juice Drink, Sparkling, Appletiser, Coca-Cola*	1 Glass/200ml	94	0	47	0	11	0	0.4
APRICOTS								
& Prunes, in Fruit Juice, Breakfast, Sainsbury's*	1 Pot/150g	134	0.2	89	1.1	21.2	0.1	0.7
Canned, in Syrup, Average	*1oz/28g*	*18*	*0*	*63*	*0.4*	*16.1*	*0.1*	*0.9*
Dried, Average	*1 Apricot/10g*	*17*	*0.1*	*171*	*3.6*	*37.4*	*0.5*	*6.3*
Dried, Soft, Average	*1 Serving/50g*	*104*	*0.2*	*208*	*2.4*	*48.5*	*0.4*	*5.2*
Halves, in Fruit Juice, Average	*1 Can/221g*	*87*	*0.1*	*40*	*0.5*	*9.2*	*0.1*	*1*
Milk Chocolate Coated, Graze*	1 Pack/35g	158	8.6	450	6.1	55.9	24.7	5
Raw, Flesh Only, Average	*1 Apricot/37g*	*19*	*0.2*	*52*	*1.5*	*12*	*0.4*	*2.2*
Raw, Weighed with Stone, Average	*1 Apricot/40g*	*19*	*0.2*	*47*	*1.4*	*10.8*	*0.4*	*1.9*
Yoghurt Coated, Graze*	1 Pack/40g	176	9	441	3.4	58.6	22.4	0
AQUAFABA								
Average	*1 Tbsp/15ml*	*3*	*0*	*18*	*1*	*2.9*	*0.2*	*0*
ARANCINI								
Aubergine, Cauldron Foods*	1 Arancini/30g	63	2.8	211	5.6	24.9	9.2	3.2
Mozzarella & Pecorino, World Cafe, Waitrose*	½ Pack/75g	223	10.9	314	8	34.8	15.3	2.5
ARCHERS*								
& Lemonade, Premixed, Canned, Archers*	100ml	86	0	86	0	13.2	0	0
Aqua, Peach, Archers*	1 Bottle/275ml	206	0	75	0.3	7.7	0	0
Peach (Calculated Estimate), Archers*	1 Shot/35ml	91	0	260	0	0	0	0
Vea, Wildberry, Schnapps, Archers*	1 Bottle/275ml	124	0	45	0	5.8	0	0
ARTICHOKE								
Chargrilled, in Olive Oil, Cooks Ingredients, Waitrose*	1 Serving/30g	54	4.9	134	1.7	2.7	12.3	2.7
Chargrilled, Italian, Drained, Sainsbury's*	1/3 Tub/43g	40	2.7	92	3.1	2.8	6.1	6.5
Fresh, Raw, Average	*1oz/28g*	*13*	*0*	*47*	*3.3*	*10.5*	*0.2*	*5.4*
Grilled, in Olive Oil, Jar, Parente*	1 Artichoke/26g	15	1	57	1.8	2.2	3.8	0
Hearts, Canned, Drained, Average	*½ Can/117g*	*35*	*0.1*	*30*	*1.9*	*5.4*	*0*	*2.2*
Hearts, Marinated & Grilled, Waitrose*	1 Serving/50g	57	5	114	3	3	10	3
Hearts, Sliced with Extra Virgin Olive Oil, Waitrose*	1 Serving/40g	24	1.6	59	1.3	4.4	4	7

	Measure INFO/WEIGHT	per Measure KCAL	FAT	Nutrition Values per 100g / 100ml KCAL	PROT	CARB	FAT	FIBRE
ARTICHOKE								
in Oil, Grilled, Cucina, Aldi*	¼ Jar/43g	41	3.7	96	1.1	2.3	8.6	2.2
in Oil, Tesco*	1 Piece/15g	18	1.6	120	2	2.2	11	7.5
Marinated, Roasted, M&S*	1 Pack/200g	300	26.6	150	1.9	5	13.3	2.3
ASAFOETIDA								
Powder, Schwartz*	1 Tbsp/0.7g	2	0	271	6.5	56.2	2.2	0
ASPARAGUS								
& Green Vegetables (Steamer Pouch), Waitrose*	½ Pack/125g	28	0.6	22	2.1	2.3	0.5	2.1
Boiled, in Salted Water, Average	*5 Spears/125g*	*16*	*0.5*	*12*	*1.6*	*0.7*	*0.4*	*0.7*
British with Butter, Tesco*	1 Serving/50g	26	2	52	2.6	1.6	4	2
Canned, Average	*1 Can/250g*	*41*	*0.4*	*16*	*2*	*1.8*	*0.2*	*1.4*
Trimmed, Raw, Average	*1 Serving/80g*	*20*	*0.4*	*24*	*2.9*	*1.9*	*0.6*	*1.7*
AUBERGINE								
Baby, Tesco*	1 Aubergine/50g	8	0.2	15	0.9	2.2	0.4	2.3
Baked Topped, M&S*	1 Serving/150g	165	11.6	110	2.4	7.4	7.7	0.9
Fried, Average	*1oz/28g*	*85*	*8.9*	*302*	*1.2*	*2.8*	*31.9*	*2.3*
in Hot Sauce, Yarden*	1 Serving/35g	96	9	273	1.5	8.8	25.8	0
Marinated & Grilled, Waitrose*	½ Pack/100g	106	10	106	1	3	10	2
Parmigiana, M&S*	1 Pack/350g	332	18.6	95	4.6	7.6	5.3	1.1
Raw, Fresh, Average	*1 Sm/250g*	*36*	*1*	*14*	*0.9*	*2.1*	*0.4*	*1.9*
Sliced, Chargrilled, Frozen, Oven Cooked, Tesco*	¼ Pack/78g	35	0.2	46	1.6	6.8	0.3	4.6
AVOCADO								
Flesh Only, Average	*1 Med/145g*	*276*	*28.3*	*190*	*1.9*	*1.9*	*19.5*	*3.4*
Weighed with Stone, Raw	*½ Avocado/101g*	*120*	*11.4*	*119*	*1.5*	*1*	*11.3*	*3.7*

	Measure INFO/WEIGHT	per Measure KCAL	FAT	Nutrition Values per 100g / 100ml KCAL	PROT	CARB	FAT	FIBRE
BACARDI*								
& Diet Cola, Bacardi*	1 Bottle/275ml	85	0	31	0	1	0	0
37.5% Volume, Bacardi*	1 Pub Shot/35ml	72	0	207	0	0	0	0
40% Volume, Bacardi*	1 Pub Shot/35ml	78	0	222	0	0	0	0
Breezer, Apple, Half Sugar, Crisp, Bacardi*	1 Bottle/275ml	121	0	44	0	3.7	0	0
Breezer, Cranberry, Bacardi*	1 Bottle/275ml	154	0	56	0	7.1	0	0
Breezer, Lime, Bacardi*	1 Bottle/275ml	182	0	66	0	9.1	0	0
Breezer, Orange, Bacardi*	1 Bottle/275ml	179	0	65	0	8.2	0	0
Breezer, Raspberry, Half Sugar, Refreshing, Bacardi*	1 Bottle/275ml	99	0	36	0	3.3	0	0
Breezer, Watermelon, Bacardi*	1 Bottle/275ml	100	0	36	0	3.2	0	0
BACON								
Back, Dry Cured, Average	*1 Rasher/31g*	*77*	*4.7*	*250*	*28.1*	*0.3*	*15.1*	*0.3*
Back, Dry Fried or Grilled, Average	*1 Rasher/25g*	*72*	*5.4*	*287*	*23.2*	*0*	*21.6*	*0*
Back, Lean, Average	*1 Rasher/33g*	*57*	*4*	*174*	*16.3*	*0.1*	*12*	*0.5*
Back, Smoked, Average	*1 Rasher/25g*	*66*	*5*	*265*	*20.9*	*0*	*19.9*	*0*
Back, Smoked, Grilled, Tesco*	2 Rashers/38g	87	7	229	16	0	18.4	0
Back, Smoked, Lean, Average	*1 Rasher/25g*	*41*	*1.2*	*163*	*28.2*	*1.1*	*5*	*0.2*
Back, Smoked, Maple Cure, Deluxe, Lidl*	1 Rasher/16g	43	3	269	22.5	1.6	19.1	0
Back, Smoked, Rindless, Average	*1 Rasher/25g*	*60*	*4.3*	*241*	*21*	*0.1*	*17.4*	*0*
Back, Tendersweet, Average	*1 Rasher/25g*	*63*	*3.6*	*250*	*29.8*	*0.4*	*14.4*	*0*
Back, Unsmoked, Average	*1 Rasher/32g*	*78*	*5.5*	*242*	*21.3*	*0.4*	*17.3*	*0*
Back, Unsmoked, Rindless, Average	*1 Rasher/23g*	*56*	*3.9*	*241*	*22.5*	*0*	*16.9*	*0*
Bits, Average	*1oz/28g*	*75*	*5.9*	*268*	*18.6*	*0.7*	*21.2*	*0.1*
Chops, Average	*1oz/28g*	*62*	*4.2*	*222*	*22.3*	*0*	*14.8*	*0*
Chops, Coated in American Style BBQ Glaze, Tesco*	1 Serving/200g	480	36.2	240	16.1	2.1	18.1	0
Chops, Freshcure, Aldi*	1 Chop/150g	324	19.5	216	25	1.1	13	0.5
Chops, in Cheese Sauce, Tesco*	1 Serving/185g	405	26.5	219	12.6	10	14.3	1.1
Collar Joint, Lean & Fat, Boiled	*1oz/28g*	*91*	*7.6*	*325*	*20.4*	*0*	*27*	*0*
Collar Joint, Lean & Fat, Raw	*1oz/28g*	*81*	*7.4*	*290*	*13.3*	*0*	*26.3*	*0*
Collar Joint, Lean Only, Boiled	*1oz/28g*	*53*	*2.7*	*191*	*26*	*0*	*9.7*	*0*
Fat Only, Cooked, Average	*1oz/28g*	*194*	*20.4*	*692*	*9.3*	*0*	*72.8*	*0*
Fat Only, Raw, Average	*1oz/28g*	*209*	*22.7*	*747*	*4.8*	*0*	*80.9*	*0*
Gammon Rasher, Lean Only, Grilled	*1oz/28g*	*48*	*1.5*	*172*	*31.4*	*0*	*5.2*	*0*
Lardons, Smoked, Freshcure, Aldi*	¼ Pack/50g	160	11.5	321	29	0.5	23	0.5
Lean Only, Fried, Average	*1 Rasher/25g*	*83*	*5.6*	*332*	*32.8*	*0*	*22.3*	*0*
Lean Only, Grilled, Average	*1 Rasher/25g*	*73*	*4.7*	*292*	*30.5*	*0*	*18.9*	*0*
Lean, Average	*1 Rasher/33g*	*47*	*2.2*	*142*	*19.6*	*0.9*	*6.7*	*0.2*
Loin Steaks, Grilled, Average	*1 Serving/120g*	*229*	*11.6*	*191*	*25.9*	*0*	*9.7*	*0*
Medallions, Average	*1 Rasher/18g*	*27*	*0.6*	*151*	*29.4*	*0.9*	*3.3*	*0.1*
Middle, Fried	*1 Rasher/40g*	*140*	*11.4*	*350*	*23.4*	*0*	*28.5*	*0*
Middle, Grilled	*1 Rasher/40g*	*123*	*9.2*	*307*	*24.8*	*0*	*23.1*	*0*
Middle, Raw	*1 Rasher/43g*	*95*	*7.9*	*222*	*14*	*0*	*18.4*	*0*
Rashers, Lean Only, Trimmed, Average	*1 Rasher/20g*	*24*	*0.8*	*119*	*20.6*	*0*	*4*	*0*
Rindless, Average	*1 Rasher/20g*	*30*	*1.7*	*150*	*18.5*	*0*	*8.5*	*0*
Smoked, 70% Reduced Fat, Grilled, NUME, Morrisons*	1 Rasher/20g	36	0.6	181	37.6	0.9	3	0
Smoked, Average	*1 Rasher/28g*	*46*	*2.1*	*166*	*24.8*	*0.2*	*7.4*	*0*
Smoked, Crispy, Cooked, Average	*1 Serving/10g*	*46*	*2.7*	*460*	*53*	*2.1*	*26.9*	*0*
Smoked, Rindless, Average	*1 Rasher/20g*	*21*	*0.6*	*106*	*19.8*	*0*	*3*	*0*
Steaks, with 3 Cheese Sauce & Mustard Crust, Asda*	½ Pack/175g	390	25.6	223	20.6	2.3	14.6	2.9
Streaky, Average	*1 Rasher/12g*	*32*	*2.5*	*266*	*19.7*	*0*	*20.7*	*0*
Streaky, Cooked, Average	*1 Rasher/20g*	*68*	*5.6*	*342*	*22.4*	*0.3*	*27.8*	*0*
Vegetarian, Deli Style, Rashers, Quorn*	1 Rasher/15g	30	2.3	199	11.8	3	15.5	5
Vegetarian, Pieces, Bacon Style, Quorn*	1 Pack/100g	103	2.5	103	15	5	2.5	5
Vegetarian, Rashers	*1 Rasher/16g*	*33*	*1.7*	*206*	*19.5*	*8.6*	*10.4*	*2.8*

INFO/WEIGHT	Measure	per Measure		Nutrition Values per 100g / 100ml				
		KCAL	FAT	KCAL	PROT	CARB	FAT	FIBRE
BACON								
Vegetarian, Rashers, Cheatin', The Redwood Co*	1 Rasher/16g	32	1.2	196	25.9	7.3	7.3	0.5
Vegetarian, Rashers, Tesco*	1 Rasher/20g	41	2.2	203	22.5	3.3	11.1	3.9
Vegetarian, Streaky Style, Rashers, Tesco*	1 Rasher/8g	17	0.8	215	23.7	5	10.6	2.2
Vegetarian, Strips, Morningstar Farms*	1 Strip/8g	30	2.3	375	12.5	12.5	28.1	6.2
BAGEL								
Bacon, & Soft Cheese, Boots*	1 Serving/148g	481	25.2	325	12	31	17	2.2
Cream Cheese, M&S*	1 Bagel/23g	79	4.9	352	7.8	31	21.8	1.8
Ham, & Pesto, COU, M&S*	1 Pack/173g	260	2.4	150	11.1	23.5	1.4	1.7
Salmon, & Cream Cheese, Smoked, M&S*	1 Bagel185g	480	18.8	260	12.3	29.5	10.2	1.9
Soft Cheese, & Salmon, Smoked, American, Sainsbury's*	1 Bagel/131g	356	16.2	272	8.3	31.8	12.4	1.7
Soft Cheese, & Salmon, Smoked, Finest, Tesco*	1 Pack/173g	396	10	229	13.1	31.2	5.8	1.7
Toasts, with White Chocolate & Blueberry Dip, Graze*	1 Punnet/25g	130	6.8	519	5.7	62	27	3.2
Turkey, & Cranberry, Bagelmania*	1 Pack/198g	325	7.3	164	9	24.5	3.7	1.1
Turkey, Pastrami & American Mustard, Shapers, Boots*	1 Bagel/146g	296	5	203	11	32	3.4	1.4
BAGUETTE								
All Day Breakfast, Darwins Deli*	1 Serving/184g	498	21.5	271	13.4	31.9	11.7	0
Beef, & Horseradish, Freshly Prepared, M&S*	1 Baguette/274g	795	31	290	12.1	37.2	11.3	2
Brie, Tomato, & Rocket, Freshly Prepared, M&S*	1 Baguette/219g	570	21.7	260	10.3	33.2	9.9	1.9
Cheese, & Ham, Snack 'n' Go, Sainsbury's*	1 Baguette/178g	383	9.1	215	12.6	29.6	5.1	1.9
Cheese, & Pickle, Fullfillers*	1 Baguette/280g	767	31.1	274	11.9	35.5	11.1	0
Cheese, & Ham, Average	***1 Baguette/203g***	***593***	***20.8***	***292***	***14***	***35.9***	***10.3***	***1.4***
Cheese, & Onion, Asda*	¼ Loaf/42g	154	7.4	366	12	39.8	17.6	1.3
Cheese, & Tomato, Tesco*	1 Baguette/108g	243	8.3	225	9.7	29.3	7.7	1.8
Cheese, Mixed, & Spring Onion, Asda*	1 Pack/190g	629	34.8	331	9.5	32.1	18.3	1.3
Cheese, Tomato, & Basil, Asda*	¼ Baguette/42g	138	5.9	329	10	40.8	14	1.3
Chicken, & Mayonnaise, Asda*	1 Pack/190g	407	16.5	214	9.7	30.5	8.7	1.3
Chicken, & Salad, Boots*	1 Baguette/132g	202	2.4	153	11	23	1.8	2
Chicken, & Spicy Tomato, Snack, Sainsbury's*	1 Baguette/160g	344	5.9	215	14.1	31.2	3.7	2.2
Chicken, & Stuffing, Hot, Sainsbury's*	1 Baguette/227g	543	16.3	239	13.7	29.6	7.2	0
Chicken, & Salad, Asda*	1 Serving/158g	326	9.5	206	9	29	6	2.1
Chicken, & Salad, Shapers, Boots*	1 Baguette/132g	222	2.6	168	11	27	2	1.5
Chicken, Honey, & Mustard, BGTY, Sainsbury's*	1 Pack/187g	340	3.7	182	11	30	2	0
Chicken, Oakham, Fresh, M&S*	1 Baguette/225g	450	10.8	200	12.4	26.7	4.8	1.5
Chicken, Tikka, Asda*	1 Pack/190g	439	17.9	231	10.4	32.8	9.4	1.3
Chicken, Tikka, Hot, Sainsbury's*	1 Pack/190g	386	11.6	203	8.5	28.4	6.1	0
Egg, & Tomato, Oldfields*	1 Pack/198g	416	15	210	8.7	27	7.6	0
Egg, Bacon, & Tomato, Freshly Prepared, M&S*	1 Baguette/182g	455	17.3	250	12.9	28	9.5	1.7
Ham, & Turkey, Asda*	1 Baguette/360g	774	18.4	215	11.6	30.7	5.1	1.3
Ham, & Cheese, Freshly Prepared, M&S*	1 Baguette/231g	555	11.3	240	13.4	35.9	4.9	2.4
Ham, & Salad, with Mustard Mayonnaise, Sainsbury's*	1 Baguette/100g	412	15.9	412	17.6	49.6	15.9	0.1
Mozzarella, Tomato, & Pesto, Darwins Deli*	1 Serving/210g	531	20.4	253	11.7	29.7	9.7	0
Prawn Mayonnaise, Asda*	1 Pack/190g	399	9.3	210	9.1	32.5	4.9	1.3
Prawn, French, Shell*	1 Baguette/63g	171	7.2	272	9.7	32.4	11.5	0
Salmon, Smoked, & Egg, Freshly Prepared	***1 Baguette/178g***	***455***	***17.3***	***255***	***13.7***	***28.4***	***9.7***	***1.6***
Steak, & Onion, Snack 'n' Go, Sainsbury's*	1 Baguette/177g	398	8.8	225	14.3	30.6	5	2.2
Tuna, Crunch, Shapers, Boots*	1 Pack/138g	315	4.8	228	14	35	3.5	3.1
Tuna, Melt, Sainsbury's*	1 Serving/204g	373	8	183	11.3	25.8	3.9	0
BAILEYS*								
Glide, Baileys*	1 Serving/200ml	212	2.4	106	0	18	1.2	0
Irish Cream, Original, Baileys*	1 Serving/50ml	164	6.5	327	3	25	13	0
BAKE								
Aubergine, & Mozzarella Cheese, BGTY, Sainsbury's*	1 Pack/360g	194	7.2	54	3	6	2	1.3
Aubergine, Tomato, & Mozzarella, Vegetarian, Tesco*	1 Pack/380g	257	10.5	71	3.6	5.9	2.9	3.2

	Measure INFO/WEIGHT	per Measure KCAL	FAT	Nutrition Values per 100g / 100ml KCAL	PROT	CARB	FAT	FIBRE
BAKE								
Bean, Mexican, Georgia's Choice*	1 Bake/115g	266	12.9	231	4.3	28.9	11.2	3.8
Beef, & Root Vegetable, Minced, COU, M&S*	1 Pack/400g	320	11.6	80	6.6	6	2.9	3
Beetroot & Goats' Cheese, Sainsbury's*	1 Bake/114g	126	5.8	111	3.9	9.7	5.1	5.2
Broccoli, & Cheese, Asda*	1 Bake/132g	269	15.4	204	5.3	19.3	11.7	2.5
Broccoli, & Cheese, M&S*	1 Pack/400g	480	31.2	120	6.5	5.4	7.8	1.6
Butternut Squash, & Mushroom, Roasted, BFY, M&S*	1 Pack/390g	339	10.5	87	6.1	8.4	2.7	2.1
Butternut Squash, & Parsnip, Tesco*	½ Pack/124g	144	7.8	116	3.3	10.5	6.3	2.1
Butternut Squash, Red Onion, & Kale, Tesco*	½ Pack/121g	63	1.8	52	0.9	7.8	1.5	1.7
Cauliflower, & Broccoli, Tesco*	½ Pack/250g	178	10.2	71	2.8	5.8	4.1	1
Cheese, & Spinach, Tesco*	1 Bake/140g	269	10.9	192	4.5	26	7.8	1.4
Chicken, & Mushroom, COU, M&S*	1 Serving/360g	324	8.3	90	7.3	10.3	2.3	1.1
Chicken, Arrabiata, M&S*	1 Pack/450g	540	13.5	120	7.6	16	3	2
Chicken, Bacon & Potato, British Classics, Tesco*	½ Pack/375g	435	16.5	116	7	12.2	4.4	1.4
Chicken, Spiralli, M&S*	1 Serving/400g	400	15.2	100	7.9	9.1	3.8	1.1
Chickpea, Courgette & Moroccan Spiced, Gosh*	1 Bake/125g	207	5.7	166	5.2	30	4.6	5.7
Cod, & Prawn, 327, Oakhouse Foods Ltd*	1 Meal/340g	466	23.5	137	8.6	10.3	6.9	0.3
Cod, & Prawn, COU, M&S*	1 Pack/400g	320	8	80	6.5	8.8	2	1
Corned Beef, 379, Wiltshire Farm Foods*	1 Bake/290g	322	11.2	111	3.8	15.2	3.9	2.1
Courgette, & Butternut Squash, Meat Free, Tesco*	1 Pack/375g	367	13.7	98	2.5	12.8	3.6	1.8
Courgette, & Tomato, Cauldron Foods*	1 Pack/285g	593	37	208	10	17	13	6.4
Duck, & Chorizo, Oven Cooked, TTD, Sainsbury's*	1 Pack/386g	459	22.8	119	7	8.2	5.9	2.7
Fish, & Vegetable, Youngs*	1 Serving/375g	446	23.6	119	5.6	10	6.3	1.3
Fish, Dinner, Light & Easy, Youngs*	1 Pack/385g	370	13.5	96	6.4	9.7	3.5	1.6
Fish, Haddock, Smoked, Light & Easy, Youngs*	1 Pack/310g	242	7.1	78	6.4	8	2.3	0.9
Fish, Three, Roast, Deluxe, Lidl*	1 Portion/300g	498	29.7	166	12.6	6.2	9.9	0.6
Haddock, Average	*1 Serving/400g*	*312*	*9.2*	*78*	*6.4*	*8*	*2.3*	*0.9*
Haddock, Smoked, Light & Easy, Youngs*	1 Pack/300g	234	6.9	78	6.4	8	2.3	0.9
Haddock, Smoked, Luxury, Light & Easy, Youngs*	1 Pack/355g	390	17	110	7.5	9.2	4.8	0.6
Lentil, Spiced, Vegetarian, TTD, Sainsbury's*	1 Bake/132g	245	8.4	186	4.8	27.3	6.4	4.2
Mushroom, Leek, & Cheddar, CBY, Asda*	½ Pack/199g	181	8.8	91	3.7	8.1	4.4	1.9
Mushroom, Leek, & Cheddar, Wiltshire Farm Foods*	1 Serving/425g	564	28.7	133	4.6	13.3	6.8	1.5
Onion, & Potato, Roast, COU, M&S*	1 Pack/450g	338	5.8	75	1.9	13.6	1.3	1.5
Parsnip, & Mulled Red Onion Roast, Festive, M&S*	½ Pack/200g	256	9.4	128	2.9	16.9	4.7	3.3
Peppercorn, Creamy, Vegetarian, Tesco*	1 Serving/140g	322	16.8	230	3.6	27	12	1.2
Potato, & Vegetable, Co-Op*	1 Bake/340g	425	27.2	125	4	11	8	1
Potato, Cheese, & Bacon, Homepride*	1 Serving/210g	277	26.2	132	1.6	3.2	12.5	0
Potato, Cheese, & Leek, Aunt Bessie's*	½ Pack/275g	300	13.8	109	3.4	12.7	5	2.7
Potato, Cheese, & Onion, Roast, Asda*	½ Pack/200g	288	16	144	4.2	14	8	1.1
Potato, Cheese, & Onion, Tesco*	1 Pack/400g	376	19.6	94	2.4	10	4.9	1
Potato, Cherry Tomato, & Mozzarella, M&S*	½ Pack/165g	140	5.6	85	2.2	11.5	3.4	2.6
Potato, Leek, & Gruyere, M&S*	½ Pack/200g	240	15.4	120	2.2	10.3	7.7	1.4
Potato, Leek, & Mushroom, M&S*	1 Serving/225g	225	13.3	100	3.5	10	5.9	2
Potato, Sweet Potato, & Kale, M&S*	½ Pack/190g	232	10.4	122	3.9	12.9	5.5	2.4
Sausage, & Tortiglioni, Tuscan, Specially Selected, Aldi*	½ Pack/400g	592	21.2	148	6.5	18	5.3	1.6
Sausage, Bacon, & Mushroom, Traybake, Easy, Waitrose*	½ Pack/292g	456	28	156	11.2	5.7	9.6	1.1
Spinach, & Ricotta, As Consumed, M Kitchen, Morrisons*	1 Bake/128g	282	16	220	6.9	18.3	12.5	3.5
Vegetable, & Lentil, Somerfield*	1 Pack/350g	318	6.3	91	4.9	13.8	1.8	2.5
Vegetable, Mediterranean, Cooked, CBY, Asda*	1 Bake/120g	279	13.2	232	8.4	22.8	11	4.2
Vegetable, Tandoori, Cooked, Tesco*	¼ Pack/95g	70	2.6	74	2	8.7	2.8	3
BAKING POWDER								
Average	*1 Tsp/2g*	*3*	*0*	*163*	*5.2*	*37.8*	*0*	*0*
BAKLAVA								
Average	*2 Pieces/50g*	*239*	*14.2*	*478*	*8*	*47.4*	*28.4*	*2.8*

B

B

	Measure INFO/WEIGHT	per Measure KCAL	FAT	Nutrition Values per 100g / 100ml KCAL	PROT	CARB	FAT	FIBRE
BALTI								
Chick Pea & Spinach, Cauldron Foods*	1 Pack/400g	356	8	89	2.3	15.5	2	1
Chicken, & Mushroom, Tesco*	1 Serving/350g	326	10.5	93	12.3	4.2	3	0.7
Chicken, & Rice, M&S*	1 Pack/400g	380	6	95	6.9	14.1	1.5	1.2
Chicken, Asda*	1 Pack/450g	324	9.9	72	8	5	2.2	0
Chicken, Ceylon, Finest, Tesco*	1 Pack/400g	588	38	147	14.4	0.9	9.5	5
Chicken, M&S*	½ Pack/175g	245	15.2	140	13	2	8.7	1.7
Chicken, Morrisons*	1 Pack/350g	441	26.6	126	12.1	2.3	7.6	1.5
Chicken, Sainsbury's*	½ Pack/200g	222	11.2	111	11.6	3.6	5.6	1.3
Chicken, Style, & Rice, Microwaved, Asda*	1 Pack/400g	498	19.9	125	3.8	15	5	2.3
Chicken, Take Away, Tesco*	½ Pack/200g	170	7.6	85	8.1	4.6	3.8	1.9
Chicken, Takeaway, Sainsbury's*	1 Pack/400g	404	18	101	10.4	4.5	4.5	1.4
Chicken, Tesco*	1 Pack/460g	662	25.8	144	6.1	17.4	5.6	1.6
Chicken, Tikka, Finest, Tesco*	½ Pack/200g	280	17.2	140	15.8	1.1	8.6	3.2
Chicken, with Garlic & Coriander Naan, Frozen, Patak's*	1 Pack/375g	431	18.8	115	6.3	11.1	5	1.1
Chicken, with Naan Bread, PB, Waitrose*	1 Pack/375g	450	13.5	120	12.1	9.7	3.6	2.8
Chicken, with Naan Bread, Sharwood's*	1 Pack/375g	529	23.2	141	7.3	14.1	6.2	2.2
Chicken, with Pilau Rice & Naan Bread, Tesco*	1 Meal/550g	660	19.8	120	6.1	15.5	3.6	1.4
Chicken, with Pilau Rice, Asda*	1 Pack/504g	625	24.7	124	5	15	4.9	1.2
Chicken, with Pilau Rice, LC, Tesco*	1 Pack/400g	440	5.2	110	6.3	17.4	1.3	1.8
Chicken, with Pilau Rice, Weight Watchers*	1 Pack/329g	306	4.3	93	6.9	13.4	1.3	1.2
Chicken, with Rice, Curry Break, Patak's*	1 Pack/220g	198	6.2	90	4.7	11.6	2.8	0
Chicken, with Rice, Patak's*	1 Pack/370g	440	13	119	6.1	16.7	3.5	1.7
Lamb, Bhuna, Tesco*	1 Pack/400g	360	14.8	90	9.2	4.8	3.7	1.1
Prawn, Budgens*	1 Pack/350g	374	24.8	107	5.6	5.2	7.1	1.3
Vegetable, & Rice, Tesco*	1 Pack/450g	378	7.2	84	2	15.6	1.6	1.3
Vegetable, Asda*	½ Can/200g	206	12	103	2.2	10	6	2.5
Vegetable, Average	*1 Serving/200g*	*182*	*8.3*	*91*	*1.9*	*11.3*	*4.1*	*1.7*
Vegetable, CBY, Asda*	1 Pack/200g	190	11.6	95	2	7.7	5.8	2
Vegetable, GFY, Asda*	1 Pack/450g	324	4	72	1.9	14	0.9	1.5
BAMBOO SHOOTS								
Canned, Average	*1 Sm Can/120g*	*10*	*0.1*	*8*	*1*	*0.8*	*0.1*	*0.8*
BANANA								
Chips, Average	*1oz/28g*	*143*	*8.8*	*511*	*1*	*59.9*	*31.4*	*1.7*
Green, Medium, Average	*1 Sm/101g*	*91*	*0*	*90*	*1*	*23*	*0*	*3*
Raw, Flesh Only, Average	*1 Med/100g*	*95*	*0.3*	*95*	*1.2*	*20.9*	*0.3*	*4.2*
Raw, Weighed with Skin, Average	*1 Med/152g*	*98*	*0.3*	*65*	*0.8*	*14.2*	*0.2*	*2.9*
Slices, Dried, Love Life, Waitrose*	1 Serving/25g	74	0.2	295	4.8	66.5	0.6	5.2
BARLEY								
Quick Cook, Wholefoods, Tesco*	1 Portion/83g	291	1.2	351	8	70.7	1.4	11.6
BARS								
All Bran, Apple, Kellogg's*	1 Bar/40g	158	7.6	395	8	48	19	5
All Bran, Honey & Oat, Kellogg's*	1 Bar/27g	99	2.2	366	6	67	8	12
All Fruit, Frusli, Passion Fruit, Jordans*	1 Bar/30g	92	0.2	307	1.3	74	0.7	5
All Fruit, Frusli, Strawberry, Jordans*	1 Bar/30g	94	0.1	313	2.3	81.3	0.3	5
Almond & Apricot, Weight Watchers*	1 Bar/34g	151	6.6	443	8.6	55.9	19.4	5.2
Almond & Cranberry, Day Break, Atkins*	1 Bar/37g	137	5.9	371	37	23	16	15
Almond, Apricot, & Mango, M&S*	1 Bar/50g	205	7.4	410	9	60.2	14.8	5
Almond, Cashew & Peanut, Eat Real*	1 Bar/40g	191	11.1	478	13.8	41.2	27.7	9.7
Almond, Madagascan Vanilla, Kind*	1 Bar/40g	203	15.6	507	16	36	39	14
Am, Breakfast Muffin, Apple & Sultana, McVitie's*	1 Bar/45g	168	7.5	373	4.4	54.9	16.7	1.6
Am, Cereal, Apple, McVitie's*	1 Bar/40g	160	5.4	400	4.3	65.4	13.5	3.1
Am, Cereal, Apricot, McVitie's*	1 Bar/30g	146	6.2	486	6.5	68.8	20.5	0.5
Am, Cereal, Fruit & Nut, McVitie's*	1 Bar/35g	167	7.5	477	6.6	64.9	21.4	3.4

BARS

	Measure INFO/WEIGHT	per Measure KCAL	FAT	Nutrition Values per 100g / 100ml KCAL	PROT	CARB	FAT	FIBRE
Am, Cereal, Orange Marmalade, McVitie's*	1 Bar/40g	151	7.2	378	4.5	53.2	18	1.8
Am, Cereal, Raisin & Nut, McVitie's*	1 Bar/35g	148	5.8	422	6.4	62.1	16.4	2.4
Am, Cereal, Strawberry, McVitie's*	1 Bar/35g	138	3.5	395	5.7	70.5	10.1	2.7
Am, Granola, Almond, Raisin & Cranberry, McVitie's*	1 Bar/35g	133	4	380	7.1	62.9	11.4	4
Am, Muesli Fingers, McVitie's*	1 Bar/35g	154	6.9	440	6	59.8	19.6	3.1
Apollo, Morrisons*	1 Bar/38g	172	6.9	451	3.6	68.1	18	1.2
Apple & Cinnamon, Breakfast Snack, Tesco*	1 Bar/38g	137	4.7	365	4.3	58.8	12.5	2
Apple & Blackberry, Fruit Bake, McVitie's*	1 Bar/35g	124	2.5	354	2.7	73.8	7.2	1.2
Apple & Blackberry, Fruit Bakes, Go Ahead, McVitie's*	1 Bar/35g	131	3	374	3.5	71.8	8.5	3.9
Apple & Raisin, Dorset Cereals*	1 Bar/30g	109	1.1	363	4	78.3	3.7	5.3
Apple & Raisin, Snack, Geobar, Traidcraft*	1 Bar/35g	127	1.7	362	3.3	76.4	4.8	2.3
Apple & Raspberry, Chewy & Crisp, Tesco*	1 Bar/27g	123	5.3	456	3.4	66.8	19.5	2.8
Apple, & Pear, Raw , The Foodie Market, Aldi*	1 Bar/30g	91	0.2	304	2.3	66	0.6	13
Apple, Fruit Bake, Go Ahead, McVitie's*	1 Bar/35g	124	2.5	354	2.7	73.8	7.2	1.2
Apple, Granola, McVitie's*	1 Bar/35g	128	3.4	366	6.6	63.1	9.7	4.3
Apple, Peanut, & Almond, Goodness Knows*	1 Bar/34g	157	6.8	462	7.7	59.6	20	4.6
Apricot & Peach, Multigrain, BGTY, Sainsbury's*	1 Bar/25g	70	0.6	282	6.6	58.2	2.5	23.1
Apricot & Almond, Eat Natural*	1 Bar/50g	202	8.1	403	11.2	53.3	16.1	0
Apricot & Almond, Truly Juicy, Raw Health*	1 Bar/45g	182	10.4	405	17	49	23	9
Apricot & Almond, Yoghurt Coated, Eat Natural*	1 Bar/35g	155	8.7	451	5.9	49.7	25.2	4.5
Apricot & Sultana Porridge Oat, Stoats*	1 Pack/85g	370	20.8	435	8.2	70.5	24.5	5.6
Apricot, Dried Fruit, Sunsweet*	1 Bar/33g	96	0	292	3.6	72.5	0.1	0
Apricot, Orange, & Ginger, Juicy, Get Fruity*	1 Bar/35g	131	4.6	375	6.6	54	13	6.8
Baked Apple Pie, Weight Watchers*	1 Bar/27g	76	0.4	283	4.4	55.7	1.5	14.7
Banana Nut, Health Warrior*	1 Bar/25g	100	5	400	12	56	20	16
Banana, Mango & Brazil, Cereal, Dove's Farm*	1 Bar/40g	196	4.6	490	6.5	63.3	11.5	5.3
Beetroot, & Walnut, Goodness, The Food Doctor*	1 Bar/40g	118	2.8	295	5.1	33.2	6.9	39.6
Berry & Seed Oaty, Weight Watchers*	1 Bar/26g	87	2	333	10	46.8	7.5	19.3
Berry Delight, GF, Nak'd*	1 Bar/35g	135	5.2	385	9	52	15	6
Berry Snack, Diet Chef Ltd*	1 Bar/27g	96	2.2	356	7.2	64	8.2	5.5
Berry, Mixed, Moist, Get Fruity*	1 Bar/35g	140	4.6	399	6	61	13	6.3
Berry, Nut Free, Get Buzzing*	1 Bar/62g	173	8.7	279	3.2	50	14	2.9
Biscuit & Raisin, Reduced Fat, Tesco*	1 Bar/22g	90	2.8	410	4.9	69.5	12.5	1.8
Biscuit, Chocolate, Mint, Penguin, McVitie's*	1 Bar/25g	133	6.9	531	5.4	65	27.7	1.5
Biscuit, Chocolate, Orange, Penguin, McVitie's*	1 Bar/25g	133	6.9	531	5.4	65	27.7	1.5
Biscuit, Chocolate, Original, Penguin, McVitie's*	1 Bar/20g	106	5.6	515	5.1	61.4	27.1	2.4
Biscuit, Groovy, Aldi*	1 Bar/27g	123	5.3	457	4.9	64.2	19.7	1.8
Biscuit, Raisin & Chocolate Hobnobs, Snack, McVitie's*	1 Bar/32g	132	3.9	420	5.5	71.1	12.5	3.6
Blue Riband, Double Choc, Nestle*	1 Bar/22g	113	5.6	513	4.8	66.4	25.3	1.1
Blueberry & Almond, Goodness Knows*	1 Bar/34g	154	6.7	452	7.7	57	19.8	5.4
Blueberry & Yoghurt Nougat, Shapers, Boots*	1 Bar/23g	85	3	369	1.8	76	13	1.7
Blueberry Chocolate, Lean Protein, Nutramino*	1 Bar/60g	209	7.8	349	33	17	13	24
Blueberry, Beond Organic, GF, Pulsin*	1 Bar/35g	166	6.7	475	8.7	46.8	19.2	4.9
Blueberry, Fruit & Grain, Asda*	1 Bar/37g	124	2.6	335	4.1	64	7	3.9
Blueberry, Weight Watchers*	1 Bar/25g	91	1.8	365	4.5	74.9	7.4	2.2
Blueberry, Yoghurt & Honey, Altu*	1 Bar/40g	129	4.7	323	12.9	45.5	11.7	12
Brazil, Goji & Chia, Protein Snack, High Five*	1 Bar/60g	292	16.2	487	20	37	27	8.1
Brazil, Sultanas, Almonds & Hazelnuts, Eat Natural*	1 Bar/50g	227	11.3	454	11.2	40	22.6	5
Breakfast with Cranberries, Asda*	1 Bar/28g	105	1.4	376	6	77	4.9	3
Breakfast, Apple Crisp, Morning Start, Atkins*	1 Bar/37g	145	7.9	392	29.2	25.4	21.4	13.8
Breakfast, Blueberry, Free From, Sainsbury's*	1 Bar/35g	163	7.8	467	3.8	62.6	22.4	0.2
Breakfast, Cherry, Oats & More, Nestle*	1 Bar/30g	109	2	363	6	70.2	6.5	3.6
Breakfast, Chocolate Chip, Crisp, Morning Start, Atkins*	1 Bar/37g	137	7	370	31.8	22.5	18.8	15

B

	Measure INFO/WEIGHT	per Measure KCAL	FAT	Nutrition Values per 100g / 100ml KCAL	PROT	CARB	FAT	FIBRE
BARS								
Breakfast, Vitality, Fruit & Fibre, Asda*	1 Bar/29g	113	2.9	390	6	69	10	4.1
Cacao Raw Fruit & Nut, Wild Trail*	1 Bar/30g	115	3.3	383	8.6	56	11	11
Cacao, Beond Organic, Pulsin*	1 Bar/35g	146	6.3	416	10.6	50.8	17.9	4.4
Caramel Crisp Bite, Tesco*	1 Bar/15g	72	3.5	483	4.3	64.4	23.1	1.3
Caramel Crisp, Go Ahead, McVitie's*	1 Bar/33g	141	4	428	4.8	75.1	12	0.8
Caramel Crunch, Go Ahead, McVitie's*	1 Bar/24g	106	3.3	440	4.7	76.6	13.8	0.8
Caramel Nougat, Soft, Shapers, Boots*	1 Bar/25g	86	2.5	343	2.9	60.4	10	0.6
Caramel, Nut Chew, Endulge, Atkins*	1 Bar/34g	130	2.7	382	5	5.9	8	6
Cashew & Cranberry, Eat Real*	1 Bar/40g	173	8.4	432	5.6	52.4	21	7.3
Cashew Cookie, Raw Fruit & Nut, GF, Nak'd*	1 Bar/35g	143	8	410	10	46	23	5
Cashew Crush, The Foodie Market, Aldi*	1 Bar/35g	158	8	451	12	46	23	7.6
Cashew, Sultana & Pumpkin Seed, Eat Real*	1 Bar/40g	165	5.9	413	8.5	59.5	14.8	10.5
Cereal & Milk, Nesquik, Nestle*	1 Bar/25g	108	3.7	433	6.2	68.5	14.9	1
Cereal, 3 Berries & Cherries, Dorset Cereals*	1 Bar/35g	127	1.7	363	5.7	73.9	4.9	5.2
Cereal, 3 Fruit, Nuts & Seeds, Dorset Cereals*	1 Bar/35g	136	3.6	389	7.4	66.6	10.3	6.2
Cereal, Apple & Raspberry, Chewy & Crisp, Tesco*	1 Bar/27g	123	5.3	456	3.3	66.7	19.6	3
Cereal, Apple & Blackberry with Yoghurt, Alpen*	1 Bar/29g	117	3.1	404	5.4	71.8	10.6	5
Cereal, Apple & Cinnamon, Fruit 'n' Grain, Asda*	1 Bar/37g	131	2.6	353	4.5	68	7	2.9
Cereal, Apple & Cinnamon, M&S*	1 Bar/24g	84	1.2	350	3.9	68.4	5.2	6.6
Cereal, Apple & Cinnamon, Tesco*	1 Bar/38g	137	4.7	365	4.3	58.9	12.5	2.1
Cereal, Apple & Raisin, Harvest, Quaker*	1 Bar/22g	87	2.5	396	5	70	11.5	4
Cereal, Apple & Sultana, Light, Alpen*	1 Bar/20g	63	0.7	330	4.1	59.4	3.6	21.7
Cereal, Apple, Chewy, BGTY, Sainsbury's*	1 Bar/25g	85	0.5	340	4.8	76	2	2
Cereal, Apricot & Yoghurt, COU, M&S*	1 Bar/21g	75	0.5	360	5.3	79.6	2.4	3.8
Cereal, Balance with Fruit, Sainsbury's*	1 Bar/25g	100	2.2	401	5.8	75.2	8.6	1.9
Cereal, Banana, Apricot, & Milk Chocolate, Eat Natural*	1 Bar/30g	108	2	362	3.7	71.8	6.7	4
Cereal, Banana, Value, Tesco*	1 Bar/21g	80	1.6	387	6	73.9	7.5	3.7
Cereal, Banoffee, Light, Alpen, Weetabix*	1 Bar/19g	66	1.3	346	4.7	54	7	24
Cereal, Banoffee, Vitality, Asda*	1 Bar/22g	73	0.6	331	6.5	69.6	2.9	13.5
Cereal, Benefit with Fruit, Aldi*	1 Bar/27g	108	2.3	401	5.8	75.2	8.6	1.9
Cereal, Blueberry Flavour, Breakfast, Sweet Mornings*	1 Bar/38g	152	4.9	399	4.5	66	13	2.5
Cereal, Brownie, COU, M&S*	1 Bar/21g	75	0.5	365	5.5	79.7	2.6	4.6
Cereal, Cheerios & Milk Bar, Nestle*	1 Bar/22g	92	3	416	7.6	66.1	13.5	2
Cereal, Cherry Bakewell, Light, Alpen*	1 Bar/19g	65	1.1	341	5.1	56	5.6	23
Cereal, Chewy & Crisp with Choc Chips, Tesco*	1 Bar/27g	125	6.3	463	9.2	54	23.4	3.8
Cereal, Chewy & Crisp with Roasted Nuts, Tesco*	1 Bar/27g	127	6.2	471	9.3	57	22.9	2.5
Cereal, Chewy Chocolate Fudge, NUME, Morrisons*	1 Bar/21g	74	1.4	353	4.7	56.8	6.8	23
Cereal, Chewy Pomegranate, Vitality, Asda*	1 Bar/22g	76	0.6	346	4.1	69.3	2.8	13.4
Cereal, Chewy, BGTY, Sainsbury's*	1 Bar/25g	85	0.5	342	4.9	75.8	2.1	1.9
Cereal, Choc Chip & Nut, Chewy & Crisp, Sainsbury's*	1 Bar/27g	129	7	476	8.8	51.8	26	4.4
Cereal, Choc Chip, Brunch, Cadbury*	1 Bar/32g	140	5.3	445	6.1	64.5	17	4.8
Cereal, Chocolate & Orange, Officially Low Fat, Fox's*	1 Bar/19g	54	0.4	286	5	61.6	2.3	17.5
Cereal, Chocolate & Banana, Lidl*	1 Bar/25g	110	4	440	6.4	67.2	16	0
Cereal, Chocolate & Crispy Rice, Organic, Dove's Farm*	1 Bar/35g	147	5.3	421	4.4	66.9	15.1	3
Cereal, Chocolate & Fudge, Light, Alpen*	1 Bar/21g	71	1.3	342	4.9	55	6.5	22
Cereal, Chocolate & Orange, Light, Alpen*	1 Bar/21g	71	1.2	339	4.8	56	5.5	23.1
Cereal, Chocolate & Orange, Tesco*	1 Bar/22g	78	1.3	355	4.5	70.2	6	10.3
Cereal, Chocolate & Raisin, Seeds of Change*	1 Bar/29g	107	2.3	370	5	69.6	7.9	3.7
Cereal, Chocolate Chip, Special Flake, Tesco*	1 Bar/21g	85	1.6	405	6.9	75.8	7.8	2.3
Cereal, Chocolate Chip, Special K, Kellogg's*	1 Bar/21g	84	1.5	401	9	76	7	1.5
Cereal, Chocolate, Dark, Le Noir, Orco*	1 Bar/21g	95	3.3	451	7.3	69.9	15.8	0
Cereal, Chocolate, Dark, with Ginger, Weight Watchers*	1 Bar/22g	82	1.5	371	4.5	67.1	6.8	11.9
Cereal, Chocolate, Geobar, Traidcraft*	1 Bar/32g	130	2.7	407	4.3	78.5	8.4	0

BARS

	Measure INFO/WEIGHT	per Measure KCAL	FAT	Nutrition Values per 100g / 100ml KCAL	PROT	CARB	FAT	FIBRE
Cereal, Chocolate, Light & Crispy, Sainsbury's*	1 Bar/24g	88	1.5	369	6	64	6.5	15
Cereal, Chocolate, Milk, & Apricot, Value, Tesco*	1 Bar/22g	90	2.8	425	6.2	69.5	13.1	3.5
Cereal, Chocolate, Milk, Double, Special K, Kellogg's*	1 Bar/20g	79	1.8	396	9	66	9	10
Cereal, Chocolate, Milk, Double, Special K, Kellogg's*	1 Bar/20g	80	2	400	10	65	10	10
Cereal, Chocolate, Milk, Oaty, Weetabix*	1 Bar/23g	80	1.5	342	6.9	51.7	6.5	24.3
Cereal, Chocolate, Mint, Kellogg's*	1 Bar/22g	88	2.2	401	4.5	74	10	3.5
Cereal, Chocolate, Oats & More, Nestle*	1 Bar/30g	118	3.2	395	6.8	68.3	10.5	3.4
Cereal, Cinnamon Grahams, Nestle*	1 Bar/25g	106	3.7	426	7.2	66.2	14.7	1.9
Cereal, Citrus Fruits, Light, Alpen*	1 Bar/21g	59	0.9	283	5.6	55.9	4.1	22.4
Cereal, Coconut, Original Crunchy, Jordans*	1 Bar/30g	141	6.8	470	6.5	60	22.7	6.2
Cereal, Cranberry & Blackcurrant, LC, Tesco*	1 Bar/25g	75	0.7	295	4.4	62.7	2.9	21.9
Cereal, Cranberry & Orange, BGTY, Sainsbury's*	1 Bar/26g	93	1.3	358	2.7	75.8	4.9	2.3
Cereal, Cranberry & Orange, Brunch, Cadbury*	1 Bar/35g	154	5.6	440	5.9	67.7	15.9	0
Cereal, Cranberry & Orange, Weight Watchers*	1 Bar/28g	102	1.1	365	4.5	77.6	4.1	2.3
Cereal, Cranberry & Strawberry, Weight Watchers*	1 Bar/22g	69	1.2	314	6.4	51.8	5.4	16.8
Cereal, Cranberry & Yoghurt, Harvest Morn, Aldi*	1 Bar/29g	117	2.6	403	6.5	71.9	9	4.1
Cereal, Cranberry, Raisin & Nut, Shapers, Boots*	1 Bar/35g	140	4.4	400	7.1	65.7	12.6	3.7
Cereal, Crunchy Granola, Apple Crunch, Nature Valley*	1 Bar/21g	92	3.2	440	7.3	69	15	5.7
Cereal, Crunchy Granola, Ginger Nut, Nature Valley*	1 Bar/42g	189	7.1	451	7.9	64.2	16.9	2.3
Cereal, Crunchy Granola, Peanut Butter, Nature Valley*	1 Bar/21g	95	4	452	9.5	64.3	19	4.8
Cereal, Date, Beloved*	1 Bar/35g	133	3.3	379	6.7	64.1	9.4	5.7
Cereal, Double Chocolate, Light, Alpen, Weetabix*	1 Bar/19g	65	1.2	344	5	56	6.2	22
Cereal, Fig & Prune, Eurodiet*	1 Bar/50g	162	5.8	324	30	31.5	11.6	7.5
Cereal, Fruit & Fibre, Asda*	1 Bar/29g	111	2.8	390	6	69	10	4.1
Cereal, Fruit & Fibre, You Count, Love Life, Waitrose*	1 Bar/25g	88	0.2	351	6	76.5	0.9	6.3
Cereal, Fruit & Nut Break, Jordans*	1 Bar/37g	138	3.8	374	7	63.2	10.4	8.1
Cereal, Fruit & Nut, Alpen*	1 Bar/28g	109	2.3	390	5.8	73	8.3	2.9
Cereal, Fruit & Nut, Chewy Trail Mix, Nature Valley*	1 Bar/30g	114	3.2	379	7.7	63.2	10.6	7.3
Cereal, Fruit & Nut, with Milk Chocolate, Alpen*	1 Bar/29g	123	3.8	425	6.4	70.5	13	2.2
Cereal, Fruit, Average	*1 Bar/34g*	*130*	*3.9*	*382*	*5.9*	*64.7*	*11.5*	*6.5*
Cereal, Frusli, Blueberry, Jordans*	1 Bar/30g	113	2.1	375	5.2	70.2	7.1	4.9
Cereal, Frusli, Cranberry & Apple, Jordans*	1 Bar/30g	113	2.1	376	5.1	75.6	7.1	5
Cereal, Frusli, Raisin & Hazelnut, Jordans*	1 Bar/30g	117	3.7	390	5.8	64.3	12.2	4.5
Cereal, Frusli, Red Berries, Jordans*	1 Bar/30g	112	2.2	374	4.8	75.1	7.2	5.4
Cereal, Granola, Alpen*	1 Bar/29g	119	3.1	410	5.9	72.4	10.7	0
Cereal, Hazelnut, Brunch, Cadbury*	1 Bar/35g	160	7.4	460	7	60.5	21.4	2.2
Cereal, Milk Chocolate Chip, Chewy, Harvest Morn, Aldi*	1 Bar/22g	95	3.1	432	5.6	68	14	4.2
Cereal, Mixed Berry, Go Ahead, McVitie's*	1 Bar/35g	134	2.2	383	4.6	77.1	6.3	3.1
Cereal, Muesli Break, Breakfast in a Bar, Jordans*	1 Bar/46g	178	5	387	5.9	66.6	10.8	4.3
Cereal, Muesli, Apple, No Added Sugar, Crownfield, Lidl*	1 Bar/25g	96	2.8	386	6.3	67.9	11.2	6.7
Cereal, Multigrain, Peach & Apricot, BGTY, Sainsbury's*	1 Bar/28g	77	0.6	274	6.4	57	2.3	24.2
Cereal, Nut & Seed, Organic, Green & Black's*	1 Bar/50g	258	16.3	516	8.4	47.2	32.6	10
Cereal, Nutty, Free From, Sainsbury's*	1 Bar/25g	114	5	454	6.8	61.8	20	2.3
Cereal, Oat & Raisin, Basics, Sainsbury's*	1 Bar/25g	98	2.2	391	5.1	72.8	8.8	3.8
Cereal, Oat & Raisin, Soft Oaties, Nutri-Grain, Kellogg's*	1 Bar/40g	173	6.4	432	6	66	16	3.5
Cereal, Oats & Berries, Crunchy & More, Nature Valley*	1 Bar/21g	95	3.5	453	7.4	64.6	16.9	6.1
Cereal, Oaty, Strawberry, Weetabix*	1 Bar/23g	69	1.4	299	6.2	54.7	6.1	24.5
Cereal, Oaty, Toffee Dazzler, Weetabix*	1 Bar/23g	80	1.5	348	6.2	54.9	6.7	21.5
Cereal, Peanut Butter & Oat, Organic, Meridian Foods*	1 Bar/50g	204	9.2	407	12.6	50.9	18.4	5
Cereal, Raisin & Apricot, Weight Watchers*	1 Bar/28g	100	1.3	358	6.8	72.2	4.6	3.2
Cereal, Raisin & Nut Snack Bar, Benecol*	1 Bar/25g	98	2.8	390	3.9	68.5	11.1	2
Cereal, Raisin & Coconut, Value, Tesco*	1 Bar/21g	84	2.4	400	5.5	67.2	11.6	5
Cereal, Raisin, Raisin, Cadbury*	1 Bar/35g	150	5.4	430	5.6	66.4	15.5	1.8

BARS

INFO/WEIGHT	Measure		per Measure		Nutrition Values per 100g / 100ml				
			KCAL	FAT	KCAL	PROT	CARB	FAT	FIBRE
Cereal, Special Flake with Cranberries, Tesco*	1 Bar/23g		90	1.4	390	4.9	78.9	5.9	1.8
Cereal, Strawberry with Yoghurt, Alpen*	1 Bar/29g		119	3.1	409	5.7	72.6	10.6	0
Cereal, Strawberry, BGTY, Sainsbury's*	1 Bar/26g		100	1.2	385	3.8	82	4.6	5.2
Cereal, Strawberry, Fitness, Nestle*	1 Bar/24g		89	1.6	378	4.9	73.8	7	4.1
Cereal, Strawberry, Fruit 'n' Grain, Asda*	1 Bar/37g		126	2.6	340	4.2	65	7	4.5
Cereal, Strawberry, Value, Tesco*	1 Bar/21g		80	1.1	382	5.5	77.8	5.4	3.3
Cereal, Summer Fruits, Light, Alpen*	1 Bar/21g		70	0.9	334	4.4	58.7	4.1	22.4
Cereal, Toffee, Basics, Sainsbury's*	1 Bar/23g		92	1.9	398	4.8	75.8	8.4	2.5
Cereal, Very Berry, Weight Watchers*	1 Bar/27g		92	2.7	340	6.6	42.6	9.9	26.8
Cereal, White Chocolate & Strawberry, Value, Tesco*	1 Bar/21g		85	1.7	405	6.2	76.2	8.1	2.4
Cereal, White Chocolate, Oaty, Weetabix*	1 Bar/23g		78	1.4	341	6.4	52.4	6.3	24.3
Cereal, Wholegrain, Choc Chunk, Special K, Kellogg's*	1 Bar/20g		78	1.9	388	7	62	9.6	14
Cherries, & Almonds, & a Yoghurt Coating, Eat Natural*	1 Bar/45g		200	9.5	444	6.6	58.8	21.1	3.6
Cherry Crunch, Protein Flapjack, Trek*	1 Bar/56g		242	11.1	432	18.3	46	19.9	3.1
Chia, Apple & Cinnamon, Health Warrior*	1 Bar/25g		100	5	400	12	56	20	16
Chia, Chocolate Peanut Butter, Health Warrior*	1 Bar/25g		100	1	400	12	52	4	16
Chia, Coffee, Health Warrior*	1 Bar/25g		100	5	400	12	52	20	12
Chia, Dark Chocolate Cherry, Health Warrior*	1 Bar/25g		100	5	400	12	56	20	16
Chia, Mango, Health Warrior*	1 Bar/25g		100	5	400	12	56	20	16
Choco & Biscuit, Milk, Choceur, Aldi*	1 Bar/33g		174	9.6	526	7.9	59	29	1.3
Choco & Biscuit, Orange, Choceur, Aldi*	1 Bar/33g		176	9.9	533	7.6	59	30	1.1
Chocolate & Caramel, Rice Krispies Squares, Kellogg's*	1 Bar/36g		155	5	430	4.5	71	14	2
Chocolate & Orange, Crispy, Shapers, Boots*	1 Bar/22g		94	2.6	425	3.6	77	12	0.8
Chocolate & Toffee, Free From, Sainsbury's*	1 Bar/30g		139	5.4	465	4.8	71	18	0.8
Chocolate Almond Fudge, Energy, Clif*	1 Bar/68g		252	6	370	13	56	8.8	7.4
Chocolate Biscuit, with Caramel, Aldi*	1 Bar/21g		104	5.1	497	5.2	63.4	24.5	0.9
Chocolate Brownie, Average	**1 Bar/68g**		**240**	**4**	**353**	**14.7**	**60.3**	**5.9**	**8.8**
Chocolate Brownie, Big Softies, to Go, Fox's*	1 Bar/25g		87	0.7	348	5.5	74.9	2.9	0
Chocolate Brownie, Essential, Waitrose*	1 Bar/26g		108	4.7	415	5.1	55.7	18.1	4.3
Chocolate Caramel Whip, Weight Watchers*	1 Bar/25g		88	2.7	353	2.7	72.4	10.8	1
Chocolate Caramel, Weight Watchers*	1 Bar/20g		80	2.5	400	5	70	12.5	0
Chocolate Chip Granola, Advantage, Atkins*	1 Bar/48g		200	8	417	35.4	37.5	16.7	12.5
Chocolate Chip Muesli, Diet Chef Ltd*	1 Bar/50g		191	6	382	5.8	59.8	11.9	6.1
Chocolate Chip, Snack, Diet Chef Ltd*	1 Bar/27g		99	2.7	367	5.8	63.6	9.9	4.5
Chocolate Cookie Caramel, Light Bites, Lighter Life*	1 Bar/30g		99	4.7	332	11.1	22.3	15.8	37.4
Chocolate Crisp, Weight Watchers*	1 Bar/25g		94	2.6	378	4.8	66.8	10.2	1.6
Chocolate Flavour, Protein, Diet Chef Ltd*	1 Bar/60g		225	7.1	375	29.3	37.5	11.9	4.2
Chocolate Hazelnut, Atkins*	1 Bar/60g		227	10.2	378	32	29.1	17	9.8
Chocolate Hazelnut, Day Break, Atkins*	1 Bar/40g		180	14	450	15	45	35	17.5
Chocolate Orange, Montana*	1 Bar/25g		131	6.8	523	7	62.2	27.4	0
Chocolate Raisin & Cereal, Morrisons*	1 Bar/30g		126	4.4	420	5.4	66.3	14.8	3.8
Chocolate Twist Shortcake, Breakaway, Nestle*	1 Bar/19g		97	4.6	510	5.6	66.7	24.2	1.5
Chocolate, & Raspberry, COU, M&S*	1 Bar/25g		90	0.7	360	5.4	78.2	2.7	3.2
Chocolate, Caramel, & Biscuit, Asda*	1 Bar/30g		150	8.3	508	8	56	28	2.5
Chocolate, Caramel, Nut Roll, Advantage, Atkins*	1 Bar/44g		170	12	386	18.2	43.2	27.3	18.2
Chocolate, Caramel, Wacko, Belmont, Aldi*	1 Bar/21g		102	4.6	485	5.3	65	22	1.7
Chocolate, Crisp, Weight Watchers*	1 Bar/25g		92	2.6	369	5.4	75.1	10.2	0.8
Chocolate, Crispy, Free From, Tesco*	1 Bar/30g		132	4.6	440	4.1	71.2	15.4	0.5
Chocolate, Dark, & Almond, Nupo*	1 Bar/29g		99	2.8	343	11.2	41	9.8	27
Chocolate, Dark, Chewy Delight, Special K, Kellogg's*	1 Bar/24g		97	3.4	404	4.5	57	14	17
Chocolate, Dark, Nuts, & Sea Salt, Kind*	1 Bar/40g		199	15.2	498	14	39	38	18
Chocolate, Decadence, Atkins*	1 Bar/60g		233	12	388	30	27.3	20	9.8
Chocolate, Double, Caramel, Crunch, Atkins*	1 Bar/44g		160	9	364	22.7	50	20.4	25

BARS

INFO/WEIGHT	Measure	per Measure KCAL	FAT	Nutrition Values per 100g / 100ml KCAL	PROT	CARB	FAT	FIBRE
Chocolate, Double, Dark, Zone Perfect*	1 Bar/45g	190	5.5	422	24.5	44.9	12.2	2
Chocolate, Fruit & Nut, M&S*	1 Bar/50g	235	12	470	6.5	57.1	24.1	2.5
Chocolate, Healthy Meal, Herbalife*	1 Bar/56g	207	5.9	370	23.9	37.5	10.6	14.5
Chocolate, Juice Plus*	1 Bar/55g	210	6.4	382	24.8	39.4	11.6	10.2
Chocolate, Milk & White, Boohbah, M&S*	1 Bar/75g	405	24.2	540	7.9	54.7	32.3	1.2
Chocolate, Milk, Belgian, Sugar Free, Sweet' N Low*	1 Bar/42g	202	14.3	480	7.1	52.7	34.1	1.8
Chocolate, Milk, Chewy Delight, Special K, Kellogg's*	1 Bar/24g	95	3.1	397	5	57	13	17
Chocolate, Milk, Crispy, Endulge, Atkins*	1 Bar/30g	141	9.6	469	13	48	32	2
Chocolate, Milkshake, Crisp, Weight Watchers*	1 Bar/21g	82	2.1	391	4.4	59.6	10	13.4
Chocolate, Polar, Sainsbury's*	1 Bar/25g	133	7.2	533	5.5	63	28.6	1.2
Chocolate, Racer, Dairyfine, Aldi*	1 Bar/38g	185	9.5	486	8.6	54	25	4.2
Chocolate, Sandwich, Seal, Aldi*	1 Bar/25g	131	7	523	5.5	60.6	28.1	3.1
Chocolate, Soya, Dairy Free, Free From, Sainsbury's*	1 Bar/50g	274	17.5	548	10.8	47.5	35	4.3
Chocolate, Toffee Pecan, M&S*	1 Bar/36g	179	9.8	498	4.9	58.3	27.3	0.7
Chocolate, Wafer, Blue Riband, 99 Calories, Nestle*	1 Bar/19g	99	4.7	514	5.5	66.5	24.6	2
Chocolate, Wafer, Caramel, Penguin, McVitie's*	1 Bar/21g	106	5.4	492	5.1	60.7	25.2	1.4
Chocolate, Wild & Whippy, Tesco*	1 Bar/18g	78	2.8	447	3.7	72	16	0.8
Chocolix, Schar*	1 Bar/22g	101	3.9	463	3.6	70	18	4.2
Club, Fruit, Jacob's*	1 Biscuit/25g	124	6.2	496	5.6	62.2	25	2.3
Club, Milk Chocolate, Jacob's*	1 Biscuit/24g	123	6.3	511	5.8	62.6	26.4	2
Club, Mint, Jacob's*	1 Biscuit/24g	124	6.5	517	5.6	62.5	27.2	1.7
Club, Orange, Jacob's*	1 Biscuit/23g	117	6.1	509	5.7	61.8	26.5	2.3
Coco Pops, & Milk, Kellogg's*	1 Bar/20g	85	2.6	423	7	70	13	1
Cocoa Brownie, Trek, The Natural Health Company*	1 Bar/68g	223	4.1	328	17	53	6	8
Cocoa Crunch, Nak'd*	1 Bar/30g	105	2.6	351	18.4	47.2	8.8	6.3
Cocoa Delight, Wholefood, GF, Nak'd*	1 Bar/35g	135	5.3	386	9.4	49.4	15.1	6.8
Cocoa Loco, Wildly Different, Nak'd*	1 Bar/30g	106	2.9	354	7.9	55.4	9.8	7.5
Cocoa Mint, GF, Raw, Wholefood, Nak'd*	1 Bar/35g	135	5.3	386	9.4	49.4	15.1	6.8
Cocoa Orange, GF, Nak'd*	1 Bar/35g	145	7	415	11	45.1	20	6.4
Coconut & Chocolate, Vitamin & Protein, Fulfil Nutrition*	1 Bar/60g	207	8.5	344	34.4	19.6	14.1	18.7
Coconut Chocolate Crisp, Weight Watchers*	1 Bar/25g	89	2.6	356	3.6	71.2	10.4	3.2
Coconut, Nutramino*	1 Bar/66g	290	14	439	30.3	33.3	21.2	2.9
Cookie, Apple Crumble, COU, M&S*	1 Bar/27g	90	0.7	335	5.8	72.6	2.6	2.3
Cookie, Oreo, Nabisco*	1 Bar/35g	180	10.2	514	2	66	29	0
Cookies & Cream, Fit Crunch*	1 Bar/88g	380	16	432	34.1	30.7	18.2	9.1
Corn Flakes, & Chocolate Milk, Kellogg's*	1 Bar/40g	176	6.4	440	9	66	16	2
Cranberry & Macadamia Porridge Oat, Stoats*	1 Bar/85g	385	22.9	453	6.9	71.8	26.9	5.9
Cranberry & Raisin, Geobar, Traidcraft*	1 Bar/35g	131	2.8	374	3.7	72.6	8	2.3
Cranberry & Roasted Almonds, Nutty, Chewy, Kellogg's*	1 Bar/35g	157	7	449	8.9	57.1	20	4.9
Cranberry, & Almond, Goodness Knows*	1 Bar/34g	153	6.7	451	7.5	56.8	19.8	6.1
Cranberry, Almond & Macadamia, Kind*	1 Bar/40g	192	12	480	10	50	30	7.2
Cranberry, Crunchy, Meal Replacement, CWP*	1 Bar/50g	174	5.8	349	24.8	30.2	11.6	14.3
Crazy Caramel, Tesco*	1 Bar/40g	192	9.2	480	3.9	64	23	1
Creme Brulee Chocolate, M&S*	1 Bar/36g	178	10.5	495	4.4	54	29.2	0.4
Creme Brulee, Wonka*	2 Pieces/20g	111	6.5	555	5.7	59.1	32.6	1.1
Crunchy Caramel, Tesco*	1 Bar/21g	98	5.2	467	4.6	56	25	1.4
Crunchy Crispy Treat, Kids, Tesco*	1 Bar/24g	109	5	453	3.6	62.5	20.9	1.5
Crunchy Nut, Chocolate Peanut Crisp, Kellogg's*	1 Bar/35g	169	8.8	483	12	53	25	3.5
Crunchy Nut, Kellogg's*	1 Bar/30g	119	1.5	397	6	82	5	2.5
Dark Chocolate & Mint Crunch, Weight Watchers*	1 Bar/23g	85	3	371	2.7	48.7	13.1	23.7
Dark Chocolate, Cranberry, Organic, Biona*	1 Bar/40g	162	5.9	405	6.2	53.5	14.7	0
Dark Chocolate, Crispy Wafer, Tasty Little Numbers*	1 Bar/20g	100	5.1	499	6.4	60.4	25.6	7
Date & Fruit, Lyme Regis Foods*	1 Bar/42g	169	6.5	402	7.3	58.2	15.5	8.9

B

BARS

INFO/WEIGHT	Measure	per Measure		Nutrition Values per 100g / 100ml				
		KCAL	FAT	KCAL	PROT	CARB	FAT	FIBRE
Date & Peanut, Eat Real*	1 Bar/40g	155	4.6	387	7.8	59.7	11.5	6.3
Date & Walnut, with Pumpkin Seeds, Eat Natural*	1 Bar/45g	218	9	434	9.1	46.6	18	4.5
Digestive, Milk Chocolate, McVitie's*	1 Bar/23g	118	5.8	511	6.6	64.6	25.1	1.9
Digestive, Milk Chocolate, Tesco*	1 Bar/19g	96	4.9	506	6.8	61.6	25.8	2.4
Digestive, Milk Chocolate, Value, Tesco*	1 Bar/19g	96	4.9	505	6.6	61.8	25.8	3
Double Chocolate, Breakfast Snack, Tesco*	1 Bar/37g	144	6.4	385	5.3	52.7	17	3.3
Echo, Mint, Fox's*	1 Bar/25g	130	6.6	518	7.9	60.7	26.6	1.6
Energize, Berry Blast, Power Bar*	1 Bar/55g	199	2	362	10.9	70.8	3.7	2
Energy, Cocoa Brownie, Natural Balance Foods*	1 Bar/68g	216	4.1	318	17	51	6	0
Energy, Cool Mint, Chocolate, Clif*	1 Bar/68g	256	5	377	14.7	63.2	7.3	7.4
Energy, Ride, Power Bar*	1 Bar/55g	213	9.1	387	18.6	40.9	16.6	7.4
Fair Break, Traidcraft*	1 Bar/22g	116	6.2	528	6	63	28	0
Fig & Mango, Wholesome, The Food Doctor*	1 Bar/35g	111	3.3	317	7.8	35.7	9.4	29.2
Flapjack, Apple & Sultana, Organic, Dove's Farm*	1 Bar/40g	178	7.8	446	4.7	61.1	19.6	3.5
Flapjack, Buttery, Traditional, Organic, Dove's Farm*	1 Bar/40g	173	7.5	432	6.1	59.4	18.8	5.7
Flapjack, Mixed Berry, Progain, Maxinutrition*	1 Bar/90g	324	7.2	360	26.5	50.1	8	2.6
Food Bar, Apple & Walnut, The Food Doctor*	1 Bar/35g	129	4.9	367	8.4	37.3	14	29.1
Forest Fruit & Raisin, LC, Tesco*	1 Bar/27.1g	95	0.7	350	4.5	76.8	2.7	3.6
Forest Fruit, Yoghurt, Breaks, Go Ahead, McVitie's*	2 Slices/36g	144	3.6	402	5.4	72.6	10	2.2
Frosties, & Milk, Kellogg's*	1 Bar/25g	102	2.8	408	7	71	11	1
Frosties, Snack Bar, Kellogg's*	1 Bar/25g	104	2.8	414	7	72	11	1
Fruit & Fibre, Coconut, Apricot, Oats, Spelt, Eat Natural*	1 Bar/40g	165	7	413	6.4	51.6	17.5	6.1
Fruit & Fibre, Plum, Peanut, Oats, Spelt, Eat Natural*	1 Bar/40g	176	7.8	441	9.4	53.3	19.6	6.8
Fruit & Grain, Apple, Harvest Morn, Aldi*	1 Bar/37g	129	3	349	4.2	65	8	4.5
Fruit & Grain, Strawberry, Harvest Morn, Aldi*	1 Bar/37g	130	2.6	349	4.2	65	7	4.5
Fruit & Nut, Eat Natural*	1 Bar/50g	223	11.2	446	11.6	49.8	22.3	5.3
Fruit & Nut, Milk Chocolate, Eat Real*	1 Bar/40g	196	11.7	490	8.1	46.3	29.3	9.3
Fruit & Nut, Organic, Eat Natural*	1 Bar/50g	244	15.3	488	10.2	42.9	30.6	0
Fruit & Nut, Yoghurt Coated, Eat Real*	1 Bar/40g	186	9.9	466	6.6	51.9	24.8	9.2
Fruit 'n' Fibre Bakes with Sultanas, Kellogg's*	1 Bar/40g	146	5.2	365	4.5	58	13	9
Fruit 'n' Fibre, Kellogg's*	1 Bar/25g	95	2.2	380	5	71	9	5
Fruit Muesli, Morning, Oat So Simple, Quaker*	1 Bar/35g	139	3.2	398	7.7	68.1	9.1	6.6
Fruit, Apple, Hellema*	1 Bar/33g	127	2.5	384	4.5	74	7.5	2
Fruit, Apple, Trimlyne*	1 Bar/27g	92	0.7	342	4.5	69.6	2.7	3.8
Fruit, Fig, Castus*	1 Bar/27g	80	1.3	300	3	60	5	0
Fruit, Nut & Seed Bars, The Village Bakery*	1 Bar/25g	93	1.6	373	5.7	73.7	6.2	0.1
Fruit, Nut & Seeds Cereal, Eat Well, M&S*	1 Bar/24g	88	2.6	365	6.1	60.8	10.9	6.9
Fruit, Strawberry, Fruitina*	1 Bar/15g	43	0.2	289	1.9	61.9	1.1	12.2
Fruity Cereal, Go, Soreen*	1 Bar/40g	143	1.8	358	6.8	72.6	4.5	0
Fudge Brownie, Carb Killa, Grenade*	1 Bar/60g	215	8	359	38.9	22.6	13.3	11.3
Fudge Mallow Delight, Whipple Scrumptious, Wonka*	1 Bar/38g	205	12	537	4.6	59.2	31.3	0.6
Ginger & Oat, Chocolate Covered, Snack, Waitrose*	1 Bar/27g	120	5	444	4.2	65	18.6	2.1
Ginger Bread, Nak'd*	1 Bar/35g	157	10.7	450	10	35.4	30.8	9.4
Gingerbread, GF, Nak'd*	1 Bar/35g	158	10.8	450	10	35	31	9.4
Goji Berries & Fax Seeds, Porridge Oat, Stoats*	1 Bar/85g	374	24.4	440	10.9	62.4	28.7	8.2
Golden Syrup, Morning, Oat So Simple, Quaker*	1 Bar/35g	142	3.5	407	8.2	67.6	10	6.8
Goodies, Cereal & Fruit, Apricot, Organic, Organix*	1 Bar/30g	122	6.1	408	7.2	55.3	20.4	6.2
Goodness, Cocoa, & Hazelnut, Go Ahead!*	1 Bar/30g	111	4	369	7.4	56	13.4	7.8
Granola with Peanut Butter, Natco*	1 Bar/29g	129	4.1	445	10	69	14.1	5.5
Granola, Almond & Raisin, McVitie's*	1 Serving/35g	133	4	380	7	62.9	11.3	4.1
Granola, Crunchy, Oats & Chocolate, Nature Valley*	1 Bar/21g	98	4.1	464	8.3	59.8	19.8	7.1
Granola, Crunchy, Roasted Almond, Nature Valley*	1 Bar/42g	193	7.6	459	8.1	65.6	18.2	3.7
Granola, Maple Syrup, Twin Pack, Tesco*	2 Bars/42g	204	9.4	485	6	64.7	22.3	4.1

BARS

INFO/WEIGHT	Measure		per Measure		Nutrition Values per 100g / 100ml				
			KCAL	FAT	KCAL	PROT	CARB	FAT	FIBRE
Granola, Oats & Hazlenuts, Nature Valley*	2 Bars/42g		195	8.4	465	8.4	58.9	20.1	7.5
Granola, Peanut Butter, Advantage, Atkins*	1 Bar/48g		210	11	438	29.2	39.6	22.9	10.4
Granola, Peanut Butter, Quaker*	1 Bar/28g		110	3.5	393	7.1	64.3	12.5	3.6
Harvest Cheweee, Apple & Raisin, Quaker*	1 Bar/22g		89	2.6	405	5.5	68	12	3
Harvest Cheweee, Choc Chip, Quaker*	1 Bar/22g		95	3.5	430	5.5	68	16	3.5
Harvest Cheweee, Toffee, Quaker*	1 Bar/22g		94	3.3	427	5	68	15	3
Harvest Cheweee, White Chocolate Chip, Quaker*	1 Bar/22g		94	3.4	425	6	67	15.5	3.5
Hazelnut & Raisin, Energy Ball, Deliciously Ella*	1 Ball/40g		152	7.5	379	6.5	49.7	18.7	5.2
Healthy Meal, Herbalife*	1 Bar/56g		207	6	369	23.7	37.1	10.7	14.7
Hobnobs, Choc & Golden Syrup, McVitie's*	1 Bar/31g		129	4	421	6.3	68.2	13.1	4.8
Honey Nut, Special K, Special K, Kellogg's*	1 Bar/22g		90	2	409	9.1	72.7	9.1	13.6
Honey Rice Crisp, Lower Fat, Go Ahead, McVitie's*	1 Bar/22g		90	2.2	411	3.9	75.8	10.2	1.1
Honeycomb, Club, Jacob's*	1 Bar/23g		116	6	512	5.7	61.9	26.3	2.3
Lemon Drizzle, Nak'd*	1 Bar/35g		133	5.4	381	6.1	51.8	15.5	5.1
Luna, Chocolate Pecan Pie, Luna*	1 Bar/48g		180	4.5	375	20.8	50	9.4	2.1
Luna, Nutz Over Chocolate, Luna*	1 Bar/48g		180	4.5	375	20.8	50	9.4	2.1
Luxury, Absolute Nut, Jordans*	1 Bar/45g		251	18.6	557	12.7	33.3	41.4	7
Macadamia & Coconut, Paleo, Aldi*	1 Bar/45g		212	12.2	470	7.6	43	27	11
Macadamia & Fruit, Eat Natural*	1 Bar/50g		242	15.4	485	7.3	44.6	30.8	0
Macaroon, Lees*	1 Bar/70g		276	4.7	395	1.2	82.5	6.7	0
Maple & Pecan, Crunchy, Jordans*	1 Bar/33g		153	7.6	464	7.7	56.8	22.9	6.5
Maple, Glazed Pecan, & Sea Salt, Kind*	1 Bar/40g		213	17.2	532	14	33	43	13
Marshmallow, Chewy, Rice Krispies Squares, Kellogg's*	1 Bar/28g		119	3.4	424	3	76	12	0.9
Meal Replacement, Chocolate & Peanut Butter, Atkins*	1 Bar/60g		240	12	400	31.7	36.7	20	16.7
Meal Replacement, Chocolate Mint, Crunchy, CWP*	1 Bar/50g		174	5.8	349	24.8	30.2	11.6	14.4
Meal Replacement, Chocolate, Ultra Slim, Tesco*	1 Bar/60g		219	6.7	365	28.5	37.3	11.1	8.2
Meal Replacement, Raspberry, Crispy, Tesco*	1 Bar/60g		216	6.7	360	22.3	42.1	11.2	7.6
Milk Choc Joy, Meal Replacement, Shake that Weight*	1 Bar/35g		130	4.1	371	24.3	39.4	11.7	6
Milk Chocolate Chip & Hazelnut, Snack, Benecol*	1 Bar/25g		99	3.3	395	4.7	64.5	13.1	2.5
Milk Chocolate Coated Orange Flavour, Energy, Boots*	1 Bar/70g		274	7	391	5.2	70	10	2.8
Milk Chocolate Whirls, Asda*	1 Bar/26g		116	4.2	447	3.7	72	16	0.8
Milk Chocolate, Crispy Wafer, Tasty Little Numbers*	1 Bar/20g		100	5	499	6.1	61.4	25.1	3
Milk Chocolate, Mint, Vitamin & Protein, Fulfil Nutrition*	1 Bar/55g		189	6.9	344	35.9	18.8	12.5	18.8
Mint Chocolate Whip, Weight Watchers*	1 Bar/20g		80	2	402	3.6	74	9.9	0.7
Mint Crunch, Guilt Free Snacking, M&S*	1 Bar/24g		143	9.2	596	4.3	56.9	38.4	2.9
Mint, Double Take, Sainsbury's*	1 Bar/20g		107	6.2	534	7.2	56.9	30.8	1.3
Mixed Berry, Trek, Natural Balance Foods*	1 Bar/68g		204	1.5	300	15.6	56.5	2.2	6
Mixed Fruit, Juice Plus*	1 Bar/55g		211	6.9	384	27.3	35.5	12.6	9.7
Mixed Nut Feast, Eat Natural*	1 Bar/50g		278	20.5	556	18.8	28	41	0
Mudslide, Atkins*	1 Bar/48g		210	10	438	31.2	39.6	20.8	10.4
Muesli & Seeds, Bountiful, Aldi*	1 Bar/30g		98	1.4	328	3	53	4.8	18
Muesli, Apricot & Almond, Carmen's*	1 Bar/45g		190	8.2	423	10.4	50.6	18.2	7.4
Muesli, Cherry & Milk, Sirius, Lidl*	1 Bar/25g		104	2.8	417	7.2	71.3	11.4	3.9
Muesli, Cookie Coach*	1 Bar/75g		289	8.3	385	6.8	65.1	11.1	0
Muesli, Peanut, No Added Sugar, Crownfield, Lidl*	1 Bar/25g		98	3.3	391	7.9	65.7	13.2	4.7
Muesli, Yogurt Coated, Slim & Save*	1 Bar/45g		160	4.5	355	27.3	37.2	9.9	11
Muffin, Cadbury*	1 Bar/68g		274	17.3	403	5.6	38	25.4	0
Multigrain, Apple & Sultana, Jordans*	1 Bar/40g		141	2.5	353	4.4	70	6.2	4.8
Multigrain, Cranberry & Raspberry, Jordans*	1 Bar/37g		135	2.4	364	4.8	71.3	6.6	4.8
Multigrain, Fruit & Nut, Jordans*	1 Bar/40g		164	6.5	410	7	59.1	16.2	5.7
Natural Energy, Cacao Crunch, Power Bar*	1 Bar/40g		156	3.8	391	8.3	65.5	9.4	5.7
Nine Bar, Mixed Seed with Hemp, Original, Wholebake*	1 Bar/40g		222	16.2	555	18.3	29.2	40.5	5.2
Nine Bar, Nutty, Wholebake*	1 Bar/50g		279	20.4	558	15.3	32.3	40.8	4.9

	Measure INFO/WEIGHT	per Measure KCAL	FAT	Nutrition Values per 100g / 100ml KCAL	PROT	CARB	FAT	FIBRE
BARS								
Noisettes & Amandes, Special K, Kellogg's*	1 Bar/21g	83	2.1	397	8	66	10	7
Nougat, Cool Mint, & Dark Chocolate, Shapers, Boots*	1 Bar/23g	83	3.2	362	2.6	70	14	1.1
Nougat, Summer Strawberry, Shapers, Boots*	1 Bar/23g	83	3	361	2.7	73	13	0.6
Nut, Dark Chocolate & Apricot, Natural, Nice & Natural*	1 Bar/35g	163	10.2	465	15.2	35.2	29.1	5.4
Nutri-Grain, Apple, Kellogg's*	1 Bar/37g	131	3.3	355	4	67	9	4
Nutri-Grain, Apple, Soft & Fruity, Kellogg's*	1 Bar/37g	133	3	359	4	70.3	8.1	4
Nutri-Grain, Blackberry & Apple, Kellogg's*	1 Bar/37g	131	3.3	355	4	67	9	4
Nutri-Grain, Blackberry & Apple, Soft & Fruity, Kellogg's*	1 Bar/37g	133	3	359	4	70.3	8.1	4
Nutri-Grain, Blueberry, Kellogg's*	1 Bar/37g	133	3	359	3.5	69	8	3.5
Nutri-Grain, Blueberry, Soft & Fruity, Kellogg's*	1 Bar/37g	133	3	359	4	70.3	8.1	4
Nutri-Grain, Chocolate Chip, Chewy, Kellogg's*	1 Bar/25g	103	3	413	4.5	73	12	2.5
Nutri-Grain, Crunchy Oat Granola, Choc Chip, Kellogg's*	1 Bar/40g	187	7.6	468	7	65	19	4.5
Nutri-Grain, Crunchy Oat Granola, Cinnamon, Kellogg's*	2 Slices/40g	186	7.6	465	8	63	19	5
Nutri-Grain, Elevenses, Choc Chip Bakes, Kellogg's*	1 Bar/45g	179	5.8	397	4	66	13	2
Nutri-Grain, Elevenses, Ginger Bakes, Kellogg's*	1 Bar/45g	168	4	373	5	68	9	3
Nutri-Grain, Elevenses, Raisin Bakes, Kellogg's*	1 Bar/45g	168	4	374	4.5	68	9	2.5
Nutri-Grain, Oat Bakes, Cherry, Kellogg's*	1 Bar/50g	204	7	408	4.5	66	14	2.5
Nutri-Grain, Oat Bakes, Totally Oaty, Kellogg's*	1 Bar/50g	206	7.5	411	5	64	15	3
Nutri-Grain, Raspberry, Kellogg's*	1 Bar/37g	131	3.3	355	4	67	9	4
Nutri-Grain, Strawberry, Kellogg's*	1 Bar/37g	133	3	359	3.5	69	8	3.5
Nutri-Grain, Strawberry, Soft & Fruity, Kellogg's*	1 Bar/37g	133	3	359	4	70.3	8.1	4
Nuts & Berry, Weight Watchers*	1 Bar/24g	92	2.9	383	5.9	52.1	11.9	12.7
Nutty Crunch Surprise, Wonka*	1 Bar/37g	202	11.9	543	4.9	58.7	32.1	0.9
Nutty Nougat Caramel, Tesco*	1 Bar/40g	200	11.1	490	8.7	52.7	27.2	3.8
Oat, Original with Golden Syrup, Quaker*	1 Bar/38g	139	3.6	366	7.1	64.5	9.5	7.9
Oat, Quaker*	1 Bar/38g	137	3.4	360	6.8	64.5	8.8	8
Oats, Sweet Potato & Orange, COU, M&S*	1 Bar/30g	111	3.9	369	7.2	53.4	12.9	5.2
Oaty with Cranberry & Blueberry, Tesco*	1 Bar/38g	141	2.8	370	5.5	69	7.5	6.2
Oaty, Cranberry & Cashew, Perkier*	1 Bar/40g	155	4.9	387	12.1	53.5	12.3	10.4
Oaty, Fruit & Nut, Weight Watchers*	1 Bar/26g	90	2.4	345	10.5	42.4	9.2	25.5
Oaty, Strawberry Crusher, Weetabix*	1 Bar/23g	79	1.4	345	6.1	55.2	6.1	22.2
Orange Crunch, Go Ahead, McVitie's*	1 Bar/23g	99	2.9	430	4.1	78	12.8	0.8
Original Muesli, Diet Chef Ltd*	1 Bar/50g	199	6.9	398	6.1	59	13.8	6.4
Original, Crunchy, Honey & Almond, Jordans*	1 Bar/30g	139	6.8	463	8.3	56.7	22.7	6.7
Original, Nut Free, Get Buzzing*	1 Bar/62g	248	12	400	6.8	51.6	19.4	3.7
Peach & Apricot, Special K, Kellogg's*	1 Bar/23g	90	1.4	383	8	75	6	2.5
Peanut & Popcorn, Dark Chocolate Chunks, Eat Natural*	1 Bar/45g	204	9.9	453	10.7	50.6	21.9	5.2
Peanut & Banana, Protein, Meridian*	1 Bar/40g	173	9.5	432	17.4	34.8	23.8	4.8
Peanut & Caramel Whip, Weight Watchers*	1 Bar/20g	76	2.7	381	4.4	73.7	13.7	1.2
Peanut Caramel, Payday, Hershey*	1 Bar/19g	88	4.8	462	13.5	51.9	25	3.8
Peanut, Mr Toms*	1 Bar/40g	210	13	525	20	42.5	32.5	2.5
Peanut, Raisin & Chocolate, Weight Watchers*	1 Bar/25g	97	2.8	388	7.6	60	11.2	12.8
Pecan Apricot & Peach, M&S*	1 Bar/50g	255	17.8	510	9.3	38.2	35.5	4.9
Pecan Pie, GF, Nak'd*	1 Bar/35g	156	10.3	477	7.6	36.4	31.4	8.9
Penguin Bigstix, McVitie's*	1 Biscuit/12.5g	64	3.2	508	6.4	62.8	25.7	2.6
Popcorn, Caffe Nero*	1 Serving/55g	312	17.5	569	6.9	62.5	31.8	1.2
Popcorn, Cranberry & Yoghurt , Nature Valley*	1 Bar/20g	85	2.9	425	4.6	62.4	14.6	12.4
Protein, Apple Pie, GF, Quest*	1 Bar/60g	202	7.2	337	33	15	12	23
Protein, Banana Nut Muffin, GF, Quest*	1 Bar/60g	197	7.8	329	33	17	13	21
Protein, Banana, Hike, Aldi*	1 Bar/55g	169	0.8	306	20	45	1.5	18
Protein, Caramel Chaos, Carb Killa, Grenade*	1 Bar/60g	214	7.9	357	38.7	22.5	13.2	11.1
Protein, Caramel Peanut, My Bar Zero, Myprotein*	1 Bar/65g	211	7.2	325	31	6.2	11	37
Protein, Chocolate & Banana, MuleBar*	1 Bar/65g	254	5.8	390	21	56	9	2

BARS

	Measure INFO/WEIGHT	per Measure		Nutrition Values per 100g / 100ml				
		KCAL	FAT	KCAL	PROT	CARB	FAT	FIBRE
Protein, Chocolate Brownie, GF, Quest*	1 Bar/60g	191	7.2	318	33	12	12	25
Protein, Chocolate Chip Cookie Dough, GF, Quest*	1 Bar/60g	206	9	344	34	12	15	23
Protein, Chocolate Peanut Butter, GF, Quest*	1 Bar/60g	185	6.6	309	33	17	11	23
Protein, Chocolate Peanut, Musclefood*	1 Bar/42g	173	4	411	35.7	33	9.5	0
Protein, Chunky Peanut, Nutramino*	1 Bar/60g	236	10.8	393	35	35	18	1.3
Protein, Cinnamon Roll, GF, Quest*	1 Bar/60g	191	7.2	318	33	16	12	23
Protein, Coconut Cashew, GF, Quest*	1 Bar/60g	202	8.4	337	33	14	14	23
Protein, Combat Crunch, MusclePharm*	1 Bar/63g	210	7	333	31.8	39.7	11.1	0
Protein, Cookies & Cream, GF, Quest*	1 Bar/60g	209	9	349	35	12	15	23
Protein, Cookies & Cream, My Bar Zero, Myprotein*	1 Bar/65g	202	6	311	32	6.5	9.2	37
Protein, Cranberry Kick, Chunks, Trek, Natural Balance*	1 Bar/60g	202	3.9	336	20.7	44	6.5	9
Protein, Double Chocolate Chunk, GF, Quest*	1 Bar/60g	191	7.8	318	33	18	13	21
Protein, Flapjack, Oat Crunch, Natural Balance Foods*	1 Bar/56g	249	12.9	444	18	43	23	3
Protein, Fudge Cookies & Cream, McVitie's*	1 Bar/100g	230	4.5	230	14	33	4.5	1
Protein, Lemon Cream Pie, GF, Quest*	1 Bar/60g	181	6	302	33	16	10	23
Protein, Mint Chocolate Chunk, GF, Quest*	1 Bar/60g	209	9	348	33	11	15	24
Protein, Mixed Berry Bliss, GF, Quest*	1 Bar/60g	209	9	349	33	13	15	23
Protein, Peanut Blast, Natural Energy, Ball, Bounce*	1 Ball/49g	210	8	429	28.6	38.8	16.3	4.1
Protein, Peanut Butter Jelly, GF, Quest*	1 Bar/60g	217	10.2	361	33	13	17	21
Protein, Peanut Chewy Crisp, Chemical Protein Pro-Xs*	1 Bar/70g	243	5.2	347	42.9	5.5	7.5	12.5
Protein, Peanut Peak, Chunks, Trek, Natural Balance*	1 Bar/60g	232	7.9	386	20.9	42	13.2	7
Protein, Premium, Ball, Bounce*	1 Ball/49g	209	9	426	30.6	40.8	18.4	2
Protein, Pumpkin Pie, GF, Limited Edition, Quest*	1 Bar/60g	220	12	366	35	12	20	20
Protein, S'mores, GF, Quest*	1 Bar/60g	197	8.4	329	33	15	14	21
Protein, Strawberry Cheesecake, GF, Quest*	1 Bar/60g	188	6.6	314	33	17	11	22
Protein, Supreme Peanut, Musclefood*	1 Bar/44g	171	6.6	388	34.1	35.2	15	3.8
Protein, Toffee Triumph, Chunks, Trek, Natural Balance*	1 Bar/60g	213	6.4	355	21	39	10.7	11
Protein, Vanilla, Low Carb, Protein Plus, Power Bar*	1 Bar/35g	131	7.4	373	16	21.5	21	26.5
Protein, Whey, Sculptress, Maxitone*	1 Bar/60g	203	5.6	339	33.9	30.6	9.3	8.5
Protein, White Chocolate Raspberry, GF, Quest*	1 Bar/60g	215	9.6	358	33	13	16	23
Protin, Crispy Chocolate Brownie, Nutramino*	1 Bar/64g	268	10.9	418	31	39	17	0.5
Raisin & Oatmeal, Breakfast Snack, Tesco*	1 Bar/38g	133	4.4	355	5.6	56.8	11.7	2.8
Raisin, Munch, Tesco*	1 Bar/30g	126	4.4	420	5.4	66.3	14.8	3.8
Raspberry & White Chocolate Crispie, Shapers, Boots*	1 Bar/24g	93	2	387	3.8	68	8.5	11
Raspberry Pie, Weight Watchers*	1 Bar/40g	122	0.4	305	4.5	55.8	1	14.8
Raspberry, Baked, Asda*	1 Bar/27g	104	2.1	385	3.4	74.2	7.6	1.8
Raspberry, Yoghurt Breaks, Go Ahead, McVitie's*	1 Pack/35g	143	3.6	408	5.4	73.6	10.2	2.3
Rice Krispies & Milk, Kellogg's*	1 Bar/20g	83	2.4	416	7	71	12	0.3
Rice Krispies, Snack, Kellogg's*	1 Bar/20g	83	2	415	7	70	10	0.5
Rich Toffee, Weight Watchers*	1 Bar/19g	68	1.7	358	2.6	51.6	9.1	30.1
Roasted Nut, Chewy & Crisp, Sainsbury's*	1 Bar/27g	120	6.6	446	10.1	46.6	24.3	3.9
Rocky Road, Rice Krispies Squares, Kellogg's*	1 Square/34g	143	3.7	420	4	76	11	1.5
Romance Me, Rocky Road, Hi-Fi, Slimming World*	1 Bar/20g	73	1.5	366	4.8	62.7	7.3	15.4
Salted Caramel Square, Fibre One*	1 Bar/24g	87	2.8	362	4	49.5	11.7	21.2
Sandwich, Chocolate Viennese, Fox's*	1 Biscuit/14g	76	4.4	542	6.9	57.4	31.6	1.6
Sandwich, Chocolate, Rik & Rok*	1 Bar/22g	105	4.2	477	6.5	70	19	0
Sandwich, Milk Chocolate Orange, Tesco*	1 Biscuit/25g	136	7.4	536	6.2	62.2	29.1	1.8
School, Apple, Fruit Bowl*	1 Bar/20g	67	0.7	337	1	72	3.6	7.1
Sesame Snaps in Chocolate, Anglo-Dal*	1 Pack/40g	211	11.9	527	9.3	55.6	29.7	0
Sesame Snaps with Coconut, Anglo-Dal*	1 Pack/30g	155	8.8	517	9.7	52.9	29.5	0
Sesame Snaps, Anglo-Dal*	1 Pack/30g	157	8.8	522	12.2	49.4	29.4	0
Special Fruit Muesli, Jordans*	1 Bar/40g	140	2.4	349	5	68.8	6	5
Special K, Apple & Pear, Kellogg's*	1 Bar/23g	92	1.8	400	8	73	8	2

	Measure INFO/WEIGHT	per Measure KCAL	FAT	Nutrition Values per 100g / 100ml KCAL	PROT	CARB	FAT	FIBRE
BARS								
Special K, Chocolate Chip, Kellogg's*	1 Bar/22g	90	1.6	401	9	76	7	1.5
Special K, Fruits of the Forest, Kellogg's*	1 Bar/22g	87	1.8	397	8	74	8	2.5
Special K, Mint Chocolate, Bliss, Special K, Kellogg's*	1 Bar/22g	88	2.2	401	4.5	74	10	3.5
Special K, Red Berry, Kellogg's*	1 Bar/23g	90	1.2	383	8	77	5	2
Special Muesli, Jordans*	1 Bar/40g	152	4.8	379	6	61.6	12.1	5.8
Strawberry & Vanilla, Vitamin & Protein, Fulfil Nutrition*	1 Bar/60g	185	4.9	309	33.4	10.1	8.2	33.1
Strawberry, Fruit Bakes, Go Ahead, McVitie's*	1 Bar/35g	131	3	375	3.5	72	8.5	4
Strawberry, Fruit, Sweet Vine, Aldi*	1 Bar/20g	67	0.8	334	1.2	73	3.9	1.7
Strawberry, Morning Shine, Atkins*	1 Bar/37g	145	8	392	28.9	24.9	21.6	14.1
Strawberry, Picked & Pressed, Fruit Bowl*	1 Bar/19g	60	0.7	317	3.5	63	3.6	10
Strawberry, Scrumptious, Get Fruity*	1 Bar/35g	141	4.6	402	5.9	62	13	5.4
Strawberry, Shapers, Boots*	1 Bar/22g	75	2.4	343	2.5	77	11	0.9
Sweet & Nutty Almond, Nature Valley*	1 Bar/30g	143	6.9	475	10	54.3	23	5.4
Sweet & Salty, Almond Crunch, Advantage, Atkins*	1 Bar/40g	200	15	500	17.5	35	37.5	12.5
Three Musketeer, Candy, Mars*	1 Bar/60g	260	8	430	3.3	76.2	13.2	1.7
Titan, Chocolate, Aldi*	1 Bar/38g	169	6.8	444	3.5	66	18	0.5
Toffee & Banana, Weight Watchers*	1 Bar/18g	67	0.7	372	6.1	77.2	3.9	1.7
Totally Chocolatey, Rice Krispies Squares, Kellogg's*	1 Bar/36g	156	5.3	439	4.5	72	15	1.5
Tracker, Breakfast, Banana, Mars*	1 Bar/37g	176	8.4	476	4.7	63.3	22.6	9.4
Tracker, Chocolate Chip, Mars*	1 Bar/37g	178	8.7	480	6.8	58	23.6	3.8
Tracker, Forest Fruits, Mars*	1 Bar/26g	123	5.8	474	4.6	64.1	22.2	0
Tracker, Roasted Nut, Mars*	1 Bar/26g	127	6.6	489	8.1	55	25.3	4.9
Trail, Big Berries, Alpen*	1 Bar/48g	180	2.7	376	6	73	5.7	4.3
Triple Chocolate, Atkins*	1 Bar/40g	160	9	400	30	42.5	22.5	12.5
Triple Dazzle, Wonka*	1 Bar/39g	195	10	504	5.9	61.9	25.9	0
Wafer Biscuit, Milk Chocolate Coated, Value, Tesco*	1 Bar/24g	126	6.7	526	6.9	61.4	28.1	1.7
Wafer, Chocolate Flavour Crisp, Carbolite*	1 Bar/25g	120	8.7	482	8.5	52.3	34.8	2
Wafer, Milk Chocolate, & Hazelnut, Favorini, Lidl*	1 Wafer/25g	136	8.6	545	7.1	49.8	34.5	3.6
White Chocolate & Hazelnuts, Porridge Oat, Stoats*	1 Bar/85g	407	22.4	479	7.6	50.1	26.3	5.9
White Chocolate, Cookie Dough, Fulfil Nutrition*	1 Bar/55g	195	7.2	355	38.6	20.2	13.2	14.2
White Chocolate, Crispy Wafer, Tasty Little Numbers*	1 Bar/20g	100	5.2	498	7	59	26	3
Yoghurt Coated, Coconut & Apricot, Eat Natural*	1 Bar/45g	203	10.2	451	4.6	44.6	22.7	10.4
Yoghurt Fruit Crunch, Meal Replacement, Slim Fast*	1 Bar/60g	218	6.8	364	25.4	26.9	11.3	18.7
Zippy Fruit, Mini Chefs, Natco*	1 Bar/20g	60	0	300	1	70	0	5
BASA								
Fillets, Chilli & Lemon Grass Butter Sauce, Birds Eye*	1 Fillet/140g	164	10.2	117	12	0.7	7.3	0
Fillets, Lemon & Herb, Tempura Battered, Gastro, Youngs*	1 Fillet/151g	279	14	185	14.2	10.6	9.3	1.1
Fillets, Lime, Chilli & Coriander, Dusted, Gastro, Youngs*	1 Fillet/152g	288	13.9	189	15.6	11	9.1	0.4
Fillets, Mediterranean Marinated, Northern Catch, Aldi*	1 Fillet/128g	147	4.7	115	18	2.8	3.7	0.5
Fillets, Rocket, Basil & Parmesan Sauce, Gastro, Youngs*	1 Serving/136g	136	4.2	100	17.7	0.2	3.1	0.2
Fillets, Sea Salt & Cracked Black Pepper, Gastro, Youngs*	1 Fillet/148g	276	12.2	187	15.8	12.1	8.3	0.6
Fillets, Skinless & Boneless, Aldi*	1 Fillet/120g	140	2.9	117	23.7	0.1	2.4	0
Fillets, Spicy Tomato & Chorizo Sauce, Gastro, Youngs*	1 Serving/133g	122	2.8	92	17.4	0.6	2.1	0.4
Tempura, Fillets, Northern Catch*	1 Fillet/160g	248	11	155	17.5	7.9	6.9	1.9
BASIL								
Dried, Ground	*1 Tsp/1.4g*	*4*	*0.1*	*251*	*14.4*	*43.2*	*4*	*0*
Fresh, Average	*1 Tbsp/5g*	*2*	*0*	*40*	*3.1*	*5.1*	*0.8*	*0*
BATTER MIX								
for Yorkshire Puddings & Pancakes, Morrisons*	1 Pudding/30g	43	0.8	143	6.4	23.1	2.8	4.1
for Yorkshire Puddings & Pancakes, Tesco*	1 Serving/17g	34	0.3	200	2.3	43.3	1.5	2.5
for Yorkshire Puddings, Baked, Aunt Bessie's*	1 Pudding/13g	48	1.1	356	9.8	34	8.1	2.3
Green's*	1 Bag/125g	296	9	237	8.7	34.3	7.2	0
Pancake, Buttermilk, Krusteaz*	3 Pancakes/16g	57	0.8	352	11.3	66	4.7	3.4

INFO/WEIGHT	Measure	per Measure KCAL	FAT	Nutrition Values per 100g / 100ml KCAL	PROT	CARB	FAT	FIBRE
BATTER MIX								
Pancake, Sainsbury's*	1 Pancake/63g	96	1.1	152	6.5	27.4	1.8	3.1
Smart Price, Asda*	1 Pack/128g	268	5.8	209	8	34	4.5	2.7
Tesco*	1 Pack/130g	467	1.8	359	12.3	74.4	1.4	7.7
BAY LEAVES								
Dried, Average	*1 Tsp/0.6g*	*2*	*0.1*	*313*	*7.6*	*48.6*	*8.4*	*0*
BEAN SPROUTS								
Mung, Raw, Average	*1oz/28g*	*9*	*0.1*	*31*	*2.9*	*4*	*0.5*	*1.5*
Mung, Stir-Fried in Blended Oil, Average	*1 Serving/90g*	*65*	*5.5*	*72*	*1.9*	*2.5*	*6.1*	*0.9*
Raw, Average	*1 Serving/150g*	*55*	*2.6*	*37*	*2.2*	*3.2*	*1.8*	*1.2*
BEANS								
& Meatballs, in Tomato Sauce, Sainsbury's*	½ Can/200g	216	7.2	108	5.5	13.3	3.6	2.6
& Seeds, Steamer, Waitrose*	1 Bag/160g	213	7.7	133	9.4	8.1	4.8	9.9
Aduki, Cooked in Unsalted Water, Average	*1 Tbsp/30g*	*37*	*0.1*	*123*	*9.3*	*22.5*	*0.2*	*5.5*
Aduki, Dried, Raw	*1 Tbsp/30g*	*82*	*0.2*	*272*	*19.9*	*50.1*	*0.5*	*11.1*
Baked, & Pork Sausages, Sainsbury's*	1 Serving/210g	248	9.2	118	5.7	13.9	4.4	3.4
Baked, & Sausage in Tomato Sauce, Smart Price, Asda*	½ Can/203g	256	12.2	126	5	13	6	0
Baked, & Jumbo Sausages, Asda*	1 Can/405g	486	17	120	6.9	11.2	4.2	5
Baked, & Sausage, Asda*	½ Can/202.5g	211	4	104	6.7	13	2	3.5
Baked, & Sausages, Basics, Sainsbury's*	1 Serving/175g	149	2.6	85	4.8	13.1	1.5	2.6
Baked, & Sausages, Meatfree, Sainsbury's*	1 Can/420g	500	16.8	119	8	12.6	4	2.7
Baked, & Sausages, Value, Tesco*	½ Can/202g	232	7.1	115	5.6	15	3.5	2.8
Baked, & Vegetarian Sausages, in Tomato Sauce, Asda*	½ Can/210g	204	4	97	7.4	12.5	1.9	8.4
Baked, Barbecue, Beanz, Heinz*	1 Can/390g	343	0.8	88	4.9	14.6	0.2	3.8
Baked, Cheesy & Sausage, Meal For One, Iceland *	1 Pack/494g	721	30.6	146	6.4	14.3	6.2	3.7
Baked, Curried, Average	*½ Can/210g*	*203*	*1.9*	*96*	*4.8*	*17.2*	*0.9*	*3.6*
Baked, Curry, Beanz, Heinz*	1 Can/390g	382	1.2	98	4.8	17	0.3	4
Baked, Five, in Tomato Sauce, Heinz*	1 Can/415g	361	0.8	87	5.4	13.6	0.2	4.3
Baked, Giant, Sainsbury's*	½ Jar/110g	169	8.2	154	5.8	12.5	7.5	6.6
Baked, Gigantes, in Tomato Sauce, Odysea *	1 Jar/355g	593	29.1	167	5.8	14.1	8.2	0
Baked, in Tomato Sauce, Average	*1 Can/400g*	*318*	*1.6*	*80*	*4.6*	*13.9*	*0.4*	*3.7*
Baked, in Tomato Sauce, Reduced Sugar & Salt	*½ Can/210g*	*159*	*0.7*	*76*	*4.6*	*13.6*	*0.3*	*3.8*
Baked, Mexican, Mean, Beanz, Heinz*	½ Can/208g	158	1	76	5	12.9	0.5	4
Baked, Peri Peri, Beanz, Heinz*	½ Can/195g	176	1.4	90	5.2	13.7	0.7	4.2
Baked, Smokey Bacon, Beanz, Heinz*	½ Can/195g	179	2.1	92	4.9	13.9	1.1	3.6
Baked, Sweet Chilli, Mean, Beanz, Heinz*	½ Can/195g	142	0.6	73	4.5	13	0.3	3.6
Baked, Virtually Fat Free, Heinz*	½ Can/207g	164	0.4	79	4.7	12.9	0.2	3.7
Baked, with Chicken Nuggets, Beanz, Heinz*	1 Can/200g	210	6.3	105	6.8	12.4	3.2	3.2
Baked, with Hidden Veg, Beanz, Heinz*	½ Can/208g	156	0.6	75	4.7	13.5	0.3	4.1
Baked, with HP Sauce, Beanz, Heinz*	½ Can/208g	158	0.6	76	4.8	13.7	0.3	3.9
Baked, with Lea & Perrins Sauce, Beanz, Heinz*	1 Can/415g	303	0.8	73	4.8	13.1	0.2	3.8
Baked, with Sausages, Branston, Crosse & Blackwell*	½ Can/202g	233	6.5	115	6.9	12.2	3.2	5
Baked, with Spicy Meatballs, Beanz, Heinz*	1 Can/400g	372	9.6	93	5.8	12	2.4	2.9
Baked, with Vegetable Sausages, Beanz, Heinz*	1 Sm Can/200g	210	7.2	105	6	12.2	3.6	2.9
Black, Cooked, Average	*1 Cup/172g*	*227*	*0.9*	*132*	*8.8*	*23.7*	*0.5*	*8.7*
Blackeye, Canned, Average	*1 Can/172g*	*206*	*1.3*	*120*	*8.4*	*19.8*	*0.8*	*3.3*
Blackeye, Dried, Raw	*1oz/28g*	*87*	*0.4*	*311*	*23.5*	*54.1*	*1.6*	*8.2*
Borlotti, Canned, Average	*1oz/28g*	*29*	*0.1*	*103*	*7.6*	*16.9*	*0.5*	*4.7*
Borlotti, Dried, Raw, Average	*1 Serving/100g*	*335*	*1.2*	*335*	*23*	*60*	*1.2*	*24.7*
Broad, Baby, Frozen, Simply, M&S*	1 Serving/80g	54	0.8	67	4.2	6.7	1	3.4
Broad, Canned, Drained, Average	*1 Can/195g*	*136*	*1.1*	*70*	*6.9*	*9.2*	*0.6*	*6.8*
Broad, Crispy, Wasabi Flavoured, Khao Shong*	1 Serving/30g	116	3	386	17	57	10	7
Broad, Dried, Raw, Average	*1oz/28g*	*69*	*0.6*	*245*	*26.1*	*32.5*	*2.1*	*27.6*
Broad, Fresh, without Pod, Boiled, Average	*1 Serving/80g*	*78*	*0.5*	*97*	*7.9*	*11.7*	*0.6*	*6.5*

B

BEANS

INFO/WEIGHT	Measure	per Measure		Nutrition Values per 100g / 100ml				
		KCAL	FAT	KCAL	PROT	CARB	FAT	FIBRE
Broad, Fried, Tesco*	½ Pack/40g	174	6.6	436	21.8	45.5	16.6	8.5
Broad, Frozen, Average	*1 Serving/80g*	*63*	*0.6*	*79*	*7.6*	*10.8*	*0.7*	*5.3*
Butter, Canned, Drained, Average	*1oz/28g*	*23*	*0.1*	*81*	*6*	*12.8*	*0.5*	*4.3*
Butter, Dried, Boiled, Average	*1oz/28g*	*30*	*0.2*	*106*	*7.2*	*18.6*	*0.6*	*5.2*
Butter, Dried, Raw, Average	*1oz/28g*	*81*	*0.5*	*290*	*19.1*	*52.9*	*1.7*	*16*
Cannellini with Chorizo & Red Peppers, Morrisons*	½ Pack/100g	155	10	155	6.9	9.2	10	2.8
Cannellini, Canned, Drained, Average	*1 Portion/80g*	*75*	*0.4*	*94*	*8.7*	*15*	*0.5*	*5.7*
Cannellini, Dried, Tesco*	1 Serving/32g	83	0.3	260	24.8	37.4	0.8	20.9
Chilli, Canned, Average	*1 Can/420g*	*381*	*3.1*	*91*	*5.2*	*15.8*	*0.7*	*4.4*
Dry Roasted, Mix, The Food Doctor*	1 Portion/25g	98	3.3	392	34	23.6	13.2	21.2
Edamame, Sainsbury's*	1 Serving/150g	212	9.6	141	12.3	6.8	6.4	4.2
Edamame, Shelled, Frozen, Yutaka*	1 Serving/80g	102	5	128	10.8	4.5	6.3	0
Edamame, with Soy Sauce, On the Go, Sainsbury's*	1 Pot/100g	119	5.8	119	11.4	20	5.8	6.5
Fajita Beanz, Heinz*	½ Can/196g	155	1.6	79	4	11.7	0.8	4.5
Flageolet, Canned, Average	*1 Can/265g*	*235*	*1.6*	*89*	*6.8*	*14*	*0.6*	*3.5*
Flageolet, Dried, Love Life, Waitrose*	1 Serving/50g	125	3.1	250	30.4	19.8	6.2	40.4
French, Boiled, Average	*1 Serving/150g*	*38*	*0*	*25*	*2.3*	*3.8*	*0*	*3.7*
French, Canned, Average	*1oz/28g*	*5*	*0.1*	*17*	*1.3*	*2.7*	*0.2*	*1.9*
French, Raw	*1oz/28g*	*6*	*0.1*	*20*	*1.6*	*2.7*	*0.4*	*1.8*
Green, Cut, Average	*1oz/28g*	*7*	*0.1*	*24*	*1.7*	*3.6*	*0.2*	*2.7*
Green, Fine, Average	*1 Serving/75g*	*18*	*0.3*	*24*	*1.8*	*3.2*	*0.4*	*2.9*
Green, Sliced, Average	*1oz/28g*	*6*	*0.1*	*23*	*1.9*	*3.5*	*0.2*	*2.1*
Green, Sliced, Frozen, Average	*1 Serving/50g*	*13*	*0*	*26*	*1.8*	*4.4*	*0.1*	*4.1*
Green, Whole, Average	*1oz/28g*	*6*	*0.1*	*22*	*1.6*	*3*	*0.4*	*1.7*
Haricot, Canned, Average	*1 Can/400g*	*307*	*2*	*77*	*6.2*	*10.7*	*0.5*	*5.9*
Haricot, Dried, Boiled in Unsalted Water	*1oz/28g*	*27*	*0.1*	*95*	*6.6*	*17.2*	*0.5*	*6.1*
Haricot, Dried, Raw	*1 Serving/100g*	*286*	*1.6*	*286*	*22.4*	*49.7*	*1.6*	*17*
Keen Bean, Mix, Graze*	1 Punnet/31g	153	10.2	486	30.5	27.6	32.5	7.1
Kidney, Curried, Rajmah, Sohna *	½ Can/225g	217	1.1	97	3.7	17.6	0.5	1.4
Kidney, Red, Canned, Drained, Average	*½ Can/120g*	*115*	*0.7*	*96*	*7.4*	*20.7*	*0.5*	*5.5*
Kidney, Red, Dried, Boiled in Unsalted Water	*1oz/28g*	*29*	*0.1*	*103*	*8.4*	*17.4*	*0.5*	*6.7*
Kidney, Red, Dried, Raw	*1oz/28g*	*74*	*0.4*	*266*	*22.1*	*44.1*	*1.4*	*15.7*
Kidney, Red, in Chilli Sauce, Sainsbury's*	1 Can/420g	365	1.7	87	5.3	15.6	0.4	4.5
Kidney, Red, in Chilli Sauce, Waitrose*	½ Can/201g	175	0.8	87	5.5	15.3	0.4	3.2
Kidney, White, Dry, Raw, Unico*	½ Cup/80g	270	0.9	338	22.5	61.2	1.1	21.2
Lupin, Avg *	1 Serving/80g	297	8	371	36	40	10	19
Mexican Style, Mix, Tinned, Asda*	1 Serving/81g	71	0.6	88	8.7	11.8	0.7	10.4
Mix, Great Fire Dragon, Graze*	1 Pack/25g	123	7	491	15	48.1	28.1	2.5
Mixed, Canned, Average	*1 Can/300g*	*300*	*3.5*	*100*	*6.8*	*15.6*	*1.2*	*4.1*
Mixed, for Salad, As Consumed, Good & Balanced, Asda*	1 Serving/50g	57	0.6	113	8	10	1.2	15
Mixed, in Mild Chilli Sauce, Sainsbury's*	1 Can/420g	328	1.3	78	4.9	13.8	0.3	3.7
Mixed, in Tomato Sauce, Canned, CBY, Asda*	½ Can/203g	196	1	97	5	15.8	0.5	4.6
Mixed, in Water, Canned, Drained, Sweet Harvest, Aldi*	½ Can/120g	125	0.6	104	7.5	12	0.5	11
Mixed, Spicy, Average	*1 Serving/140g*	*108*	*0.7*	*78*	*4.8*	*13.4*	*0.5*	*3.9*
Mixed, with Lentils, Waitrose*	1 Pack/300g	399	21.9	133	5.1	11.6	7.3	3.1
Mixed, with Passata, Tesco*	1 Can/300g	237	2.1	79	6	12.1	0.7	3.9
Mung, Whole, Dried, Boiled in Unsalted Water	*1oz/28g*	*25*	*0.1*	*91*	*7.6*	*15.3*	*0.4*	*3*
Mung, Whole, Dried, Raw	*1oz/28g*	*78*	*0.3*	*279*	*23.9*	*46.3*	*1.1*	*10*
Pinto, Dried, Boiled in Unsalted Water	*1oz/28g*	*38*	*0.2*	*137*	*8.9*	*23.9*	*0.7*	*0*
Pinto, Dried, Raw	*1oz/28g*	*92*	*0.4*	*327*	*21.1*	*57.1*	*1.6*	*14*
Pinto, in Water, Canned, Drained, Asda*	1 Can/175g	170	1	97	6.5	13	0.6	7.1
Refried, Average	*1 Serving/215g*	*162*	*1.5*	*76*	*4.6*	*12.7*	*0.7*	*1.8*
Refried, Tesco*	¼ Can/100g	81	0.6	81	4.8	11.7	0.6	4.8

	Measure INFO/WEIGHT	per Measure KCAL	FAT	Nutrition Values per 100g / 100ml KCAL	PROT	CARB	FAT	FIBRE
BEANS								
Runner, Average	*1 Serving/80g*	*15*	*0.3*	*19*	*1.3*	*2.8*	*0.4*	*2.2*
Six, Mix, Cooks' Ingredients, Waitrose*	¼ Pack/100g	77	0.4	77	4.2	11.8	0.4	4.5
Smoky & Spicy Mighty, in a Tomato Sauce, Jamie Oliver*	½ Pouch/125g	154	6.8	123	5	11	5.4	4.6
Soya, Black, in Filtered Water, Nature Organic*	1 Serving/200g	240	6.4	120	8.8	14.2	3.2	6.2
Soya, Dried, Average	*1oz/28g*	*104*	*5.1*	*370*	*34.2*	*15.4*	*18.3*	*19.6*
Soya, Dried, Boiled in Unsalted Water	*1oz/28g*	*39*	*2*	*141*	*14*	*5.1*	*7.3*	*6.1*
Soya, Frozen, Birds Eye*	1 Serving/80g	98	5.1	123	12.4	4	6.4	4.2
Soya, Shelled, Frozen, Raw, Average	*1 Serving/80g*	*99*	*4.3*	*124*	*12.2*	*6.9*	*5.3*	*4.4*
Soya, Tesco*	1 Pack/200g	240	11.6	120	10.2	6.7	5.8	2
Tuscan, Beanz, Heinz*	½ Can/195g	178	3.3	91	4.9	12	1.7	4.1
Wasabi, Mix, Whitworths*	1 Serving/25g	108	3.4	430	30.9	40.1	13.7	10.7
White, Campo Largo, Lidl*	½ Jar/200g	180	1	90	7.1	11.2	0.5	0
BEEF								
Brisket, Boiled, Lean	*1 Serving/100g*	*225*	*11*	*225*	*31.4*	*0*	*11*	*0*
Brisket, Boiled, Lean & Fat	*1 Serving/100g*	*268*	*17.4*	*268*	*27.8*	*0*	*17.4*	*0*
Brisket, Braised, Lean	*1 Serving/100g*	*280*	*17.4*	*280*	*29*	*0*	*17.4*	*0*
Brisket, Raw, Lean	*1oz/28g*	*39*	*1.7*	*139*	*21.1*	*0*	*6.1*	*0*
Brisket, Raw, Lean & Fat	*1oz/28g*	*60*	*4.4*	*216*	*18.2*	*0*	*15.8*	*0*
Brisket, Red Wine Sauce, Slow Cooked, Appleby's, Aldi*	½ Pack/160g	249	7.6	155	26	2.8	4.7	0.5
Brisket, Slow Cooked, BBQ Mustard Sauce, Morrisons*	½ Pack/128g	164	3.2	128	18.8	7.4	2.5	0.3
Brisket, with Gravy, Slow Cooked, M Kitchen, Morrisons*	1 Pack/300g	318	7.8	106	19	1.7	2.6	0
Carpaccio Del Lago, Dry Cured, Unearthed*	½ Pack/35g	41	0.5	116	26	0.5	1.4	0.5
Cheeks, Ox, Aberdeen Angus, Waitrose*	1 Serving/100g	123	4.6	123	22	0	4.6	0
Diced, Casserole, Lean, Average	*1oz/28g*	*35*	*1.1*	*126*	*23*	*0*	*3.8*	*0*
Escalope, Healthy Range, Average	*1 Serving/170g*	*233*	*6.7*	*137*	*24.2*	*1.2*	*4*	*0.4*
Flank, Pot-Roasted, Lean	*1oz/28g*	*71*	*3.9*	*253*	*31.8*	*0*	*14*	*0*
Flank, Pot-Roasted, Lean & Fat	*1oz/28g*	*85*	*6.1*	*303*	*26.6*	*0*	*21.9*	*0*
Flank, Raw, Lean	*1oz/28g*	*49*	*2.6*	*175*	*22.7*	*0*	*9.3*	*0*
Flank, Raw, Lean & Fat	*1oz/28g*	*74*	*5.8*	*266*	*19.7*	*0*	*20.8*	*0*
Fore Rib, Lean & Fat, Average	*1oz/28g*	*40*	*1.8*	*144*	*21.7*	*0*	*6.2*	*0.2*
Fore Rib, Raw, Lean	*1oz/28g*	*41*	*1.8*	*145*	*21.5*	*0*	*6.5*	*0*
Fore Rib, Roasted, Lean	*1oz/28g*	*66*	*3.2*	*236*	*33.3*	*0*	*11.4*	*0*
Fore Rib, Roasted, Lean & Fat	*1oz/28g*	*84*	*5.7*	*300*	*29.1*	*0*	*20.4*	*0*
Grill Steak, Average	*1 Steak/170g*	*501*	*39.5*	*295*	*19.3*	*2.1*	*23.2*	*0.1*
Grill Steak, Peppered, Average	*1 Serving/172g*	*419*	*24.4*	*244*	*23.6*	*5.2*	*14.2*	*0.3*
Joint, for Roasting, Average	*1oz/28g*	*38*	*1*	*134*	*24.5*	*1.4*	*3.4*	*0*
Joint, Sirloin, Roasted, Lean	*1oz/28g*	*53*	*1.8*	*188*	*32.4*	*0*	*6.5*	*0*
Joint, Sirloin, Roasted, Lean & Fat	*1oz/28g*	*65*	*3.5*	*233*	*29.8*	*0*	*12.6*	*0*
Mince, Cooked, Average	*1 Serving/75g*	*214*	*15.3*	*286*	*24*	*0*	*20.3*	*0*
Mince, Extra Lean, Raw, Average	*1 Serving/100g*	*124*	*5*	*124*	*21.2*	*0.1*	*5*	*0*
Mince, Extra Lean, Stewed	*1oz/28g*	*50*	*2.4*	*177*	*24.7*	*0*	*8.7*	*0*
Mince, Lean, Raw, Average	*1oz/28g*	*48*	*2.8*	*172*	*20.8*	*0*	*10*	*0.1*
Mince, Raw, Average	*1oz/28g*	*68*	*5.1*	*242*	*19.6*	*0.2*	*18.1*	*0*
Mince, Raw, Frozen, Average	*1 Serving/100g*	*176*	*10*	*176*	*20.4*	*0*	*10*	*0*
Mince, Steak, Extra Lean, Average	*1oz/28g*	*37*	*1.6*	*131*	*20.5*	*0.4*	*5.6*	*0*
Mince, Steak, Raw, Average	*1 Serving/125g*	*318*	*25*	*254*	*17.2*	*0*	*20*	*0*
Mince, Stewed	*1oz/28g*	*59*	*3.8*	*209*	*21.8*	*0*	*13.5*	*0*
Peppered, Sliced, Average	*1 Slice/20g*	*26*	*1.1*	*129*	*18.2*	*1.3*	*5.6*	*1*
Potted, Binghams*	1 Serving/30g	76	6.6	254	13.8	1	22	0.6
Roast, Sliced, Average	*1 Slice/35g*	*48*	*1.3*	*136*	*26.1*	*0.4*	*3.6*	*0.2*
Salt, Average	*1 Serving/70g*	*80*	*1.7*	*114*	*21.7*	*1*	*2.5*	*0.1*
Salted, Dried, Raw	*1oz/28g*	*70*	*0.4*	*250*	*55.4*	*0*	*1.5*	*0*
Silverside, Pot-Roasted, Lean	*1oz/28g*	*54*	*1.8*	*193*	*34*	*0*	*6.3*	*0*

B

	Measure INFO/WEIGHT	per Measure KCAL	FAT	Nutrition Values per 100g / 100ml KCAL	PROT	CARB	FAT	FIBRE
BEEF								
Silverside, Pot-Roasted, Lean & Fat	1oz/28g	69	3.8	247	31	0	13.7	0
Silverside, Raw, Lean	1oz/28g	38	1.2	134	23.8	0	4.3	0
Silverside, Raw, Lean & Fat	1oz/28g	60	4.1	213	20.2	0	14.7	0
Silverside, Salted, Boiled, Lean	1oz/28g	52	1.9	184	30.4	0	6.9	0
Silverside, Salted, Boiled, Lean & Fat	1oz/28g	63	3.5	224	27.9	0	12.5	0
Silverside, Salted, Raw, Lean	1oz/28g	39	2	140	19.2	0	7	0
Silverside, Salted, Raw, Lean & Fat	1oz/28g	64	5	227	16.3	0	18	0
Sliced, Cooked, From Supermarket, Average	1 Slice/35g	47	1.2	135	23.6	2	3.5	0.5
Steak, 8oz Rump & Chips	1 Serving/466g	870	41.1	187	10.7	16.2	8.8	0
Steak, Braising, Braised, Lean	1oz/28g	63	2.7	225	34.4	0	9.7	0
Steak, Braising, Braised, Lean & Fat	1oz/28g	69	3.6	246	32.9	0	12.7	0
Steak, Braising, Lean, Raw, Average	1oz/28g	40	1.4	144	24.8	0	5	0
Steak, Braising, Raw, Lean & Fat	1oz/28g	44	2.4	158	20.5	0	8.5	0
Steak, Economy, Average	1oz/28g	53	2.4	190	26.9	1.2	8.7	0.4
Steak, Fillet, Cooked, Average	1oz/28g	54	2.4	191	28.6	0	8.5	0
Steak, Fillet, Lean, Average	1oz/28g	42	2	150	21	0	7.3	0
Steak, Fillet, Lean, Cooked, Average	1oz/28g	52	2.2	186	28.6	0	8	0
Steak, Frying, Average	1 Steak/110g	128	2.7	116	23.7	0	2.5	0
Steak, Hache, Peri Peri, Musclefood*	1 Steak/170g	233	6.3	137	21.1	6.3	3.7	1
Steak, Pink Peppercorn Crusted, Easy, Waitrose*	1 Steak/125g	195	6.6	156	18.4	8.6	5.3	1.1
Steak, Rump, Cooked, Average	1oz/28g	69	4	246	29.1	0.5	14.1	0
Steak, Rump, Grilled, Rare, Lean	1 Steak/227g	381	15.6	168	26.5	0	6.9	0
Steak, Rump, Lean, Cooked, Average	1oz/28g	50	1.7	179	31	0	6.1	0
Steak, Rump, Raw, Lean & Fat	1oz/28g	49	2.8	174	20.7	0	10.1	0
Steak, Rump, Raw, Lean, Average	1 Steak/175g	219	7.2	125	22	0	4.1	0
Steak, Sirloin, Fried, Rare, Lean	1oz/28g	53	2.3	189	28.8	0	8.2	0
Steak, Sirloin, Fried, Rare, Lean & Fat	1oz/28g	65	3.9	231	26.5	0	13.9	0
Steak, Sirloin, Grilled, Medium-Rare, Lean	1oz/28g	49	2.2	176	26.6	0	7.7	0
Steak, Sirloin, Grilled, Medium-Rare, Lean & Fat	1oz/28g	59	3.5	211	24.6	0	12.5	0
Steak, Sirloin, Grilled, Rare, Lean	1oz/28g	46	1.9	166	26.4	0	6.7	0
Steak, Sirloin, Grilled, Rare, Lean & Fat	1oz/28g	60	3.6	216	25.1	0	12.8	0
Steak, Sirloin, Grilled, Well-Done, Lean	1oz/28g	63	2.8	225	33.9	0	9.9	0
Steak, Sirloin, Grilled, Well-Done, Lean & Fat	1oz/28g	71	4	254	31.5	0	14.3	0
Steak, Sirloin, Raw, Lean & Fat	1oz/28g	56	3.6	201	21.6	0	12.7	0
Steak, Sirloin, Raw, Lean, Average	1 Steak/150g	202	6.8	135	23.5	0	4.5	0
Steak, Smoked Paprika & Garlic, Grilled, Tesco*	1 Steak/45g	81	1.6	179	29.4	7.2	3.6	0
Steaks, British, Louisiana Inspired, BBQ, Waitrose*	1 Steak/112g	197	6.3	176	28	3.1	5.6	0.7
Stewed Steak, Average	1 Serving/220g	258	10.1	117	15.8	3.3	4.6	0
Stewed Steak, Canned, Morrisons*	½ Can/200g	205	5	103	17	2.6	2.5	0.9
Stewing Steak, Lean & Fat, Raw, Average	1 Serving/100g	136	4.3	136	24.2	0.1	4.3	0.1
Stewing Steak, Raw, Lean	1oz/28g	34	1	122	22.6	0	3.5	0
Stewing Steak, Stewed, Lean	1oz/28g	52	1.8	185	32	0	6.3	0
Stewing Steak, Stewed, Lean & Fat	1oz/28g	57	2.7	203	29.2	0	9.6	0
Stir Fry Strips, Raw, Average	1 Serving/125g	149	3.8	119	23	0	3	0.2
Topside, Lean & Fat, Raw, Average	1oz/28g	55	3.6	198	20.4	0	12.9	0
Topside, Raw, Lean	1oz/28g	32	0.8	116	23	0	2.7	0
Vegetarian, Mince, Frozen & Chilled, Quorn*	1 Serving/87g	91	1.7	105	14.5	4.5	2	5.5
Vegetarian, Pieces, Beef Style, Quorn*	½ Pack/75g	69	1.7	92	13.5	4.5	2.2	5
Vegetarian, Slices, Peppered Style, Quorn*	¼ Pack/25g	29	0.5	115	14.5	7.6	2.1	4
Vegetarian, Steak Strips, Frozen, Quorn*	¼ Pack/75g	75	1.8	100	14.3	4.3	2.4	6
Vegetarian, Steaks, Peppered, Quorn*	1 Steak/98g	123	3.9	126	13.6	5.7	4	6.9
Wafer Thin Sliced, Cooked, Average	1 Slice/10g	13	0.3	129	24.5	0.5	3.2	0.2

	Measure INFO/WEIGHT	per Measure KCAL	FAT	Nutrition Values per 100g / 100ml KCAL	PROT	CARB	FAT	FIBRE
BEEF &								
Ale, with Yorkshire Pudding, Ovenbaked, G&C, Asda*	1 Pack/337g	391	9.8	116	8.3	13	2.9	2.4
Beer, Princes*	½ Can/205g	215	6.2	105	14	5.5	3	0
Black Bean with Rice, Weight Watchers*	1 Pack/320g	288	4.2	90	5	14.6	1.3	0.1
Black Bean, Sizzling, Oriental Express*	1 Pack/400g	420	8.4	105	7.2	14	2.1	2.1
Chips, Steak, HE, Tesco*	1 Pack/450g	472	12.2	105	6.3	13.8	2.7	0.5
Mashed Potato, Braised, Sainsbury's*	1 Pack/434g	425	14.3	98	7.6	9.4	3.3	0.8
Onions with Gravy, Minced, Lean, Sainsbury's*	1 Sm Can/198g	285	13.9	144	17	3.1	7	0.2
Onions, Minced, Asda*	½ Can/196g	314	19.6	160	13	4.6	10	0.1
Potatoes, Minced, LC, Tesco*	1 Pack/450g	400	9.5	80	4.3	10.3	1.9	2.3
BEEF BOURGUIGNON								
Finest, Tesco*	½ Pack/300g	247	7.8	82	9.9	4.8	2.6	0.5
BEEF BRAISED								
& Gravy, My Fit Lifestyle, Tesco*	1 Pack/375g	263	3.8	70	6.2	8.8	1	0.9
& New Potatoes, GFY, Asda*	1 Pack/448g	242	6.3	54	8.1	2.2	1.4	3.1
Braised, in Ale, & Butternut Mash, Tesco*	1 Pack/450g	248	2.2	55	5.8	6.9	0.5	2
Braised, Red Wine, & Roast Potatoes, BGTY, Sainsbury's*	1 Pack/400g	428	9.2	107	9.1	11.4	2.3	2.2
Classic Steak & Mash, CBY, Asda*	1 Pack/453g	358	11.3	79	7.6	5.7	2.5	1.8
in Ale with Mash & Baby Onions, COU, M&S*	1 Pack/400g	380	9.2	95	7.4	11	2.3	1.4
Steak & Mash, Tastes of Home, M Kitchen, Morrisons*	1 Meal/250g	209	6	87	6.4	9.1	2.5	1.1
Steak, & Cabbage, COU, M&S*	1 Pack/380g	323	9.9	85	8.3	6.7	2.6	1.9
Steak, & Carrots, Mini Favourites, M&S*	1 Serving/200g	140	5	70	8	4.2	2.5	1.3
Steak, & Mash, GFY, Asda*	1 Pack/400g	260	3.2	65	3.4	11	0.8	0.7
Steak, & Mash, HL, Tesco*	1 Pack/450g	418	12.2	93	7	10.2	2.7	0.7
Steak, Braised, & Mash, British, Meal for One, M&S*	1 Meal/450g	369	11.2	82	6.7	7.3	2.5	1.9
Steak, with Root Vegetable Crush, British, COU, M&S*	1 Pack/380g	243	3.8	64	7.1	5.9	1	1.4
Tender, Pub Specials, Birds Eye*	1 Pack/450g	243	3.6	54	5.5	6.1	0.8	1.8
BEEF CRISPY CHILLI								
Cantonese, Chilled, Sainsbury's*	1 Pack/250g	682	38.8	273	11.4	22.1	15.5	1.9
Chinese, Oven Baked, Iceland*	½ Box/100g	297	15.2	297	11.7	28	15.2	0.6
Oriental, Ken Hom, Tesco*	1 Pack/250g	712	28.8	285	6	38.1	11.5	0.7
Sainsbury's*	½ Pack/125g	242	10.4	194	9.2	20	8.3	1
Tesco*	1 Pack/250g	472	17.2	189	10.8	21	6.9	0.5
BEEF DINNER								
Roast with Trimmings	*1 Dinner/840g*	*1310*	*63*	*156*	*6.1*	*17.7*	*7.5*	*2.3*
Roast, Iceland*	1 Serving/340g	354	12.6	104	8.5	9.1	3.7	1.6
Roast, Sainsbury's*	1 Pack/400g	356	6.8	89	6.5	12	1.7	1.9
Roast, Yorkshire Pudding, Potatoes, Veg, & Gravy, Iceland*	1 Pack/413g	429	5.4	104	6.2	15.8	1.3	2.4
BEEF HOT & SOUR								
Chef's Selection, M&S*	1 Pack/329g	395	17.4	120	9.2	8.4	5.3	1.3
with Garlic Rice, BGTY, Sainsbury's*	1 Pack/400g	428	6.8	107	5.9	17	1.7	0.6
with Vegetable Rice, COU, M&S*	1 Pack/400g	360	5.6	90	5.5	14.4	1.4	0.6
BEEF IN								
Ale Gravy, Chunky, Birds Eye*	1 Pack/340g	272	6.8	80	7.4	8.3	2	1.5
Ale with Mushrooms, BGTY, Sainsbury's*	1 Pack/251g	193	3.8	77	10.2	5.6	1.5	0.4
Ale, Diet Chef Ltd*	1 Meal/300g	201	3.6	67	8.2	6	1.2	2.1
Black Bean Sauce, CBY, Asda*	1 Pack/450g	378	14	84	6.3	7.4	3.1	0.7
Black Bean Sauce, CBY, Asda*	1 Pack/375g	368	12.4	98	8.5	8.2	3.3	0.8
Black Bean Sauce, Chinese Takeaway, Morrisons*	½ Pack/168g	234	11.3	139	10.3	8.3	6.7	2.3
Black Bean Sauce, Chinese, Tesco*	1 Pack/400g	396	12.4	99	9.1	8.7	3.1	0.5
Black Bean Sauce, GF, Ilumi*	1 Bag/250g	242	10.2	97	8.2	6.2	4.1	1.3
Black Bean Sauce, M&S*	1 Pack/350g	402	22.4	115	8.9	5.7	6.4	1.1
Black Bean with Egg Noodles, M&S*	1 Pack/400g	460	6	115	8.6	16.7	1.5	1.8
Black Pepper Sauce & Egg Fried Rice, Tesco*	1 Pack/451g	622	24.8	138	7	15.2	5.5	1.2

	Measure INFO/WEIGHT	per Measure KCAL	FAT	Nutrition Values per 100g / 100ml KCAL	PROT	CARB	FAT	FIBRE
BEEF IN								
Burgundy Red Wine, GFY, Asda*	1 Pack/405g	348	8.1	86	8	9	2	1.1
Creamy Peppercorn Sauce, Steak, Tesco*	1 Steak/150g	189	8.2	126	16.5	2.6	5.5	0.1
Gravy, Roast, Birds Eye*	1 Pack/227g	177	3.9	78	13.4	2.2	1.7	0
Gravy, Sliced, Iceland*	1 Pack/200g	172	3.2	86	12.1	5.9	1.6	0.3
Gravy, Sliced, Sainsbury's*	1 Serving/125g	100	2.2	80	13.5	2.6	1.8	0.2
Gravy, Sliced, Tesco*	1 Serving/200g	152	4.2	76	11.3	3.1	2.1	0.2
Madeira & Mushroom Gravy, Sliced, Finest, Tesco*	1 Pack/400g	536	24.8	134	15.2	4.3	6.2	1
Peppercorn Sauce, & Mashed Potato, Weight Watchers*	1 Pack/400g	312	8	78	5	10	2	1
Red Wine Sauce, Milson's Kitchen, Aldi*	1 Pack/400g	256	6	64	5.6	9.6	1.5	2.1
Red Wine Sauce, Simply Bistro, Aldi*	1 Pack/400g	316	6	79	5.6	9.2	1.5	2.1
Rich Ale Gravy, Slow Cooked Brisket, COU, M&S*	1 Pack/350g	242	6.7	69	8.4	3.7	1.9	1.6
Velvet Porter with Potatoes, Look What We Found*	1 Pack/300g	201	3.6	67	8.2	6	1.2	2.1
BEEF RAGU								
with Rigatoni Pasta, Chianti, Balanced for You, M&S*	1 Pack/400g	484	12.4	121	10.3	12.1	3.1	1.5
BEEF SZECHUAN								
Sizzling Hot Spicy, Oriental Express*	1 Pack/400g	380	7.6	95	6.4	13.2	1.9	2
BEEF TERIYAKI								
Sizzler, As Consumed, Fresh Ideas, Morrisons*	½ Pack/142g	183	5.2	129	18.2	5.4	3.7	0.6
with Noodles, BGTY, Sainsbury's*	1 Pack/400g	320	4	80	7.7	10.1	1	1
BEEF WELLINGTON								
As Prepared, Waitrose*	1/6 Pack/267g	635	33.6	238	13	17.9	12.6	0.6
Average	*1 Serving/200g*	*530*	*33.3*	*265*	*12.4*	*17*	*16.6*	*1*
Extra Special, Asda*	1 Serving/218g	605	37.1	277	11	20	17	0.9
Mini, Party, Waitrose*	1 Parcel/18g	62	4	346	9	27.3	22.2	0.5
BEEF WITH								
Black Bean Sauce, Chilli, Sainsbury's*	1 Pack/300g	336	14.4	112	8.7	8.6	4.8	1
Black Bean Sauce, Rice Bowl, Uncle Ben's*	1 Pack/350g	368	4.9	105	5.6	17.4	1.4	0
Diane Sauce, Rump Steak, Tesco*	1 Steak/165g	182	8.1	110	15.1	1.1	4.9	0.3
Horseradish Dressing, Slow Cooked, HL, Tesco*	1 Pack/356g	285	10.3	80	5.4	7.5	2.9	1.4
Onion & Gravy, Minced, Princes*	1 Serving/200g	342	24.4	171	9.9	5.5	12.2	0
Onions & Gravy, Minced, Tesco*	1 Can/198g	224	10.1	113	14	2.8	5.1	0.8
Oyster Sauce, Ooodles of Noodles, Oriental Express*	1 Pack/425g	378	5.5	89	4.9	14.2	1.3	1.5
Peppercorn Sauce, Steak, Fried, Simply Cook, Tesco*	½ Pack/125g	215	9.1	172	24.8	1.7	7.3	0.4
Peppercorn Sauce, Steak, Just Cook, Sainsbury's*	½ Pack/128g	174	7.3	136	17.7	3.4	5.7	1.2
Red Wine Sauce, Rump Steak, Tesco*	1 Serving/150g	180	8.6	120	17.2	0.1	5.7	3.3
Steak, Rump with a Peppercorn Sauce, Waitrose*	½ Pack/180g	189	5.9	105	17.9	0.9	3.3	0.2
Steak, Rump, with Peppercorn Sauce, M&S*	½ Pack/213g	281	8.7	132	19.4	4.2	4.1	0.1
Steak, Sirloin, Medallion, with Roquefort Butter, Waitrose*	1 Pack/210g	491	26.2	234	30	0.4	12.5	0.1
Vegetables & Gravy, Minced, Birds Eye*	1 Pack/178g	155	6.1	87	9.1	5.1	3.4	0.6
BEER								
Ale, 1698, Kentish Strong, Shepherd Neame*	1 Bottle/500ml	285	0	57	0.4	4.8	0	0
Ale, Bottled, Old Speckled Hen*	1 Bottle/330ml	124	0.3	38	0.2	1.8	0.1	0.2
Ale, Freeminer, Organic, Fairtrade, Co-Op*	1 Bottle/480ml	240	0.5	50	0.2	2.7	0.1	0
Ale, Gingerbread, Wychwood, Marstons PLC*	1 Bottle/500ml	304	0	61	0.3	3	0	0
Ale, Goliath, Wychwood, Marstons PLC*	1 Bottle/500ml	191	0	38	0.4	2.8	0	0
Ale, Honey Dew, Fullers*	1 Bottle/500ml	232	0	46	0	4.6	0	0
Ale, Hopped Bourbon, Cask, Innis & Gunn*	1 Bottle/330ml	201	0	61	0.3	4.9	0	0
Ale, Hopping Hare, Hall & Woodhouse Ltd*	1 Bottle/500ml	189	0	38	0.4	3	0	0
Ale, Old Peculiar, Theakstons*	1 Serving/500ml	250	0	50	0	4.6	0	0
Ale, Old Speckled Hen*	1 Pint/568ml	185	0.6	32	0.2	1.6	0.1	0.2
Ale, Pale, Alcohol Free, Innis & Gunn*	1 Can/330ml	66	0	20	0.5	4.7	0	0
Ale, Pale, IPA, Greene King*	1 Pint/568ml	157	0.1	28	0.2	1.6	0	0.1
Ale, Pale, IPA, Innis & Gunn*	1 Bottle/330ml	162	0	49	0.3	4.6	0	0

	Measure INFO/WEIGHT	KCAL	FAT	Nutrition Values per 100g / 100ml				
				KCAL	PROT	CARB	FAT	FIBRE
BEER								
Ale, Pale, IPA, TTD, Sainsbury's*	½ Bottle/250ml	128	0	51	0.5	4.4	0	0.5
Ale, Pale, Sierra Nevada*	1 Bottle/350g	175	0	50	0.4	4	0	0
Ale, Scarecrow, Wychwood, Marstons PLC*	1 Bottle/500ml	214	0	43	0.4	4.3	0	0
Ale, Wychcraft, Wychwood, Marstons PLC*	1 Bottle/500ml	210	0	42	0.3	4.2	0	0
Becks Blue Lemon, No Alcohol, Beck & Co*	1 Bottle/1196ml	275	0.1	23	0.2	6	0	0
Bitter, Average	*1 Can/440ml*	*141*	*0*	*32*	*0.3*	*2.3*	*0*	*0*
Bitter, Banks, Marstons PLC*	1 Pint/568ml	193	0.1	34	0.3	3.4	0	0
Bitter, Cask, Draught, London Pride, Fullers*	1 Pint/568ml	201	0	35	0	0	0	0
Bitter, Draught, Average	*1 Pint/568ml*	*182*	*0*	*32*	*0.3*	*2.3*	*0*	*0*
Bitter, Keg, Average	*1 Pint/568ml*	*176*	*0*	*31*	*0.3*	*2.3*	*0*	*0*
Bitter, Low Alcohol, Average	*1 Pint/568ml*	*74*	*0*	*13*	*0.2*	*2.1*	*0*	*0*
Bitter, Original, Tetley's*	1 Can/440ml	140	0	32	0.2	4.6	0	0
Bitter, Oxford Gold, Brakspear*	1 Bottle/500ml	161	0	32	0	0	0	0
Bitter, Strong, Broadside, Adnams*	1 Bottle/500ml	285	0	57	0	0	0	0
Brown Ale, Bottled, Average	*1 Bottle/330ml*	*99*	*0*	*30*	*0.3*	*3*	*0*	*0*
Especial, Modelo*	1 Bottle/355ml	145	0	41	0	1.1	0	0
Guinness Extra Stout, Bottled*	*1 Bottle/500ml*	*215*	*0*	*43*	*4*	*0*	*0*	*0*
Guinness, Draught*	*1 Can/440ml*	*158*	*0.2*	*36*	*0.3*	*3*	*0*	*0*
Guinness, Stout*	*1 Pint/568ml*	*205*	*0*	*36*	*0.3*	*3*	*0*	*0*
Kilkenny, Diageo*	1 Pint/568ml	210	0	37	0.3	3	0	0
Low Calorie, Low Carb, Cobra*	1 Bottle/330ml	96	0	29	0.1	1.3	0	0
Mackeson, Stout	*1 Pint/568ml*	*205*	*0*	*36*	*0.4*	*4.6*	*0*	*0*
Mild, Draught, Average	*1 Pint/568ml*	*136*	*0*	*24*	*0.2*	*1.6*	*0*	*0*
Non Alcoholic, Zero, Cobra*	1 Bottle/330ml	79	0	24	0.8	2	0	0
Oak Aged, Original, Innis & Gunn*	1 Bottle/330ml	182	0	55	0.3	4.7	0	0
Raspberry, Framboise, Lindemans*	1 Serving/355ml	185	0	52	0	8.8	0	0
Rum Finish, Oak Aged, Innis & Gunn*	1 Bottle/330ml	188	0	57	0.3	4.8	0	0
Stout, Coopers*	1 Pint/375ml	191	0	51	0	2.9	0	0
Ultra, Michelob*	1 Bottle/275ml	88	0	32	0	0.9	0	0
Weissbier, Alcohol Free, Erdinger*	1 Bottle/500ml	125	0	25	0.4	5.3	0	0
Wheat, Tesco*	1 Bottle/500ml	155	0	31	0.5	0.4	0	0
BEETROOT								
Baby, Pickled, Average	*1 Beetroot/12.5g*	*5*	*0*	*37*	*1.7*	*7.2*	*0.1*	*1.2*
Cooked, Boiled, Drained, Average	*1 Serving/100g*	*44*	*0.2*	*44*	*1.7*	*10*	*0.2*	*2*
Golden, Spaghetti, Tesco*	½ Pack/125g	54	0.1	43	1.7	7.3	0.1	2.8
Grated, Tesco*	1 Serving/80g	34	0.1	42	1.7	7.2	0.1	2.8
Pickled, in Sweet Vinegar, Average	*1oz/28g*	*16*	*0*	*57*	*1.2*	*12.8*	*0.1*	*1.5*
Pickled, in Vinegar, Average	*1 Serving/50g*	*18*	*0*	*36*	*1.6*	*7.3*	*0.1*	*1.2*
Raw, Unprepared, Average	*1oz/28g*	*8*	*0*	*29*	*1.4*	*5.4*	*0.1*	*1.7*
Rosebud, M&S*	½ Pack/90g	45	0.3	50	1.9	8.9	0.3	3.2
Rosebud, Sweet Chilli Marinated, M&S*	1 Serving/80g	52	0.2	65	1.5	12.3	0.3	3.6
Spiralized, Sweet & Aromatic, Waitrose*	1 Serving/50g	31	0.1	62	1.5	12.4	0.2	2.2
Sweet Chilli, Diced, The Lincolnshire Beetroot Co*	1 Serving/50g	32	0.1	65	1.4	12.9	0.2	2.4
Sweet Smoky, Shredded, TTD, Sainsbury's*	½ Pack/100g	77	0.5	77	1.4	16	0.5	2.1
Sweetened Vinegar, Pomegranate, & Cumin, Waitrose*	½ Pack/90g	70	0.6	78	1.1	15.8	0.7	1.9
Tagliatelle, Tesco*	1 Pack/250g	108	0.2	43	1.7	7.3	0.1	2.8
with Balsamic Vinaigrette, Side Salad, M&S*	1 Pack/225g	146	2.9	65	0.7	12.4	1.3	2.2
BERRIES								
Medley, Grapes, Strawberry, Blueberry, Blackberry, Tesco*	1/2 Pack/120g	67	0.2	56	0.6	12.2	0.2	1
Mixed, Raspberry, Blackcurrant & Blackberry, Waitrose*	1 Serving/80g	30	0.2	38	1.1	5.5	0.2	5.3
Mixed, Strawberries, Raspberries & Blueberries, Tesco*	½ Pack/150g	102	0.4	68	0.7	14.5	0.3	2.4
Mixed, Summer Fruits, Frozen, Tesco*	1 Serving/80g	30	0.2	37	1.1	6.2	0.2	3.2

B

	Measure INFO/WEIGHT	per Measure KCAL	FAT	Nutrition Values per 100g / 100ml KCAL	PROT	CARB	FAT	FIBRE
BHAJI								
Aubergine, & Potato, Fried in Vegetable Oil, Average	*1oz/28g*	*36*	*2.5*	*130*	*2*	*12*	*8.8*	*1.7*
Cabbage, & Pea, Fried in Vegetable Oil, Average	*1oz/28g*	*50*	*4.1*	*178*	*3.3*	*9.2*	*14.7*	*3.4*
Cauliflower, & Paneer, Waitrose*	1 Pack/88g	218	14.7	248	7.6	11.6	16.7	10.1
Cauliflower, Fried in Vegetable Oil, Average	*1oz/28g*	*60*	*5.7*	*214*	*4*	*4*	*20.5*	*2*
Cauliflower, from 8 Snack Pack, Takeaway, Tesco*	1 Bhaji/18g	30	1.1	170	7.1	20.6	6.3	4.7
Indian Snack Selection, Chef Select, Lidl*	1 Serving/50g	125	7.2	250	5.6	22.1	14.3	5.3
Mango Chutney, Ovenbaked, Asda*	1 Bhaji/20g	52	1.7	255	5.9	36	8.5	5.3
Mushroom, Fried in Vegetable Oil, Average	*1oz/28g*	*46*	*4.5*	*166*	*1.7*	*4.4*	*16.1*	*1.3*
Okra, Bangladeshi, Fried in Butter Ghee, Average	*1oz/28g*	*27*	*1.8*	*95*	*2.5*	*7.6*	*6.4*	*3.2*
Onion, Asda*	1 Bhaji/49g	96	4.9	196	6	20	10	2
Onion, CBY, Asda*	1 Bhaji/30g	76	3.9	254	6	26	13	4.5
Onion, Fried in Vegetable Oil, Takeaway, Average	*1 Bhaji/70g*	*190*	*10.3*	*270*	*9.8*	*24.6*	*14.7*	*5.6*
Onion, Indian Meal for One, Tesco*	1 Bhaji/100g	204	7.3	204	5.5	29.2	7.3	1.3
Onion, Indian Starter Selection, M&S*	1 Bhaji/22g	57	3.7	260	5.7	19.3	17	3.5
Onion, Indian, Mini, Asda*	1 Bhaji/18g	33	1.8	186	4.9	19	10	6
Onion, Mini Indian Selection, Tesco*	1 Bhaji/23g	40	2.2	172	6.1	15.4	9.5	4.6
Onion, Mini, Asda*	1 Bhaji/35g	63	2.8	179	4.8	22	8	4.4
Onion, Mini, Snack Selection, Sainsbury's*	1 Bhaji/22g	49	3.4	226	4.1	17.4	15.5	3.5
Onion, Mini, Tesco*	1 Bhaji/23g	48	1.9	210	7.3	26.7	8.2	1.3
Onion, Sainsbury's*	1 Bhaji/38g	93	5.1	245	6.5	24.7	13.4	6.4
Onion, Tesco*	1 Bhaji/47g	85	4.9	181	5.7	16.2	10.4	4.3
Onion, Waitrose*	1 Bhaji/45g	124	9.4	276	4.7	17.5	20.8	2.5
Onion, with Tomato & Chilli Dip, M&S*	1 Bhaji/54g	111	6.3	205	4.1	21.1	11.7	3.6
Potato, & Onion, Fried in Vegetable Oil, Average	*1oz/28g*	*45*	*2.8*	*160*	*2.1*	*16.6*	*10.1*	*1.6*
Potato, Onion & Mushroom, Fried, Average	*1oz/28g*	*58*	*4.9*	*208*	*2*	*12*	*17.5*	*1.5*
Potato, Spinach & Cauliflower, Fried, Average	*1oz/28g*	*47*	*4.2*	*169*	*2.2*	*7.1*	*15.1*	*1.4*
Spinach, & Potato, Fried in Vegetable Oil, Average	*1oz/28g*	*53*	*3.9*	*191*	*3.7*	*13.4*	*14.1*	*2.3*
Spinach, Fried in Vegetable Oil, Average	*1oz/28g*	*23*	*1.9*	*83*	*3.3*	*2.6*	*6.8*	*2.4*
Vegetable, Fried in Vegetable Oil, Average	*1oz/28g*	*59*	*5.2*	*212*	*2.1*	*10.1*	*18.5*	*2.4*
Vegetable, from 8 Snack Pack, Takeaway, Tesco*	1 Bhaji/21g	36	1.9	175	6	16.8	9.1	4.9
BHUNA								
Chicken, & Rice, Sainsbury's*	1 Pack/501g	696	31.5	139	7.3	13.3	6.3	1.5
Chicken, Curry, Tesco*	1 Serving/300g	396	22.8	132	11.4	4.5	7.6	0.5
Chicken, Hyderabadi, Sainsbury's*	1 Pack/400g	472	20.8	118	12.6	5.2	5.2	1.3
Chicken, Indian Takeaway, Tesco*	1 Pack/350g	438	27.6	125	8.3	4.6	7.9	2.2
Chicken, Tikka, Tesco*	1 Pack/350g	438	23.4	125	11.3	5	6.7	0.9
Chicken, with Naan Bread, Sharwood's*	1 Pack/375g	465	19.1	124	6.8	12.8	5.1	2.8
Chicken, with Rice, Ready Meal, Average	*1 Pack/350g*	*444*	*20.8*	*127*	*9.4*	*8.9*	*5.9*	*1.4*
Lamb, & Rice, Sainsbury's*	1 Pack/500g	619	26.5	124	7.4	11.6	5.3	2
Prawn, Co-Op*	1 Pack/400g	300	16	75	3	6	4	1
Prawn, King, CBY, Asda*	1 Pack/375g	296	17.2	79	4.4	4.3	4.6	1.4
Prawn, King, M&S*	1 Pack /350g	262	13.3	75	6.7	3.3	3.8	1.5
Prawn, King, Morrisons*	1 Pack/350g	301	20.6	86	6.5	1.8	5.9	0.5
Prawn, Tandoori, Indian, Sainsbury's*	½ Pack/200g	152	8	76	5.5	4.5	4	1.7
BILBERRIES								
Fresh, Raw	*1oz/28g*	*8*	*0.1*	*29*	*0.6*	*6.8*	*0.2*	*1.8*
BILTONG								
Average	*1 Serving/25g*	*64*	*1*	*256*	*50*	*0*	*4*	*0*
BIRYANI								
Chicken Tikka, & Lentil Pilau, Fuller Longer, M&S*	1 Pack/400g	440	11.6	110	9.5	12	2.9	2.3
Chicken Tikka, Northern Indian, Sainsbury's*	1 Pack/450g	698	25.6	155	9.4	16.5	5.7	1.2
Chicken, & Basmati Rice, Fresh Ideas, Morrisons*	1 Pot/371g	505	19.3	136	5.8	15.1	5.2	2.7
Chicken, CBY, Asda*	1 Pack/401g	505	18.4	126	7.5	12.5	4.6	2.4

INFO/WEIGHT	Measure	per Measure		Nutrition Values per 100g / 100ml				
		KCAL	FAT	KCAL	PROT	CARB	FAT	FIBRE

BIRYANI

	Measure	KCAL	FAT	KCAL	PROT	CARB	FAT	FIBRE
Chicken, Indian, Asda*	1 Pack/450g	778	22.5	173	9	23	5	0.7
Chicken, LC, Tesco*	1 Serving/450g	495	10.3	110	7	15	2.3	3.4
Chicken, Ready Meal, Average	*1 Pack/400g*	*521*	*17.1*	*130*	*7.5*	*15.2*	*4.3*	*1.6*
Chicken, Ready Meal, Healthy Range, Average	*1 Pack/400g*	*369*	*5.5*	*92*	*7.4*	*12.6*	*1.4*	*0.9*
Chicken, Tikka, Ready Meal, Average	*1 Pack/400g*	*460*	*11.5*	*115*	*7.3*	*14.8*	*2.9*	*1.5*
Chicken, Vegetarian, Linda McCartney*	½ Pack/180g	300	11.7	167	8.6	17	6.5	3.3
Chicken, Weight Watchers*	1 Pack/330g	308	3.7	93	6.2	14.6	1.1	0.6
Lamb, Average	*1 Serving/200g*	*390*	*19.4*	*195*	*7.3*	*20.9*	*9.7*	*0*
Lamb, HL, Tesco*	1 Pack/400g	560	17.6	140	5.1	19	4.4	3.1
Lamb, Ready Meal, Average	*1 Pack/400g*	*535*	*18.9*	*134*	*6*	*16.6*	*4.7*	*2.2*
Seafood, M&S*	1 Pack/450g	619	25.7	138	7.1	14.4	5.7	1.7
Vegetable, & Rice, Sainsbury's*	½ Pack/125g	229	5	183	4.4	32.4	4	0.7
Vegetable, Curry, Microwaved, Slimzone, Asda*	1 Pack/459g	395	2.3	86	3.3	16	0.5	2.9
Vegetable, HL, Tesco*	1 Pack/450g	454	9.4	101	2.7	17.9	2.1	1.6
Vegetable, Sainsbury's*	1 Serving/225g	328	17.8	146	2.4	16.3	7.9	1.1
Vegetable, Waitrose*	1 Pack/450g	521	19.8	116	2.4	14.9	4.4	3.6
Vegetable, with Rice, Patak's*	½ Pack/125g	194	1.9	155	3.6	32.9	1.5	1.2
Vegetarian, Chicken Style, Lunch Pot, Quorn*	1 Pot/300g	300	13	100	3.5	10.9	4.4	1.7

BISCUITS

	Measure	KCAL	FAT	KCAL	PROT	CARB	FAT	FIBRE
Breakfast, Fruit & Seed, Weight Watchers *	2 Biscuits/36g	159	5.4	442	8	64.7	15.1	7.9
Abbey Crunch, McVitie's*	1 Biscuit/9g	43	1.6	477	6	72.8	17.9	2.5
Abernethy, Simmers*	1 Biscuit/12g	61	2.7	490	5.7	69.2	21.9	0
Ace Milk Chocolate, McVitie's*	1 Biscuit/24g	122	5.9	510	6.1	66.2	24.5	1.6
Aero, Nestle*	1 Bar/19g	99	5.4	534	6.4	59.4	29.4	2.1
Aero, Orange, Aero, Nestle*	1 Biscuit/19g	101	5.6	534	6	60.6	29.3	1.7
After Eight, Nestle*	1 Biscuit/5g	26	1.4	525	6.5	62.6	27.7	1.5
All Butter, Tesco*	1 Biscuit/9g	44	2.1	486	6.3	63.5	23	1.9
Almond & Chocolate, Biscotti, TTD, Sainsbury's*	1 Biscuit/30g	132	4.8	440	8.4	65.6	16	3.1
Almond Butter Thins, Extra Special, Asda*	1 Biscuit/4g	15	0.5	375	5	60	12.5	2.5
Almond Fingers, Tesco*	1 Finger/46g	180	6.8	391	6.2	58.4	14.7	1
Almond Thins, Continental, Tesco*	1 Biscuit/3g	15	0.5	450	6.7	72.8	14.7	3.1
Almond Thins, Sainsbury's*	1 Biscuit/3g	13	0.3	430	7	80.3	9	1
Almond, Artisan Bakery, Extra Special, Asda*	1 Biscuit/19g	103	6.1	548	7.9	54.3	32.3	4.2
Almond, Thins, TTD, Sainsbury's*	1 Biscuit/4g	16	0.5	450	6.7	72.8	14.7	3.1
Amaretti, Average	*1 Biscuit/5g*	*22*	*0.8*	*434*	*8.1*	*66.4*	*15.4*	*2.8*
Amaretti, Doria*	1 Biscuit/4g	17	0.3	433	6	84.8	7.8	0
Amaretti, M&S*	1 Biscuit/6g	30	1.1	480	9.6	71.3	17.2	3.8
Amaretti, Sainsbury's*	1 Biscuit/6g	27	0.7	450	6.5	80.5	11.3	1.1
Amaretti, Soft, Arden & Amici*	1 Biscuit/10g	47	2.5	470	13	46	25	5
Anzac, Bitesmart*	1 Biscuit/20g	84	4.6	420	5.1	46.8	23	0
Apple & Blackberry, Oat Squares, Go Ahead, McVitie's*	1 Bar/40g	137	3.8	343	4.5	63.8	9.5	4.2
Apple & Cinnamon Thins, Finest, Tesco*	1 Biscuit/5g	22	0.8	470	5.9	71.7	17.5	1.5
Apple & Raisin, Slices, G&C, Asda*	1 Pack/29g	109	1.3	382	6	77	4.5	4.5
Apple Crumble, Officially Low Fat, Fox's*	1 Biscuit/23g	85	0.6	365	5.4	80.4	2.4	2.5
Apricot & Yoghurt, Coupland's Bakeries*	1 Biscuit/30g	145	7.6	483	1.5	62.4	25.5	0
Apricot, Low Fat, M&S*	1 Biscuit/23g	79	1	343	6.1	69.6	4.4	7.8
Arrowroot, Thin, Crawfords*	1 Biscuit/7g	35	1.2	450	6.9	71.4	15.2	2.8
Baked Bites, Cheddar, Mini, Cathedral City*	1 Pack/22g	115	6.4	521	12.2	51.4	29.2	2.6
Belgian Chocolate Chip, Walkers Shortbread Ltd*	2 Biscuits/25g	124	6.1	494	5.1	63.3	24.5	2.2
Belgian Chocolate, Selection, Finest, Tesco*	1 Biscuit/10g	52	2.7	515	6	62	27	3
Belgian Chocolate, Thins, Extra Special, Asda*	1 Biscuit/9g	44	2	503	7	67	23	0.2
Belgian Milk Chocolate, M&S*	1 Biscuit/12g	60	2.5	490	6.2	70.1	20.3	2.5
Berry GI, Diet Chef Ltd*	1 Biscuit/20g	87	3.2	435	7	65.2	16.1	7.2

BISCUITS

	Measure INFO/WEIGHT	per Measure KCAL	FAT	Nutrition Values per 100g / 100ml KCAL	PROT	CARB	FAT	FIBRE
Bisc & Twix, Master Foods*	1 Bar/27g	140	7.6	520	5.2	61.1	28.3	0
Biscbits, Honeycomb Crunch, Cadbury*	7 Pieces/25g	120	5.2	480	6	67.3	20.9	1.4
Biscotti, Almond, Kate's Cakes Ltd*	1 Biscotti/36g	137	5.5	381	8.8	51.7	15.4	3.1
Biscotti, Chocolate Chip, Kate's Cakes Ltd*	1 Biscotti/36g	134	4.6	372	6.5	57.9	12.7	2.7
Biscotti, Chocolate, Heinz*	1 Biscuit/20g	80	1.7	398	8.5	72	8.7	5.8
Biscuits, Digestive, Thins, Capuccino, Mcvitie's*	1 Biscuit/6g	31	1.5	508	6.9	64	24.2	3.1
Black Forest Gateau, Moments , Special K, Kellogg's*	2 Biscuits/25g	95	2.2	381	5.2	72	9	2.4
Blackcurrant with Wheat Bran, Bisca*	1 Biscuit/7.5g	32	0.9	420	6	72	12	5.5
Blueberry & Vanilla, Oaty, Weight Watchers*	1 Biscuit/19g	86	3.3	452	7.3	62.1	17.6	8
Blueberry, Biscuit Moments, Special K, Kellogg's*	2 Biscuits/25g	99	2.3	394	4.5	73	9	1.5
Bn, Chocolate Flavour, McVitie's*	1 Biscuit/18g	83	3	460	6.6	71	16.7	2.6
Bn, Strawberry Flavour, McVitie's*	1 Biscuit/18g	71	1.2	395	5.6	78	6.8	0
Bn, Vanilla Flavour, McVitie's*	1 Biscuit/18g	85	3	470	5.9	74	16.6	1.2
Bourbon Creams, Asda*	1 Biscuit/14g	67	3.1	482	5	66	22	3.4
Bourbon Creams, Sainsbury's*	1 Biscuit/13g	60	2.4	476	5.7	70.4	19.1	1.7
Bourbon Creams, Tesco*	1 Biscuit/14g	68	3	485	5.4	66.2	21.6	3.4
Bourbon Creams, Value, Multipack, Tesco*	1 Biscuit/13g	62	2.9	494	5.9	68	22.8	1.7
Bourbon, Average	*1 Biscuit/13g*	*63*	*2.8*	*488*	*5.7*	*68.2*	*21.3*	*2.1*
Bourbon, Gluten & Wheat Free, Lovemore*	1 Biscuit/15g	70	2.9	469	4.1	67.9	19.1	4.7
Bourbon, Trufree*	1 Biscuit/12.5g	61	2.8	486	7.5	62.6	22.6	1.1
Bournville, Cadbury*	1 Biscuit/16g	85	5	520	6	54.9	30.7	1.4
Brandy Snap, Askeys*	1 Basket/20g	98	4.3	490	1.9	72.7	21.3	0
Brandy Snaps, Average	*1 Biscuit/15g*	*69*	*2.2*	*460*	*2.7*	*79.8*	*14.4*	*0.5*
Breakfast, Apricot, Crunchy, Belvita*	1 Pack/50g	198	4.8	395	7.5	65	9.5	12
Breakfast, Choc Chips, Crunchy, Belvita*	1 Pack/50g	208	6	415	8	63	12	12
Breakfast, Choc Chips, Soft Bakes, Belvita*	1 Pack/50g	202	7.5	405	5.7	61	15	6.9
Breakfast, Choco Hazlenut, Tops, Belvita*	1 Pack/50g	230	8	460	7.2	69	16	4.9
Breakfast, Cocoa, & Creamy Live Yoghurt, Belvita*	1 Pack/51g	228	7.6	450	7.5	68	15	4.4
Breakfast, Cocoa, Chocolate Chip, Belvita*	1 Pack/50g	220	7.5	440	7.8	66	15	7.1
Breakfast, Coconut & Yoghurt, Sainsbury's*	2 Biscuits/46g	203	7.3	437	7.6	62.1	15.7	8.7
Breakfast, Forest Fruit, Belvita*	1 Pack/50g	225	8	450	7.5	68	16	4.6
Breakfast, Fruit & Fibre, Belvita*	1 Pack/50g	215	7	430	7.3	64.5	14	8.5
Breakfast, Golden Grain, Soft Bakes, Belvita*	1 Pack/50g	192	6	385	5.9	63	12	6.7
Breakfast, Golden Oats, Belvita*	1 Pack/50g	220	7.5	440	7.7	67	15	5.7
Breakfast, Hazlenuts, Crunchy, Belvita*	1 Pack/50g	210	6	420	8.7	63	12	12
Breakfast, Honey & Nuts, Belvita*	1 Pack/50g	228	7.5	455	7.6	69	15	4.4
Breakfast, Honey & Oat, Eat Well, M&S*	2 Biscuits/20g	88	3	442	9	65.6	15	4.3
Breakfast, Milk & Cereals, Belvita*	1 Pack/50g	220	7.2	440	7.9	67	14.5	6.5
Breakfast, Mixed Berry, Soft Bakes, Belvita*	1 Pack/50g	200	7	400	6	66	14	8
Breakfast, Original, All Bran, Kellogg's*	1 Pack/40g	176	8	440	8	49	20	16
Breakfast, Porridge Oats & Blueberries , McVitie's*	1 Slice/20g	80	2.1	402	7.3	67.1	10.4	6.5
Breakfast, Porridge Oats, Oats & Honey, McVitie's*	4 Biscuits/50g	226	7	452	9.6	69.5	14	4.6
Breakfast, Porridge Oats, Raspberry & Yoghurt, Mcvities*	2 Biscuits/51g	248	10.8	487	9.1	63.5	21.1	3.2
Breakfast, Porridge Oats, Red Berries , McVitie's*	4 Biscuits/50g	226	6.9	452	9.6	71	13.8	5.1
Breakfast, Red Berries, Soft Bakes, Belvita*	1 Pack/50g	190	5.5	380	5.5	65	11	6.6
Breakfast, Strawberry, Tops, Belvita*	1 Pack/50g	208	5.5	415	6.6	72.5	11	4.2
Butter, Covered in Dark 70% Chocolate, Green & Black's*	1 Biscuit/12g	62	3.5	520	7.1	5.6	29.4	0.1
Butter, Crinkle Crunch, Fox's*	1 Biscuit/11g	50	1.9	460	5.8	69.8	17.5	2.4
Butter, Dark Chocolate, Momento, Aldi*	1 Biscuit/14g	69	3.2	491	6.2	63.5	22.6	4.2
Cadbury Creme Egg, Cadbury*	1 Biscuit/18g	80	3.7	435	5	58.3	20.1	1.3
Cafe Noir, with Coffee Flavour Icing, McVitie's*	1 Biscuit/6g	27	0.8	458	4.9	76	14	1.7
Cantucci with Honey, Loyd Grossman*	1 Biscuit/7g	32	1.1	450	9.5	66.3	16.3	0.9
Cantuccini with Almonds, Average	*1 Biscotti/30g*	*130*	*5*	*433*	*10*	*60*	*16.7*	*3.3*

BISCUITS

	Measure INFO/WEIGHT	per Measure KCAL	per Measure FAT	Nutrition Values per 100g / 100ml KCAL	PROT	CARB	FAT	FIBRE
Cantuccini, Sainsbury's*	1 Biscotti/8g	35	1.3	440	10.4	63.1	16.2	4.4
Caramac, Breakaway, Breakaway *	1 Biscuit/19g	100	5.2	524	6.5	61.7	27.4	1.9
Caramel Crunch, Go Ahead, McVitie's*	1 Bar/24g	106	3.3	440	4.7	76.6	13.8	0.8
Caramel Squares, Thorntons*	2 Biscuits/32g	150	6.4	470	6.2	65	20	2.4
Caramel, Treat Size, Asda*	1 Bar/21g	97	4.8	463	4.6	59	23	0.9
Caramelised, Biscoff, Lotus*	1 Biscuit/8g	38	1.5	484	4.9	72.7	19	1.3
Caramels, Milk Chocolate, McVitie's*	1 Serving/17g	81	3.6	478	5.6	65.8	21.4	2.3
Cheese Melts, Carr's*	1 Biscuit/4g	21	1	493	10.8	59.6	22.9	2.5
Cheese Sandwich, Ritz*	1 Biscuit/9g	50	2.8	530	9.5	55	30.2	2
Cheese Savouries, Sainsbury's*	1 Serving/50g	268	15.3	536	11.6	53.3	30.6	2.5
Cheese, & Chutney, Delicious, Boots*	1 Pack/134g	290	14.7	217	9	19	11	2.3
Cheese, Baked, Cheddars, Jacob's*	1 Cheddar/4g	20	1.2	525	10.8	47	31.8	2.9
Cherry Bakewell, Handfinished, M&S*	1 Biscuit/40g	200	9.7	495	5.9	62.1	24	0.5
Choc Chip, Paterson's*	1 Biscuit/17g	79	3.6	474	5.6	64	21.6	3.1
Chockas, Original, Fox's*	1 Biscuit/24g	85	1	355	1.1	10.4	4.2	0.4
Choco & Caramel, Pick Up, Bar, Bahlsen*	1 Bar/28g	140	6.7	501	6	64	24	0
Choco Leibniz, Dark Chocolate, Bahlsen*	1 Biscuit/14g	69	3.6	493	6.8	59	26	5.1
Choco Leibniz, Milk, Bahlsen*	1 Biscuit/14g	72	3.6	515	7.9	63.4	25.5	2.4
Choco Leibniz, Orange Flavour, Bahlsen*	1 Biscuit/14g	70	3.7	504	7.9	58.5	26.4	0
Chocolate & Coconut, Duchy Originals*	1 Biscuit/13g	68	4.3	543	6.3	52.1	34.4	2.6
Chocolate & Hazelnut, Quirks, McVitie's*	1 Biscuit/13g	66	3.6	511	5	58.4	28	2.6
Chocolate Chip & Peanut, Trufree*	1 Biscuit/11g	55	2.6	496	4	66	24	2
Chocolate Chip GI, Diet Chef Ltd*	1 Pack/20g	90	3.6	450	7.4	64.4	17.9	6.4
Chocolate Fingers, Milk, Cadbury*	1 Biscuit/6g	31	1.6	515	6.8	60.8	27.1	1.7
Chocolate Fingers, Milk, Extra Crunchy, Cadbury*	1 Biscuit/5g	25	1.2	505	6.6	66.2	23.6	0
Chocolate Fingers, Plain, Cadbury*	1 Biscuit/6g	30	1.6	508	6.2	60.6	26.8	0
Chocolate Fingers, Salted Peanut Crunch, Cadbury*	4 Fingers/21g	100	5.5	478	6.6	52.9	26.5	1.4
Chocolate Flavour, Taillefine, Lu*	1 Biscuit/8g	33	0.9	408	5.8	70.8	10.8	5.8
Chocolate Florentine, M&S*	1 Serving/39g	195	9.7	500	7.4	64.5	24.9	1.7
Chocolate Ginger, Organic, Duchy Originals*	1 Biscuit/12g	64	3.6	518	4.6	59.7	29	2.1
Chocolate Ginger, Thorntons*	1 Biscuit/19g	96	5.3	512	5.9	58.2	28.4	0
Chocolate Kimberley, Jacob's*	1 Biscuit/20g	86	3.4	428	3.9	64.4	17.2	1.1
Chocolate Mini Shorties, McVitie's*	1 Pack/25g	131	7.1	524	6	61.2	28.3	2
Chocolate Seville, Thorntons*	1 Biscuit/19g	97	5.3	512	5.7	59	28.1	0
Chocolate Toffee, Crunch, Moments, McVitie's*	1 Biscuit/17g	89	4.7	520	5.6	62.3	27.6	1.7
Chocolate Viennese, Fox's*	1 Biscuit/16g	85	4.9	530	6.7	56.6	30.7	1.7
Chocolate, Belgian Chocolate, Weight Watchers*	1 Biscuit/18g	87	4.1	481	7.1	61.8	22.8	4.5
Chocolate, Breakaway, Nestle*	1 Bar/19g	99	4.9	511	6.1	63.5	25.2	3
Chocolate, Chunky, Eat Me, Aldi*	1 Biscuit/24g	122	6	510	6	64	25	2.7
Chocolate, Fingers, Average	*1 Biscuit/6g*	*31*	*1.6*	*514*	*6.7*	*61.4*	*26.8*	*1.5*
Chocolate, Golden Crunch, Free From Milk, Tesco*	1 Biscuit/16.6g	85	4.9	510	4.2	57.2	29.4	4.6
Chocolate, Mint, Round, Tower Gate, Lidl*	1 Round/14g	74	4.1	529	4.3	60.7	29.3	0
Chocolinis, Milk Chocolate, Go Ahead, McVitie's*	1 Biscuit/12g	56	1.7	466	7.7	77.2	14	2
Chocolinis, Plain Chocolate, McVitie's*	1 Biscuit/12g	56	1.8	468	6.9	77	14.7	2.6
Christmas Shapes, Assorted, Sainsbury's*	1 Biscuit/15g	77	4.3	525	5.2	59	29.8	1.7
Classic, Creams, Fox's*	1 Biscuit/14g	72	3.6	516	4.4	65.2	25.8	1.7
Classic, Milk Chocolate, Fox's*	1 Biscuit/13g	67	3.1	517	6.1	64.9	24	1.6
Coconut Cream, Hill Biscuits Ltd*	1 Biscuit/12g	64	3	505	4.9	67	24	1.6
Coconut Crinkle, Sainsbury's*	1 Biscuit/11g	54	2.8	500	6.4	59.6	26.2	3.7
Coconut Crinkles, Fox's*	1 Biscuit/11g	53	2.5	487	5.2	63.8	22.6	3.7
Coconut Rings, Tesco*	1 Biscuit/9g	44	2	485	6.2	66.1	21.7	2.6
Coconut, Ring, Average	*1 Biscuit/9g*	*44*	*2*	*490*	*6.1*	*67.4*	*21.8*	*2.6*
Coffee, GF, Barkat*	2 Biscuits/15g	72	2.8	479	2	75	19	0

BISCUITS

	Measure INFO/WEIGHT	per Measure KCAL	FAT	Nutrition Values per 100g / 100ml KCAL	PROT	CARB	FAT	FIBRE
Cookies 'n Cream, Eat Me, Aldi*	1 Biscuit/12g	58	2.1	467	5.4	72	17	2.9
Cornish Fairings, Original, Furniss Of Cornwall*	1 Biscuit/17g	75	2.5	448	5.1	72.9	15.1	0
Cracked Black Pepper, Savoury, Weight Watchers*	1 Serving/16g	71	3.1	446	8.3	59.2	19.5	9.4
Cranberry & Pumpkin Seed, BGTY, Sainsbury's*	1 Biscuit/17g	68	2.8	410	7.2	56.6	17.1	13.9
Cranberry & Sunflower Seed, Oaty, Weight Watchers*	1 Biscuit/19g	87	3.7	457	7.9	58	19.3	10
Cranberry, Crispy Slices, LC, Tesco*	1 Biscuit/14.5g	54	0.6	370	6	76	3.9	5.5
Crinkles, Classics, Milk Chocolate, Fox's*	1 Biscuit/14g	67	3.1	487	5.7	65.2	22.7	2.7
Crispy Fruit Slices, Apple, Sultana, Go Ahead, McVitie's*	1 Slice/13g	50	0.9	388	5.4	74	7.1	2.9
Crispy Fruit Slices, Forest Fruit, Go Ahead, McVitie's*	1 Biscuit/13g	49	0.9	380	5.4	73.7	7	3
Crispy Slices, Raspberry, Go Ahead, McVitie's*	1 Slice/13g	50	0.9	385	5.3	74	7	2.8
Crispy Slices, Red Cherry, Go Ahead, McVitie's*	3 Slices/39g	147	2.7	380	5.5	73.9	7	2.9
Crunch Creams, Double Choc, Fox's*	1 Biscuit/15g	77	3.8	511	4.7	65	25	2.7
Crunchers, Salted, Savoury, Crackers, Sainsbury's*	1 Cracker/5g	22	1	448	6.1	59.4	20.4	1.4
Crunchie, Cadbury*	1 Biscuit/13g	64	3.1	495	4.8	65.7	23.6	0.9
Crunchy Caramel, Tesco*	1 Bar/21g	98	5.2	467	4.6	56	25	1.4
Custard Cream, Giant, Tesco*	1 Biscuit/90g	436	20.3	484	4.7	64.7	22.5	2.1
Custard Cream, Gluten & Wheat Free, Lovemore*	1 Biscuit/15g	71	2.5	475	0	33	16.8	0
Custard Creams, 25% Less Fat, Sainsbury's*	1 Biscuit/13g	59	2.2	469	5.8	72.7	17.3	1.3
Custard Creams, 25% Less Fat, Tesco*	1 Biscuit/13g	59	2.2	473	5.8	72.2	17.9	1.2
Custard Creams, Asda*	1 Biscuit/12g	59	2.7	495	5	67	23	2
Custard Creams, BGTY, Sainsbury's*	1 Biscuit/12g	56	2.1	473	5.8	72.2	17.9	1.2
Custard Creams, Crawfords*	1 Biscuit/11g	57	2.7	517	5.9	69.2	24.1	1.5
Custard Creams, Everyday Value, Tesco*	1 Biscuit/13g	62	2.6	495	5.6	69.7	20.9	1.7
Custard Creams, Jacob's*	1 Biscuit/16g	77	3.3	481	5.3	68	20.9	1.6
Custard Creams, Sainsbury's*	1 Biscuit/13g	67	3	514	5.5	70.4	23.4	1.6
Custard Creams, Smart Price, Asda*	1 Biscuit/13g	61	2.6	486	6	69	21	1.6
Custard Creams, Tesco*	1 Biscuit/13g	65	2.9	505	5.4	68.3	22.5	1.6
Custard Creams, Trufree*	1 Biscuit/12g	60	2.8	504	8.7	65	23	1
Custard Creams, Value, Tesco*	1 Biscuit/11g	51	1.6	450	7.2	72.5	14.3	3
Dark Chocolate All Butter, M&S*	1 Biscuit/15g	72	4.1	480	6.9	52.4	27.2	11.4
Dark Chocolate Ginger, M&S*	1 Biscuit/21g	105	5.7	505	5	58.8	27.6	4.2
Dark Chocolate Gingers, Border*	1 Biscuit/17g	74	3.4	445	4.4	61.4	20.1	2.9
Diet Fibre, Gullon*	2 Biscuits/16g	65	2.6	405	6.5	48.7	16.4	23
Digestive with Wheatgerm, Hovis*	1 Biscuit/12g	57	2.4	475	8.3	65	20	3.3
Digestive, 25% Less Fat, Asda*	1 Biscuit/16g	73	2.6	455	7.3	69.8	16.3	2.6
Digestive, 25% Less Fat, Tesco*	1 Biscuit/14g	65	2.3	462	7.3	71	16.5	3.8
Digestive, BGTY, Sainsbury's*	1 Biscuit/15g	70	2.6	468	7.4	71	17.2	3.8
Digestive, Caramels, Milk Chocolate, McVitie's*	1 Biscuit/17g	81	3.7	478	5.6	65.1	21.7	2.3
Digestive, Caramels, Plain Chocolate, McVitie's*	1 Biscuit/17g	82	3.8	481	5.7	65.5	22.1	2.1
Digestive, Chocolate	**1 Biscuit/17g**	**84**	**4.1**	**493**	**6.8**	**66.5**	**24.1**	**2.2**
Digestive, Chocolate Chip, Asda*	1 Biscuit/14g	68	3.2	491	6	65	23	2.9
Digestive, Chocolate, Free From, Co-Op*	1 Biscuit/11g	54	2.3	495	6.3	69	21	2.9
Digestive, Cracker Selection, Tesco*	1 Biscuit/12g	56	2.3	464	7.1	65.2	19.4	4.3
Digestive, Crawfords*	1 Biscuit/12g	58	2.4	484	7.1	68.8	20	3.4
Digestive, Creams, McVitie's*	1 Biscuit/12g	60	2.8	502	5.6	68.2	23	2.1
Digestive, Dark Chocolate, McVitie's*	1 Biscuit/17g	83	4.1	495	6	60.8	24.2	4.2
Digestive, Dark Chocolate, Thins, McVitie's*	1 Biscuit/6g	31	1.5	499	6	60.9	24.7	4.7
Digestive, Economy, Sainsbury's*	1 Biscuit/13g	65	3	498	6.8	66.3	22.8	3.3
Digestive, Everyday Value, Tesco*	1 Biscuit/16g	80	3.4	490	6.7	66.5	21	3
Digestive, Fingers, Morrisons*	1 Finger/8g	39	1.8	482	6.8	63.6	22.2	3.2
Digestive, GF, Barkat*	1 Biscuit/15g	56	2.7	378	3.4	49.3	18.5	18.4
Digestive, GFY, Asda*	1 Biscuit/14g	65	2.4	461	6	71	17	3.6
Digestive, Gluten & Wheat Free, Lovemore*	1 Biscuit/14.5g	55	2.7	378	3.4	49.3	18.5	18.4

BISCUITS

INFO/WEIGHT	Measure		per Measure		Nutrition Values per 100g / 100ml				
			KCAL	FAT	KCAL	PROT	CARB	FAT	FIBRE
Digestive, Happy Shopper*	1 Biscuit/13g		64	2.9	498	6.8	66.3	22.8	3.3
Digestive, High Fibre, Reduced Sugar, M&S*	1 Biscuit/13g		60	2.8	460	6.5	59.3	21.7	9.4
Digestive, Hovis*	1 Biscuit/6g		27	1.1	447	10.2	60	18.5	4.4
Digestive, Jacob's*	1 Biscuit/14g		67	3	479	6.6	65.7	21.1	3.4
Digestive, Lemon & Ginger, McVitie's*	1 Biscuit/15g		72	3.1	480	6.7	66.7	20.7	2.7
Digestive, Light, McVitie's*	1 Biscuit/15g		66	2.1	444	7.3	69.5	14.4	3.6
Digestive, McVitie's*	1 Biscuit/15g		70	3.2	470	7.2	62.7	21.5	3.6
Digestive, Milk Chocolate Mint, McVitie's*	1 Biscuit/16.6g		81	3.9	487	6.7	62.6	23.4	2.9
Digestive, Milk Chocolate, 25% Reduced Fat, McVitie's*	1 Biscuit/17g		78	2.9	459	7.2	68.6	17.3	3.2
Digestive, Milk Chocolate, Basics, Sainsbury's*	1 Biscuit/14g		71	3.4	496	6.5	62.9	23.7	2.9
Digestive, Milk Chocolate, Cadbury*	1 Biscuit/16g		80	3.8	490	7.4	61.3	23.3	3.9
Digestive, Milk Chocolate, GFY, Asda*	1 Biscuit/17g		78	2.9	457	7	69	17	3.2
Digestive, Milk Chocolate, Homewheat, McVitie's*	1 Biscuit/17g		83	4.1	486	6	61.5	24	4
Digestive, Milk Chocolate, M&S*	1 Biscuit/17g		85	4.4	505	6.1	62.2	26	2.6
Digestive, Milk Chocolate, McVitie's*	1 Biscuit/17g		84	4	488	6.7	62.7	23.4	2.9
Digestive, Milk Chocolate, Mini, McVitie's*	1 Bag/25g		124	6.2	496	6.6	61.9	24.7	2.9
Digestive, Milk Chocolate, Mini, Tesco*	1 Pack/30g		153	8.1	510	6.6	59.8	27.1	1.8
Digestive, Milk Chocolate, Sainsbury's*	1 Biscuit/17g		87	6.3	511	6.9	65.9	36.8	2.5
Digestive, Milk Chocolate, Tesco*	1 Biscuit/17g		85	4.1	498	6.6	62.8	23.9	3.1
Digestive, Milk Chocolate, Thins, McVitie's*	1 Biscuit/6g		32	1.5	508	6.9	64.3	24.1	3.1
Digestive, Milk Chocolate, Trufree*	1 Biscuit/12g		63	3	521	4	70	25	2
Digestive, Munch Bites, McVitie's*	1 Pack/40g		205	10.2	512	6.5	64.5	25.5	2
Digestive, Oat, Weight Watchers*	1 Biscuit/11g		50	2.1	457	6	66.3	18.6	6.9
Digestive, Organic, Sainsbury's*	1 Biscuit/12g		60	2.9	483	6.6	60.9	23.7	5.8
Digestive, Plain Chocolate, Asda*	1 Biscuit/17g		84	4	500	7	64	24	3.2
Digestive, Plain Chocolate, Tesco*	1 Biscuit/17g		85	4.1	499	6.2	63.5	24.4	2.8
Digestive, Plain Chocolate, Value, Tesco*	1 Biscuit/19g		97	4.9	510	6.4	61.5	26	2.9
Digestive, Plain, Average	*1 Biscuit/14g*		*67*	*2.9*	*480*	*7.1*	*65.6*	*20.5*	*3.5*
Digestive, Plain, M&S*	1 Biscuit/16g		80	3.9	490	6.5	62.7	23.8	3.3
Digestive, Reduced Fat, McVitie's*	1 Biscuit/15g		70	2.4	467	7.1	72.8	16.3	3.4
Digestive, Reduced Fat, Tesco*	1 Biscuit/16g		70	2.6	453	7	69.1	16.6	3.4
Digestive, Smart Price, Asda*	1 Biscuit/14g		67	2.9	465	6	65.3	20	3.1
Digestive, Sugar Free, Gullon*	1 Biscuit/13g		57	2.1	430	6.2	68	16	6.5
Digestive, Sweetmeal, Asda*	1 Biscuit/14g		68	3.1	499	7	66	23	3.5
Digestive, Sweetmeal, Sainsbury's*	1 Biscuit/14g		72	3.3	498	6	66.4	23.1	3.3
Digestive, Sweetmeal, Tesco*	1 Biscuit/18g		80	2.6	444	8.4	70	14.5	3.1
Digestive, Value, Tesco*	1 Biscuit/15g		74	3.4	490	6.9	64	22.4	3.3
Digestive, Whole Wheat, Organic, Dove's Farm*	1 Biscuit/12.5g		56	2.4	446	5.9	61.6	19.5	7.8
Digestives, Chocolate, Belmont Biscuit Co, Aldi*	1 Biscuit/17g		85	4	499	6.5	63.3	23.8	2.9
Digestives, Double Chocolate, Mcvitie's*	1 Biscuit/17g		83	4.1	497	6.5	60.9	24.3	3.6
Double Choc Chip, Trufree*	1 Biscuit/11g		58	3	523	3	67	27	1.8
Extremely Chocolatey Mini Rings, M&S*	1 Biscuit/13g		67	3.5	515	7.4	60.2	27.2	1.9
Extremely Chocolatey Orange, M&S*	1 Biscuit/24g		120	6.2	510	7.5	59.9	26.5	2.7
Extremely Chocolatey, Dark Chocolate Rounds, M&S*	1 Biscuit/19g		97	5.6	510	6.2	55.7	29.3	6.3
Fig Roll, Tesco*	1 Biscuit/19g		70	1.6	375	4	69.3	8.8	3.1
Florentines, Decadent Dark Chocolate, Thomas J Fudge*	1 Florentine/19g		107	7.1	565	8	46.8	37.3	0
Florentines, Sainsbury's*	1 Florentine/8g		40	2.5	506	10	47.2	30.8	7
for Cheese, Oat & Chive, Waitrose*	1 Biscuit/5.4g		26	1.2	483	10.8	57.5	22.4	4.1
Forest Fruit Slices, , Harvest Morn, Aldi*	1 Biscuit/14g		54	1	387	5.3	75	6.8	2.8
Forest Fruits, Benefit Delights , Aldi*	2 Biscuits/25g		97	1.6	388	5	77	6.2	2.2
Fruit & Spice Oat, Diet Chef Ltd*	2 Biscuits/20g		85	2.9	425	7.8	65.3	14.7	7.6
Fruit Bake, Organic, Tesco*	1 Biscuit/12g		53	2.1	453	7.5	65.1	18.1	5.6
Fruit Shortcake, McVitie's*	1 Biscuit/8g		37	1.5	462	5.6	65.9	18.9	3.1

B

B

BISCUITS

	Measure INFO/WEIGHT	per Measure KCAL	FAT	Nutrition Values per 100g / 100ml KCAL	PROT	CARB	FAT	FIBRE
Fruit Shortcake, Sainsbury's*	1 Biscuit/8g	39	1.6	483	5.9	69.6	20.1	2.1
Fruit Shortcake, Tesco*	1 Biscuit/9g	43	1.7	473	5.8	70.1	18.8	1.9
Fruit Slices, Apple, Raisin & Currant, Belmont, Aldi*	1 Biscuit/15g	57	1	379	7	72.8	6.4	1.3
Fruit, All Butter, Sainsbury's*	1 Biscuit/9g	45	2	477	5.6	66	21.2	1.9
Fruit, Oat, GI, Diet Chef Ltd*	1 Biscuit/20g	85	2.9	425	7.8	65.3	14.7	7.6
Fruity Iced, Blue Parrot Cafe, Sainsbury's*	1 Pack/20g	83	1.4	415	6	82	7	1.1
Fruity Oat, Organic, Dove's Farm*	1 Biscuit/12g	53	2.1	453	7.5	65.1	18.1	5.6
Galettes, Chocolate Butter, Bonne Maman*	2 Biscuits/28g	146	7.6	521	7.1	61.1	27.1	3.6
Galettes, Lemon & Poppy Seed, Butter, Bonne Maman*	2 Biscuits/28g	142	7.3	506	6.4	62	26	2
Garibaldi, Asda*	1 Biscuit/10g	39	0.9	375	4.7	68.5	9.1	2.2
Garibaldi, Sainsbury's*	1 Biscuit/9g	35	1	389	5.7	67.1	10.9	3.3
Garibaldi, Tesco*	1 Biscuit/10g	40	0.9	400	4.7	74	9.1	2.2
Ginger Crinkle Crunch, Fox's*	1 Biscuit/12g	50	1.4	435	4.7	75.3	12.5	1.6
Ginger Crinkle, Sainsbury's*	1 Biscuit/11g	53	2.5	486	6.2	63.8	22.9	2.9
Ginger Crunch Creams, Fox's*	1 Biscuit/15g	77	3.5	501	4.1	68	23	1.6
Ginger Crunch, Hand Baked, Border*	1 Biscuit/12g	54	2.3	470	4.7	71.4	20.4	0
Ginger Crunches, Organic, Against the Grain*	1 Biscuit/15g	71	3.4	474	2.8	65.6	23	1.2
Ginger GI, Diet Chef Ltd*	1 Biscuit/20g	87	3	435	8.8	65.6	15.2	6.1
Ginger Nuts, CBY, Asda*	1 Biscuit/10g	46	1.5	452	5.4	73.5	14.7	2.1
Ginger Nuts, McVitie's*	1 Biscuit/10g	46	1.5	452	5.4	73.5	14.7	2.1
Ginger Nuts, Milk Chocolate, McVitie's*	1 Biscuit/14g	68	2.8	489	5.8	71.8	19.9	1.5
Ginger Nuts, Tesco*	1 Biscuit/10g	46	1.5	450	5.3	73.2	14.7	2.2
Ginger Nuts, Value, Tesco*	1 Biscuit/12g	55	1.9	460	5.2	74.2	15.8	1.6
Ginger Snap, BGTY, Sainsbury's*	1 Biscuit/12g	51	1.2	427	6.5	78.2	9.8	1.8
Ginger Snap, Fox's*	1 Biscuit/8g	35	1	443	4.6	77.1	12.8	1.5
Ginger Snap, Less Than 10% Fat, Sainsbury's*	1 Biscuit/12g	51	1.1	424	6.5	78.9	9.1	1.9
Ginger Snap, Sainsbury's*	1 Biscuit/11g	47	1.6	445	5.3	73	14.7	2.2
Ginger Snaps, Hand Baked, Ringtons *	1 Biscuit/15g	69	2.4	458	5	73.9	16.2	0
Ginger Snaps, Trufree*	1 Biscuit/11g	51	1.9	467	2.5	76	17	1.5
Ginger Thins, Anna's*	1 Biscuit/5g	24	1	480	6	70	20	2
Ginger Thins, Asda*	1 Biscuit/5g	23	0.8	462	6	73	16	1.9
Ginger, Belgian Dark Chocolate, Thins, Waitrose*	1 Biscuit/10g	48	2.2	481	6.2	61.2	22.5	4.6
Ginger, Snap, 35% Reduced Fat, Sainsbury's*	1 Biscuit/10g	42	0.9	421	6.8	77.1	9	2.4
Ginger, Traditional, Fox's*	1 Biscuit/8g	33	1	404	4.4	70.1	11.7	1.4
Ginger, Value, Morrisons*	1 Biscuit/12g	55	1.9	459	5.3	74	15.8	1.7
Gingerbread Man, Gluten & Wheat Free, Lovemore*	1 Biscuit/37g	179	7.6	485	4.7	70.1	20.5	1.7
Gingerbread Shapes, Milk Chocolate, Favorina, Lidl*	1 Shape/28g	105	2.5	376	5.2	67.8	8.8	0
Gingernut	***1 Biscuit/11g***	***50***	***1.7***	***456***	***5.6***	***79.1***	***15.2***	***1.4***
Golden Crunch Creams, Fox's*	1 Biscuit/15g	75	3.8	515	4.7	64.8	26.3	1.2
Golden Crunch, Bronte*	1 Biscuit/14.6g	69	3.3	474	5.1	62.5	22.6	0
Golden Crunch, Go Ahead, McVitie's*	1 Biscuit/9g	38	0.9	419	7.7	75.2	9.7	2.1
Golden Crunch, Paterson's*	1 Biscuit/15g	69	3.3	474	5.1	62.5	22.6	4.8
Golden Shortie, Jacob's*	1 Biscuit/11g	54	2.6	492	6	64.9	23.2	0
Golden Syrup, McVitie's*	1 Biscuit/12g	63	3	508	5.1	67.3	24.2	2.2
Gouda Cheese, & Chive, Buiteman*	1/3 Pack/25g	129	8	516	16	40	32	4
Gruyere & Spinach Twists, Savoury, Ardens*	1 Twist/7g	33	1.4	466	13	56	20	5
Happy Faces, Jacob's*	1 Biscuit/16g	78	3.6	485	4.8	66.1	22.3	1.6
Hazelnut Crispies, Occasions, Sainsbury's*	1 Biscuit/7g	36	1.8	518	6	64.3	26.3	0
Hazelnut Meringue, Sainsbury's*	1 Biscuit/6g	24	1.4	404	5	43	23.5	1.1
Hobnobs, Chocolate Creams, McVitie's*	1 Biscuit/12g	60	3.1	503	6.7	60.3	26.1	4
Hobnobs, Light, 25% Reduced Fat, McVitie's*	1 Biscuit/14g	62	2.3	435	8.1	64.6	16.1	6.2
Hobnobs, McVitie's*	1 Biscuit/15g	72	3.2	473	7	61.8	20.7	5.4
Hobnobs, Milk Chocolate, McVitie's*	1 Biscuit/19g	92	4.5	479	6.8	60.7	23.3	4.5

BISCUITS

	Measure INFO/WEIGHT	per Measure KCAL	FAT	Nutrition Values per 100g / 100ml KCAL	PROT	CARB	FAT	FIBRE
Hobnobs, Milk Chocolate, Mini, McVitie's*	1 Pack/25g	121	5.9	483	6.6	61.3	23.5	4.4
Hobnobs, Plain Chocolate, McVitie's*	1 Biscuit/16g	81	3.9	498	6.7	63.3	24.3	4.2
Hobnobs, Vanilla Creams, McVitie's*	1 Biscuit/12g	60	3	501	6.1	62.3	25.2	3.6
Iced Gems, Jacob's*	1 Bag/25g	98	0.8	393	5	86.3	3.1	2
Jaffa Cakes, Asda*	1 Cake/12g	43	1	368	4.7	67.5	8.8	1.9
Jaffa Cakes, Basics, Sainsbury's*	1 Jaffa Cake/11g	44	1.1	385	4.6	69.7	9.7	2.5
Jaffa Cakes, Belmont Biscuit Co, Aldi*	1 Biscuit/13g	52	1.3	400	3.7	72.8	10.2	1
Jaffa Cakes, Dark Chocolate, M&S*	1 Cake/11g	45	1.5	395	3.7	64.9	13.2	2.8
Jaffa Cakes, Dark Chocolate, Mini, M&S*	1 Cake/5g	20	0.8	410	3.9	62.8	15.8	1.9
Jaffa Cakes, Free From, Asda*	1 Cake/12g	42	0.9	340	5.8	62.6	7.4	8
Jaffa Cakes, Lunch Box, McVitie's*	1 Cake/7g	26	0.6	395	4.2	74.3	9	1.4
Jaffa Cakes, McVitie's*	1 Cake/12g	46	1	380	4.9	70.8	8	2.2
Jaffa Cakes, Mini Roll XI, McVitie's*	1 Cake/44g	169	5	384	3.5	66.9	11.4	0
Jaffa Cakes, Mini Roll, McVitie's*	1 Cake/30g	108	3.5	407	4.2	66.9	13.3	2.9
Jaffa Cakes, Mini, Asda*	1 Cake/5g	21	0.8	412	3.9	63	16	1.9
Jaffa Cakes, Mini, Bags, McVitie's*	1 Cake/5g	20	0.7	396	4.2	65	13.1	3.5
Jaffa Cakes, Mini, Orange Pods, McVitie's*	1 Cake/40g	150	3.4	380	4.3	71.2	8.7	3.5
Jaffa Cakes, Mini, Tesco*	1 Cake/5g	19	0.6	380	4	64	12	2
Jaffa Cakes, Plain Chocolate, Sainsbury's*	1 Cake/13g	50	1.1	384	4.4	73.3	8.1	1.3
Jaffa Cakes, Sainsbury's*	1 Cake/11g	41	1	373	4.3	69.3	8.8	2
Jaffa Cakes, Smart Price, Asda*	1 Cake/11.5g	43	1	374	4.3	69	9	2
Jaffa Cakes, Value, Tesco*	1 Cake/11g	42	1	370	4.8	67.6	8.8	1.9
Jam & Cream, Belmont Biscuit Co, Aldi*	1 Biscuit/16g	78	3.6	490	5.9	65.8	22.3	1.2
Jam Creams, Jacob's*	1 Biscuit/15g	75	3.4	486	5	67.4	21.8	1.6
Jam Rings, Crawfords*	1 Biscuit/12g	56	2.1	470	5.5	73	17.2	1.9
Jam Sandwich Creams, M&S*	1 Biscuit/17g	80	3.7	485	5.7	64.5	22.6	1.8
Jam Sandwich Creams, Sainsbury's*	1 Biscuit/16g	77	3.4	486	5	67	21.8	1.6
Jammie Dodgers, Minis, Lunchbox, Burton's*	1 Pack/20g	90	2.9	452	5.5	72.7	14.7	2.5
Jammie Dodgers, Original, Burton's*	1 Biscuit/19g	83	3	437	5.1	69.5	15.9	1.9
Jammy Wheels, GF, Prewett's*	1 Biscuit/24g	95	5.6	394	5	60.1	23.2	4.7
Jestives, Milk Chocolate, Cadbury*	1 Biscuit/17g	86	4.2	506	6.4	64.4	24.8	0
Key Lime Pie, Crunch Creams, Fox's*	1 Biscuit/16g	78	3.7	507	4.1	67.5	24.2	1.7
Kimberley, Bolands*	1 Biscuit/16g	72	1.7	449	5.1	82.6	10.9	1.4
Lebkuchen, Sainsbury's*	1 Biscuit/10g	39	0.8	400	5.7	76.1	8	1.3
Lemon Butter, Thins, Sainsbury's*	1 Biscuit/13g	65	3.5	515	5.3	60.7	27.9	2.2
Lemon Curd Sandwich, Fox's*	1 Biscuit/14g	69	3.3	494	4.7	66.2	23.4	1.3
Lemon Puff, Jacob's*	1 Biscuit/13g	69	4.1	533	4.3	58.8	31.2	2.8
Lemon Thins, Sainsbury's*	1 Biscuit/10g	47	1.7	468	5.6	72.3	17.3	1.7
Lemon, All Butter, Half Coated, Finest, Tesco*	1 Biscuit/17g	84	4.5	505	5.6	60.4	26.9	3.6
Lincoln, McVitie's*	1 Biscuit/8g	41	1.9	514	6.3	69	23.6	2
Lincoln, Sainsbury's*	1 Biscuit/8g	40	1.7	479	7.2	66.1	20.6	2.1
Malt, Basics, Sainsbury's*	1 Biscuit/8g	36	1.2	470	7.1	73.6	15.7	0
Malted Milk, Asda*	1 Biscuit/8g	39	1.8	490	7	66	22	2
Malted Milk, Average	*1 Biscuit/8.5g*	*42*	*1.9*	*490*	*7*	*65.6*	*22.2*	*1.8*
Malted Milk, Chocolate, Tesco*	1 Biscuit/10g	52	2.5	500	6.7	64.4	24	1.9
Malted Milk, Milk Chocolate, Asda*	1 Biscuit/11g	56	2.8	509	7	64	25	1.7
Malted Milk, Sainsbury's*	1 Biscuit/8g	40	1.8	488	7.1	65.5	21.9	2
Malted Milk, Tesco*	1 Biscuit/9g	44	1.9	495	6.6	66.8	21.8	2
Maple Leaf, M&S*	1 Biscuit/13g	50	1.9	395	5.1	59.8	14.8	2
Maria, Gullon*	1 Biscuit/6g	24	0.7	408	7	75	11	4.5
Marie, Crawfords*	1 Biscuit/7g	33	1.1	475	7.5	76.3	15.5	2.3
Melts, Sesame with Chive, Carr's*	1 Biscuit/5g	23	1.2	498	8.2	57.4	26.2	3.5
Mikado, Jacob's*	1 Biscuit/13.4g	53	1.6	397	4.2	67.7	12.1	2.5

INFO/WEIGHT	Measure	per Measure		Nutrition Values per 100g / 100ml				
		KCAL	FAT	KCAL	PROT	CARB	FAT	FIBRE

BISCUITS

	Measure INFO/WEIGHT	KCAL	FAT	KCAL	PROT	CARB	FAT	FIBRE
Milk Chocolate Digestive, Everyday Value, Tesco*	1 Biscuit/17g	82	3.7	494	7.2	65.4	22.3	1.7
Milk Chocolate, All Butter, M&S*	1 Biscuit/14g	70	3.6	490	7.9	57.4	25.5	1.4
Milk Chocolate, Assortment, Cadbury*	1 Serving/10g	51	2.6	510	6.8	61	26.4	0
Milk Chocolate, Tesco*	1 Biscuit/25g	135	7.3	535	6.4	62.1	29	1.8
Mini Assortment, M&S*	1 Biscuit/2.5g	12	0.6	480	6.1	63.9	22.5	2.8
Mini Clotted Cream, Fosters Traditional Foods*	1 Biscuit/13g	66	3.6	507	5.4	59.5	27.4	0
Mint, Viscount*	1 Biscuit/13g	73	3.8	552	5.1	60.6	28.8	1.3
Mixed Berry, Oat Square, Go Ahead, McVitie's*	1 Bar/40g	137	3.7	342	4.6	64.4	9.2	4.2
Mixed Seed & Honey, Oaty, Weight Watchers*	1 Biscuit/22g	106	5.1	482	9.2	59	23.2	4.9
Morning Coffee, Asda*	1 Biscuit/5g	22	0.7	455	8	72	15	2.4
Morning Coffee, Tesco*	1 Biscuit/5g	22	0.7	450	7.6	72.3	14.5	2.4
Nice Creams, Fox's*	1 Biscuit/13g	64	3	505	5	67	24	2
Nice, Asda*	1 Biscuit/8g	38	1.7	480	6	68	21	2.4
Nice, Average	*1 Biscuit/7.5g*	*36*	*1.6*	*484*	*6.3*	*67.3*	*21*	*2.5*
Nice, Belmont, Aldi*	1 Biscuit/8g	39	1.6	489	6.2	68.9	20.4	2.3
Nice, Cream, Tesco*	1 Serving/13g	65	3.1	510	4.9	67	24	2
Nice, Fox's*	1 Biscuit/9g	39	1.7	450	6.3	62.4	19.4	5
Nice, Jacob's*	1 Biscuit/7g	33	1.3	471	6.1	68.5	19.2	1.8
Nice, Sainsbury's*	1 Biscuit/8g	39	1.9	490	5.8	63.1	23.8	3.8
Nice, Sainsbury's*	1 Biscuit/8g	40	1.7	486	5.9	68.3	20.9	2.7
Nice, Value, Multipack, Tesco*	1 Biscuit/8g	39	1.7	485	6.5	68	20.8	2.4
Nice, Value, Tesco*	1 Biscuit/5g	24	1.1	489	6.9	64.6	22.6	2.4
Oat & Wholemeal, Crawfords*	1 Biscuit/14g	67	3	482	7.7	64.2	21.6	4.8
Oat & Chocolate Chip, Cadbury*	1 Biscuit/16.5g	80	3.9	485	6.9	60.2	23.9	4.2
Oat & Walnut, M&S*	2 Biscuits/12g	59	3.1	492	10.8	54.2	25.8	2.5
Oat & Wholemeal, Dbc Foodservice*	1 Biscuit/14g	67	3.1	466	7.1	60.8	21.7	5.5
Oat Bites, Caramelised Onion, Diet Chef Ltd*	1 Pack/23g	99	3.9	430	7.5	64.2	16.8	6
Oat Bites, Cheese, Diet Chef Ltd*	1 Pack/23g	99	3.6	430	15	57.4	15.8	4.9
Oat Bites, Chilli, Diet Chef Ltd*	1 Pack/23g	128	3.1	556	8.1	68.4	13.3	7.2
Oat Crisps, Orange, Swedish, Gille*	1 Biscuit/8g	40	2	500	4.7	63.8	25	0
Oat Crumbles, Border*	1 Biscuit/15g	66	3.1	443	5.3	58.9	20.7	1.8
Oat Crunch, M&S*	1 Biscuit/14.4g	65	2.7	450	7.8	62	18.7	6.1
Oat Crunch, Weight Watchers*	1 Biscuit/11.5g	52	2.1	448	7.4	65.2	17.8	6.1
Oat Digestives, Nairn's*	1 Biscuit/11.4g	50	2	437	12	57.8	17.5	7.8
Oat Digestives, TTD, Sainsbury's*	1 Biscuit/12.5g	56	2.3	448	9.8	56.4	18.5	8.5
Oat, Black Sesame & Seaweed, 1, Waitrose*	1 Biscuit/5g	27	1.3	487	10.5	55.5	23.1	7.8
Oat, Fruit & Spice, Nairn's*	1 Biscuit/10g	43	1.5	425	7.8	65.3	14.7	7.6
Oat, Mixed Berries, Nairn's*	1 Biscuit/10g	43	1.5	427	7.5	64.8	15.3	7.1
Oat, Stem Ginger, Nairn's*	1 Biscuit/10g	43	1.5	434	8.8	65.6	15.2	6.1
Oaten, Organic, Duchy Originals*	1 Biscuit/16g	71	2.7	441	9.8	62.3	16.9	5.3
Oatie Crumbles, CBY, Asda*	1 Biscuit/14g	68	2.9	483	6.6	65.6	20.6	4.5
Oaties, Belmont Biscuit Co, Aldi*	1 Biscuit/15g	71	3.1	475	7.8	66.7	20.4	3.3
Oaties, Oatland, Tesco*	1 Biscuit/15g	70	3.1	470	6.5	64.9	20.5	4.5
Oatmeal Crunch, Jacob's*	1 Biscuit/8g	37	1.5	458	6.8	65.9	18.6	3.6
Oatmeal, Asda*	1 Biscuit/12g	54	2.5	470	6	62	22	6
Oaty Thins, Rude Health*	1 Thin/6g	23	0.3	380	11.5	68.5	4.7	8.7
Oaty, 4 Seed, Rude Health*	1 Biscuit/13g	57	2.6	455	11.1	50.8	21	9.4
Orange Chocolate, Organic, Duchy Originals*	1 Biscuit/13g	64	3.5	509	5.5	60	28	3
Orange Sultana, Go Ahead, McVitie's*	1 Biscuit/15g	58	1.2	400	5.1	75.7	8.1	3
Oreo, Chocolate Cream, Thins, Mondelez*	4 Biscuits/24g	117	4.8	488	5.4	69	20	3.5
Oreo, Thins, Mondelez*	4 Biscuits/24g	118	5.1	490	4.8	69	21	2.6
Parmesan Cheese, Sainsbury's*	1 Biscuit/3g	18	1	553	14.7	56.4	29.9	1.8
Party Rings, Iced, Fox's*	1 Biscuit/6g	29	0.9	459	5.1	75.8	15	0

BISCUITS

	Measure INFO/WEIGHT	per Measure KCAL	per Measure FAT	Nutrition Values per 100g / 100ml KCAL	PROT	CARB	FAT	FIBRE
Peanut Butter Cups, Mini, Hershey*	1 Cup/8g	44	2.4	564	10.3	56.4	30.8	2.6
Peanut Butter, American Style, Sainsbury's*	1 Biscuit/13g	63	2.9	504	5.2	68.7	23.1	2.2
Petit Beurre, Stella Artois*	1 Biscuit/6g	26	0.9	440	9	73	15	0
Pink Wafers, Crawfords*	1 Biscuit/7g	36	1.9	521	2.5	68.6	26.5	1.1
Pink Wafers, Eat Me, Aldi*	1 Biscuit/8g	44	2.6	552	4.2	58.4	32.9	2.9
Pink Wafers, Sainsbury's*	1 Biscuit/8g	36	1.8	486	4.6	64.2	23.4	1.7
Puffin, Chocolate, Asda*	1 Biscuit/25g	133	7.2	533	5	63	29	1.2
Puffin, Orange, Asda*	1 Biscuit/25g	133	7.3	529	5	62	29	2.2
Raspberry & Cream Viennese, Melts, Fox's*	1 Biscuit/16g	84	4.5	521	4	62.1	28.1	1.7
Redcurrant Puffs, Eat Well, M&S*	1 Biscuit/7g	32	1.4	470	5.6	67.7	19.8	2
Rich Shorties, Asda*	1 Biscuit/10g	50	2.3	486	6	66	22	2
Rich Tea, 25% Less Fat, Tesco*	1 Biscuit/10g	44	1.1	435	7.1	77	11	1.3
Rich Tea, Average	*1 Biscuit/10g*	*45*	*1.5*	*451*	*6.8*	*72.8*	*14.5*	*2.5*
Rich Tea, Basics, Sainsbury's*	1 Biscuit/8g	35	1.2	450	7.1	71.3	15.2	2.9
Rich Tea, Belmont Biscuit Co, Aldi*	1 Biscuit/8g	37	1.2	464	7.4	74	15	3.2
Rich Tea, BGTY, Sainsbury's*	1 Biscuit/10g	43	1.1	430	7.8	75.9	10.6	2.4
Rich Tea, CBY, Asda*	1 Biscuit/7.6g	34	1	447	7.2	72.9	13.4	3
Rich Tea, Classic, McVitie's*	1 Biscuit/8g	38	1.3	453	7.1	71.2	15.5	2.9
Rich Tea, Essential, Waitrose*	1 Biscuit/8g	36	1.2	452	7.1	71.1	15.2	2.9
Rich Tea, Finger, Essential, Waitrose*	1 Biscuit/5g	22	0.7	450	7.2	72.5	14.3	3
Rich Tea, Finger, Tesco*	1 Finger/5g	23	0.7	451	7.4	72.9	14.4	2.3
Rich Tea, Fingers, Morrisons*	1 Finger/4g	22	0.7	550	10	90	17.5	5
Rich Tea, Light, McVitie's*	1 Biscuit/8g	36	0.9	436	7.6	75.3	10.7	3.1
Rich Tea, Low Fat, M&S*	1 Biscuit/9g	40	1	435	8.3	76.7	10.5	2.4
Rich Tea, Lower Fat, M&S*	1 Biscuit/10g	42	0.9	425	8.1	77.1	8.6	3.2
Rich Tea, Milk Chocolate Covered, Cadbury*	1 Biscuit/12g	60	2.6	490	6.6	67.6	21.4	0
Rich Tea, Milk Chocolate, Sainsbury's*	1 Biscuit/13g	66	3	504	6.3	68.5	22.7	2.1
Rich Tea, Plain Chocolate, Sainsbury's*	1 Biscuit/13g	65	3	497	6.6	66	23	2.6
Rich Tea, Sainsbury's*	1 Biscuit/8g	34	1	440	7.2	72.7	13.4	3
Rich Tea, Tesco*	1 Biscuit/10g	43	1.3	451	7.2	72.8	14	2.7
Rich Tea, Value, Tesco*	1 Biscuit/8g	35	1.2	453	7.2	72.4	15	2.3
Rocky, Chocolate & Caramel, Fox's*	1 Biscuit/21g	107	4.1	507	6.9	60.3	19.3	15.5
Rocky, Chocolate, Fox's*	1 Biscuit/21g	106	5.4	505	5.7	62.4	25.7	2.4
Rocky, Rounds, Caramel, Fox's*	1 Biscuit/15g	72	3.4	480	6.2	62.3	22.9	1.1
Rocky, Rounds, Chocolate, Fox's*	1 Biscuit/6g	31	1.7	517	7.2	58.5	28.3	1.6
Rosemary & Raisin, M&S*	1 Biscuit/7g	35	1.7	490	5.1	62.5	24.1	1.8
Rosemary & Thyme, Oaten, Duchy Originals, Waitrose*	1 Biscuit/12g	58	2.7	467	8.5	56.8	21.5	6
Roundie, Milk Chocolate Covered Wafer, Cadbury*	1 Biscuit/30g	161	9.3	536	6.8	56	31	2.8
Savoury Oat, with Thyme, Rick Stein*	1 Biscuit/10g	46	2.1	460	9.8	66.9	21.4	10.4
Savoury, Gluten, Wheat & Dairy Free, Sainsbury's*	1 Biscuit/17g	77	2.9	467	11.7	65.1	17.7	2.4
Savoury, Organic, M&S*	1 Biscuit/7g	28	1	395	7	58.4	14.6	8.7
Scotch Finger, Arnotts Australia*	1 Biscuit/18g	88	3.9	489	6.6	65.8	21.5	0
Scottish Sweet Oatie, Organic, Daylesford Organic*	1 Biscuit/23g	119	7.1	516	6.1	53.9	30.7	4.7
Sea Salt & Black Pepper, for Cheese, TTD, Sainsbury's*	3 Biscuits/19.5g	93	4.3	484	8.8	60.1	22.4	3.8
Shortbread, All Butter, Fingers, Walkers Shortbread Ltd*	2 Fingers/48g	256	14.5	533	5.6	58.4	30.3	2.1
Shortcake with Real Milk Chocolate, Cadbury*	1 Biscuit/15g	75	3.5	500	6.3	65.8	23.5	0
Shortcake, Asda*	1 Biscuit/14g	73	3.6	518	5	66	26	2
Shortcake, Average	*1 Biscuit/11g*	*55*	*3*	*501*	*6.3*	*66.1*	*27.1*	*2.1*
Shortcake, Caramel, Mini, Festive, Thorntons*	1 Cake/14g	71	4.3	508	4	52.5	30.8	0.6
Shortcake, Caramel, Mini, Finest, Tesco*	1 Biscuit/15g	74	4.2	493	4.3	56.3	27.8	1
Shortcake, Caramel, Mini, Thorntons*	1 Biscuit/14.5g	71	4.6	492	4.8	46.3	31.9	0.6
Shortcake, Caramel, Mr Kipling*	1 Biscuit/36g	182	10.4	506	4.2	57.6	28.8	1.3
Shortcake, Caramel, Squares, M&S*	1 Square/40g	190	9.6	475	5.5	59.7	23.9	1

B

BISCUITS

INFO/WEIGHT	Measure	per Measure		Nutrition Values per 100g / 100ml				
		KCAL	FAT	KCAL	PROT	CARB	FAT	FIBRE
Shortcake, Caramel, Squares, Tesco*	1 Square/54g	274	16.4	507	4.6	54.1	30.4	0.4
Shortcake, Caramel, The Handmade Flapjack Company*	1 Biscuit/75g	383	23	511	4.6	54.3	30.6	0
Shortcake, Crawfords*	1 Biscuit/10g	52	2.5	504	6.2	63.5	24.4	2.6
Shortcake, Dairy Milk Chocolate, Cadbury*	1 Bar/49g	252	13.5	515	7.5	59.2	27.5	0
Shortcake, Dutch, M&S*	1 Biscuit/17g	90	5.1	540	5.4	59	30.8	2.5
Shortcake, Fruit, Crawfords*	1 Biscuit/8g	34	1.5	419	5.4	55.9	19.3	2.4
Shortcake, Jacob's*	1 Biscuit/10g	48	2.2	485	6.7	65.6	21.8	2
Shortcake, Mini Pack, Paterson's*	1 Biscuit/17g	82	4.2	490	5.5	60.8	25	3.2
Shortcake, Organic, Waitrose*	1 Biscuit/13g	64	3.2	495	5.8	63	24.4	1.8
Shortcake, Ring, Creations, Fox's*	1 Biscuit/20g	105	5.6	515	7.8	59.1	27.4	1
Shortcake, Rounds, Value, Tesco*	1 Biscuit/22g	120	7	540	5.5	58.8	31.4	2.1
Shortcake, Sainsbury's*	1 Biscuit/11g	53	5.2	479	6.1	65.3	47.2	2.5
Shortcake, Snack, Cadbury*	2 Biscuits/15g	70	3.7	475	7	54.5	25	1.7
Shortcake, Value, Tesco*	1 Biscuit/10g	49	2.1	486	7.1	66.5	21.2	2.1
Shorties, Cadbury*	1 Biscuit/15g	77	3.6	511	6.5	67.3	24	0
Shorties, Fruit, Value, Tesco*	1 Serving/10g	46	1.7	457	5.7	69.3	17.4	3
Shorties, Rich Highland, Tesco*	1 Biscuit/10g	48	2.2	485	6.1	65.3	21.7	2.6
Shorties, Rich, Tesco*	1 Biscuit/10g	48	2.2	484	6.4	65.6	21.8	2
Shorties, Sainsbury's*	1 Biscuit/10g	50	2.2	500	6.4	69.8	21.8	2
Signature Collection, Cadbury*	1 Biscuit/15g	80	4.4	530	6.2	60.1	29.5	0
Snappy, Milk Chocolate Finger, Tesco*	2 Fingers/21g	113	6.1	528	6.5	60.8	28.3	2
Speculaas, Large, Hema*	1 Biscuit/23g	106	4.8	459	5.4	61.2	20.8	2.6
Spiced, German, Christmas, Favorina, Lidl*	1 Biscuit/10g	47	1.9	472	5.8	70.2	18.7	0
Spiced, Whole Wheat, Prodia*	1 Biscuit/5g	17	1	339	7.1	41.4	19.4	8.5
Sports, Fox's*	1 Biscuit/8.5g	41	1.7	483	6.7	67	20	2
Stem Ginger, Brakes*	1 Biscuit/12.5g	62	3.1	495	5.6	62.6	24.7	0
Stornoway, Water, Stag Bakeries Ltd*	1 Biscuit/9g	31	1.2	341	6.5	47.9	13.6	1.7
Strawberry, Biscuit Moments, Special K, Kellogg's*	2 Biscuits/25g	98	2	391	5	74	8	1.5
Strawberry, Cream Tease, McVitie's*	1 Biscuit/19g	97	4.8	510	4.8	65.9	25.2	1.2
Sugar Wafers, Vanilla, Flavoured, Triunfo*	1 Biscuit/10.4g	53	2.5	511	4.1	70.1	24.3	0.6
Sultana & Cinnamon, Weight Watchers*	1 Biscuit/11.5g	51	1.7	441	4.3	72.3	15	3
Tangy Jaffa Viennese, Creations, Fox's*	1 Biscuit/17g	76	3.3	447	5	63.5	19.2	0.9
Tangy Stilton Wafers, Thomas J Fudge*	1 Wafer/3g	18	1.1	529	15.8	42.2	32.4	0
Tasties, Jam & Cream, Sandwich, Mcvitie's*	1 Biscuit/15g	74	3.4	488	4.8	65.6	22.4	2.2
Taxi, McVitie's*	1 Biscuit/27g	134	6.9	504	4.2	63.3	26	0.7
Teddy Bear, Mini, M&S*	1 Biscuit/17g	80	3.8	475	5.4	62.6	22.7	3.2
The Oaty, Wheat Free, Rude Health*	1 Biscuit/12g	55	2.2	437	9	57.2	17.5	7.9
Toffee Apple Crumbles, Border Biscuits Ltd*	1 Biscuit/18g	77	3.7	427	5	56.7	20.4	2.3
Toffee Chip Crinkle Crunch, Fox's*	1 Biscuit/11g	51	2	460	4.6	69.6	18.2	0
Toffee Dodgers, Burton's*	1 Biscuit/18g	84	3.2	468	5.7	71.4	17.5	1.1
Tostada, Opey, Lidl*	1 Biscuit/6g	26	0.6	435	6.9	78.3	10.1	1.7
Treacle Crunch Creams, Fox's*	1 Biscuit/13g	65	3.2	502	4.5	65.3	24.8	1.4
Triple Chocolate, Caramel Shortcakes, Thorntons*	1 Bite/14g	62	3.2	445	4.6	54.8	22.7	0
Triple Chocolate, Fox's*	1 Biscuit/21g	100	5.2	478	5.7	57.3	25.1	2.5
Twix, Caramel Slice, McVitie's*	1 Slice/29g	142	7.8	491	4.5	57.3	26.8	1.4
Viennese Creams, Raspberry, M&S*	1 Biscuit/17g	90	4.9	520	4.6	60.4	28.6	1.3
Viennese Creams, Strawberry, M&S*	1 Biscuit/17g	80	3.7	485	6.4	63	22.2	1.7
Viennese Finger, Belmont Biscuit Co, Aldi*	1 Biscuit/16g	84	4.7	521	4.8	61	29	1.5
Viennese Finger, Mr Kipling*	1 Finger/32g	167	10.2	523	4.3	54.9	31.8	0
Viennese Whirl, Chocolate, Border*	1 Biscuit/19g	96	4.3	512	6.5	61.9	23.2	0
Viennese Whirl, Fox's*	1 Biscuit/25g	130	7	518	6.7	60.1	27.8	0
Viennese, Bronte*	1 Biscuit/25g	106	6.2	424	4.4	45.6	24.8	0
Viennese, Chocolate, Melts, Fox's*	1 Biscuit/12g	64	3.4	526	6.1	60.5	28.3	2.4

	Measure INFO/WEIGHT	KCAL per Measure	FAT	KCAL Nutrition Values per 100g / 100ml	PROT	CARB	FAT	FIBRE

BISCUITS

	Measure INFO/WEIGHT	per Measure KCAL	FAT	KCAL	PROT	CARB	FAT	FIBRE
Viennese, Jaffa, M&S*	1 Biscuit/17g	80	3.7	465	5.9	61.1	21.7	0.9
Viennese, Mini Pack, Paterson's*	1 Biscuit/20g	106	6.2	527	5.4	67.1	30.8	1.6
Viennese, Sandwich, Chocolate, M&S*	1 Biscuit/15g	80	4.6	535	7.2	58	30.6	1.7
Viennese, with Milk Chocolate Filling	*1 Biscuit/15g*	*81*	*4.5*	*533*	*6.5*	*59.6*	*29.4*	*2.1*
Wafer, Vanilla, Loacker*	1 Pack/45g	231	12.6	514	7.5	58	28	0
Water, Asda*	1 Biscuit/6g	25	0.5	412	10	75	8	3.3
Water, Average	*1 Biscuit/5.5g*	*24*	*0.7*	*440*	*10.8*	*75.8*	*12.5*	*3.1*
Water, High Bake, Jacob's*	1 Biscuit/5g	22	0.4	414	10.5	76.4	7.4	3
Water, High Bake, Sainsbury's*	1 Biscuit/5g	21	0.4	412	9.8	76.3	7.5	3.2
Water, High Baked, Tesco*	1 Biscuit/5g	20	0.4	405	10.1	75	7.1	4.2
Water, Table, Carr's*	1 Biscuit/3g	14	0.3	417	10.1	74.7	7.6	4.2
Water, Table, Large, Carr's*	1 Biscuit/8g	31	0.6	408	9.9	73.1	7.5	4.1
Water, Table, Small, Carr's*	1 Biscuit/3g	14	0.3	406	10.1	80	7.6	4.2
White, Chocolate, Coated, Bakery Instore, Lidl*	1 Biscuit/8g	41	2	509	6	64	25	2
Wholemeal Brans, Fox's*	1 Biscuit/20g	90	4	451	8.5	58.8	20.2	7.5
Yoghurt Break, Blueberry, Go Ahead, McVitie's*	1 Slice/18g	72	1.8	401	5.5	72.1	10	2.2
Yoghurt Break, Plain, Go Ahead, McVitie's*	1 Slice/18.3g	72	2.1	394	6.5	66	11.5	3.3
Yoghurt Break, Red Cherry, Go Ahead, McVitie's*	1 Slice/18g	72	1.8	407	5.5	73.4	10.1	2.2
Yoghurt Break, Strawberry, Go Ahead, McVitie's*	1 Slice/18.1g	72	2	397	5.9	68	11.1	2.1
Yoghurt Break, Tropical, Go Ahead, McVitie's*	1 Slice/18g	77	2	430	5.9	76.3	11	2.3
Yorkie, Nestle*	1 Biscuit/25g	128	6.7	510	6.7	60.4	26.8	1.3

BISON

	Measure INFO/WEIGHT	per Measure KCAL	FAT	KCAL	PROT	CARB	FAT	FIBRE
Raw	*1oz/28g*	*31*	*0.5*	*109*	*21.6*	*0*	*1.8*	*0*

BITES

	Measure INFO/WEIGHT	per Measure KCAL	FAT	KCAL	PROT	CARB	FAT	FIBRE
All Butter, Chocolate, M&S*	1 Biscuit/10g	55	3.1	530	7.9	57	30.1	3.5
Banana & Cocoa, Super, Good4U*	1 Pack/40g	153	6.1	383	10.8	46.9	15.2	7.7
Blueberry & Yoghurt Clusters, Mini, M&S*	1 Bite/13g	60	2.7	465	5	64.4	20.7	4.7
Caramel Crispy, Crunchy & Tempting, Mini, Waitrose*	1 Bite/13g	54	1.7	412	4	69.9	12.7	1.2
Caramel Crispy, Extremely Chocolatey, Mini, M&S*	1 Bite/11g	50	2	455	4.7	68.2	17.9	2.8
Caramel Shortcake, Mini, Bakers Selection, Asda*	1 Bite/12g	60	3.1	499	5.6	60	26	1.4
Cheese & Garlic, M&S*	1 Bite/11g	40	3.1	350	8.3	17.2	27.3	5.8
Cheese, Mrs Crimble's*	1 Bag/60g	263	8.4	439	17	61	14	1
Cherry & Almond, with a Citrus Green Tea, Graze*	1 Punnet/30g	102	4.2	339	13	39	14	3.7
Chocolate Caramel, Mini, M&S*	1 Bite/21g	95	5.1	460	5.6	53.5	24.6	1.6
Chocolate Cornflake, Mini, M&S*	1 Bite/11.8g	55	2.4	470	6.2	66.3	20.1	3.6
Chocolate Orange, Mini, M&S*	1 Bite/22g	95	4.8	430	5.5	54.6	21.6	1.8
Ciabatta, Garlic & Herb, Occasions, Sainsbury's*	1 Bite/12g	48	2.6	398	8.9	42.2	21.5	3.2
Cocoa & Orange, with Citrus Green Tea, Graze*	1 Punnet/30g	97	3.9	322	12	37	13	3.8
Egg & Bacon, Mini, Savoury, Tesco*	1 Bite/18g	55	3.8	305	8.8	20.2	21	2.7
Extremely Chocolatey, Mini, M&S*	1 Bite/20g	90	4.9	450	5.7	52.4	24.6	1.6
Flapjack, Mini, M&S*	1 Bite/14g	70	3.5	500	6.4	62.1	25	3.6
Honeycomb Clusters, Rich & Chocolatey, Mini, Waitrose*	1 Bite/11g	50	2	456	4.8	66.2	18.5	2.9
Milk Chocolate, Mini, Luxury, Holly Lane*	1 Mini Bite/15g	72	3.9	479	5.1	55.5	26.3	2.5
Protein, Honey & Seed, Oat Squares, Graze*	1 Square/30g	140	8.1	465	15	42	27	4.4
Raspberry, Mini, COU, M&S*	1 Pack/25g	85	0.7	340	3.8	74.9	2.7	4.5
Rocky Road, Mini, M&S*	1 Bite/12.2g	50	1.6	410	5.2	66.9	13.3	2.5
Salted Caramel Popcorn, Mini, Extremely Indulgent, M&S*	1 Bite/9g	42	1.7	481	5.1	69.9	19.8	1.6

BITTER LEMON

	Measure INFO/WEIGHT	per Measure KCAL	FAT	KCAL	PROT	CARB	FAT	FIBRE
Fever-Tree*	1 Glass/200ml	77	0	38	0	9.2	0	0
Low Calorie, Tesco*	1 Glass/200ml	6	0.2	3	0.1	0.3	0.1	0.1
Sainsbury's*	1 Glass/250ml	45	0.2	18	0.1	4.4	0.1	0.1
Schweppes*	1 Glass/250ml	85	0	34	0	8.2	0	0

	Measure INFO/WEIGHT	per Measure KCAL	 FAT	Nutrition Values per 100g / 100ml KCAL	 PROT	 CARB	 FAT	 FIBRE
BLACK GRAM								
Urad Gram, Dried, Raw	*1oz/28g*	*77*	*0.4*	*275*	*24.9*	*40.8*	*1.4*	*0*
BLACK PUDDING								
Average, Uncooked	*1 Serving/40g*	*101*	*6*	*252*	*10.2*	*19*	*14.9*	*0.6*
BLACKBERRIES								
Fresh, Raw, Average	*1oz/28g*	*7*	*0.1*	*25*	*0.9*	*5.1*	*0.2*	*5.3*
Frozen, Average	*1 Serving/80g*	*37*	*0.1*	*46*	*0.9*	*9.6*	*0.2*	*5.3*
in Fruit Juice, Average	*½ Can/145g*	*52*	*0.3*	*36*	*0.6*	*7.9*	*0.2*	*1.3*
in Light Syrup, Canned, Tesco*	½ Can/145g	70	0.1	48	0.5	10.6	0.1	1.5
BLACKCURRANTS								
Dried, Graze*	1 Pack/30g	95	0.3	317	3.3	79	1	0
Fresh, Raw, Average	*1 Serving/80g*	*22*	*0*	*27*	*0.9*	*6.5*	*0*	*3.5*
in Fruit Juice, Average	*1 Serving/30g*	*11*	*0*	*38*	*0.6*	*8.6*	*0.2*	*2.4*
in Light Syrup, British, Canned, Tesco*	½ Can/145g	71	0.1	49	0.5	10.4	0.1	2.1
Stewed with Sugar	*1oz/28g*	*16*	*0*	*58*	*0.7*	*15*	*0*	*2.8*
Stewed without Sugar	*1oz/28g*	*7*	*0*	*24*	*0.8*	*5.6*	*0*	*3.1*
BLANCMANGE								
Chocolate Flavour, Made Up, Pearce Duff*	1 Serving/140g	137	5.6	98	3.3	12.3	4	0
Raspberry Flavour, Pearce Duff*	1 Serving/138g	123	2.5	89	3.1	15	1.8	0
Strawberry Flavour, Pearce Duff*	1 Serving/138g	123	2.5	89	3.1	15	1.8	0
Vanilla Flavour, Pearce Duff*	1 Serving/138g	123	2.5	89	3.1	15	1.8	0
BLUEBERRIES								
Chocolate Covered, Waitrose*	1 Serving/25g	120	5.6	481	4	65.6	22.4	3
Dried, Love Life, Waitrose*	1 Serving/30g	107	0.2	358	1.1	80.1	0.8	3.6
Dried, Wholefoods, Tesco*	1 Serving/20g	66	0.2	329	2	77.9	1	3.2
Frozen, Average	*1 Serving/80g*	*41*	*0.2*	*51*	*0.6*	*13.8*	*0.2*	*4.4*
Raw, Average	*50 Berries/68g*	*39*	*0.2*	*57*	*0.7*	*14.5*	*0.3*	*2.4*
BOAR								
Wild, Raw, Average	*1 Serving/200g*	*244*	*6.7*	*122*	*21.5*	*0*	*3.3*	*0*
BOILED SWEETS								
Average	*1 Sweet/6.5g*	*21*	*0*	*327*	*0*	*87.1*	*0*	*0*
Blackcurrant & Liquorice, Co-Op*	1 Sweet/8g	32	0.4	405	0.9	91	5	0
Cherry Drops, Bassett's*	1 Sweet/5g	18	0	390	0	98.1	0	0
Clear Fruits, Sainsbury's*	1 Sweet/7g	26	0	372	0.1	92.9	0	0
Fruit Drops, Co-Op*	1 Sweet/6g	24	0	395	0.2	98	0	0
Fruit Sherbets, Assorted, M&S*	1 Sweet/9g	35	0.4	405	0.3	91.6	4.3	0.1
Lockets, Mars*	1 Pack/43g	165	0	383	0	95.8	0	0
Mentho-Lyptus, Cherry, Sugar Free, Hall's*	1 Lozenge/3.6g	8	0	234	0	62.4	0	0
Mentho-Lyptus, Extra Strong, Hall's*	1 Lozenge/4g	14	0	389	0	96.9	0	0
Pear Drops, Bassett's*	1 Sweet/4g	16	0	390	0	96.4	0	0
Pear Drops, Sugar Free, Sula*	1 Sweet/3g	7	0	235	0.1	97	0.1	0
Soothers, Blackcurrant, Hall's*	1 Lozenge/4.5g	16	0	365	0	91.4	0	0
Soothers, Cherry, Hall's*	1 Pack/45.2g	165	0	365	0	91.3	0	0
Soothers, Strawberry Flavour, Hall's*	1 Sweet/5g	19	0	385	0	96	0	0
BOK CHOY								
Tesco*	1 Serving/100g	11	0.2	11	1	1.4	0.2	1.2
BOLOGNESE								
Al Forno, Weight Watchers*	1 Pack/354g	312	6.7	88	6.6	10.3	1.9	1.8
Beanfeast, Dry, Batchelors*	1 Pack/120g	362	6.7	302	23.9	39	5.6	13.5
Beef, Asda*	1 Pack/392g	412	19.6	105	8	7	5	0
Courgetti, BGTY, Sainsbury's*	1 Pack/380g	224	6.8	59	5.9	4.1	1.8	1.4
Fusilli, Pasta Vita, Dolmio*	1 Serving/300g	333	5.1	111	5.3	17.9	1.7	0
Meatless, Granose*	1 Pack/400g	400	16	100	8	8	4	0
Pappardelle, Cooked, Stir Your Senses, Birds Eye*	1 Serving/350g	610	23	174	6.9	20.9	6.6	2.4

	Measure INFO/WEIGHT	per Measure KCAL	FAT	Nutrition Values per 100g / 100ml KCAL	PROT	CARB	FAT	FIBRE
BOLOGNESE								
Pasta Pot, Prepared, NutriPot*	1 Pot/314g	300	3	96	6.6	14	1	2.1
Pasta, Diet Chef Ltd*	1 Pack/300g	255	10.2	85	7.9	5.8	3.4	4.4
Pasta, Diet Chef Ltd*	1 Serving/300g	288	10.2	96	7.9	5.8	3.4	4.4
Pasta, Goodness, Tesco*	1 Pack/280g	324	8.4	116	7.1	15.1	3	1.8
Pasta, Medaglioni, Rich Red Wine, Waitrose*	½ Pack/125g	266	7	213	12.5	28.1	5.6	2.6
Pasta, Mugfull, As Consumed, Batchelors*	1 Portion/245g	197	1.2	80	2.7	15.9	0.5	0.8
Penne, Heinz*	1 Pack/300g	213	2.7	71	3.8	11.8	0.9	0.6
Ragu, Slimfree, Aldi*	1 Pack/450g	234	4.5	52	5.8	4.1	1	1.5
Spaghetti, Al Forno, Sainsbury's*	1 Pack/400g	460	19.6	115	7.8	10	4.9	1.1
Spaghetti, As Consumed, Savers, Morrisons*	1 Pack/300g	338	10.4	120	4.5	16.3	3.7	1.6
Spaghetti, BGTY, Sainsbury's*	1 Pack/400g	416	9.2	104	6.3	14.4	2.3	1.1
Spaghetti, Canned, Asda*	½ Can/205g	174	5.7	85	4.2	10.7	2.8	0.6
Spaghetti, CBY, Asda*	1 Pack/100g	108	2	108	6	15.6	2	2
Spaghetti, Co-Op*	1 Pack/300g	285	12	95	4	11	4	1
Spaghetti, Cook*	1 Portion/430g	636	24.9	148	7.6	16.2	5.8	1
Spaghetti, Egg Pasta in Rich Beef Sauce, Waitrose*	1 Pack/400g	404	10.4	101	7.6	11.7	2.6	1
Spaghetti, Frozen, Tesco*	1 Pack/450g	472	9	105	5.8	15	2	1.8
Spaghetti, GFY, Asda*	1 Pack/400g	352	6.4	88	4.9	13.4	1.6	2.2
Spaghetti, Healthy Choice, Iceland*	1 Pack/400g	428	4	107	6.8	17.8	1	1.1
Spaghetti, Hidden Veg, Heinz*	1 Can/400g	312	6.4	78	3.4	12.6	1.6	0.9
Spaghetti, HL, Tesco*	1 Pack/360g	360	7.6	100	7.5	12	2.1	1.2
Spaghetti, Italian Inspirations, Co-Op*	1 Pack/400g	500	18.4	125	7.5	13	4.6	1.2
Spaghetti, Italian, Chilled, Tesco*	1 Pack/400g	520	17.2	130	6.5	15.9	4.3	1.5
Spaghetti, Italian, Microwaved, Morrisons*	1 Pack/400g	398	9.1	101	6.5	12.7	2.3	1.6
Spaghetti, Italiano, Pro-Cuisine, Pro Cuisine*	1 Pack/600g	522	11.4	87	5.7	11.7	1.9	0
Spaghetti, Lean Cuisine, Findus*	1 Pack/320g	275	7.4	86	4.5	11.5	2.3	1.1
Spaghetti, M&S*	1 Pack/400g	380	8.4	95	7.5	11.7	2.1	1.7
Spaghetti, Noodle Box, Slim Fast*	1 Box/250g	76	1.8	30	2	2.8	0.7	2.7
Spaghetti, PB, Waitrose*	1 Pack/400g	380	6.8	95	6.7	13.4	1.7	1.1
Spaghetti, Quick Pasta, Dry, Sainsbury's*	1 Serving/63g	231	2.8	367	10.8	71	4.4	3.3
Spaghetti, Ready to Cook, Musclefood*	1 Pack/390g	433	14	111	8.1	10.1	3.6	3.2
Spaghetti, Sainsbury's*	1 Pack/400g	525	18.8	131	6.1	16	4.7	2.2
Spaghetti, Weight Watchers*	1 Meal/320g	353	6.7	110	6.6	15.7	2.1	1
Tagliatelle, Weight Watchers*	1 Serving/300g	300	5.4	100	5.5	15.4	1.8	0.1
Tortellini, Beef, Rich, Italian, Giovanni Rana*	½ Pack/125g	222	9	178	7.6	20.6	7.2	4.1
Turkey, Microwaved, Slimzone, Asda*	1 Pack/419g	381	3.8	91	7.2	12	0.9	2.4
Vegetarian, M&S*	1 Pack/360g	360	12.6	100	4.5	12.5	3.5	2.1
Vegetarian, Pasta, Lunch Pot, Quorn*	1 Pot/300g	285	6	95	5.2	13	2	2
Vegetarian, Spaghetti, Meat Free, Heinz*	1 Serving/200g	162	3.4	81	3.3	13.1	1.7	0.6
Vegetarian, Spaghetti, Quorn*	1 Pack/300g	255	1.8	85	4.4	14.8	0.6	1.5
Vegetarian, Spaghetti, Sainsbury's*	1 Pack/450g	346	5	77	4.9	11.9	1.1	1.8
Vegetarian, Spaghetti, Tesco*	1 Pack/340g	374	13.3	110	5.1	13.7	3.9	1.2
Vegetarian, Vegelicious, Tesco*	1 Pack/400g	420	10.8	105	4.6	14.9	2.7	2
BOMBAY MIX								
Average	*1oz/28g*	*141*	*9.2*	*503*	*18.8*	*35.1*	*32.9*	*6.2*
BON BONS								
Apple, Lemon & Strawberry, Co-Op*	¼ Bag/50g	202	2.5	405	1	88	5	0
Bassett's*	1 Sweet/7g	28	0.5	417	1.1	85.4	7.5	0
Fruit, Bassett's*	1 Serving/7g	25	0	380	0.1	94.2	0	0
Lemon, Bassett's*	1 Sweet/7g	30	0.7	425	0	83.7	9.8	0
Mixed Fruit Flavour, Vimto, Tangerine Confectionery Ltd*	1 Sweet/5g	20	0.3	409	0.1	85.8	6.7	0.6
BOOST								
Standard Bar, Cadbury*	1 Bar/49g	250	13.8	515	5.8	58.6	28.5	1.5

B

INFO/WEIGHT	Measure	per Measure		Nutrition Values per 100g / 100ml				
		KCAL	FAT	KCAL	PROT	CARB	FAT	FIBRE
BOOST								
Treat Size, Cadbury*	1 Bar/24g	130	7.4	535	5.3	59.6	30.5	0
with Glucose & Guarana, Cadbury*	1 Bar/61g	314	18	515	5.5	56.7	29.5	0
with Glucose, Cadbury*	1 Bar/61g	315	17.8	521	5.6	58	29.4	4
BOUILLABAISSE								
Average	*1 Serving/400g*	*556*	*38.8*	*139*	*11.2*	*2*	*9.7*	*0.4*
BOUILLON								
Powder, Miso, Marigold*	1 Tsp/5g	12	0.5	248	7	34	9.3	1.4
Powder, Swiss Vegetable, Green Tub, Marigold*	1 Tsp/5g	12	0.4	243	10.5	29.4	8.1	0.7
Vegetable, Benedicta*	1fl oz/30ml	30	0.1	101	7.5	17	0.3	0
BOUNTY								
Dark, Mars*	1 Funsize/29g	141	7.9	493	3.6	55.8	27.5	0
Milk, Mars*	1 Funsize/29g	139	7.3	487	3.7	58.9	25.7	0
BOUQUET GARNI								
Handtied, Fresh, Asda*	1 Bunch/2.4g	11	0.2	455	8.3	69.4	7.9	31.6
BOURNVITA*								
Powder, Made Up with Semi-Skimmed Milk	*1 Mug/227ml*	*132*	*3.6*	*58*	*3.5*	*7.8*	*1.6*	*0*
Powder, Made Up with Whole Milk	*1 Mug/227ml*	*173*	*8.6*	*76*	*3.4*	*7.6*	*3.8*	*0*
BOVRIL*								
Beef Extract, Drink, Made Up with Water, Bovril*	1 Serving/12g	22	0.1	184	38.9	4.6	1.2	0
Chicken Savoury Drink, Bovril*	1 Serving/13g	16	0.2	129	9.7	19.4	1.4	2.1
BRANDY								
37.5% Volume, Average	*1 Pub Shot/35ml*	*72*	*0*	*207*	*0*	*0*	*0*	*0*
40% Volume, Average	*1 Pub Shot/35ml*	*78*	*0*	*224*	*0*	*0*	*0*	*0*
Cherry, Average	*1 Pub Shot/35ml*	*89*	*0*	*255*	*0*	*32.6*	*0*	*0*
BRAWN								
Average	*1 Serving/100g*	*153*	*11.5*	*153*	*12.4*	*0*	*11.5*	*0*
BRAZIL NUTS								
Average	*6 Whole/20g*	*136*	*13.7*	*682*	*15.3*	*2.8*	*68.4*	*5.4*
Milk Chocolate, Tesco*	1 Nut/8g	47	3.5	585	9.9	38	43.7	1.9
BREAD								
50/50, Wholemeal & White, Med Sliced, Kingsmill*	1 Slice/40g	94	0.9	235	9.9	41.2	2.3	4.9
Ancient Grain, Pave, Bakery, Tesco*	1 Serving/94g	237	2.3	252	9.9	46.3	2.4	2.8
Apple Sourdough, Gail's*	1 Slice/50g	118	0.4	236	7.5	43.9	0.7	4.3
Apricot & Sesame Seed, Lifefibre*	1 Slice/43g	148	4.4	344	8.1	55	10.3	6.2
Arabic, El Amar Bakery*	1 Serving/110g	318	1.3	289	11.6	57.9	1.2	0
Bagel, 4 Everything, Finest, Tesco*	1 Bagel/100g	268	1.8	268	11.1	51.9	1.8	2.5
Bagel, Baked with Marmite, Marmite*	1 Bagel/85g	240	2.6	282	12.9	49.3	3.1	2.8
Bagel, Caramelised Onion & Poppyseed, Waitrose*	1 Bagel/86g	222	2.2	258	9.7	49.2	2.5	2.4
Bagel, Caramelised Onion & Poppy Seed, Tesco*	1 Bagel/85g	221	2.1	260	10.9	47.6	2.5	3.8
Bagel, Cinnamon & Raisin, Morrisons*	1 Bagel/85g	215	1.7	253	7.7	51.1	2	4.5
Bagel, Cinnamon & Raisin, New York Bagel Co*	1 Bagel/90g	231	1	257	10.1	49.9	1.1	3.6
Bagel, Cinnamon & Raisin, Tesco*	1 Bagel/85g	230	1.4	270	10.4	51.3	1.7	3.8
Bagel, Cranberry & Orange, New York Bakery Co*	1 Bagel/90g	246	2.3	273	9.6	51	2.5	3.9
Bagel, Fruit & Spice, Sainsbury's*	1 Bagel/85g	234	1.8	275	9.7	54.3	2.1	3.8
Bagel, Fruit & Fibre, Kingsmill*	1 Bagel/85g	225	1.2	265	9.8	50.8	1.4	5.2
Bagel, Granary, Bagel Factory*	1 Bagel/100g	288	2.1	288	11.9	57.4	2.1	4.5
Bagel, Mini, Sainsbury's*	1 Bagel/25g	67	0.4	268	11.2	52.4	1.6	2.8
Bagel, Multi Seed, BFree*	1 Bagel/80g	186	2	232	4.1	51.4	2.5	6.5
Bagel, Multi Seed, New York Bagel Co*	1 Bagel/90g	244	4.3	271	12.4	41.6	4.8	5.8
Bagel, Multigrain, Sainsbury's*	1 Bagel/113g	293	3.5	259	10	49.6	3.1	2
Bagel, Onion & Poppy Seed, Average	*1 Bagel/85g*	*225*	*2.8*	*264*	*9*	*50.5*	*3.3*	*3.2*
Bagel, Onion, New York Bagel Co*	1 Bagel/85g	222	1.6	261	10.6	50.4	1.9	3.1
Bagel, Onion, Tesco*	1 Bagel/85g	233	2	274	10.5	52.4	2.4	1.9

BREAD

	Measure INFO/WEIGHT	per Measure KCAL	FAT	Nutrition Values per 100g / 100ml KCAL	PROT	CARB	FAT	FIBRE
Bagel, Original, Organic, New York Bagel Co*	1 Bagel/85g	220	1.2	259	9.3	52.2	1.4	4.1
Bagel, Plain	**1 Bagel/104g**	**290**	**2**	**279**	**10.6**	**53.8**	**1.9**	**2.9**
Bagel, Plain, Asda*	1 Bagel/85g	226	2	265	15	46	2.3	2.9
Bagel, Plain, Average	**1 Bagel/78g**	**202**	**1.5**	**259**	**10.1**	**50.4**	**1.9**	**3.1**
Bagel, Plain, Bagel Factory*	1 Bagel/150g	318	1.3	212	9.4	41.6	0.9	2.1
Bagel, Plain, Free From, Tesco*	1 Bagel/80g	215	5.5	270	3.4	47.7	6.9	4.7
Bagel, Plain, GFY, Asda*	1 Bagel/84g	218	1.8	259	10	50	2.1	1.8
Bagel, Plain, New York Bagel Co*	1 Bagel/90g	230	1.7	255	9.1	50.4	1.9	2.9
Bagel, Plain, Organic, Tesco*	1 Bagel/85g	216	2.3	254	9	48.4	2.7	3.6
Bagel, Plain, So Organic, Sainsbury's*	1 Bagel/85g	216	2.3	254	9	48.4	2.7	3.6
Bagel, Plain, Tesco*	1 Bagel/85g	220	1.8	259	9.8	50.2	2.1	1.8
Bagel, Red Onion & Chive, New York Bakery Co.*	1 Bagel/90g	225	1.2	250	10.4	47.2	1.3	3.8
Bagel, Rye, Bagel Factory*	1 Bagel/85g	279	1.3	329	14.5	64.3	1.6	6.2
Bagel, Sesame Seed, Essential, Waitrose*	1 Bagel/85g	243	2.7	286	9.6	54.6	3.2	3.6
Bagel, Sesame Seed, GFY, Asda*	1 Bagel/84g	227	2.1	271	11	51	2.5	2.6
Bagel, Sesame, M&S*	1 Bagel/87g	240	2.8	275	10.2	51.2	3.2	2.1
Bagel, Sesame, New York Bagel Co*	1 Bagel/85g	226	2.6	266	10.3	49.2	3.1	4
Bagel, Sesame, New York Bakery*	1 Bagel/91g	241	2.6	265	10.5	47.3	2.9	4.4
Bagel, Thins, Plain, New York Bakery Co*	1 Thin/48g	133	0.6	277	9.4	55.8	1.2	2.7
Bagel, Thins, Seeded, Sliced, New York Bakery Co*	1 Thin/45g	129	1.5	286	10	52.1	3.4	3.9
Bagel, Thins, Sesame, Warburton's*	1 Thin/50g	130	1.7	260	10.1	46.8	3.4	3.6
Bagel, Wee Soda, Genesis Crafty*	1 Bagel/65g	148	2.5	227	6.9	41.3	3.9	2.9
Bagel, White, Asda*	1 Bagel/86g	227	2.7	264	10	49	3.1	0
Bagel, White, Original, Weight Watchers*	1 Bagel/67g	158	0.5	236	9.5	42.4	0.8	10.7
Bagel, Wholemeal, & White, Mini, New York Bakery Co*	1 Bagel/45g	114	1	254	10.8	45.2	2.2	5.1
Bagel, Wholemeal, Average	**1 Bagel/90g**	**235**	**2.7**	**261**	**12.7**	**44.6**	**3**	**7.7**
Bagel, Wholemeal, Multiseed, M&S*	1 Bagel/84g	215	5.6	255	13.1	35.4	6.6	8.3
Bagel, Wholemeal, New York Bagel Co*	1 Bagel/90g	223	2.1	248	11.4	41.5	2.3	7.5
Baguette, Bake At Home, Tesco*	1 Baguette/75g	216	0.9	289	8.6	59.1	1.2	3.5
Baguette, Budgens*	1 Baguette/125g	335	1.5	268	8.5	55.7	1.2	2.3
Baguette, Crusty Brown, M&S*	½ Loaf/71g	160	1.1	225	9.8	42.7	1.6	6.3
Baguette, French, Tesco*	1 Serving/60g	144	0.7	240	7.8	49.5	1.2	3.4
Baguette, Garlic, Slices, Frozen, CBY, Asda*	1 Slice/26g	92	4.7	355	8.2	38.3	18.1	2.8
Baguette, Granary, Co-Op*	1 Serving/60g	150	1.5	250	20	46	2.5	6
Baguette, Harvester, French Style, Somerfield*	1 Serving/110g	276	2.1	251	10.6	47.9	1.9	3.7
Baguette, Homebake, Half, Tesco*	1 Serving/75g	217	0.9	289	8.6	49.1	1.2	3.5
Baguette, Multiseed, Mini, GF, Fria*	1 Baguette/70g	203	6	290	3.5	47	8.5	6
Baguette, Part Baked, Classique, Deli France, Delifrance*	1 Pack/250g	745	3	298	9.8	54.8	1.2	2.7
Baguette, Part Baked, Half, Tesco*	½ Baguette/75g	180	0.9	240	7.8	49.5	1.2	3.4
Baguette, Paysanne, Stonebaked, Asda*	1/6 Loaf/46g	119	1.4	259	10	48	3	3.3
Baguette, Ready to Bake, Sainsbury's*	½ Baguette/62g	150	0.8	242	7.8	49.7	1.3	2.8
Baguette, Sourdough, la Brea Bakery*	1 Serving/60g	160	0.4	266	8.8	56.1	0.7	1.8
Baguette, White, Half, Crusty, M&S*	1 Baguette/162g	420	1.8	260	8.4	53.5	1.1	2.3
Baguette, White, Homebake, Tesco*	1 Baguette/150g	434	1.8	289	8.6	59.1	1.2	3.5
Baguette, White, Ready to Bake, Asda*	1 Serving/60g	168	1.1	280	10	56	1.8	2.6
Baguette, White, Sainsbury's*	1 Serving/50g	132	0.8	263	9.3	53.1	1.5	2.7
Baguette, White, Sandwich, Somerfield*	1 Serving/60g	155	0.8	259	9.4	52.1	1.4	1.7
Baguette, Wholemeal, Part Baked, Asda*	½ Baguette/75g	176	1	235	8.2	47.7	1.3	3
Baguette, Wholemeal, Part Baked, Mini, Landgut*	½ Baguette/25g	56	0.2	223	7.5	46	1	0
Banana, with Dates & Hazelnuts, Graze*	1 Slice/19g	59	2.7	309	4.8	38.7	14.4	2.7
Bap, Brown, Large, G H Sheldon*	1 Bap/64g	169	4.3	264	5.3	47.5	6.7	4
Baps, Brown, Large, Asda*	1 Bap/58g	140	0.9	242	10	47	1.6	0
Baps, Brown, Malted Grain, Large, Tesco*	1 Bap/93g	228	3.1	245	9.9	42.7	3.3	5.3

BREAD

INFO/WEIGHT	Measure	per Measure		Nutrition Values per 100g / 100ml				
		KCAL	FAT	KCAL	PROT	CARB	FAT	FIBRE
Baps, Cheese Top, Sainsbury's*	1 Bap/75g	218	6.4	291	12.1	41.6	8.5	2
Baps, Cheese Topped, Baker's Soft, Tesco*	1 Bap/65g	180	3.7	275	10.2	45.8	5.6	2.2
Baps, Cheese Topped, Country Choice*	1 Bap/64g	194	5.6	303	12	43	8.8	2.5
Baps, Cheese Topped, G H Sheldon*	1 Roll/70g	197	5.8	282	12.4	38.6	8.3	1.4
Baps, Cheese Topped, White, Tesco*	1 Bap/65g	179	3.6	275	10.2	45.8	5.6	0.7
Baps, Floured, M&S*	1 Bap/60g	168	3.7	280	11.5	46.8	6.2	2
Baps, Giant Malted, Sainsbury's*	1 Bap/109g	282	5.2	260	8.6	45.7	4.8	5.7
Baps, Malted, Large, Co-Op*	1 Bap/85g	208	2.6	245	10.2	44.3	3.1	5
Baps, Multigrain, Tesco*	1 Bap/98g	238	3.1	244	8.7	45.1	3.2	1.9
Baps, White Sandwich, Kingsmill*	1 Bap/80g	209	3.2	261	10.1	46.2	4	2.2
Baps, White Soft, Giant, Somerfield*	1 Bap/105g	262	4	249	9.1	44.7	3.8	2.3
Baps, White, Average	**1 Bap/65g**	**167**	**2.3**	**257**	**9.5**	**47**	**3.5**	**1.9**
Baps, White, Floured, Waitrose*	1 Bap/60g	147	1.2	244	8	48.6	2	1.1
Baps, White, Giant, Sainsbury's*	1 Bap/86g	235	3.2	273	8.3	51.7	3.7	3.4
Baps, White, Giant, Waitrose*	1 Bap/104g	260	3.7	250	9.5	45	3.6	4.8
Baps, White, Large, Tesco*	1 Bap/95g	252	4.3	265	8.7	46.2	4.5	2.4
Baps, White, Sliced, Large, Asda*	1 Bap/58g	148	1	255	10	50	1.7	0
Baps, White, Soft, Floured, M&S*	1 Bap/61g	175	3.4	285	11.5	46.6	5.5	2.8
Baps, White, Super Soft, The Bakery, M&S*	1 Roll/60g	161	2.8	268	8.4	46.6	4.7	3
Baps, White, Warburton's*	1 Bap/57g	144	2.5	252	9.8	43.4	4.3	2.7
Baps, Wholemeal, Brace's*	1 Bap/58.5g	137	2.6	234	10.5	42.5	4.4	4.3
Baps, Wholemeal, Country Oven*	1 Bap/40g	92	1.3	231	9.5	41	3.3	4.1
Baps, Wholemeal, Giant, Rathbones*	1 Bap/110g	230	2.1	209	9.4	39	1.9	8
Baps, Wholemeal, Giant, Sainsbury's*	1 Bap/86g	230	3.5	268	9.7	48.1	4.1	7.7
Baps, Wholemeal, Tesco*	1 Bap/46g	104	2.4	227	9.6	41.4	5.3	5.6
Baps, Wholemeal, Waitrose*	1 Bap/63g	148	3.3	235	11	35.9	5.3	7.7
Best of Both, Farmhouse, Hovis*	1 Slice/44g	99	1.4	226	9.5	40	3.1	4.9
Best of Both, Med Sliced, Eat Well, M&S*	1 Slice/36g	83	0.8	229	9.4	41.2	2.2	3.5
Best of Both, Medium, Hovis*	1 Slice/38g	87	0.8	233	5.2	40.4	2.2	5.2
Best of Both, Thick Sliced, Hovis*	1 Slice/50g	113	0.9	224	9	40.4	1.8	5
Black Olive, Finest, Tesco*	1 Serving/72g	184	4.6	255	9.7	39.7	6.4	2.9
Bloomer, Brown, Slices, GF, Made Without Wheat, M&S*	1 Slice/53g	131	2.9	247	4.3	41.4	5.4	7.8
Bloomer, COU, M&S*	1 Slice/33g	78	0.5	235	9.5	45.5	1.5	3.6
Bloomer, Multi Seed, Organic, Sainsbury's*	1 Serving/60g	160	4.1	266	10.9	40.3	6.8	8.8
Bloomer, Multi Seed, Sliced, M&S*	1 Slice/54g	150	3.9	280	10.5	43.6	7.2	3.1
Bloomer, Multiseed, Average	**1 Slice/50g**	**120**	**2.4**	**240**	**11.8**	**37.2**	**4.9**	**7.7**
Bloomer, Multiseed, Finest, Tesco*	1 Slice/50g	145	3.8	290	9.8	40.2	7.6	7.4
Bloomer, Multiseed, TTD, Sainsbury's*	1 Slice/50g	119	1.8	239	12	39.7	3.6	8.8
Bloomer, Soft Grain, M&S*	1 Slice/34g	80	0.5	235	9.5	45.5	1.5	3.6
Bloomer, White, Crusty, Bakery, Tesco*	1 Serving/100g	244	1.7	244	8.3	47.2	1.7	3.3
Bloomer, White, Sliced, Waitrose*	1 Slice/50g	130	0.9	259	8.5	52.1	1.8	2.6
Bloomer, Wholemeal, Organic, M&S*	1 Slice/50g	110	2.1	220	10.2	35.5	4.2	6.4
Both in One, Village Bakery, Aldi*	1 Slice/40g	95	1	237	8.5	43	2.5	4.3
Breadcakes, Big Brown, Morrisons*	1 Cake/63g	154	2.1	245	9	44.6	3.4	4.3
Brioche, Apple, & Custard, Mini, Maitre Jean Pierre, Lidl*	1 Brioche/50g	148	4.3	296	6.8	48	8.6	4
Brioche, Burger Buns, Luxury, Specially Selected, Aldi*	1 Bun/50g	159	3.7	317	9.5	52	7.3	3.1
Brioche, Burger Buns, Signature, Morrisons*	1 Bun/55g	156	2.3	284	9.4	51	4.2	2.2
Brioche, Chocolate & Custard, Rolls, Mini, Lidl*	1 Roll/50g	152	4.5	305	7	48	9	2
Brioche, French Marble, with Vanilla, Bon Appetit, Aldi*	1 Serving/50g	132	3.4	264	6.6	42.6	6.7	1.8
Brioche, Loaf, Butter, Sainsbury's*	1/8 Loaf/50g	174	5.2	347	8	55	10.5	2.2
Brioche, Loaf, Hand Plaited, Aldi*	1 Slice/50g	178	5.5	355	8.1	50	11	1.7
Brioche, Loaf, Sliced, Tesco*	2 Slices/42g	151	5	360	7.3	54.8	11.9	2
Brioche, Rolls, Chocolate Chip, Tesco*	1 Serving/35g	131	5.6	374	8.6	49.1	16	6

BREAD

Measure INFO/WEIGHT	per Measure KCAL	FAT	Nutrition Values per 100g / 100ml KCAL	PROT	CARB	FAT	FIBRE
Brown, Ciabatta, Rolls, GF, Dietary Specials* — 1 Roll/50g	137	4	274	5.8	36.9	8.1	8.9
Brown, Danish, Weight Watchers, Warburton's* — 1 Slice/20g	48	0.4	233	10.3	40.7	1.8	6.2
Brown, Deli Sub, Roll, Asda* — 1 Roll/60g	142	1.9	236	0	35	3.2	0
Brown, Farmhouse, GF, Newburn, Warburton's* — 1 Slice/35g	82	1.9	234	7.8	35.8	5.4	5.7
Brown, Farmhouse, Linwoods* — 1 Slice/25g	56	0.4	225	7.3	44.4	1.7	5.8
Brown, GF, Genius * — 1 Slice/35g	97	4.7	277	6.7	42.2	13.3	9.5
Brown, Gluten & Wheat Free, Sliced — 1 Slice/25g	56	1.3	224	3.4	41	5.2	9.4
Brown, Granary Malted, thick Sliced, Waitrose* — 1 Slice/40g	95	0.9	238	9.4	44.8	2.3	5.1
Brown, High Fibre, Ormo* — 1 Slice/24g	57	0.6	239	9.2	42.9	2.6	7.5
Brown, Irwin's Bakery* — 1 Slice/64g	137	0.4	214	10.4	41.8	0.6	6.1
Brown, Kingsmill Gold, Seeds & Oats, Kingsmill* — 1 Slice/45g	126	4.4	280	12.2	35.6	9.8	4.9
Brown, Malted, Average — **1 Thin Slice/25g**	**60**	**0.6**	**242**	**9.4**	**45.5**	**2.4**	**4.2**
Brown, Malted, Farmhouse Gold, Morrisons* — 1 Slice/38g	94	0.5	248	8.2	49.6	1.4	3
Brown, Med Slice, Smart Price, Asda* — 1 Slice/36.7g	77	0.6	210	8	41	1.6	6
Brown, Med Sliced — **1 Slice/34g**	**74**	**0.7**	**218**	**8.5**	**44.3**	**2**	**3.5**
Brown, Med Sliced, Asda* — 1 Slice/36g	78	0.6	216	8	42	1.8	4.1
Brown, Med Sliced, Bettabuy, Morrisons* — 1 Slice/31g	66	0.4	212	8.6	42	1.3	3.6
Brown, Med Sliced, Sainsbury's* — 1 Slice/36g	81	0.7	225	8.2	43.8	1.9	3.9
Brown, Med Sliced, Tesco* — 1 Slice/36g	78	0.8	218	8	41.6	2.2	4.5
Brown, Mixed Grain, Original, Vogel* — 1 Slice/45g	102	0.6	227	9.8	47.1	1.2	6.4
Brown, Multi Grain, Wheat Free, GF — 1 Slice/33g	76	1.7	229	5.1	40.8	5.1	5.6
Brown, Premium, Med Sliced, Warburton's* — 1 Slice/24g	61	0.9	258	10.6	43.2	3.7	4.3
Brown, Sainsbury's* — 1 Slice/34g	81	0.7	239	8.4	46.8	2.1	4.2
Brown, Sandwich Bread, GF, Udi's* — 1 Slice/37g	79	1.1	216	5.2	39.2	2.9	6.3
Brown, Seeded, Bloomer, Sliced, BFree* — 1 Slice/30g	68	1.7	228	5.1	33.3	5.7	11.7
Brown, Sliced, By Brennans, Weight Watchers* — 1 Slice/20g	51	0.4	257	9.5	45.4	2.1	6.8
Brown, Sliced, Free From, Tesco* — 1 Slice/42g	81	1.7	194	5.6	29.5	4	8.8
Brown, Soda, M&S* — 1 Slice/40g	92	1.4	229	9.2	43.6	3.6	4.9
Brown, Soft, Farmhouse , Warburton's* — 1 Slice/42g	104	1.1	246	9.9	42.8	2.7	5.3
Brown, Sunflower & Barley, Vogel* — 1 Slice/42g	100	1.9	239	9.4	40.3	4.5	6.7
Brown, Thick Slice, Tesco* — 1 Serving/50g	110	1.2	219	10.3	38.9	2.5	5.3
Brown, Thin Sliced, Sainsbury's* — 1 Slice/29g	65	0.5	225	8.2	43.8	1.9	3.9
Brown, Toasted, Average — **1 Med Slice/24g**	**65**	**0.5**	**272**	**10.4**	**56.5**	**2.1**	**4.5**
Brown, Toastie, Thick Sliced, Kingsmill* — 1 Slice/44g	101	1.4	230	9.5	40.5	3.3	4.7
Brown, Very Dark, Albert Heijn* — 1 Slice/35g	84	1.4	240	12	35	4	7.4
Bruschettine, Italian, Toasted, Crosta & Mollica* — 1 Portion/10.7g	41	1.9	382	10.1	66.2	17.6	0
Buckwheat, Artisan* — 1 Loaf/400g	736	7	184	6.1	38.1	1.8	4.3
Buns, Burger Seeded, Sliced, Warburton's* — 1 Roll/60g	158	3.2	264	9	43.6	5.3	2.7
Buns, Burger, American Style, Sainsbury's* — 1 Bun/50g	131	2.1	261	10.5	45.6	4.1	3.6
Buns, Burger, Cheese & Onion Topped, Finest, Tesco* — 1 Serving/105g	309	10	294	10.2	41.9	9.5	2.8
Buns, Burger, GF, Made Without Wheat, M&S* — 1 Bun/80g	201	5	251	4.8	38.9	6.2	10.4
Buns, Burger, Giant, Sainsbury's* — 1 Bun/95g	249	4.9	262	8.7	45.2	5.2	2.9
Buns, Burger, M&S* — 1 Bun/58g	162	3.3	280	10.1	45.7	5.7	2.5
Buns, Burger, Sainsbury's* — 1 Bun/56g	154	2.9	275	9.2	47.8	5.2	4.1
Buns, Burger, Sesame, American Style, Sainsbury's* — 1 Bun/60g	162	3.8	270	7.3	46.2	6.3	2.2
Buns, Burger, Sesame, Sliced, Tesco* — 1 Bun/60g	168	4	280	7.9	47.3	6.6	2.1
Buns, White, Burger, Waitrose* — 1 Serving/64g	169	2.5	264	10	47.2	3.9	2.7
Buns, White, Stay Fresh, Tesco* — 1 Bun/56g	152	3.7	271	7.5	45.5	6.6	0
Butterbread, Nature's Own* — 1 Slice/30g	70	0.6	231	11.5	46.2	1.9	0
Challah, Average — **1 Slice/50g**	**143**	**3.6**	**286**	**8.9**	**53.6**	**7.1**	**3.6**
Cheese & Garlic, Pizza Style, Sainsbury's* — ¼ Bread/63g	199	8.1	318	10.7	39.7	13	2.2
Cheese & Garlic, Stonebaked, Morrisons* — ¼ Bread/68.8g	228	9.9	331	10.9	39.5	14.4	1.9
Cheese & Onion, Tear & Share, Sainsbury's* — ¼ Bread/71g	202	6.6	285	9.8	40.6	9.3	1.9

BREAD

INFO/WEIGHT	Measure		per Measure		Nutrition Values per 100g / 100ml				
			KCAL	FAT	KCAL	PROT	CARB	FAT	FIBRE
Cheese & Tomato, Tear & Share, Sainsbury's*	¼ Bread/72g		211	9.5	293	8	35.7	13.2	1.5
Cheese & Onion, Toastie, Warburton's*	1 Slice/42g		120	5.8	286	7.5	33.1	13.7	0
Cheese Topped, Baton, Bakery, Tesco*	½ Baton/100g		292	4.5	292	10.7	51.2	4.5	2
Cheese, Morrisons*	1 Serving/96g		297	13.6	311	9.9	35.9	14.2	3
Cheese, Onion & Garlic, Tear & Share, Waitrose*	¼ Bread/112g		326	14.6	290	9.4	33.9	13	2.1
Cheese, Onion Mustard Seed, Cluster, Sainsbury's*	1 Cluster/100g		276	8.1	276	10	40.6	8.1	3.1
Cheese, Tear & Share, Tesco*	¼ Loaf/72.5g		225	7.8	310	8.8	44	10.7	0.8
Cholla, Average	**1/10 Loaf/154g**		**421**	**14.3**	**274**	**6.9**	**40.8**	**9.3**	**1**
Ciabatta Stick, Organic, M&S*	1 Stick/140g		315	2	225	8.9	48.5	1.4	4.2
Ciabatta, Black Olive, Part Baked, Sainsbury's*	¼ Ciabatta/67g		172	2.5	257	8.6	46.8	3.8	2.4
Ciabatta, Finest, Tesco*	1/6 Ciabatta/45g		124	2.7	275	10.4	44.8	5.9	2.7
Ciabatta, Gluten & Wheat Free, Average	**1 Slice/55g**		**136**	**1.6**	**248**	**2**	**52.4**	**2.9**	**4.2**
Ciabatta, Green Olive, Tesco*	¼ Ciabatta/70g		155	3.1	222	7.4	38.2	4.4	1.9
Ciabatta, Half, M&S*	1 Ciabatta/135g		354	5.5	262	10.3	48.1	4.1	2.1
Ciabatta, Half, Organic, Sainsbury's*	½ Ciabatta/63g		152	0.6	241	9.1	48.7	1	2.3
Ciabatta, Half, Part Baked, TTD, Sainsbury's*	¼ Pack/67g		173	3.3	257	8.6	44.6	4.9	3.5
Ciabatta, Half, Tesco*	1 Ciabatta/135g		351	4.7	260	8.9	47.7	3.5	2.2
Ciabatta, Italian Style, Waitrose*	1 Ciabatta/89g		231	1.2	260	10.7	51.2	1.4	2.2
Ciabatta, Olive & Rosemary, Mini, Tesco*	1 Pack/75g		319	8.2	425	17.8	63	10.9	3.6
Ciabatta, Organic, Tesco*	1/3 Ciabatta/100g		240	3.6	240	8.7	43.2	3.6	2.4
Ciabatta, Part Baked, Half, Sainsbury's*	½ Ciabbatta/67g		174	2.5	260	8.9	47.7	3.7	2.2
Ciabatta, Plain, Half, Two, Waitrose*	1 Roll/80g		248	5.8	310	10	51.3	7.2	2.2
Ciabatta, Plain, Tesco*	¼ Ciabatta/73g		174	2.8	240	9.8	41.5	3.9	2.4
Ciabatta, Ready to Bake, M&S*	1 Serving/150g		393	6.1	262	10.3	48.1	4.1	2.1
Ciabatta, Ready to Bake, Sainsbury's*	½ Ciabatta/66g		172	2.4	260	8.9	47.7	3.7	2.2
Ciabatta, Spicy Topped, Finest, Tesco*	1 Serving/73g		163	4	223	9.2	34	5.5	1.7
Ciabatta, Square, Bake at Home, Part Baked, Asda*	1 Roll/60g		157	2.1	262	8.4	49.1	3.5	2.1
Ciabatta, Sun Dried Tomato & Basil, Tesco*	¼ Ciabatta/75g		193	4.3	257	8.9	42.4	5.7	2.4
Ciabatta, Sweet Pepper, HE, Tesco*	1 Serving/50g		135	1.4	270	11.8	49.5	2.7	2.8
Ciabatta, Tomato & Basil, GFY, Asda*	1 Serving/55g		143	1.2	260	9	51	2.2	0
Ciabatta, Tomato & Mozzarella, Iceland*	1 Ciabatta/150g		374	15.2	249	10	29.6	10.1	3.3
Ciabatta, TTD, Sainsbury's*	¼ Pack/68g		185	4	274	10.4	44.8	5.9	2.7
Cinnamon & Fruit Swirl, Genesis Crafty*	1 Slice/40g		133	4.1	332	6.8	53.8	10.2	0
Cinnamon Swirl, Asda*	1 Serving/25g		87	3.2	349	6	52	13	1.6
Cob, Cheese & Chutney, Bakery, Tesco*	1 Slice/50g		124	2.2	249	11.3	39.7	4.4	2.5
Corn, with Sunflower Seed & Mixed Spice, Bakery, Tesco*	1 Slice/50g		131	2	262	9.9	45	4.1	2.6
Cottage Loaf, Stonebaked, Asda*	1 Serving/67g		155	0.9	232	10	45	1.3	3.2
Cranberry Raisin & Cashew, Bloomer, Bakery, Tesco*	1 Serving/70g		211	5	302	9.8	47.6	7.2	3.9
Crostini, Olive Oil, TTD, Sainsbury's*	1 Roll/4g		16	0.3	409	11.4	72.2	8.3	3.3
Farina, Seeded, Crosta & Mollica*	1 Pack/360g		878	9.4	244	9.5	43.4	2.6	4.1
Farl, Irish Soda, Irwin's Bakery*	1 Farl/150g		334	5.1	223	4	44	3.4	2.3
Farmhouse Soft Grained, Sliced, Warburton's*	1 Slice/42.3g		109	1.7	258	10.2	44.6	4	5
Farmhouse with Oatmeal, Batch, Finest, Tesco*	1 Slice/44g		110	1.4	240	9.8	43.2	3.1	5.2
Farmhouse, Batch, Multiseed, Love Life, Waitrose*	1 Slice/50g		130	3.5	259	9.9	39.2	7	7.2
Farmhouse, Poppy Seed, Crusty, Loaf, M&S*	1 Slice/40g		104	1.3	260	9.4	47.6	3.3	2.3
Farmhouse, Wholemeal, Average	**1 Slice/43g**		**94**	**1.4**	**219**	**10.7**	**36.2**	**3.3**	**7.3**
Ficelle, Mixed Olive, Waitrose*	1/5 Stick/50g		133	1.4	267	7.5	51.1	2.8	3.4
Fig & Almond, BrÃf¶derna Cartwright*	4 Slices/100g		267	7.5	267	9.2	39.7	7.5	0
Fig & Hazelnut, Loaf, M&S*	1 Serving/100g		285	8.2	285	11	38.9	8.2	5.4
Flat, Italian, Piada Sfogliata, Italiamo, Lidl*	1 Piece/130g		402	12.5	309	7.9	45.9	9.6	2
Flatbread, Folded, Lge Plain, by, Sainsbury's*	1 Flatbread/65g		192	3.4	295	8.5	51.4	5.3	4.1
Flatbread, Garlic & Herb, Tear & Share, Sainsbury's*	¼ Bread/68g		201	6.3	297	10.9	42.5	9.3	3.7
Flatbread, Garlic, BGTY, Sainsbury's*	¼ Bread/56g		177	5.7	316	9.6	46.6	10.1	2.7

BREAD

	Measure INFO/WEIGHT	KCAL	FAT	Nutrition Values per 100g / 100ml KCAL	PROT	CARB	FAT	FIBRE
Flatbread, Garlic, Tesco*	1 Serving/83g	249	8.6	302	6.7	45.3	10.4	3
Flatbread, Khobez, White, Dina Foods Ltd*	1 Bread/56g	158	0.6	282	10.5	57.5	1.1	3
Flatbread, Multi Seed, Tower Gate, Lidl*	1 Bread/8g	34	1.1	430	13.1	57.4	13.9	11.2
Flatbread, Multiseed, Folded, Tesco*	1 Flatbread/35g	107	2.4	305	10.4	47.8	6.8	5.3
Flatbread, Super Seeded, Folded, Village Bakery, Aldi*	1 Flatbread/35g	123	4.6	352	9.7	47	13	5.5
Flatbread, Tomato, & Garlic, Sainsbury's*	1/3 Bread/73g	191	4.9	261	8.4	41.7	6.7	3.4
Focaccia, Cherry Tomato, Basil & Puglian Pesto, Graze*	1 Punnet/40g	120	6.5	301	7.2	31.6	16.2	3.2
Focaccia, Harissa Peperonata, Bake at Home, M&S*	1 Bun/114g	282	8.3	247	7.9	35.8	7.3	3.2
Focaccia, Onion & Herb, Tesco*	½ Pack/190g	547	23.8	288	8.7	35.2	12.5	3.7
Focaccia, Roast Cherry Tomato & Olive, GFY, Asda*	½ Pack/148g	350	6	237	9	41	4.1	2.8
Focaccia, Roasted Onion & Cheese, M&S*	1 Serving/89g	240	4.1	270	10.4	45.7	4.6	2.8
French Stick, Average	*1 Serving/60g*	*147*	*0.2*	*245*	*8.7*	*52.2*	*0.4*	*2.1*
French, Sliced, Parisian*	2 Slices/39g	100	1	256	5.1	48.7	2.6	0
Fruit & Cinnamon Loaf, Finest, Tesco*	1 Slice/37g	134	4.9	363	6.4	54.6	13.2	1.5
Fruit Loaf, Apple & Cinnamon, Soreen*	1 Serving/10g	31	0.4	307	6.9	60.5	4.2	0
Fruit Loaf, Apple, M&S*	1 Slice/39g	100	0.6	255	8.5	51.9	1.5	3.3
Fruit Loaf, Banana, Soreen*	1 Slice/25g	78	1	313	6.6	61.2	4.1	2.6
Fruit Loaf, Cinnamon & Raisin, Soreen*	1/8 Loaf/25g	77	1	308	7.7	54.1	4	4.1
Fruit Loaf, Fresh, Free From, Sainsbury's*	1 Slice/33g	93	2.5	279	3.2	45.5	7.5	8.1
Fruit Loaf, Fruity Five, Snack Pack, Soreen*	1 Pack/61g	200	5.5	329	7.1	54.9	9	2.7
Fruit Loaf, Luxury, Christmas, Soreen*	1 Serving/28g	85	0.6	303	4.5	66.6	2.1	0
Fruit Loaf, Mixed Berry, Weight Watchers*	1 Slice/34g	79	0.9	231	7.6	44.3	2.6	7.7
Fruit Loaf, Plum, Lincolnshire, Soreen*	1 Slice/25g	65	0.8	261	8.4	49.3	3.4	2.1
Fruit Loaf, Sliced, Bakers Selection, Asda*	1 Serving/36g	100	1.5	278	8.2	50	4.2	3.6
Fruit Loaf, Sliced, Sainsbury's*	1 Slice/40g	104	1.4	260	8.9	47.9	3.6	2.4
Fruit Loaf, Sliced, Tesco*	1 Slice/36g	100	1.8	278	6.9	51.2	5.1	3.7
Fruit Loaf, Sultana & Cherry, Sainsbury's*	1 Slice/50g	178	6.1	357	2.7	59	12.2	1.7
Fruit, Loaf, Banana, Lunchbox, Soreen*	1 Bar/30g	100	1.3	332	8.2	63.3	4.4	2.9
Fruit, Loaf, Toasted, Cafe Instore, Asda*	1 Slice/33g	89	1.2	269	8	51	3.7	2.9
Fruit, Raisin Swirl, Sun-Maid*	1 Slice/33g	95	1.9	287	8.3	50.4	5.8	2.6
Fruited, Malt Loaf, Weight Watchers*	1 Serving/23g	68	0.4	294	8.9	60.2	1.9	3.6
Garlic & Cheese, Slices, Tesco*	1 Slice/30g	114	5	380	11.7	43.9	16.8	2
Garlic & Gruyere, Fougasse, TTD, Sainsbury's*	¼ Bread/76g	219	6.8	288	9.5	42.6	8.9	2.9
Garlic & Herb, Ciabatta, GFY, Asda*	¼ Ciabatta/60g	137	1.4	230	8.8	43.2	2.4	1
Garlic & Herb, Tear & Share, CBY, Asda*	¼ Portion /63g	185	6.7	295	9.2	39	10.7	2.7
Garlic with Cheese, Asda*	1 Slice/34g	130	6.1	382	11	44	18	0
Garlic, & Cheese, Tesco*	1 Serving/143g	490	24	343	9.4	38.5	16.8	2
Garlic, & Herb, Giant Feast, Sainsbury's*	1 Serving/50g	158	6.4	317	8	42.1	12.9	2.6
Garlic, & Herb, Tear & Share, Tesco*	1 Serving/73g	218	9.2	300	6.3	40	12.7	1.7
Garlic, & Parsley, Tesco*	1 Loaf/230g	699	26.7	304	9	41	11.6	2.7
Garlic, & Red Onion, Somerfield*	1 Serving/60g	177	6.7	295	9.6	38.9	11.1	2.1
Garlic, & Tomato, Pizza, Italiano, Tesco*	½ Bread/140g	405	15.1	289	7.5	40.5	10.8	2.5
Garlic, 25% Less Fat, Sainsbury's*	½ Baguette/85g	268	11.9	315	7.8	39.4	14	3.1
Garlic, 30% Less Fat, Morrisons*	1 Serving/80g	231	7.4	289	7.9	43.8	9.2	2.7
Garlic, Average	*1 Serving/100g*	*327*	*13.8*	*327*	*8.1*	*43.7*	*13.8*	*1.4*
Garlic, Baguette, 50% Less Fat, Asda*	¼ Baguette/43g	123	3	287	10	46	7	2.5
Garlic, Baguette, Average	*1 Slice/20g*	*66*	*2.8*	*330*	*7.8*	*43.1*	*14.2*	*1.8*
Garlic, Baguette, Extra Strong, Italiano, Tesco*	¼ Baguette/52.5g	178	8.7	340	7.9	39.8	16.6	2.8
Garlic, Baguette, Extra Strong, Sainsbury's*	½ Baguette/85g	278	12.6	327	8.4	40	14.8	3.4
Garlic, Baguette, Frozen, GFY, Asda*	¼ Baguette/48g	132	4.3	277	7	42	9	2.7
Garlic, Baguette, GFY, Asda*	¼ Baguette/42.6g	106	2.7	249	8.1	39.9	6.3	2.1
Garlic, Baguette, Good Choice, Iceland*	1/3 Baguette/54g	158	4.6	292	8.7	45.1	8.5	2.9
Garlic, Baguette, Italian, Asda*	¼ Baguette/48g	173	9.5	364	7	39	20	3.4

B

BREAD

	Measure INFO/WEIGHT	per Measure KCAL	FAT	Nutrition Values per 100g / 100ml KCAL	PROT	CARB	FAT	FIBRE
Garlic, Baguette, Italiano, Tesco*	¼ Baguette/52.5g	186	9.9	355	6.9	39.2	18.8	2.4
Garlic, Baguette, LC, Tesco*	¼ Baguette/52g	130	2.9	250	7	42.2	5.5	2.4
Garlic, Baguette, Mediterranean Herb, Tesco*	¼ Baguette/54g	181	8.8	335	6.9	40.3	16.3	2.3
Garlic, Baguette, Morrisons*	½ Baguette/95g	295	14.2	311	6.3	37.8	15	1.5
Garlic, Baguette, Organic, Tesco*	1 Serving/60g	192	8.1	320	8.5	41.1	13.5	2.5
Garlic, Baguette, Reduced Fat, Asda*	¼ Loaf/43g	107	2.7	249	8.1	39.9	6.3	2.7
Garlic, Baguette, Reduced Fat, Average	*¼ Baguette/40g*	*102*	*2.6*	*256*	*7.9*	*41.6*	*6.4*	*2.6*
Garlic, Baguette, Reduced Fat, Waitrose*	½ Baguette/85g	230	6.8	270	8.1	41.5	8	2.7
Garlic, Baguette, Sainsbury's*	½ Baguette/85g	342	16.3	403	8.9	48.6	19.2	2.3
Garlic, Baguette, Slices, Tesco*	1 Serving/60g	187	9.2	312	9.8	33.8	15.3	1.7
Garlic, Baguette, Trattoria Alfredo, Lidl*	¼ Baguette/44g	136	6.9	312	6.7	35.1	15.8	1.4
Garlic, Baguette, Value, Tesco*	½ Baguette/85g	270	11.1	318	8.1	42	13.1	2.3
Garlic, Baguette, Waitrose*	½ Baguette/85g	290	15.2	341	7.1	37.8	17.9	0
Garlic, Baguette, White, Homebake, Tesco*	1/3 Baguette/55g	160	5.5	290	7	43.1	10	1.9
Garlic, Baguette, with Cheese, HL, Tesco*	1 Serving/50g	114	1.1	229	9.4	43	2.2	2.1
Garlic, Ciabatta with Herbs, Weight Watchers*	1 Pack/88g	216	3.5	245	9.2	43	4	2.9
Garlic, Ciabatta, & Herb Butter, Sainsbury's*	½ Ciabatta/105g	345	16.3	329	8.5	38.8	15.5	0
Garlic, Ciabatta, BGTY, Sainsbury's*	½ Ciabatta/105g	306	13	291	8.7	36.2	12.4	2.7
Garlic, Ciabatta, Finest, Tesco*	1 Serving/65g	205	8.9	316	8.1	40.1	13.7	2.4
Garlic, Ciabatta, Hand Stretched, Sainsbury's*	¼ Pack/75g	244	10.6	325	8.4	41	14.1	2.9
Garlic, Ciabatta, Italian, Sainsbury's*	1 Serving/145g	454	17.1	313	10	41.6	11.8	2.9
Garlic, Ciabatta, Italiano, Tesco*	1 Ciabatta/65g	211	9.4	324	7.7	40.9	14.4	2.2
Garlic, Ciabatta, Mini, Italiano, Tesco*	½ Ciabatta/47g	150	6.9	320	8.2	38.5	14.6	2.8
Garlic, Ciabatta, TTD, Sainsbury's*	1 Serving/67g	199	8.1	298	8.3	38.7	12.2	3.1
Garlic, Finest, Tesco*	¼ Loaf/60g	187	7.9	311	7.7	40.3	13.2	1.8
Garlic, Focaccia, & Onion, GFY, Asda*	¼ Focaccia/55g	150	2.2	272	12	47	4	0
Garlic, Focaccia, & Rosemary, Sainsbury's*	¼ Focaccia/75g	219	7.4	292	8	43	9.8	2.8
Garlic, Focaccia, & Herb, Italian Style, Morrisons*	1/6 Focaccia/76g	259	10.9	341	8.5	44.7	14.3	2.5
Garlic, Foccacia, & Rosemary, Tesco*	¼ Loaf/73g	193	4.9	266	9	42.1	6.8	3.7
Garlic, Homebake, Tesco*	1 Serving/60g	209	12.3	348	7.1	33.7	20.5	1.5
Garlic, Italian Style Stone Baked, Morrisons*	½ Pack/115g	420	22	365	7.9	40.4	19.1	1.9
Garlic, Organic, Waitrose*	1 Baguette/170g	536	23.3	315	8.7	39.1	13.7	1.8
Garlic, Pizza Bread, Co-Op*	1 Pizza/240g	756	31.2	315	8	41	13	2
Garlic, Reduced Fat, Waitrose*	1 Pack/170g	551	18.7	324	6.9	49.4	11	0.9
Garlic, Slices, 50 % Less Fat, Asda*	1 Slice/29g	75	1.1	262	7.9	47.1	3.9	3.2
Garlic, Slices, Asda*	1 Slice/27g	88	3.3	328	8	46.2	12.4	2.8
Garlic, Slices, BGTY, Sainsbury's*	1 Slice/30g	86	2.3	285	7.2	45.5	7.7	2.6
Garlic, Slices, Chilled, Sainsbury's*	1 Pack/368g	1369	60	372	9.1	47.3	16.3	3.2
Garlic, Slices, GFY, Asda*	1 Slice/31g	80	1	259	8.9	48.1	3.3	3
Garlic, Slices, HL, Tesco*	1 Slice/52g	131	2.2	251	8.6	44.6	4.2	2.6
Garlic, Slices, LC, Tesco*	1 Slice/30g	75	1.7	250	7.3	42.3	5.7	2.9
Garlic, Slices, LC, Tesco*	1 Slice/30g	75	1.7	250	7.3	42.3	5.7	2.9
Garlic, Slices, Morrisons*	1 Slice/30g	82	2.7	272	7.3	40.2	9.1	2.6
Garlic, Stonebaked, M&S*	1 Loaf/85g	264	10.1	310	9.3	41.4	11.9	3.1
Garlic, to Share, M&S*	¼ Loaf/82g	230	10.7	280	6.5	33.2	13	1.3
GF, Burger Buns, Wellfoods*	1 Bun/95g	226	3.6	238	1.5	49.2	3.8	1.2
GF, Loaf, Unsliced, Wellfoods*	2 Slices/100g	216	2.3	216	1.6	47.1	2.3	1.5
GF, Rolls, Wellfoods*	1 Roll/70g	157	1.5	224	1.9	48.8	2.2	1.5
Grained, Soft, Farmhouse, Warburton's*	1 Slice/42g	109	1.7	258	10.2	44.6	4	5
Granary Rolls, Homebake, Hovis*	1 Roll/75g	194	1.6	259	10.2	47.7	2.2	3.6
Granary White, Hovis*	1 Slice/44g	102	1.5	233	9.7	40.8	3.5	5.6
Granary, Average	*1 Med Slice/35g*	*85*	*1*	*242*	*9.8*	*44*	*2.8*	*4.8*
Granary, Baps, Large, Asda*	1 Bap/64g	143	1.4	224	10	41	2.2	4.3

BREAD

INFO/WEIGHT	Measure	per Measure KCAL	FAT	Nutrition Values per 100g / 100ml KCAL	PROT	CARB	FAT	FIBRE
Granary, Country, Multiseeded, Hovis*	1 Slice/44g	104	1.1	236	10.6	39.8	2.4	6.8
Granary, M&S*	1 Slice/30g	75	0.9	250	9.5	46.4	3.1	3.2
Granary, Malted, Med Brown, Asda*	1 Slice/35g	81	0.9	231	9	43	2.6	3.3
Granary, Oatmeal, Hovis*	1 Slice/44g	104	0.9	236	9.2	45.3	2.1	3.1
Granary, Original, All Sizes, Hovis*	1 Thin Slice/33g	84	0.8	256	10.6	46.4	2.4	3.7
Granary, Seeded, Sunflower, Hovis*	1 Slice/44g	119	2.5	271	10.1	44.9	5.7	2.9
Granary, Thick Slice, COU, M&S*	1 Slice/25g	60	0.6	240	10.5	44.1	2.2	6
Granary, Waitrose*	1 Slice/40g	88	1	220	9.4	39.9	2.5	4.3
Granary, White, Seeded, Med Sliced, Hovis*	1 Slice/44g	109	1.8	248	10.9	41.7	4.2	3.8
Granary, Wholemeal, Average	*1 Slice/35g*	*80*	*0.9*	*228*	*10.8*	*38.4*	*2.6*	*6.6*
Granary, Wholemeal, Seeded, Med Sliced, Hovis*	1 Slice/44g	104	1.1	237	10.6	39.8	2.4	6.8
Half & Half, Medium, Warburton's*	1 Slice/40g	95	0.8	240	8.8	44.2	2	5
Half & Half, Toastie, Warburton's*	1 Slice/47g	112	0.9	240	8.8	44.2	2	5
Half Wheat Rye, The Polish Bakery, Tesco*	1 Slice/40g	93	0.6	233	5.7	51.1	1.5	6.6
Hamburer Rolls, Gluten & Wheat Free	*1 Roll/55g*	*137*	*1.9*	*249*	*2*	*52.4*	*3.4*	*4*
Herby, Basket, Snack, Graze*	1 Punnet/20g	101	5	503	8	61	25	3
Herby, Basket, Snack, Retail, Graze*	1 Punnet/18g	90	4.3	500	8.1	61	24	3.5
Heyford Sliced Bloomer, Waitrose*	1 Slice/50g	104	1.6	208	10.1	35	3.1	6.6
Hi Bran, M&S*	1 Slice/26g	55	0.8	210	12.6	32.5	3	6.3
Hi Fibre, Seed, Lifefibre*	1 Slice/35g	109	3.5	313	12.5	43.6	10.1	2.7
High Bran, Loaf, M&S*	2 Slices/62g	143	2.4	230	13.1	31.7	3.9	7.7
Hot Cross Bun, Loaf, Warburton's*	1 Slice/35g	94	1.3	269	8.3	50.4	3.7	2.9
Irish Barm Brack, Tesco*	1 Serving/75g	232	5.2	310	16	47.6	6.9	3
Irish Brown Soda, Tesco*	1 Serving/50g	110	1.9	219	9.2	36.2	3.8	6.4
Irish Cottage Wheaten, Loaf, Tesco*	1 Serving/50g	116	1.3	231	8.6	41.4	2.6	4.2
Irish Sliced Fruit Soda, Irwin's Bakery*	2 Slices/80g	218	4.2	273	2.4	53.8	5.3	2.5
Jalapeno Chilli, & Three Cheese, Bloomer, Bakery, Tesco*	1 Serving/82g	214	3.6	261	12.5	41.1	4.4	3.7
Juvela*	1 Slice/25g	60	0.8	240	3.3	50	3	1.7
Loaf, Tasty Grains & Seeds, Warburton's*	1 Slice/38g	100	1.6	264	10.6	45.6	4.3	5.2
Low Carb, Protein Rich, Carbzone*	1 Slice/50g	132	6.5	264	22	7.5	13	14
Low GI, Multiseed, Percy Ingle*	1 Med Slice/35g	99	3.1	283	0	0	8.9	6
Malt Loaf, Buttered, 2 Slices, Soreen*	1 Pack/45g	150	3.9	333	7.5	54.2	8.6	4.4
Malt Loaf, Chocolatey, Soreen*	1/8 Loaf/28g	95	1.7	344	8	58.7	6.3	5.1
Malt Loaf, Family, Asda*	1 Serving/20g	54	0.3	270	8	56	1.5	5
Malt Loaf, Fruited, Sliced, Weight Watchers*	1 Slice/23g	68	0.4	294	8.9	60.2	1.9	3.6
Malt Loaf, Fruity, Sliced, Soreen*	1 Slice/33g	101	0.7	303	7.6	62.1	2.2	3.8
Malt Loaf, Organic, Tesco*	1 Slice/28g	82	0.6	292	7.2	61.2	2	2.3
Malt Loaf, Original, Low Fat, Soreen*	1 Slice/22g	63	0.4	288	7.5	60	1.6	2
Malt Loaf, Tesco*	1 Slice/50g	146	1.4	291	8.6	58	2.7	4.8
Malted Brown, Slice, BGTY, Sainsbury's*	1 Slice/22g	53	0.6	239	12.1	41.4	2.8	5.8
Malted Brown, Thick Sliced, Organic, Tesco*	1 Slice/44.4g	111	0.9	249	8.9	48.8	2	3.5
Malted Grain, Baton, Tesco*	¼ Baton/57g	143	0.5	251	10.5	47.6	0.9	5
Malted Grain, Co-Op*	1 Slice/43g	99	0.9	230	8	46	2	3
Malted Grain, Good As Gold, Kingsmill*	1 Slice/46.9g	114	1.2	243	9.5	45.4	2.6	4.2
Malted Oat, Duchy Originals*	1 Serving/80g	195	3	244	8.8	43.6	3.8	3.7
Malted Wheatgrain, Roberts Bakery*	1 Slice/30g	80	1	265	11	48	3.3	3.6
Malted, & Seeded, Batch, Organic, Waitrose*	1 Slice/50g	118	2	236	10.9	39.5	3.9	6.2
Malted, Crusty, Sainsbury's*	1 Slice/42g	109	1.4	259	8.6	48.6	3.3	4.4
Malted, Danish, Weight Watchers, Warburton's*	1 Slice/20g	51	0.3	249	11.8	45.1	1.5	4.2
Malted, Farmhouse, Morrisons*	1 Serving/40g	94	0.7	235	9.1	45.6	1.8	4.7
Malted, Wheat Loaf, Crusty, Finest, Tesco*	1 Slice/50g	115	0.8	230	9.8	44.2	1.5	4.4
Mediterranean Olive, Waitrose*	1 Slice/30g	82	2.8	273	7.4	40.1	9.2	4.9
Mediterranean Style, M&S*	1/6 Loaf/48g	150	5.3	315	10.9	42.5	11.1	1.2

GENERAL FOODS AND DRINKS A-Z

BREAD

	Measure INFO/WEIGHT	per Measure KCAL	FAT	Nutrition Values per 100g / 100ml KCAL	PROT	CARB	FAT	FIBRE
Mediterranean Style, Stonebaked Tomato Batard, Tesco*	¼ Loaf/100g	256	3.1	256	9.8	45.5	3.1	3.5
Mixed Seed, Organic, Duchy Originals*	1 Slice/42.5g	114	3.4	269	10.9	39.1	8.1	5.3
Multi Seed, Somerfield*	1 Slice/44.7g	105	1.7	235	11	38.2	3.7	8.1
Multi Seeded Loaf, Gluten & Wheat Free, Lovemore*	1 Serving/35g	102	4.3	291	0	3	12.3	0
Multigrain, Batch, Finest, Tesco*	1 Slice/50g	117	1.4	235	10.8	40.4	2.9	5.5
Multigrain, Brennans*	1 Slice/40g	110	1.3	275	8.8	48	3.3	6.3
Multigrain, Brown, Farmhouse Baker's, M&S*	1 Slice/51g	115	2.8	225	13	31.2	5.4	5.1
Multigrain, Crusty, Finest, Tesco*	1 Slice/40g	98	1.4	245	9	44.7	3.4	5
Multigrain, GF, Sainsbury's*	1 Slice/17g	39	0.8	229	5.1	40.8	5	5.6
Multigrain, Sliced, Fresh And Easy*	1 Slice/40g	110	1	275	10	52.5	2.5	5
Multigrain, Soft Batch, Sainsbury's*	1 Slice/44g	106	2.9	242	11.3	34.5	6.5	5.6
Multigrain, Sub Rolls, Asda*	1 Sub/150g	357	6.3	238	0	0	4.2	0
Multigrain, Sunblest*	1 Slice/30g	76	0.8	254	9	47	2.5	4.5
Multigrain, Tesco*	1 Slice/31g	66	1	214	11.1	36.8	3.2	8.9
Multigrain, Thick Sliced, Tesco*	1 Slice/50g	112	1.2	225	8.4	42.2	2.5	3.9
Multiseed Farmhouse Batch, Finest, Tesco*	1 Slice/44g	108	1.9	245	9.9	40.4	4.4	7.5
Multiseed, Farmhouse, Finest, Tesco*	1 Slice /50g	135	3.8	270	12.5	37	7.7	5.8
Multiseed, Sliced, Free From, Tesco*	1 Slice/29g	85	3.4	294	6.7	34.8	11.8	10.7
Multiseeded, Bloomer, TTD, Sainsbury's*	1 Slice/50g	128	1.8	256	12	39.7	3.6	8.8
Naan, Asda*	1 Naan/130g	308	2.3	237	7.7	47.4	1.8	2.2
Naan, Average	*1 Naan/130g*	*344*	*5.6*	*264*	*8.3*	*48.5*	*4.3*	*2*
Naan, Bombay Brassiere, Sainsbury's*	1 Naan/140g	372	4.3	266	9.8	49.6	3.1	2.9
Naan, Chilli & Mango, Finest, Tesco*	½ Naan/90g	230	5.1	255	8.4	41.9	5.7	3.2
Naan, Fresh, BGTY, Sainsbury's*	1 Serving/150g	368	4.6	245	9.4	44.9	3.1	2.2
Naan, Garlic & Coriander, Free From, Tesco*	1 Naan/89.6g	215	6	240	5.1	38.7	6.7	4.9
Naan, Garlic & Coriander, Large, TTD, Sainsbury's*	¼ Pack/70g	194	3.8	277	9.4	47.7	5.4	2.2
Naan, Garlic & Coriander, Mild, Patak's*	1 Naan/140g	452	15.1	323	9	47.5	10.8	0
Naan, Garlic & Coriander, Tesco*	½ Naan/82.5g	235	6.4	285	7.6	45.6	7.7	2.6
Naan, Garlic & Coriander, TTD, Sainsbury's*	1 Serving/70g	215	8.1	307	7	43.9	11.5	2.9
Naan, Garlic & Coriander, M&S*	1 Naan/150g	375	2.1	250	9.8	50.1	1.4	2
Naan, Garlic & Coriander, Mini, Asda*	1 Naan/110g	320	12.5	291	6.9	40.2	11.4	2.5
Naan, Garlic & Coriander, Mini, Finest, Tesco*	1 Naan/50g	160	6.8	320	6.7	42.4	13.5	0.8
Naan, Garlic & Coriander, Mini, Sainsbury's*	1 Naan/50g	140	2	280	8.2	51.2	4.1	2.6
Naan, Garlic & Coriander, Mini, Sharwood's*	1 Naan/65g	196	4.2	302	8	51.5	6.5	2.8
Naan, Garlic & Coriander, Mini, Tesco*	1 Naan/65g	185	5	285	7.6	45.6	7.7	2.6
Naan, Garlic & Coriander, Mini, Weight Watchers*	1 Naan/40g	100	1	250	9.3	47.6	2.5	4.2
Naan, Garlic & Coriander, Sainsbury's*	1 Serving/130g	373	10	287	8.7	45.8	7.7	2.4
Naan, Garlic & Coriander, Weight Watchers*	1 Naan/60g	155	2.6	259	8.9	46	4.3	3.4
Naan, Indian Meal for One, BGTY, Sainsbury's*	1 Serving/45g	115	1.9	257	10.3	44.2	4.3	2.1
Naan, Indian Meal for Two, Sainsbury's*	1 Naan/125g	357	9.3	285	8.7	45.9	7.4	1.9
Naan, LC, Tesco*	1 Naan/71g	181	1.6	255	7.5	50.7	2.2	2.3
Naan, Mini, LC, Tesco*	1 Naan/65g	150	1.8	230	8.1	42.5	2.8	2.9
Naan, Ocado*	½ Naan/75g	194	1.7	258	8.4	48.3	2.3	5.3
Naan, Onion & Mint, M&S*	½ Naan/135g	351	11.7	260	8.9	35.8	8.7	2.5
Naan, Onion Bhaji, Sharwood's*	1 Pack/130g	378	9.9	291	7.3	48.4	7.6	2.2
Naan, Peshwari, Apple & Coconut, Mini, Sharwood's*	1 Naan/65g	179	3.1	275	7.5	47.1	4.8	6.7
Naan, Peshwari, Finest, Tesco*	1 Naan/130g	338	7.3	260	8.6	43.7	5.6	4.9
Naan, Peshwari, M&S*	1 Serving/127g	394	12.8	310	9.2	45.8	10.1	1.9
Naan, Peshwari, Mega, Asda*	1 Naan/220g	680	26.4	309	7.1	43.1	12	2.7
Naan, Peshwari, Mini, Bilash, Aldi*	1 Naan/58g	212	9.5	366	7	45.1	16.4	4.9
Naan, Peshwari, Sainsbury's*	1 Naan/166g	511	18.3	308	7.1	45.1	11	4.7
Naan, Peshwari, Sharwood's*	1 Naan/130g	334	6.9	257	7.2	45.1	5.3	2.5
Naan, Peshwari, Tesco*	1 Naan/215g	684	26.7	318	7.5	48.9	12.4	4.8

B

BREAD

INFO/WEIGHT	Measure	per Measure		Nutrition Values per 100g / 100ml				
		KCAL	FAT	KCAL	PROT	CARB	FAT	FIBRE
Naan, Plain, Average	*1 Naan/160g*	*437*	*10.5*	*273*	*8*	*45.7*	*6.5*	*2.1*
Naan, Plain, Indian, Mini, Asda*	1 Naan/110g	329	12.6	299	6.6	42.2	11.5	2.1
Naan, Plain, Large, Sainsbury's*	½ Naan/70g	191	4.6	273	7.1	46.2	6.6	3
Naan, Plain, Mega, Indian Takeaway, Asda*	1 Naan/222g	572	8.4	258	7	49	3.8	2.5
Naan, Plain, Mini, Asda*	1 Naan/58g	156	2.7	269	8	49	4.6	2.3
Naan, Plain, Mini, BGTY, Sainsbury's*	1 Naan/50g	113	1.1	226	8.2	43.2	2.2	3.3
Naan, Plain, Mini, BGTY, Sainsbury's*	1 Naan/50g	124	0.6	248	7.6	49.8	1.3	3.3
Naan, Plain, Mini, Weight Watchers*	1 Naan/44g	108	1.1	245	9.1	46.5	2.5	4.9
Naan, Plain, Sharwood's*	1 Naan/120g	326	8.9	272	8.5	42.9	7.4	2.4
Naan, Plain, Tesco*	1 Naan/150g	392	6.9	261	8.4	46.4	4.6	2.3
Naan, Plain, Value, Tesco*	1 Naan/135g	363	9.7	269	8.1	42.9	7.2	1.6
Naan, Smart Price, Asda*	1 Naan/100g	233	1.9	233	8.7	45.3	1.9	2.8
Naan, Take Away, Tesco*	1 Naan/39g	97	1.3	248	8.7	45.6	3.4	1.7
Naan, Tandoori Baked, Waitrose*	1 Naan/140g	372	4.3	266	9.8	49.6	3.1	2.9
Naan, Tandoori, Sharwood's*	1 Naan/130g	330	6.5	254	7.3	45	5	2
Oatmeal, Farmhouse, Extra Special, Asda*	1 Slice/44g	102	1.1	231	11	41	2.6	6
Oatmeal, Farmhouse, Soft, M&S*	1 Slice/45g	110	2	245	11.1	39.5	4.4	5.2
Oatmeal, Farmhouse, Waitrose*	1 Slice/40g	110	2.1	276	9.4	47.9	5.2	4.6
Oatmeal, Sliced Loaf, Tesco*	1 Slice/50g	111	1.7	222	7.4	40.5	3.4	2.8
Olive, Waitrose*	1 Slice/28g	86	3	306	9	43.6	10.6	2
Oliven Ringbrot, Rewe*	1 Portion/100g	247	3.2	247	8.5	44.1	3.2	2.8
Pain Au Raisin, M&S*	1 Pain/74g	215	9.5	290	5.3	38.7	12.8	1.2
Paleo, Almond, GF, Non GMO, Julian Bakery*	1 Slice/43g	60	3	140	16.3	14	7	11.6
Pane Pugliese, Italian, Toasting, Crosta & Mollica*	1 Slice/69g	184	0.8	267	8.6	55.5	1.2	0.2
Pave, Walnut, Sainsbury's*	1 Serving/50g	140	4.8	280	9	40	9.5	3.5
Petit Pain, Homebake, Mini, Tesco*	1 Roll/50g	120	0.6	240	7.8	48.5	1.2	3.4
Petit Pain, Organic, Tesco*	1 Roll/100g	235	0.8	235	7.8	49.1	0.8	1.2
Petit Pain, Part Bake, Weight Watchers*	1 Roll/50g	111	0.4	223	6.8	43.5	0.9	6.8
Petit Pain, White, Soft, Somerfield*	1 Roll/68g	186	1.2	274	8.5	56.1	1.7	2.1
Petits Pains, Mini, Homebake, Tesco*	1 Roll/45g	110	0.6	245	7.8	49.7	1.3	2.5
Pitta, 159, Pride Valley*	1 Pitta/63g	159	1.2	252	10.1	51.2	1.9	2.6
Pitta, Bakersfield*	1 Pitta/67g	167	0.7	250	7	52	1	1.5
Pitta, Brown, Organic, Waitrose*	1 Pitta/53g	124	0.5	234	8.5	43.9	1	7.4
Pitta, Free From, Sainsbury's*	1 Pitta/65g	164	2.5	252	4.1	50	3.9	2.9
Pitta, Garlic & Herb, Tesco*	1 Pitta/60g	134	1.2	223	9.6	44.6	2	3
Pitta, Garlic & Coriander, Asda*	1 Pitta/55g	116	0.5	212	7	44	0.9	1.8
Pitta, Garlic, Morrisons*	1 Pitta/60g	149	1.1	249	9.7	51.1	1.8	0
Pitta, Mediterranean Style, The Bakery, M&S*	1 Pitta/85g	247	3.7	291	6.7	54.9	4.3	2.8
Pitta, Mexican, Santa Maria*	1 Pitta/66g	165	0.7	250	7.5	52	1	0
Pitta, Multi Seed & Cereal, The Food Doctor*	1 Pitta/70g	157	1.9	224	10.1	39.9	2.7	10.2
Pitta, Organic, Tesco*	1 Pitta/60g	124	0.8	206	8.3	40.2	1.4	5.7
Pitta, Pockets, Pride Valley*	1 Pitta/63g	151	0.6	239	9.3	48.4	0.9	3.2
Pitta, Pockets, Sainsbury's*	1 Pitta/75g	188	0.8	250	8.5	52	1	3.5
Pitta, Sd Tomato, Olive & Oregano, Extra Special, Asda*	1 Pitta/75g	194	0.8	259	7.1	55.2	1.1	1.6
Pitta, Seeded, HL, Tesco*	1 Pitta/60g	153	3.6	255	10.8	39.4	6	12.8
Pitta, Spelt, Albert Heijn*	1 Pitta/80g	196	0.8	245	2.5	48	1	0
Pitta, Tex Mex Style, Mini, Morrisons*	1 Pitta/18g	43	0.2	240	9.2	48.7	0.9	3.3
Pitta, White Picnic, Waitrose*	1 Pitta/30g	75	0.4	249	10.3	49.3	1.2	3.5
Pitta, White, Average	*1 Pitta/75g*	*191*	*1.1*	*255*	*9.2*	*50.8*	*1.5*	*2.7*
Pitta, White, Basics, Sainsbury's*	1 Pitta/47.5g	124	0.6	261	8.8	52.7	1.2	2
Pitta, White, Essential, Waitrose*	1 Pitta/60g	157	0.5	262	9	53.4	0.9	2.3
Pitta, White, Free From, Tesco*	1 Pitta/55g	140	1.2	255	6.5	52.6	2.1	5.5
Pitta, White, Greek Style, Asda*	1 Pitta/50g	126	1	253	8	51	1.9	0

BREAD

	Measure INFO/WEIGHT	per Measure KCAL	FAT	Nutrition Values per 100g / 100ml KCAL	PROT	CARB	FAT	FIBRE
Pitta, White, Large, Tesco*	1 Pitta/90g	252	1.9	280	9.8	55.1	2.1	3.4
Pitta, White, M&S*	1 Pitta/61g	146	1.2	240	9.3	46.9	2	3.6
Pitta, White, Mini, Sainsbury's*	1 Pitta/20g	54	0.2	268	8.8	54.6	1.2	2
Pitta, White, Mini, Tesco*	1 Pitta/30g	84	0.6	280	9.8	55.1	2.1	3.4
Pitta, White, Organic, Sainsbury's*	1 Pitta/59g	150	0.6	254	10.3	50.7	1.1	2.5
Pitta, White, Sainsbury's*	1 Pitta/60g	161	0.8	269	9	54.1	1.3	2.5
Pitta, White, Soft, Sandwich, Warburton's*	½ Pitta/36g	81	0.9	228	9.8	41.4	2.6	1.8
Pitta, White, Somerfield*	1 Pitta/56g	146	1.1	262	10.1	51.2	1.9	2.6
Pitta, White, Speciality Breads, Waitrose*	1 Pitta/60g	149	0.7	249	10.3	49.3	1.2	3.5
Pitta, White, Tesco*	1 Pitta/58g	146	0.5	251	8.9	50.3	0.9	3.1
Pitta, White, Weight Watchers*	1 Pitta/44.5g	106	0.3	238	8.7	45.9	0.7	6.7
Pitta, Wholemeal with Extra Virgin Olive Oil, Tesco*	1 Pitta/60g	135	1.6	225	8.3	41.5	2.6	5.5
Pitta, Wholemeal, Acropolis, Lidl*	1 Pitta/57g	136	0.9	238	12	44	1.6	6
Pitta, Wholemeal, Asda*	1 Pitta/56g	133	0.9	238	12	44	1.6	6
Pitta, Wholemeal, Average	*1 Pitta/64g*	*154*	*1.1*	*241*	*11*	*45.8*	*1.7*	*6.4*
Pitta, Wholemeal, Essential, Waitrose*	1 Pitta/60g	159	0.7	264	9.7	50.1	1.2	7.2
Pitta, Wholemeal, Healthy Eating, Co-Op*	1 Pitta/63g	135	1.3	215	12	37	2	9
Pitta, Wholemeal, Hollyland Bakery*	1 Pitta/20g	48	0.3	242	13.1	43.7	1.6	6
Pitta, Wholemeal, M&S*	1 Pitta/60g	155	1.6	255	10	45	2.6	5.5
Pitta, Wholemeal, Mini, M&S*	1 Pitta/18g	44	0.4	247	10.3	45.8	2.5	5.6
Pitta, Wholemeal, Mini, Sainsbury's*	1 Pitta/30g	69	0.5	231	10	43.8	1.7	6.2
Pitta, Wholemeal, Mini, Tesco*	1 Pitta/30g	76	0.5	255	11.8	48.2	1.7	4.2
Pitta, Wholemeal, Sainsbury's*	1 Pitta/57g	154	0.9	271	10.9	49.7	1.5	7.4
Pitta, Wholemeal, Simple & Versatile, As Sold, Tesco*	1 Pitta/58g	145	0.7	250	9.6	46.2	1.2	7.8
Pitta, Wholemeal, So Organic, Sainsbury's*	1 Pitta/60g	140	1	233	9.8	44.8	1.6	8.1
Pitta, Wholemeal, Tesco*	1 Pitta/58g	139	0.7	240	9.5	44.5	1.2	6.4
Pitta, Wholemeal, Waitrose*	1 Pitta/60g	145	0.5	242	12.4	46	0.9	3.1
Pitta, Wholemeal, Weight Watchers*	1 Pitta /46g	106	0.6	229	8.7	44.5	1.2	7.6
Potato & Rosemary, M&S*	1 Serving/40g	108	2.7	270	9.4	42.2	6.8	2.3
Potato Farls, Irish, Rankin Selection, Irwin's Bakery*	1 Farl/60g	110	2.2	184	2.3	34.4	3.6	2.5
Potato Farls, M&S*	1 Farl/55g	79	0.2	144	4.2	33.8	0.4	4.7
Potato Farls, Sunblest*	1 Farl/100g	156	0.9	156	3.8	33.2	0.9	1.9
Pumpernickel, Average	*1 Slice/50g*	*96*	*0.6*	*191*	*5.5*	*37.9*	*1.1*	*7.8*
Pumpernickel, Organic, Bavarian Pumpernickel*	1 Slice/50g	90	0.5	180	6	38	1	10
Pumpernickel, Organic, Biona*	1 Slice/80g	158	1.4	197	4.6	36	1.7	9.6
Pumpernickel, Rye, Kelderman*	1 Slice/50g	92	0.5	185	6	38	1	0
Pumpkin Seed, Raisin & Sunflower Seed, Sainsbury's*	1 Slice/30g	76	0.8	255	11.6	45.9	2.8	3.4
Pure Grain, Heart of Nature, Pure Nature*	1 Slice/55g	172	9.1	313	9.7	24.8	16.6	7.9
Pure Grain, with Prunes, Pure Nature*	1 Slice/50g	169	10.4	338	8	28.3	20.8	9
Raisin & Pumpkin Seed, Organic, Tesco*	1 Slice/30g	76	1.7	253	9.7	40.6	5.8	3.8
Raisin Loaf with Cinnamon, Warburton's*	1 Slice/36g	96	1.3	267	7.2	51.1	3.7	3.2
Roasted Onion, M&S*	1 Slice/50g	125	1.6	250	9	46.7	3.3	2.1
Rolls, American Style Deli, Tesco*	1 Roll/65g	162	2.2	249	7.8	46.8	3.4	1.6
Rolls, Best of Both, Hovis*	1 Roll/62g	148	2.9	239	9.8	39.7	4.6	5
Rolls, Brioche, Average	*1 Roll/49g*	*177*	*6.9*	*361*	*8.8*	*50.1*	*14.1*	*1.5*
Rolls, Brioche, Brialys*	1 Roll/35g	121	3.9	347	8.8	52.8	11.2	1.5
Rolls, Brioche, Butter, Tesco*	1 Serving/35g	124	4	355	8.8	53.3	11.4	2
Rolls, Brioche, Continental Classics*	1 Roll/35g	122	3.3	349	8.2	58.3	9.3	0
Rolls, Brioche, Finest, Tesco*	1 Roll/52g	207	11.6	398	10.8	38.3	22.4	2
Rolls, Brioche, French Milk, Bon Appetit, Aldi*	1 Roll/35g	116	2.7	330	8.3	56	7.8	2.2
Rolls, Brioche, Hot Dog, Specially Selected, Aldi*	1 Roll/45g	142	3.4	316	9.4	52	7.5	2
Rolls, Brioche, La Boulangere, Lidl*	1 Roll/35g	122	3.6	350	8.2	55.5	10.2	1.8
Rolls, Brioche, Plain Chocolate Chip, Sainsbury's*	1 Roll/35g	131	5.6	374	8.5	49	16	5.9

BREAD

INFO/WEIGHT	Measure	per Measure KCAL	per Measure FAT	Nutrition Values per 100g / 100ml KCAL	PROT	CARB	FAT	FIBRE
Rolls, Brioche, Sainsbury's*	1 Roll/35g	123	3.9	352	8.1	53.5	11.3	1.8
Rolls, Brioche, Tesco*	1 Roll/26g	92	2.9	349	8.5	54	11	0
Rolls, Brown, bake at Home, Aldi*	1 Roll/45g	131	1.5	291	10	52	3.3	5.8
Rolls, Brown, Carb Control, Tesco*	1 Roll/45g	98	2.7	218	20.5	20.7	5.9	10.7
Rolls, Brown, Ciabatta, Schar*	1 Roll/50g	138	4.1	274	5.8	40	8.1	8.9
Rolls, Brown, Crusty	*1 Roll/50g*	*128*	*1.4*	*255*	*10.3*	*50.4*	*2.8*	*3.5*
Rolls, Brown, Free From, Tesco*	1 Roll/65g	174	5.3	268	5.4	43.2	8.2	3.6
Rolls, Brown, Large, Asda*	1 Roll/57g	138	0.9	242	10	47	1.6	0
Rolls, Brown, M&S*	1 Roll/105g	242	6.4	230	9.2	37.3	6.1	4.4
Rolls, Brown, Malted Grain, Tesco*	1 Roll/58g	144	1.9	248	8.7	46.2	3.2	1.9
Rolls, Brown, Mini, M&S*	1 Roll/33g	80	2.5	245	9.8	35.5	7.6	3.8
Rolls, Brown, Morning, Farmfoods*	1 Roll/50g	134	1.8	269	12	47	3.7	4.2
Rolls, Brown, Old Fashioned, Waitrose*	1 Roll/63g	152	2.6	241	9.6	41.3	4.1	4.7
Rolls, Brown, Part Baked, Sunnyhills, Aldi*	1 Roll/50g	129	1.5	258	9.3	45.3	3	6.3
Rolls, Brown, Seeded, Organic, Sainsbury's*	1 Roll/70g	166	3.2	237	9.9	39.1	4.6	6.5
Rolls, Brown, Snack, Allinson*	1 Roll/44g	119	2.9	270	10.8	41.6	6.7	5.6
Rolls, Brown, Soft, Average	*1 Roll/50g*	*134*	*1.9*	*268*	*10*	*51.8*	*3.8*	*3.5*
Rolls, Brown, Soft, Organic, Sainsbury's*	1 Roll/70g	166	3.2	237	9.9	39.1	4.6	6.6
Rolls, Brown, Soft, Tesco*	1 Roll/50g	118	1.8	235	9	41.6	3.6	4.5
Rolls, Brown, Square, M&S*	1 Roll/105g	242	6.4	230	9.2	37.3	6.1	4.4
Rolls, Cheese & Tomato, Seeded, White, M&S*	1 Pack/160g	480	25	300	13.7	26.1	15.6	2.1
Rolls, Cheese Topped, Sandwich, Warburton's*	1 Roll/62g	168	4	270	12.1	40.7	6.5	2.6
Rolls, Cheese Topped, Village Green*	1 Roll/56g	159	4.1	284	13.1	41.2	7.4	4.8
Rolls, Chunky Cheese, Tesco*	1 Roll/80g	197	4.8	247	12.8	41.1	6	2
Rolls, Ciabatta, Cheese Topped, Mini, Finest, Tesco*	1 Roll/30g	85	2.4	282	11.5	40.9	8.1	3.8
Rolls, Ciabatta, Garlic, Asda*	1 Roll/93g	333	16.7	358	9	40	18	2.3
Rolls, Ciabatta, GF, Schar*	1 Roll/50g	109	0.9	213	4.1	41	1.8	8.3
Rolls, Ciabatta, M&S*	1 Roll/80g	210	3.3	262	10.3	48.1	4.1	2.1
Rolls, Ciabatta, Mini, Finest, Tesco*	1 Roll/30g	89	2	297	9.9	49.1	6.8	4.1
Rolls, Ciabatta, Sun Dried Tomato, Mini, Finest, Tesco*	1 Roll/30g	79	1.9	262	8.7	42.3	6.4	2.6
Rolls, Ciabatta, Tesco*	1 Roll/80g	208	2.5	260	8.6	48.2	3.1	3.3
Rolls, Country Grain, Mini, M&S*	1 Roll/31g	85	3	275	10.2	38.9	9.7	3.8
Rolls, Crisp, Original, Organic, Kallo*	1 Roll/9g	34	0.5	390	11	74	5.6	3
Rolls, Crusty, Booths*	1 Roll/50g	124	0.6	247	8.7	50.3	1.2	2.6
Rolls, Crusty, French, M&S*	1 Roll/65g	159	0.8	245	8.1	50.5	1.2	3.3
Rolls, Crusty, Part-Baked, Budgens*	1 Roll/50g	148	0.7	296	9.4	61.4	1.4	2.5
Rolls, Finger, Morrisons*	1 Roll/46g	119	0.8	259	10.7	50	1.8	2.3
Rolls, Finger, White, Sainsbury's*	1 Roll/40g	96	1	240	9	45.2	2.6	3.2
Rolls, Focaccia, Tesco*	1 Roll/75g	226	7	302	8.7	45.6	9.4	3.8
Rolls, GF, Antoinette Savill*	1 Roll/70g	157	1.5	224	1.9	48.8	2.2	1.5
Rolls, Granary Malted Wheatgrain, Soft, M&S*	1 Roll/80g	208	3.1	260	9.3	47.2	3.9	2.3
Rolls, Granary, Average	*1 Roll/70g*	*176*	*2.7*	*251*	*9.6*	*45.2*	*3.9*	*3.3*
Rolls, Granary, Bakers Premium, Tesco*	1 Roll/65g	158	0.8	243	9.9	47.8	1.3	2.3
Rolls, Granary, Mini, Tesco*	1 Roll/34g	92	2.2	271	10	43.5	6.5	3.8
Rolls, Granary, Original, Hovis*	1 Roll/70g	180	2.9	257	10.7	44.3	4.1	5.3
Rolls, Granary, Waitrose*	1 Roll/59g	160	3.8	271	10	47.2	6.4	3.8
Rolls, Green Olive, M&S*	1 Roll/75g	210	4.5	280	11.2	44	6	1.8
Rolls, Half & Half, Warburton's*	1 Roll/55g	144	2.5	261	10.4	42.7	4.5	4
Rolls, Heyford Wholemeal, Soft & Grainy, Waitrose*	1 Roll/75g	164	1.3	219	11.2	36.7	1.7	5.8
Rolls, Hot Dog, Sliced, Asda*	1 Roll/84g	197	2.8	234	7	44	3.3	0
Rolls, Hot Dog, Tesco*	1 Roll/85g	200	2.8	235	7.3	44	3.3	1.9
Rolls, Hot Dog, Value, Tesco*	1 Roll/40g	93	0.8	232	8.7	45	1.9	2.2
Rolls, Hot Dog, White, Warburton's*	1 Roll/55g	142	2.1	259	8.8	46.4	3.9	1.6

BREAD

INFO/WEIGHT	Measure	per Measure KCAL	FAT	Nutrition Values per 100g / 100ml KCAL	PROT	CARB	FAT	FIBRE
Rolls, Malted Grain, Sainsbury's*	1 Roll/68g	190	2.9	280	8.7	51.6	4.3	4.2
Rolls, Malted Grain, Submarine, M&S*	1 Roll/109g	300	4.7	275	8.9	53.6	4.3	3
Rolls, Malted Wheat, Sub, Organic, Tesco*	1 Serving/108g	279	4.4	258	10.1	45.2	4.1	4.8
Rolls, Malted, Whole Grain Rolls, Batched, Soft, M&S*	1 Roll/80g	180	3.6	225	7.8	38.5	4.5	3.1
Rolls, Mini Submarine, M&S*	1 Roll/23g	63	1.1	275	11.4	47.7	4.9	1.1
Rolls, Morning, Scottish, Warburton's*	1 Roll/50g	138	0.4	276	10.9	56.2	0.8	2.1
Rolls, Morning, Tesco*	1 Roll/48g	117	1.2	243	10.4	44.8	2.5	4.7
Rolls, Multi Seed, Free From, Free From, Tesco*	1 Roll/70g	214	8.3	305	5.4	44.2	11.8	6.3
Rolls, Multigrain, Pain Rustique, Homebake, Finest, Tesco*	1 Roll/60g	162	4.3	270	12.7	38.4	7.1	9.6
Rolls, Multigrain, Torpedo, Sainsbury's*	1 Roll/112g	328	7.5	293	10.5	47.7	6.7	6.3
Rolls, Nut & Raisin, Bakery, Tesco*	1 Serving/120g	426	11.2	355	9	56.8	9.3	4
Rolls, Oatmeal, Co-Op*	1 Roll/70g	175	3.2	250	10.1	42.6	4.6	5.6
Rolls, Oatmeal, Ploughman's, GFY, Asda*	1 Roll/72g	181	3.2	252	10	43	4.4	3.9
Rolls, Oatmeal, Soft, M&S*	1 Roll/83g	224	3.9	270	12.3	43.4	4.7	3.4
Rolls, Panini, Sainsbury's*	1 Roll/90g	249	5.6	276	11	44.1	6.2	3
Rolls, Panini, White, Tesco*	1 Roll/75g	210	4.6	280	10.1	45.2	6.1	2.7
Rolls, Part Baked, Mini, Tesco*	1 Roll/50g	120	0.6	240	7.8	49.5	1.2	3.4
Rolls, Poppy Seed, Vienna, Bakery, Tesco*	1 Roll/90g	278	5.1	309	10.3	52.8	5.7	2.5
Rolls, Poppy Seeded Knot, Waitrose*	1 Roll/60g	169	3.2	282	10.3	48.3	5.3	2.2
Rolls, Pumpkin Seed, Lidl*	1 Roll/80g	271	9	339	15	42.5	11.2	3.8
Rolls, Rye, Toasting, Good & Hot*	1 Roll/65g	143	0.7	220	7.3	44.6	1.1	7.1
Rolls, Scottish Morning, Morrisons*	1 Roll/60g	157	1.3	261	11.3	51.4	2.2	2.4
Rolls, Seed Sensations, Deli, Hovis*	1 Roll/70g	184	6	263	10.3	36.5	8.5	10.6
Rolls, Seeded, Deli, Rowan Hill Bakery, Lidl*	1 Roll/75g	243	8.2	324	11.4	42.2	11	5.4
Rolls, Seeded, Mixed Mini Loaf Pack, M&S*	1 Roll/76g	220	7.3	290	10.6	39.7	9.6	4
Rolls, Seeded, Oval Bite, Gregg's *	1 Roll/79g	220	4.5	278	10.1	44.3	5.7	0
Rolls, Seeded, Sandwich, Warburton's*	1 Roll/77g	242	6.7	314	13.3	41.2	8.7	6
Rolls, Seeded, Soft, GF, Newburn, Warburton's*	1 Roll/65g	176	6.2	270	9	33.8	9.5	6.7
Rolls, Seeded, Three Seeds, Sandwich, Warburton's*	1 Roll/77g	242	6.7	314	13.3	41.2	8.7	6
Rolls, Snack, Mini, Tesco*	1 Roll/35g	95	2.1	271	19	43	6	4
Rolls, Soft, White, Rowan Hill Bakery, Lidl*	1 Roll/66g	157	1.6	238	8.5	44	2.5	2.8
Rolls, Soft, Wholemeal, Finger, M&S*	1 Roll/66g	145	1.3	220	12.6	38	2	5.8
Rolls, Stone Baked, Bakery Instore, Lidl*	1 Roll/100g	292	1.5	292	9.5	58.4	1.5	3.5
Rolls, Sub, White, Batch, Warburton's*	1 Roll/80g	215	3.5	269	11	45	4.4	2.4
Rolls, Sub, Wholemeal, Warburton's*	1 Roll/94g	231	4.1	246	10.9	40.6	4.4	6.3
Rolls, Submarine, Sainsbury's*	1 Roll/117g	305	4.6	261	9.1	47.4	3.9	2.4
Rolls, Sun Dried Tomato, Homebake, Tesco*	1 Roll/50g	123	1.5	246	11.3	44	3	0
Rolls, Sunflower Seed, Toasting, Good & Hot*	1 Roll/65g	162	3.2	250	8.5	41	5	8
Rolls, Tiger, Crusty, Baked by Us, Morrisons*	1 Roll/63g	143	1.8	227	6.3	46	2.9	2.5
Rolls, Tomato & Basil, Sub, COU, M&S*	1 Roll/33g	86	0.9	265	11	48.7	2.7	2.4
Rolls, Triple Seeded, Genius *	1 Roll/75g	242	9.8	322	5.6	38	13	7.1
Rolls, White with Mixed Seeds & Bran, Wheatfield Bakery*	1 Roll/76g	190	3.9	250	8.5	41.6	5.1	6.1
Rolls, White, 4 Pack, Warburton's*	1 Roll/58g	145	2.5	253	9.7	42.6	4.3	2.4
Rolls, White, 50/50, Soft, Kingsmill*	1 Roll/63g	154	2.4	245	9.3	41.2	3.8	4.4
Rolls, White, Basics, Somerfield*	1 Roll/44g	107	0.7	243	8.9	48.2	1.6	2.1
Rolls, White, BGTY, Sainsbury's*	1 Roll/50g	114	0.5	227	9.1	45.3	1	3
Rolls, White, Cheese Topped, Asda*	1 Roll/46g	121	2	264	10	46	4.4	2
Rolls, White, Cheese Topped, Sainsbury's*	1 Roll/75g	218	6.4	291	12.1	41.6	8.5	2
Rolls, White, Chunky, Hovis*	1 Roll/73g	173	2.4	237	9.4	41.7	3.3	2.5
Rolls, White, Crusty, Average	***1 Roll/50g***	***140***	***1.2***	***280***	***10.9***	***57.6***	***2.3***	***1.5***
Rolls, White, Crusty, Home Bake, Tesco*	1 Roll/68.5g	185	1	270	9.3	54.2	1.4	2.9
Rolls, White, Crusty, Morning, M&S*	1 Roll/65g	176	0.8	270	8.8	53.8	1.3	2.7
Rolls, White, Dinner, Village Bakery, Aldi*	1 Roll/70g	183	0.9	262	8.8	52	1.3	3

BREAD

	Measure INFO/WEIGHT	per Measure KCAL	per Measure FAT	Nutrition Values per 100g / 100ml KCAL	PROT	CARB	FAT	FIBRE
Rolls, White, Finger, Smart Price, Asda*	1 Roll/50g	121	0.8	242	9	48	1.6	2.1
Rolls, White, Finger, Tesco*	1 Roll/68g	170	2.4	250	8.5	45.8	3.5	2.1
Rolls, White, Finger, Value, Tesco*	1 Roll/50g	116	1	232	8.7	45	1.9	2.2
Rolls, White, Floured, Batch, Tesco*	1 Roll/76g	193	2.5	254	8.8	47.3	3.3	2.2
Rolls, White, Floury Batch, Sainsbury's*	1 Roll/68g	168	1.9	247	8.3	47.2	2.8	2.2
Rolls, White, Floury, Roberts Bakery*	1 Roll/63g	160	1.6	254	8.4	49.5	2.5	2
Rolls, White, Hot Dog, Jumbo, Sainsbury's*	1 Roll/85g	239	5.2	281	7.5	49.1	6.1	2.9
Rolls, White, Hot Dog, Tesco*	1 Roll/65g	169	2.4	260	9.6	46.1	3.7	3.2
Rolls, White, Large, Warburton's*	1 Roll/88g	229	3.1	259	10.2	44.3	3.5	2.5
Rolls, White, Low Price, Sainsbury's*	1 Roll/44g	107	0.7	243	8.9	48.2	1.6	2.1
Rolls, White, Mini, Submarine, M&S*	1 Roll/30g	86	1.5	285	11.4	47.7	4.9	1.1
Rolls, White, Morning, Co-Op*	1 Roll/47g	134	1.4	285	12	53	3	2
Rolls, White, Old Fashioned, Waitrose*	1 Roll/64g	176	2.9	275	8.8	49.8	4.5	2.8
Rolls, White, Organic, Sainsbury's*	1 Roll/65g	170	2	262	8.7	49.9	3	1
Rolls, White, Part Baked, Morrisons*	1 Roll/75g	227	1	303	9.6	63	1.4	2.6
Rolls, White, Ploughman's, Sainsbury's*	1 Roll/65g	185	2.5	285	8.6	54.1	3.8	2.3
Rolls, White, Premium Soft, Rathbones*	1 Roll/65g	190	3.9	293	9.3	50.3	6	2.7
Rolls, White, Premium, Brown Hill Bakery*	1 Roll/74g	206	2.2	279	11	51.5	3	2.3
Rolls, White, Premium, Hovis*	1 Roll/70g	180	3.1	257	9.5	44.8	4.4	3
Rolls, White, Scottish, Tesco*	1 Roll/48g	117	1.2	243	10.4	44.8	2.5	4.7
Rolls, White, Seeded, Sainsbury's*	1 Roll/80g	217	4.7	271	10.9	43.4	5.9	4.8
Rolls, White, Seeded, Soft, M&S*	1 Roll/75g	214	4.3	285	11.7	46.2	5.7	2.8
Rolls, White, Sliced, Warburton's*	1 Roll/55g	145	2.5	263	9.7	44.6	4.5	2.4
Rolls, White, Snack, Sainsbury's*	1 Roll/67g	159	0.7	237	7.9	49.2	1	2.3
Rolls, White, Soft, Average	*1 Sm Roll/45g*	*114*	*1.5*	*253*	*9.2*	*46.5*	*3.3*	*2.2*
Rolls, White, Soft, COU, M&S*	1 Roll/37g	94	1	255	10.7	47.1	2.7	1.5
Rolls, White, Soft, Dietary Specials*	1 Roll/75g	130	2.9	172	2.2	29.8	3.8	4.7
Rolls, White, Soft, Farmhouse, TTD, Sainsbury's*	1 Slice/47g	111	0.8	235	8.1	45.4	1.7	2.9
Rolls, White, Soft, GF, Newburn Bakehouse, Warburton's*	1 Roll/65g	159	4	244	7.3	37.1	6.2	5.4
Rolls, White, Soft, Hovis*	1 Roll/70g	180	3.1	257	9.5	44.8	4.4	3
Rolls, White, Soft, Kingsmill*	1 Roll/62g	156	1.7	252	8.9	46.7	2.8	2.4
Rolls, White, Soft, M&S*	1 Roll/60g	150	1.9	250	10.3	45.2	3.1	2.7
Rolls, White, Soft, Morrisons*	1 Roll/42g	100	0.8	238	9.1	46.4	1.9	2.4
Rolls, White, Soft, Tesco*	1 Roll/72g	175	1.8	243	7.6	46.7	2.5	2.8
Rolls, White, Softgrain, GFY, Asda*	1 Roll/54g	128	1	237	9	46	1.9	2.9
Rolls, White, Split, Asda*	1 Roll/45g	113	1.5	251	10	45	3.4	2.8
Rolls, White, Submarine, M&S*	1 Roll/109g	300	5.4	275	11	47	5	1
Rolls, White, Super Soft, Bakers Selection, Asda*	1 Roll/64g	173	2.9	272	7.5	49	4.6	2.5
Rolls, White, Tesco*	1 Roll/65g	180	2.5	277	8.7	52	3.8	2.7
Rolls, White, Tesco*	1 Roll/30g	79	0.7	262	9.7	50.5	2.3	2.9
Rolls, Wholemeal	*1 Roll/45g*	*108*	*1.3*	*241*	*9*	*48.3*	*2.9*	*5.9*
Rolls, Wholemeal & White, Kingsmill*	1 Roll/60g	151	2.5	251	9.5	43.7	4.2	3.5
Rolls, Wholemeal with Cracked Wheat, Allinson*	1 Roll/58g	134	2.3	231	11	38	3.9	7
Rolls, Wholemeal, Asda*	1 Roll/58g	130	1.6	225	11	39	2.8	6
Rolls, Wholemeal, COU, M&S*	1 Roll/110g	226	3.1	205	11.3	33.4	2.8	7.1
Rolls, Wholemeal, Deli, Tesco*	1 Serving/65g	156	3.1	240	9	40.2	4.8	5.7
Rolls, Wholemeal, Finest, Tesco*	1 Roll/75g	182	2.6	243	11.3	39	3.4	5.9
Rolls, Wholemeal, Finger, Six, Bakers Selection, Asda*	1 Roll/49g	112	0.7	228	9.5	41	1.4	6.6
Rolls, Wholemeal, Floury Batch, Sainsbury's*	1 Roll/68g	152	2.3	223	9.9	37.8	3.4	6.5
Rolls, Wholemeal, Golden, Hovis*	1 Roll/50g	112	2	223	10.5	36.5	3.9	6.8
Rolls, Wholemeal, High Protein, High Fibre, Warburton's*	1 Roll/68g	156	2.9	229	14	30	4.2	7.7
Rolls, Wholemeal, HL, Tesco*	1 Roll/67.5g	155	1.4	230	10.4	41.3	2.1	6.6
Rolls, Wholemeal, Mini, Assorted, Waitrose*	1 Roll/35g	86	2.1	244	9.7	37.9	6	7.3

	Measure INFO/WEIGHT	per Measure KCAL	FAT	Nutrition Values per 100g / 100ml KCAL	PROT	CARB	FAT	FIBRE

BREAD

	Measure INFO/WEIGHT	per Measure KCAL	FAT	KCAL	PROT	CARB	FAT	FIBRE
Rolls, Wholemeal, Morrisons*	1 Roll/67g	155	2.7	231	10.2	38.6	4	6.3
Rolls, Wholemeal, Oat Topped, Deli, Tesco*	1 Roll/65g	170	3.5	260	10.9	38.3	5.3	6.7
Rolls, Wholemeal, Oat Topped, Tesco*	1 Roll/65g	166	2.9	255	11.3	42.2	4.5	5.1
Rolls, Wholemeal, Oatbran, HL, Tesco*	1 Roll/56g	115	1.4	205	11.4	33.6	2.5	7.4
Rolls, Wholemeal, Old Fashioned, Waitrose*	1 Roll/57g	135	2.7	236	11.1	37.2	4.8	6.6
Rolls, Wholemeal, Organic, Sainsbury's*	1 Roll/66g	152	1.8	230	10.7	41	2.7	6.6
Rolls, Wholemeal, Organic, Tesco*	1 Roll/65g	177	4	273	10.3	44.1	6.2	5.5
Rolls, Wholemeal, Sainsbury's*	1 Roll/65g	153	2.1	236	10.7	40.8	3.3	7.4
Rolls, Wholemeal, Seeded, The Country Miller, Waitrose*	1 Roll/74.5g	190	7.7	255	13.6	26.9	10.3	7.6
Rolls, Wholemeal, Sliced, Hovis*	1 Roll/60g	150	3.5	250	10.6	38.7	5.9	6.8
Rolls, Wholemeal, Sliced, Sandwich, Warburton's*	1 Roll/56g	130	2.2	233	10.5	35.8	3.9	6.6
Rolls, Wholemeal, Soft, Average	**1 Roll/65g**	**151**	**2.7**	**233**	**10.8**	**37.3**	**4.1**	**6.3**
Rolls, Wholemeal, Soft, Batch Baked, Warburton's*	1 Roll/65g	158	2.1	245	10.7	37.3	3.2	6.1
Rolls, Wholemeal, Soft, Sainsbury's*	1 Roll/60g	133	2	221	9.9	37.8	3.4	6.5
Rolls, Wholemeal, Soft, Seeded, Sainsbury's*	1 Roll/75g	193	5.6	257	11.8	35.6	7.4	6.2
Rolls, Wholemeal, Submarine, Tesco*	1 Roll/100g	221	3.1	221	9.3	39	3.1	5.2
Rolls, Wholemeal, Submarine, Wheatfield Bakery*	1 Roll/100g	230	3.4	230	10.4	39	3.4	6.2
Rolls, Wholemeal, Sunflower & Honey, Sainsbury's*	1 Roll/85g	225	4.3	265	9.2	45.4	5.1	4.5
Rolls, Wholemeal, Super Soft, Bakers Selection, Asda*	1 Roll/65g	181	2.5	280	9.8	48	3.9	6.9
Rolls, Wholemeal, Tasty, Kingsmill*	1 Roll/68g	171	2.5	251	10.7	39.1	3.7	6.5
Rolls, Wholemeal, Tesco*	1 Roll/46g	115	1.8	250	10.9	41.8	4	7.5
Rolls, Wholemeal, The Best, Morrisons*	1 Roll/72g	174	2.1	242	10.5	39.7	2.9	7.6
Rolls, Wholemeal, Village Bakery, Aldi*	1 Roll/63g	144	0.9	228	10	40	1.5	5.3
Rolls, Wholmeal, Deli, Tesco*	1 Roll/65g	156	3.1	240	9	40.2	4.8	5.7
Roti, Tesco*	1 Bread/95g	256	5.2	269	8.4	46.4	5.5	3.2
Rye, & Flax, Organic, Profusion*	1 Slice/50g	120	4.4	241	20.1	14.4	8.9	11.4
Rye, Artisan Bread Organic*	1 Slice/50g	80	0.7	160	5	28.4	1.4	7.1
Rye, Average	**1 Slice/25g**	**55**	**0.4**	**219**	**8.3**	**45.8**	**1.7**	**4.4**
Rye, Dark, Sliced, Trianon*	1 Slice/41g	74	0.6	180	6.5	35	1.5	0
Rye, German Style, Bolletje*	1 Slice/60g	114	1.2	190	6	35	2	9.5
Rye, German Style, Kelderman*	1 Slice/64g	122	1.3	190	6	35	2	9.5
Rye, German Style, Loaf, Bakery in Store, M&S*	2 Slices/50g	112	0.6	225	9.5	40.8	1.1	6.3
Rye, Light, Finest, Tesco*	1 Slice/20g	47	0.4	237	10.4	44.3	2	3.7
Rye, Organic with Coriander, Village Bakery*	1 Thin Slice/30g	63	0.8	209	4.9	49.9	2.7	8.5
Rye, Seeded, Organic, The Village Bakery*	1 Slice/50g	107	1.6	214	5	37.8	3.2	7.2
Rye, Swedish Style, Kelderman*	1 Slice/50g	92	1.6	185	7.2	31.5	3.2	4.3
Rye, Vitality, Organic, Biona*	1 Slice/71g	147	1.4	207	5.3	37	2	9.9
Rye, Wholegrain , Sliced, Rowan Hill Bakery, Lidl*	1 Slice/56g	118	1	210	5.8	38	1.8	9.3
Rye, Wholegrain, with Sunflower Seeds, Rowan Hill*	1 Slice/56g	126	2.6	225	6.3	35	4.6	9.3
Rye, Wholemeal with Sunflower Seeds, Organic, Biona*	1 Slice/72g	150	2.9	210	7	36	4	6
Rye, Wholemeal, Organic, House Of Westphalia*	1 Slice/71g	131	0.9	184	4.5	34.2	1.2	9.2
Rye, with Pumpkin Seed, Organic, Lindale*	1 Slice/71g	150	2.9	211	6.1	32.1	4.1	10.6
Rye, with Seeds, Organic, The Village Bakery Melmerby*	1 Slice/42g	80	1	190	6.9	35.6	2.3	9.4
Rye, with Sprouted Seeds, Yeast Free, Biona Organic*	1 Slice/35g	71	0.7	204	5.3	36.6	2	9.9
Rye, with Sunflower Seeds, Organic, Schneider Brot*	1 Slice/72g	138	2.6	191	6.2	33.4	3.6	7.9
Rye, with Sunflower Seeds, Organic, Sunnyvale*	1 Slice/25g	50	1.6	198	5.1	30.3	6.3	7.9
Sandwich Thins, 50/50, Kingsmill*	1 Thin/37g	99	1	266	10.6	46.2	2.8	5.2
Sandwich Thins, Brown, Warburton's*	1 Thin/42g	100	1.1	239	9.9	48	2.6	5.4
Sandwich Thins, Seeded, Free From, Tesco*	1 Thin/50g	125	3.8	250	7.8	32.3	7.6	10.8
Sandwich Thins, Seeded, GF, Warburton's*	1 Thin/43g	122	3.5	284	6.5	43.1	8.1	6.5
Sandwich Thins, White, CBY, Asda*	1 Thin/55g	141	2.2	257	9.3	44.3	4	3.1
Sandwich Thins, White, GF, Warburton's*	1 Thin/58g	143	3.7	247	6	38.7	6.3	5.7
Sandwich Thins, White, Kingsmill*	1 Thin/40g	99	1	248	9.4	45.6	2.5	2.9

BREAD

INFO/WEIGHT	Measure	per Measure KCAL	FAT	Nutrition Values per 100g / 100ml KCAL	PROT	CARB	FAT	FIBRE
Sandwich Thins, White, Warburton's*	1 Thin/42g	100	1	239	9.2	47.1	2.5	3.8
Sandwich Thins, Wholemeal, Good Inside, Hovis*	1 Thin/45g	114	2.3	254	11.1	37.5	5.2	7.1
Sandwich Thins, Wholemeal, Kingsmill*	1 Thin/41g	98	1.2	240	10.3	39.8	3	6.1
Sandwich Thins, Wholemeal, Protein & Fibre, Warburton's*	1 Thin/50g	121	2.8	241	14.7	29.6	5.5	7.3
Seeded Farmhouse, Organic, Cranks*	2 Slices/94g	232	3.5	247	10.1	39.9	3.7	6.9
Seeded, Batch, Finest, Tesco*	1 Slice/65g	168	4	259	9.3	41.8	6.1	6.1
Seeded, Farmhouse, GF, Warburton's*	1 Slice/35g	92	3.2	262	8.7	33	9.1	6.5
Seeded, Farmhouse, Loaf, Extra Special, Asda*	1 Slice/44.4g	92	0.5	207	11	38	1.2	8
Seeded, Farmhouse, Roberts Bakery*	1 Slice/37g	89	1.1	240	10.6	49	2.9	6.7
Seeded, Free From, Gluten, Wheat, & Milk, Tesco*	1 Slice/42g	95	3.7	227	7	25.7	8.8	8.7
Seeded, Free From, Tesco*	1 Slice/42g	90	3.3	214	6.4	24.8	7.9	9.2
Seeded, Med Sliced, Average	*1 Slice/44g*	*116*	*2.9*	*262*	*11.3*	*38.6*	*6.5*	*5.6*
Seeded, Mighty, GF, Mini Loaf, Warburton's*	1 Slice/27g	75	2.9	277	7.7	33.5	10.9	7
Seeded, Rye, Loaf, la Brea Bakery*	1 Slice/55g	120	0.6	218	7	42.5	1	5.7
Seriously Seeded, Gold, Kingsmill*	1 Slice/50g	136	3.4	272	10.9	41.6	6.9	6.4
Sesame Seed, la Brea Bakery*	1 Slice/35g	85	0.8	244	8.8	47.1	2.3	2
Soda	*1oz/28g*	*72*	*0.7*	*258*	*7.7*	*54.6*	*2.5*	*2.1*
Soda Farls, M&S*	1 Farl/110g	267	3	243	9.6	50.1	2.7	2.3
Soda Farls, Tesco*	1 Farl/142g	325	4.5	229	7.1	42.2	3.2	2.6
Soda, Fruit, M&S*	1 Slice/40g	105	1.9	260	5.9	51.3	4.6	2.5
Soda, M&S*	1 Slice/40g	82	0.6	205	8.7	39.2	1.6	4.2
Softgrain, Med Sliced, GFY, Asda*	1 Slice/35g	79	0.5	226	7	46	1.5	3.7
Softgrain, Mighty White*	1 Slice/36g	81	0.5	224	7.2	45.5	1.5	3.7
Sourdough, Bloomer, Bakery, Tesco*	1 Serving/80g	190	1.4	238	8.1	46.2	1.7	2.7
Sourdough, Average	*1 Med Slice/50g*	*144*	*0.9*	*289*	*11.8*	*56.4*	*1.8*	*2.4*
Sourdough, Loaf, Finest, Tesco*	1 Slice/33g	86	1.8	262	9.6	41.9	5.5	3.3
Sourdough, White, Cob, Free From, Tesco*	1 Slice/50g	92	1.4	184	5.1	31	2.7	7.4
Soy & Linseed, 500g Loaf, Burgen*	1 Slice/42g	117	3.9	278	7.8	37.8	9.3	5.7
Soya & Linseed, Vogel*	1 Slice/42g	95	2.1	227	11.7	34.1	4.9	6.8
Spelt, & Seed, Sliced, Lifefibre*	1 Slice/42g	141	5.8	335	11.6	32.2	13.7	9.2
Spelt, Healthguard, T & W Bakeries*	1 Slice/40g	80	0.7	201	6.2	36.5	1.7	7.2
Spinach, & Goats Cheese, Twist, Waitrose*	1 Twist/45g	114	2.9	253	11.8	34.7	6.5	4.3
Sprouted Grain, Ezekiel *	1 Slice/34g	80	0.5	235	11.8	44.1	1.5	0.9
Sprouted Spelt with Raisins, Everfresh Bakery*	¼ Loaf/100g	230	1.9	230	9.2	43.9	1.9	6.6
Stoneground, Sm Loaf, Organic, Sainsbury's*	1 Slice/24g	50	0.5	208	10	37.9	2.1	7.9
Stoneground, Wholemeal, Thick, Love Life, Waitrose*	1 Slice/40g	86	1.1	214	10.1	36.5	2.8	7.9
Sunflower & Honey, M&S*	1 Serving/67g	206	9	308	12.9	34	13.4	5.6
Sunflower & Honey, Organic, Cranks*	1 Slice/30g	64	0.9	215	11.6	37.2	3	8.3
Sunflower & Pumpkin Seed, Batched, Organic, Tesco*	1 Slice/30g	73	2.2	243	11	33.1	7.4	5.2
Sunflower & Pumpkin Seed, So Organic, Sainsbury's*	1 Slice/30g	76	1.6	254	11.4	40	5.4	12.9
Sunflower & Pumpkin, Cob, Sliced, Finest, Tesco*	1 Slice/40g	120	4.4	299	12.3	34.7	10.9	6.6
Sunflower Seed, Bolletje, Delhaize*	1 Slice/44g	106	3.1	240	7.5	35	7	6
Sunflower Seed, Organic, Natural, Mestemacher*	1 Slice/75g	162	3	216	5.6	34.7	4	9.4
Sunflower, Bakers Selection, Asda*	1 Slice/60g	162	5.9	270	11.3	50	9.8	8.3
Sunflower, Multi-Grain, Allinson*	1 Slice/47g	113	2.2	240	9.8	39.6	4.7	3.9
Tandoori Rustic Marble, Graze*	1 Punnet/36g	117	5	324	8.7	41.2	13.8	4.8
Ten Seed, Organic, The Village Bakery*	1 Slice/25g	66	1.4	263	9	43.8	5.7	3.8
The Really Seeded One, Kingsmill*	1 Slice/44g	118	3.2	268	10.4	37.3	7.3	5.5
The White, Toastie, Loved by Us, Co-Op*	1 Slice/50g	120	1.2	240	7.9	45.4	2.4	2.6
Thins, Seeded, Kingsmill*	1 Thin/40g	106	1.8	264	9.6	43.6	4.6	4.8
Three Cheese, Bloomer, Bakery, Tesco*	1 Slice/30g	77	1.8	257	12.8	36.9	6	1.9
Three Grain, Organic, Schneider Brot*	1 Slice/72g	142	1.6	199	5.3	34.5	2.3	9.3
Tiger Baton, Bakery, Tesco*	½ Baton/100g	299	3.6	299	9.2	56.5	3.6	2

B

BREAD

INFO/WEIGHT	Measure	per Measure KCAL	FAT	Nutrition Values per 100g / 100ml KCAL	PROT	CARB	FAT	FIBRE
Tiger Loaf, Bloomer, Bakery, Tesco*	1 Slice/50g	133	1.6	266	8.4	49.2	3.2	3.2
Tiger, White, Warburton's*	1 Slice/32g	90	0.7	280	10.1	52	2.3	2.9
Toaster, White, Rathbones*	1 Slice/38g	92	0.5	243	9.1	48.6	1.3	2.3
Toastie Pockets, Brown, Easy Fill, Warburtons*	1 Pocket/55g	134	1.6	243	9.8	42.2	3	4.2
Tomato & Garlic, Italian Style, Morrisons*	½ Pack/155g	355	12.4	229	5.8	33.4	8	2.5
Tomato & Chilli, BGTY, Sainsbury's*	¼ Bread/65g	155	3.1	238	11.9	36.9	4.7	2.8
Tomato & Herb, Tear & Share, Tesco*	¼ Pack/73g	164	3.2	226	6.3	40.2	4.4	2.1
Tortilla, Flour, Soft, Mini, Stand n Stuff, Old El Paso*	1 Tortilla/12g	36	0.6	296	8.5	52.5	5.2	2.7
Tortilla, Flour, Stand n Stuff, Old El Paso*	1 Tortilla/24g	71	1.2	296	8.5	52.5	5.2	2.7
Tortilla, Whole Wheat, Stand n Stuff, Old El Paso*	1 Tortilla/24g	71	1.2	294	8.9	50.3	5.2	6
Veda Malt, St Michael*	1 Serving/45g	99	0.5	219	7.1	45.3	1.1	2.2
Walnut, Waitrose*	1/8 Loaf/50g	170	7.6	339	10	40.6	15.2	5.9
Wheat	*1 Slice/25g*	*65*	*1*	*260*	*9.1*	*47.2*	*4.1*	*4.3*
Wheat, & Wholemeal Spelt, & Seeds, Love Life, Waitrose*	1 Slice/34g	88	2.6	267	10.5	33.5	7.9	9.9
Wheat, Golden, Warburton's*	1 Slice/40g	100	1	249	9.4	45.2	2.4	4.3
Wheat, Spelt, & Rye, Loaf, Baked by Us, Morrisons*	1 Serving/70g	165	1.4	236	11.3	39.9	2	6.6
Wheat, Tasty, Kingsmill*	1 Serving/38g	84	1.3	221	10.1	37.6	3.4	6.8
Wheaten Loaf, Sliced, No Added Sugar, Genesis Crafty*	1 Slice/40g	86	1	214	7.5	40.2	2.6	3.6
Wheaten, Big Slice	*1 Slice/65g*	*139*	*1.7*	*214*	*7.5*	*40.2*	*2.6*	*3.6*
Wheaten, Loaf, Sliced, Genesis*	1 Slice/40g	86	1	214	7.5	40.2	2.6	3.6
Wheaten, M&S*	1 Slice/33g	74	1.2	225	9.3	42.9	3.5	3.9
Wheaten, Sliced, Healthy, Irwin's Bakery*	1 Slice/40g	76	0.8	190	9	40.5	1.9	6.2
Wheatgerm, Hovis, Soft, Sliced, M&S*	1 Slice/23g	50	0.7	220	10.1	38.5	3	4.6
White Loaf, Gluten & Wheat Free, Lovemore*	1 Serving/35g	111	3.8	316	0	3.4	10.9	0
White, Average	*1 Thick Slice/40g*	*94*	*0.8*	*235*	*8.4*	*49.3*	*1.9*	*1.5*
White, Batch Loaf, Extra Special, Asda*	1 Slice/47g	109	0.9	233	9	45	1.9	2.2
White, Batch, Warburton's*	1 Slice/42g	98	0.9	233	9.8	43.6	2.1	2.7
White, Baton, Bakery, Tesco*	½ Baton/100g	276	0.8	276	9.3	56.7	0.8	2.6
White, Ciabatta, Roll, GF, Dietary Specials*	1 Roll/50g	106	0.9	213	4.1	40.9	1.8	8.3
White, Classic, Med Sliced, Hovis*	1 Slice/38g	91	0.9	240	11.4	40.3	2.3	2.5
White, Classic, Thick Sliced, Hovis*	1 Slice/50g	120	2.2	240	9.2	40.5	4.5	3.1
White, Commercially Prepared, Average	*1oz/28g*	*74*	*0.9*	*266*	*7.6*	*50.6*	*3.3*	*2.4*
White, Commercially Prepared, Toasted, Average	*1oz/28g*	*82*	*1.1*	*293*	*9*	*54.4*	*4*	*2.5*
White, Country Maid*	1 Slice/33g	76	0.7	229	8.5	44.1	2.1	3
White, Crusty, Fresh, Finest, Tesco*	1 Slice/52g	130	1	250	8.6	48.5	1.9	2.4
White, Crusty, Gold, Kingsmill*	1 Slice/27g	70	0.8	258	9.4	48.5	2.9	2.7
White, Crusty, Hovis*	1 Slice/44g	103	1	233	8.8	44.3	2.2	2.1
White, Crusty, Premium, Warburton's*	1 Slice/31g	77	0.7	254	10.6	46.5	2.3	2.6
White, Crusty, Sliced Loaf, Tesco*	1 Slice/50g	116	1	233	7.4	46	2.1	2
White, Crusty, Sliced, Premium, Budgens*	1 Slice/50g	121	1.1	242	8.8	46.9	2.2	2.2
White, Crusty, Split Tin, Bakery, Tesco*	1 Slice/50g	134	0.8	268	9.4	52.6	1.5	3.3
White, Danish Style, Thick Sliced, Light, Tesco*	1 Slice/21.5g	55	0.6	255	9.4	47.3	2.9	2.7
White, Danish, Lighter, Warburton's*	1 Slice/26g	63	0.3	243	10.5	45.8	1.2	2.6
White, Danish, Med Sliced, BFY, Morrisons*	1 Slice/17g	42	0.3	245	10.2	49.1	1.8	2.2
White, Danish, Med Sliced, Soft, Somerfield*	1 Slice/21g	48	0.3	229	8.6	44.8	1.4	2.4
White, Danish, Med Sliced, Tesco*	1 Slice/20g	47	0.3	234	9.4	45.4	1.7	3.3
White, Danish, Soft & Light, Thick Cut, Asda*	1 Slice/26g	60	0.4	230	9	45	1.6	2.1
White, Danish, Soft, Weight Watchers, Warburton's*	1 Slice/21g	50	0.3	243	9.8	46.5	1.3	2.9
White, Danish, Thick Sliced, Tesco*	1 Slice/24g	60	0.6	250	9.7	47.4	2.3	2.9
White, Extra Thick Sliced, Kingsmill*	1 Slice/58g	135	1.4	232	8.8	43.8	2.4	2.8
White, Farmhouse Crusty, M&S*	1 Slice/34g	82	0.7	240	8.9	46.6	2.2	3
White, Farmhouse Gold Premium, Morrisons*	1 Slice/38g	90	0.5	236	8.9	47.4	1.2	2.2
White, Farmhouse, GF, Newburn, Warburton's*	1 Slice/35g	83	2.1	236	6.8	35.6	6.1	5.5

BREAD

INFO/WEIGHT	Measure	per Measure KCAL	FAT	Nutrition Values per 100g / 100ml KCAL	PROT	CARB	FAT	FIBRE
White, Farmhouse, Hovis*	1 Thick Slice/44g	103	1	234	8.7	44.6	2.3	2.4
White, Farmhouse, Seeded, Waitrose*	1 Serving/75g	192	4.1	256	10.8	40.9	5.5	5.6
White, Farmhouse, Sliced, Bakery, Tesco*	1 Slice/50g	130	0.6	259	9.4	51.1	1.2	3.3
White, Farmhouse, Soft, 400g Loaf, Warburton's*	1 Slice/27g	66	0.7	245	10.1	43.7	2.6	2.8
White, Farmhouse, Soft, 800g Loaf, Warburton's*	1 Slice/43g	103	1.1	241	9.9	43.4	2.5	2.7
White, Fibre, Morrisons*	1 Slice/40g	96	0.7	240	8	48.4	1.7	0.3
White, Fried in Blended Oil	*1 Slice/28g*	*141*	*9*	*503*	*7.9*	*48.5*	*32.2*	*1.6*
White, Gluten & Wheat Free, Free From, Sainsbury's*	1 Slice/33g	75	2.8	227	1.9	35.5	8.6	1
White, Gold Seeded, Kingsmill*	1 Slice/44g	108	2.5	245	9.7	38.8	5.7	3.5
White, Golden, Square Cut, M&S*	1 Slice/40g	85	0.8	215	8.9	40.7	2.1	6.1
White, Harvest Crust Premium, Ormo*	1 Slice/40g	92	0.6	229	9.4	47.4	1.5	2.7
White, Invisible Crust, Hovis*	1 Slice/40g	90	0.6	226	8.8	44.1	1.6	2.4
White, Loaf, Danish, Asda*	1 Serving/23g	53	0.5	236	9	45	2.2	2
White, Low Carb, Sliced, Tesco*	1 Slice/16g	35	0.4	211	11.3	36.4	2.2	6.9
White, Med Sliced, Asda*	1 Slice/36.7g	80	0.6	218	8	43	1.5	3.3
White, Med Sliced, Average	*1 Slice/39g*	*93*	*0.6*	*238*	*7.5*	*48.5*	*1.6*	*1.8*
White, Med Sliced, Basics, Sainsbury's*	1 Slice/36g	83	0.5	231	8	46.4	1.5	2.1
White, Med Sliced, Brace's*	1 Slice/32g	75	0.4	235	9.5	46.6	1.2	2.6
White, Med Sliced, Great Everyday, Kingsmill*	1 Slice/40g	93	0.8	232	9	44.6	2	2.7
White, Med Sliced, Long Life, Asda*	1 Slice/36g	82	0.6	228	8	45	1.8	2.7
White, Med Sliced, Mother's Pride*	1 Slice/36g	82	0.6	229	8	45.6	1.6	3
White, Med Sliced, Sainsbury's*	1 Slice/36g	78	0.7	216	8.7	41.1	1.9	7.1
White, Med Sliced, Smart Price, Asda*	1 Slice/36g	81	0.5	226	7	46	1.5	2.8
White, Med Sliced, Stay Fresh, Tesco*	1 Slice/36g	88	0.7	250	8.9	47.7	2	2.9
White, Med Sliced, Superlife, Morrisons*	1 Slice/30g	79	1.2	263	9.6	47.4	3.9	2.5
White, Med Sliced, Tesco*	1 Slice/36g	86	0.5	240	8.2	47.8	1.5	3
White, Med Sliced, Value, Tesco*	1 Slice/36g	81	0.4	225	7.9	46.1	1	2.1
White, Medium, 400g Loaf, Warburton's*	1 Slice/24g	58	0.5	244	10.3	45.1	1.9	2.4
White, Medium, Round Top, Kingsmill*	1 Slice/42g	97	1	232	8.8	43.8	2.4	2.8
White, Medium, Warburton's*	1 Slice/40g	96	0.8	239	10.3	45.1	1.9	2.4
White, Mega Thick, Roberts Bakery*	1 Slice/66g	154	1.2	233	8.3	46.2	1.8	2.2
White, Mighty, GF, Mini Loaf, Warburton's*	1 Slice/27g	67	1.8	249	6.7	37.9	6.5	5.8
White, Milk Roll, Warburton's*	1 Slice/18g	47	0.5	254	11	45	2.8	2.4
White, Oaten, Rolls, Love Life, Waitrose*	1 Roll/70g	183	3.4	261	8.1	46.4	4.8	3.2
White, Old English, Warburton's*	1 Slice/40g	99	1.2	248	9.8	44.3	2.9	2.8
White, Organic, Sainsbury's*	1 Slice/36g	84	0.6	234	8.9	45.5	1.8	2.3
White, Plain, Scottish, Sunblest*	1 Slice/57g	133	1.5	233	10.1	42.3	2.6	2.8
White, Premium Farmhouse, Lidl*	1 Slice/44g	99	0.7	225	7.4	45.4	1.5	2.5
White, Premium, M&S*	1 Slice/40g	95	0.8	235	8.5	45.8	1.9	2.7
White, Sandwich, Bakery, Sainsbury's*	1 Slice/50g	121	0.3	242	10.3	49	0.6	2.9
White, Sandwich, Kingsmill*	1 Slice/42g	97	1	232	8.8	43.8	2.4	2.8
White, Scottish Plain, Mother's Pride*	1 Med Slice/50g	114	0.8	227	8.7	44.6	1.5	3
White, Sea Salt & Black Pepper, Bloomer, Bakery, Tesco*	1 Slice/50g	131	0.8	262	10.1	50.4	1.6	3
White, Seeded, Batch, Loaf, Truly Irresistible, Co-Op*	1 Slice/47g	129	3.4	275	11.6	41.1	7.2	4.3
White, Seeds, Oats, & Honey, TTD, Sainsbury's*	1 Slice/50g	154	5.4	308	12.1	36.7	10.9	7.1
White, Sliced, Free From, Tesco*	1 Slice/47g	89	1.9	190	5.2	29.7	4	7.3
White, Sliced, GF, Free From, Tesco*	1 Slice/42g	80	1.7	190	5.2	29.7	4	7.3
White, Sliced, Roberts Bakery*	1 Slice/35g	87	0.7	249	10	48	2.1	2.5
White, Sm Loaf, Classic, Hovis*	1 Slice/33g	75	0.8	228	11.4	40.3	2.3	6.5
White, Soft Batch, Sliced, Sainsbury's*	1 Slice/44.0g	102	0.8	232	8.2	45.4	1.9	2.3
White, Soft Crusty, M&S*	1 Slice/25g	64	0.6	256	9.3	49	2.5	2.4
White, Soft, Batch Loaf, Sliced, Tesco*	1 Slice/50g	116	1	233	7.5	46.1	2.1	2.1
White, Soft, Burger, Thins, Kingsmill*	1 Thin/44g	112	1.1	254	9.1	47	2.6	3

BREAD

	Measure INFO/WEIGHT	per Measure KCAL	FAT	Nutrition Values per 100g / 100ml KCAL	PROT	CARB	FAT	FIBRE
White, Soft, Farmhouse, Loaf, M&S*	1 Slice/50g	130	2	259	9.9	44.4	4	3
White, Soft, Gold, Kingsmill*	1 Slice/47g	112	1.5	239	8.2	44.5	3.1	2.7
White, Soft, Hovis*	1 Slice/40g	94	0.9	234	8.7	44.6	2.3	2.4
White, Soft, M&S*	1 Slice/47g	105	0.8	225	7.3	46.1	1.7	2.4
White, Soft, Sandwich, Loaf, BFree*	1 Slice/30g	60	0.3	200	7.7	35.7	1.1	8.4
White, Soft, Sliced, Hovis*	1 Thin Slice/25g	58	0.6	234	8.7	44.6	2.3	2.4
White, Sourdough, Country, Oval, la Brea Bakery*	1 Slice/60g	143	0.4	239	8.8	49.4	0.6	1.6
White, Sourdough, Waitrose*	1 Slice/50g	119	0.6	237	9	45.9	1.2	3.3
White, Square, Extra Thick Sliced, Hovis*	1 Slice/67g	155	1.3	231	8.5	44.7	2	2.6
White, Square, Med Sliced, Hovis*	1 Slice/40g	92	0.8	231	8.5	44.7	2	2.6
White, Square, Thick Sliced, Hovis*	1 Slice/50g	116	1	231	8.5	44.7	2	2.6
White, Superior English Quality, Thin Cut, Hovis*	1 Slice/73g	169	1.1	232	9.2	42.8	1.5	3.8
White, Thick Sliced, Bakers Gold, Asda*	1 Slice/44g	101	0.8	229	8	45	1.9	2.3
White, Thick Sliced, Brace's*	1 Slice/38g	90	0.5	235	9.5	46.6	1.2	2.6
White, Thick Sliced, Budgens*	1 Slice/40g	89	0.5	223	7.4	45.3	1.3	2.5
White, Thick Sliced, Fine Lady*	1 Slice/44g	113	0.5	254	7.8	53.1	1.2	2.3
White, Thick Sliced, Golden Sun, Lidl*	1 Slice/44g	100	0.7	228	7.5	46.1	1.5	2.4
White, Thick Sliced, Healthy, Warburton's*	1 Slice/38g	84	0.7	222	10.3	41.2	1.8	4.1
White, Thick Sliced, M&S*	1 Slice/42g	96	0.5	228	7.3	46.7	1.3	2.8
White, Thick Sliced, Organic, Tesco*	1 Slice/44g	108	0.9	245	8.5	46.8	2.1	3.1
White, Thick Sliced, Sainsbury's*	1 Slice/44g	95	0.8	216	8.7	41.1	1.9	7.1
White, Thick Sliced, Square Cut, Asda*	1 Slice/44g	101	0.7	230	8	46	1.5	2.1
White, Thick Sliced, Sunblest*	1 Slice/40g	91	0.6	228	8	45.7	1.5	2.8
White, Thick Sliced, Super Toastie, Morrisons*	1 Slice/50g	128	1.5	257	8.7	48.9	3	2.1
White, Thick Sliced, Tesco*	1 Slice/44g	106	0.7	240	8.2	47.8	1.5	3
White, Thick, So Organic, Sainsbury's*	1 Slice/44g	102	1	231	8.2	44.6	2.2	3.1
White, Thick, Super Soft, M&S*	1 Slice/48g	115	1.2	240	8.7	45.3	2.6	2.5
White, Thickest, Warburton's*	1 Slice/58g	137	1.2	239	9.9	43.8	2	2.6
White, Thin Sliced, Sainsbury's*	1 Slice/29g	66	0.4	228	7.1	46.4	1.5	2.8
White, Thin Sliced, Tesco*	1 Slice/30g	68	0.4	228	9.5	44.5	1.3	3.4
White, Toast, Gamle MÃƒ‚ lle*	1 Slice/32g	83	0.6	260	8	52	2	3
White, Toasted, Average	*1 Slice/33g*	*87*	*0.5*	*265*	*9.3*	*57.1*	*1.6*	*1.8*
White, Toastie, 400g Loaf, Warburton's*	1 Slice/29g	70	0.5	244	10.3	45.1	1.9	2.4
White, Toastie, Thick Cut, Hovis*	1 Slice/50g	115	1	230	8.5	44.8	2	2.5
White, Toastie, Thick, Love to Toast, Kingsmill*	1 Slice/50g	116	1	232	9	44.6	2	2.7
White, Toastie, Warburton's*	1 Slice/47g	113	0.9	239	9.9	43.8	2	2.6
White, Trio of Olive, Bloomer, Bakery, Tesco*	1 Serving/82g	199	4	243	6.8	41.3	4.9	3
White, Whole, Extra Thick, Kingsmill*	1 Slice/57g	130	1.4	228	9	42.3	2.5	4
White, Whole, Kingsmill*	1 Slice/38g	87	1	230	9	42.9	2.5	3.4
White, Wholesome, Loaf, Sainsbury's*	1 Serving/36g	81	0.7	224	9.4	42.5	1.8	4.4
White, Wholesome, Med Sliced, Asda*	1 Slice/35g	78	0.9	223	7	43	2.6	5
White, Wholesome, Thick Sliced, Tesco*	1 Serving/80g	177	1.5	221	10.5	40.5	1.9	4.8
Whole Seed, Cob, Crusty, Bakery, Tesco*	1 Slice/50g	179	6.1	359	13.7	45.7	12.3	5.2
Wholegrain, & Rye, Schneider Brot*	1 Slice/50g	98	0.6	197	5.9	36.6	1.2	8.2
Wholegrain, & Oats, Warburton's*	1 Slice/40g	98	1.4	245	11.7	38.8	3.5	5.9
Wholegrain, Average	*1 Thick Slice/44g*	*117*	*1.9*	*265*	*13.4*	*43.3*	*4.2*	*7.4*
Wholegrain, Batch, Finest, Tesco*	1 Slice/44g	112	1.2	254	9.8	47.7	2.7	4.2
Wholegrain, Brennans*	1 Slice/39g	79	0.6	203	9	40	1.5	4.9
Wholegrain, Med Sliced, Irish Pride*	1 Slice/38g	90	0.8	237	9.2	46.6	2.1	7.6
Wholegrain, Soft, M&S*	1 Slice/51g	115	2.8	225	13	31.2	5.4	8.2
Wholegrain, Toasted, Average	*1 Thick Slice/40g*	*117*	*1.9*	*288*	*14.5*	*47.1*	*4.6*	*8.1*
Wholegrain, with Sunflower Seeds, Landgut*	1 Slice/83g	183	4.2	221	7	37	5	29
Wholemeal & Oat, Loaf, Vogel*	1 Slice/42g	86	0.6	205	8.7	34.3	1.5	9.7

BREAD

INFO/WEIGHT	Measure	per Measure KCAL	FAT	Nutrition Values per 100g / 100ml KCAL	PROT	CARB	FAT	FIBRE
Wholemeal & Tasty Spelt, Sliced, Hovis*	1 Slice/47g	108	1	230	11.1	38.4	2.1	6.7
Wholemeal Loaf, British Farmers, Hovis*	1 Slice/47g	108	1.3	229	10	37.9	2.8	6.8
Wholemeal Oatbran, Sliced, Tesco*	1 Slice/45g	90	0.7	200	10.1	35.3	1.6	7.4
Wholemeal, & Oat Flakes, Gold, Kingsmill*	1 Slice/47g	103	1.6	220	10	37.3	3.4	7
Wholemeal, & Rye, Farmhouse,, Extra Special, Asda*	1 Slice/50g	112	1.2	225	11	36	2.5	7.3
Wholemeal, 7 Seed Sensation, Hovis*	1 Slice/44g	109	2.5	249	11.9	31.4	5.6	12.4
Wholemeal, 7 Seeded, Irwin's Bakery*	1 Slice/38g	90	2	237	9.5	33.4	5.2	9.4
Wholemeal, American Sandwich, Harry's*	1 Slice/43g	110	2.1	259	9	45	5	5
Wholemeal, Average	*1 Thick Slice/40g*	*88*	*1*	*215*	*9.2*	*41.6*	*2.5*	*5.8*
Wholemeal, Baker`s Soft, Medium, Tesco*	1 Slice/40g	94	1.1	235	10.8	37.8	2.8	6.9
Wholemeal, Batch, Sliced, Organic, Duchy, Waitrose*	1 Slice/50g	121	1.2	242	10.2	41.8	2.3	6.8
Wholemeal, BGTY, Sainsbury's*	1 Slice/20g	41	0.2	207	12.6	36.8	1	7.3
Wholemeal, Brennans*	1 Slice/33g	78	1.4	236	11.2	38.4	4.2	7.7
Wholemeal, Brown, Med Sliced, 400g, Hovis*	1 Slice/29g	64	0.8	221	10	37.8	2.8	6.8
Wholemeal, COU, M&S*	1 Slice/21g	45	0.5	213	13.6	33.7	2.6	7
Wholemeal, Crusty, Finest, Tesco*	1 Slice/50g	103	0.8	206	10.8	37	1.7	6.9
Wholemeal, Crusty, Kingsmill*	1 Slice/42g	104	1.8	247	11.2	41.1	4.2	7
Wholemeal, Danish, BFY, Morrisons*	1 Slice/17g	39	0.3	228	11.2	47.9	1.8	6.2
Wholemeal, Economy, Sainsbury's*	1 Slice/28g	61	0.7	217	10.3	38.4	2.5	6.5
Wholemeal, Farmhouse, Bakery in Store, M&S*	1 Slice/35g	80	1	229	11.4	35.3	3	7.9
Wholemeal, Farmhouse, Hovis*	1 Slice/44g	91	1	207	11	36	2.2	7.1
Wholemeal, Farmhouse, Soft, Tesco*	1 Slice/44g	99	1	224	11.1	36.4	2.2	6.9
Wholemeal, Fh, Stoneground, Batch, Finest, Tesco*	1 Slice/50g	108	1.4	215	10.3	36.1	2.8	6.9
Wholemeal, Gold, Kingsmill*	1 Slice/44g	95	1.3	217	10.9	36.8	2.9	7
Wholemeal, Golden Crust, Ormo*	1 Slice/38g	83	0.8	218	10.4	36.1	2	7
Wholemeal, Golden Wheat, Kingsmill*	1 Slice/44g	97	1.3	221	10.9	37.8	2.9	6
Wholemeal, Healthy Range, Pat The Baker*	1 Slice/27g	58	0.5	215	10	36.4	1.8	6.6
Wholemeal, High Protein, High Fibre, Warburton's*	1 Slice/29g	66	1	227	13.5	32	3.3	7.8
Wholemeal, Light, Irish Pride*	1 Slice/28g	68	0.4	241	13.3	44.1	1.3	4.5
Wholemeal, Little Brown Loaf, Unsliced, Hovis*	1 Slice/40g	86	1.1	216	10	37.8	2.7	6.8
Wholemeal, Live Good, Hovis*	1 Slice/26g	67	0.4	258	10	46.9	1.5	6.9
Wholemeal, Loaf, 400g, Kingsmill*	1 Slice/29g	68	0.8	234	10.2	39	2.8	6.2
Wholemeal, Loaf, Sliced, Medium, 800g, Hovis*	1 Slice/40g	88	1.1	221	10	37.8	2.7	6.8
Wholemeal, Loaf, Sliced, Thick, 800g, Hovis*	1 Slice/47g	104	0.8	221	10	37.8	1.8	6.8
Wholemeal, Longer Life, Med Sliced, Sainsbury's*	1 Slice/35g	78	1.3	222	10.9	36.2	3.7	6.5
Wholemeal, Longer Life, Sainsbury's*	1 Slice/36g	85	1.2	237	10.7	41	3.4	6.2
Wholemeal, Longer Life, Thick Slice, Sainsbury's*	1 Slice/45g	101	1.6	224	10.6	37.4	3.6	5.9
Wholemeal, Lower Carb , Hovis*	1 Slice/36g	84	1.3	234	16	27	3.7	14.4
Wholemeal, Med Sliced, Great Everyday, Kingsmill*	1 Slice/40g	91	1.5	227	10.5	37.7	3.8	6.2
Wholemeal, Med Sliced, Little Big Loaf, Kingsmill*	1 Slice/39g	93	1.5	239	10.5	37.7	3.8	6.2
Wholemeal, Med Sliced, M&S*	1 Slice/40g	80	1.2	200	10.5	32.7	3.1	6.7
Wholemeal, Med Sliced, Morrisons*	1 Slice/33g	72	0.5	216	9.6	38	1.4	6.5
Wholemeal, Med Sliced, Organic, Tesco*	1 Slice/27g	55	0.7	209	9.2	37.2	2.8	6
Wholemeal, Med Sliced, Premium, Tesco*	1 Slice/36g	71	0.2	196	9.8	37.8	0.6	7.2
Wholemeal, Med Sliced, Roberts Bakery*	1 Slice/37g	86	0.6	233	10.9	38.1	1.5	6.6
Wholemeal, Med Sliced, Sainsbury's*	1 Slice/36g	77	0.9	214	10.3	37.8	2.4	7.4
Wholemeal, Med Sliced, The Village Bakery*	1 Slice/33g	69	0.7	209	9.8	38	2	6
Wholemeal, Med Sliced, Waitrose*	1 Slice/36g	76	0.9	213	10.1	37.6	2.4	7
Wholemeal, Medium, 400g Loaf, Warburton's*	1 Slice/24g	55	0.7	231	10.6	37.8	2.8	6.4
Wholemeal, Medium, 800g Loaf, Warburton's*	1 Slice/45g	103	1.3	231	10.6	37.8	2.8	6.4
Wholemeal, Medium, Sliced, Everyday Essentials, Aldi*	1 Slice/36g	83	0.9	231	9.6	39	2.5	7
Wholemeal, Multi Seeded, TTD, Sainsbury's*	1 Slice/47g	110	3.4	234	11.7	30.7	7.2	8.1
Wholemeal, Multigrain, Sliced, Finest, Tesco*	1 Slice/50g	123	2	246	10.1	42.1	4.1	6.5

BREAD

	Measure INFO/WEIGHT	per Measure KCAL	FAT	Nutrition Values per 100g / 100ml KCAL	PROT	CARB	FAT	FIBRE
Wholemeal, Multigrain, Soft Batch, Sainsbury's*	1 Slice/44g	106	2.9	242	11.3	34.5	6.5	5.6
Wholemeal, Multiseed, Batch, So Organic, Sainsbury's*	1 Slice/30g	79	2.2	263	11.8	30.9	7.4	12.9
Wholemeal, Oat Topped, TTD, Sainsbury's*	1 Slice/47g	109	1.3	232	10	38.5	2.8	0.3
Wholemeal, Organic, Hovis*	1 Slice/44g	92	1.3	209	10.2	35.6	2.9	7.6
Wholemeal, Premium, Med Slice, M&S*	1 Slice/33g	65	1	200	10.5	32.9	3.1	6.7
Wholemeal, Premium, Thick Slice, M&S*	1 Slice/50g	95	1.5	190	9.8	30.8	3	6.4
Wholemeal, Rolls, Mini Loaves, Hovis*	1 Loaf/70g	175	4.1	250	10.6	38.7	5.9	6.8
Wholemeal, Rustic, Tin, Tesco*	1 Slice/37g	92	1.3	249	12.2	44	3.5	3.1
Wholemeal, Sandwich Loaf, Brennans*	1 Slice/40g	88	0.7	221	9.8	38.5	1.7	8
Wholemeal, Seeded Batch, Truly Irresistible, Co-Op*	1 Slice/47g	115	1.9	245	11.5	36.2	4	6.6
Wholemeal, Seeded, High Protein, Low Carb, Hi-Lo*	1 Slice/33g	86	2.9	260	24.7	15.6	8.7	10.2
Wholemeal, Seeded, Roll, Love Life, Waitrose*	1 Roll/72g	192	6.3	266	12.6	34.1	8.8	6.4
Wholemeal, Seeded, Rowan Hill Bakery, Lidl*	1 Slice/33g	86	1.9	261	12.7	34.9	5.8	9
Wholemeal, Seeded, Signature, Allinson*	1 Slice/46g	118	4	256	11.1	28.9	8.7	8.9
Wholemeal, Sliced, Loaf, Average	***1 Slice/40g***	***90***	***0.9***	***224***	***9.9***	***38.8***	***2.4***	***6.9***
Wholemeal, Sliced, McCambridge*	1 Slice/38g	90	0.7	237	7.9	44.7	1.8	0
Wholemeal, Sliced, Medium, Tesco*	1 Slice/40g	94	1.2	235	11.5	36.9	3	7.1
Wholemeal, Sliced, Organic, Harvestime*	1 Slice/44g	95	1.2	216	9	38.8	2.7	5.6
Wholemeal, Soft Crusty, M&S*	1 Slice/25g	58	0.8	230	11.4	39.1	3.1	6.5
Wholemeal, Soft, Thick, Rowan Hill Bakery, Lidl*	1 Slice/44g	103	1.3	235	11.5	36.9	3	7.1
Wholemeal, Square Cut, Thick Sliced, Asda*	1 Slice/44g	91	1	208	10	37	2.2	6
Wholemeal, Stayfresh, Tesco*	1 Slice/36g	81	0.8	225	11	39.1	2.2	6
Wholemeal, Stoneground, Batch Baked, Warburton's*	1 Slice/45g	101	1.2	224	10.3	35.7	2.6	6.9
Wholemeal, Stoneground, Organic, Waitrose*	1 Sm Slice/25g	57	0.9	228	10.8	38.2	3.6	7.1
Wholemeal, Stoneground, Thick Sliced, Sainsbury's*	1 Slice/44g	92	0.8	210	10.2	37.9	1.9	7.8
Wholemeal, Supersoft, Eat Well, M&S*	1 Slice/33g	81	1.1	245	10.9	40	3.3	6.7
Wholemeal, Tasty, Medium, Kingsmill*	1 Slice/40g	96	1.5	239	10.5	37.7	3.8	6.2
Wholemeal, Tasty, Thick, Kingsmill*	1 Slice/44g	105	1.7	239	10.5	37.7	3.8	6.2
Wholemeal, Thick Slice, Brennans*	1 Slice/27g	69	0.6	257	9.2	45.4	2.1	6.8
Wholemeal, Thick Sliced, Bakers Gold, Asda*	1 Slice/44g	99	1.4	225	12	37	3.2	6
Wholemeal, Thick Sliced, Great Everyday, Kingsmill*	1 Slice/44g	100	1.7	227	10.5	37.7	3.8	6.2
Wholemeal, Thick Sliced, Sainsbury's*	1 Slice/48g	102	1.2	213	10.1	37.4	2.6	8.5
Wholemeal, Thick Sliced, Stephenson's Bakery*	1 Slice/40g	84	0.8	209	10.7	37.3	1.9	6.2
Wholemeal, Thick Sliced, Tesco*	1 Slice/40g	96	1.1	240	9.5	40.9	2.7	6.8
Wholemeal, Thick Sliced, Waitrose*	1 Slice/44g	94	1.1	213	10.1	37.6	2.4	7
Wholemeal, Thick, Weight Watchers, Warburton's*	1 Slice/29g	72	0.8	250	9.2	43.6	2.9	6.5
Wholemeal, Toasted, Average	***1 Med Slice/26g***	***58***	***0.6***	***224***	***8.6***	***42.3***	***2.2***	***5.8***
Wholemeal, Unsliced, Organic, Dove's Farm*	1 Med Slice/35g	77	0.9	221	11.4	37.9	2.6	8.3
Wholemeal, with Rye, Rich & Tasty, Warburton's*	1 Slice/45g	109	1.1	246	9.9	40.6	2.4	7.5
Wholemeal. Medium, Brace's*	1 Med Slice/32g	72	0.7	226	10.2	44.3	2.2	6
Wholewheat, 100%, Stoneground, Maxwell House*	1 Slice/27g	60	0.5	222	11.1	44.4	1.9	7.4
Wholewheat, Harvest	1 Serving/42g	90	1	214	7.1	45.2	2.4	7.1
Wholewheat, Nature's Own*	1 Slice/28g	66	1	236	14.3	39.3	3.6	10.7
Wholewheat, No Crusts, Harry's*	1 Slice/25g	58	1.1	233	8	40	4.5	5.5
Wholewheat, Soft, Trader Joe's*	1 Slice/37g	70	1	189	10.8	37.8	2.7	5.4
Wrap, Brown, Soft, Easy Roll, Warburton's*	1 Wrap/65g	190	2.9	292	12	49.3	4.5	3.2
Wrap, Half & Half, Warburton's*	1 Wrap/41g	121	1.8	296	12.8	49.6	4.4	3.8
Wrap, Mediterranean Herb, Soft, Village Bakery, Aldi*	1 Wrap/64g	188	2.6	294	8	54.7	4.1	2
Wrap, Seeded, GF, Newburn Bakehouse, Warburton's*	1 Wrap/60g	178	4.5	297	5.5	48.1	7.5	7.4
Wrap, Tortilla, 8 Pack, Asda*	1 Tortilla/50g	143	3	286	8	50	6	1.9
Wrap, Tortilla, 8 Pack, LC, Tesco*	1 Tortilla/50g	135	1	270	7.1	53.2	2.1	3.5
Wrap, Tortilla, Ancient Grain, Blue Menu*	1 Tortilla/34g	100	2	294	8.8	50	5.9	5.9
Wrap, Tortilla, BGTY, Sainsbury's*	1 Tortilla/50g	136	1.4	271	7.9	53.7	2.7	1.9

BREAD

INFO/WEIGHT	Measure	per Measure KCAL	per Measure FAT	Nutrition Values per 100g / 100ml KCAL	PROT	CARB	FAT	FIBRE
Wrap, Tortilla, Both in One, Sunnyhills, Aldi*	1 Wrap/64g	184	2.9	287	8.1	52	4.5	3
Wrap, Tortilla, Bueno*	1 Tortilla/63g	171	3.6	272	6.9	48.2	5.7	2
Wrap, Tortilla, Deli, Multigrain, Mission Deli*	1 Tortilla/61g	202	6.1	330	7.9	50.5	10	3
Wrap, Tortilla, Flour, Soft, Old El Paso*	1 Tortilla/41g	123	2.1	299	8.5	53.7	5.2	1.9
Wrap, Tortilla, from Tex Mex Meal, Tesco*	2 Wraps/61g	190	4.7	310	8.5	50.4	7.6	1.6
Wrap, Tortilla, Garlic, & Parsley, Sainsbury's*	1 Tortilla/60g	166	3.7	277	7.2	48	6.2	1.8
Wrap, Tortilla, GF, Lovemore*	1 Wrap/50g	150	4.2	299	1.8	48.1	8.3	4.1
Wrap, Tortilla, Healthy 'n' White, Wrap 'n' Roll, Discovery*	1 Tortilla/40g	161	3.5	288	8	49.7	6.3	2.6
Wrap, Tortilla, Large, Essential, Waitrose*	1 Tortilla/64g	190	3.7	297	7.2	52.5	5.8	3.1
Wrap, Tortilla, LC, Tesco*	1 Tortilla/64g	166	1.3	260	7.1	53.2	2.1	3.5
Wrap, Tortilla, Less Than 3% Fat, BGTY, Sainsbury's*	1 Tortilla/51g	128	1.1	250	7.8	50.1	2.2	2.9
Wrap, Tortilla, Low Carb, Carbzone*	1 Wrap/65g	182	8.4	280	18	10	13	26
Wrap, Tortilla, Low Fat, M&S*	1 Serving/180g	225	4	125	6.3	20.6	2.2	1.9
Wrap, Tortilla, Mediterranean Herb, Rowan Hill, Lidl*	1 Wrap/64g	178	2.2	278	7.3	53	3.5	2.5
Wrap, Tortilla, Mexican, Asda*	1 Tortilla/34g	100	2.8	295	7.9	47.2	8.3	3.9
Wrap, Tortilla, Morrisons*	1 Serving/60g	132	2.1	220	6.2	42	3.5	1.7
Wrap, Tortilla, Multiseed, Discovery*	1 Tortilla/57g	160	2.8	280	8.7	50.1	5	3.6
Wrap, Tortilla, Organic, Sainsbury's*	1 Tortilla/56g	167	4.3	298	8.6	48.8	7.7	2.1
Wrap, Tortilla, Plain , Ocado*	1 Wrap/53g	154	4.4	291	6.7	45.7	8.4	3.1
Wrap, Tortilla, Plain, HL, Tesco*	1 Wrap/67g	188	1.9	280	8.5	54.2	2.8	3.3
Wrap, Tortilla, Plain, Mini, Morrisons*	1 Tortilla/34g	91	1.4	267	8.1	48.9	4	2.8
Wrap, Tortilla, Plain, Nannak*	1 Wrap/80g	134	3.5	167	8.9	62.2	4.4	0
Wrap, Tortilla, Plain, Ready to Eat, Sunnyhills, Aldi*	1 Wrap/64g	181	2.2	283	7.1	54.5	3.4	3
Wrap, Tortilla, Plain, Sainsbury's*	1 Wrap/64g	182	2.9	285	7.8	51.2	4.5	4.3
Wrap, Tortilla, Plain, Tesco*	1 Tortilla/64g	182	3.2	284	8.1	49.7	5	3.8
Wrap, Tortilla, Plain, Village Bakery, Aldi*	1 Wrap/65g	194	4.9	298	7.8	49.6	7.6	2.7
Wrap, Tortilla, Quinoa, & Chia Seed, BFree*	1 Wrap/42g	105	2.4	250	7.6	36	5.7	11.4
Wrap, Tortilla, Rice, Mountain Bread*	1 Wrap/25g	68	0.3	272	10	53	1.3	2.6
Wrap, Tortilla, Seeded, Love Life, Waitrose*	1 Tortilla/64g	185	3.6	290	8.8	46.6	5.7	4.3
Wrap, Tortilla, Seeded, Tesco*	1 Wrap/64g	170	1.4	266	7.7	51.2	2.2	4.2
Wrap, Tortilla, Soft, M&S*	1 Wrap/64g	186	3.8	290	8	49.7	6	2.5
Wrap, Tortilla, Soft, Mini, Old El Paso*	1 Tortilla/25g	80	2.1	319	7.7	51	8.5	2.4
Wrap, Tortilla, Spicy Tomato, Morrisons*	1 Tortilla/55g	158	3.1	288	8.6	50.5	5.7	0.7
Wrap, Tortilla, Spicy Tomato, Tesco*	1 Tortilla/63g	175	3.5	278	7.8	49.2	5.6	2.4
Wrap, Tortilla, Sweet Chilli, Mission Deli*	1 Wrap/62g	193	4.2	311	7.5	52.8	6.8	4.1
Wrap, Tortilla, Sweet Chilli, Tesco*	1 Wrap/64g	184	2.9	288	7.4	53.1	4.5	2.7
Wrap, Tortilla, Sweet Potato, GF, BFree*	1 Wrap/42g	95	0.9	227	4.6	41.7	2.2	11
Wrap, Tortilla, Tomato, & Herb, Tesco*	1 Serving/63g	165	3.5	262	7.9	45.1	5.5	2.1
Wrap, Tortilla, Value, Tesco*	1 Wrap/47g	129	2.4	275	8.5	49.1	5	4.3
Wrap, Tortilla, Weight Watchers*	1 Wrap/42g	107	0.4	254	7.1	50.7	1	6.7
Wrap, Tortilla, White, Bakers Selection, Asda*	1 Tortilla/62g	181	2.9	290	7.9	53	4.6	2.5
Wrap, Tortilla, White, M&S*	1 Tortilla/64g	170	2.4	265	7.9	49	3.8	1.6
Wrap, Tortilla, Whole & White, HL, Tesco*	1 Wrap/64g	182	1.7	284	8.5	54.1	2.7	4.5
Wrap, Tortilla, Whole 'n' White, Goodness, Kids, Tesco*	1 Wrap/27g	72	1.2	265	8.3	47.6	4.5	5.8
Wrap, Tortilla, Whole, & White, Mini, Kids, Sainsbury's*	1 Tortilla/26g	67	1.4	258	9.2	42.9	5.5	6.2
Wrap, Tortilla, Wholemeal , M&S*	1 Wrap/64g	160	2.4	250	11.2	42.5	3.8	6.5
Wrap, Tortilla, Wholemeal, Bakers Selection, Asda*	1 Wraps/63g	177	4.1	283	8	46	6.5	4
Wrap, Tortilla, Wholemeal, Discovery*	1 Wrap/40g	109	3.3	273	9.2	40.4	8.3	6.4
Wrap, White, GF, Newburn Bakehouse, Warburton's*	1 Wrap/60g	167	3.4	279	4.5	49	5.7	7
Wrap, White, Soft, Easy Roll, Warburton's*	1 Wrap/65g	192	2.8	296	11.7	51.6	4.3	2
Wrap, Wholegrain, GF, Mini, Warburton's*	1 Wrap/35g	101	2.3	288	9.2	44.7	6.6	6.7
Wrap, Wholemeal, High Protein & Fibre, Warburton's*	1 Wrap/68g	184	3.3	271	15	38.4	4.8	7.3

	Measure INFO/WEIGHT	per Measure KCAL	FAT	Nutrition Values per 100g / 100ml KCAL	PROT	CARB	FAT	FIBRE
BREAD & BUTTER PUDDING								
Average	*1 Serving/250g*	*400*	*19.5*	*160*	*6.2*	*17.5*	*7.8*	*0.3*
BGTY, Sainsbury's*	1 Serving/125g	126	2.9	101	6.3	13.4	2.3	5.4
Finest, Tesco*	1 Serving/153g	379	22	248	4.9	24.6	14.4	0.9
Individual, M&S*	1 Pudding/130g	280	16.4	215	4.4	21.4	12.6	0.5
Low Fat, Individual, BGTY, Sainsbury's*	1 Pack/125g	125	2.9	100	6.3	13.4	2.3	5.4
Sainsbury's*	½ Pudding/115g	223	11.2	194	4.8	21.9	9.7	0.4
Seville Orange Marmalade, Luxury, Baked, Iceland*	1/3 Pudding/156g	443	25.9	284	5.2	28.1	16.6	0.6
Tesco*	½ Pack/198g	494	31.8	250	5	20.8	16.1	0.4
BREAD MIX								
Brown, Sunflower, Sainsbury's*	1 Serving/60g	151	3.7	251	10	38.9	6.1	4
Chia & Hemp, Free From, Baked, Sukrin*	1 Slice/30g	49	2.7	163	9.3	3.5	8.9	18.2
Ciabatta, Made Up with Water & Olive Oil, Wrights*	1 Slice/45g	113	1.8	251	10	43.6	4	1.8
Crusty White, Made Up, Tesco*	1 Slice/126g	316	2.3	251	9.4	49.3	1.8	2.5
Focaccia, Garlic & Herb, Asda*	1 Serving/125g	385	10	308	11	48	8	3.3
Italian Ciabatta, Sainsbury's*	1 Slice/45g	96	0.9	213	8.7	40	2	2.4
Mixed Grain, Sainsbury's*	1 Serving/45g	103	0.7	228	7.7	46	1.5	4.4
Multiseed, Baked, Sainsbury's*	1 Slice/44g	112	4.3	252	10.8	30.5	9.6	6.8
Pain De Compagne, Made Up, Francine*	2 Slices/100g	237	2.5	237	9.7	42.3	2.5	0
Parmesan & Sun Dried Tomato, Made Up, Wrights*	1 Slice/45g	103	0.6	229	9.3	46	1.3	2.4
White Loaf, Asda*	1 Slice/60g	128	0.2	213	7.9	43	0.3	3.5
Wholemeal, CBY, Asda*	1 Slice/45g	93	0.3	207	9.6	37.5	0.6	6.5
Wholemeal, Hovis*	1 Serving/65g	148	3.1	227	10	35.8	4.8	6.8
Wholemeal, Made Up, M&S*	1 Loaf/600g	1410	14.4	235	11	42	2.4	5.3
BREADCRUMBS								
Average	*1oz/28g*	*98*	*0.5*	*350*	*10.8*	*74.8*	*1.9*	*2.6*
BREADFRUIT								
Raw	*1oz/28g*	*19*	*0.1*	*67*	*0.9*	*16.4*	*0.2*	*0*
BREADSTICKS								
Asda*	1 Serving/5g	21	0.4	412	12	73	8	2.9
Bruschetta, Olive & Rosemary, Graze*	1 Punnet/29g	138	7.5	480	13.4	53	26	4.1
Chive & Onion Twists, Tesco*	3 Twists/24g	115	5.3	480	11.6	57.6	22.1	2.2
Classic, Somerfield*	1 Breadstick/6g	24	0.2	396	10	82.5	2.9	1
Grissini, Italian, Sainsbury's*	1 Breadstick/5g	20	0.4	408	11.6	72.9	7.8	2.9
Grissini, Thin with Olive Oil, Forno Bianco*	1 Stick/5g	21	0.4	420	11	77	7.5	0
Grissini, Waitrose*	1 Breadstick/6g	25	0.4	397	12	72.5	6.2	3.1
Italian Original, Tesco*	1 Stick/5.5g	23	0.4	410	11.6	72.9	7.8	2.9
Mini Grissini, Traditional Italian, Lupa*	6 Sticks/10g	39	0.7	393	13.9	65.3	6.6	8.2
Mini, CBY, Asda*	1 Pack/22g	89	1.8	405	12	69	8	4.5
Mini, Sainsbury's*	4 Breadsticks/5g	20	0.4	404	15.6	68.7	7.4	4.8
Olive Oil & Rosemary, Finest, Tesco*	2 Sticks/9.8g	42	1.2	427	13.9	64.4	12.6	4.1
Olive, Italian, Finest, Tesco*	1 Stick/40g	170	5.4	424	10.5	65	13.6	4.8
Original, Italian, Tesco*	1 Stick/5.5g	23	0.4	410	11.6	72.9	7.8	2.9
Original, Organic, Kallo*	1 Breadstick/6g	24	0.5	393	11.8	69.5	7.6	4.7
PB, Waitrose*	1 Breadstick/5g	20	0.1	378	13.7	77.3	1.6	3.8
Plain, Asda*	1 Stick/5g	21	0.4	412	12	73	8	2.9
Plain, You Count, Love Life, Waitrose*	1 Breadstick/5g	17	0.1	349	13.4	70.1	1.7	5.6
Rosemary, Asda*	1 Breadstick/6.6g	29	1	439	12	64	15	3.5
Salted, Asda*	1 Stick/8g	36	1.4	445	13	60	17	4.3
Sesame Seed Grissini, Sainsbury's*	1 Breadstick/5g	21	0.6	419	12.7	65.5	11.8	3.2
Thin, Healthy Eating, D'oro, Primo*	1 Breadstick/3g	11	0.2	400	10	75	6.5	1.1
BREAKFAST CEREAL								
3 in One, Strawberry, Jordans*	1 Serving/50g	181	2.9	362	9.4	68	5.8	11.9
Advantage, Weetabix*	1 Serving/30g	105	0.7	350	10.2	72	2.4	9

BREAKFAST CEREAL

	Measure INFO/WEIGHT	per Measure KCAL	FAT	Nutrition Values per 100g / 100ml KCAL	PROT	CARB	FAT	FIBRE
All Bran, Asda*	1 Serving/40g	110	1.4	276	15	46	3.5	27
All Bran, Bran Flakes, & Fruit, Kellogg's*	1 Serving/40g	143	2.4	358	8	68	6	9
All Bran, Bran Flakes, Chocolate, Kellogg's*	1 Serving/30g	106	1.8	354	10	65	6	13
All Bran, Fruit 'n' Fibre, Kellogg's*	1 Serving/30g	114	1.8	380	8	69	6	9
All Bran, Fruitful, Kellogg's*	1 Serving/40g	136	3	340	12.5	57.5	7.5	0
All Bran, Golden Crunch, Kellogg's*	1 Serving/45g	182	5	405	8	62	11	13
All Bran, High Fibre, Morrisons*	1 Serving/40g	109	1.4	272	14.8	45.5	3.5	27
All Bran, Muesli, Cranberry & Sultana, Kellogg's*	1 Serving/45g	158	2.5	350	10	58	5.5	14
All Bran, Original, High Fibre, Kellogg's*	1 Serving/40g	134	1.4	334	14	48	3.5	27
All Bran, Yoghurty Flakes, As Sold, Kellogg's*	1 Serving/30g	112	1.2	372	10	68	4	12
Almond, Oats & More, Nestle*	1 Serving/30g	119	2.7	398	10.7	68.7	8.9	5.5
Almond, Pecan & Cashew Muesli, Kellogg's*	1 Serving/45g	188	6.3	418	11	62	14	8
Alpen*, Crunchy Bran*	1 Serving/40g	120	1.9	299	11.8	52.3	4.7	24.8
Amaranth, Flakes, Organic, Gillian McKeith*	1 Serving/50g	198	2	396	10	80	4	3
Apple & Cinnamon Flakes, M&S*	1 Serving/30g	111	0.6	370	6	82.7	1.9	3.4
Apple & Cinnamon, Crisp, Sainsbury's*	1 Serving/50g	216	7.4	433	6.2	69.1	14.7	3.4
Apple & Cinnamon Crisp, Tesco*	1 Serving/50g	217	6.6	433	8.7	67.1	13.1	6.1
Apple & Cinnamon, Oat & Fruit Breakfast, Quaker*	1 Sachet/200g	172	3.6	86	2.3	14	1.8	2.3
Apple & Cinnamon, Quaker*	1 Sachet/38g	136	2.1	358	8	68	5.5	2.5
Apple & Raisin, Additions, Weetabix*	2 Biscuits/43g	149	0.8	344	9.5	66	1.8	13
Apple Spice, Oats & Chia, The Chia Co*	1 Serving/45g	184	7	409	9.6	47.4	15.6	13.6
Apple, Spelt & Chia, Ancient Legends, Kellogg's*	1 Serving/45g	171	2.1	380	10	70	4.7	8.6
Apricot Wheats, Harvest Morn, Aldi*	1 Serving/30g	101	0.4	337	7.6	72.3	1.4	8
Apricot Wheats, Whole Grain, Tesco*	1 Serving/40g	130	0.6	326	7.6	70.6	1.4	8
Balance, Sainsbury's*	1 Serving/30g	111	0.4	370	11.4	77.7	1.5	3.2
Banana & Toffee Crisp, Mornflake*	1 Serving/30g	133	4.8	443	5.7	68.8	16.1	5.4
Banana & Mango, Oats & Chia, The Chia Co*	1 Serving/45g	187	7	414	9.7	50.3	15.4	11.2
Banana, Papaya & Honey Oat, Crunchy, Waitrose*	1 Serving/40g	170	4.8	426	9.6	69.8	12	5.5
Benefit Flakes, Original, Harvest Morn, Aldi*	1 Serving/40g	154	0.5	384	12	80	1.3	2.2
Berry Granola, Rude Health*	1 Serving/40g	178	6.4	446	10	61	16	7
Bircher Muesli, Love Life, Waitrose*	1 Serving/45g	153	3.5	341	8.8	57.7	7.7	6.8
Biscuit, with Coconut & Raisin, Additions, Weetabix*	2 Biscuits/43g	157	2.5	363	9.5	62	5.7	13
Biscuit, Baked with Golden Syrup, Weetabix*	2 Biscuits/44g	158	0.8	363	10.3	72	1.9	8.2
Biscuit, with Apple & Raisin, Additions	*2 Biscuits/43g*	*149*	*0.8*	*344*	*9.5*	*66*	*1.8*	*13*
Bitesize Wheats, Crownfield, Lidl*	1 Serving/40g	142	0.8	356	10.6	67	1.9	14
Bitesize, Weetabix*	1 Serving/40g	135	0.8	338	11.5	68.4	2	10
Bixies, Wheat Biscuits, Wholegrain, Crownfield, Lidl*	2 Biscuits/40g	145	0.8	362	10.8	70.3	1.9	10
Blueberry Wheats, Tesco*	1 Serving/50g	168	0.8	336	7.5	71.6	1.5	8.5
Bran Crunch, Raisin, Kellogg's*	1 Pack/80g	280	1.5	350	6.2	83.8	1.9	7.5
Bran Flakes, Asda*	1 Serving/47g	157	1.5	333	11	65	3.2	14
Bran Flakes, Harvest Home, Nestle*	1 Serving/30g	99	0.7	331	10.2	67.1	2.4	14.1
Bran Flakes, Honey Nut, Tesco*	1 Serving/40g	143	1.8	358	9.6	70	4.4	11
Bran Flakes, Kellogg's*	1 Serving/30g	108	1	359	12	63	3.2	15
Bran Flakes, Organic, Asda*	1 Serving/30g	99	0.7	330	10	67	2.4	14
Bran Flakes, Organic, Sainsbury's*	1 Serving/30g	100	0.7	332	10.2	67.4	2.4	14.1
Bran Flakes, Sainsbury's*	1 Serving/30g	100	0.8	333	10.3	67.5	2.5	14.3
Bran Flakes, Sultana Bran, Kellogg's*	1 Serving/40g	138	0.8	344	8	67	2	13
Bran Flakes, Sultana, Dry, Sainsbury's*	1 Serving/30g	98	0.6	325	8.3	68.6	1.9	12.1
Bran Flakes, Tesco*	1 Bowl/50g	178	1.2	356	10.8	64.3	2.4	16.8
Bran Flakes, Wholegrain, Essential, Waitrose*	1 Serving/30g	107	0.7	356	10.8	64.7	2.4	16
Bran Flakes, Wholegrain, Sainsbury's*	1 Serving/30g	110	0.6	365	10.5	69.4	2	13.8
Bran, High Fibre, Tesco*	1 Serving/40g	140	1.6	350	13.7	54	3.9	22.1
Bran, Natural, Sainsbury's*	1 Serving/30g	64	1.5	212	14.7	27	5	36

BREAKFAST CEREAL

	Measure INFO/WEIGHT	per Measure KCAL	FAT	Nutrition Values per 100g / 100ml KCAL	PROT	CARB	FAT	FIBRE
Breakfast Biscuits, Aldi*	4 Biscuits/60g	213	1.5	355	13.7	69.5	2.5	7.5
Caribbean Crunch, Alpen*	1 Serving/40g	155	3.6	388	8.8	67.9	9	4.6
Cheerios, Chocolate, Dry, Nestle*	1 Serving/30g	115	1	384	8	73.4	3.5	2.2
Cheerios, Honey Nut, Nestle*	1 Serving/30g	112	1.1	374	7	78.3	3.7	5.2
Cheerios, Honey, Nestle*	1 Serving/50g	184	1.4	369	6.6	79.2	2.8	5.8
Cheerios, Low Sugar, As Sold, Nestle*	1 Bowl/30g	120	2.3	399	11.1	67.4	7.6	8.5
Cheerios, Nestle*	1 Serving/30g	114	1.1	381	8.6	74.5	3.8	7.1
Cheerios, Oat Crisp, Nestle*	1 Portion/40g	154	2.1	385	11	70	5.2	8.5
Choc & Nut Crisp, Tesco*	1 Serving/40g	185	8	462	8.3	62.5	19.9	4.8
Choco Crackles, Morrisons*	1 Serving/30g	115	0.7	383	5.5	84.8	2.4	1.9
Choco Flakes, Asda*	1 Serving/50g	187	0.4	374	6	86	0.7	2.6
Choco Flakes, Kellogg's*	1 Serving/30g	114	0.9	380	5	84	3	2.5
Choco Hoops, Aldi*	1 Serving/30g	116	1.4	385	7	79.1	4.5	0
Choco Hoops, Asda*	1 Serving/40g	154	1.8	385	7	79	4.5	4
Choco Hoops, Tesco*	1 Serving/30g	116	1.2	385	7.5	75	4	8
Choco Snaps, Asda*	1 Serving/30g	115	0.7	382	5	85	2.4	1.9
Choco Squares, Asda*	1 Serving/30g	130	4.2	434	10	67	14	4
Chocolate Crisp, Minis, Weetabix*	1 Serving/36g	134	1.9	371	9	71.7	5.3	8.5
Chocolate Hoops, Average	**1 Serving/30g**	**116**	**1.3**	**386**	**7.2**	**79.3**	**4.4**	**3.4**
Chocolate Rice, Puffed, Average	**1 Serving/30g**	**117**	**1.2**	**389**	**5.7**	**81**	**4.1**	**3.2**
Chocolate Wheats, Kellogg's*	1 Serving/40g	148	3.6	369	10	62	9	12
Chocolate, Granola, Diet Chef Ltd*	1 Serving/40g	195	11.5	488	10.7	45	28.7	13
Cinnamon Grahams, Nestle*	1 Serving/40g	164	3.9	411	4.7	76.1	9.8	4.2
Cinnamon, Puffins, Barbara's Bakery*	1 Serving/30g	100	1	333	6.7	86.7	3.3	20
Clusters, Nestle*	1 Serving/30g	111	1.4	371	9.3	72.6	4.8	7.4
Coco Pops, Crunchers, Kellogg's*	1 Serving/30g	114	1	380	7	81	3.5	3
Coco Pops, Kellogg's*	1 Serving/30g	116	0.8	387	5	85	2.5	2
Coco Rice, GF, Nestle*	1 Serving/30g	115	0.7	382	6.2	82	2.4	3.1
Coco Shreddies with 125ml Semi Skimmed Milk, Nestle*	1 Serving/40g	210	2.7	525	18	90.2	6.7	8.7
Coco Snaps, Value, Tesco*	1 Serving/30g	117	0.7	390	7	84.1	2.4	2.4
Coconut & Wheat Flakes, Toasted, Dorset Cereals*	1 Serving/45g	171	3.6	381	8.2	54	8	8
con Salvado de Trigo, Hacendado*	1 Serving/50g	159	1.8	318	14	44	3.5	28
Cookie Crunch, Nestle*	1 Serving/40g	154	1.1	385	4.6	85.3	2.8	1.8
Corn Flakes, Asda*	1 Serving/30g	111	0.2	370	7	84	0.7	3
Corn Flakes, Banana Crunch, Kellogg's*	1 Serving/40g	163	3.2	408	6	78	8	3
Corn Flakes, Crispy Nut, Asda*	1 Serving/30g	117	1.3	390	7	81	4.2	2.5
Corn Flakes, Hint of Honey, Kellogg's*	1 Serving/30g	113	0.2	377	6	87	0.6	2.5
Corn Flakes, Honey Nut & Cranberries, Sainsbury's*	1 Serving/40g	166	4	416	7.4	74.4	9.9	3.1
Corn Flakes, Honey Nut, Average	**1 Serving/30g**	**118**	**1.3**	**393**	**7**	**81.4**	**4.3**	**2.4**
Corn Flakes, Honey Nut, Harvest Home, Nestle*	1 Serving/30g	118	1.3	392	7.4	81.1	4.2	2.5
Corn Flakes, Kellogg's*	1 Serving/30g	113	0.3	378	7	84	0.9	3
Corn Flakes, Morrisons*	1 Serving/30g	111	0.2	371	7.3	83.8	0.7	3
Corn Flakes, Organic, Lima*	1 Serving/50g	178	0.5	355	8.3	77.7	1	6.4
Corn Flakes, Organic, Whole Earth*	1 Serving/40g	154	0.4	386	8.6	84.2	1	3
Corn Flakes, Sainsbury's*	1 Serving/25g	93	0.2	371	7.3	83.8	0.7	3
Corn Flakes, Tesco*	1 Serving/25g	93	0.2	371	7.3	83.8	0.7	3
Corn Flakes, Value, Tesco*	1 Serving/30g	111	0.4	370	7.3	82.4	1.2	3.5
Cornflakes, Essential, Waitrose*	1 Serving/30g	116	0.3	385	7.4	84.8	1.1	3.1
Cornflakes, GF, Nestle*	1 Serving/30g	115	0.3	384	7.4	84.6	1.1	3.1
Cornflakes, Honey, GF, Nestle*	1 Serving/30g	114	0.2	381	5.6	86.2	0.8	3.5
Country Crisp with Real Raspberries, Jordans*	1 Serving/50g	214	7.9	429	7.5	64.1	15.8	7.1
Country Crisp with Real Strawberries, Jordans*	1 Serving/50g	214	7.8	428	7.5	64.1	15.7	7.1
Country Crisp, Four Nut Combo, Jordans*	1 Serving/50g	240	12.4	480	8.9	55.4	24.7	6.9

BREAKFAST CEREAL

	Measure INFO/WEIGHT	per Measure KCAL	FAT	Nutrition Values per 100g / 100ml KCAL	PROT	CARB	FAT	FIBRE
Country Crisp, Wild About Berries, Jordans*	1 Serving/50g	222	7.8	443	7.5	68	15.7	5.7
Cranberry Wheats, Tesco*	1 Serving/50g	160	0.8	320	7.6	72	1.5	8
Cranberry Wheats, Whole Grain, Sainsbury's*	1 Serving/50g	162	0.7	325	7.3	70.9	1.4	7.7
Crispix Krispies, Kellogg's*	1 Serving/30g	110	0	367	6.7	86.7	0	0
Crispy Minis, Banana, Weetabix*	1 Serving/40g	156	2	389	9.3	72	4.9	9.7
Crispy Minis, Strawberry, Weetabix*	1 Serving/40g	150	0.9	375	9.4	74.1	2.3	10
Crispy Rice & Wheat Flakes, Asda*	1 Serving/50g	185	0.8	370	11	78	1.5	3.2
Crunchy Bran Muesli, Diet Chef Ltd*	1 Serving/40g	164	3.8	409	8.1	68.4	9.5	8.9
Crunchy Bran, Weetabix*	1 Serving/40g	140	1.4	350	11.9	57.6	3.6	20
Crunchy Choco, Crisp & Square, Tesco*	1 Serving/50g	212	7	423	8	66.3	14	6
Crunchy Chocolate, Carrefour*	1 Serving/40g	176	6.8	440	9	62	17	8
Crunchy Nut, Clusters, Honey & Nut, Kellogg's*	1 Serving/40g	161	2	402	6	82	5	2.5
Crunchy Nut, Clusters, Milk Chocolate Curls, Kellogg's*	1 Serving/40g	183	7.2	458	8	66	18	4
Crunchy Nut, Clusters, Summer Berries, Kellogg's*	1 Serving/40g	176	6	439	8	68	15	5
Crunchy Nut, Corn Flakes, Kellogg's*	1 Serving/30g	118	1.2	392	6	83	4	2.5
Crunchy Nut, Oat Granola, with Chocolate, Kellogg's*	1 Serving/45g	224	11.2	497	8	57	25	6
Crunchy Nut, Red, Kellogg's*	1 Serving/40g	138	0.8	346	10	72	2	9
Crunchy Oat with Raisins, Almonds & Fruit, Tesco*	1 Serving/50g	202	6.3	403	8.5	63.8	12.6	6.6
Crunchy Oat with Tropical Fruits, Tesco*	1 Serving/35g	146	4.8	417	7.8	65.3	13.8	6.1
Crunchy Oat, Golden Sun, Lidl*	1 Serving/50g	206	6.4	411	8.6	65	12.9	6.2
Crunchy Rice & Wheat Flakes, Co-Op*	1 Serving/30g	111	0.6	370	11	78	2	3
Curiously Cinnamon, Nestle*	1 Serving/30g	124	3	412	4.9	75.9	9.9	4.1
Fibre 1, Nestle*	1 Serving/40g	107	1	267	10.8	50.2	2.6	30.5
Fibre Flakes, GF, Organic, Dove's Farm*	1 Serving/30g	105	0.4	351	7.1	69.7	1.5	15
Fitnesse & Fruits, Nestle*	1 Serving/40g	148	0.4	370	6.6	83.4	1.1	3.4
Flakes & Grains, Exotic Fruit, BGTY, Sainsbury's*	1 Serving/30g	113	1.5	377	6.8	76.4	4.9	5.9
Flakes & Orchard Fruits, BGTY, Sainsbury's*	1 Serving/40g	154	0.5	385	13	80.6	1.2	4.5
Flakes & Clusters, Tesco*	1 Serving/50g	220	8.5	440	11.2	55.4	17	10.5
Flakes, 7 Cereal, De Halm*	1 Serving/40g	139	1.3	347	11.3	66.7	3.4	9
Froot Loops, 30g, & 125ml Semi Skimmed, Kellogg's*	1 Serving/30g	176	3.5	587	23.3	100	11.7	3.3
Frosted Flakes, Sainsbury's*	1 Serving/30g	114	0.2	381	4.9	88	0.6	2
Frosted Flakes, Tesco*	1 Serving/30g	112	0.1	374	4.9	87.8	0.4	2.4
Frosted Wheats, Kellogg's*	1 Serving/30g	104	0.6	346	10	72	2	9
Frosties, Caramel, Kellogg's*	1 Serving/30g	113	0.2	377	5	88	0.6	2
Frosties, Kellogg's*	1 Serving/30g	112	0.2	375	4.5	87	0.6	2
Fruit & Fibre, Flakes, Waitrose*	1 Serving/40g	143	2.5	357	8.2	67.2	6.2	9.9
Fruit & Fibre, Morrisons*	1 Serving/30g	110	2.2	366	8.8	66.5	7.2	8.5
Fruit & Fibre, Organic, Sainsbury's*	1 Serving/40g	147	1.6	367	10	72.4	4.1	7.8
Fruit & Fibre, Somerfield*	1 Serving/40g	144	2.4	361	8.1	68.7	6	8.9
Fruit & Fibre, Value, Tesco*	1 Serving/40g	144	2.2	359	11.4	65.7	5.6	8
Fruit & Fibre, Whole Grain, Sainsbury's*	1 Serving/30g	108	1.8	361	8.1	68.7	6	8.9
Fruit & Nut Crisp, Minis, Weetabix*	1 Serving/40g	144	1.8	359	9.3	70	4.6	8.9
Fruit & Fibre, Asda*	1 Serving/40g	146	2.6	366	8.2	68.4	6.6	8.5
Fruit & Fibre, Harvest Morn, Aldi*	1 Serving/30g	105	1.5	349	8.5	67.6	4.9	10.1
Fruit 'n' Fibre, Kellogg's*	1 Serving/40g	152	2.4	380	8	69	6	9
Fruit, Nuts & Flakes, M&S*	1 Serving/30g	117	2.6	391	9.1	69.6	8.5	3.5
Golden Balls, Asda*	1 Serving/30g	112	0.4	374	5	85	1.5	1.5
Golden Grahams, Nestle*	1 Serving/30g	112	0.9	375	6	81	3	3.4
Golden Honey Puffs, Tesco*	1 Serving/30g	115	0.4	382	6.6	86.3	1.2	3
Golden Nuggets, Nestle*	1 Serving/40g	152	0.3	381	6.2	87.4	0.7	1.5
Golden Puffs, Sainsbury's*	1 Serving/28g	107	0.3	383	6.6	86.3	1.2	3
Granola	**1 Serving/45g**	**194**	**8.7**	**430**	**17.5**	**48.8**	**19.4**	**16.8**
Granola & Strawberries with Bio Yoghurt, Rumblers*	1 Pot/168g	267	9.7	159	4.3	22.4	5.8	1.1

B

INFO/WEIGHT	Measure	per Measure		Nutrition Values per 100g / 100ml				
		KCAL	FAT	KCAL	PROT	CARB	FAT	FIBRE

BREAKFAST CEREAL

	Measure INFO/WEIGHT	per Measure KCAL	FAT	KCAL	PROT	CARB	FAT	FIBRE
Granola, 5 Ways, Honey, Almonds & Seeds, Nutri Brex*	1 Serving/40g	165	5.9	413	12.4	54.1	14.7	7
Granola, Cherry Bakewell, 1, Waitrose*	1 Serving/40g	176	6	440	10	62.2	15.1	7.5
Granola, Chocolate, Dorset Cereals*	1 Serving/40g	206	12	515	8.8	47.2	30	10.5
Granola, Chocolate, Sante*	1 Serving/50g	220	7.5	440	7	66	15	6.2
Granola, Cranberry & Honey Nut, Topper, Graze*	1 Punnet/35g	157	7.1	447	11	56.2	20.3	8
Granola, Crunchy Nut Glorious Oat, Kellogg's*	1 Serving/45g	212	9.4	470	7	61	21	4.5
Granola, Crunchy Oat, Raisin, Almond, Harvest Morn, Aldi*	1 Serving/40g	166	4.6	416	8.2	66.9	11.4	6.4
Granola, Crunchy Oat, Tropical Fruits, Harvest Morn, Aldi*	1 Serving/40g	174	5.2	436	9.4	66	13	7.4
Granola, Fruit, Simply Sumptuous, Lidl*	1 Bowl/45g	198	8.1	440	10	56	18	7.1
Granola, High Protein, Lizi's*	1 Serving/40g	180	6.8	450	27	44	17	6.7
Granola, Honey, Dorset Cereals*	1 Serving/40g	204	12	511	13	44	30	7.4
Granola, Low Fat, Home Farm*	1 Serving/55g	180	3	328	7.3	69	5.4	9
Granola, Multigrain Nutty, Good & Balanced, Asda*	1 Serving/40g	162	6	406	9.9	54	15	7.6
Granola, Nut, Simply Nut, Dorset Cereals*	1 Serving/40g	200	10.8	500	11	48	27	8.3
Granola, Nuts, Pumpkin Seeds, & Fruit, Aldi*	1 Serving/45g	210	8.6	466	27	45	19	5
Granola, Oat Clusters, Apple & Cinnamon, Quaker*	1 Pack/48g	193	3.8	403	8	70.2	8	9.4
Granola, Oat, Simply Oat, Dorset Cereals*	1 Serving/40g	177	6.8	443	8.8	60	17	7.4
Granola, Organic, Lizi's, The GoodCarb Food Company*	1 Serving/50g	246	14	493	11.3	48.6	28.1	7.4
Granola, Original, Diet Chef Ltd*	1 Pack/50g	248	14.6	496	10.9	46.2	29.3	10.6
Granola, Original, Lizi's, The GoodCarb Food Company*	1 Serving/50g	248	14.6	496	10.9	46.2	29.3	10.6
Granola, Pink Apple & Cinnamon, Diet Chef Ltd*	1 Pack/40g	193	10.7	483	10.1	49.3	26.8	11.2
Granola, Quaker*	1 Serving/48g	210	7	438	10.4	72.9	14.6	6.2
Granola, Seed & Nut, The Natural Low Carb store*	1 Portion/30g	151	11.5	504	19.4	5.4	38.4	29.9
Granola, Summer Fruits, Pomegranate Infused, M&S*	1 Serving/50g	200	6.4	400	8.6	63.2	12.7	5.8
Granola, Super Fruity, Jordan's*	1 Serving/45g	194	5.6	431	9.5	66.6	12.4	7.5
Granola, Super Nutty, Aldi*	1 Serving/45g	217	9.9	483	11	56	22	7.2
Granola, Superfoods, Jordans*	1 Serving/50g	208	6.7	415	9	64.7	13.4	8.6
Granola, Toffee & Pecan, Jane Plan*	1 Portion/40g	200	11.1	500	10	48.2	27.8	11
Granola, Treacle & Pecan, Diet Chef Ltd*	1 Pack/40g	196	11.3	490	9.7	47.6	28.3	11.3
Granola, Tropical Twist, Paleo, Planet Organic*	1 Serving/35g	197	14.3	536	16	36	39	7.8
Granola, Yacon, Organic, Pertwood Farm*	1 Serving/50g	234	12	469	10.9	51	23.9	9.3
Grape Nuts, Kraft*	1 Serving/45g	158	0.9	350	10.9	81.9	2	11.9
Harvest Crunch, Nut, Quaker*	1 Serving/40g	184	7.8	459	8	62.5	19.5	6
Harvest Crunch, Real Red Berries, Quaker*	1 Serving/50g	224	8.5	447	7	66	17	4.5
Harvest Crunch, Soft Juicy Raisins, Quaker*	1 Serving/50g	221	8	442	6	67	16	4
Hawaiian Crunch, Asda*	1 Serving/50g	224	7.6	448	8	69.6	15.3	7
Hawaiian Crunch, Mornflake*	1 Serving/60g	247	7.4	411	8.1	66.8	12.4	6.8
High Bran, CBY, Asda*	1 Serving/40g	136	1.5	341	13.6	49.5	3.8	27.1
High Fibre Bran, Co-Op*	1 Serving/40g	110	1.6	275	15	46	4	27
High Fibre Bran, Sainsbury's*	1 Serving/40g	134	1.5	335	14.3	48.4	3.7	25.4
High Fruit Muesli, BGTY, Sainsbury's*	1 Serving/50g	164	1	328	6.7	71	1.9	6.6
Honey & Nut Crisp, Mini, Weetabix*	1 Serving/40g	150	0.8	375	9.4	75.1	2	9.3
Honey Cheerios with 125ml Semi Skimmed Milk, Nestle*	1 Serving/30g	174	2.9	580	21	99.7	9.7	5.7
Honey Hoops, Harvest Morn, Aldi*	1 Serving/30g	117	1	389	6.5	81	3.4	4
Honey Loops, Kellogg's*	1 Serving/30g	110	0.9	367	8	77	3	6
Honey Numbers, Harvest Morn, Aldi*	1 Serving/30g	114	1	379	6.9	78.7	3.3	3.3
Honey Raisin & Almond, Crunchy, Waitrose*	1 Serving/40g	170	4.8	425	10.5	68.8	12	5.7
Honey, Crisp Minis, Weetabix*	1 Serving/40g	150	0.8	375	9.5	75	2	9.2
Honey, Oats & More, Nestle*	1 Serving/30g	114	1.6	379	9.7	73.1	5.3	5.9
Hooplas, Sainsbury's*	1 Serving/30g	112	1.1	375	6.5	78.6	3.8	4.6
Hoops, Multigrain, Asda*	1 Serving/30g	113	1.2	376	6.5	78.4	4	4.6
Hoops, Multigrain, Tesco*	1 Serving/30g	112	1.1	375	6.5	78.6	3.8	4.6
Hot Oat, Aldi*	1 Serving/40g	142	3.3	356	11.6	58.8	8.3	8.9

BREAKFAST CEREAL

INFO/WEIGHT	Measure		Nutrition Values per 100g / 100ml				
	per Measure KCAL	FAT	KCAL	PROT	CARB	FAT	FIBRE
Hot Oats, Instant, Tesco*	1 Serving/30g	108	2.6	360	11.8	58.4	8.7	7.9
Instant Oats, Dry Weight	*1 Sachet/36g*	*129*	*3.1*	*359*	*11.5*	*59.1*	*8.5*	*8.3*
Just Right, Kellogg's*	1 Serving/40g	148	0.8	371	7	79	2	4.5
Kashi, Crunch, Seven Whole Grains, Original, Kellogg's*	1 Serving/40g	162	3.6	405	8	73	9	5
Krave, Chocolate & Hazelnut, Kellogg's*	1 Serving/30g	136	4.8	452	7.2	68	16	3.4
Krave, Milk Chocolate, Kellogg's*	1 Serving/30g	134	4.5	445	7.1	69	15	3
Lion, Nestle*	1 Serving/40g	166	3.1	415	7.2	76.9	7.7	4.3
Luxury Muesli, Diet Chef Ltd*	1 Pack/40g	166	4.7	414	10.6	61	11.8	10.9
Malted Wheaties, CBY, Asda*	1 Serving/40g	146	0.8	366	10.3	72.7	1.9	8.2
Malted Wheats, Waitrose*	1 Serving/32g	110	0.6	343	9.7	71.7	1.9	9.9
Malties, Sainsbury's*	1 Serving/40g	137	1.2	343	10	72.9	2.9	10
Malty Flakes with Red Berries, Tesco*	1 Serving/30g	111	0.6	369	9.9	78.1	1.9	3.1
Malty Flakes, Tesco*	1 Serving/40g	148	0.6	371	11	78.4	1.5	4.3
Maple & Pecan Crisp, Sainsbury's*	1 Serving/50g	226	9.8	452	7.9	61.3	19.5	5.4
Maple & Pecan Crisp, Tesco*	1 Serving/50g	215	7.6	430	10.5	62.5	15.2	10.2
Maple & Pecan, Crisp, Asda*	1 Serving/30g	135	5.7	451	8	62	19	6
Millet Rice Oatbran Flakes, Nature's Path*	1 Serving/56g	204	3.2	365	11.3	67	5.8	10
Milo Duo, Nestle*	1 Serving/30g	116	1.7	386	8.2	75.6	5.6	4.9
Mini Wheats, Original, Frosted, Kellogg's*	21 Biscuits/54g	190	1	352	9.3	83.3	1.8	11.1
Mini Wheats, Sainsbury's*	1 Serving/45g	157	1	348	11.8	69.9	2.3	11.8
Minibix, Weetabix*	1 Serving/40g	134	1.5	335	8.8	71.2	3.8	8.1
Mixed Berry, Oats & Chia, The Chia Co*	1 Serving/45g	188	7.2	417	10.6	47.1	16	12.7
Muesli Base, Wholesome, Waitrose*	1 Portion/50g	125	4.2	250	11.5	31.8	8.4	5
Muesli Mix, Perfect Start, Organic, The Food Doctor*	1 Serving/50g	196	7.1	392	12.1	55.5	14.2	7.1
Muesli, Apricot, Traidcraft*	1 Serving/30g	103	1.8	344	8	68	6	5
Muesli, Base, Nature's Harvest*	1 Serving/50g	179	2.6	358	11	71.2	5.1	7.4
Muesli, Basics, Sainsbury's*	1 Serving/50g	178	2.6	355	11.2	61.5	5.1	9.2
Muesli, Beeren Bircher, Mymuesli*	1 Serving/60g	213	5.4	355	11	53	9	11
Muesli, Berry, & Cherry, Luscious, Dorset Cereals*	1 Serving/45g	149	0.9	332	7	67	2.1	8.3
Muesli, Carb Control, Tesco*	1 Serving/35g	154	9.3	439	25	25	26.6	13.8
Muesli, COU, M&S*	1 Serving/60g	201	1.5	335	7.6	70.2	2.5	8.1
Muesli, Creamy Tropical Fruit, Finest, Tesco*	1 Serving/80g	283	4.5	354	7.2	68.8	5.6	6.9
Muesli, Crunchy, Organic, Sainsbury's*	1 Serving/40g	168	5.8	420	10.6	62	14.4	9.2
Muesli, De Luxe, No Added Salt or Sugar, Sainsbury's*	1 Serving/40g	161	5.6	403	11.9	57.6	13.9	8.4
Muesli, Fantastically Fruity, Roast & Toast, Dorset Cereals*	1 Bowl/60g	251	10.1	418	11.9	54.7	16.8	7.4
Muesli, Flahavans*	1 Serving/52g	187	2.8	360	10.4	72.1	5.3	5.5
Muesli, Fruit & Nut, 55%, Asda*	1 Serving/40g	151	5.6	378	9	54	14	7
Muesli, Fruit & Nut, COU, M&S*	1 Serving/40g	128	1.1	320	7.4	74.5	2.8	7.4
Muesli, Fruit & Nut, Luxury, Co-Op*	1 Serving/40g	150	4	375	8	64	10	6
Muesli, Fruit & Nut, Luxury, Lidl*	1 Serving/57g	205	5.6	360	8	60	9.8	7.5
Muesli, Fruit & Nut, Luxury, Simply Sumptuous, Lidl*	1 Serving/45g	179	6.2	398	8	57.6	13.8	5.8
Muesli, Fruit & Nut, Luxury, Waitrose*	1 Serving/40g	145	3.8	363	9	60.3	9.5	6.5
Muesli, Fruit & Nut, M&S*	1 Serving/40g	128	1.1	320	7.4	74.5	2.8	7.4
Muesli, Fruit & Nut, Organic, M&S*	1 Serving/50g	166	3	333	8.2	61.6	6	7.6
Muesli, Fruit & Nut, Tesco*	1 Serving/50g	190	5.6	380	8.4	60.3	11.3	5.3
Muesli, Fruit & Nut, Whole Wheat, Organic, Asda*	1 Serving/50g	172	3.5	343	10	60	7	7
Muesli, Fruit & Seeds, Organic, Pertwood Farm*	1 Serving/50g	164	3.4	328	11.4	55.5	6.7	12.6
Muesli, Fruit & Nut, Essential, Waitrose*	1 Serving/45g	173	6.1	384	8.6	51.5	13.5	11
Muesli, Fruit & Nut, Jordans*	1 Serving/50g	180	4.7	361	8	61.2	9.4	7.5
Muesli, Fruit & Nut, Luxury, Sainsbury's*	1 Serving/50g	178	4.6	355	10.3	57.9	9.1	11.3
Muesli, Fruit & Nut, Sainsbury's*	1 Serving/30g	114	3.1	379	9.5	58.7	10.3	6.9
Muesli, Fruit Nut & Seed, Organic, Dorset Cereals*	1 Serving/70g	251	6.9	358	10.8	56.6	9.8	8.4
Muesli, Fruit Rush, Saffola*	1 Serving/30g	112	1.6	373	9	78.5	5.5	6.7

BREAKFAST CEREAL

INFO/WEIGHT	Measure	per Measure		Nutrition Values per 100g / 100ml				
		KCAL	FAT	KCAL	PROT	CARB	FAT	FIBRE
Muesli, Fruit Sensation, M&S*	1 Serving/50g	158	1.5	315	6	66	3	7.4
Muesli, Fruit, Luxury, Weight Watchers*	1 Serving/40g	127	0.8	318	7.2	67.7	2	8.1
Muesli, Fruit, Nuts & Seeds, Dorset Cereals*	1 Serving/70g	265	8	379	10.6	58.4	11.4	6.1
Muesli, Fruit, Sainsbury's*	1 Serving/40g	132	1.8	330	8.1	64.3	4.5	9.6
Muesli, Fruit, Somerfield*	1 Serving/50g	164	2	329	6.4	66.5	4.1	4.8
Muesli, Fruit, Waitrose*	1 Serving/30g	101	1.4	338	7.2	66.8	4.7	6.8
Muesli, GF, Nature's Harvest, Holland & Barrett*	1 Serving/60g	234	7.8	390	14.1	54.1	13	3.3
Muesli, Golden Sun, Lidl*	1 Serving/40g	144	3.9	360	8	60	9.8	7.5
Muesli, High Fibre, Neal's Yard*	1 Serving/50g	182	1	364	7.6	72.7	1.9	12.9
Muesli, High Fibre, You Count, Love Life, Waitrose*	1 Serving/45g	155	1.3	344	7.7	67.4	2.9	8.8
Muesli, HL, Tesco*	1 Serving/40g	126	0.9	315	7.6	64.3	2.3	7.5
Muesli, Light & Crispy, Jordans*	1 Serving/50g	172	2.5	343	7.7	66.7	5	9.5
Muesli, Lite n Natural, Saffola*	1 Serving/30g	114	1.6	381	10.2	78.7	5.5	6
Muesli, Luxury Fruit, Harvest Morn, Aldi*	1 Serving/50g	179	2.3	358	7.2	69	4.6	5.6
Muesli, Luxury, Finest, Tesco*	1 Serving/50g	197	6.6	394	8.3	60.8	13.1	5.4
Muesli, Luxury, Sainsbury's*	1 Serving/40g	144	4.3	359	8.5	57.1	10.7	7.7
Muesli, Natural, No Added Sugar or Salt, Jordans*	1 Serving/45g	161	2.2	357	9.5	63.7	5	9.7
Muesli, No Added Sugar Or Salt, Organic, Jordans*	1 Serving/50g	175	4.4	350	9.2	58.4	8.8	9.3
Muesli, No Added Sugar, Morrisons*	1 Serving/50g	166	2.6	331	11.2	64.7	5.1	6.3
Muesli, No Added Sugar, Waitrose*	1 Serving/40g	146	2.5	364	12	64.9	6.3	6.7
Muesli, Nuts & Seeds , Tesco*	1 Serving/50g	195	5.5	390	10.9	57.2	11	9.2
Muesli, Nutty Crunch, Saffola*	1 Serving/30g	113	1.8	378	9	78.2	6	6.3
Muesli, Organic, Waitrose*	1 Serving/50g	188	0.8	375	10.3	59.6	1.6	8.3
Muesli, Original, Holland & Barrett*	1 Serving/30g	105	2.5	351	11.1	61.2	8.4	7.1
Muesli, Original, Raisins, Hazelnuts, & Almonds, Alpen*	1 Serving/40g	144	2.3	359	10.5	66.6	5.8	7.3
Muesli, Original, Simply, Hubbards*	1 Serving/50g	212	6.7	424	11.8	59.4	13.4	9.2
Muesli, Really Nutty, Dorset Cereals*	1 Serving/70g	253	6.1	362	9.8	61.1	8.7	6.3
Muesli, Really Nutty, Simply Sumptuous, Lidl*	1 Serving/45g	167	3.9	371	9.5	59.2	8.7	8.9
Muesli, Rich, Nature's Harvest*	1 Serving/40g	143	3.7	358	10	60.5	9.2	7.6
Muesli, Seriously Nutty, Mornflake*	1 Bowl/45g	202	10.1	449	14.5	43.4	22.5	7.6
Muesli, Simply Delicious, Dorset Cereals*	1 Serving/45g	160	3.3	356	9.9	58.1	7.4	8.9
Muesli, Simply Fruity, As Sold, Dorset Cereals*	1 Serving/45g	152	1.1	337	7.3	68	2.4	6.8
Muesli, Simply Sumptuous, Luxury Fruit, Lidl*	1 Serving/45g	154	1.5	343	6.5	68.7	3.3	6.2
Muesli, Special, Fruit, Jordans*	1 Serving/50g	162	1.4	323	6.6	68	2.7	8.4
Muesli, Special, Jordans*	1 Serving/50g	183	5.4	366	7.9	59.5	10.7	8.5
Muesli, Special, Luxury Fruit & Nut, Goody*	1 Serving/50g	193	6.9	386	8	57.6	13.8	8
Muesli, Super Berry, Jordans*	1 Serving/50g	174	3.8	348	9	60.8	7.6	8.1
Muesli, Super High Fibre, Dorset Cereals*	1 Serving/70g	250	6.6	357	8	60.1	9.4	8.4
Muesli, Superfoods, Jordans*	1 Serving/50g	173	3.6	346	9.2	60.9	7.3	10.2
Muesli, Swiss Style with Fruit, Tesco*	1 Serving/40g	144	2.1	360	10.4	67.4	5.3	7.4
Muesli, Swiss Style, Aldi*	1 Serving/50g	180	3.2	359	9.8	65.3	6.5	8.3
Muesli, Swiss Style, Bettabuy, Morrisons*	1 Serving/50g	170	2.5	340	11	62.8	5	9.4
Muesli, Swiss Style, Co-Op*	1 Serving/40g	148	2.4	370	11	67	6	6
Muesli, Swiss Style, No Added Salt or Sugar, Sainsbury's*	1 Serving/50g	178	3	357	10.9	64.9	6	6
Muesli, Swiss Style, No Added Salt or Sugar, Tesco*	1 Serving/50g	182	3.2	364	11	61	6.4	9.6
Muesli, Swiss Style, No Added Sugar or Salt, Asda*	1 Serving/50g	182	3.5	363	11	64	7	8
Muesli, Swiss Style, No Added Sugar, Lidl*	1 Serving/30g	111	1.8	371	10.9	64.5	6	7.8
Muesli, Swiss Style, Organic, Whole Earth*	1 Serving/50g	172	3.6	344	9.2	60.8	7.1	11.3
Muesli, Swiss Style, Smart Price, Asda*	1 Serving/60g	222	3.6	370	9	70	6	10
Muesli, The Ultimate, Organic, Rude Health*	1 Serving/50g	163	4.5	326	10.8	50.5	9	12.3
Muesli, Toasted Spelt, Barley, Oat Flakes, Dorset Cereals*	1 Serving/40g	148	4.5	371	9.5	57.9	11.3	7.4
Muesli, Toasted, GF with Buckwheat, Eat Natural*	1 Serving/50g	230	11.4	461	11.7	53.2	22.8	2
Muesli, Tropical Fruit, Holland & Barrett*	1 Serving/60g	197	1.9	328	7.5	69.8	3.2	5.1

BREAKFAST CEREAL

	Measure INFO/WEIGHT	per Measure KCAL	FAT	Nutrition Values per 100g / 100ml KCAL	PROT	CARB	FAT	FIBRE
Muesli, Tropical Fruits, Jordans*	1 Serving/50g	164	1.4	329	6.9	68.7	2.9	7.1
Muesli, Tropical, Sainsbury's*	1 Serving/50g	182	3.4	365	6.5	69.4	6.8	6.4
Muesli, Tropical, Tesco*	1 Serving/50g	173	2.4	346	7.8	68.2	4.7	9.1
Muesli, Twelve Fruit & Nut, Sainsbury's*	1 Serving/50g	166	2.4	332	8.1	64.2	4.7	7.8
Muesli, Unsweetened, M&S*	1 Serving/40g	129	1.1	322	8.1	68	2.7	9.4
Muesli, Whole Wheat, Co-Op*	1 Serving/40g	140	2.8	350	11	61	7	7
Muesli, Whole Wheat, No Added Sugar & Salt, Tesco*	1 Serving/40g	154	5	386	9.5	59.1	12.4	7.4
Muesli, Wholewheat, Asda*	1 Serving/45g	150	3.5	333	8	57.9	7.7	9.7
Muesli, with Berries, Swiss, Dry, Love Life, Waitrose*	1 Serving/45g	172	4.3	383	13.5	55.7	9.6	9.8
Muesli, with Toasted Nuts & Seeds, Eat Natural*	1 Portion/50g	219	11.1	438	11.5	38.9	22.2	7.9
Multigrain Boulders, Tesco*	1 Serving/30g	112	0.4	375	8.2	82.3	1.3	3.6
Multigrain Flakes with Fruit & Nuts, Aldi*	1 Serving/30g	108	0.7	360	7.5	77.1	2.4	4.5
Multigrain Flakes, Protiflake, Fuel 10K*	1 Serving/30g	112	0.4	373	23.8	65.9	1.2	1.9
Multigrain Flakes, with Fruit, Tesco*	1 Serving/40g	147	0.9	367	7.2	77.3	2.2	4.7
Multigrain Wheelies, CBY, Asda*	1 Serving/30g	115	1	384	8.9	76	3.5	6.5
Multigrain, Balanced Lifestyle, Aldi*	1 Serving/30g	108	0.7	360	7.5	77.1	2.4	4.5
Multigrain, Fitnesse, Nestle*	1 Serving/30g	109	0.4	363	8	79.8	1.3	5.1
Multigrain, Hoops, Average	*1 Serving/30g*	*112*	*1.1*	*374*	*6.6*	*77.4*	*3.6*	*6.1*
Museli, Premium, Lidl*	1 Bowl/45g	165	3.3	367	8.4	62.5	7.4	8.3
Nesquik, Chocolatey Corn & Rice, Nestle*	1 Serving/30g	114	1.2	380	7.2	79.1	3.9	5.1
Nutri Brex, Biscuits, GF, Nutri Brex*	3 Biscuits/46g	174	1.7	378	12.3	70	3.6	6.8
Nutty Crunch, Alpen*	1 Serving/40g	159	4.5	398	10.7	63.6	11.2	6.5
Nutty Crunch, Deliciously, M&S*	1 Serving/50g	238	11.2	476	8.8	59.6	22.5	4.4
Oat & Bran Flakes, Sainsbury's*	1 Serving/30g	97	1.7	324	12.2	56	5.7	17.7
Oat Bran, Hodgson Mill*	1 Serving/40g	48	1.2	120	6	23	3	6
Oat Clusters, Triple Chocolate Crunch, M&S*	1 Serving/45g	212	8.9	471	8.5	61.9	19.8	5.6
Oat Crunchy, Blueberry & Cranberry, Waitrose*	1 Serving/60g	259	9.1	432	8	65.9	15.2	8.5
Oat Granola, Quaker*	1 Serving/50g	206	4.4	411	8.6	73	8.8	5.2
Oat Granola, Raisin, Quaker*	1 Serving/45g	188	4.1	418	8	70.9	9.1	6.9
Oat Krunchies, Quaker*	1 Serving/30g	118	2.1	393	9.5	72	7	5.5
Oat Meal, Medium, Heart's Content, Mornflake*	1 Serving/30g	108	2.4	359	11	60.4	8.1	8.5
Oat So Easy, Banana & Toffee, Jungle*	1 Pack/50g	187	4.6	374	1.8	74.7	9.2	5.1
Oat, Crunchy, Sainsbury's*	1 Serving/50g	226	10.2	453	8.2	59.3	20.3	6.6
Oat, Raisin, Nut & Honey, Crunchy, Dry, Sainsbury's*	1 Serving/50g	201	7	402	8.5	60.2	14.1	7.6
Oatbran & Oatgerm, Prewett's*	1 Serving/30g	104	2.9	345	14.8	49.7	9.7	15.2
Oatbran 100%, Pure & Simple, Mornflake*	1 Serving/40g	146	3.8	364	13.4	47.3	9.4	18.2
Oatbran Flakes, Nature's Path*	1 Serving/30g	124	1.4	414	8.7	83	4.7	6.7
Oatbran Flakes, Original, Mornflake*	1 Serving/40g	149	2.1	372	11.9	63.2	5.2	12.4
Oatbran Sprinkles, Mornflake*	1 Serving/40g	146	3.8	364	13.4	47.3	9.4	18.2
Oatbran, Original Pure, Mornflake*	1 Serving/30g	104	2.9	345	14.8	49.7	9.7	15.2
Oatbran, Very Berry, Flakes, Mornflake*	1 Serving/40g	149	2	372	11.7	63.8	5.1	12
Oatibix, Flakes, Weetabix*	1 Serving/50g	190	2.8	381	9.5	73.2	5.6	3.5
Oatibix, Original, Bitesize, Weetabix*	1 Serving/36g	133	2.4	370	10.6	66.5	6.8	10.1
Oatibix, Weetabix*	2 Biscuits/48g	189	3.8	394	12.5	64.3	8	7.3
Oatmeal, Coarse, Prewett's*	1 Serving/40g	137	4.2	343	14.3	47.6	10.6	16
Oatmeal, Instant, Cinnamon, Weight Control, Quaker*	1 Pack/45g	160	3	356	15.6	64.4	6.7	13.3
Oatmeal, Instant, Heart to Heart, Kashi*	1 Serving/43g	150	2	349	7	76.7	4.6	9.3
Oatmeal, Quick Oats, Dry, Quaker*	1 Serving/30g	114	2	380	14	66.7	6.7	10
Oatmeal, Raw	*1oz/28g*	*112*	*2.4*	*401*	*12.4*	*72.8*	*8.7*	*6.8*
Oatmeal, Scottish, Hamlyns of Scotland*	1 Portion/40g	157	3.7	392	11.2	66	9.2	7.1
Oats, Ginger Bread, Bench Press, Instant, Oomf*	1 Pot/75g	296	3.4	395	28.3	57.1	4.5	6.7
Oats, Golden Syrup Flavour, Instant, Hot, Waitrose*	1 Serving/39g	153	2.3	393	7.8	77.4	5.8	6
Oats, Jumbo, Organic, Waitrose*	1 Serving/50g	180	4	361	11	61.1	8.1	7.8

	Measure INFO/WEIGHT	per Measure KCAL	FAT	Nutrition Values per 100g / 100ml KCAL	PROT	CARB	FAT	FIBRE
BREAKFAST CEREAL								
Oats, Original, Instant, Hot, Waitrose*	1 Sachet/27g	97	2.2	359	11	60.4	8.1	8.5
Oats, Pure, Free From, Sainsbury's*	1 Serving/40g	164	3.2	410	14.9	64	8	11
Oats, Strawberry & Banana, Toasted, Crunch, White's*	1 Serving/40g	175	5.5	437	7.7	67.3	13.8	6.2
Oats, Superfast, Mornflake*	1 Serving/40g	147	3.4	367	12.1	56.1	8.4	9.1
Oats, Tesco*	1 Serving/40g	142	3.2	356	11	60	8	8
Oats, Wholegrain, Organic, Quaker*	1 Serving/25g	89	2	356	11	60	8	9
Optivita, Berry Oat Crisp, Kellogg's*	1 Serving/30g	107	1.5	357	10	68	5	9
Organic, Weetabix*	2 Biscuits/38g	134	0.7	358	11.5	68.6	2	10
Original, Crunchy, Raisins & Almonds, Jordans*	1 Serving/50g	204	6.4	407	8.7	64	12.9	6.6
Original, Crunchy, Tropical Fruits, Jordans*	1 Serving/50g	212	7.2	423	8.1	65.1	14.5	6.7
Perfect Balance, Weight Watchers*	1 Serving/30g	90	0.5	300	7.8	63.3	1.7	15.6
Perfekt, Granola, Ultimate, Organic, GranoVita*	1 Serving/40g	190	6.6	474	13.3	40.6	16.4	11.8
Pomegranate & Raspberry, Wheats, Tesco*	1 Serving/45g	151	0.6	335	7.5	71.8	1.4	8.2
Porage Oats, Old Fashioned, Dry, Scotts*	1 Serving/40g	142	3.2	355	11	60	8	9
Porage Oats, Original, Dry, Scotts*	1 Serving/40g	149	3.2	372	11	60	8	9
Porage Oats, Original, So-Easy, Dry, Scotts*	1 Serving/30g	109	2.6	364	11	60	8.5	9
Porage Oats, Syrup Swirl, So-Easy, Dry, Scotts*	1 Sachet/37g	135	2.2	366	8	70	6	6.5
Porridge 5 Grain, 5 Seed, Rude Health*	1 Serving/50g	176	4.1	351	12.2	57.1	8.2	12.4
Porridge Oats, & Bran, Co-Op*	1 Serving/40g	141	2.8	353	12.5	60	7	12
Porridge Oats, & Bran, Somerfield*	1 Serving/40g	154	2.8	385	12	68	7	0
Porridge Oats, Co-Op*	1 Serving/40g	144	3.2	360	12	61	8	9
Porridge Oats, Dry Weight, Value, Tesco*	1 Serving/50g	180	4	359	11	60.4	8.1	8.5
Porridge Oats, Honey Flavour, Paw Ridge, Quaker*	1 Sachet/28.5g	103	2	361	9.6	64.7	7	7.9
Porridge Oats, Mornflake*	1 Serving/50g	180	4	359	11	60.4	8.1	8.5
Porridge Oats, Organic, Evernat*	1 Serving/40g	167	3.8	418	13	69	9.6	7.4
Porridge Oats, Organic, Tesco*	1 Serving/50g	184	4.2	368	12.1	56.1	8.4	10
Porridge Oats, Original, Dry, Quaker*	1 Serving/45g	160	3.6	356	11	60	8	4
Porridge Oats, Original, Paw Ridge, Quaker*	1 Sachet/25g	89	2	356	11	60	8	9
Porridge Oats, Rolled, Tesco*	1 Serving/50g	180	4	359	11	60.4	8.1	8.5
Porridge Oats, Scottish, Organic, Sainsbury's*	1 Serving/45g	172	2.2	383	10	74.4	5	7.9
Porridge Oats, Scottish, Tesco*	1 Serving/50g	180	4	359	11	60.4	8.1	8.5
Porridge Oats, Sprouted, Organic, Rude Health*	1 Serving/10g	38	0.6	375	16	64	6.5	10
Porridge Oats, with Bran, Scottish, Sainsbury's*	1 Serving/50g	190	2.5	380	9.6	74.1	5	10.3
Porridge Oats, with Grains & Seeds, Tesco*	1 Serving/50g	198	5.6	395	12.1	56.5	11.1	10.5
Porridge Oats, with Oat & Wheat Bran, HL, Tesco*	1 Sachet/30g	105	1.8	350	10.8	62.3	6.1	9.2
Porridge Oats, with Oatbran & Wheatbran, Tesco*	1 Portion/50g	187	4.1	375	11	58.3	8.3	11.4
Porridge Oats, with Wheat Bran, Tesco*	1 Serving/50g	167	3.6	334	12.3	55	7.2	13
Porridge Oats, with Wheatbran, Essential, Waitrose*	1 Serving/50g	168	3.8	336	11.2	55.8	7.6	13
Porridge, Apple & Cinnamon, Express, Dry, Sainsbury's*	1 Sachet/36g	138	2.1	383	8.6	70.3	5.9	7.2
Porridge, Apple & Cinnamon, Variety Box, Graze*	1 Bag/67g	240	3.4	356	8	68	5	10
Porridge, Apple & Pear, Variety Box, Graze*	1 Bag/63g	226	3.7	359	9.4	65	5.9	11
Porridge, Apple, Sultana & Cinnamon, M&S*	1 Sachet/40g	144	3	360	10.3	62.3	7.5	8.6
Porridge, Banana, Ready Brek, Weetabix*	1 Serving/40g	146	2.6	365	8.9	68	6.4	6.7
Porridge, Berry Burst, Oat So Simple, Quaker*	1 Serving/39g	144	2.3	370	8	70	6	6.5
Porridge, Blueberry, Cranberry, Guava, Made Up, Quaker*	1 Serving/35g	201	5.1	574	24.8	83.4	14.6	9.1
Porridge, Caramel, Instant, Pot, Oat So Simple, Quaker*	1 Pot/57g	208	3.2	365	10.5	67.7	5.6	6.3
Porridge, Chocolate, Instant, Grasshopper*	1 Pot/60g	221	3	368	15	68.3	5	0
Porridge, Chocolate, Oatibix, Weetabix*	1 Pack/40g	149	3.9	372	9.9	61.3	9.7	6.2
Porridge, Chocolate, Ready Brek, Weetabix*	1 Serving/30g	114	2.4	380	10	63.6	8	7
Porridge, Coconut & Date, Graze*	1 Punnet/45g	176	5.9	391	8	57	13	9
Porridge, Country Honey, Oat So Simple, Quaker*	1 Serving/36g	134	2.3	373	8.5	69	6.5	6
Porridge, Cranberry & Raspberry, Fruity, Dorset Cereals*	1 Sachet/30g	99	1.8	330	10.2	58.7	6	12.3
Porridge, Flakes, Organic, Barkat*	1 Serving/30g	109	0.9	362	8.5	74.1	3	0

BREAKFAST CEREAL

	Measure INFO/WEIGHT	per Measure KCAL	per Measure FAT	Nutrition Values per 100g / 100ml KCAL	PROT	CARB	FAT	FIBRE
Porridge, Free From, Sainsbury's*	1 Serving/50g	174	1.5	348	8.6	72	3	3.4
Porridge, Fresh, Double Cream, & Demerara Sugar, M&S*	1 Pot/200g	254	15.2	127	4.3	9.7	7.6	1.3
Porridge, Fruit & Nut, Fruity, Dorset Cereals*	1 Serving/70g	242	5.6	346	9.4	59	8	8.2
Porridge, Golden Honey, Oatibix, Weetabix*	1 Serving/40g	145	2.6	363	9.2	66.7	6.6	7
Porridge, Golden Syrup, Dry, Oat So Simple, Quaker*	1 Sachet/36g	137	2.2	380	8.4	68.7	6.2	6.8
Porridge, Golden Syrup, Instant, As Consumed, Slim Fast*	1 Sachet/29g	99	1.3	340	17.4	53.2	4.6	7.9
Porridge, Golden Syrup, Prepared, Oatilicious, Lidl*	1 Sachet/39g	140	1.5	358	8.8	69	3.9	6
Porridge, Honey & Vanilla, Express Pot, Quaker*	1 Pot/57g	213	2.9	374	15.1	64.1	5.1	5.5
Porridge, Instant, Sweet Cinnamon, Harvest Morn, Aldi*	1 Pot/57g	211	2.6	371	15	64	4.5	7.8
Porridge, Made with Semi Skimmed Milk, Waitrose*	1 Serving/50g	277	7.5	554	24.6	80.4	15	8.6
Porridge, Maple & Pecan, Oat So Simple, Quaker*	1 Pack/35g	132	2.3	376	8.4	66.6	6.5	8.8
Porridge, Maple Syrup Flavour, Pot, As Sold, M&S*	1 Pot/70g	260	2.6	371	11.6	70.7	3.7	4.3
Porridge, Mealpak, All About Weight*	1 Mealpak/42g	153	5	364	39.5	21.1	11.9	7.4
Porridge, Mixed Berries, Fruity, Dorset Cereals*	1 Serving/70g	243	4.2	347	10.8	62.6	6	7.9
Porridge, Morning Glory, Rude Health*	1 Bowl/50g	176	4.1	351	12.2	57.1	8.2	12.4
Porridge, Multigrain, Jordans*	1 Serving/40g	134	2.2	335	10.4	60.9	5.5	10
Porridge, Oats, 100% Whole Grain, Rolled, Jumbo, Quaker*	1 Serving/40g	150	3.2	374	11	60	8	9
Porridge, Oats, 100% Whole Grain, Rolled, Quaker*	1 Portion/40g	150	3.2	374	11	60	8	9
Porridge, Oats, Dry, Smart Price, Asda*	1 Serving/50g	186	4	372	11	60	8	8
Porridge, Oats, Everyday Essentials, Aldi*	1 Portion/30g	118	2.3	392	11	66	7.7	7.1
Porridge, Oats, GF, Organic, Scottish, Alara *	1 Serving/40g	148	2.2	369	11.8	67.9	5.5	7.5
Porridge, Oats, Golden Syrup, Sainsbury's*	1 Sachet/39g	143	2.1	367	6.3	73.6	5.3	6.7
Porridge, Oats, Original, Instant, As Consumed, Tesco*	1 Serving/255g	207	3.3	81	3.1	13.5	1.3	1.6
Porridge, Oats, Twice the Fibre, M&S*	1 Portion/60g	230	3.5	384	10.4	62.6	5.9	19.5
Porridge, Oats, Whole, Chunky, Traditional, Jordans*	1 Serving/40g	143	2.7	358	6.7	63.6	6.8	7.9
Porridge, Original, As Sold, Moma Foods*	1 Pot/70g	257	4.2	367	15.6	59	6	7.6
Porridge, Original, Diet Chef Ltd*	1 Sachet/40g	157	2.5	392	12	67	6.3	9.8
Porridge, Original, Dry, Oat So Simple, Quaker*	1 Sachet/27g	100	2.1	370	11	58.9	7.7	10.5
Porridge, Original, Express, Sachet, Sainsbury's*	1 Pack/27g	100	2.2	370	11	58	8	10.8
Porridge, Original, Oatibix, Weetabix*	1 Sachet/30g	104	2.5	347	12.5	55.6	8.3	10.1
Porridge, Original, Ready Brek, Weetabix*	1 Serving/40g	149	3.5	373	11.7	57.9	8.7	7.9
Porridge, Original, Simply, Sachet, Asda*	1 Sachet/27g	96	2.2	356	11	60	8	8
Porridge, Original, Super Goodness, Quaker*	1 Serving/31g	114	2.8	372	14.1	56.7	9.1	9.9
Porridge, Perfectly, Dorset Cereals*	1 Sachet/30g	107	2.5	356	11.8	58.2	8.4	11
Porridge, Plain, Instant, Quaker*	1 Serving/34g	124	2.9	364	11	60	8.5	9
Porridge, Raspberry & Cranberry, Made Up, Quaker*	1 Sachet/39g	217	5.6	564	26	81.6	14.6	9.4
Porridge, Ready Oats, CBY, Asda*	1 Serving/40g	149	3.5	374	12	58	8.7	7.9
Porridge, Red Berry, Instant, As Consumed, Slim Fast*	1 Sachet/29g	99	1.3	341	17.2	53.1	4.5	7.9
Porridge, Rice & Buckwheat, Free From, Sainsbury's*	1 Serving/50g	179	0.4	358	6.8	81.1	0.7	1.4
Porridge, Spelt, Sharpham Park*	1 Serving/50g	159	1.6	318	11.3	7	3.3	9.5
Porridge, Spiced Apple, Sultana, Oatibix, Weetabix*	1 Sachet/40g	138	2.3	345	9.7	65.4	5.7	8.5
Porridge, Strawberry, Diet Chef Ltd*	1 Serving/40g	159	3.1	398	11.2	65.9	7.7	10.6
Porridge, Superfoods, Jordans*	1 Serving/40g	145	3.6	362	10.4	59.8	9	8.3
Porridge, Vanilla & Banana, Diet Chef Ltd*	1 Pack/40g	151	2.2	378	10.7	70.6	5.6	9.8
Porridge, with Apple & Cinnamon, Diet Chef Ltd*	1 Pack/40g	150	1.9	375	8.9	69.5	4.7	9
Porridge, with Blueberries, Cranberries, & Nuts, Alpen*	1 Sachet/40g	154	3.4	385	10.8	62.6	8.5	7.3
Porridge, with Cocao Nib, Diet Chef Ltd*	1 Pack/40g	164	3.5	410	10.9	67.3	8.8	9.5
Protein Crunch, Chocolate, Weetabix*	1 Serving/30g	114	1	379	20	64	3.2	7
Protein Crunch, Weetabix*	1 Serving/30g	114	0.8	379	20	66	2.5	6.1
Protein, Big Biscuit, Weetabix*	1 Biscuit/20g	72	0.4	360	19	62	1.9	9.6
Protioats, Fuel 10K*	1 Pot/60g	229	4	381	19.3	61.2	6.7	5.8
Puffed Rice, Average	*1 Serving/30g*	*115*	*0.8*	*382*	*7.1*	*82.2*	*2.8*	*3*
Puffed Rice, Honey, Organic, Kallo*	1 Serving/25g	98	0.9	392	5	85	3.5	2.1

BREAKFAST CEREAL

	Measure INFO/WEIGHT	per Measure KCAL	FAT	Nutrition Values per 100g / 100ml KCAL	PROT	CARB	FAT	FIBRE
Puffed Rice, Organic, Natural, Kallo*	1 Bowl/25g	92	0.5	370	7	81	2	3
Puffed Rice, Wholegrain, Brown, Original, Organic, Kallo*	1 Serving/25g	95	0.8	380	8	80	3	9
Puffed Wheat, Quaker*	1 Serving/15g	49	0.2	328	15.3	62.4	1.3	5.6
Puffed Wheat, Tesco*	1 Serving/28g	104	0.9	373	13.9	72.2	3.2	5.7
Raisin & Almond, Crunchy, Jordans*	1 Serving/56g	230	7	411	8.4	66	12.5	5
Raisin Oats & More, & 125ml Semi Skimmed Milk, Nestle*	1 Serving/40g	207	3.9	518	19.8	88	9.8	6.2
Raisin Wheats, Kellogg's*	1 Serving/45g	104	0.6	345	9	69	2	9
Raisin Wheats, Sainsbury's*	1 Serving/50g	166	0.8	332	8.2	71.5	1.5	8
Raisin, Bran Flakes, Asda*	1 Serving/50g	166	1.5	331	7	69	3	10
Raisin, Oats & More, Nestle*	1 Serving/30g	112	1.4	373	8.9	73.7	4.7	5.8
Red Berries, Special K, Kellogg's*	1 Serving/30g	112	0.4	374	14	76	1.5	3
Red Berry, & Almond, Luxury Crunch, Jordans*	1 Serving/40g	176	7.4	441	8.2	60.5	18.5	6.6
Rice & Wheat Flakes, Toasted, Love Life, Waitrose*	1 Serving/30g	115	0.4	382	11.7	79.7	1.3	2.2
Rice Krispies, Honey, Kellogg's*	1 Serving/30g	114	0.2	380	4	89	0.7	1
Rice Krispies, Kellogg's*	1 Serving/30g	115	0.3	383	6	87	1	1
Rice Krispies, Multi-Grain, Shapes, Kellogg's*	1 Serving/30g	111	0.8	370	8	77	2.5	8
Rice Pops, Blue Parrot Cafe, Sainsbury's*	1 Serving/30g	111	0.4	370	7.2	82.3	1.3	2.2
Rice Pops, GF, Nestle*	1 Serving/30g	116	0.4	385	7.5	85	1.2	1.5
Rice Pops, Organic, Dove's Farm*	1 Serving/30g	107	0.2	357	6.8	86.1	0.8	2
Rice Pops, Sainsbury's*	1 Serving/25g	98	0.4	391	6.7	87.1	1.4	1.7
Rice Snaps, Asda*	1 Serving/28g	105	0.4	376	7	84	1.3	1.5
Rice Snaps, Everyday Value, Tesco*	1 Serving/30g	115	0.3	380	7.5	84.5	0.9	1.4
Ricicles, Kellogg's*	1 Serving/30g	114	0.2	381	4.5	89	0.8	0.8
Right Balance, Morrisons*	1 Serving/50g	181	1.1	362	6.9	78.6	2.2	5.3
Shredded Wheat, Average	*2 Biscuits/45g*	*157*	*0.8*	*348*	*9*	*77*	*1.8*	*10*
Shredded Wheat, Bitesize, Nestle*	1 Serving/40g	148	0.9	369	11.8	69.6	2.2	11.8
Shredded Wheat, Fruitful, No Added Salt, Nestle*	1 Serving/40g	142	2	354	8.3	68.7	5.1	8.9
Shredded Wheat, Honey Nut, Nestle*	1 Serving/40g	151	2.6	378	11.2	68.8	6.5	9.4
Shreddies, Coco Orange Flavoured, Nestle*	1 Serving/40g	150	0.8	374	8.5	76.2	2	8.6
Shreddies, Coco, Nestle*	1 Serving/45g	161	0.9	358	8.4	76.5	2	8.6
Shreddies, Crunchy Cranberry & Oat Granola, Nestle*	1 Serving/45g	181	3.1	403	13	68	7	7.2
Shreddies, Frosted, Kellogg's*	1 Serving/50g	162	0.9	323	0.7	78.5	1.8	4.7
Shreddies, Frosted, Nestle*	1 Serving/45g	164	0.7	365	7.4	80.7	1.5	6.4
Shreddies, Frosted, Variety Pack, Nestle*	1 Pack/45g	163	0.6	363	6.7	81.1	1.3	6.8
Shreddies, Honey, Nestle*	1 Serving/45g	169	0.7	375	8.2	78.1	1.5	8.1
Shreddies, Malt Wheats, Tesco*	1 Serving/45g	169	0.9	375	10.3	73.8	2	8.2
Shreddies, Nestle*	1 Serving/45g	186	1	371	10	73.7	1.9	9.9
Smoothies, Strawberry, Quaker*	1 Sachet/29g	117	3.5	402	6.5	67	12	5.5
Special Flakes, Gluten, Wheat, & Milk, Free From, Tesco*	1 Serving/30g	115	0.6	382	6.5	83	2	3
Special Flakes, Tesco*	1 Serving/20g	74	0.3	371	11	78.4	1.5	4.3
Special Flakes, with Red Berries, Crownfield, Lidl*	1 Serving/30g	113	0.5	377	6.5	81	1.6	6.4
Special K, Bliss, Creamy Berry Crunch, Kellogg's*	1 Serving/30g	114	0.8	379	13	76	2.5	2.5
Special K, Bliss, Strawberry & Chocolate, Kellogg's*	1 Serving/30g	115	0.9	383	13	76	3	2.5
Special K, Choco, Kellogg's*	1 Serving/40g	160	2.8	400	14	70	7	3.5
Special K, Clusters, Honey, Kellogg's*	1 Serving/45g	175	1.4	389	9	80	3	3.5
Special K, Kellogg's*	1 Serving/30g	114	0.4	379	14	76	1.5	2.5
Special K, Oats & Honey, Kellogg's*	1 Serving/30g	114	0.9	381	9	77	3	5
Special K, Peach & Apricot, Kellogg's*	1 Serving/30g	112	0.3	373	14	77	1	2.5
Special K, Protein Plus, Kellogg's*	1 Serving/29g	100	3	345	34.5	31	10.3	17.2
Special K, Purple Berries, Kellogg's*	1 Serving/30g	112	0.3	374	13	77	1	3.5
Special K, Yoghurty, Kellogg's*	1 Serving/30g	115	0.9	383	14	75	3	2.5
Start, Kellogg's*	1 Serving/30g	117	1	390	8	79	3.5	5
Strawberry & Almond Crunch, M&S*	1 Serving/40g	186	7.4	465	8	66	18.6	4.9

BREAKFAST CEREAL	Measure INFO/WEIGHT	per Measure		Nutrition Values per 100g / 100ml				
		KCAL	FAT	KCAL	PROT	CARB	FAT	FIBRE
Strawberry Crisp, Asda*	1 Serving/45g	194	7	431	8.1	64.7	15.5	5.9
Strawberry, Alpen*	1 Serving/40g	144	1.9	359	9.4	69.5	4.8	7.9
Sugar Puffs, Quaker*	1 Serving/30g	114	0.5	379	5.3	85.8	1.6	3.7
Sultana Bran, Co-Op*	1 Serving/40g	130	1.2	325	9	66	3	11
Sultana Bran, HL, Tesco*	1 Serving/30g	98	0.6	325	8.2	68	1.9	12
Sultana Bran, Morrisons*	1 Serving/30g	98	0.9	325	8.8	65.8	3	11.4
Sultana Bran, Waitrose*	1 Serving/30g	97	0.6	324	8.2	68.6	1.9	11.6
Toffee Crisp, Nestle*	1 Serving/30g	126	3	421	6.5	73.8	10	5
Vitality, Asda*	1 Serving/30g	111	0.4	370	11	78	1.5	3.2
Vitality, with Red Fruit, Asda*	1 Serving/30g	110	0.5	366	11	77	1.6	3.8
Weet Bix, Oat Bran, Sanitarium*	2 Biscuits/40g	156	1	390	12.8	71.9	2.5	11.7
Weet Bix, Sanitarium*	2 Biscuits/30g	106	0.4	352	12	67	1.4	10.5
Weetabix, Banana, Weetabix*	1 Serving/44g	157	0.9	357	10	70.4	2	9.8
Weetabix, Chocolate, Weetabix*	2 Biscuits/45g	166	1.8	368	10.1	67.9	4	10
Weetaflakes, Weetabix*	1 Serving/30g	102	0.4	340	8.9	72.9	1.4	11
Weetos, Chocolate, Weetabix*	1 Serving/30g	113	1.5	378	8.4	75.1	4.9	5.8
Wheat Biscuits, As Sold, Savers, Morrisons*	2 Biscuits/36g	127	0.6	353	10.8	67.6	1.8	11.6
Wheat Biscuits, Average	**2 Biscuits/37.5g**	**130**	**0.8**	**347**	**11.7**	**68.4**	**2.2**	**9.9**
Wheat Bisks, Banana, Mini, Asda*	1 Serving/50g	190	2.7	380	9.7	73.1	5.4	7.4
Wheat Bisks, Chocolate, Asda*	2 Biscuits/43g	158	1.5	367	10	69	3.4	10
Wheat Bisks, Harvest Morn, Aldi*	2 Biscuits/38g	136	0.8	358	11.5	68.6	2	10
Wheat Pillows, Wholegrain, Tesco*	1 Biscuit/45g	151	0.9	335	10.6	67.6	2.1	11.3
Wheat Shreds, Harvest Morn, Aldi*	2 Biscuits/45g	156	0.8	346	13	64	1.8	13
Wheats, Mini, Maple & Brown Sugar, Sainsbury's*	1 Serving/52g	99	0.5	190	4	44	1	5
Whole Wheat Biscuits, Organic, Dove's Farm*	1 Serving/30g	99	0.8	329	11	65	2.8	11
Wholegrain Hoops, Goldenvale, Aldi*	1 Serving/30g	111	0.8	371	6.9	74	2.6	10.7
Wholegrain, Apricot, Wheats, Sainsbury's*	1 Serving/50g	160	0.8	320	7.9	71.6	1.5	8.2
Wholegrain, Fruit & Fibre, Sainsbury's*	1 Serving/30g	109	1.8	363	8.1	69.1	6	8.9
Wholegrain, Mini Wheats, Sainsbury's*	1 Serving/40g	144	0.7	359	11.8	68.2	1.8	11.2
Wholegrain, Minis, Weetabix*	1 Serving/40g	149	0.8	372	10.2	73.2	2	10
Wholegrain, Sultana Bran, Sainsbury's*	1 Serving/30g	98	0.6	325	8.3	68.6	1.9	12.1
Wholesome Crunch, Granola, Pecan & Brazil Nut, Quaker*	1 Serving/45g	189	5	420	11.1	61.8	11.1	13.2
Wholesome Crunch, Granola, Goji & Blueberry, Quaker*	1 Serving/45g	181	3.6	402	11	64.5	7.9	13.5
Yoghurt & Raspberry, Crisp, Sainsbury's*	1 Serving/45g	191	6.7	424	7.5	65.2	14.8	6.4
BRESAOLA								
Della Valtellina, Air Dried Beef, Deluxe, Lidl*	1 Pack/80g	130	2.4	163	33.5	0.5	3	0
Della Valtellina, Sainsbury's*	1 Slice/14g	23	0.4	163	34.7	0.1	2.6	0.1
Finest, Tesco*	1 Serving/35g	64	1.4	182	36	0.5	4	0
BROCCOLI								
& Cauliflower, Floret Mix, Fresh, Tesco*	1 Serving/80g	27	0.7	34	3.9	2.5	0.9	2.7
& Cauliflower, Floret Mix, Iceland*	1 Serving/80g	24	0.7	30	3	1.6	0.9	2
Chinese, Kai Lan, Cooked	**1 Serving/80g**	**18**	**0.6**	**22**	**1.4**	**3.8**	**0.7**	**2.5**
Courgette & Peppers, COU, M&S*	1 Pack/283g	156	11.6	55	1.7	2.7	4.1	1.7
Green, Boiled, Average	**1 Serving/80g**	**19**	**0.6**	**24**	**3.1**	**1.1**	**0.8**	**2.3**
Green, Raw, Average	**1 Serving/80g**	**24**	**0.7**	**30**	**3.7**	**1.6**	**0.8**	**2.5**
Purple Sprouting, Boiled, Average	**1 Serving/80g**	**15**	**0.5**	**19**	**2.1**	**1.3**	**0.6**	**2.3**
Purple Sprouting, Raw	**1oz/28g**	**10**	**0.3**	**35**	**3.9**	**2.6**	**1.1**	**3.5**
Rice, Cooked, Sainsbury's*	½ Pack/150g	64	0.7	43	4.1	3.5	0.5	3.8
Steamed, Average	**1 Serving/100g**	**24**	**0.8**	**24**	**3.1**	**1.1**	**0.8**	**2.3**
Tenderstem, Average	**1 Serving/80g**	**28**	**0.4**	**35**	**4.1**	**2.9**	**0.6**	**2.3**
BROCCOLI CHEESE								
Morrisons*	1 Pack/350g	406	24.8	116	6.2	6.6	7.1	0.8

	Measure INFO/WEIGHT	per Measure KCAL	FAT	Nutrition Values per 100g / 100ml KCAL	PROT	CARB	FAT	FIBRE
BROWNIES								
Average	*1 Brownie/60g*	*243*	*10.1*	*405*	*4.6*	*0*	*16.8*	*0*
Chocolate, & Caramel Fudge, Sea Salted, Morrisons*	1 Brownie/94g	410	20.3	438	5.4	54.1	21.7	2.2
Chocolate, & Pecan, Gu*	1 Brownie/40g	188	11.6	471	7.2	47.6	29.1	2.5
Chocolate, Average	*1 Serving/100g*	*446*	*22.3*	*446*	*5.9*	*55.6*	*22.3*	*2.2*
Chocolate, Bites, Mini, Weight Watchers*	1 Brownie/9g	29	0.5	325	5.3	63.7	5.5	2.2
Chocolate, Cadbury*	1 Brownie/36g	145	5.7	403	6.1	59.7	15.8	0
Chocolate, Chewy, M&S*	1 Brownie/29g	130	6	455	6.5	59.8	21.1	2
Chocolate, Chunky, Belgian, M&S*	1 Brownie/55g	242	11.2	440	6.2	57.7	20.3	2.5
Chocolate, Double, Iced, Otis Spunkmeyer*	1 Brownie/57g	250	6.8	439	3.5	61.4	12	1.8
Chocolate, Double, Mini Bites, Sainsbury's*	1 Brownie/15g	49	2.5	326	5.8	38.9	16.4	1.6
Chocolate, Double, Un-Iced, Otis Spunkmeyer*	1 Brownie/57g	250	12	439	3.5	61.4	21	1.8
Chocolate, Fudge, Mini, Thorntons*	1 Bite/14g	61	2.8	435	5.6	57.4	20	0
Chocolate, Fudgy, M&S*	1 Brownie/87g	400	21.9	460	4.8	56.9	25.2	3
Chocolate, Mini Bites, Asda*	1 Brownie/15g	62	3	420	5	55	20	1.4
Chocolate, Orange, Organic, The Village Bakery*	1 Brownie/30g	126	6.7	421	5	50.5	22.2	0.9
Chocolate, Sainsbury's*	1 Brownie/60g	265	13.6	442	4.6	55	22.6	1.6
Chocolate, Slices, M&S*	1 Brownie/36g	158	8.7	440	5.3	51.1	24.1	1.3
Chocolate, Tray Bake, Tesco*	1 Brownie/37g	155	6.8	420	5.5	57.1	18.4	5.7
Chocolate, Waitrose*	1 Brownie/45g	192	8.9	426	6.3	55.6	19.8	2.7
Chocolate, Weight Watchers*	1 Brownie/47g	143	1.8	304	4.8	62.5	3.8	3.2
Chocolate, Wheat & GF, Mrs Crimble's*	1 Slice/47.5g	180	9.6	379	4.2	47.9	20.3	1.5
Praline, Mini, Finest, Tesco*	1 Brownie/12g	59	3.1	492	4.2	60	25.8	0.8
The Graze Brownie, Graze*	1 Portion/30g	110	5.4	368	7.1	50.5	17.9	3.8
BRUSCHETTA								
Cheese & Tomato, Asda*	1 Bruschetta/38g	68	1.7	180	8.6	26	4.6	2.9
Pane Italia*	1 Serving/75g	367	18.8	489	12.4	53.6	25.1	1.4
Red Pepper & Onion, Brunchetta, Golden Vale*	1 Pack/90g	266	17.1	296	14.6	17	19	1.3
Soft Cheese & Cranberry, Brunchetta, Golden Vale*	1 Pack/95g	200	8.6	211	8.2	24.8	9	1.3
Toasted, Olive Oil & Sea Salt, Tesco*	1 Serving/30g	126	4.6	420	11.5	58.7	15.5	4.5
BRUSSELS SPROUTS								
& Sweet Chestnuts, Asda*	1 Serving/100g	73	1.7	73	3.1	11	1.7	4.2
Boiled, Average	*1 Serving/80g*	*27*	*1*	*33*	*3*	*3*	*1.2*	*3.3*
Button, Raw, Average	*1 Serving/80g*	*28*	*1*	*36*	*3.3*	*2.8*	*1.3*	*3*
Canned, Drained	*1oz/28g*	*5*	*0.2*	*17*	*1.6*	*1.5*	*0.6*	*1.6*
Frozen, Morrisons*	1 Serving/200g	70	2.6	35	3.5	2.5	1.3	4.3
Raw, Average	*1 Serving/80g*	*28*	*0.8*	*35*	*3.3*	*3.1*	*1*	*2.9*
Red, Limited Selection, Waitrose*	1 Serving/80g	41	1.1	51	3.5	4.1	1.4	3.8
Steamed, Average	*1 Serving/100g*	*35*	*1.3*	*35*	*3.1*	*3.2*	*1.3*	*3.5*
BUBBLE & SQUEAK								
Aunt Bessie's*	1 Serving/100g	145	7.1	145	2.7	17.5	7.1	1.3
Crush, Finest, Tesco*	½ Pack/163g	160	4.9	98	2.1	14.8	3	2.1
Fried in Vegetable Oil	*1oz/28g*	*35*	*2.5*	*124*	*1.4*	*9.8*	*9.1*	*1.5*
Tesco*	½ Pack/325g	292	12.7	90	1.6	11.3	3.9	0.9
with Butter & Parsley, As Prepared, Waitrose*	½ Pack/145g	113	3.3	78	2.1	11.3	2.3	2.1
with Chicken, Frozen, Stir Fried, Iceland*	½ Pack/400g	392	16.2	104	5.9	9.6	4.3	1.9
BUCKWHEAT								
Average	*1oz/28g*	*102*	*0.4*	*364*	*8.1*	*84.9*	*1.5*	*2.1*
BUFFALO								
Mince, Raw, Lean, Abel & Cole*	1 Serving/100g	95	0.7	95	21.7	0.4	0.7	0
BULGUR WHEAT								
Dry Weight, Average	*1oz/28g*	*99*	*0.5*	*353*	*9.7*	*76.3*	*1.7*	*8*
Quinoa & Rainbow Vegetables, As Prepared, Waitrose*	1 Pack/300g	372	11.4	124	3.1	17.6	3.8	3.6

	Measure INFO/WEIGHT	per Measure		Nutrition Values per 100g / 100ml				
		KCAL	FAT	KCAL	PROT	CARB	FAT	FIBRE
BULGUR WHEAT								
Wholefoods, Tesco*	1 Serving/50g	180	0.8	360	9.7	76.3	1.7	9.1
with Chick Peas, & Quinoa, Ready to Eat, Sainsbury's*	½ Pack/125g	239	4.1	191	7.7	30	3.3	4.7
BUNS								
Bath, M&S*	1 Bun/71g	217	5.7	305	8.3	49.8	8	1.9
Bath, Tesco*	1 Bun/80g	262	8.9	328	8	48.9	11.1	5.8
Belgian, Asda*	1 Bun/133g	464	19.9	350	4.8	49	15	2.2
Belgian, Co-Op*	1 Bun/118g	413	15.3	350	5	54	13	2
Belgian, Dairy Cream, Somerfield*	1 Serving/121g	400	13.4	331	5.2	52.6	11.1	2
Belgian, Iced, CBY, Asda*	1 Bun/115g	375	6.8	327	6.1	62.3	5.9	2.9
Belgian, Sainsbury's*	1 Bun/110g	398	11.3	362	6.1	61.3	10.3	1.9
Belgian, Tesco*	1 Bun/123g	438	15.7	356	5.2	54.9	12.8	2.2
Chelsea	*1 Bun/78g*	*285*	*10.8*	*366*	*7.8*	*56.1*	*13.8*	*1.7*
Chelsea, Sainsbury's*	1 Bun/85g	239	4.4	281	6.9	51.6	5.2	2.9
Chelsea, Tesco*	1 Bun/85g	269	6.5	316	7.9	53.9	7.6	2.3
Choux, Caramel, Asda*	1 Bun/189g	745	51	394	4.3	33.5	27	1.3
Choux, Custard, M&S*	1 Bun/85g	234	18.7	275	4.2	15	22	0.3
Choux, Fresh Cream, Tesco*	1 Bun/95g	340	23.7	358	4.9	28.5	24.9	0.9
Choux, M&S*	1 Bun/78g	247	17.3	317	5.4	25.6	22.2	0.3
Cinnamon, Tear & Share, Bakery, Tesco*	¼ Bun/108g	363	10.7	334	6.9	52.9	9.8	3.3
Currant	*1 Bun/60g*	*178*	*4.5*	*296*	*7.6*	*52.7*	*7.5*	*0*
Currant, HE, Tesco*	1 Bun/62g	157	1.6	253	6.6	50.8	2.6	3.2
Currant, Sainsbury's*	1 Bun/72g	197	3.7	274	7	50	5.1	2.8
Dairy Cream, Somerfield*	1 Bun/98g	304	10.7	310	6	46.9	10.9	0
Fruit, Waitrose*	1 Bun/54g	155	2.3	287	8.1	54	4.3	1.6
Hot Cross	*1 Bun/50g*	*156*	*3.5*	*312*	*7.4*	*58.5*	*7*	*1.7*
Hot Cross, 25% Reduced Fat, Asda*	1 Bun/61g	153	1.4	253	9	49	2.3	3
Hot Cross, Apple & Cinnamon, Large, Finest, Tesco*	1 Bun/117g	342	8.2	292	7.3	49.9	7	3.6
Hot Cross, Asda*	1 Bun/60g	190	3.8	317	10	55	6.3	3.3
Hot Cross, Best of Both, Hovis*	1 Bun/65g	185	4.3	285	9.1	47.3	6.6	4.4
Hot Cross, BGTY, Sainsbury's*	1 Bun/70g	189	1.8	270	6.7	53.7	2.6	2.4
Hot Cross, Bramley Apple & Cinnamon, Waitrose*	1 Bun/70g	194	2.7	277	7.7	52.2	3.8	1.5
Hot Cross, Chocolate & Raisin, Mini, Tesco*	1 Bun/40g	127	4.4	318	8.1	47	10.9	2.8
Hot Cross, Chocolate & Orange, Mini, M&S*	1 Bun/28g	86	2.3	307	8.2	48.2	8.2	3.9
Hot Cross, Chocolate, Coles*	1 Bun/86g	296	9	344	7	53.4	10.5	0
Hot Cross, Chocolate, Mini, Sainsbury's*	1 Bun/39g	127	4.4	325	7.7	48.1	11.3	2.5
Hot Cross, Classics, M&S*	1 Bun/65g	159	1.2	245	8.5	49.1	1.8	2.2
Hot Cross, Co-Op*	1 Bun/60g	165	3.6	275	8	47	6	3
Hot Cross, Extra Spicy, M&S*	1 Bun/76g	175	1.4	230	8.6	44.1	1.9	4.2
Hot Cross, Finest, Tesco*	1 Bun/75g	210	4	280	7.8	49.5	5.4	2.8
Hot Cross, Golden Wholemeal, Sainsbury's*	1 Bun/65g	180	4	277	9.9	45.4	6.2	4.3
Hot Cross, HE, Tesco*	1 Bun/60g	155	1.5	258	8.6	50.3	2.5	2.6
Hot Cross, HL, Tesco*	1 Bun/70g	176	1.9	251	6.7	50.3	2.7	2.6
Hot Cross, Less Than 3% Fat, M&S*	1 Bun/70g	175	1.3	250	8.1	49.8	1.8	2.2
Hot Cross, Lightly Fruited, M&S*	1 Bun/63.5g	165	3.4	260	8.1	45.1	5.4	4.7
Hot Cross, Luxury, Cafe, M&S*	1 Bun/78g	199	3.1	255	8.6	46.2	4	2.1
Hot Cross, Luxury, M&S*	1 Bun/79g	201	3.2	255	8.6	46.2	4	2.1
Hot Cross, Luxury, Rowan Hill Bakery, Lidl*	1 Bun/75g	204	3.5	272	8.3	47	4.7	4
Hot Cross, Mini, M&S*	1 Bun/41g	110	1.4	265	7.8	51.4	3.4	3.7
Hot Cross, Mini, Tesco*	1 Bun/36g	99	2	274	7.9	48.1	5.5	2.7
Hot Cross, Morrisons*	1 Bun/72g	178	1.4	247	7.4	49.9	2	3.3
Hot Cross, Reduced Fat, GFY, Asda*	1 Bun/63g	156	1.6	248	8.4	47.9	2.5	3.7
Hot Cross, Reduced Fat, Waitrose*	1 Bun/67g	171	1.4	255	8.1	54.3	2.1	3.3
Hot Cross, Sticky Toffee, The Best, Morrisons*	1 Bun/77g	222	3.5	288	6.8	52.8	4.6	4

B

	Measure INFO/WEIGHT	per Measure KCAL	FAT	Nutrition Values per 100g / 100ml KCAL	PROT	CARB	FAT	FIBRE
BUNS								
Hot Cross, Tesco*	1 Bun/70g	186	1.9	265	7.4	51.8	2.7	3.6
Hot Cross, The Village Bakery*	1 Bun/70g	178	1.5	254	7.2	50	2.2	2.9
Hot Cross, TTD, Sainsbury's*	1 Bun/75g	200	4.2	267	7.2	47	5.6	3.8
Hot Cross, White, Kingsmill*	1 Bun/70g	186	2.4	266	8.7	48	3.5	3.6
Hot Cross, White, LC, Tesco*	1 Bun/70g	185	1.4	260	8.3	50.3	1.9	3.8
Hot Cross, White, Sainsbury's*	1 Bun/70g	199	3.4	284	7.9	50.6	4.8	3.4
Hot Cross, White, Waitrose*	1 Bun/68g	174	2.1	258	8.1	49.5	3.1	3.9
Hot Cross, Wholemeal, Asda*	1 Bun/70g	182	4.2	262	9	43	6	6
Hot Cross, Wholemeal, Organic, Tesco*	1 Bun/55g	140	2.7	254	7.6	44.8	4.9	4.5
Hot Cross, Wholemeal, Waitrose*	1 Bun/64g	177	4.3	276	8.8	45.2	6.7	4.9
Hot Cross, You Count, Love Life, Waitrose*	1 Bun/70g	195	3.2	278	6.8	51.5	4.5	2.3
Iced Finger, Lemon, Aldi*	1 Bun/40g	130	3.4	325	6.4	55	8.5	2
Iced Finger, Sainsbury's*	1 Bun/40g	130	3.3	326	7	55.4	8.2	1.4
Iced Finger, Sticky, CBY, Asda*	1 Finger/40g	132	2.4	330	7.1	62	5.9	2.7
Iced Finger, Tesco*	1 Bun/40g	135	3.6	338	6.2	57.2	9	1.9
Iced Lemon, Tesco*	1 Bun/48g	156	4.2	325	5.2	56.5	8.7	1.9
Iced, Filled with Raspberry Jam, M&S*	1 Bun/48g	155	3.2	320	6.4	58.9	6.6	1.9
Iced, Finger, Average	*1 Bun/40g*	*130*	*3.1*	*325*	*7.2*	*57*	*7.7*	*2.3*
Iced, Finger, Coconut, Genesis Crafty*	1 Bun/64g	210	6.9	328	7.7	52.4	10.8	2.4
Iced, Spiced Fruit, M&S*	1 Bun/90g	270	3.3	300	7	60.3	3.7	1.5
Iced, Tesco*	1 Bun/35g	117	3.4	334	7	54.8	9.6	2.5
Marlborough, M&S*	1 Bun/70.5g	215	6.3	305	6.2	43.4	8.9	2.2
Raspberry, Iced, Aldi*	1 Bun/40g	133	3.6	332	6.5	55	9	2
Saffron, Somerfield*	1 Bun/70g	266	11.7	380	6.4	50.9	16.7	1.9
Spiced, PB, Waitrose*	1 Bun/65g	177	2.2	272	8	52.3	3.4	2.9
Vanilla Iced, Soft, M&S*	1 Bun/39g	125	3.1	320	7.6	54.9	8	2.9
BURGERS								
American Style, Asda*	1 Burger/42g	156	10.8	374	25	10	26	1.1
American Style, Tesco*	1 Burger/125g	250	9.1	200	13	20.4	7.3	3.9
Beef, & Caramelised Red Onion, Steak, TTD, Sainsbury's*	1 Burger/133g	287	15.3	216	20.2	7.8	11.5	0.5
Beef, & Mature Cheddar, Asda*	1 Burger/80g	178	10	223	21.5	6.2	12.5	0.5
Beef, & Onion, Grilled, Asda*	1 Burger/81g	201	11.5	248	23.1	6.9	14.2	0.5
Beef, 100%, Average	*1 Burger/52g*	*148*	*11.6*	*286*	*20.5*	*0.6*	*22.3*	*0.1*
Beef, 100%, Birds Eye*	1 Burger/41g	120	10.2	292	17.3	0	24.8	0
Beef, 100%, Half Pounders, Sainsbury's*	1 Burger/148g	462	33.1	313	26	1.7	22.4	0.2
Beef, 100%, Organic, Waitrose*	1 Burger/56.7g	140	9.6	247	23.6	0	16.9	0
Beef, 100%, Pure, Ross*	1 Burger/56g	128	9.6	229	17.1	1.4	17.1	0
Beef, 100%, Quarter Pounders, Aldi*	1 Burger/114g	320	23.3	282	24.3	0.1	20.5	1.3
Beef, 100%, Quarter Pounders, Ross*	1 Burger/74g	222	18.8	301	16.8	1.1	25.5	0
Beef, 100%, Sainsbury's*	1 Burger/44g	133	10.4	302	21.4	0.9	23.6	0.9
Beef, 100%, Somerfield*	1 Burger/114g	328	27.2	289	17	1	24	0
Beef, 100%, with Seasoning, No Onion, Birds Eye*	1 Burger/41g	134	11.9	326	16.1	0.2	29	0
Beef, 30 Day Dry Aged Hereford, 1, Waitrose*	1 Burger/130g	300	17.7	231	24.1	2.7	13.6	0.6
Beef, 97%, Grilled, Heck*	1 Burger/113g	246	12.5	217	26.9	3.4	11	0
Beef, Aberdeen Angus, Asda*	1 Burger/112g	249	13.3	222	22.2	6.7	11.8	0.9
Beef, Aberdeen Angus, Fresh, Waitrose*	1 Burger/113g	269	21	238	16.4	1.2	18.6	0
Beef, Aberdeen Angus, Frozen, Waitrose*	1 Serving/57g	145	11.6	255	18.1	0	20.3	1.1
Beef, Aberdeen Angus, Gourmet, Finest, Tesco*	1 Burger/118.4g	225	13.4	190	18.9	2	11.3	1
Beef, Aberdeen Angus, M&S*	1 Burger/142g	298	18.9	210	18.3	4.1	13.3	0.1
Beef, Aberdeen Angus, Quarter Pounder, TTD, Sainsbury's*	1 Serving/91g	258	15.6	284	29.9	2.4	17.2	0.5
Beef, Aberdeen Angus, Scotch, Deluxe, Lidl*	1 Burger /170g	430	30.4	253	21.9	0.7	17.9	0.6
Beef, Aberdeen Angus, Virgin Trains*	1 Burger/240g	695	37.6	290	13.5	23.8	15.7	0
Beef, Asda*	1 Burger/114g	304	18.6	267	26.8	3.2	16.3	0.7

BURGERS

INFO/WEIGHT	Measure per Measure		Nutrition Values per 100g / 100ml				
	KCAL	FAT	KCAL	PROT	CARB	FAT	FIBRE
Beef, Barbecue, Tesco*	1 Burger/114g	295	22.7	260	15.6	3.5	20	0.5
Beef, BGTY, Sainsbury's*	1 Burger/110g	177	6	161	20.8	7.1	5.5	1.1
Beef, British, Cooked, Savers, Morrisons*	1 Burger/39g	79	4.2	203	0.3	7.2	10.7	0.5
Beef, British, Grilled, Finest, Tesco*	1 Burger/95g	185	11.8	195	17.2	3.3	12.4	0.9
Beef, British, Organic, Waitrose*	1 Burger/85g	226	16.6	266	19	3.5	19.5	1
Beef, British, Waitrose*	1 Burger/113g	279	21	247	18.6	1.2	18.6	0
Beef, Chargrill, Tesco*	1 Burger/114g	246	18.4	217	17	0.8	16.2	2.5
Beef, Cheese & Caramelised Onion Melt, Waitrose*	1 Burger/165g	378	26.6	229	14.2	6.9	16.1	0.5
Beef, Economy, Value, Tesco*	1 Burger/41g	105	5.9	255	21.6	8.5	14.5	0.3
Beef, Farmfoods*	1 Burger/50g	128	9.8	255	14.4	5.4	19.6	0.1
Beef, Filled with Gorgonzola, M&S*	1 Burger/167g	384	26.9	230	16.5	4.9	16.1	0.5
Beef, Flame Grilled, Feasters*	1 Burger/58g	164	13.5	282	19.3	2.6	23.2	0
Beef, Giant, Chargrilled, Farmfoods*	1 Burger/170g	352	21.8	207	17.3	5.6	12.8	1.2
Beef, in a Bun, HE, Tesco*	1 Pack/189g	282	2.5	149	13.6	20.7	1.3	2.1
Beef, Morrisons*	1 Burger/57g	169	14.3	298	12.3	5.5	25.2	0.6
Beef, New York Style, Grilled, Tesco*	1 Burger/35g	80	5.2	229	18.6	5.7	14.9	0.6
Beef, Organic, M&S*	1 Burger/110g	239	17.6	217	18.2	0	16	0.2
Beef, Original, & Best, Birds Eye*	1 Burger/45.6g	115	8.9	252	14.1	5.1	19.5	0.4
Beef, Original, with Onion, Grilled, Birds Eye*	1 Burger/38g	110	9.5	287	13.4	2.6	24.8	0.3
Beef, Quarter Pounders, BGTY, Sainsbury's*	1 Burger/113.5g	188	9.3	166	16.9	6.1	8.2	1
Beef, Quarter Pounders, Chilled, Morrisons*	1 Burger/115g	228	13.9	198	17.2	4.4	12.1	0.2
Beef, Quarter Pounders, Farmfoods*	1 Burger/113g	289	22.1	256	14.4	5.4	19.6	0.1
Beef, Quarter Pounders, Flame Grilled, Rustlers*	1 Burger/190g	557	28.7	293	14.9	24.3	15.1	0
Beef, Quarter Pounders, Flame Grilled, Tesco*	1 Burger/88g	246	20.4	280	13.1	4.8	23.2	0.8
Beef, Quarter Pounders, GF, Butchers Selection, Asda*	1 Burger/93g	210	13.1	225	16	8.5	14	0.5
Beef, Quarter Pounders, Good Intentions, Somerfield*	1 Burger/96g	184	11.6	191	18.9	1.9	12	0.8
Beef, Quarter Pounders, Morrisons*	1 Burger/114g	338	28.6	298	12.3	5.5	25.2	0.6
Beef, Quarter Pounders, Reduced Fat, Tesco*	1 Burger/95g	171	12.4	180	14	1.8	13	0.8
Beef, Quarter Pounders, Scotch, Sainsbury's*	1 Burger/114g	255	15.4	225	22.2	3.5	13.6	0.5
Beef, Quarter Pounders, Scotch, The Best, Morrisons*	1 Burger/97g	223	13.9	230	21	4	14.3	0.5
Beef, Quarter Pounders, Somerfield*	1 Burger/114g	295	20.6	259	20.9	3	18.1	0
Beef, Quarter Pounders, Steak Country, Lidl*	1 Burger/68g	188	15.1	276	16.3	2.4	22.2	0.1
Beef, Quarter Pounders, Tesco*	1 Burger/113g	292	23.1	258	17.8	0.7	20.4	1.3
Beef, Quarter Pounders, with Onion, BGTY, Sainsbury's*	1 Burger/83g	171	7.8	205	26.6	3.8	9.3	0.9
Beef, Quarter Pounders, with Onion, Birds Eye*	1 Burger/114g	286	22.1	252	14.1	5.1	19.5	0.4
Beef, Quarter Pounders, with Onion, Cooked, Birds Eye*	1 Burger/100g	230	16	230	16	5.9	16	0.4
Beef, Quarter Pounders, with Onion, Sainsbury's*	1 Burger/113g	306	22.4	271	18	5.1	19.8	1.5
Beef, Red Onion & Cheese, Butchers Selection, Asda*	1 Burger/114g	243	13.7	213	21	5	12	0.5
Beef, Sainsbury's*	1 Burger/57g	152	9.1	267	29.6	1.3	15.9	1.5
Beef, Scotch, Ultimate, TTD, Sainsbury's*	1 Burger/119g	265	15.8	223	25.3	0.5	13.3	1
Beef, Steak, 95%, British, Grilled, TTD, Sainsbury's*	1 Burger/110g	276	19.2	250	21.6	1.8	17.4	0.5
Beef, Steak, British, Cooked, TTD, Sainsbury's*	1 Burger/93g	191	11.9	205	21	1.5	12.8	0.5
Beef, Steak, British, Tesco*	1 Burger/80g	184	10.9	230	24.8	2.2	13.6	0.1
Beef, Steak, Extra Lean, Musclefood*	1 Burger/113g	160	5.4	142	19.6	5.7	4.8	1.3
Beef, Steak, Full of Flavour, Finest, Tesco*	1 Burger/86g	200	12.6	233	22.6	2.3	14.6	0.5
Beef, Steak, Smoked Garlic, Finest, Tesco*	1 Burger/80g	178	12.6	223	18	2	15.8	0.5
Beef, Steak, TTD, Sainsbury's*	1 Burger/170g	389	24.3	229	24.5	0.5	14.3	0.5
Beef, Steak, Ultimate, TTD, Sainsbury's*	1 Burger/136g	355	24.1	261	25.3	0.1	17.7	0.5
Beef, Sweet Chilli, Skinniburger, Aldi*	1 Burger/113g	125	1	111	18.9	6.7	0.9	0
Beef, Sweetflame Red Chilli, Steak, TTD, Sainsbury's*	1 Burger/134g	245	11.5	183	21.6	4.2	8.6	1
Beef, Wagyu, Grilled, Specially Selected, Aldi*	1 Burger/150g	332	22.5	221	18	4	15	0.5
Beef, Wagyu, Specially Selected, Aldi*	1 Burger/150g	420	30	280	19	5.1	20	0.5
Beef, with Cheese Melt, COOK!, M&S*	1 Burger/182g	400	28.9	220	17.9	1.3	15.9	1.2

	Measure INFO/WEIGHT	per Measure KCAL	FAT	Nutrition Values per 100g / 100ml KCAL	PROT	CARB	FAT	FIBRE

BURGERS

	Measure INFO/WEIGHT	per Measure KCAL	FAT	KCAL	PROT	CARB	FAT	FIBRE
Beef, with Fresh Garden Herbs, Raw, TTD, Sainsbury's*	1 Burger/142g	280	14.8	197	21.5	4.4	10.4	1.3
Beef, with Herbs, Finest, Tesco*	1 Burger/105g	200	11.8	190	17.3	4.5	11.2	0.7
Beef, with Jalapeno Chilli, Finest, Tesco*	1 Burger /205g	379	22.3	185	17	3.4	10.9	0.4
Beef, with Mediterranean Tomato & Basil, M&S*	1 Burger/169g	304	18.6	180	15.7	5.1	11	1.4
Beef, with Onion, Sainsbury's*	1 Burger/42g	102	6.2	243	20.7	6.9	14.8	1
Beef, with Red Onion, & Mustard, Finest, Tesco*	1 Burger/130g	308	24.2	237	17.2	0.2	18.6	2.6
Beef, with West Country Cheddar, TTD, Sainsbury's*	1 Burger/112g	252	13.7	225	26.4	2.3	12.2	0
Cheeseburger	*1 Serving/275g*	*706*	*29*	*257*	*13.7*	*25.6*	*10.6*	*1.8*
Cheeseburger, American, Tesco*	1 Burger/275g	660	26.3	240	13.6	24.9	9.6	1.6
Cheeseburger, Bacon with Bun, Chargrilled, Tesco*	1 Burger/265g	726	42.1	274	13	19.6	15.9	1
Cheeseburger, Micro Snack, Tesco*	1 Burger/115g	309	14.5	269	12.6	26.4	12.6	0
Cheeseburger, Smart Price, Asda*	1 Burger/150g	374	14	249	13.3	28	9.3	1.4
Cheeseburger, with Sesame Seed Bun, Tesco*	1 Burger/275g	644	32.2	234	12.2	20.1	11.7	2
Chicken, Average	*1 Burger/46g*	*111*	*5.6*	*242*	*14.9*	*18.7*	*12.1*	*1*
Chicken, Breaded, Value, Tesco*	1 Burger/57g	165	10.8	290	10.5	19.2	19	1.4
Chicken, Cajun, Fillets, Birds Eye*	1 Pack/180g	275	8.8	153	21.5	5.8	4.9	0.3
Chicken, Cooked, Butcher's Choice, Sainsbury's*	1 Burger/97g	142	4.8	147	20	5.5	5	0.5
Chicken, Crunch & Fries, M&S*	1 Pack/425g	915	47.6	215	8.8	20.8	11.2	2.1
Chicken, Crunch Crumb, Tesco*	1 Burger/57g	161	10.8	282	12.3	15.6	18.9	0
Chicken, Fillets, Weight After Cooking, Birds Eye*	1 Burger/90g	126	4.1	140	20	5.1	4.6	0.2
Chicken, Fresh, Non Coated, Waitrose*	1 Burger/100g	141	4	141	16	10.4	4	0.9
Chicken, Golden Breadcrumbs, Frozen, Birds Eye*	1 Burger/56g	130	6.9	232	13.8	16.4	12.4	0.3
Chicken, Italia, Grilled, Heck*	1 Burger/114g	121	2.6	106	18.7	1.5	2.3	0
Chicken, Quarter Pounders, Birds Eye*	1 Burger/117g	280	16.1	239	13.5	15.2	13.8	0.6
Chicken, Sainsbury's*	1 Burger/46g	115	7	247	15.6	12.2	15.1	1.3
Chicken, Souther Fried, Microwavable, Snack'In, Iceland*	1 Pack/129g	321	7.5	249	11.8	36.4	5.8	1.8
Chicken, Southern Fried, Sainsbury's*	1 Burger/52g	154	10.3	297	12.6	17.2	19.8	1.3
Chicken, Spar*	1 Burger/67g	163	7.5	244	16.1	20.8	11.2	1.5
Chicken, with Sesame Seed Bun, Breaded, Tesco*	1 Burger/205g	588	32.2	287	10.2	26.2	15.7	2.9
Chicken, Zesty, Grilled, Heck*	1 Burger/114g	165	2.2	145	25.2	8.1	1.9	0
Crocodile, Exotic Meat Feast, Kezie, Iceland*	1 Burger/110g	187	9.7	170	15.2	7.5	8.8	0
Economy, Smart Price, Asda*	1 Burger/49g	142	10.2	293	14	12	21	1.1
Fish Fillet, Hot & Spicy, Oven Baked, Birdseye*	1 Burger/116g	234	9	202	12.2	20.3	7.8	0.9
Lamb, Minted, Asda*	1 Burger/100g	234	14	234	22	4.9	14	0.3
Lamb, Minted, Average	*1 Burger/56g*	*125*	*7.4*	*223*	*20.6*	*5.5*	*13.2*	*0.2*
Lamb, Minted, Grilled, Specially Selected, Aldi*	1 Burger/92g	223	14.7	242	17	6.4	16	0.5
Lamb, Minted, Quarter Pounders, Asda*	1 Burger/113.5g	241	14	212	19.2	6.1	12.3	0
Lamb, Moroccan Spiced, Waitrose*	1 Burger/88g	215	13.2	245	16.9	10.5	15	0.1
Lamb, Quarter Pounder, Average	*1 Burger/113g*	*283*	*19.3*	*250*	*17.4*	*5.2*	*17.1*	*0.8*
Lamb, Quarter Pounders, Asda*	1 Burger/85g	213	13.9	251	20.9	5.2	16.3	0.9
Lamb, Quarter Pounders, Birds Eye*	1 Burger/112g	232	16.9	207	13.9	3.8	15.1	0.3
Lamb, Waitrose*	1 Burger/66.9g	99	4.7	148	15.7	5.4	7	0.9
Mushroom & Spinach, Cooked, Love Veg, Sainsbury's*	1 Burger/76g	192	11	254	5.2	22.7	14.6	5.6
Nacho, Chicken & Sweetcorn, Asda*	½ Pack/144g	249	13	173	14	9	9	2.3
Ostrich, Quarter Pounder, Oslinc*	1 Burger/113g	132	1.5	117	22.9	3.5	1.3	1.1
Pork, Free Range, Waitrose*	1 Burger/115g	306	19.9	266	19.3	7.7	17.3	1
Pork, & Apple, Grilled, Finest, Tesco*	1 Burger/88g	251	18.4	285	14.3	9.6	20.9	1.2
Pork, & Apple, Quarter Pounder, Grilled, Asda*	1 Burger/80g	147	6.4	184	23.9	4.1	8	0.5
Pork, Chorizo Sliders, Cooked, TTD, Sainsbury's*	1 Burger/36g	134	8.5	377	17.2	22.3	23.8	2.2
Pork, Hog Roast, Waitrose*	1 Burger/190g	481	29.8	253	17.2	9.9	15.7	1.8
Pork, Quarter Pounders, Birds Eye*	1 Burger/122g	292	23.2	239	13.9	3.2	19	0.2
Quarter Pounders, Chargrilled, BGTY, Sainsbury's*	1 Burger/114g	184	6.3	161	20.8	7.1	5.5	1.1
Quarter Pounders, Chilli, Asda*	1 Burger/88g	221	14	252	25	2	16	0

BURGERS	Measure INFO/WEIGHT	per Measure KCAL	FAT	Nutrition Values per 100g / 100ml KCAL	PROT	CARB	FAT	FIBRE
Quarter Pounders, Chilli, Farmfoods*	1 Burger/115g	285	23.3	248	13.5	2.9	20.3	0.9
Quarter Pounders, Chilli, Iceland*	1 Burger/84g	265	20.1	316	18.6	6.5	23.9	0.4
Quarter Pounders, Iceland*	1 Burger/83g	253	18.8	305	20.4	5.1	22.6	0.6
Quarter Pounders, Loved by Us, Co-Op*	1 Burger/114g	301	23.9	265	19	0.5	21	0
Quarter Pounders, Steak, Deluxe, Lidl*	1 Burger/98g	237	17.6	242	18	2.1	18	0
Quarter Pounders, with Cheese & Buns, Sainsbury's*	1 Burger/198g	471	22.8	238	15.6	19.1	11.5	1.4
Quarter Pounders, with Cheese, Flame Grilled, Feasters*	1 Burger/200g	550	19.8	275	17.2	22.1	9.9	0.9
Quarter Pounders, with Onion, Tesco*	1 Burger/87g	213	16.2	245	16	3	18.6	0.5
Salmon, Quarter Pounders, Tesco*	1 Burger/114g	145	2.7	128	15.9	10.6	2.4	1.2
Salmon, Smoky BBQ, The Grill, M&S*	1 Burger/90g	175	8.4	194	16.4	10.3	9.3	1.7
Salmon, Tesco*	1 Burger/100g	101	3	101	18.2	0.3	3	0
Spicy Bean, Ainsley Harriott*	1 Burger/200g	302	7.5	151	7.2	23.5	3.8	5.2
Spicy Bean, in Herby Nacho Crumb, Morrisons*	1 Burger/102g	185	8.1	181	5.2	19.5	7.9	5.5
Spicy Bean, Sainsbury's*	1 Burger/110g	262	13.5	240	5	27.1	12.4	2
Steak, Peppered, M&S*	1 Burger/114g	310	24.4	272	18.8	0.8	21.4	0.7
Steak, Rump, The Grill, M&S*	1 Burger/169g	330	20.6	195	18.7	2.6	12.2	1.1
Steak, Scotch, Quarter Pounder, Grilled, Deluxe, Lidl*	1 Burger/93g	236	16	254	21.5	3.3	17.2	0
Steak, with Cheese Melt, COOK!, M&S*	1 Burger/196g	480	35.7	245	18.4	2.3	18.2	0.2
Turkey, Cheeseburgers, Tesco*	1 Burger/105g	252	14.8	240	15.4	12.8	14.1	1.3
Turkey, Crispy Crumb, Bernard Matthews*	1 Burger/60g	158	9.5	263	12.6	17.5	15.8	1.8
Turkey, Harvestland*	1 Burger/112g	179	9	160	23	1	8	0
Turkey, Sea Salt & Pepper, Butchers Selection, Asda*	1 Burger/96g	141	4.4	147	23	3.2	4.6	0.5
Venison, & Sweet Onion, M&S*	1 Burger/142g	163	5	115	19.3	1.4	3.5	0.5
Venison, As Sold, Tesco*	1 Burger/113g	149	4	132	19.3	5.5	3.5	0.5
Venison, British Food, Sainsbury's*	1 Burger/64g	130	6.1	203	22.6	6	9.6	0.8
Venison, Finnebrougue Estate*	1 Burger/142g	170	7	120	19.9	4.2	4.9	0.5
Venison, Grilled, Extra Special, Asda*	2 Burgers/227g	331	8.2	146	21.5	5.3	3.6	3.2
Venison, Grilled, Tesco*	1 Burger/96g	149	4	155	22.8	6.2	4.2	0.5
Venison, Lightly Seasoned, As Consumed, Waitrose*	1 Burger/95g	159	6.2	168	23.8	3.3	6.6	0.1
Venison, Spirit of Summer, M&S*	1 Burger/90g	121	5.1	134	17.8	2.8	5.6	0.5
Venison, TTD, Sainsbury's*	1 Burger/150g	224	6.3	149	20.4	6.5	4.2	3.2
Zebra, Cooked, Kezie*	1 Burger/110g	160	3.8	145	25.3	2.2	3.5	0
BURGERS VEGETARIAN								
Aubergine & Feta, Aromatic & Minty, Waitrose*	1 Burger/105g	238	12.9	235	5.2	22.3	12.7	5.3
Bean, Spicy Veg, with Chipotle Chilli, Good Life*	1 Burger/109g	219	9.6	201	5.2	22	8.8	6.4
Bean, Sweetcorn & Roasted Red Pepper, Vegan, Tesco*	1 Burger/115g	201	8.4	175	4.8	19	7.3	7.2
Bean, Zesty, As Consumed, M Kitchen, Morrisons*	1 Burger/124g	207	8.1	167	4.7	18.4	6.5	7.9
Beetroot & Root Vegetable, Vegetarian, Asda*	½ Pack/107g	158	8.8	148	3.7	11	8.2	7.2
Black Bean Beetroot, Bean Supreme*	1 Burger/85g	127	4.2	149	6.7	16.2	4.9	6.7
Black Bean, Organic, Cauldron Foods*	1 Burger/87.5g	169	10.1	193	9.2	13.1	11.5	8.5
Cheese & Spring Onion, Tesco*	1 Burger/87.3g	178	10.3	204	4.4	20	11.8	3.2
Chicken Style, Quorn*	1 Burger/67g	149	8.1	222	10.5	16	12	4
Chilli Bean, Crisp & Spicy, Frozen, Cooked, Waitrose*	1 Burger/95g	226	8.3	238	5.8	31	8.7	6.1
Crisp & Golden, Vegetable Quarter Pounders, Waitrose*	1 Burger/113g	236	8.8	209	4.8	28.2	7.8	3.4
Falafel, Quinoa & Fresh Cilantro, Fry's*	1 Burger/65g	128	5	197	7.8	19.8	7.7	8.8
Flame Grilled, Linda McCartney*	1 Burger/60g	104	3.1	174	17.9	13.8	5.2	3.3
Fry's*	1 Patty/80g	120	3.5	150	15.8	12.2	4.4	0.6
Goat's Cheese, Gourmet, as Sold, Heck*	1 Burger/114g	290	14.6	254	9	28.3	12.8	4.9
Hot & Spicy, Vegan, Quorn*	1 Burger/66g	118	2.6	179	10.9	23	4	3.7
Lamb Style, Minted, Quorn*	1 Burger/80g	86	3.2	108	12	6	4	4
Lentil, & Beetroot, Veggie, M&S*	1 Burger/120g	191	5.9	159	12	13.4	4.9	6.8
Manhattan, Amy's Kitchen*	1 Burger/68g	88	2.9	129	3.8	18	4.2	1.8
Meat Free, Asda*	1 Burger/60g	138	6	230	24	11	10	0.3

B

INFO/WEIGHT	Measure	per Measure		Nutrition Values per 100g / 100ml				
		KCAL	FAT	KCAL	PROT	CARB	FAT	FIBRE

BURGERS VEGETARIAN

Meat Free, Average	**¼ Pounder/113g**	**195**	**8.8**	**172**	**17.5**	**7.9**	**7.8**	**3**
Meat Free, Sainsbury's*	1 Burger/57g	92	4.2	161	19.6	3.9	7.4	4.8
Meat Free, Sainsbury's*	1 Burger/57g	86	2.8	151	22	4.4	5	3.4
Meat Free, Spicy, Bean & Nacho, Cooked, Asda*	1 Burger/113g	247	9.6	218	5.3	27.7	8.5	4.7
Mexican Bean, Tomato Salsa, Love Life, Waitrose*	1 Burger/163g	173	4.6	106	4.1	16.2	2.8	3.8
Mexican Style, Bean, Meat Free, Tesco*	1 Burger/106g	238	10.9	225	6.2	22.7	10.3	8.3
Mushroom & Spinach, Grilled, Linda McCartney*	1 Burger/104g	188	7.8	181	13.6	11.3	7.5	6.9
Mushroom & Wensleydale Cheese, Cauldron Foods*	1 Burger/87.2g	156	9.6	179	9	11	11	4
Mushroom, Cauldron Foods*	1 Burger/88g	125	5.5	143	5.5	16.1	6.3	2.6
Mushroom, Crunchy Quinoa, Parsley, Pepper, Tesco*	1 Burger/123g	230	4	188	8.1	25.8	3.3	11.2
Mushroom, Portobello, Creamy, Smoky, Waitrose*	1 Burger/120g	130	8.2	108	5	6	6.8	1.4
Peri Peri, Frozen, Linda McCartney*	1 Burger/113g	251	9.7	222	20.8	14.7	8.6	4.1
Pulled Pork, Quarter Pounder, Grilled, Linda McCartney*	1 Burger/97g	150	4.5	154	16.1	11.1	4.6	2
Quarter Pounder, Average	**1 Burger/113g**	**210**	**9.8**	**186**	**9.1**	**17.7**	**8.6**	**3.2**
Quarter Pounder, Mexican Style, Quorn*	1 Burger/113g	180	6.3	159	18.3	8.9	5.6	3.8
Quarter Pounder, Quorn*	1 Burger/113.5g	170	6.8	150	14.4	7.7	6	4
Quarter Pounders, Beef Style, Sainsbury's*	1 Burger/114g	216	10.8	190	20	6	9.5	2.5
Quarter Pounders, Chargrilled, Tesco*	1 Burger/114g	186	9.1	164	16	7	8	2.5
Savoury, Cauldron Foods*	1 Burger/87.5g	145	8	166	108	7.9	9.2	2.4
Sizzling, Quorn*	1 Burger/80g	123	4.8	154	18	7	6	3
Smoked Chilli & Lime, Chef's Selection, Quorn*	1 Burger/90g	147	6.3	163	17	6.6	7	3
Spicy Bean, Average	**1 Burger/56g**	**125**	**6.8**	**223**	**5.6**	**24.3**	**12.2**	**4.8**
Spicy Bean, BGTY, Sainsbury's*	1 Burger/85g	123	2.3	145	6.9	23.3	2.7	3.1
Spicy Bean, Cauldron Foods*	1 Burger/87.5g	203	9.8	232	5.4	27.4	11.2	6.2
Spicy Bean, Linda McCartney*	1 Burger/85g	190	9.5	223	4.3	26.2	11.2	2.9
Spicy Bean, Quarter Pounder, Dalepak*	1 Burger/115g	237	12.5	206	4.6	22.3	10.9	2.6
Spicy Bean, Quarter Pounder, Mae's Kitchen, Aldi*	1 Burger/105g	234	9.9	223	5.9	26	9.4	6.3
Sweet Potato & Edamame, Meat Free, Morrisons*	1 Burger/88g	144	8	164	6.4	10.6	9.1	7.2
Sweet Potato & Blackbean, Coles*	1 Burger/125g	229	1.2	183	7.1	33	1	5.9
Sweet Potato, with Piri Piri Glaze, Frozen, Iceland*	1 Burger/140g	264	9.1	188	3.8	24.6	6.5	8.1
Sweetcorn, & Chickpea, M&S*	1 Burger/120g	200	5.2	167	5.7	21.8	4.3	9.1
Tesco*	1 Burger/56g	92	4.5	164	16	7	8	2.5
Vegan, Onion Bhaji, Frozen, As Consumed, Tesco*	1 Burger/117g	167	8.5	143	3.5	12.3	7.3	7.1
Vegeburger, Linda McCartney*	1 Burger/50g	62	1.4	124	15.8	10.7	2.9	5.8
Vegeburger, Retail, Grilled	**1oz/28g**	**55**	**3.1**	**196**	**16.6**	**8**	**11.1**	**4.2**
Vegetable, Average	**1 Burger/56g**	**100**	**4.5**	**179**	**4.4**	**22.4**	**8**	**2.3**
Vegetable, Captains, Birds Eye*	1 Burger/48g	96	4.2	200	4.7	25.5	8.8	2
Vegetable, Organic, Goodlife*	1 Burger/67g	114	3.9	170	3.2	26.3	5.8	2.6
Vegetable, Organic, Tesco*	1 Burger/90g	108	3.9	120	2.6	17.6	4.3	2.1
Vegetable, Quarter Pounders, Crunchy, Birds Eye*	1 Burger/114g	240	11.6	211	4.8	24.9	10.2	1.8
Vegetable, Quarter Pounders, Dalepak*	1 Burger/113.5g	227	9.6	200	4.8	26.3	8.5	1.8
Vegetable, Quarter Pounders, Meat Free, Vegan, Tesco*	1 Burger/108g	204	8.5	190	3.7	24.2	7.9	3.6
Vegetable, Spicy, Asda*	1 Burger/56g	108	6.2	193	3.4	20	11	0

BURRITO

Beef	**1 Serving/225g**	**536**	**20.2**	**238**	**12**	**27**	**9**	**2.2**
Beef, Chilli, As Consumed, Morrisons*	½ Pack/200g	368	16	184	8.9	17.7	8	2.7
Beef, Chilli, Cooked, World Cafe, Waitrose*	½ Pack/87g	169	5.5	195	8.8	24.4	6.3	2.5
Beef, Chilli, with Sour Cream, Good to Go, Waitrose*	1 Pack/241g	431	12.8	179	7.5	23.7	5.3	3.2
Beef, Mix, Vegetarian, Linda McCartney*	1 Serving/200g	240	7.8	120	6.2	12.7	3.9	4.5
Black Bean, Chilli, Everdine*	1 Serving/450g	594	14.4	132	4.2	19.4	3.2	4.5
Chicken, On the Go, Sainsbury's*	1 Burrito/310g	511	15.5	165	8.1	21	5	2
Pork, Pulled, BBQ, Scratch, Waitrose*	½ Pack/404g	654	18.6	162	10.1	18.2	4.6	0
Veg Medley, Bowl, Musclefood*	1 Serving/435g	344	7.8	79	5.6	8.4	1.8	3.6

	Measure INFO/WEIGHT	per Measure KCAL	FAT	Nutrition Values per 100g / 100ml KCAL	PROT	CARB	FAT	FIBRE
BUTTER								
Brandy, Average	*1 Serving/10g*	*56*	*3.8*	*556*	*0.2*	*46.2*	*38.4*	*0.1*
Brandy, with Courvoisier, Sainsbury's*	1 Serving/10g	61	4.6	609	0.5	42.6	46.2	0.5
Cashew, Pip & Nut*	1 Serving/15g	87	6.6	580	18	27	44	0
Coconut, Artisana*	2 Tbsp/32.4g	186	18	574	6.2	21.6	55.5	15.4
Creamery, Average	*1 Serving/10g*	*74*	*8.1*	*736*	*0.5*	*0.4*	*81.4*	*0*
Fresh, Average	*1 Thin Spread/7g*	*51*	*5.7*	*735*	*0.6*	*0.4*	*81.3*	*0*
Garlic, Crushed, Lurpak*	1 Serving/10g	69	7.5	692	1.3	3.7	75	0
Goat's, St Helen's Farm*	1 Thin Spread/7g	56	6.2	794	0.5	0	88	0
Granules, Butter Buds*	1 Tsp/1.4g	5	0.1	368	1.8	77.9	6.5	2.3
Reduced Fat, Fresh, Average	*1 Thin Spread/7g*	*26*	*2.8*	*368*	*2.3*	*1.2*	*39.4*	*0.2*
Salted, Average	*1 Thin Spread/7g*	*51*	*5.7*	*729*	*0.4*	*0.3*	*81.1*	*0*
Spreadable, Fresh, Average	*1 Thin Spread/7g*	*51*	*5.7*	*730*	*0.4*	*0.3*	*80.8*	*0*
Spreadable, Reduced Fat, Average	*1 Thin Spread/7g*	*38*	*4.2*	*540*	*0.5*	*0.5*	*60*	*0*
with Chilli & Lime, Infusions, Lurpak*	1 Thin Spread/7g	44	4.8	633	0.7	1.4	69	0
with Olive Oil, Lighter, Spreadable, Lurpak*	1 Thin Spread/7g	38	4.2	543	0.3	0.4	60	0
with Sea Salt, & Pink Peppercorn, Infusions, Lurpak*	1 Thin Spread/7g	47	5.2	677	0.7	1.8	74	0
with Smoked Chipotle, Infusions, Lurpak*	1 Thin Spread/7g	45	4.8	642	1.4	3.1	69	0
BUTTERMILK								
Average	*1 Mug/400ml*	*177*	*1.3*	*44*	*4.2*	*5.9*	*0.3*	*0*
BUTTERNUT SQUASH								
& Chargrilled Halloumi, Roasted, M&S*	1 Pack/370g	445	15.5	120	6.2	10.9	4.2	5.3
& Red Onion, Quick Roast, M&S*	1 Pack/340g	109	0.3	32	1	6	0.1	1.5
& Sweet Potato, Lets Cook, Aldi*	1 Portion/100g	102	5.3	102	1.1	11	5.3	0
Chips, Crinkle Cut, Cooked, Sainsbury's*	½ Pack/95g	71	1.4	75	0.8	12.8	1.5	3.5
Chunks, Frozen, Scratch Cook, Asda*	1 Serving/80g	33	0.4	41	0.9	7.4	0.5	1.4
Frozen, Tesco*	1 Serving/80g	34	0.1	42	1.1	8.3	0.1	1.6
Fusilli, Tesco*	1 Pack/250g	98	0.2	39	1.1	7.7	0.1	1.6
Lasagne Sheets, Tesco*	¼ Pack/100g	40	0.1	40	1.1	7.9	0.1	1.6
Noodles, Ready Prepared, Sainsbury's*	½ Pack/152g	50	0.8	33	1.1	5.8	0.5	1.4
Spaghetti, Tesco*	1 Serving/80g	31	0.1	39	1.1	7.7	0.1	1.6
Squaffles, Cooked, Sainsbury's*	½ Pack/150g	114	2.6	76	1.7	12.4	1.7	2
Wedges, Moroccan Spiced, M&S*	½ Pack/200g	140	5.6	70	2.4	7.1	2.8	2.6
Wedges, Tesco*	1 Pack/300g	108	0.3	36	1.1	7.7	0.1	1.6
Winter, Boiled, Flesh Only	*1 Serving/80g*	*27*	*0.1*	*34*	*0.7*	*8.8*	*0.1*	*2.6*
Winter, Butternut, Baked, Average	*1 Serving/100g*	*32*	*0.1*	*32*	*0.9*	*7.4*	*0.1*	*1.4*
Winter, Butternut, Raw, Prepared, Average	*1 Serving/80g*	*29*	*0.1*	*36*	*1.1*	*8.3*	*0.1*	*1.6*
Winter, Butternut, Raw, Unprepared, Average	*1 Serving/80g*	*24*	*0.1*	*30*	*0.9*	*6.8*	*0.1*	*1.3*
BUTTONS								
Milk Chocolate, Asda*	1 Bag/70g	368	21	526	7	57	30	1.5
Milk Chocolate, Giant, Dairy Milk, Cadbury*	1 Button/2g	11	0.6	530	7.6	56.5	30.5	0.7
Milk Chocolate, M&S*	1 Pack/75g	375	19	500	8.6	59.8	25.3	1.9
Milk Chocolate, Somerfield*	1 Pack/75g	390	21	520	8	58	28	0
Milk Chocolate, Tesco*	1 Bag/70g	359	19.3	513	7.1	59.1	27.6	2.1
White Chocolate, Co-Op*	½ Pack/35g	186	9.8	530	7	64	28	0
White Chocolate, Dairy Milk, Cadbury*	1 Pack/32g	174	9.5	540	4.7	63	29.5	0
White Chocolate, Milkybar, Nestle*	1 Bag/30g	164	9.5	546	7.5	58.1	31.6	0
White Chocolate, Tesco*	1 Bag/70g	388	23.4	554	5.1	58	33.5	0

B

	Measure INFO/WEIGHT	per Measure KCAL	FAT	Nutrition Values per 100g / 100ml KCAL	PROT	CARB	FAT	FIBRE
CABBAGE								
& Leek, Crunchy Mix, Ready to Cook, Sainsbury's*	1 Serving/125g	34	0.6	27	1.9	3.7	0.5	2.6
& Bacon, Medly, in a Herb Butter, Waitrose*	1 Pack/225g	250	17.6	111	4	4.7	7.8	3.2
& Leek, Ready for Use, Cooked, Sainsbury's*	1 Bag/200g	68	1	34	1.5	4.9	0.5	3.2
& Leek, Ready Sliced, Sainsbury's*	1 Pack/240g	53	1.2	22	1.1	2.2	0.5	2.1
& Leek, Ready Sliced, Sainsbury's*	1 Pack/240g	53	1.2	22	1.1	2.2	0.5	2.1
& Leek, Sliced, Tesco*	1/3 Pack/100g	32	0.6	32	2.1	3.4	0.6	2.6
Boiled, Average	**1 Serving/90g**	**14**	**0.3**	**15**	**1**	**2.2**	**0.3**	**1.7**
Creamed, Cooked, Sainsbury's*	½ Pack/150g	95	6.8	67	2	2.6	4.8	2.5
Greens, Trimmed, Average	**1oz/28g**	**8**	**0.1**	**28**	**2.9**	**3**	**0.5**	**3.4**
Medley, Washed, Ready to Cook, Tesco*	1 Pack/200g	60	1.2	30	2.3	3.7	0.6	2.8
Raw, Average	**1 Serving/100g**	**21**	**0.4**	**21**	**1.3**	**3.2**	**0.4**	**1.8**
Red, & Beetroot, Mash Direct*	1 Serving/88g	67	2.1	76	1.2	12.4	2.4	2.6
Red, Average	**1 Serving/90g**	**19**	**0.2**	**21**	**1**	**3.7**	**0.3**	**2.2**
Red, Braised with Red Wine, M&S*	½ Pack/150g	180	7.2	120	1.4	17.1	4.8	1
Red, Pickled, Average	**1 Serving/50g**	**13**	**0.1**	**26**	**0.9**	**4.6**	**0.2**	**1.6**
Red, Spiced, Morrisons*	¼ Pack/95g	154	2.2	162	1.1	32.4	2.3	3.7
Red, Spiced, Steamer, Sainsbury's*	½ Pack/150g	105	3.3	70	1	10.5	2.2	2.9
Red, with Apple, Bramley, Aunt Bessie's*	1 Serving/125g	72	1.1	58	0.9	10	0.9	2.7
Red, with Apple, Bramley, British, Sainsbury's*	1 Pack/300g	213	1.5	71	1.2	14.9	0.5	2.3
Red, with Apple, Dawtona *	1 Portion/80g	27	0	33	1	6.1	0	2.4
Red, with Apple, Finest, Tesco*	½ Pack/150g	177	8.8	118	1.6	14.7	5.9	4.6
Red, with Apple, Frozen, Sainsbury's*	1 Serving/75g	38	0	50	1.8	10.8	0	2.2
Red, with Apple, Microwaved, Iceland*	¼ Pack/100g	73	4.1	73	0.9	7.2	4.1	1.9
Red, with Apple, Onions & Redcurrant Jelly, M&S*	½ Pack/150g	112	3.3	75	0.9	12.4	2.2	2
Savoy, Boiled in Salted Water, Average	**1 Serving/90g**	**15**	**0.4**	**17**	**1.1**	**2.2**	**0.5**	**2**
Savoy, Raw, Average	**1 Serving/90g**	**24**	**0.4**	**27**	**2.1**	**3.9**	**0.5**	**3.1**
Spring Greens, Boiled, Average	**1 Serving/80g**	**16**	**0.6**	**20**	**1.9**	**1.6**	**0.7**	**2.6**
Spring Greens, Raw, Average	**1 Serving/80g**	**22**	**0.7**	**28**	**2.5**	**2.6**	**0.8**	**2.9**
Steamed, Average	**1 Serving/100g**	**15**	**0.3**	**15**	**1**	**2.2**	**0.3**	**1.7**
Sweetheart, Raw	**1 Serving/100g**	**26**	**0.6**	**26**	**2.1**	**3.2**	**0.6**	**2.8**
White, Raw, Average	**1oz/28g**	**8**	**0.1**	**27**	**1.4**	**5**	**0.2**	**2.1**
CAKE								
Action Man, Birthday, Memory Lane Cakes*	1/12 Cake/83g	322	13.6	388	3	57	16.4	0.8
Alabama Chocolate Fudge, Farmfoods*	1/6 Cake/61g	201	5.9	329	4.7	55.7	9.7	2.7
Alabama Chocolate Fudge, Morrisons*	1/6 Cake/58g	195	6.4	337	4.5	55.1	11	2.3
Almond Flavoured Rounds, Country Garden Cakes*	1 Cake/45g	183	6.7	403	4.3	62.4	14.7	2.3
Almond Slices, Mr Kipling*	1 Slice/32.5g	131	4.6	403	6.3	63.4	14	2
Almond Slices, Sainsbury's*	1 Serving/27g	120	7.1	444	5.9	45.9	26.3	1.5
Almond Slices, Weight Watchers*	1 Slice/26g	95	2.6	365	5.2	63.8	9.9	2.4
Angel Layer, Somerfield*	1 Serving/37.0g	146	7	395	4.1	51.9	19	0.6
Angel Layer, Tesco*	1 Serving/25g	101	4.3	403	4.5	57.4	17.3	0.9
Angel Slices, Mr Kipling*	1 Slice/33g	145	6.1	431	3	63.4	18.2	0.6
Angel Slices, Snap Packs, Mr Kipling*	1 Slice/34g	148	6.6	417	2.7	60.1	18.5	0.6
Angel, Average	**1 Slice/44g**	**175**	**7.9**	**397**	**4.2**	**54.9**	**17.9**	**0.8**
Angel, Sainsbury's*	1/8 Cake/41g	171	8.1	417	4.1	55.7	19.8	0.8
Apple & Cinnamon, Oat Break, Go Ahead, McVitie's*	1 Serving/35g	122	2.3	349	5.2	67.2	6.6	2.6
Apple & Blackcurrant, Crumble, Graze*	1 Punnet/33g	121	7.5	365	6.1	34.5	22.7	3.1
Apple & Blackcurrant, The Best, Morrisons*	1/6 Cake/66g	254	10.9	384	3.1	55.5	16.5	0.6
Apple Bakes, Go Ahead, McVitie's*	1 Cake/35g	126	2.7	361	2.6	70	7.8	2
Apple Crumble, Slices, Weight Watchers*	1 Slice/26g	90	2	346	4.5	64.8	7.7	2.3
Apple Slice, Delightful, Mr Kipling*	1 Slice/29g	92	1.1	317	4.4	66.2	3.9	1.3
Apple, Bramley, & Blackberry Crumble, M&S*	1/8 Cake/56g	221	10	395	4.4	54.1	17.9	1.5
Apple, Home Style, M&S*	1 Cake/54g	189	7.9	350	5.3	49.4	14.7	1.5

CAKE

	Measure INFO/WEIGHT	per Measure KCAL	FAT	Nutrition Values per 100g / 100ml KCAL	PROT	CARB	FAT	FIBRE
Apricot & Apple, Trimlyne*	1 Cake/50g	134	1.4	267	4.3	58.4	2.7	1.9
Bakewell Slice, Weight Watchers*	1 Slice/26g	84	0.6	324	3.7	71	2.4	2
Bakewell Slices, Mr Kipling*	1 Slice/36g	163	7.3	454	4.2	63.4	20.4	1.2
Bakewell, Lemon, Average	*1 Cake/42g*	*173*	*6.4*	*411*	*3.7*	*64.6*	*15.2*	*1.3*
Bakewell, The Handmade Flapjack Company*	1 Cake/75g	311	17.1	415	4.5	47.4	22.8	0
Banana Loaf, Waitrose*	1 Slice/70g	236	7.5	337	5	55.2	10.7	1.7
Banana, Iced, Waitrose*	1/6 Cake/55g	190	5.9	345	4.2	58	10.7	2.7
Banana, Loaf, The Best, Morrisons*	1 Serving/75g	273	13.4	364	5.7	44.1	17.9	2
Banana, Organic, Loaf, Respect Organics*	¼ Pack/65g	254	13.6	391	3.9	48.6	21	1.5
Banana, The Handmade Flapjack Company*	1 Cake/75g	290	10.8	387	5.3	59.2	14.4	0
Banana, with An Afternoon Tea Infusion, Graze*	1 Punnet/18g	55	2.5	307	5	39	14	3
Banoffee Slices, Dessert Classics, Mr Kipling*	1 Slice/34g	140	6.2	414	2.9	59	18.4	0.6
Bar, Iced Rich Fruit, Finest, Tesco*	1 Serving/100g	360	10.7	360	3.8	61.3	10.7	4.2
Bara Brith, Tan Y Castell*	1 Serving/100g	261	1	261	4	58.8	1	1.5
Battenberg, Asda*	1 Slice/25g	104	3	418	6	71.1	12.2	0.8
Battenberg, Mini, Mr Kipling*	1 Cake/33g	134	3.4	410	4.2	74.2	10.4	1.2
Battenberg, Mr Kipling*	1 Serving/38g	161	4.6	421	5	73.3	12	1.6
Belgian Chocolate, Slices, Weight Watchers*	1 Slice/25g	86	2.4	344	6.5	57.6	9.8	2.9
Belgian Chocolate, Waitrose*	1 Slice/47g	223	12.6	474	4.8	53.1	26.9	1.9
Birthday Present, Tesco*	1 Serving/79g	347	13.9	439	3.5	66.6	17.6	0.4
Birthday, M&S*	1 Serving/60g	240	7.1	400	2.3	70.9	11.9	0.8
Bites, Caramel, Mr Kipling*	1 Cake/14g	68	3.8	492	5.9	55.3	27.4	0.8
Bites, Chocolate Roll, Mini, Tesco*	1 Bite/18g	78	3.6	435	6	58	19.8	1.9
Bites, Coconut, Sainsbury's*	1 Bite/80g	339	16.9	424	5.3	53	21.2	4.2
Blackcurrant Delice, Specially Selected, Aldi*	1/6 Cake/74g	152	6.9	206	2.6	28	9.3	0.8
Brilliant Banana Bread, Graze*	1 Cake/23g	72	3.6	312	5.2	40.4	15.6	3
Butterfly, Mr Kipling*	1 Cake/29g	114	6.4	392	4.4	43.4	22.2	0.6
Buttons, Happy Birthday, Cadbury*	1 Slice/50g	235	13.6	470	4.1	52.8	27.1	0
Caramel Crunchy, Devondale*	1 Cake/80g	359	19.2	449	2.9	56.3	24	1.3
Caramel Shortbread, Devondale*	1 Cake/75g	356	18.6	474	3	57	24.8	0.8
Caramel Shortcake Slices, McVitie's*	1 Slice /31.6g	146	7.7	463	4.3	56.5	24.4	1.6
Caramel Slice, M&S*	1 Slice/64g	304	16.1	475	4.9	60.4	25.2	2.6
Caramel, Milk Chocolate, Holly Lane*	1 Cake/25g	110	5.1	441	6.9	57.6	20.3	1.1
Carrot & Orange Slices, GFY, Asda*	1 Serving/23g	77	0.6	334	3.4	74	2.7	1
Carrot & Orange Slices, Good Intentions, Somerfield*	1 Cake/27g	85	0.8	315	4.1	68	3	1.5
Carrot & Orange, Extra Special, Asda*	1/6 Cake/65g	240	11.7	369	4.7	47	18	0.9
Carrot & Orange, Finest, Tesco*	1/8 Cake/50g	205	10.2	410	4.6	51.2	20.5	2.1
Carrot & Orange, Waitrose*	1/6 Cake/47g	164	7.4	350	5.3	46.8	15.7	1.8
Carrot & Pecan, M&S*	1 Slice/90g	330	14.6	365	6.4	48.7	16.2	2.3
Carrot & Walnut, Layered, Asda*	1 Serving/42g	172	8	409	4.6	55	19	1
Carrot & Walnut, Mini Classics, Mr Kipling*	1 Cake/39g	172	9.8	440	4.5	48.6	25.2	1
Carrot & Walnut, Aldi*	¼ Cake/100g	409	23	409	5.1	44	23	2.2
Carrot Slices, Less Than 3% Fat, BGTY, Sainsbury's*	1 Slice/30g	94	0.8	313	3.4	68.7	2.7	2.4
Carrot Slices, Weight Watchers*	1 Slice/27g	84	0.2	311	2.8	73	0.8	0.9
Carrot Wedge, Tesco*	1 Pack/175g	532	27.6	304	3.9	36.6	15.8	1.5
Carrot, Average	*1 Slice/56g*	*211*	*10.4*	*377*	*4.6*	*47.6*	*18.6*	*1.4*
Carrot, Entenmann's*	1 Serving/40g	156	8.2	391	4.1	47.4	20.5	1.5
Carrot, GF , Finest, Tesco*	1 Serving/50g	204	10.4	407	3.4	50.4	20.9	1.9
Carrot, Handmade, Delicious, Boots*	1 Slice/75g	292	13.5	389	4.1	53	18	1.4
Carrot, Iced, Tesco*	1 Serving/61g	246	12	404	3.1	53.7	19.6	1.6
Carrot, Lidl*	1/6 Cake/71g	280	13.7	394	4.7	48.9	19.3	3
Carrot, Made Without Wheat, M&S*	1 Serving/50g	196	10.6	391	3.1	46.3	21.3	0.8
Carrot, McVitie's*	1/9 of Cake/24g	87	3.5	360	4.8	52.8	14.4	2.3

C

CAKE

	Measure INFO/WEIGHT	per Measure KCAL	FAT	Nutrition Values per 100g / 100ml KCAL	PROT	CARB	FAT	FIBRE
Carrot, Mini, Weight Watchers*	1 Cake/31g	120	3.3	388	3.7	68.9	10.8	2.7
Carrot, Organic, Respect Organics*	1 Slice/45g	179	10.1	398	3.1	47.4	22.4	1.5
Carrot, Slices, Asda*	1 Slice/80g	302	13.2	377	3.4	53.8	16.5	1.7
Carrot, Slices, Eat Smart, Morrisons*	1 Cake/27g	84	0.6	312	3	70	2.2	2.3
Carrot, Slices, Inspirations, Mr Kipling*	1 Slice/34g	139	6.3	411	3.5	57.7	18.5	1.3
Carrot, Square, Margaret's Country Kitchen*	1 Cake/80g	307	13.5	384	3.6	54.4	16.9	2.4
Carrot, The Best, Morrisons*	1/6 Cake/64g	260	12.9	406	3.9	51.3	20.1	1.9
Carrot, TTD, Sainsbury's*	1 Slice/72g	287	13.7	398	4.5	51.1	19	2.5
Celebration, Sainsbury's*	1/12 Cake/100g	265	9.2	265	2.1	43.6	9.2	0.3
Cherry Bakewell, Co-Op*	1 Cake/47g	205	8	435	3.7	67.2	16.9	1.8
Cherry Bakewell, GF, Bakers Delight*	1 Cake/50g	211	8.2	422	2.9	66.1	16.3	0.4
Cherry Bakewell, M&S*	1 Cake/44g	185	7.8	420	4.5	61.7	17.7	1
Cherry Bakewell, Mini, Sainsbury's*	1 Cake/27g	101	3.3	370	3.4	62.2	12	0.4
Cherry Bakewell, Sainsbury's*	1 Cake/46g	200	8.1	436	3.1	66.3	17.6	1.4
Cherry Bakewell, Slices, GFY, Asda*	1 Slice/29g	98	0.7	337	3.4	75.4	2.4	0.7
Cherry Bakewell, Smart Price, Asda*	1 Cake/38g	157	6.8	413	2.7	60	18	2.6
Cherry Bakewell, Tesco*	1 Cake/39g	171	7.5	439	3.2	63.3	19.2	1.1
Cherry Bakewell, Waitrose*	1 Cake/44g	184	8.5	419	3.8	57.4	19.3	2.1
Cherry Bakewells, Delightful, Mr Kipling*	1 Cake/45g	176	5.8	390	3.9	66.4	12.9	1.2
Cherry Bakewells, Mr Kipling*	1 Cake/45g	193	8.3	428	3.9	61.3	18.5	1.4
Cherry Shortbread, Devondale*	1 Cake/75g	340	18	453	3.9	52	24	1.3
Cherry, Asda*	1 Slice/37g	131	4.5	351	4.7	56	12	0.6
Cherry, Co-Op*	1/8 Cake/47g	190	8.5	405	4	57	18	0.8
Cherry, Linda Kearns*	1 Serving/100g	265	14.2	265	12.1	29.9	14.2	4.2
Cherry, M&S*	1 Serving/75g	285	9.5	380	5	60.6	12.7	0.8
Chewy Rice Pop & Chocolate, Dove's Farm*	1 Bar/35g	156	7.1	447	3.9	69.9	20.2	2.3
Chocolate	***1oz/28g***	***128***	***7.4***	***456***	***7.4***	***50.4***	***26.4***	***1.7***
Chocolate & Orange Slices, GFY, Asda*	1 Serving/30g	95	0.8	315	3.2	70	2.5	1.3
Chocolate & Sweetest, Beetroot, Battle Bakehouse*	1/6 Cake/49g	185	8.7	379	5.2	48.6	17.9	4
Chocolate & Caramel Tiffin Bites, Gu*	1 Tiffin/35g	168	9.9	480	3.8	51.9	28.3	2.8
Chocolate & Madeira, Marble Loaf, M&S*	1/6 Cake/88g	380	20.4	430	5	50	23.1	1
Chocolate & Orange Rolls, M&S*	1 Cake/60g	228	17	380	3.6	27	28.4	1.3
Chocolate Box, Asda*	1 Serving/60g	263	13.8	439	5	53	23	0.7
Chocolate Brownie, Devondale*	1 Cake/60g	246	12.9	410	4.4	51	21.5	2.1
Chocolate Brownie, Fudge, Entenmann's*	1/8 Cake/55g	168	2.4	306	4	62.7	4.4	1.5
Chocolate Brownie, Gluten & Wheat Free, Lovemore*	1 Slice/36g	127	4.6	352	3.7	56.1	12.8	0.2
Chocolate Button, Cakes for the Connoisseur*	1 Cake/30g	145	9.8	485	5.2	42.1	32.8	2.3
Chocolate Chip, Co-Op*	1/6 Cake/63g	275	16.9	440	5	44	27	0.5
Chocolate Chip, The Cake Shop*	1 Cake/35g	178	11	508	4.7	50.2	31.5	1.1
Chocolate Crunch, Tray Bake, Kate's Cakes Ltd*	1 Serving/80g	400	23	500	4.8	53.4	28.8	3.7
Chocolate Flavour Slices, GFY, Asda*	1 Slice/27.5g	71	0.7	257	4.3	54	2.6	1.4
Chocolate Fudge	***1 Serving/110g***	***415***	***19.1***	***377***	***4.4***	***50.4***	***17.4***	***1.4***
Chocolate Fudge Slice, Waitrose*	1 Slice/60g	230	9.7	383	4.7	54.6	16.2	1.5
Chocolate Fudge, & Vanilla Cream, M&S*	1/6 Cake/69g	310	17.9	450	5.2	49.8	26	1.3
Chocolate Fudge, Belgian, TTD, Sainsbury's*	1 Slice/66g	278	14.3	423	4.4	52.5	21.7	2.5
Chocolate Fudge, Classics, M&S*	1 Serving/71g	195	7.5	275	2.8	42.8	10.6	1.1
Chocolate Fudge, Sainsbury's*	1/8 Cake/98g	402	21.9	410	5.5	47.3	22.3	1.9
Chocolate Fudge, Tea Time Treats, Asda*	1 Cake/37.0g	157	8.1	424	3.6	53	22	1.7
Chocolate Heaven, Extra Special, Asda*	1/6 Cake/66g	255	13.1	388	4	48	20	1
Chocolate Indulgence, Finest, Tesco*	1 Slice/51g	207	9.1	405	4.8	55.9	17.9	1.2
Chocolate Log, Fresh Cream, Finest, Tesco*	1 Slice/85g	301	15.4	354	4.5	43.2	18.1	1.4
Chocolate Orange, Sponge, Asda*	1 Serving/70g	298	18.2	425	4.9	42.9	26	3
Chocolate Party, M&S*	1 Serving/61g	240	12.6	395	4.6	46.9	20.8	1.1

	Measure INFO/WEIGHT	per Measure KCAL	FAT	Nutrition Values per 100g / 100ml KCAL	PROT	CARB	FAT	FIBRE

CAKE

	Measure INFO/WEIGHT	KCAL	FAT	KCAL	PROT	CARB	FAT	FIBRE
Chocolate Rice Crispy, Knightsbridge, Lidl*	1 Cake/24g	88	4.2	368	3.9	48.7	17.5	0.1
Chocolate Roll, Sainsbury's*	1 Slice/50g	210	10.2	420	5	54	20.4	3.3
Chocolate Sensation, Sainsbury's*	1 Serving/92g	320	17.7	348	3.7	40	19.2	2.3
Chocolate Slice, Go Ahead, McVitie's*	1 Slice/32g	94	2.6	293	4.5	49.4	8.2	1.9
Chocolate Slices, Mr Kipling*	1 Slice/32.5g	132	6.7	406	5.6	50.4	20.6	2.7
Chocolate Sponge, Budgens*	1/6 Cake/76g	297	13.6	392	3.8	55.9	18	2.1
Chocolate Sponge, Morrisons*	1 Serving/59g	179	7.6	303	4.4	42.5	12.8	0.7
Chocolate Sponge, Tesco*	1 Serving/37g	129	3.6	358	5.1	60.8	10.1	1.7
Chocolate Tiffin, Devondale*	1 Cake/100g	513	27	513	2.8	54	27	1.7
Chocolate Truffle, Extra Special, Asda*	1 Serving/103g	402	26.8	390	5	34	26	1.8
Chocolate Truffle, Mini, Finest, Tesco*	1 Cake/28g	125	6.6	448	5.9	52.9	23.7	0.3
Chocolate Truffle, So Good, Somerfield*	1 Slice/80g	328	18.6	410	6.4	44	23.2	1
Chocolate Victoria Sponge, Co-Op*	1 Slice/61g	201	9.8	330	5	42	16	1
Chocolate with Butter Icing, Average	*1oz/28g*	*135*	*8.3*	*481*	*5.7*	*50.9*	*29.7*	*0*
Chocolate with White Chocolate, The Cake Shop*	1 Cake/29g	146	9.3	503	4.6	49.2	32	1.2
Chocolate, Big, Tesco*	1 Slice/79g	311	13.1	396	7.4	54.1	16.7	1.8
Chocolate, Birthday, Tesco*	1 Serving/54g	229	13.2	425	5.9	45.5	24.4	2.1
Chocolate, Caterpillar, Tesco*	1 Serving/53g	248	13.2	468	5.7	55.3	24.9	1.1
Chocolate, Cup, Mini, Weight Watchers*	1 Cake/17g	72	3.6	422	6.1	52	21.1	1.8
Chocolate, Fondants, Weight Watchers*	1 Cake/19g	70	2.3	368	6.1	59	12	3.2
Chocolate, Fudge, The Cake Shop*	1 Cake/37g	178	10.8	480	3.7	50.5	29.2	1.3
Chocolate, Happy Birthday, Tesco*	1 Serving/58g	241	13.2	415	4.7	46.9	22.7	2.9
Chocolate, Iced, Tesco*	1 Serving/40g	158	6.3	395	4.7	58.5	15.8	1.8
Chocolate, Individual with Mini Eggs, Cadbury*	1 Cake/26g	119	6.1	455	4.6	57.5	23.1	1.3
Chocolate, Large, Happy Birthday, Tesco*	1/18 Cake/63g	249	12.2	396	6.2	49.3	19.3	1.8
Chocolate, Loaf, Moist, McVitie's*	1 Slice/30g	119	6.1	398	4.8	49	20.3	1.9
Chocolate, Morrisons*	1/6 of Cake/83g	339	19.5	407	5.5	42.5	23.4	2
Chocolate, Party, Tesco*	1 Slice/62g	244	13.1	394	4.6	46.3	21.2	0.9
Chocolate, Sainsbury's*	1 Serving/30g	118	5.6	395	4.1	52.6	18.5	1.3
Chocolate, Sara Lee*	¼ Cake/88g	339	14.8	385	4.1	54.3	16.8	0
Chocolate, Slices, HE, Tesco*	1 Slice/25g	78	0.6	314	4.7	65.5	2.4	3.7
Chocolate, Smarties, Celebration, Large, Nestle*	1/16 Cake/71g	308	17.4	432	5.4	48.9	24.4	1.2
Chocolate, The Best, Morrisons*	1/6 Cake/69g	294	15	426	4.3	52.5	21.7	1.5
Chocolate, The Handmade Flapjack Company*	1 Cake/75g	303	16.2	404	12.5	39.8	21.6	0
Chocolate, Thorntons*	1 Serving/87g	408	25.1	469	5.2	47.1	28.8	0.6
Chocolate, Triple Layer, Celebration, Tesco*	1/24 of cake/79g	345	18.8	430	5	47.7	23.4	2.8
Chocolate, White Star, Traybake, Asda*	1/15 Portion/47g	28	1.1	405	4.4	60	16	1.7
Chocolate, White Button, Asda*	1 Cake/30g	117	6.3	390	5	44	21	2
Chorley, Asda*	1 Cake/60g	269	12.6	449	6	59	21	2.2
Christmas Slices, Mr Kipling*	1 Slice/43g	159	3.8	368	3	68.4	8.8	1.4
Christmas, Bites, M&S*	1 Bite/21g	75	1.7	359	4	66.5	8.3	1.1
Christmas, Connoisseur, M&S*	1 Slice/60g	216	5.5	360	4.1	64.7	9.2	3.3
Christmas, Fruit, Iced, Bar, Bakers Selection, Asda*	1 Serving/67g	233	5.3	349	3.8	64	7.9	2.5
Christmas, Iced Fruit, Decorative, Bakers Selection, Asda*	1/12 Cake/76g	276	8.3	365	4.6	62	11	1.4
Christmas, Iced Rich Fruit, Finest, Tesco*	1/8 Cake/50g	183	4.3	366	4.3	66.4	8.6	3.3
Christmas, Iced, Slices, Tesco*	1 Slice/45g	168	4.4	369	2.9	67.6	9.6	1.2
Christmas, Rich Fruit, Free From, Tesco*	1/12 Cake/75g	284	6.4	376	3	71	8.5	1.6
Christmas, Rich Fruit, Organic, Tesco*	1 Serving/76g	282	7.6	374	3.9	67.1	10	2
Christmas, Rich Fruit, Tesco*	1 Serving/75g	261	7.2	348	3.8	60.6	9.6	2.1
Christmas, Royal Iced, Waitrose*	1/6 Cake/75g	270	4.6	360	3.7	71.3	6.2	2
Christmas, Top Iced, Rich Fruit, Essential, Waitrose*	1 Slice/75g	278	5.8	368	3.6	69.6	7.7	2.9
Cinnamon, Cannelle Zimt, Pagen*	1 Roll/21g	78	2.9	370	7	53	14	0
Classic Lemon Drizzle, M&S*	1/6 Cake/68g	253	10.3	375	4.7	55	15.3	0.6

C

CAKE

INFO/WEIGHT	Measure	per Measure KCAL	FAT	Nutrition Values per 100g / 100ml KCAL	PROT	CARB	FAT	FIBRE
Classic, Selection, Bakers Selection, Asda*	1 Slice/91g	249	10	275	2.5	41	11	1.2
Coconut	*1 Slice/70g*	*304*	*16.7*	*434*	*6.7*	*51.2*	*23.8*	*2.5*
Coconut & Raspberry, M&S*	1 Serving/52g	231	13.9	445	5	45.5	26.8	2.3
Coconut Delight, Burton's*	1 Cake/21g	89	3.5	424	4	63	16.9	2
Coconut Snowball, Bobby's*	1 Cake/18g	80	4	436	2.2	57.3	22.1	0
Coconut Snowballs, Tunnock's*	1 Cake/30g	134	6.2	446	4.2	56.7	20.8	3.6
Coconut Sponge, Memory Lane*	1/6 Cake/42g	172	7.5	406	4.1	57.1	17.6	1.5
Coconut Sponge, Mini Classics, Mr Kipling*	1 Cake/38g	155	8.7	409	3.7	47	22.9	0.9
Coffee & Walnut Slices, HE, Tesco*	1 Slice/23g	69	0.5	301	4.4	65.7	2.3	2.8
Coffee & Walnut, Mrs Beeton's*	1 Slice/54g	219	13.5	405	3.7	41.4	25	0.3
Coffee Sponge Roll, M&S*	1/6 Roll/41.6g	160	7.4	385	3.1	53.1	17.8	1.4
Coffee, Iced, M&S*	1 Slice/33g	135	6.5	410	4.4	54.5	19.6	1.6
Coffee, The Best, Morrisons*	1/6 Cake/69g	296	13.5	429	3.8	59.1	19.5	0.8
Coffee, TTD, Sainsbury's*	1 Slice/68g	294	16.4	430	4.3	49.1	24	2.6
Colin the Caterpillar, M&S*	1 Slice/60g	234	12.8	390	5.3	57.2	21.3	1.3
Corn Flake, Chocolate, Mini Bites, Tesco*	1 Bite/14g	62	2.5	446	7.1	64.1	17.9	5.9
Cornflake, Average	*1 Cake/18g*	*83*	*3.7*	*464*	*5.2*	*64.6*	*20.4*	*2*
Cornflake, Bobby's*	1/6 Cake/45g	207	9.2	461	3.9	65.5	20.4	0
Cornflake, Chocolate Clusters, Asda*	1 Cake/14g	64	2.6	460	8.2	65.2	18.5	2.7
Country Farmhouse, Waitrose*	1 Serving/80g	308	12.1	385	4.7	57.5	15.1	1.4
Country Slices, Asda*	1 Serving/27g	111	5.1	411	3.9	56	19	2.4
Country Slices, Good Intentions, Somerfield*	1 Cake/22g	70	0.4	318	5.5	70	1.8	1.8
Courgette & Feta Quinoa, Everdine*	1 Serving/450g	508	18	113	1.8	16.1	4	2.9
Cranberry, Linda Kearns*	1 Serving/100g	265	14.2	265	12	29.9	14.2	5.2
Cream Oysters, M&S*	1 Cake/72g	227	15.3	315	3.6	27.5	21.2	3
Cream Slices, M&S*	1 Slice/80g	310	18.3	387	2.3	45.7	22.9	0.6
Crispy Chocolate Clusters, Mini, Tesco*	1 Cluster/7.9g	37	1.5	470	7	67.8	18.7	2.5
Date & Walnut Loaf, Sainsbury's*	1/10 Slice/40g	148	8.2	371	6.7	40.1	20.4	1
Date & Walnut Slices, GFY, Asda*	1 Slice/22.1g	62	0.3	281	5	61.8	1.5	1.8
Date, Linda Kearns*	1 Serving/100g	269	16.8	269	12.7	24.4	16.8	4.4
Double Chocolate Ganache, M&S*	1/12 Cake/61g	281	16.8	460	5.9	46.1	27.6	2.5
Eccles, Fresh Baked	*1 Cake/45g*	*171*	*7.6*	*381*	*4.3*	*56.3*	*17*	*1.5*
Eccles, Weight Watchers*	1 Cake/48g	190	7.9	396	4.5	57.5	16.5	2
Fairy, Average	*1 Cake/23g*	*96*	*4.6*	*416*	*5.1*	*53*	*20.2*	*1.5*
Fairy, Holly Lane*	1 Cake/26g	118	6.7	460	3.7	52.5	26.1	3.5
Fairy, Iced, Average	*1 Cake/23g*	*91*	*3.4*	*394*	*4.2*	*60.8*	*14.8*	*0.9*
Fairy, Lemon Iced, Average	*1 Cake/23g*	*90*	*3.1*	*393*	*4.4*	*63.2*	*13.6*	*1.1*
Fairy, Mini, Kids, Tesco*	1 Cake/12g	54	2.8	435	5.3	53.3	22.3	1.1
Fairy, Mini, Tesco*	1 Cake/13g	53	2.5	424	6.1	54.6	20.1	1.3
Fairy, Plain, Average	*1 Cake/23g*	*95*	*4.6*	*413*	*5.5*	*51.1*	*20.2*	*1.5*
Fairy, Plain, Sainsbury's*	1 Cake/20g	84	4.3	422	4.9	46.4	21.5	1.2
Fairy, Plain, Value, Tesco*	1 Cake/15g	52	1.3	348	5.3	62.4	8.6	0.9
Fairy, Smart Price, Asda*	1 Cake/15g	66	3.3	438	6	54	22	1
Fairy, Snowman, Christmas, Tesco*	1 Cake/24g	114	6.8	471	4.6	49.8	28.1	2.9
Fairy, Strawberry Iced, Tesco*	1 Cake/24g	94	3.2	392	4.9	62.9	13.4	1.4
Fairy, Vanilla Iced, Average, Tesco*	1 Cake/23g	89	2.8	388	4.4	65.1	12.2	1.2
Farmhouse Slice, Weight Watchers*	1 Slice/23g	73	0.9	317	5.5	64.9	4	1.3
Flake, Cadbury*	1 Cake/20g	90	4.5	445	6.3	54.5	22.3	0
Fondant Fancies, Lemon, Waitrose*	1 Cake/40g	176	7.1	441	2.5	67.9	17.7	0.6
Fondant Fancies, Sainsbury's*	1 Cake/27g	95	2.4	353	2.4	65.7	9	0.4
Fondant, Dark Chocolate, Graze*	1 Pack/40g	157	5.8	393	3.5	66.2	14.5	0
Fondants with Chocolate, Mini, Delhaize*	1 Cake Mini/20g	88	6.2	440	4.6	36.3	30.8	3.8

CAKE	Measure INFO/WEIGHT	per Measure		Nutrition Values per 100g / 100ml				
		KCAL	FAT	KCAL	PROT	CARB	FAT	FIBRE
French Fancies, Average	*1 Cake/27g*	*100*	*2.5*	*371*	*2.7*	*69.6*	*9.1*	*0.8*
French Fancies, Lemon, Average	*1 Cake/28g*	*106*	*2.7*	*378*	*2.5*	*69.9*	*9.8*	*0.5*
French Fancies, Lemon, Mr Kipling*	1 Cake/28g	106	2.7	378	2.5	69.9	9.8	0.5
French Fancies, M&S*	1 Cake/25g	91	2	365	2.7	70.6	8.1	1.3
French Fancies, Mr Kipling*	1 Cake/28g	106	2.8	378	2.6	69.7	9.9	0.6
French Fancies, Strawberry, Mr Kipling*	1 Cake/28g	106	2.7	379	2.5	70.6	9.6	0.4
Friday Feeling, Crunchie, Cadbury*	1 Serving/43g	200	9.8	455	4.2	58.4	22.3	1.7
Fruit & Nut Cluster, Finest, Tesco*	1 Slice/77g	262	10.3	338	4.5	50.1	13.3	2.7
Fruit & Nut Cluster, TTD, Sainsbury's*	1 Slice/62.4g	239	9.2	383	5.7	56.8	14.8	4.2
Fruit Cake with Marzipan & Icing, Asda*	1/12 Slice/76g	280	6.8	369	3.9	68	9	0
Fruit Slices, Rich, Iced, Finest, Tesco*	1 Slice/41g	152	3.4	370	3.2	69.4	8.3	2.1
Fruit, Iced, Slices, Tesco*	1 Slice/44g	165	4.1	375	3.2	68.6	9.3	2.1
Fruit, Luxury, Fully Iced Slice, The Best, Morrisons*	1 Serving/50g	178	3.8	356	3.7	66.6	7.6	3.1
Fruit, Parisienne, Rich, Finest, Tesco*	1 Serving/69g	262	9.7	380	4.7	55.2	14.1	1.9
Fruit, Plain, Average	*1 Slice/90g*	*319*	*11.6*	*354*	*5.1*	*57.9*	*12.9*	*0*
Fruit, Rich, Average	*1 Slice/70g*	*225*	*8.8*	*322*	*4.9*	*50.7*	*12.5*	*1.7*
Fruit, Rich, Iced	*1 Slice/70g*	*249*	*8*	*356*	*4.1*	*62.7*	*11.4*	*1.7*
Fruit, Rich, M&S*	1 Serving/50g	158	3.2	315	3.1	60.9	6.5	4.3
Fruit, Slices, Gluten & Wheat Free, Lovemore*	1 Slice/40g	122	3.8	304	2.3	51.1	9.4	1.5
Fruit, Slices, Value, Tesco*	1 Slice/23g	84	4	372	4	48.7	17.7	1.3
Fudge Brownie, The Handmade Flapjack Company*	1 Cake/75g	286	9.2	381	4.9	62.8	12.3	0
Fudgy Chocolate Slices, COU, M&S*	1 Slice/36g	95	0.8	265	4.6	66.4	2.2	2.1
Genoa, Tesco*	1 Serving/44g	150	3.9	340	3.7	59.1	8.8	3.1
Ginger Drizzle, Iced, Co-Op*	1/6 Cake/64.5g	226	7.7	350	3	58	12	1
Glitzy Bag, Birthday, Tesco*	1 Serving/81g	314	6.9	388	2.1	75.9	8.5	0.6
Granola Square, All Butter, Finest, Tesco*	1 Square/72g	328	16.5	455	7.7	53.1	22.9	3
Granola Square, M&S*	1 Square/72g	330	18.1	464	7.9	49.3	25.5	5
Happy Birthday, Sainsbury's*	1 Slice/50g	207	8	414	2.8	64.5	16.1	0.6
Holly Hedgehog, Tesco*	1 Serving/55g	227	7.9	413	2	69	14.3	0.8
Hot Chocolate Fudge, Sainsbury's*	1/8 Cake/91.2g	343	15.6	376	5.1	50.3	17.1	3.5
Iced Fruit Slice, Gluten & Wheat Free, Lovemore*	1 Slice/44g	141	3.3	321	1.6	60	7.6	1.1
Iced Madeira, Sainsbury's*	1/8 Cake/47g	182	6.6	388	3.6	61.6	14.1	0.7
Jamaica Ginger with Lemon Filling, McVitie's*	1 Cake/33g	143	8.2	434	4	48.3	25	0.8
Jamaica Ginger, McVitie's*	1/9 Cake/26g	92	2.6	362	3.7	63.1	10.4	1.6
La Madeleine, Bonne Maman*	1 Cake/25g	112	6.8	449	6.4	44	27	2.3
Lardy, Warings The Bakers*	1 Slice/120g	379	14.8	316	0	48	12.3	0
Lemon & Orange, Finest, Tesco*	1 Serving/53g	216	10.7	410	4.5	52.4	20.3	1.1
Lemon & Raspberry, Loaf , Morrisons*	1 Cake/305g	1174	47.9	385	4.7	56	15.7	0.6
Lemon Bakewell, CBY, Asda*	1 Cake/42g	181	7.3	432	3.8	64.4	17.4	1.4
Lemon Bakewell, Mr Kipling*	1 Cake/43g	185	7.4	430	3.6	64.4	17.3	1
Lemon Buttercream & Lemon Curd, The Cake Shop*	1 Cake/28g	124	7.8	444	3.5	43.4	27.8	0.6
Lemon Drizzle Cake, Asda*	1 Serving/50g	150	6	299	2.8	45	12	0.4
Lemon Drizzle Slices, LC, Tesco*	1 Slice/23g	67	0.5	290	4.8	62.7	2	2.8
Lemon Drizzle, M&S*	1/6 Cake/63g	230	8.8	365	4.2	55.8	13.9	1.4
Lemon Drizzle, The Best, Morrisons*	1/6 Cake/72g	287	11.8	398	3.2	59.1	16.3	1.1
Lemon Madeira, Half Moon, Dan Cake*	1 Slice/50g	215	10	430	3.5	59	20	0
Lemon Slice, Iced, Tesco*	1 Slice/29g	114	4.9	394	3	56.1	17.1	2
Lemon Slices, BGTY, Sainsbury's*	1 Slice/26g	84	0.4	323	3.7	74	1.4	1.3
Lemon Slices, Eat Smart, Morrisons*	1 Slice/26g	81	0.7	312	3.8	68.1	2.7	1.9
Lemon Slices, Low Fat, Weight Watchers*	1 Slice/26.1g	79	0.5	303	3.1	68.1	2	2.2
Lemon Slices, Mr Kipling*	1 Slice/27g	109	4.5	405	4.1	59.4	16.7	0.7
Lemon, Average	*1 Slice/81g*	*320*	*14.5*	*396*	*4.1*	*54.8*	*18*	*0.6*
Lemon, Half Moon, Bobby's*	1/6 Cake/60g	244	11	406	4.1	55.7	18.4	0

CAKE

	Measure INFO/WEIGHT	per Measure KCAL	FAT	Nutrition Values per 100g / 100ml KCAL	PROT	CARB	FAT	FIBRE
Lemon, Loaf, M&S*	1 Slice/47g	190	8.8	400	2.1	55.8	18.6	0.6
Lemon, Mini, Weight Watchers*	1 Cake/27g	90	3	333	3.7	66.7	11.1	11.1
Leo the Lion, Birthday, Asda*	1 Slice/81g	325	12.9	402	2.6	62	16	0.5
Madeira	*1 Slice/40g*	*157*	*6.8*	*393*	*5.4*	*58.4*	*16.9*	*0.9*
Madeira, All Butter, Sainsbury's*	1 Serving/30g	116	5.9	388	5.2	47.4	19.7	0.8
Madeira, Cherry, Tesco*	¼ Cake/100g	342	11.2	342	4.3	55.9	11.2	2.6
Madeira, Iced, Tesco*	1/16 Cake/56g	218	6.8	389	2.6	67.2	12.2	0.4
Madeira, Lemon Iced, Co-Op*	1 Cake/290g	1131	52.2	390	4	53	18	0.6
Madeira, Lemon Iced, Tesco*	1 Slice/30g	122	5.2	407	4.5	57.8	17.5	0.9
Madeira, Lightly Fruited, Yorkshire Baking Company*	1 Portion/54g	261	12.7	484	6.3	60.3	23.5	1.3
Madeira, Party, Sainsbury's*	1 Slice/75g	321	15.2	427	4.1	56.8	20.2	1.1
Madeira, Tesco*	1 Serving/50g	197	7.8	394	5.5	57.9	15.6	1.2
Manor House, Mr Kipling*	1 Serving/69g	277	13.8	400	5.3	49.7	20	1.4
Marble, Tesco*	1/8 Cake/45g	184	8.4	410	4.4	55.9	18.7	1.5
Melting Butterscotch, Hot, Cadbury*	1 Cake/50g	225	10.4	445	4.9	59.6	20.6	2.2
Melting Double Chocolate, Hot, Cadbury*	1 Cake/50g	225	10.6	445	5.6	57.3	20.9	2.4
Mini Log, Chocolate, Free From, Sainsbury's*	1 Slice/45g	202	10.8	450	5.6	51	24	3
Mini Rolls, Blackcurrant, Bite, Trick Or Treat , Cadbury*	1 Mini Roll/28g	122	5.5	435	4.4	59.3	19.5	1.9
Mini Rolls, Blackforest, Weight Watchers*	1 Cake/24g	89	3.4	374	5.3	58.9	14.2	4.4
Mini Rolls, Cadbury*	1 Roll/27g	120	6.1	445	4.4	56.4	22.5	1.3
Mini Rolls, Chocolate, Average	*1 Cake/27g*	*122*	*6.2*	*453*	*4.8*	*56.9*	*22.9*	*0.9*
Mini Rolls, Chocolate, Tesco*	1 Roll/29g	135	6.7	465	5.5	58.1	23.1	1.3
Mini Rolls, Cola, Chocolate, Cadbury*	1 Roll/27g	115	6.1	435	4.8	50.4	23.1	2.3
Mini Rolls, Jaffa, Average	*1 Cake/29g*	*111*	*3.3*	*382*	*3.5*	*67.2*	*11.2*	*1.4*
Mini Rolls, Jam, Average	*1 Cake/29g*	*115*	*4.5*	*395*	*3.8*	*59.8*	*15.6*	*1.8*
Mini Rolls, Jammy Strawberry, Cadbury*	1 Cake/29g	119	4.8	411	4.9	59.8	16.5	0.5
Mini Rolls, Juicy Orange, Cadbury*	1 Cake/28g	110	4.7	390	5	55	16.8	0
Mini Rolls, Lemon, Average	*1 Cake/29g*	*125*	*5.8*	*430*	*4.8*	*58.6*	*19.9*	*0.9*
Mini Rolls, Milk Chocolate, Cadbury*	1 Roll/27g	120	6	445	4.4	56.5	22.2	0
Mini Rolls, Mint, Cadbury*	1 Roll/27g	123	6.2	455	5	55.4	23.1	1.4
Mini Rolls, Raspberry Ripple , Cadbury*	1 Roll/29g	126	5.7	435	4.5	59	19.6	1.4
Mint Aero, Celebration, Nestle*	1 Slice/58g	232	11.8	400	4	49.7	20.3	1.7
Mint Bar, Devondale*	1 Cake/85g	371	19.6	436	4.3	49.7	23	2
Orange & Cranberry, Mini Classics, Mr Kipling*	1 Cake/36g	164	7.3	455	4.5	42.2	20.2	0.7
Orange Marmalade Loaf, Aldi*	1 Slice/33.0g	88	0.7	267	4.5	57.4	2.2	1.8
Orange Marmalade, M&S*	1 Slice/50g	195	9.2	390	3.6	53.2	18.3	1.8
Pandoro, Italian	*1/8 Cake/87g*	*357*	*18.2*	*408*	*7.1*	*47.2*	*20.8*	*1.6*
Panettone, Amaretti & Amaretto, Finest, Tesco*	1/8 Cake/93g	344	14.9	367	6.2	48.7	15.9	2.2
Panettone, Average	*1 Portion/90g*	*345*	*15.3*	*383*	*8*	*52*	*17*	*0*
Panettone, Classic, Sainsbury's*	1 Slice/63g	227	8.2	363	7.4	53.3	13.1	1.2
Panettone, Finest, Tesco*	1/8 Cake/93g	318	11.8	339	6.1	49.1	12.6	2.5
Panettone, Luxury, Christmas, Tesco*	1 Serving/83g	307	11.6	370	7	53.5	14	2.5
Panettone, Prosecco Maron Glace, TTD, Sainsbury's*	1 Slice/85g	328	14.6	386	6.6	50.1	17.2	2.2
Party Bake, M&S*	1/15 Cake/60g	230	12.1	385	4	46.6	20.2	0.9
Party, Asda*	1 Serving/57g	238	9	421	2.3	67	16	0.4
Perfect Pumpkin & Ginger, Graze*	1 Punnet/34g	101	5.1	298	6.1	38.6	15	4
Petit Cakes Aux Fruits, Bonne Maman*	1 Cake/30g	122	6.3	407	5.4	48	21	0
Piece of Cake, Birthday, M&S*	1 Serving/85g	395	24.4	465	4.3	39.7	28.7	0.9
Plum & Ginger, Crumble, Graze*	1 Punnet/33g	119	9.1	361	6.2	35.1	27.6	3.3
Pumpkin Patch, Cadbury*	1 Cake/31g	149	7.1	480	5.3	61.7	22.9	2.4
Punschrulle Punsch Roll, Delicato*	1 Roll/40g	173	8	433	5	59	20	0
Raisin Fruit Slab, Basics, Sainsbury's*	1 Slice/50g	183	6.2	367	5.3	57.3	12.5	1.9
Raisin, Tesco*	1 Cake/38g	158	7.6	417	5.6	53.8	19.9	1.4

CAKE	Measure INFO/WEIGHT	per Measure KCAL	FAT	Nutrition Values per 100g / 100ml KCAL	PROT	CARB	FAT	FIBRE
Raspberry Flavour Sponge, Value, Tesco*	1 Slice/39g	130	4.6	334	3.4	53.4	11.9	0.7
Red Velvet, Delicious, Boots*	1 Pack/65g	285	14.9	439	4.5	52	23	1.4
Red Velvet, The Best, Morrisons*	1/6 Cake/63g	277	13.2	440	3.7	58.8	20.9	0.8
Red Velvet, TTD, Sainsbury's*	1 Slice/71g	302	16	428	2.8	52.8	22.7	0.8
Rich Chocolate, Christmas, Tesco*	1 Slice/82g	300	13.5	367	7	47.5	16.5	1.6
Rich Fruit Slices, Free From, Sainsbury's*	1 Slice/40g	144	5	361	4.5	57.4	12.6	3.7
Rich Fruit, Golden Bow, TTD, Sainsbury's*	1 Slice/85g	324	7.7	381	3.3	70.3	9	2.7
Rich Fruit, Iced, Finest, Tesco*	1 Slice/57g	191	4.7	335	3.6	61.2	8.3	4.4
Rich Fruit, Top Iced, Sainsbury's*	1 Slice/75g	268	5.3	357	3	69.3	7.1	2.2
Rock	**1 Sm Cake/40g**	**158**	**6.6**	**396**	**5.4**	**60.5**	**16.4**	**1.5**
Rock, Tesco*	1 Serving/87g	311	8.4	357	7.4	60.1	9.7	1.6
Salted Caramel, The Best, Morrisons*	1/6 Cake/63g	262	12.2	416	3.9	56.2	19.4	0.5
Seriously Chocolatey Celebration, Sainsbury's*	1/8 Cake/77g	336	19.8	437	6.3	45	25.7	0.3
Seriously Chocolatey, Large, Sainsbury's*	1/24 Cake/77g	352	19.5	457	5.4	51	25.3	3
Shrek Birthday, Tesco*	1/16 Cake/72g	248	8.8	344	3.3	64	12.2	0.5
Simnel Slices, Mr Kipling*	1 Slice/47g	177	5.9	379	2.9	63.4	12.6	1.2
Slice, Chocolate Brownie, Kate's Cakes Ltd*	1 Bar/60g	258	13	430	4.9	52.9	21.7	1.5
Slices, Carrot & Orange, LC, Tesco*	1 Slice/30g	93	0.7	310	3.2	68.5	2.2	1.9
Snowballs, Sainsbury's*	1 Snowball/18g	80	4.1	445	2.5	55.6	23	3.6
Snowballs, Tesco*	1 Snowball/18g	79	4	432	2.5	55.8	22.1	5.4
Sponge	**1 Slice/53g**	**243**	**13.9**	**459**	**6.4**	**52.4**	**26.3**	**0.9**
Sponge Roll, Chocolate, M&S*	¼ Cake/66g	251	12.1	380	3.9	50.5	18.4	1.8
Sponge with Butter Icing	**1 Slice/65g**	**318**	**19.9**	**490**	**4.5**	**52.4**	**30.6**	**0.6**
Sponge, Fatless	**1 Slice/53g**	**156**	**3.2**	**294**	**10.1**	**53**	**6.1**	**0.9**
Sponge, Fresh Cream & Strawberry, Asda*	1/12 Cake/60g	170	6	284	4.6	44	10	1.1
Sponge, Jam Filled	**1 Slice/65g**	**196**	**3.2**	**302**	**4.2**	**64.2**	**4.9**	**1.8**
St. Clements, Finest, Tesco*	1 Serving/49g	194	10.5	395	3.1	47.2	21.5	0.4
Stem Ginger, Loaf , Waitrose*	1 Slice/35g	134	4.8	384	3.7	60.1	13.7	2.6
Stem Ginger, Mrs Crimble's*	1 Slice/48g	158	1.1	329	2.7	73.3	2.2	2.7
Sticky Golden Lemon, Pudding, McVitie's*	1 Slice/25g	91	2.5	358	3.6	63.8	10	1.8
Stollen, Bites, Finest, Tesco*	1 Bite/17g	68	3.2	398	5	50.9	18.8	4.4
Stollen, Bites, Waitrose*	1 Bite/18g	71	3.1	395	4.6	54.5	17.1	2.2
Stollen, Chocolate & Rum, Finest, Tesco*	1/8 Cake/68g	262	9.5	381	5.3	57	13.8	3.9
Stollen, Kuchenmeister*	1 Serving/80g	357	16	446	5	61.2	20	2.5
Stollen, Marzipan Butter, Mini, Favorina, Lidl*	1 Stollen/18g	81	4.2	452	9.5	49.2	23.3	0
Stollen, Marzipan, Marzipan, Finest, Favorina, Lidl*	1 Slice/50g	206	9.3	412	6.2	53.4	18.6	0
Stollen, Slices, Average	**1 Slice/42g**	**160**	**6.3**	**381**	**5.5**	**55.8**	**15**	**3.1**
Stollen, Slices, Finest, Tesco*	1 Slice/33g	130	5.8	394	5.2	52.5	17.6	2.5
Stollen, Slices, Waitrose*	1 Slices/35g	143	5.8	402	4.7	57.3	16.3	3.8
Strawberry Milkshake, Slices, Mr Kipling*	1 Slice/34g	139	5.5	402	3.3	61.1	16	0.6
Strawberry Sponge Roll, M&S*	1/6 Cake/49g	160	4.6	330	2.8	58	9.5	0.8
Sultana & Cherry, Tesco*	1 Cake/37g	124	4	334	4.7	54.4	10.8	2.5
Sultana Fingerellas, Mrs Crimble's*	2 Cakes/25g	102	4	410	5.7	80	16	1.8
Sultana, Apple & Cranberry, 99% Fat Free, Trimlyne*	1/6 Cake/66.6g	130	0.6	195	4.6	45.5	0.9	3.3
Sultana, Fair Trade, Co-Op*	1/8 Cake/45g	155	4	345	5	60	9	1
Summer Fruit Cream, GFY, Asda*	1 Serving/74g	165	3.6	223	3.6	41	4.9	2.5
Summer Strawberry Bakes, Go Ahead, McVitie's*	1 Bar/35g	128	2.8	367	2.7	75.1	8	1
Super Carrot, Graze*	1 Punnet/31g	102	4.9	330	4.1	46.5	15.7	3.5
Swiss Roll, Average	**1oz/28g**	**77**	**1.2**	**276**	**7.2**	**55.5**	**4.4**	**0.8**
Swiss Roll, Butter Cream, M&S*	1/6 Roll/46g	162	4.3	354	2.9	63.9	9.5	0.5
Swiss Roll, Chocolate Flavour, Value, Tesco*	1 Slice/20g	79	3.9	394	5.5	49.2	19.5	1.4
Swiss Roll, Chocolate, Individual	**1 Roll/26g**	**88**	**2.9**	**337**	**4.3**	**58.1**	**11.3**	**0**
Swiss Roll, Chocolate, Lyons*	1 Serving/50g	190	9.6	379	4.3	47	19.3	0.9

C

C

	Measure INFO/WEIGHT	per Measure KCAL	FAT	Nutrition Values per 100g / 100ml KCAL	PROT	CARB	FAT	FIBRE
CAKE								
Swiss Roll, Chocolate, M&S*	1 Serving/46g	168	11.1	365	4.6	32.6	24.2	1.2
Swiss Roll, Chocolate, Morrisons*	1/6 Roll/26g	103	4.9	401	4.4	56.4	18.9	3.1
Swiss Roll, Chocolate, Value, Tesco*	1 Serving/20g	81	3.7	404	5	54.1	18.7	2.1
Swiss Roll, Raspberry & Vanilla, Morrisons*	1 Serving/28g	98	2.7	350	4.2	61.8	9.5	0
Swiss Roll, Raspberry Jam, Mr Kipling*	1/6 Cake/52g	184	5.3	355	2.8	63	10.2	1
Swiss Roll, Raspberry, Average	*1 Slice/35g*	*107*	*1.2*	*305*	*3.8*	*64.8*	*3.5*	*0.6*
Swiss Roll, Raspberry, Lyons*	1 Roll/175g	485	2.4	277	5.2	60.6	1.4	0
Syrup & Ginger, Tesco*	1 Serving/32g	134	7	420	4.5	51.4	21.8	0.7
Tangy Lemon Trickle, M&S*	1 Slice/75g	281	14.1	375	4.7	47.4	18.8	1.1
Tea Loaf, Rowan Hill Bakery, Lidl*	1 Slice/50g	135	0.4	270	3.8	63.3	0.9	3.4
The Ultimate Carrot Passion, Entenmann's*	1 Slice/52g	210	12.6	403	4.6	42.4	24.3	1
Tiffin, Chocolate, Sainsbury's*	1 Cake/61g	184	11.6	301	2.7	29.8	19	1.3
Toffee & Pecan Slices, M&S*	1 Slice/36g	160	8.5	445	4.7	54	23.7	1.3
Toffee Apple, McVitie's*	1 Slice/29g	104	3.2	354	3.5	60.2	11	1.5
Toffee Flavour Slices, Low Fat, Weight Watchers*	1 Slice/27g	80	0.7	297	4.2	63.9	2.6	3.2
Toffee Fudge, Entenmann's*	1 Serving/65g	274	14.1	421	3.4	53	21.7	0.5
Toffee Temptation, Tesco*	1 Slice/67g	228	12.8	340	2.9	39.1	19.1	0.3
Toffee Terror Whirls, Mr Kipling*	1 Whirl/28g	141	7.9	509	3.9	58.3	28.7	1.2
Toffee, Iced, Tesco*	1 Serving/35g	132	5.2	376	3.3	57.2	14.9	1.6
Toffee, Slices, BGTY, Sainsbury's*	1 Slice/27g	88	0.7	327	4.3	71.7	2.5	1.8
Toffee, The Handmade Flapjack Company*	1 Cake/75g	346	18.8	462	5.1	54	25.1	0
Toffee, Thorntons*	1/6 Cake/70g	302	16.8	431	4.6	49.2	24	0.8
Trifle Bakewells, Mr Kipling*	1 Tart/45g	193	8	423	3.7	62.2	17.5	1.1
Triple Chocolate Roll, Cadbury*	1 Serving/40g	165	6.7	410	4.3	60.1	16.6	1.5
Turkish Delight, Fry's*	1 Cake/26g	96	2.8	371	4.5	62.4	10.8	0.5
Twinkie, Hostess*	1 Serving/77g	270	8.1	351	2.3	62.8	10.5	0
Vanilla & Chocolate, St Michel Biscuits*	1 Cake/25g	111	5.5	443	4.7	55	22	2.1
Vanilla Sponge, Fresh Cream, Sainsbury's*	1 Slice/50g	152	5.1	304	7.5	45.6	10.2	0.4
Victoria Fairy, Sainsbury's*	1 Cake/50g	218	10.8	436	3.7	56.1	21.5	1.3
Victoria Sandwich, Average	*1 Slice/68g*	*267*	*12.9*	*392*	*4.4*	*50.9*	*19*	*1*
Victoria Sandwich, Individual, M&S*	1 Pack/75g	299	13.1	399	3.6	55.8	17.5	1.8
Victoria Sponge, Free From, Finest, Tesco*	1 Slice/60g	234	9.7	389	3.3	57.4	16.1	0.8
Victoria Sponge, Fresh Cream, Value, Tesco*	1 Serving/50g	168	8.7	337	4.4	40.7	17.4	0.6
Victoria Sponge, Lemon, Co-Op*	1 Slice/42g	151	8	360	4	44	19	0.7
Victoria Sponge, Mini, Bobby's*	1 Cake/35g	164	9.6	469	4	51.3	27.5	0.2
Victoria Sponge, Mini, Mr Kipling*	1 Cake/36g	152	6.9	420	3.9	58.5	19	0.8
Victoria Sponge, Mini, Weight Watchers*	1 Cake/30g	103	2.5	343	5.7	57.2	8.3	8.4
Victoria, Sponge, TTD, Sainsbury's*	1 Slice/57g	229	11	401	5	51.8	19.3	1.4
Viennese Whirl, Average	*1 Cake/28g*	*131*	*6.9*	*467*	*4.1*	*56.7*	*24.8*	*1.1*
Viennese Whirl, Chocolate, Mr Kipling*	1 Whirl/27.7g	134	7.8	484	4.6	53.1	28	2.1
Viennese Whirl, Lemon, Mr Kipling*	1 Cake/28g	115	4.5	409	4.2	62.2	15.9	0.7
Viennese Whirl, Mr Kipling*	1 Cake/28g	145	8.5	514	3.8	56.2	30.2	1.3
Viennese, M&S*	1 Cake/51g	250	14.1	495	4.1	58.9	28	2.8
Walnut Layer, Somerfield*	¼ Cake/77.5g	295	15.5	381	6	45	20	0
Walnut, Sandwich, Sainsbury's*	1/8 Cake/48g	182	8.3	379	5.4	53.8	17.3	1.3
Wedding, Rich Fruit, with Cognac, Iced, Sainsbury's*	1 Slice/55g	212	5.5	385	3.8	68.9	10	2
Welsh, Average	*1oz/28g*	*121*	*5.5*	*431*	*5.6*	*61.8*	*19.6*	*1.5*
Yorkshire Parkin, Bakers Delight*	1oz/28g	111	4.1	395	5.1	60.3	14.8	1.5
CAKE BAR								
Blueberry, Trimlyne*	1 Cake/50g	142	1.1	283	3.9	64	2.2	2.2
Boost, Cadbury*	1 Bar/40g	190	10.8	475	5.3	52.8	26.9	1.1
Caramel, Tesco*	1 Cake/26g	103	4.9	395	5.1	50.8	19	8.2
Carrot, Tesco*	1 Bar/68g	239	12.6	351	4.7	41.4	18.5	2.4

	Measure INFO/WEIGHT	per Measure KCAL	FAT	Nutrition Values per 100g / 100ml KCAL	PROT	CARB	FAT	FIBRE
CAKE BAR								
Chocolate & Orange, Go Ahead, McVitie's*	1 Cake/33g	109	2	330	4.3	64.9	6	1
Chocolate Chip, Average	*1 Cake/28g*	*428*	*21.6*	*428*	*6.3*	*51.9*	*21.6*	*1.6*
Chocolate Chip, HL, Tesco*	1 Serving/37g	109	1	295	4.8	63.6	2.6	0.6
Chocolate Chip, Mr Kipling*	1 Bar/32g	151	8.4	472	5.3	53.5	26.3	1.2
Chocolate Chip, Sainsbury's*	1 Cake/25g	108	5.6	430	6.1	51.2	22.3	0.6
Chocolate Chip, Tesco*	1 Cake/30g	124	5.9	415	7	51.4	19.7	2.3
Chocolate Chip, Value, Tesco*	1 Cake/28g	115	5.5	410	6.3	52.2	19.5	1.7
Chocolate Dream, Go Ahead, McVitie's*	1 Bar/36g	141	4.8	391	4.6	63.2	13.4	0.9
Chocolate, Average	*1 Cake/28g*	*125*	*6.2*	*446*	*5.6*	*56.3*	*22.1*	*1.9*
Chocolate, High Lights, Cadbury*	1 Bar/25g	95	3.5	380	5.5	58.8	14	1.1
Chocolate, Snack Cakes, Penguin, McVitie's*	1 Bar/24g	122	7.2	510	4.8	54.6	30.2	1.6
Chocolate, Squidgy, Minis, Soreen*	1 Cake/30g	99	1.8	330	9.2	59.5	6	3.4
Cinder Toffee, Cadbury*	1 Cake Bar/32g	149	8.4	465	4.2	53.4	26.2	0.9
Double Chocolate, Free From, Sainsbury's*	1 Cake/50g	196	7.9	391	4.2	58.2	15.7	1
Double Chocolate, Free From, Tesco*	1 Serving/45g	190	9.1	425	4.2	55.6	20.3	4.1
Flake, Cadbury*	1 Cake/25g	120	6.2	470	4.8	56.5	24.4	1.9
Fudge, Cadbury*	1 Pack/52g	220	9.2	420	5.7	60.3	17.6	0
Golden Syrup, McVitie's*	1 Cake/33g	127	4.8	385	3.6	60.2	14.4	1.2
Jaffa Cakes, Spooky, McVitie's*	1 Bar/25g	96	3.5	390	3.2	62.1	14.2	2.7
Jaffa, McVitie's*	1 Bar/25g	94	3.5	385	3.2	61.1	14.2	2.4
Jamaica Ginger, McVitie's*	1 Cake/33g	128	4.9	388	3.5	60.2	14.7	1.2
Lemon Meringue, Indulgence, Weight Watchers*	1 Bar/24g	21	0.3	86	1.1	7.1	1.3	0
Milk Chocolate & Orange, Crispy, Asda*	1 Bar/22g	91	2.2	413	4.8	75.6	10.2	2
Milk Chocolate Orange, Sandwich Bar, Lyons*	1 Bar/28g	142	8	516	5	62	29	0
Milk Chocolate, Cadbury*	1 Bar/35g	150	7.6	430	5.6	53.3	21.7	1.2
Milky Way, McVitie's*	1 Cake/26g	124	6.2	476	5.1	58.5	23.6	1.2
Rich Chocolate, Trimlyne*	1 Serving/40g	115	1.7	288	5.2	59.2	4.2	2.2
Toffee, Squidgy, Minis, Soreen*	1 Bar/30g	95	1.3	317	7.7	59.7	4.2	5.9
CAKE DECORATIONS								
Chocolate Chips, Plain, Bake Stable, Tesco*	1 Bag/100g	500	26.1	500	5.4	56.5	26.1	8.9
Sprinkles, Chocolate, Renshaw*	1 Serving/1g	4	0.1	438	2.4	79	12	0
CAKE MIX								
Carrot Cake, Betty Crocker*	¼ Pack/125g	504	8.4	403	5.8	78.9	6.7	1.4
Cheesecake, Original, Made Up, Asda*	1/6 Cake/85g	228	10.2	268	4.1	36	12	1.4
Cheesecake, Tesco*	1 Serving/76g	199	7.9	262	4.1	38	10.4	1.6
Sponge, Value, Tesco*	1 Slice/55g	181	4.8	329	4.6	57.9	8.8	1.4
Yellow, Super Moist, Betty Crocker*	1 Cake/128.0g	517	9.5	404	3.3	81.6	7.4	1.1
CALLALOO								
Leaves, Raw, Unprepared	*1 Cup/28g*	*6*	*0.1*	*23*	*2.5*	*4*	*0.3*	*0*
CALZONE								
Bolognese, Weight Watchers*	1 Calzone/88g	178	3	202	11.7	31.2	3.4	4.3
Cream Cheese & Pepperonata, Waitrose*	½ Pizza/165g	383	15.8	232	7	29.4	9.6	1.5
Ham & Gruyere, Asda*	1 Serving/280g	661	22.4	236	10	31	8	2.7
Ham & Mushroom, Waitrose*	½ Pizza/145g	362	13.5	250	10	31.6	9.3	1.6
Speciale, Ristorante, Dr Oetker*	½ Pizza/145g	381	20.3	263	11	23	14	0
Three Cheese, Waitrose*	1 Pizza/265g	747	31.8	282	10.4	33	12	1.4
Vegan, Laura's Idea*	1 Calzone/270g	394	17.3	146	3.3	13.8	6.4	2.3
CANAPES								
Aegean Tomato, Finest, Tesco*	1 Canape/15g	45	2.2	300	7.2	34.3	14.7	2.1
Caponata, Puff Pastry, Occasions, Sainsbury's*	1 Square/12g	30	1.9	249	4.1	22.9	15.7	2.1
Salmon & Dill, Finest, Tesco*	1 Canape/15g	47	2.4	315	9.2	32.7	16.1	1.9
Smoked Salmon, Youngs*	1 Canape/10g	21	1.5	210	15.9	2	15.2	0.7

C

	Measure INFO/WEIGHT	per Measure KCAL	FAT	Nutrition Values per 100g / 100ml KCAL	PROT	CARB	FAT	FIBRE
CANNELLONI								
Beef & Red Wine, Waitrose*	½ Pack/170g	355	16	209	17.5	13.8	9.4	1
Beef, As Prepared, Waitrose*	1 Pack/360g	501	26.7	139	6.2	11.5	7.4	1
Beef, Great Value, Asda*	1 Pack/400g	384	10.8	96	6	12	2.7	1.6
Beef, Italian, Sainsbury's*	1 Pack/400g	498	26.2	124	5.9	10.5	6.6	1.6
Beef, Italian, Tesco*	1 Pack/400g	520	26.8	130	5.3	11.6	6.7	0.9
Beef, Ready Meal	**1 Serving/335g**	**501**	**21.8**	**149**	**8.4**	**14.1**	**6.5**	**1.4**
Butternut Squash, with Spinach & Goats' Cheese, Tesco*	1 Pack/350g	490	29.4	140	5.1	10.7	8.4	1.9
Chicken, & Pesto, Italian, Sainsbury's*	1 Pack/450g	675	33.8	150	6.1	14.4	7.5	1.1
Mushroom, Italian, Sainsbury's*	1 Pack/450g	598	31	133	5.2	12.5	6.9	0.5
Salmon, & Spinach, Smoked, Sainsbury's*	1 Pack/450g	598	27.9	133	5.7	13.5	6.2	0.4
Spinach, & Cheese, Finest, Tesco*	1 Pack/350g	532	31.8	152	5.4	12.1	9.1	1.5
Spinach, & Ricotta, Charlie Bigham's*	½ Pack/330g	489	30.4	148	5.9	10.5	9.2	0.7
Spinach, & Ricotta, Fresh, Ready Meal, Average	**1 Serving/300g**	**393**	**22**	**131**	**5**	**10.8**	**7.4**	**1.2**
Spinach, & Ricotta, Italian Style, Co-Op*	1 Pack/450g	540	27	120	5	12	6	2
Spinach, & Ricotta, Low Fat, COU, M&S*	1 Pack/400g	340	7.6	85	4.8	11.4	1.9	1.7
Spinach, & Ricotta, Ready Meal, Average	**1 Serving/300g**	**426**	**22**	**142**	**5.6**	**13.3**	**7.3**	**1.4**
Spinach, & Ricotta, Sainsbury's*	1 Pack/400g	520	27.2	130	4.9	11.6	6.8	1.4
Spinach, & Wild Mushroom, Linda McCartney*	1 Pack/340g	381	13.6	112	4.9	14.1	4	1.7
Tubes, Dry, Average	**1oz/28g**	**101**	**1**	**361**	**12.5**	**69.1**	**3.6**	**1.2**
Vegetable, Mediterranean, Waitrose*	1 Serving/170g	330	15.3	194	9.7	18.7	9	1.9
Vegetarian, Tesco*	1 Pack/400g	552	34.4	138	5.3	9.8	8.6	1.5
CAPERS								
Caperberries, Spanish, Waitrose*	1 Serving/55g	9	0.3	17	1.1	2.1	0.5	2.5
in Vinegar, Average	**1 Tsp/5g**	**2**	**0**	**34**	**1.7**	**3**	**0.6**	**0**
CAPPELLETTI								
Goats Cheese & Red Pesto, Waitrose*	½ Pack/125g	374	10.9	299	11.6	43.5	8.7	2.2
Meat, Italian, Somerfield*	½ Pack/125g	331	7.9	265	13.6	38.5	6.3	2.4
Parma Ham, Fresh, Waitrose*	½ Pack/125g	368	11.5	294	14.1	38.6	9.2	2.2
CAPRI SUN								
Orange	**1 Pouch/200ml**	**90**	**0**	**45**	**0**	**11**	**0**	**0**
Orange, 100%, Juice	**1 Pouch/200ml**	**75**	**0**	**38**	**0.5**	**9.2**	**0**	**0.1**
CARAMAC								
Nestle*	1 Bar/30g	174	11	571	5.9	55.5	36.1	0
CARAMBOLA								
Average	**1oz/28g**	**9**	**0.1**	**31**	**0.5**	**7.1**	**0.3**	**1.3**
CARAWAY								
Seeds, Schwartz*	1 Pack/38g	170	8.1	448	23.3	40.9	21.2	0
CARBONARA								
Chicken, & Asparagus, Spaghetti, Sainsbury's*	1 Pack/450g	657	27.4	146	6.6	16.2	6.1	1.1
Chicken, & Bacon, Balanced for You, M&S*	1 Pack/375g	484	10.5	129	10.7	14.7	2.8	1.1
Chicken, Mushroom, & Ham, Spaghetti, Asda*	1 Pack/700g	686	14	98	10	10	2	1.5
Mushroom, Spaghetti, Everdine*	1 Serving/450g	369	13.5	82	3.6	8.1	3	4.1
Pasta, Diet Chef Ltd*	1 Pack/300g	243	10.8	81	3.5	8.6	3.6	0.1
Pasta, GFY, Asda*	½ Pack/174g	240	4.7	138	5.2	23.1	2.7	1.5
Pasta, Pasta Vita, Dolmio*	1 Pack/270g	322	10.3	119	3.8	17.1	3.8	0.7
Rigatoni, Tesco*	1 Serving/205g	236	11.9	115	5.2	10.6	5.8	1.2
Spaghetti, 887, Oakhouse Foods Ltd*	1 Serving/400g	800	47.6	200	8.2	14.5	11.9	0.8
Spaghetti, COU, M&S*	1 Pack/330g	346	7.2	105	6.1	15.7	2.2	0.8
Spaghetti, Creamy, Mini Meals, Heinz*	1 Sm Can/200g	130	2.7	65	3.8	9	1.4	0.6
Spaghetti, GFY, Asda*	1 Pack/400g	406	7.6	102	5.5	15.3	1.9	0.7
Spaghetti, Heated, HL, Tesco*	1 Pack/365g	372	5.1	102	6	16	1.4	0.8
Spaghetti, Italian Quisine, Microwaved, Aldi*	1 Pack/400g	669	33.4	174	7.1	16	8.7	1.5
Spaghetti, Italian, Chilled, Sainsbury's*	1 Pack/400g	492	15.6	123	5.5	16.1	3.9	1.4

INFO/WEIGHT	Measure	per Measure		Nutrition Values per 100g / 100ml				
		KCAL	FAT	KCAL	PROT	CARB	FAT	FIBRE
CARBONARA								
Spaghetti, Italian, Fresh, Chilled, Tesco*	1 Pack/430g	606	26.2	141	7.6	13.9	6.1	1.3
Spaghetti, Italian, Tesco*	1 Pack/450g	608	26.6	135	5.4	14.1	5.9	0.6
Spaghetti, LC, Tesco*	1 Pack/400g	460	9.6	115	6.9	15.7	2.4	1.2
Spaghetti, M&S*	1 Pack/400g	660	36	165	6.5	14.2	9	0.6
Spaghetti, M&S*	1 Pack/400g	560	27.2	140	5.2	14	6.8	0.9
Spaghetti, Ready Meal, Average	*1 Pack/400g*	*524*	*21.5*	*131*	*5.9*	*14.4*	*5.4*	*1.1*
Tagliatelle, Italiano, Tesco*	1 Serving/325g	757	37.4	233	8.6	23.8	11.5	1.2
Tagliatelle, Naturally Less 5% Fat, Asda*	1 Pack/400g	440	9.6	110	4.2	18	2.4	0.8
Tagliatelle, PB, Waitrose*	1 Pack/350g	357	12.6	102	5.3	12.1	3.6	0.7
Tagliatelle, Ready Meal, Average	*1 Serving/400g*	*460*	*13.4*	*115*	*5.5*	*15.8*	*3.3*	*1*
Tagliatelle, TTD, Sainsbury's*	1 Pack/405g	644	25.9	159	7.8	17.6	6.4	1.6
Tortelloni, Sainsbury's*	½ Pack/210g	405	12.6	193	8.4	26.3	6	2.2
CARDAMOM								
Black, Ground, Average	*1 Tsp/2g*	*6*	*0.1*	*311*	*10.8*	*68.5*	*6.7*	*28*
CAROB POWDER								
Average	*1 Tsp/2g*	*3*	*0*	*159*	*4.9*	*37*	*0.1*	*0*
CARP								
Fillet, Raw, Average	*1 Fillet/218g*	*244*	*10.2*	*112*	*17.5*	*0*	*4.7*	*0*
CARROT & SWEDE								
Diced, for Mashing, Average	*½ Pack/250g*	*58*	*0.7*	*23*	*0.6*	*4.7*	*0.3*	*1.9*
Mash, From Supermarket, Average	*1 Serving/150g*	*138*	*7.5*	*92*	*1.3*	*10.4*	*5*	*1.3*
Mash, Healthy Range, Average	*1 Serving/150g*	*98*	*4.2*	*66*	*1.3*	*8.6*	*2.8*	*2.1*
CARROTS								
& Cauliflower, M&S*	1 Serving/335g	74	1.3	22	0.6	4.4	0.4	2.3
& Peas, Sainsbury's*	1 Serving/200g	100	1	50	3.3	8.3	0.5	3.8
& Houmous Dip, Tesco*	1 Pack/120g	96	4.9	80	1.9	7.1	4.1	3.6
& Swede, Crush, Sainsbury's*	¼ Pack/150g	126	9	84	1.7	4.9	6	1.6
Baby with Fine Beans, Tesco*	1 Pack/200g	58	1	29	1.3	4.7	0.5	2.3
Baby, Canned, Average	*1 Can/195g*	*40*	*0.5*	*21*	*0.5*	*4.2*	*0.3*	*2.1*
Baby, Fresh, Average	*1 Serving/80g*	*28*	*0.1*	*35*	*0.6*	*8.2*	*0.1*	*2.9*
Batons & Sliced Runner Beans, Sainsbury's*	1 Serving/200g	40	1	20	1	3.2	0.5	3.2
Batons, Fresh, Average	*½ Pack/150g*	*41*	*0.4*	*28*	*0.6*	*5.7*	*0.3*	*2.6*
Boiled, Average	*1oz/28g*	*6*	*0.1*	*22*	*0.6*	*4.4*	*0.4*	*2.3*
Canned, Average	*1oz/28g*	*6*	*0.1*	*20*	*0.5*	*4*	*0.2*	*1.9*
Chantenay, Frozen, Morrisons*	1 Serving /80g	28	0.3	35	0.4	6.7	0.4	3.2
Chantenay, Steamer, Sainsbury's*	½ Pack/125g	60	2.1	48	0.5	7.7	1.7	2.2
Chantenay, Wood Farm, Raw, Aldi*	1 Serving/80g	34	0.4	42	0.6	7.9	0.5	2.4
Raw, Scrubbed, Average	*1 Serving/80g*	*24*	*0.4*	*30*	*0.7*	*6*	*0.5*	*2.4*
Roasting, with Honey & Ginger Glaze, Aunt Bessie's*	1 Serving/133g	80	4.1	60	0.7	6.1	3.1	2.5
Sliced, Canned, Average	*1 Serving/180g*	*36*	*0.2*	*20*	*0.7*	*4.1*	*0.1*	*1.5*
Sliced, Fresh, Average	*1 Serving/60g*	*17*	*0.2*	*28*	*0.7*	*5.7*	*0.3*	*2*
Whole, Raw, Peeled, Average	*1 Carrot/75g*	*21*	*0.2*	*29*	*0.6*	*6.4*	*0.3*	*2.2*
with Parsley & English Butter, M&S*	½ Pack/100g	65	3.9	65	0.6	7.1	3.9	2.4
CASHEW NUTS								
BBQ, Graze*	1 Pack/26g	142	10.8	546	13.9	37	41.7	0
Ca-shew! Bless You, Graze*	1 Punnet/40g	146	5.8	365	6.1	57.2	14.5	0
Caramel, Sesame Coated, , Eat Real*	1 Serving/25g	149	8.8	531	13.3	51.1	31.4	4
Cheese Flavour, Graze*	1 Pack/26g	140	10.8	540	15.3	35.7	41.5	0
Chili, Holland & Barrett*	1 Bag/250g	1450	118.8	580	19.4	20.1	47.5	3.5
Cracking Black Pepper, Graze*	1 Punnet/36g	216	16.6	600	19	26	46	4
Honey Glazed, Itsu*	1 Pack/30g	167	10.4	557	13.6	46.3	34.8	2.3
Honey, Graze*	½ Pack/13g	67	4.2	516	10.5	53	32.2	0
Hot Chilli, Graze*	1 Box/26g	139	10.9	535	14.5	33.6	41.8	0

	Measure INFO/WEIGHT	per Measure KCAL	FAT	Nutrition Values per 100g / 100ml KCAL	PROT	CARB	FAT	FIBRE
CASHEW NUTS								
Hot Chilli, Graze*	1 Pack/26g	139	10.9	535	14.5	33.6	41.8	0
Mexican Chilli, Graze*	1 Pack/26g	140	10.8	539	14.3	34.9	41.6	0
Plain, Average	*½ Pack/25g*	*146*	*12.2*	*584*	*15.7*	*18.8*	*48.9*	*3.4*
Roasted & Salted, Average	*1 Serving/50g*	*306*	*25.6*	*612*	*18.8*	*19.6*	*51.1*	*3.1*
Salt & Pepper, Morrisons*	1 Pack/100g	595	46.3	595	20.9	20.4	46.3	6.6
Wasabi, Roasted, Vitasia, Lidl*	1 Serving/30g	185	14.6	616	17.5	25.6	48.6	0
CASSAVA								
Baked, Average	*1oz/28g*	*43*	*0.1*	*155*	*0.7*	*40.1*	*0.2*	*1.7*
Boiled in Unsalted Water, Average	*1oz/28g*	*36*	*0.1*	*130*	*0.5*	*33.5*	*0.2*	*1.4*
Gari, Average	*1oz/28g*	*100*	*0.1*	*358*	*1.3*	*92.9*	*0.5*	*0*
CASSEROLE								
Bean & Lentil, Morrisons*	1 Can/410g	287	1.6	70	4.1	12.5	0.4	0
Bean Cassoulet, Organic, Free & Easy*	1 Tin/400g	256	1.2	64	3.4	11.9	0.3	2.3
Bean, Spicy, BGTY, Sainsbury's*	1 Pack/300g	171	2.7	57	3	9.1	0.9	4.2
Beef	*1 Serving/336g*	*490*	*23*	*146*	*16.3*	*4.6*	*6.8*	*0.6*
Beef, & Ale with Dumplings, Sainsbury's*	1 Pack/450g	711	32.8	158	7.7	15.4	7.3	0.6
Beef, & Ale with Mashed Potato, HL, Tesco*	1 Pack/450g	364	11.2	81	5.1	10.9	2.5	0.6
Beef, & Ale, Finest, Tesco*	½ Pack/300g	234	4.2	78	11.5	5	1.4	1.1
Beef, & Dumplings, M Kitchen, Morrisons*	1 Pack/450g	596	28	132	7.3	11	6.2	1.7
Beef, & Dumplings, Minced, Smart Price, Asda*	1 Pack/299g	320	12.6	107	4.5	12.7	4.2	2.3
Beef, & Kidney, 153, Oakhouse Foods Ltd*	1 Meal/400g	384	16.8	96	6.7	7.2	4.2	0.7
Beef, & Red Wine, BGTY, Sainsbury's*	1 Pack/300g	192	1.8	64	8	6.7	0.6	0.9
Beef, & Red Wine, Fuller Longer, M&S*	1 Pack/420g	355	11.7	85	7.2	6.9	2.8	1.7
Beef, & Red Wine, Weight Watchers*	1 Pack/330g	254	9.2	77	4.3	8.6	2.8	0.3
Beef, & Ale, Average	*1 Serving/300g*	*251*	*6.8*	*84*	*9.4*	*6.5*	*2.2*	*1.3*
Beef, & Dumplings, Heated, Free From, Tesco*	1 Pack/413g	472	14.1	114	5.5	14.9	3.4	1.1
Beef, & Parsnip Mash, Ovenbaked, Slimzone, Asda*	1 Pack/487g	336	6.3	69	7.4	6.1	1.3	1.8
Beef, & Red Wine, Average	*1 Serving/350g*	*290*	*7.3*	*83*	*7.2*	*8.2*	*2.1*	*1.5*
Beef, Diet Chef Ltd*	1 Pack/300g	177	3	59	7.8	4.7	1	2.4
Beef, Meal for One, Tesco*	1 Pack/450g	425	18.9	94	3.6	10.6	4.2	1.7
Beef, Mini Favourites, M&S*	1 Pack/200g	210	8.4	105	7.1	9.3	4.2	1.4
Beef, with Dumplings, GFY, Asda*	1 Pack/400g	416	8.8	104	11	10	2.2	0.9
Beef, with Dumplings, Ready Meal, Average	*1 Serving/350g*	*464*	*21.1*	*132*	*9.5*	*10.1*	*6*	*1.5*
Beef, with Herb Potatoes, Ready Meal, Average	*1 Serving/475g*	*504*	*17.1*	*106*	*6.8*	*11.5*	*3.6*	*1.6*
Beef, with Herb Potatoes, Tesco*	1 Serving/475g	504	17.1	106	6.8	11.5	3.6	1.6
Chicken, & Asparagus in White Wine, Finest, Tesco*	1 Pack/350g	683	42.4	195	10	11.6	12.1	0.3
Chicken, & Asparagus in White Wine, Tesco*	½ Pack/300g	444	23.7	148	11.5	7.7	7.9	0.8
Chicken, & Asparagus, HL, Tesco*	1 Serving/450g	342	10.3	76	6.3	8.3	2.3	0.5
Chicken, & Dumpling, 548, Wiltshire Farm Foods*	1 Serving/440g	485	22.5	110	5.2	11	5.1	0.8
Chicken, & Dumplings, Sainsbury's*	1 Serving/450g	612	32.4	136	6.8	11	7.2	0.6
Chicken, & Red Wine, Duchy Originals*	½ Pack/175g	187	7.5	107	14	5.1	4.3	1.6
Chicken, & Tomato, Asda*	¼ Pack/273g	569	41	208	16	2.2	15	0.5
Chicken, & Vegetable, Apetito*	1 Pack/330g	286	9.9	87	6.3	9.4	3	1.6
Chicken, & Vegetable, Hearty, 142, Wiltshire Farm Foods*	1 Serving/510g	338	7.2	66	5.7	7	1.4	0
Chicken, & Vegetable, Long Life, Sainsbury's*	1 Pack/300g	186	4.5	62	4.6	7.4	1.5	0.8
Chicken, & Vegetable, Ready Meal, Healthy Range	*1 Serving/330g*	*265*	*11.9*	*80*	*4.7*	*7.6*	*3.6*	*1.1*
Chicken, & White Wine, BGTY, Sainsbury's*	1 Serving/300g	216	6.6	72	7.2	5.9	2.2	1.3
Chicken, & White Wine, Ready Meal, Healthy Range	*1 Serving/300g*	*234*	*7.4*	*78*	*7.7*	*6.3*	*2.4*	*1.2*
Chicken, Classic, Pack, Ashfield Farm, Aldi*	1/3 Pack/333g	659	36.6	198	21	3.2	11	1.3
Chicken, Leek & Mushroom, Tesco*	1 Pack/350g	382	22	109	4.5	8.6	6.3	1
Chicken, Mediterranean, Tesco*	1 Pack/400g	260	9.2	65	6.7	4.5	2.3	0.9
Chicken, PB, Waitrose*	1 Pack/400g	392	14.4	98	6.6	9.8	3.6	1.2
Chicken, with Dumplings, M&S*	½ Pack/227g	261	10	115	9.7	9	4.4	0.9

INFO/WEIGHT	Measure	per Measure		Nutrition Values per 100g / 100ml				
		KCAL	FAT	KCAL	PROT	CARB	FAT	FIBRE

CASSEROLE

	Measure INFO/WEIGHT	KCAL	FAT	KCAL	PROT	CARB	FAT	FIBRE
Chicken, You Count, Love Life, Waitrose*	1 Pack/400g	297	4.8	74	7.4	7.9	1.2	1.2
Cowboy, Iceland*	1 Pack/400g	500	26	125	5.8	10.9	6.5	1.7
Fish, Mediterranean, 612, Apetito*	1 Pack/420g	336	8	80	4.9	8.8	1.9	0
Ham Hock & Mash, Tesco*	1 Pack/250g	225	8	90	6.1	9	3.2	0.8
Lamb, & Rosemary, Eat Well, M&S*	1 Pack/380g	325	11	86	7.6	7	2.9	2.2
Lamb, Braised, British Classics, Tesco*	1 Pack/350g	332	18.2	95	7.5	4.6	5.2	1.2
Lamb, COU, M&S*	1 Pack/390g	254	6.6	65	5.9	6.7	1.7	1.6
Lamb, Ready Meal, Healthy Range, Average	*1 Serving/300g*	*273*	*9.9*	*91*	*10.5*	*4.9*	*3.3*	*1*
Lamb, with Dumplings, & Vegetables, Minced, M&S*	1 Pack/200g	260	12.8	130	7	11.6	6.4	1.2
Lamb, with Mint Dumplings, Minced, Sainsbury's*	1 Pack/450g	558	30.6	124	5.4	10.4	6.8	1.1
Pork, & Leek, Sausage, 387, Wiltshire Farm Foods*	1 Serving/280g	307	17.3	110	4.6	7.8	6.2	1
Pork, Normandy Style, Finest, Tesco*	1 Pack/450g	405	21.6	90	7.6	4.1	4.8	2.3
Rabbit, Average	*1oz/28g*	*29*	*1.4*	*102*	*11.6*	*2.6*	*5.1*	*0.4*
Red Lentil & Mixed Bean, Cook*	1 Portion/290g	258	7	89	4.7	12.1	2.4	3.9
Sausage, & Potato, M&S*	1 Serving/200g	190	11.8	95	3.3	7.5	5.9	0.9
Sausage, 154, Oakhouse Foods Ltd*	1 Meal/400g	484	28	121	4.8	10	7	0.7
Sausage, CBY, Asda*	1 Pot/400g	240	15.2	60	3.6	1.9	3.8	2.1
Sausage, Pork, Diet Chef Ltd*	1 Pack/300g	303	18.3	101	6.6	4.9	6.1	1.4
Seafood, Mediterranean, HL, Tesco*	1 Pack/344g	292	6.9	85	5.8	10.5	2	3.2
Steak, & Kidney, Mini, Favourites, M&S*	1 Pack/200g	240	10.8	120	7.9	9.5	5.4	1.5
Steak, & Mushroom, 214, Wiltshire Farm Foods*	1 Pack/360g	322	16.2	89	5	7.2	4.5	1.3
Steak, & Mushroom, 305, Wiltshire Farm Foods*	1 Serving/410g	328	9	80	5	8	2.2	1.4
Steak, & Mushroom, Asda*	½ Pack/304g	411	30.4	135	7	4.2	10	0.3
Steak, & Ale, Average	*1 Serving/275g*	*324*	*14.4*	*118*	*9*	*8.8*	*5.2*	*1*
Steak, & Mushroom, Average	*1 Serving/275g*	*274*	*15.5*	*100*	*6.2*	*6*	*5.6*	*1*
Vegetable, & Lentil, Canned, Granose*	1 Can/400g	272	8	68	3.5	9	2	3
Vegetable, Tesco*	1 Serving/220g	66	0.7	30	0.8	6.1	0.3	1.5
Venison, Scottish Wild, & Beaujolais, Tesco*	1 Pack/425g	366	8.9	86	11.9	4.9	2.1	0.6

CASSEROLE MIX

	Measure INFO/WEIGHT	KCAL	FAT	KCAL	PROT	CARB	FAT	FIBRE
Bean, As Sold, Growers Selection, Asda*	1 Pack/600g	540	18	90	3.8	10	3	3.6
Beef & Ale, Colman's*	1 Pack/45g	144	0.9	320	9.2	66.3	2	2.3
Beef, Colman's*	1 Pack/40g	123	0.6	308	7.5	66	1.5	2.5
Beef, Recipe, Colman's*	1 Pack/42g	142	0.5	338	9.1	13.1	1.1	4
Beef, Recipe, Schwartz*	1 Pack/43g	123	0.9	287	7	56.6	2.1	6.6
Chicken Chasseur, Asda*	1 Pack/80g	273	0.8	341	9	74	1	1.4
Chicken, Authentic, Schwartz*	1 Pack/36g	131	1.5	363	10.4	70.7	4.3	2
Chicken, Recipe, As Sold, Colman's*	1 Pack/40g	131	1	328	6.2	68.2	2.6	3.1
Chicken, Traditional, Colman's*	1 Pack/40g	124	0.5	311	5.7	69.4	1.3	1.5
Farmhouse Sausage, Schwartz*	1 Pack/39g	124	1.1	317	8.1	64.6	2.9	0.5
Honey Chicken, Colman's*	1 Pack/50g	128	0.6	257	3.4	58.3	1.1	1.8
Lamb, Authentic, Schwartz*	1 Pack/35g	116	1.2	332	7.7	68	3.3	1.3
Moroccan Lamb, As Sold, Schwartz*	1 Pack/35g	114	0.9	327	5.5	67.4	2.6	5.8
Peppered Beef, Schwartz*	1 Pack/40g	129	2	323	7	62.9	4.9	7.3
Pork, As Sold, Colman's*	1 Pack/38g	125	0.8	330	8	68	2	5
Sausage, As Sold, Colman's*	1 Pack/39g	136	1	350	10	70	2.5	6
Sausage, Asda*	¼ Pack/25g	80	1	321	6	65	4.1	3
Sausage, Classic, Schwartz*	1 Pack/35g	96	0.9	275	12.4	50.1	2.7	14.9
Somerset Pork, Colman's*	1 Pack/45g	144	0.6	321	7.1	70.2	1.3	2.2
Somerset Pork, Schwartz*	1 Pack/36g	115	1.4	320	9.4	61.9	3.8	7.7
Spicy Chicken, Colman's*	1 Pack/45g	151	0.8	336	6.5	73.4	1.8	1.5
Turkey, Colman's*	1 Pack/50g	156	1	313	5.9	68	1.9	3.5

CASSOULET

	Measure INFO/WEIGHT	KCAL	FAT	KCAL	PROT	CARB	FAT	FIBRE
Lamb, & Spinach, High in Protein, Asda*	1 Pack/400g	340	10.4	85	7.2	4	2.6	4.5

	Measure INFO/WEIGHT	per Measure KCAL	FAT	Nutrition Values per 100g / 100ml KCAL	PROT	CARB	FAT	FIBRE
CATFISH								
Cooked, Steamed, Weighed with Bone, Average	*1 Serving/100g*	*101*	*3.1*	*101*	*18.2*	*0*	*3.1*	*0.7*
Raw, Average	*1oz/28g*	*27*	*0.8*	*96*	*17.6*	*0*	*2.8*	*0*
CAULIFLOWER								
& Coconut, Spiced, Meal Pot, Co-Op*	1 Pot/275g	221	7.4	80	2.7	9.4	2.7	3.8
& Parsley, Rice, Natures Pick, Aldi*	1 Serving/80g	27	0.7	34	2.9	2.1	0.9	2.7
& Red Onion, Spiced, Quick Roast, M&S*	½ Pack/150g	63	0.9	42	2.2	5.8	0.6	2.3
Boiled, Average	*1 Serving/80g*	*22*	*0.7*	*28*	*2.9*	*2.1*	*0.9*	*1.6*
Cous Cous, Ready to Cook, As Sold, Morrisons*	1 Pack/330g	129	3	39	3.6	2.8	0.9	2.6
Raw, Average	*1 Serving/80g*	*25*	*0.7*	*31*	*3.2*	*2.7*	*0.8*	*1.6*
Spiced, Roasted, Tesco*	½ Pack/70g	59	4.4	84	2.2	3.9	6.2	1.8
Sprouting, Biancoli Spears, M&S*	1 Serving/80g	20	0.2	25	1.9	4.7	0.3	1.9
Steamed, Average	*1 Serving/100g*	*28*	*0.9*	*28*	*2.9*	*2.1*	*0.9*	*1.6*
CAULIFLOWER CHEESE								
& Bacon, Gastropub, M&S*	1 Pack/300g	318	21	106	6.3	4.5	7	1
& Broccoli, Sainsbury's*	1 Serving/130g	83	2.1	64	4.8	7.6	1.6	2.7
& Broccoli, Average	*1 Serving/200g*	*127*	*6.4*	*64*	*3.8*	*4.6*	*3.2*	*2*
Asda*	1 Pack/450g	486	36	108	4.6	4.3	8	1.5
Average	*1 Meal/400g*	*362*	*23.3*	*90*	*4.5*	*4.6*	*5.8*	*1.3*
Basics, Sainsbury's*	1 Pack/300g	180	12	60	3	3	4	1.6
BFY, Morrisons*	1 Pack/300g	231	12.3	77	4.5	5.4	4.1	1.2
Birds Eye*	1 Pack/330g	248	13.9	75	4	4.9	4.2	0.9
Budgens*	1 Pack/450g	284	18.9	63	5.3	4	4.2	1
Cook*	1 Pack/300g	333	11.1	111	6.1	12.7	3.7	1
Eat Smart, Morrisons*	1 Pack/300g	192	6	64	4.9	6.7	2	1.5
Florets in a Cheese Sauce, As Prepared, Sainsbury's*	1 Pack/200g	145	7.7	75	4.8	3.3	4	3.2
Fresh, Oven Heated, Tesco*	½ Pack/170g	158	8.2	93	5.7	6.2	4.8	1.1
Frozen, Iceland*	1 Serving/200g	190	12	95	4	5.5	6	1.6
Frozen, Tesco*	1 Pack/450g	428	30.2	95	4.2	4.3	6.7	1.3
Great Value, Asda*	1 Pack/396g	352	23.8	89	3.9	4.9	6	0.8
Grills, Grassington's Food Co*	1 Grill/92g	157	4.6	171	6.1	25.3	5	2.6
Grills, Meat Free, Tesco*	1 Grill/91.4g	160	7.4	175	5.3	20	8.1	2.9
Grills, Tesco*	1 Grill/92g	207	10.9	225	6.5	22.2	11.9	4
Heated, Finest, Tesco*	½ Pack/168g	209	13.8	124	5.7	6.4	8.2	1.4
Less Than 3% fat, BGTY, Sainsbury's*	½ Pack/200g	98	3.4	49	3.3	5.3	1.7	1
Loved by Us, Co-Op*	1 Serving/150g	120	7.4	80	3.7	4.5	4.9	1.4
M&S*	1 Serving/150g	150	9.2	100	5.5	5.9	6.1	1.1
Made with Half Fat Cheese, HL, Tesco*	1 Pack/500g	285	13	57	6.5	2	2.6	2.2
Made with Semi-Skimmed Milk	*1oz/28g*	*28*	*1.8*	*100*	*6*	*5.2*	*6.4*	*1.3*
Made with Skimmed Milk	*1oz/28g*	*27*	*1.7*	*97*	*6*	*5.2*	*6*	*1.3*
Made with Whole Milk	*1oz/28g*	*29*	*1.9*	*105*	*6*	*5.2*	*6.9*	*1.3*
Morrisons*	½ Pack/225g	200	14.6	89	3.3	4.4	6.5	1
Topped with Vegetarian Cheddar Cheese, Tesco*	½ Pack/175g	163	8.4	93	5.7	6.2	4.8	1.1
TTD, Sainsbury's*	½ Pack/186g	284	22.5	153	5.8	5.3	12.1	1
with Crispy Bacon, Finest, Tesco*	1/3 Pack/166g	211	14.1	127	6.5	6.1	8.5	0.4
with Wexford Mature Cheddar, M&S*	½ Pack/150g	176	11.7	117	6.7	4.3	7.8	1.3
CAVIAR								
Average	*1oz/28g*	*25*	*1.3*	*89*	*11.6*	*0.5*	*4.6*	*0*
CELERIAC								
Boiled in Salted Water, Average	*1oz/28g*	*5*	*0.1*	*18*	*0.9*	*1.9*	*0.4*	*3.2*
Raw, Average	*1 Serving/80g*	*17*	*0.3*	*21*	*1*	*1.9*	*0.4*	*3.2*
CELERY								
Boiled in Salted Water	*1 Serving/50g*	*4*	*0.2*	*8*	*0.5*	*0.8*	*0.3*	*1.2*
Raw, Trimmed, Average	1 Stalk/40g	3	0.1	7	0.5	0.9	0.2	1.1

	Measure INFO/WEIGHT	per Measure KCAL	FAT	Nutrition Values per 100g / 100ml KCAL	PROT	CARB	FAT	FIBRE
CHAMPAGNE								
Average	*1 Glass/125ml*	*95*	*0*	*76*	*0.3*	*1.4*	*0*	*0*
CHANNA MASALA								
Indian, Sainsbury's*	1 Serving/149g	165	7.3	111	4.2	12.4	4.9	3.3
M&S*	1 Pack/225g	360	23.7	160	5.6	11.2	10.5	8.2
Waitrose*	1 Pack/300g	300	18.3	100	3.7	7.4	6.1	7.9
CHAPATIS								
Brown Wheat Flour, Waitrose*	1 Chapati/42g	128	3.4	305	8.6	49.4	8	4.6
Elephant Atta*	1 Chapati/45g	129	2.9	287	7.5	53.1	6.4	3.2
Indian Style, Asda*	1 Chapati/43g	95	0.4	221	8	45	1	2.9
Made with Fat	*1 Chapati/60g*	*197*	*7.7*	*328*	*8.1*	*48.3*	*12.8*	*0*
Made without Fat	*1 Chapati/55g*	*111*	*0.6*	*202*	*7.3*	*43.7*	*1*	*0*
Morrisons*	1 Chapati/40g	108	2.8	269	8.6	49.8	6.9	0
Plain, Original, Wrap, Patak's*	1 Chapati/42g	115	3.2	273	9.4	48.8	7.5	0
Wholemeal, Patak's*	1 Chapati/42g	130	4	310	11.2	44.9	9.5	9
CHARD								
Average	*1 Serving/80g*	*15*	*0.2*	*19*	*1.4*	*3.3*	*0.2*	*0.8*
Silverbeet, Fresh, Steamed	*1 Serving/100g*	*15*	*0*	*15*	*1.9*	*1.3*	*0*	*3.3*
Swiss, Boiled in Unsalted Water	*1oz/28g*	*6*	*0*	*20*	*1.9*	*4.1*	*0.1*	*2.1*
Swiss, Raw	*1oz/28g*	*5*	*0.1*	*17*	*1.7*	*3.4*	*0.2*	*1.5*
CHEDDARS								
Baked, Mini, Cheese & Ham Flavour, McVitie's*	1 Bag/30g	160	8.9	534	11	55.5	29.8	2
Baked, Mini, Chilli Beef Flavour, Jacob's*	1 Pack/50g	262	15	522	9	52.2	29.9	2.7
Baked, Mini, Red Leicester, Jacob's*	1 Pack/25g	132	7.9	530	8.7	50.2	31.8	2.5
Baked, Mini, Stilton, Jacob's*	1 Pack/25g	132	7.9	530	8.8	50.3	31.8	2.5
Cheese, Baked, Mini, Original, Jacobs*	1 Bag/25g	128	7.3	512	10.6	50.1	29.2	2.5
McVitie's*	1 Cracker/4g	20	1.2	526	10.9	47.2	31.9	2.9
Mini, Average	*1 Bag/26g*	*134*	*7.8*	*516*	*11.2*	*50.8*	*29.9*	*2.4*
Smokey BBQ, McVitie's*	1 Sm Pack/30g	155	8.9	516	9.3	52.8	29.8	2.6
CHEESE								
Appenzeller, Extra, Strength 6, Waitrose*	1 Serving/30g	126	9.6	420	32	1	32	0
Appenzeller, Swiss, TTD, Sainsbury's*	1 Serving/30g	116	9.5	386	25.4	0	31.6	0
Babybel, Cheddar Variety, Mini, Fromageries Bel*	1 Cheese/20g	75	6.2	375	24	0	31	0
Babybel, Emmental, Fromageries Bel*	1 Serving/20g	63	4.9	316	23	1	24.5	0
Babybel, Goat's Variety, Mini, Fromageries Bel*	1 Cheese/20g	65	5.4	327	21	0	27	0
Babybel, Gouda Variety, Mini, Fromageries Bel*	1 Cheese/20g	68	5.6	340	22	0	28	0
Babybel, Light, Mini, Fromageries Bel*	1 Babybel/20g	42	2.4	208	25	0	12	0
Babybel, Original, Mini, Fromageries Bel*	1 Cheese/20g	61	4.8	304	22	0.1	24	0
Bavarian, Smoked with Ham, Sainsbury's*	1 Serving/30g	89	7.2	298	19.4	0.8	24.1	0
Bavarian, Smoked, Slices, Asda*	1 Slice/18g	50	4.1	277	17	0.4	23	0
Berthaut's, Epoisses, Strength 6, 1, Waitrose*	1 Serving/30g	86	7.2	285	17	1	23.7	0
Bites, Quattro Formaggi, Specially Selected, Aldi*	½ Pack/35g	185	10.5	528	20	44	30	3.1
Bleu D' Auvergne, Sainsbury's*	1 Serving/25g	84	6.6	335	22	2	26.5	0
Blue D'affinois, Waitrose*	1 Serving/30g	126	12.3	421	12	1	41	0
Blue, Castello, Soft, Castello*	¼ Pack/37.5g	162	15.6	432	14	0.5	41.5	0
Blue, French, CBY, Asda*	1 Serving/30g	90	7.4	301	20	0	24.5	0
Blue, Saint Agur*	1 Serving /30g	109	9.9	363	16	0.2	33	0
Blue, Savers, Morrisons*	1 Portion/30g	99	8.1	331	22	0.1	27	0
Blue, Sliced for Burger, Castello*	1 Slice/25g	100	9.2	400	17	0.5	37	0
Brie, Average	*1 Serving/25g*	*74*	*6*	*296*	*19.7*	*0.3*	*24*	*0*
Brie, Breaded, Bites, Frozen, Tesco*	1 Bite/17g	54	3.4	319	8.6	24.2	20.2	2.8
Brie, Reduced Fat, Average	*1 Serving/50g*	*99*	*5.7*	*198*	*23*	*0.8*	*11.4*	*0*
Caerphilly, Average	*1 Serving/50g*	*187*	*15.6*	*374*	*23*	*0.1*	*31.3*	*0*
Cambazola, Tesco*	1 Serving/30g	128	12.3	425	13.5	0.5	41	0

	Measure INFO/WEIGHT	per Measure KCAL	FAT	Nutrition Values per 100g / 100ml KCAL	PROT	CARB	FAT	FIBRE
CHEESE								
Camembert, Average	*1 Serving/50g*	*141*	*11.1*	*283*	*20.5*	*0.1*	*22.2*	*0*
Camembert, Breaded, Average	*1 Serving/90g*	*307*	*20.9*	*342*	*16.6*	*14.2*	*23.2*	*0.4*
Cantal, French, Sainsbury's*	1 Serving/30g	106	8.7	353	23	0.1	29	0
Cashel Blue, Waitrose*	1 Serving/28g	94	7.6	336	17.6	1.2	27.2	0
Cheddar, & Mozzarella, Spicy, Grated, Tesco*	1 Serving/40g	140	10.5	350	26	2.5	26.2	0
Cheddar, Average	*1 Serving/30g*	*123*	*10.3*	*410*	*25*	*0.1*	*34.4*	*0*
Cheddar, Canadian, Average	*1 Serving/30g*	*123*	*10.3*	*409*	*25*	*0.1*	*34.3*	*0*
Cheddar, Davidstow, Mature, Average	*1 Serving/28g*	*115*	*9.6*	*410*	*25*	*0.1*	*34.4*	*0*
Cheddar, Extra Mature, Average	*1 Serving/30g*	*123*	*10.3*	*410*	*25.1*	*0.1*	*34.4*	*0*
Cheddar, Grated, Average	*1 Serving/50g*	*206*	*17.2*	*413*	*24.4*	*1.5*	*34.3*	*0*
Cheddar, Mature, Average	*1 Serving/30g*	*123*	*10.3*	*410*	*25*	*0.1*	*34.4*	*0*
Cheddar, Mature, Grated, Average	*1 Serving/28g*	*113*	*9.3*	*404*	*24.7*	*1.6*	*33.2*	*0*
Cheddar, Mature, Reduced Fat, Average	*1 Serving/25g*	*68*	*4.2*	*271*	*30*	*0.1*	*16.7*	*0*
Cheddar, Medium, Average	*1 Serving/30g*	*123*	*10.4*	*411*	*24.9*	*0.2*	*34.5*	*0*
Cheddar, Mild, Average	*1 Serving/30g*	*123*	*10.3*	*409*	*25*	*0.1*	*34.3*	*0*
Cheddar, Reduced Fat, Average	*1 Serving/30g*	*76*	*4.2*	*255*	*32.2*	*0.1*	*14*	*0*
Cheddar, Scotch Bonnet, Slices, Tesco*	1 Slice/28g	110	9	394	20.3	4.8	32.2	1.7
Cheddar, Smoked, Average	*1 Serving/30g*	*123*	*10.3*	*411*	*25.2*	*0.1*	*34.4*	*0*
Cheddar, West Country Farmhouse, Average	*1 Serving/28g*	*115*	*9.6*	*410*	*25*	*0.1*	*34.4*	*0*
Cheddar, Wexford, Average	*1 Serving/20g*	*82*	*6.9*	*410*	*25*	*0.1*	*34.4*	*0*
Cheddar, with Caramelised Onion, Sainsbury's*	1 Serving/28g	109	8.7	391	22.8	5.1	31	0
Cheddar, with Caramelised Onion, Tesco*	1 Serving/50g	183	14	366	21.4	7.1	28	0.4
Cheddar, with Onion & Chives, Davidson*	1 Serving/25g	100	8.3	400	24.3	0.6	33.3	0
Cheddar, with Pickled Onion Relish, Christmas, Tesco*	¼ Cheese/50g	191	15.5	382	23	2.7	31	0.1
Chedds, Bricks, Cathedral City, Dairy Crest Ltd*	1 Brick/18g	75	6.3	416	25.4	0.1	34.9	0
Chedds, Nibbles, Cathedral City, Dairy Crest Ltd*	1 Mini Bag/16g	67	5.6	416	25.4	0.1	34.9	0
Cheshire	*1oz/28g*	*106*	*8.8*	*379*	*24*	*0.1*	*31.4*	*0*
Chevre Pave D'affinois, Finest, Tesco*	1 Pack/150g	404	32.6	269	18.5	0	21.7	0
Cottage, Low Fat, 2% Fat, Natural, Average	*1 Serving/75g*	*68*	*1.4*	*90*	*13.7*	*3.6*	*1.9*	*0*
Cottage, Plain, Average	*1 Tbsp/20g*	*19*	*0.7*	*93*	*12*	*3.3*	*3.5*	*0.1*
Cottage, Plain, Reduced Fat, Average	*100g*	*85*	*1.9*	*85*	*12.3*	*4.4*	*1.9*	*0.1*
Cottage, Virtually Fat Free, Average	*1 Tbsp/20g*	*16*	*0.2*	*79*	*13*	*4.5*	*1*	*0*
Cottage, Whole Milk, Natural, Average	*1 Serving/75g*	*77*	*3.4*	*103*	*12.5*	*2.7*	*4.5*	*0*
Cottage, with Black Pepper, HE, Tesco*	1 Pot/125g	101	2.2	81	12.1	4	1.8	0
Cottage, with Chives, Low Fat, Westacre*	1 Pot/100g	81	1.4	81	13.7	3.5	1.4	1.2
Cottage, with Chives, Virtually Fat free, Longley Farm*	½ Pot/125g	88	0.1	70	14.3	2.9	0.1	0
Cottage, with Cucumber & Mint, HE, Tesco*	½ Pot/125g	91	2.1	73	10.7	3.8	1.7	0.1
Cottage, with Grilled Pepper & Pesto, LC, Tesco*	1 Portion/60g	45	0.9	75	10.2	4.3	1.5	0.5
Cottage, with Mango & Pineapple, BGTY, Sainsbury's*	½ Pot/125g	112	0.9	90	10.7	10.4	0.7	0.2
Cottage, with Onion & Chive, GFY, Asda*	¼ Tub/75g	50	1	66	9.3	3.8	1.4	0.5
Cottage, with Onion & Chive, Iceland*	½ Pot/100g	81	1.3	81	8.5	8.9	1.3	0.3
Cottage, with Onion & Chive, HL, Tesco*	1 Serving/60g	40	0.2	67	10.1	56	0.3	0.5
Cottage, with Pineapple, 70% Less fat, CBY, Asda*	¼ Tub/75g	70	1	93	8.4	11.9	1.3	0
Cottage, with Pineapple, GFY, Asda*	1 Pot/227g	193	2.3	85	9	10	1	0.5
Cottage, with Sweet Chilli, & Red Pepper, CBY, Asda*	½ Tub/150g	118	2	79	9.9	7.1	1.3	0.3
Cottage, with Tomato & Cracked Black Pepper, Asda*	½ Pot/113g	86	2.4	76	10	3.1	2.1	1.3
Cottage, with Tuna & Sweetcorn, HL, Tesco*	1 Serving/150g	136	3.2	91	12.8	4.8	2.1	0.4
Cream, Average	*1 Portion/30g*	*132*	*14.2*	*439*	*3.1*	*0*	*47.4*	*0*
Cream, Garlic & Herbs, Light, Boursin*	1 Portion/20g	26	1.8	131	8	4.5	9	0
Cream, Reduced Fat, Average	*1 Serving/20g*	*23*	*1.1*	*117*	*13*	*4*	*5.3*	*0.1*
Cream, with Onion & Chives, Morrisons*	1 Serving/20g	38	3	190	11	3	15	0
Cream, with Pineapple, Asda*	1 Serving/40g	77	5.2	193	8	11	13	0
Cream, with Red Peppers & Onion, GFY, Asda*	1 Serving/32g	42	1.9	130	13	6	6	0

CHEESE

INFO/WEIGHT	Measure	per Measure KCAL	FAT	Nutrition Values per 100g / 100ml KCAL	PROT	CARB	FAT	FIBRE
Creme de Saint Agur, Saint Agur*	1 Serving/10g	28	2.5	285	13.5	2.3	24.7	0
Dairylea, Light, Slices, Kraft*	1 Slice/25g	44	1.9	177	16	8.2	7.6	1.6
Danish Blue, Average	*1 Serving/30g*	*106*	*8.7*	*352*	*20.8*	*0*	*29.1*	*0*
Demi Pont L'eveque, Finest, Tesco*	1 Serving/46g	138	10.6	301	21.1	0.4	23	0
Dolcelatte, Average	*1 Serving/30g*	*110*	*9.7*	*366*	*17.8*	*0.4*	*32.3*	*0.4*
Double Gloucester with Onion & Chives, Sainsbury's*	1 Serving/30g	110	8.5	365	22.2	5.5	28.2	0
Double Gloucester, Average	*1 Serving/30g*	*121*	*10.2*	*404*	*24.5*	*0.1*	*34*	*0*
Doux De Montagne, Average	*1 Serving/25g*	*88*	*7.1*	*352*	*22.9*	*1.5*	*28.3*	*0*
Edam, Average	*1 Serving/10g*	*33*	*2.5*	*326*	*25.3*	*0*	*24.9*	*0*
Edam, Dutch, Garlic & Herb Wedge, Asda*	1 Serving/60g	197	15	329	26	0	25	0
Edam, Reduced Fat, Average	*1 Serving/30g*	*69*	*3.3*	*230*	*32.4*	*0.1*	*11.1*	*0*
Edam, Slices, Average	*1 Slice/30g*	*96*	*7.2*	*320*	*25*	*0.4*	*24.1*	*0*
Emmental, Average	*1 Serving/10g*	*37*	*2.8*	*368*	*28.4*	*0*	*28.4*	*0*
Emmental, Light, Slices, President*	1 Slice/20g	60	3.6	298	34	0	18	0
Emmental, Spreadable, Low Low, Kerry*	1 Serving/20g	40	2.7	200	13	6.7	13.5	0
Feta, Apetina, Light, 10 % Fat, Arla*	1 Serving/30g	52	3	173	18.4	0.6	10.1	0
Feta, Average	*1 Serving/30g*	*79*	*6.4*	*262*	*16.3*	*1*	*21.5*	*0*
Feta, Lemon, Asda*	1 Serving/25g	76	6.8	302	13.2	1	27.2	0.6
Feta, Light, Greek, Salad, 40% Reduced Fat, Attis*	1 Portion/30g	51	3.6	170	20	0.6	12	0
Fondue, Original, Fromalp*	1 Pack/400g	888	68	222	15	2.5	17	0
Fondue, Swiss, Easy Cook, Tesco*	¼ Pack/100g	235	17	235	15.5	4	17	0
Fondue, Traditionnelle, Co-Op*	1 Serving/100g	409	34	409	26	0.9	34	0
Fontina, Average	*1 Serving/28g*	*109*	*9*	*389*	*25*	*0*	*32.1*	*0*
for Pizza, Grated	*1 Serving/50g*	*163*	*12.2*	*326*	*25*	*1.6*	*24.4*	*0*
Goats, Average	*1 Tsp/10g*	*26*	*2.1*	*262*	*13.8*	*3.8*	*21.2*	*0*
Goats, Breaded, Bites, Sainsbury's*	1 Bite/25g	84	6.2	337	13	15.1	25	0.8
Goats, Breaded, Cheese Emporium, Aldi*	1 Portion/25g	78	5.5	312	10.8	17.2	22	2
Goats, French, Mild, Average	*1 Serving/30g*	*49*	*3.5*	*163*	*11.2*	*3*	*11.8*	*0*
Goats, Premium, Average	*1 Serving/30g*	*98*	*7.8*	*327*	*20.5*	*0.6*	*26.1*	*0*
Goats, Soft, Average	*1 Serving/30g*	*79*	*6.3*	*262*	*16.7*	*1.8*	*20.8*	*0.5*
Goats, with Garlic & Chives, Welsh, Tesco*	1 Serving/32g	93	7.7	290	15.1	3.3	24.1	0.1
Goats, with Herbs, Welsh, Sainsbury's*	1 Serving/30g	90	7.4	299	15.3	3.6	24.8	0.1
Gorgonzola, Average	*1 Serving/30g*	*100*	*8.1*	*334*	*20*	*0*	*27*	*0*
Gouda, Average	*1 Serving/30g*	*113*	*9.4*	*376*	*24*	*0*	*31.5*	*0*
Gran Padano, Reserva, Deluxe, Lidl*	1 Serving/10g	39	2.8	388	33	0	28.4	0
Grana Padano, Italian Cheese, Waitrose*	1 Serving/14g	54	4	388	33	0	28.4	0
Greek Style, for Salad, Weight Watchers*	1 Serving/30g	34	0.8	113	18	4.3	2.7	0
Greek Style, Salad Cheese, Everyday Value, Tesco*	1 Serving/30g	80	6.2	270	17.2	1.9	21	0
Gruyere	*1oz/28g*	*115*	*9.3*	*409*	*27.2*	*0*	*33.3*	*0*
Halloumi, Average	*1 Serving/80g*	*253*	*19.7*	*316*	*20.8*	*1.6*	*24.7*	*0*
Halloumi, Light Average	*1 Serving/100g*	*245*	*15.3*	*245*	*24.7*	*1.7*	*15.3*	*0*
Halum, Milky*	1 Serving/30g	70	7.6	234	21.8	0	25.5	0
Havarti, Slices, Tesco*	1 Slice/25g	85	6.5	340	24	1.4	26	0
Havarti, Slices, Tesco*	1 Slice/25g	85	6.5	340	24	1.4	26	0
Healthy Range, Average	*1 Slice/20g*	*39*	*2.1*	*197*	*20.6*	*5.2*	*10.4*	*0*
Healthy Range, Slices, Average	*1 Slice/25g*	*45*	*2.2*	*180*	*19.5*	*5.4*	*9*	*0*
Iberico, Sainsbury's, Ttd*	1 Serving/30g	133	11.1	443	25.4	2.2	37	0
Italian Hard, Basics, Sainsbury's*	1 Portion/30g	122	9.6	408	28.1	1.8	32	0.1
Italian, Grated, Average	*1 Serving/30g*	*144*	*10*	*481*	*44*	*1.1*	*33.4*	*0*
Jarlsberg, Slices, Average	*1 Slice/15g*	*54*	*4*	*360*	*27*	*0*	*27*	*0*
Lactose Free, Arla*	1 Serving/30g	103	8.1	344	25.3	1	27	0
Lactose Free, Semi Hard, Lactofree, Arla*	1 Portion/30g	103	8.1	344	25.3	1	27	0
Lancashire	*1oz/28g*	*104*	*8.7*	*373*	*23.3*	*0.1*	*31*	*0*

CHEESE

INFO/WEIGHT	Measure	per Measure KCAL	FAT	Nutrition Values per 100g / 100ml KCAL	PROT	CARB	FAT	FIBRE
Leerdammer, Lighter, Sliced, M&S*	1 Slice/23g	62	3.9	271	29.5	0.1	17	0
Manchego	**1 Serving/70g**	**340**	**30.8**	**485**	**22.2**	**0.1**	**44**	**0**
Marscapone, Lighter, Tesco*	½ Tub/125g	306	26.9	245	9.5	3	21.5	0
Mascarpone, 25% Less Fat, Sainsbury's*	1 Portion/30g	95	9	316	6.7	4.8	30	0
Mascarpone, Average	**1 Serving/30g**	**131**	**13.1**	**437**	**5.6**	**4.1**	**43.6**	**0**
Mature, Half Fat, Average	**1 Serving/25g**	**66**	**3.9**	**265**	**29.9**	**0.4**	**15.6**	**0.1**
Mild, Reduced Fat, Grated, Average	**1 Serving/30g**	**70**	**3.3**	**235**	**31.5**	**2.2**	**11.1**	**0**
Monterey Jack, Iga*	1 Serving/28g	110	9	393	25	0	32.1	0
Monterey Jack, Shredded, Kraft*	¼ Cup/28g	101	8.1	360	22	3.6	28.8	0
Morbier, Sainsbury's*	1 Serving/10g	33	2.4	330	28	0.1	24.2	0
Mozzarella, Average	**½ Ball/62.5g**	**172**	**12.9**	**275**	**21.2**	**1.2**	**20.6**	**0**
Mozzarella, Reduced Fat, Average	**½ Ball/62.5g**	**115**	**6.4**	**184**	**21.2**	**1**	**10.2**	**0**
Mozzarella, Sticks, Ovenbaked, Iceland*	½ Pack/90g	280	17.4	311	12.9	20.4	19.3	2.2
NeufchÃf¢tel, Soft, Average	**1 Serving/30g**	**76**	**6.9**	**253**	**9**	**3.6**	**23**	**0**
Norvegia, Sliced Light, Tine*	1 Slice/10g	27	1.6	272	32	0	16	0
Ossau-Iraty, Average	**1 Serving/30g**	**120**	**10.2**	**400**	**22.3**	**0.2**	**34**	**0**
Parlick Fell, Hard, Sheeps, Sainsbury's*	1 Serving/30g	109	9.1	364	22.6	0	30.4	0
Parmesan, Average	**1 Tbsp/10g**	**40**	**2.9**	**401**	**35.2**	**0**	**29.4**	**0**
Pecorino, Italian, Tesco*	1 Serving/30g	119	9.9	397	22	0	33	0
Poivre, Boursin*	1oz/28g	116	11.8	414	7	2	42	0
Port Salut, M&S*	1oz/28g	90	7.3	322	21	1	26	0
Provolone Piccante, Italiamo, Lidl*	1 Serving/30g	112	9	372	25	0.5	30	0.5
Quark, Average	**1 Serving/20g**	**13**	**0**	**66**	**11.9**	**4**	**0.2**	**0**
Quark, Natural, with Mango & Passion Fruit, Nutrii*	1 Pot/180g	139	0.7	77	0.1	7.4	0.4	0.3
Raclette, Richsmonts*	1 Slice/28g	100	8	357	25	0	28.6	0
Reblochon	**1 Serving/30g**	**95**	**8**	**318**	**19.7**	**0**	**26.6**	**0**
Red Hot Dutch, Deli, Morrisons*	1 Serving/30g	102	8.5	341	19.8	1.3	28.4	0.6
Red Leicester, Average	**1 Serving/30g**	**120**	**10.1**	**400**	**23.8**	**0.1**	**33.7**	**0**
Red Leicester, Reduced Fat, Average	**1 Serving/30g**	**78**	**4.6**	**261**	**30.2**	**0.1**	**15.4**	**0**
Red, & Mozzarella, Grated, Low Low, Kerry*	1 Serving/30g	90	6.6	301	26	0.6	22	0
Ricotta, Average	**1 Serving/50g**	**67**	**4.8**	**134**	**9.3**	**2.9**	**9.5**	**0**
Roquefort, Average	**1oz/28g**	**105**	**9.2**	**375**	**19.7**	**0**	**32.9**	**0**
Roule, French, Sainsbury's*	1 Serving/30g	96	9.2	321	8.5	3	30.5	0
Roule, Garlic & Parsley, Light, BGTY, Sainsbury's*	1 Serving/30g	51	3.2	171	16.4	2.6	10.6	0
Roule, Garlic, & Herb, Lidl*	1 Serving/30g	90	8.4	301	7.3	5	28	0
Sage Derby	**1oz/28g**	**113**	**9.5**	**402**	**24.2**	**0.1**	**33.9**	**0**
Seriously Strong, Lighter, Spreadable, Mclelland*	1 Serving/25g	56	4.2	225	15.5	2.5	17	0
Shropshire, Blue, Average	**1 Serving/50g**	**196**	**17.1**	**391**	**21**	**0**	**34.2**	**0**
Slices, Average	**1 Slice/23g**	**82**	**6.6**	**358**	**24**	**0.8**	**28.6**	**0**
Slices, Red Leicester, Tesco*	1 Slice/30g	120	10.1	400	23.7	0	33.7	0
Slices, Smoked with Ham, Aldi*	1 Slice/21g	66	5.2	313	21	1	25	0.1
Soft with Onion & Chives, Lighter, Asda*	1 Serving/30g	32	1.3	105	11.6	4.5	4.3	0.2
Soft, & Creamy with Onions & Garlic, GFY, Asda*	1 Serving/25g	32	1.5	126	13	5	6	0
Soft, & Smooth, Extra Light, HL, Tesco*	1 Serving/30g	39	1.8	130	14.2	3.7	6	0
Soft, 50% Lighter, NUME, Morrisons*	1 Serving/30g	51	3.8	169	9.7	4.2	12.5	0.5
Soft, Extra Light, Average	**1 Serving/20g**	**25**	**1.2**	**125**	**14.3**	**3.6**	**5.9**	**0.1**
Soft, Fruit & Rum Halo, Discover*	1 Serving/25g	104	8.5	414	8.6	11.7	34.1	0
Soft, Full Fat, Average	**1 Serving/50g**	**156**	**15.2**	**312**	**8.2**	**1.7**	**30.3**	**0**
Soft, Full Fat, Original, Lactose Free, Kraft*	1 Serving/30g	84	8.2	280	4.5	2.7	27.5	0.3
Soft, Garlic & Herb, Extra Light, LC, Tesco*	1 Serving/38g	49	2.4	130	12.3	5.1	6.3	0.3
Soft, Garlic & Herb, Roulade, M&S*	1 Portion/100g	295	27.3	295	7.8	4.1	27.3	1.3
Soft, Garlic & Herbs, Light, Med Fat, Philadelphia*	1 Serving/20g	30	2.1	149	7.3	5.4	10.5	0.5
Soft, Greek Style, Philadelphia*	1 Serving/30g	34	2.1	114	7.7	4.3	7.1	0.2

CHEESE

INFO/WEIGHT	Measure			Nutrition Values per 100g / 100ml				
		KCAL	FAT	KCAL	PROT	CARB	FAT	FIBRE
CHEESE								
Soft, Light, Average	*1 Tbsp/30g*	*54*	*3.9*	*179*	*12.1*	*3.2*	*13.1*	*0*
Soft, Med Fat, Average	*1 Serving/30g*	*62*	*5.4*	*207*	*8.4*	*3*	*17.9*	*0*
Soft, Mediterranean Herbs, Full Fat, Philadelphia*	1 Serving/30g	64	5.7	213	5	4.1	19	0.3
Soft, Pineapple Halo, Discover*	1 Serving/25g	101	8.2	404	7.2	16.6	32.6	1.2
Soft, Salmon & Dill, Light, Med Fat, Philadelphia*	1 Serving/20g	28	2	142	7.3	5.1	10	0.5
Soft, Smoked Ham, Light, Med Fat, Philadelphia*	1 Serving/20g	29	1.9	143	7.4	5.9	9.7	0.4
Soft, Sweet Chilli, Light, Med Fat, Philadelphia*	1 Serving/20g	30	2	148	6.8	7.3	10	0.5
Soft, White, Lactofree, Arla*	1 Serving/30g	59	5	197	8.6	3	16.5	0
Soft, with Black Pepper, Light, Sainsbury's*	½ Pack/100g	205	16.5	205	11	3	16.5	0
Soft, with Chives, Light, Med Fat, Philadelphia*	1 Serving/20g	30	2.2	151	7.4	5.2	11	0.6
Soft, with Garlic & Herbs, Full Fat, Deli, Boursin*	1 Serving/28g	84	8.3	299	3.5	5	29.5	0
Soft, with Garlic & Herbs, Light, Sainsbury's*	2 Servings/100g	157	11.4	157	10.6	3.1	11.4	0
Stilton, Average	*1 Serving/30g*	*123*	*10.6*	*410*	*22.4*	*0.1*	*35.5*	*0*
Stilton, Blue, Average	*1 Serving/30g*	*124*	*10.7*	*412*	*22.8*	*0.1*	*35.7*	*0*
Stilton, White & Apricot, M&S*	1oz/28g	94	6.5	337	13.8	18.5	23.1	0
Stilton, White with Apricot, Somerfield*	1oz/28g	103	8.4	369	16	8	30	0
Stilton, White with Cranberries, Tesco*	1 Serving/50g	184	14.8	368	15.8	9.5	29.7	0.7
Stilton, White with Mango & Ginger, Tesco*	1/3 Pack/65g	228	14	350	13.1	25.8	21.6	0.6
Stilton, White, Average	*1oz/28g*	*101*	*8.8*	*362*	*19.9*	*0.1*	*31.3*	*0*
Substitute, Mozzarella Style, Grated, Value, Tesco*	1 Serving/40g	120	8.4	300	25	2.5	21.1	0
Sussex Slipcote, Soft, Creamy, High Weald Dairy*	1 Serving/25g	60	4.7	238	14	3	18.9	0.7
Taleggio D.o.p., Finest, Tesco*	1 Serving/30g	89	7.5	297	18	0	25	0
Twisted, Cheestrings*	1 String/20g	61	4.5	305	23	2.5	22.5	0
Vacherin Badoz, Waitrose*	1 Serving/30g	87	7.2	289	17.6	0.7	24	0
Wedge, Leerdammer*	1 Serving/30g	107	8.3	357	27	0	27.7	0
Wedges, Camembert, Breaded, Morrisons*	1 Wedge/25g	88	5.6	352	15.1	22.9	22.2	2
Wensleydale, & Ginger, Truckle, Morrisons*	1 Truckle/90g	330	23.7	367	18	14	26.3	1.1
Wensleydale, Average	*1 Serving/25g*	*92*	*7.8*	*369*	*22.4*	*0.1*	*31*	*0*
Wensleydale, with Blueberries, M&S*	1 Portion/30g	111	7.9	370	18.7	13.4	26.4	0.9
Wensleydale, with Cranberries, Sainsbury's*	1 Serving/50g	180	13.9	359	20.7	6.4	27.8	0
CHEESE ALTERNATIVE								
Cheezly, Cream, Original Flavour, The Redwood Co*	1 Pack/113g	357	34.5	316	5.6	4.8	30.5	0
Cheezly, Feta Style in Oil, The Redwood Co*	1 Serving/25g	119	11.8	475	2.5	10.6	47	0
Cheezly, Mozzarella Style, The Redwood Co*	1 Portion/25g	69	6.4	274	5.4	5.9	25.4	1
Chive & Garlic, Spread, Vegan, Go Veggie*	1 Mini Tub/37g	100	10	270	5.4	2.7	27	0
Herbs & Chives, Creamy Smooth, Tofutti*	1 Serving/18g	51	4.9	283	3.3	6.7	27	0
Mozzarella, Slices, Dairy Free	*1 Slice/19g*	*80*	*6*	*420*	*10.5*	*10.5*	*31.5*	*0*
Original, Violife*	1 Slice/20g	57	4.6	285	0	20	23	0
Vegetarian, Average	*1 Serving/30g*	*110*	*8.4*	*368*	*28.2*	*0*	*28.1*	*0*
CHEESE ON TOAST								
Average	*1 Slice/130g*	*494*	*34.2*	*380*	*13.8*	*23.8*	*26.3*	*0.7*
CHEESE PUFFS								
Average	*1 Bag/25g*	*129*	*7.4*	*517*	*7.8*	*54.8*	*29.5*	*1.5*
Cheeky, Tesco*	1 Bag/20g	108	7	542	6.7	50.2	34.9	0
Morrisons*	1 Bag/25g	136	8.7	542	6.7	50.2	34.9	1.1
Sainsbury's*	1 Pack/100g	530	32	530	9.1	51.4	32	1.9
Shapers, Boots*	1 Bag/16g	80	3.8	500	7.1	64	24	0.9
Value, Tesco*	1 Pack/16g	84	4.6	525	6.2	60	28.8	0.6
CHEESE SPREAD								
Average	*1 Serving/30g*	*76*	*6.4*	*254*	*9.4*	*5.9*	*21.4*	*0.1*
Cheese & Ham, Primula*	1 Squeeze/25g	50	3.8	200	12.3	3.1	15	4.9
Dairylea, Light, Tub, Kraft*	1 Serving/30g	47	2.2	158	16.5	5.2	7.2	0
Dairylea, Tub, Kraft*	1 Serving/25g	60	4.9	240	11	5.3	19.5	0

INFO/WEIGHT	Measure	per Measure KCAL	FAT	Nutrition Values per 100g / 100ml KCAL	PROT	CARB	FAT	FIBRE

CHEESE SPREAD

	Measure	KCAL	FAT	KCAL	PROT	CARB	FAT	FIBRE
Flavoured	*1oz/28g*	*72*	*5.7*	*258*	*14.2*	*4.4*	*20.5*	*0*
Healthy Range, Average	*1 Serving/30g*	*31*	*1*	*102*	*14.3*	*3.8*	*3.2*	*0.9*
with Chives, Primula*	1 Squeeze/25g	48	3.6	190	12.5	2.9	14.2	4.5
with Prawn, Primula*	1 Squeeze/25g	48	3.6	190	12.5	3.3	14.4	3.6

CHEESE STRAWS

& Bacon, Party, Tesco*	1 Straw/12.5g	40	2.6	321	10.5	23.8	20.4	2.1
Cheddar, M&S*	1 Straw/11g	59	3.8	535	14.9	40.1	34.9	2.4
Cheese Twists, Tesco*	1 Serving/20g	99	5.6	494	14	46.4	28	4.2
Finest, Tesco*	1 Straw/7g	39	2.6	558	13.3	41.5	37.6	1.5
Homemade or Bakery, Average	*1 Straw/41g*	*173*	*12.6*	*422*	*12*	*24.2*	*30.7*	*0.7*
Mature Cheddar, Puffed, Thomas J Fudge*	1 Straw/10g	53	3.2	532	12.3	46.8	31.9	0
Selection, Sainsbury's*	1 Straw/7g	41	2.9	558	16.6	34.5	39.3	2.8

CHEESE TRIANGLES

Average	*1 Triangle/14g*	*33*	*2.2*	*238*	*10.3*	*14.2*	*15.6*	*0.2*
Dairylea, Light, Kraft*	1 Triangle/17.5g	36	2.2	205	15.5	6.3	12.5	0
Light, Extra, The Laughing Cow, Fromageries Bel*	1 Triangle/18g	19	0.4	108	17	5.5	2	0
Light, with Blue Cheese, The Laughing Cow*	1 Triangle/16g	24	1.4	151	13	5.5	8.5	0
Reduced Fat, Average	*1 Triangle/18g*	*27*	*1.2*	*154*	*15.4*	*7*	*7*	*0*

CHEESE TWISTS

All Butter, M&S*	1 Pack/125g	625	33.4	500	14.2	50.2	26.7	3.2
Asda*	1 Twist/8g	42	2.4	500	14	48	28	5
Gruyere & Poppy Seed, Truly Irresistible, Co-Op*	1 Twist/8g	42	2.4	520	13.2	48.8	30.1	2.5
Gruyere & Poppy Seed, TTD, Sainsbury's*	1 Serving/8g	41	2.3	509	13.7	50.5	28	2.6
Parmesan, All Butter, TTD, Sainsbury's*	1 Serving/8g	38	2	487	13.8	51	25.3	2.8
Pre Packed, Average	*1 Twist/8g*	*41*	*2.2*	*515*	*13.7*	*47.9*	*27.7*	*2.3*

CHEESECAKE

After Noon, Mango & Passionfruit, 3 Pack, Gu*	1 Portion/45g	155	11.3	345	3.4	26.5	25.2	0.4
American Red White & Blueberry, Sainsbury's*	1/6 Cake/83g	264	15.4	318	3.8	35.1	18.5	0.4
Apple & Cinnamon, Baked, M&S*	1 Serving/116g	390	22	335	3.7	39.7	18.9	2.1
Apricot, Co-Op*	1 Cake/100g	230	11	230	4	29	11	0.9
Apricot, HL, Tesco*	1 Pot/100g	179	2.3	179	4.9	34.7	2.3	1.6
Autumn Berry, Waitrose*	1 Slice/92g	316	20.3	343	4.4	31.5	22.1	2
Average	*1 Slice/115g*	*490*	*40.8*	*426*	*3.7*	*24.6*	*35.5*	*0.4*
Belgian Chocolate, M&S*	1 Slice/100g	385	23.9	385	5.3	39.2	23.9	2.5
Belgian Chocolate, Tesco*	1/6 Cake/90g	392	25.8	436	5.1	37.9	28.7	2.8
Blackcurrant Devonshire, McVitie's*	1/6 Cake/67g	193	11.5	288	3.8	29.7	17.1	1.7
Blackcurrant Swirl, Heinz*	1/5 Cake/87g	241	13.4	277	4.1	30.3	15.4	3.6
Blackcurrant, Average	*1 Serving/90g*	*237*	*11.9*	*263*	*3.6*	*32.3*	*13.2*	*2.4*
Blackcurrant, Healthy Range, Average	*1 Serving/90g*	*182*	*4.7*	*203*	*4.7*	*33.6*	*5.3*	*2.1*
Blackcurrant, PB, Waitrose*	1/6 Cake/99g	212	3.6	214	4	39.6	3.6	2.4
Blackcurrant, Value, Tesco*	1 Serving/70g	174	8.6	248	2.8	31.4	12.3	1
Blackcurrant, Weight Watchers*	1 Cake/103g	191	2.9	185	4.6	35.4	2.8	3.5
Blueberry & Lemon Flavour Wedges, Sainsbury's*	1 Serving/80g	262	16.9	327	5.1	29.2	21.1	1.2
Blueberry & Vanilla, TTD, Sainsbury's*	1 Serving/95g	353	24.8	372	5.4	28.9	26.1	2.1
Caramel Swirl, Cadbury*	1 Slice/91g	373	23.5	410	6	40.1	25.8	0
Cherry, BGTY, Sainsbury's*	1 Serving/91g	181	3.9	199	4.6	35.5	4.3	0.5
Cherry, Healthy Range, Average	*1 Serving/90g*	*172*	*3*	*191*	*3.7*	*36.4*	*3.3*	*1.1*
Chocolate & Hazelnut, Sara Lee*	1 Serving/65g	224	13.9	345	6.5	31.2	21.4	1.2
Chocolate & Hazlenut, Gold, Sara Lee*	1 Slice/65g	205	12.8	316	5.9	28.7	19.7	1.1
Chocolate & Honeycomb, Slice, Sainsbury's*	1 Slice/98g	333	20.3	340	3.7	33.7	20.7	2.4
Chocolate & Irish Cream Liqueur, Tesco*	1 Serving/93g	385	28	414	5	30.7	30.1	0.8
Chocolate & Vanilla, Gu*	1 Pot/90g	379	27.1	421	4.1	34.6	30.1	1.6
Chocolate & Vanilla, Reduced Fat, M&S*	1 Serving/114g	319	13.7	280	7	37.9	12	1.5

CHEESECAKE

	Measure INFO/WEIGHT	per Measure KCAL	FAT	Nutrition Values per 100g / 100ml KCAL	PROT	CARB	FAT	FIBRE
Chocolate & Vanilla, Tesco*	1 Serving/90g	330	19.4	365	5.2	37.1	21.5	1.6
Chocolate Orange, Aldi*	1/6 Pack/83g	262	16.6	316	4.4	29	20	1.1
Chocolate Truffle, HL, Tesco*	1 Slice/96g	250	13.2	260	10.3	23.7	13.8	6.5
Chocolate, Average	*1 Serving/75g*	*265*	*15.7*	*353*	*5.7*	*35.6*	*20.9*	*1.9*
Chocolate, Pure Indulgence, Thorntons*	1 Serving/75g	308	17.6	410	5.6	44.3	23.4	0.6
Chocolate, Tesco*	1 Serving/91g	317	17.4	348	6.2	37.8	19.1	1.5
Chocolate, Weight Watchers*	1 Cake/95g	143	3.8	151	7.5	20.7	4	0.7
Citrus, Good Choice, Mini, Iceland*	1 Cake/111g	198	4.7	178	3.5	31.6	4.2	0.4
Commercially Prepared	*1/6 Cake/80g*	*257*	*18*	*321*	*5.5*	*25.5*	*22.5*	*0.4*
Creamy Vanilla, New York, Slices, Tesco*	1 Slice/106g	371	26.7	350	4.6	25.9	25.2	2.2
Devonshire Strawberry, McVitie's*	1/6 Cake/66g	192	10.7	291	4.4	31.8	16.2	3.6
Double Chocolate Wedge, Sainsbury's*	1 Serving/75g	327	24.8	436	5.7	29	33	1.7
Eton Mess, Pizza Express*	1 Serving/155g	555	35	358	3.7	35.1	22.6	0.7
Fruit, Average	*1 Serving/75g*	*207*	*10.9*	*276*	*5.3*	*32.3*	*14.5*	*1.6*
Fudge, Tesco*	1 Serving/102g	384	23.6	376	4.6	37.5	23.1	0.5
Gorgeous Blueberry, Cooked, Aunt Bessie's*	1 Portion/75g	225	6.1	300	3.9	33.5	8.2	0.9
Indulgent with Liqueur, Average	*1 Serving/90g*	*366*	*23.4*	*406*	*5*	*38.2*	*26*	*0.8*
Irish Cream, McVitie's*	¼ Slice/190g	616	36.9	324	4.4	33	19.4	0.4
Lemon Creamy & Light, M&S*	1/6 Cake/68g	236	13.8	350	3.5	32.3	20.4	0.4
Lemon Meringue, Tesco*	1 Slice/94g	352	25	375	3.8	30.1	26.6	0.3
Lemon Swirl, Individual, Sainsbury's*	1 Pot/125g	380	23	304	3	31.1	18.4	0.9
Lemon Swirl, Sainsbury's*	1/6 Cake/95g	350	21	369	4.8	37.2	22.1	1
Lemon, Asda*	1 Slice/90g	319	21.2	354	4.3	31.2	23.5	1.1
Lemon, Average	*1 Serving/90g*	*307*	*19.5*	*341*	*4.1*	*33*	*21.6*	*1.8*
Lemon, BGTY, Sainsbury's*	1/6 Cake/71g	142	2.7	200	4.4	37	3.8	0.5
Lemon, Sainsbury's*	1 Serving/180g	650	37.1	361	4	39.9	20.6	1.3
Lemon, Sicilian, Slices, Finest, Tesco*	1 Slice/100g	351	21	351	3	36.8	21	1.2
Lemon, Swirl, Asda*	1 Pack/125g	445	29.9	356	3.1	32.1	23.9	1.8
Lemon, Tesco*	1 Slice/93g	315	21	339	5.2	28.6	22.6	0.3
Lemon, Value, Tesco*	1 Serving/79g	221	11.8	281	4.3	32.2	15	4.2
Madagascan Vanilla, Finest, Tesco*	1 Serving/90g	335	20.9	372	5.1	35.3	23.2	0.8
Mandarin, Co-Op*	1 Slice/99g	297	16.8	300	4	32	17	0.3
Mandarin, GFY, Asda*	1/6 Cake/92g	178	4	194	3.6	35	4.4	1.2
Mandarin, Low Fat, Tesco*	1 Serving/70g	145	3.3	207	3.3	37	4.7	1.4
Mandarin, Morrisons*	1 Serving/135g	335	16.9	248	3.8	32.2	12.5	0.8
Mandarin, Weight Watchers*	1 Cake/103g	180	2.9	175	4.6	32.9	2.8	1.5
Milk Chocolate, Belgian, Specially Selected, Aldi*	1/6 Cake/93g	386	25.1	415	5.8	37	27	1.6
New York, Baked, Waitrose*	1/12 Cake/83g	317	22.6	380	5.1	28.3	27.1	1.2
New York, Mini, Iceland*	1 Cake/22g	86	5.1	385	3.6	40.7	23	0.5
Pecan, Seriously Nutty, Waitrose*	1 Serving/91g	341	21	376	5.8	35.7	23.2	1
Praline, Asda*	1/8 Cake/62g	226	14.9	364	7	30	24	3.2
Raspberry & Strawberry, M&S*	1 Slice/104.6g	340	21.1	325	3.9	33.4	20.2	1.2
Raspberry & Mascarpone, Best, Morrisons*	1 Cake/84g	257	14	306	3.9	34.8	16.7	1
Raspberry & Vanilla, Slices, M&S*	1 Slice/100g	300	17.5	300	4.4	30.4	17.5	1.7
Raspberry Rapture, Slices, Tesco*	1 Slice/110g	341	20.4	310	4.2	30.8	18.5	1.8
Raspberry Ripple, Sainsbury's*	1 Portion/95g	348	21.3	366	4.7	36	22.4	0.8
Raspberry, BGTY, Sainsbury's*	1 Pot/94.5g	154	2.5	163	6.6	28.2	2.6	2.8
Raspberry, LC, Tesco*	1 Cake/95g	185	4.1	195	4.3	34.7	4.3	1.3
Raspberry, M&S*	1 Slice/105g	331	21.5	315	5	32.2	20.5	1
Red Berry, Waitrose*	1 Slice/101g	350	22.5	346	4.6	31.3	22.2	1.4
Rhubarb Crumble, Sainsbury's*	1 Serving/114g	268	10.6	235	3.1	34.8	9.3	2.4
Rocky Road, CBY, Asda*	1 Serving/75g	302	17.3	402	4.5	43.4	23.1	1.4
Salted Caramel, Mini, Iceland*	1 Cake/22g	85	4.7	380	3.2	44.5	20.9	0.6

	Measure INFO/WEIGHT	per Measure KCAL	FAT	Nutrition Values per 100g / 100ml KCAL	PROT	CARB	FAT	FIBRE
CHEESECAKE								
Sticky Toffee, Tesco*	1 Slice/66g	248	16	375	4	35.3	24.2	0.5
Strawberries & Cream, Finest, Tesco*	1 Serving/104g	325	22.4	312	4.3	25.3	21.5	0.5
Strawberry Shortcake, Sara Lee*	1/6 Slice/68g	230	15.7	337	4.9	27.6	23	0.5
Strawberry, Creamy, Weight Watchers*	1 Cake/105g	187	2.6	178	4.7	34.2	2.5	2.2
Strawberry, Finest, Tesco*	1 Slice/113g	383	25.1	339	4.8	30.1	22.2	0.9
Strawberry, Fresh, M&S*	¼ Cake/125g	300	19.2	240	2.8	23.1	15.4	1.1
Strawberry, Frozen, Sainsbury's*	1/6 Cake/84g	277	14.2	332	4.3	40.4	17	2.3
Summerfruit, GFY, Asda*	1/6 Cake/92g	175	3.8	191	3.7	34.5	4.2	1.4
The Ultimate New York Baked, Entenmann's*	1 Cake/100g	347	21.3	347	4.2	35.7	21.3	0.9
Toffee & Pecan, Wedge, Sainsbury's*	1 Serving/75g	296	21.8	395	5.4	28.1	29	3.1
Toffee Apple, Tesco*	1/6 Cake/80g	233	11	291	4	37.7	13.7	0.6
Toffee, American Style, Asda*	1 Serving/75g	269	15.8	359	4.5	38	21	3.8
Toffee, Asda*	1 Cake/87g	295	19.1	339	4.3	31	22	3.5
Toffee, Lidl*	1 Pot/100g	275	12.3	275	3	37.6	12.3	1
Toffee, M&S*	1 Serving/105g	357	22.6	340	5.2	37.2	21.5	0.9
Toffee, Mini, Asda*	1 Cake/20g	57	2.4	286	4.6	40	12	2.1
Toffee, Tesco*	1 Serving/100g	265	12.9	265	4.3	33.1	12.9	0.8
Vanilla	*1 Serving/100g*	*395*	*26.2*	*395*	*5.3*	*42.8*	*26.2*	*1.1*
Vanilla Chocolate, Baked, Slice, Sainsbury's*	1 Slice/90g	349	23	388	5.7	33.8	25.6	2.7
Vanilla, & Berry, Weight Watchers*	1 Dessert/85g	156	3	184	3.6	34	3.5	1.8
Vanilla, Tesco*	1 Serving/115g	417	28.4	363	5.7	29.4	24.7	0.6
with Belgian Chocolate, Rhokett*	1 Slice/100g	332	21.2	332	5	31.2	21.2	1.6
Zesty Lemon, M&S*	1/6 Cake/97g	325	18.9	335	4	38.7	19.5	2.6
CHERRIES								
Black in Syrup, Average	*1 Serving/242g*	*160*	*0*	*66*	*0.6*	*16*	*0*	*0.7*
Black, Fresh, Average	*1 Serving/80g*	*41*	*0.1*	*51*	*0.9*	*11.5*	*0.1*	*1.6*
Black, in Kirsch, Drained, Opies*	1 Jar/250g	155	0.5	62	0.5	15	0.2	1.1
Dark, Sweet, Pitted, Frozen, Essential, Waitrose*	1 Serving/80g	44	0.1	55	0.9	11.5	0.1	2.1
Dried, Wholefoods, Tesco*	1 Serving/25g	86	0.2	345	1.9	81.6	0.8	4.6
Glace, Average	*1oz/28g*	*79*	*0*	*280*	*0.4*	*71.2*	*0.2*	*1.1*
Morello, Dried, Graze*	1 Pack/30g	100	0.4	335	4.5	82	1.5	0
Picota, Average	*1 Serving/80g*	*42*	*0.1*	*52*	*0.9*	*11.4*	*0.1*	*1.2*
Raw, Average	*1oz/28g*	*14*	*0*	*49*	*0.9*	*11.2*	*0.1*	*1.4*
Stewed with Sugar, Average	*1oz/28g*	*23*	*0*	*82*	*0.7*	*21*	*0.1*	*0.7*
Stewed without Sugar, Average	*1oz/28g*	*12*	*0*	*42*	*0.8*	*10.1*	*0.1*	*0.8*
CHERRYADE								
Barr's*	1 Serving/200ml	32	0	16	0	4	0	0
No Added Sugar, Morrisons*	1 Glass/250ml	2	0	1	0	0.1	0	0
Sugar Free, Tesco*	1 Glass/200ml	2	0	1	0	0	0	0
CHESTNUTS								
Average	*1 Serving/100g*	*174*	*2.3*	*174*	*2.9*	*31*	*2.3*	*8.9*
Candied, Marrons Glace, Wholefoods Online*	1 Piece/20g	65	0.2	325	0.8	76.4	0.8	4.8
Roasted, Peeled, Average	*1 Nut/10g*	*17*	*0.3*	*170*	*2*	*36.6*	*2.7*	*4.1*
CHEWING GUM								
Airwaves, Sugar Free, Wrigleys*	1 Pack/15g	23	0	155	0	62	0	0
Doublemint, Wrigleys*	1 Stick/3g	10	0	370	0	74.1	0	0
Extra, Cool Breeze, Wrigleys*	1 Piece/2g	3	0	153	0	64	0	0
Extra, Peppermint, Sugar Free, Wrigleys*	1 Piece/2g	3	0	155	0	39	0	0
Peppermint, Sugar Free, Active, Aldi*	2 Pieces/3g	4	0	146	0	61	0	0
Spearmint, Extra, Wrigleys*	1 Piece/1g	1	0	143	0	64.3	0	0
Spearmint, Wrigleys*	1 Piece/3g	9	0	295	0	73	0	0
Splash, Raspberry & Peach, Trident*	1 Piece/2g	4	0	180	1.6	68.5	0.5	0

	Measure INFO/WEIGHT	per Measure KCAL	FAT	Nutrition Values per 100g / 100ml KCAL	PROT	CARB	FAT	FIBRE
CHICK PEAS								
Canned, Drained, Average	*1 Can/240g*	*276*	*6*	*115*	*7.4*	*15.2*	*2.5*	*4.6*
Dried, Average	*1 Serving/100g*	*319*	*5.4*	*319*	*21.7*	*47.4*	*5.4*	*8*
Dried, Boiled, Average	*1 Serving/75g*	*85*	*1.7*	*114*	*7.3*	*16.4*	*2.2*	*2.6*
in Salted Water, Canned, Average	*1 Can/179g*	*204*	*5.2*	*114*	*7.2*	*14.9*	*2.9*	*4.1*
in Water, Canned, Average	*1 Can/250g*	*282*	*6.6*	*113*	*7.2*	*15.3*	*2.6*	*4.8*
Thai Sweet Chilli Flavour, Dry Roasted, Garbanzo*	1 Bag/65g	88	1.3	135	10.2	23.8	2	7.4
CHICKEN								
Bites, Hot & Spicy, Tesco*	1 Pack/110g	143	1.8	130	18.9	9.6	1.6	2.5
Bites, Hot And Spicy, Fridge Raiders, Mattessons*	1 Bag/60g	131	7.3	218	21.1	5.4	12.2	1.1
Bites, Southern Fried, Fridge Raiders, Mattessons*	1 Bag/60g	133	8.5	221	18.8	4.2	14.2	0.8
Bites, Southern Fried, Tesco*	1 Pack/300g	720	33.3	240	18.1	16.9	11.1	2.1
Bites, Tikka, Average	*1 Serving/50g*	*96*	*5.3*	*193*	*20.7*	*3.8*	*10.5*	*1.9*
Breast, Chargrilled, Premium, Average	*1 Piece/10g*	*13*	*0.3*	*134*	*25.9*	*0.6*	*2.6*	*0.3*
Breast, Chargrilled, Sliced, Average	*1 Slice/19g*	*24*	*0.5*	*124*	*24.4*	*0.5*	*2.7*	*0.4*
Breast, Diced, Average	*1 Serving/188g*	*242*	*4.4*	*129*	*26.9*	*0.1*	*2.4*	*0.1*
Breast, Fillet, Flame Grilled, Mini, Co-Op*	1 Pack/100g	144	2.8	144	30	0.5	2.8	0.5
Breast, Fillet, Pesto Breaded, Finest, Tesco*	½ Pack/151g	293	10.9	194	21.5	10.5	7.2	0.5
Breast, Fillets, Breaded, Average	*1 Fillet/112g*	*246*	*11.6*	*220*	*17.6*	*14*	*10.4*	*1.3*
Breast, Fillets, Breaded, Lemon & Pepper, Average	*1 Fillet/89g*	*133*	*2*	*150*	*22*	*10.1*	*2.3*	*1.3*
Breast, Fillets, Cajun, Average	*1 Fillet/93g*	*124*	*2.6*	*134*	*23.6*	*3.5*	*2.8*	*0.3*
Breast, Fillets, Chargrilled, Average	*1 Serving/100g*	*120*	*1.1*	*120*	*27.3*	*0.3*	*1.1*	*0.3*
Breast, Fillets, Garlic & Herb, Tesco*	1 Fillet/135g	290	12.2	215	18.9	14.4	9	1.3
Breast, Fillets, Korma Style, Average	*1 Serving/100g*	*132*	*2.8*	*132*	*27.4*	*0.8*	*2.8*	*0.6*
Breast, Fillets, Mini, Raw, Average	*1oz/28g*	*34*	*0.4*	*121*	*26.9*	*0.2*	*1.5*	*0.1*
Breast, Fillets, Organic, Average	*1 Serving/150g*	*153*	*1.1*	*102*	*24*	*0*	*0.8*	*0*
Breast, Fillets, Skinless & Boneless, Raw, Average	*1 Breast/100g*	*129*	*2*	*129*	*27.7*	*0*	*2*	*0*
Breast, Grilled, Average	*1 Breast/130g*	*174*	*2.8*	*134*	*29*	*0.1*	*2.2*	*0*
Breast, Meat & Skin, Raw, Average	*1 Serving/145g*	*249*	*13.4*	*172*	*20.8*	*0*	*9.2*	*0*
Breast, Meat & Skin, Weighed with Bone, Raw, Average	*1oz/28g*	*39*	*2.1*	*138*	*16.7*	*0*	*7.4*	*0*
Breast, Meat Only, Fried	*1 Serving/50g*	*68*	*1.7*	*137*	*24.4*	*0.4*	*3.4*	*0*
Breast, Pieces, BBQ, Sainsbury's*	½ Pack/70g	93	0.8	132	23.8	6.3	1.2	0.5
Breast, Pieces, Tikka, Average	*1 Serving/100g*	*154*	*3.4*	*154*	*28.2*	*2.8*	*3.4*	*0.4*
Breast, Roast, Sliced, From Supermarket, Average	*1 Slice/13g*	*17*	*0.4*	*139*	*25*	*1.8*	*3.5*	*0.2*
Breast, Roast, without Skin, Average	*1oz/28g*	*41*	*1.3*	*146*	*24.8*	*1*	*4.6*	*0.2*
Breast, Short Sliced, Mexican, Sainsbury's*	1 Pack/130g	177	2.9	136	26.4	2.5	2.2	0.1
Breast, Slices, Chargrill Style, Asda*	1 Slice/28g	31	0.6	112	22.7	0.8	2	0
Breast, Slices, Maple, Dulano, Lidl*	1 Slice/9g	10	0.2	111	20	3	2	0.5
Breast, Smoked, Sliced, Average	*1 Slice/20g*	*22*	*0.5*	*110*	*20.7*	*0.9*	*2.6*	*0.1*
Breast, Strips, Raw, Average	*1 Serving/280g*	*358*	*5.7*	*128*	*27.1*	*0.4*	*2*	*0.3*
Breast, Tandoori Style, Average	*1 Serving/180g*	*237*	*6.8*	*132*	*22.3*	*2.3*	*3.8*	*1*
Breast, Tikka, Sliced, Average	*1oz/28g*	*34*	*0.5*	*120*	*24.9*	*2*	*1.7*	*0.6*
Butter Basted, TTD, Sainsbury's*	1 Slice/30g	44	1.9	147	22.8	0	6.2	0.6
Dippers, Crispy, Average	*5 Dippers/93g*	*231*	*14.3*	*249*	*13.2*	*14.4*	*15.4*	*0.6*
Drumsticks, BBQ Flavour, Average	*1 Serving/200g*	*348*	*16*	*174*	*22.6*	*3.1*	*8*	*0.4*
Drumsticks, Breaded, Fried, Average	*1oz/28g*	*66*	*3.9*	*237*	*18.7*	*9.4*	*13.9*	*0.6*
Drumsticks, Chinese Style, Average	*1 Drumstick/100g*	*178*	*8.1*	*178*	*22.6*	*3.6*	*8.1*	*0.7*
Drumsticks, Meat & Skin, Weighed with Bone, Raw	*1 Drumstick/133g*	*188*	*11*	*141*	*15.7*	*0.1*	*8.3*	*0*
Drumsticks, Meat Only, Weighed with Bone, Raw	*1 Drumstick/122g*	*159*	*9.3*	*130*	*14.4*	*0.1*	*7.6*	*0*
Drumsticks, Meat Only, Weighed with Bone, Roast	*1 Serving/100g*	*116*	*5.5*	*116*	*16*	*0.3*	*5.5*	*0.1*
Drumsticks, with Skin, Average	*1 Piece/125g*	*268*	*16.6*	*215*	*22.1*	*1.8*	*13.3*	*0.3*
Escalope, Breaded, Average	*1 Escalope/128g*	*361*	*21.6*	*282*	*13.4*	*19.1*	*16.9*	*0.7*
Escalope, Plain, Breast, Average	*1 Serving/100g*	*110*	*2.2*	*110*	*22.3*	*0.7*	*2.2*	*0.5*
Fillet Strips, Barbeque, Birds Eye*	4 Strips/100.6g	180	8.7	179	18.9	6.5	8.6	0.2

CHICKEN

INFO/WEIGHT	Measure	per Measure KCAL	per Measure FAT	Nutrition Values per 100g / 100ml KCAL	PROT	CARB	FAT	FIBRE
Fillets, Battered, Average	*1 Fillet/90g*	*199*	*10.4*	*221*	*16.1*	*13.3*	*11.5*	*0.5*
Fillets, Breaded, Average	*1 Piece/98g*	*214*	*10.5*	*219*	*14.2*	*15.9*	*10.7*	*1.9*
Fillets, Cajun, Ashfield Farm, Aldi*	1 Fillet/122g	161	3.3	132	26	0.7	2.7	0.5
Fillets, Chinese Style, Average	*1oz/28g*	*37*	*0.5*	*132*	*24.4*	*4.6*	*1.8*	*0.5*
Fillets, Honey & Mustard, Average	*1 Serving/100g*	*138*	*3.7*	*138*	*18.4*	*7.5*	*3.7*	*0.8*
Fillets, Hot & Spicy, Average	*1oz/28g*	*58*	*3.1*	*206*	*16.4*	*10.5*	*11*	*1.1*
Fillets, Lime & Coriander, Mini, Average	*1 Fillet/42g*	*49*	*0.5*	*118*	*24.3*	*2.6*	*1.3*	*0.6*
Fillets, Mini, Sweet & Smokey, Eat Well, M&S*	½ Pack/60g	70	0.2	117	25.5	2.9	0.4	0.1
Fillets, Red Thai, Mini, Average	*1oz/28g*	*36*	*0.6*	*128*	*21.7*	*5.4*	*2*	*0.6*
Fillets, Roast, Sweet Chilli, Mini, British, Waitrose*	½ Pack/88g	119	0.9	136	23.5	8	1	0.5
Fillets, Southern Fried, Meat Only, Average	*1 Piece/100g*	*222*	*12*	*222*	*16.4*	*12.2*	*12*	*1.1*
Fillets, Sweet Chilli, Mini, Sainsbury's*	½ Pack/100g	119	1.1	119	21.8	5.4	1.1	0.9
Fillets, Tandoori Style, Mini, Average	*1 Serving/100g*	*128*	*2*	*128*	*24.7*	*2.6*	*2*	*0.4*
Fillets, Tikka, Average	*1 Serving/100g*	*141*	*5*	*141*	*22.4*	*1.7*	*5*	*1.1*
Fillets, Tikka, Mini, Average	*1oz/28g*	*35*	*0.6*	*124*	*25.1*	*1.3*	*2.2*	*1.2*
Fingers, Average	*1 Serving/75g*	*188*	*9.9*	*250*	*13.7*	*18.8*	*13.2*	*1.2*
Goujons, Breaded, Average	*1 Serving/114g*	*293*	*17.1*	*258*	*15.8*	*15.2*	*15*	*1*
Goujons, Breast, Fresh, Average	*1oz/28g*	*36*	*0.5*	*127*	*28*	*0*	*1.6*	*0*
Hunter's, Asda*	½ Pack/190g	348	14.1	183	19.1	10.1	7.4	0
Hunters, with Spicy Rice, Weight Watchers*	1 Serving/300g	311	3.6	104	7.8	14.3	1.2	2.3
Leg or Thigh, Hot & Spicy, Average	*1oz/28g*	*50*	*3*	*179*	*19.4*	*1*	*10.8*	*0.4*
Leg Portion, Roast, weighed with Bone, without Skin	*1 Portion/114g*	*175*	*11*	*153*	*30.9*	*0*	*9.6*	*0*
Leg Portion, Roasted Dry, with Skin, without Bone	*1 Portion/120g*	*188*	*11.8*	*156*	*16.7*	*0.2*	*9.8*	*0.2*
Leg, Meat Only, Raw, Average	*1oz/28g*	*34*	*1.1*	*120*	*20.1*	*0*	*3.8*	*0*
Leg, Meat Only, Raw, Weighed with Skin & Bone	*1oz/28g*	*21*	*0.7*	*76*	*12.8*	*0*	*2.4*	*0*
Leg, Meat Only, Stewed with Bone & Skin, Average	*1oz/28g*	*31*	*1.4*	*111*	*15.8*	*0*	*4.8*	*0*
Leg, with Skin, Raw, Average	*1oz/28g*	*48*	*2.9*	*172*	*19.1*	*0*	*10.4*	*0*
Leg, with Skin, Roasted, Weighed with Bone, Average	*1oz/28g*	*47*	*3.3*	*166*	*15.3*	*0.1*	*11.6*	*0*
Light Meat, Raw	*1oz/28g*	*30*	*0.3*	*106*	*24*	*0*	*1.1*	*0*
Light Meat, Roasted	*1oz/28g*	*43*	*1*	*153*	*30.2*	*0*	*3.6*	*0*
Meat & Skin Portions, Deep Fried, Average	*1oz/28g*	*73*	*4.7*	*259*	*26.9*	*0*	*16.8*	*0*
Meat & Skin, Roasted, Average	*1oz/28g*	*60*	*3.9*	*216*	*22.6*	*0*	*14*	*0*
Meat, Roasted, Average	*1oz/28g*	*50*	*2.1*	*177*	*27.3*	*0*	*7.5*	*0*
Mexican Chilli, Sliced, Eat Well, M&S*	1 Pack/130g	169	3.4	130	25.9	0.8	2.6	0.5
Mince, Average	*1oz/28g*	*39*	*1.7*	*140*	*20.9*	*0.1*	*6*	*0.2*
Nuggets, Battered, Average	*1 Nugget/20g*	*50*	*2.9*	*251*	*13.5*	*16.9*	*14.4*	*0.9*
Nuggets, Breaded, Average	*1 Nugget/14g*	*37*	*2*	*263*	*14.8*	*19.8*	*13.8*	*1.9*
Nuggets, Free From Gluten & Wheat, Sainsbury's*	1 Nugget/19g	47	2.5	251	13.4	19.7	13.2	0.8
Pieces, Barbeque, Chunky, Ready to Eat, Tesco*	1 Pack/200g	290	4	145	25.4	5.3	2	0.5
Pieces, Boneless, Breaded, Fried, From Restaurant	*1 Piece/17g*	*51*	*3.3*	*301*	*17*	*14.4*	*19.4*	*0*
Pieces, Flame Grilled, Waitrose*	1 Pack/130g	168	2.3	129	27.9	0.2	1.8	0.2
Pieces, Vegan, Quorn*	1 Serving/100g	104	1.4	104	16	4.3	1.4	5.3
Roll, Breast, Average	*1 Slice/10g*	*17*	*1*	*167*	*16.1*	*3.2*	*10*	*0.2*
Roll, Value, Tesco*	1 Slice/13g	30	2.2	223	15.4	3.9	16.2	0.1
Schnitzel, As Prepared, Easy to Cook, Waitrose*	½ Pack/99g	168	5.4	170	27	2.4	5.5	1.3
Shashlik, Patak's*	1 Serving/250g	203	3.6	81	12.4	4.4	1.4	0
Skewers, Indian Style, Party Bites, Sainsbury's*	1 Skewer/10g	18	0.4	182	27.3	9.2	3.9	0.5
Skewers, Marinated, Asda*	1 Skewer/35g	50	0.4	142	24.9	8	1.2	0.9
Skewers, with Choizo, Moordale, Lidl*	1 Skewer/74g	110	3.5	148	22.1	4.3	4.7	0.5
Skewers, Yakitori, M&S*	1 Box/65g	125	4.5	192	20.9	11.2	6.9	0.6
Skin, Dry, Roasted or Grilled, Average	*1 Serving/100g*	*501*	*46.1*	*501*	*21.5*	*0*	*46.1*	*0*
Skin, Moist, Roasted or Grilled, Average	*1 Serving/100g*	*452*	*42.6*	*452*	*17*	*0*	*42.6*	*0*
Sliced, Cooked, Average	*1 Slice/15g*	*18*	*0.4*	*118*	*22.4*	*1.6*	*2.4*	*0.1*

INFO/WEIGHT	Measure	per Measure		Nutrition Values per 100g / 100ml				
		KCAL	FAT	KCAL	PROT	CARB	FAT	FIBRE
CHICKEN								
Spatchcock, Poussin, Sainsbury's*	1 Serving/122g	168	6.6	138	21.1	0.1	5.4	0.2
Steaks, Average	*1 Serving/100g*	*205*	*9.4*	*205*	*21.1*	*9*	*9.4*	*0.7*
Strips or Tenders, Chinese Style, Average	*1oz/28g*	*41*	*1.1*	*145*	*19.6*	*8*	*4.1*	*1*
Strips, Mexican, Sliced, M&S*	½ Pack/70g	77	0.4	110	24.3	2.3	0.6	0.5
Thigh, Meat & Skin, Casseroled, Average	*1oz/28g*	*65*	*4.6*	*233*	*21.5*	*0*	*16.3*	*0*
Thigh, Meat & Skin, Raw, Average	*1 Serving/100g*	*218*	*14.7*	*218*	*21.4*	*0*	*14.7*	*0*
Thigh, Meat & Skin, Weighed with Bone, Raw, Average	*1 Serving/100g*	*186*	*14.1*	*186*	*13.8*	*0.2*	*14.1*	*0*
Thigh, Meat Only, Diced, Casseroled	1oz/28g	50	2.4	180	25.6	0	8.6	0
Thigh, Meat Only, Raw, Average	*1 Thigh/90g*	*113*	*4.9*	*126*	*19.4*	*0*	*5.4*	*0*
Thigh, Roast, Average	*1 Serving/100g*	*238*	*15.6*	*238*	*23.8*	*0.4*	*15.6*	*0*
Vegetarian, Dippers, Quorn*	4 Dippers/92g	195	8	212	11.1	21.2	8.7	2.4
Vegetarian, Fillets, Breaded, Mini, Quorn*	1 Fillet/30g	59	2.9	196	10.2	15	9.6	4.5
Vegetarian, Fillets, Crispy, Quorn*	1 Fillet/100g	192	8.5	192	12.5	14.2	8.5	4
Vegetarian, Fillets, Garlic & Herb, Quorn*	1 Fillet/100g	208	9.8	208	13.9	16.1	9.8	4.1
Vegetarian, Nuggets, Crispy, Chicken Style, Quorn*	1 Nugget/17g	33	2	198	12	8	12	4.8
Vegetarian, Roast Style, Quorn*	1/5 Roast/90.6g	96	1.8	106	15	4.5	2	4.9
Vegetarian, Roast, Family, Frozen, Cooked, Quorn*	1 Serving/91g	132	5.5	145	16.6	3.6	6	5.3
Vegetarian, Slices, Deli, Chicken Style, Quorn*	1 Slice/12.5g	13	0.3	107	16.3	4.5	2.6	6
Vegetarian, Slices, Wafer Thin, Chicken Style, Quorn*	¼ Pack/25g	30	0.7	119	16.3	4.5	2.6	5.9
Wafer Thin, Average	*1 Slice/10g*	*12*	*0.4*	*120*	*19*	*2.8*	*3.6*	*0.2*
Whole, Garlic & Herb, Lidl*	3 Slices/150g	261	16.5	174	18	0.6	11	0.5
Whole, Roast, Average	*½ Chicken/685g*	*910*	*57.7*	*133*	*13.4*	*0.9*	*8.4*	*0.1*
Wing Quarter, Meat Only, Casseroled	*1oz/28g*	*46*	*1.8*	*164*	*26.9*	*0*	*6.3*	*0*
Wing, Breaded, Fried, Average	*1oz/28g*	*77*	*4.8*	*273*	*17.1*	*13*	*17.2*	*0.4*
Wing, Meat & Skin, Cooked, Average	*1oz/28g*	*67*	*4.4*	*241*	*23.3*	*1.9*	*15.6*	*0.3*
Wings, BBQ Flavour, Average	*3 Wings/150g*	*330*	*18.7*	*220*	*20.3*	*6.6*	*12.4*	*0.6*
Wings, Chinese Style, Average	*1oz/28g*	*72*	*4.3*	*256*	*24.2*	*5.1*	*15.5*	*0.6*
Wings, Chinese Style, M&S*	½ Pack /175g	388	22.8	222	22.8	3.3	13	0.1
Wings, Hot & Spicy, Average	*1oz/28g*	*65*	*3.8*	*231*	*21.8*	*5.2*	*13.6*	*0.8*
Wings, Meat & Skin, Raw, Average	*1oz/28g*	*52*	*3.3*	*184*	*19*	*0.5*	*11.8*	*0.2*
Wings, Piri Piri, Mixed, Frozen, As Consumed, Tesco*	1 Wing/18g	41	2.5	229	22.4	3.3	13.9	0.5
CHICKEN &								
Bacon, Forestiere, As Prepared, 1, Waitrose*	½ Pack/200g	250	9.2	133	18.6	3.4	4.9	0.6
Black Bean Noodles, Sainsbury's*	1 Serving/130g	155	0.9	119	4.3	23.9	0.7	0.8
Black Bean Sauce, with Egg Fried Rice, Ready Meal	*1 Serving/400g*	*390*	*6.1*	*97*	*6.5*	*14.5*	*1.5*	*0.8*
Black Bean with Noodles, Tesco*	1 Pack/475g	470	7.6	99	7.6	13.6	1.6	0.2
Black Bean with Rice, Chinese, Tesco*	1 Serving/450g	459	9.5	102	5.3	15.4	2.1	0.5
Black Bean, Chinese Takeaway, Tesco*	1 Serving/200g	190	6.6	95	8.3	8	3.3	0.5
Butternut Squash, Curry Pot, Weight Watchers*	1 Pot/250g	232	3.5	93	6.6	12.5	1.4	1.6
Cashew Nuts, Chinese, Cantonese, Sainsbury's*	½ Pack/175g	172	8.8	98	8.4	4.9	5	1.3
Cashew Nuts, Chinese, Ready Meal, Average	*1 Serving/400g*	*497*	*24*	*124*	*9.2*	*7.5*	*6*	*1.2*
Cashew Nuts, Oriental, HL, Tesco*	1 Pack/450g	436	4.5	97	7	15.1	1	0.7
Chorizo Paella, Go Cook, Asda*	½ Pack/475g	591	10.5	124	10.2	15.9	2.2	2.6
Cous Cous, HE, Tesco*	1 Pack/351g	263	1.8	75	10.3	7.3	0.5	1.4
Fries, Southern Fried Style, Tesco*	1 Pack/500g	930	40	186	11.5	16	8	1.4
Gravy, COU, M&S*	1 Pack/300g	216	3.9	72	7.2	7.8	1.3	1.6
King Prawn Special Fried Rice, Finest, Tesco*	1 Pack/450g	734	32	163	7.7	17	7.1	0.7
Mushroom with Rice, Egg Fried, Average	*1 Serving/400g*	*421*	*10.1*	*105*	*6.3*	*14.4*	*2.5*	*0.8*
Mushroom, Al Forno, Charlie Bigham's*	½ Pack/324g	509	29.2	157	7.2	11.2	9	0.6
Mushroom, Chinese, Sainsbury's*	½ Pack/175g	116	3.5	66	7.6	4.4	2	0.9
Mushroom, Chinese, Tesco*	1 Pack/460g	474	12.9	103	5.7	13.8	2.8	1
Peppers in a Black Bean Sauce, M&S*	1 Pack/320g	256	4.8	80	9.4	7.3	1.5	1.2

	Measure INFO/WEIGHT	per Measure KCAL	FAT	Nutrition Values per 100g / 100ml KCAL	PROT	CARB	FAT	FIBRE
CHICKEN &								
Pineapple, Chilled, Tesco*	1 Pack/350g	364	8.4	104	9.6	11.1	2.4	5.5
Roasted Potatoes, Spanish, Charlie Bigham's*	½ Pack/387g	479	25.9	124	7.2	9.8	6.7	0
Stuffing, Roast, HL, Tesco*	1 Serving/17g	19	0.2	111	23.3	1.3	1.4	0.2
Tomato & Basil, COU, M&S*	½ Pack/200g	180	4.6	90	14.3	3.4	2.3	0.8
CHICKEN ALFREDO								
Average	*1 Pack/400g*	*416*	*10*	*104*	*12.2*	*8.2*	*2.5*	*0.8*
CHICKEN ARRABIATA								
Bistro, Waitrose*	½ Pack/175g	156	5.2	89	12.9	2.5	3	0.5
COU, M&S*	1 Meal/360g	396	6.5	110	8.4	14.5	1.8	1.3
Easy Steam, HL, Tesco*	1 Pack/400g	284	3.2	71	8.4	7.6	0.8	1.2
GFY, Asda*	1 Pack/447.7g	394	3.1	88	5.2	15.1	0.7	1.1
HL, Tesco*	1 Pack/387g	341	1.5	88	7.3	13.3	0.4	1.2
Italian Kitchen, Tesco*	1 Pack/370g	411	11.5	111	7.6	12.4	3.1	1.5
Italian, Microwaved, Iceland*	1 Pack/366g	421	8.1	115	7	16.2	2.2	1.3
Meal for One, M&S*	1 Pack/400g	528	20.8	132	7.9	12.5	5.2	1.9
with Spiralized Vegetables, Balanced for You, M&S*	1 Pack/370g	229	5.9	62	6.8	3.9	1.6	2.4
CHICKEN BANG BANG								
Waitrose*	1 Pack/350g	368	17.2	105	9.4	5.9	4.9	1.2
CHICKEN BUTTER								
with Rice, Average	*1 Serving/400g*	*561*	*27.6*	*140*	*10.6*	*8.9*	*6.9*	*1.4*
CHICKEN CAJUN								
& Potato Hash, HL, Tesco*	1 Pack/450g	428	6.3	95	6.5	14.1	1.4	1.5
Breast, Chargrilled, Iceland*	1 Serving/80g	114	1.5	142	27.4	3.9	1.9	0
Breast, Morrisons*	½ Pack/180g	328	16.9	182	16.6	7.7	9.4	2
CHICKEN CANTONESE								
& Rice, Sizzler, Tesco*	1 Serving/450g	639	25.6	142	7.7	14.9	5.7	0.9
Breast, Fillets, Sainsbury's*	1 Serving/154g	168	2.3	109	20.3	3.6	1.5	0.6
Chinese, Tesco*	½ Pack/175g	196	6.5	112	10.3	9.4	3.7	0.4
Honey, Sesame, Sainsbury's*	1/3 Pack/135g	116	3.6	86	9.8	5.5	2.7	0.8
CHICKEN CARIBBEAN								
Fruity with Rice & Peas, New, BGTY, Sainsbury's*	1 Pack/400g	352	3.6	88	6.9	13.1	0.9	2.2
with Rice & Beans, One Pot, Cook*	1 Pot/300g	387	19.2	129	6.7	7.4	6.4	7.4
with Rice & Peas, HL, Tesco*	1 Pack/360g	434	3.6	121	8.5	16.7	1	5.4
CHICKEN CHAR SUI								
Shredded, Ready To Eat, Tesco*	½ Pack/65g	77	0.8	119	20.4	5.8	1.3	1
CHICKEN CHASSEUR								
Average	*1 Serving/400g*	*363*	*9.2*	*91*	*12.2*	*4.9*	*2.3*	*0.9*
Breast Fillets, Morrisons*	1 Pack/380g	384	11.4	101	15.7	2.9	3	0.8
Finest, Tesco*	½ Pack/200g	200	6.4	100	14.3	2.4	3.2	1.1
CHICKEN CHILLI								
Sweet & Egg Fried Rice, HL, Tesco*	1 Serving/450g	446	8.1	99	5.7	15	1.8	0.4
Sweet with Noodles, Frozen, HL, Tesco*	1 Pack/330g	291	3.6	88	7.4	11.4	1.1	1.4
Sweet, CBY, Asda*	½ Pack/170g	253	6.8	149	19.1	8.9	4	0.7
Sweet, Just Cook, Sainsbury's*	½ Pack/190.5g	200	1.3	105	15.2	9.4	0.7	0.5
Sweet, Pieces, Morrisons*	1 Pack/200g	282	5	141	25.5	4.1	2.5	0.5
Sweet, With Noodles, Ready Meal, Average	*1 Serving/400g*	*404*	*5.8*	*101*	*6.5*	*15.5*	*1.4*	*1.4*
CHICKEN CHINESE								
& Prawns, Sizzler, House Special, Tesco*	1 Serving/450g	684	23.4	152	7.5	18.8	5.2	1.2
Balls, M&S*	1 Ball/16g	45	2.2	280	10.8	29.2	13.6	2.1
Crispy Aromatic, Half, Tesco*	1 Serving/233g	524	24.2	225	16.3	16.7	10.4	1.2
Fillets, with Sweet Chilli Sauce, Tesco*	1 Serving/350g	592	22	169	8.8	19.2	6.3	0.7
Stir Fry, Morrisons*	1 Serving/319g	341	5.4	107	5.7	17	1.7	1.5
Style Sauce, Breast Fillets, Morrisons*	½ Pack/200g	162	2	81	13.5	4.6	1	1.2

INFO/WEIGHT	Measure			Nutrition Values per 100g / 100ml				
		KCAL	FAT	KCAL	PROT	CARB	FAT	FIBRE
CHICKEN CHINESE								
with Ginger & Spring Onion, Tesco*	1 Serving/350g	299	10.1	85	7.6	7.3	2.9	0.6
CHICKEN CORONATION								
M&S*	1 Serving/200g	420	26.4	210	12.6	10.6	13.2	1.3
CHICKEN DINNER								
Cooked, Eat Smart, Morrisons*	1 Pack/355g	245	4.3	69	8.2	4.4	1.2	4.1
Ovenbaked, Slimzone, Asda*	1 Pack/452g	285	2.7	63	8.9	4.6	0.6	2
Roast, Mini, As Consumed, Fresh Ideas, Morrisons*	½ Pack/209g	310	13.6	148	18.7	3.3	6.5	1
Tesco*	1 Serving/400g	388	7.2	97	9.2	10.9	1.8	1.2
CHICKEN EN CROUTE								
Charlie Bigham's*	½ Pack/230g	568	36.8	247	11.1	14.1	16	0.6
Chef Select, Lidl*	½ Pack/206g	558	34.8	271	12.8	16.1	16.9	1.7
Just Cook, Sainsbury's*	1 Serving/180g	481	27.2	267	16.8	15.9	15.1	0.4
with Cheddar & Ham, Oven Baked, CBY, Asda*	½ Pack/209g	568	33.4	272	16	15.1	16	1.7
CHICKEN IN								
Barbeque Sauce, Breasts, COU, M&S*	1 Pack/350g	420	6.7	120	8.5	20.6	1.9	0.6
BBQ Sauce, Breast, Sainsbury's*	1 Serving/170g	199	1.2	117	14.5	13.1	0.7	1.3
Black Bean Sauce with Rice, Asda*	1 Pack/400g	500	7.6	125	7	20	1.9	0.6
Black Bean Sauce with Rice, Iceland*	1 Pack/400g	388	6	97	5.1	15.8	1.5	0.8
Black Bean Sauce, Asia, Aldi*	1 Pack/375g	364	10.9	97	10.9	6.1	2.9	1.3
Black Bean Sauce, M&S*	1 Pack/350g	298	7	85	8.7	8	2	1.1
Black Bean Sauce, Sainsbury's*	1 Pack/465g	484	7.9	104	5	17.3	1.7	0.3
Black Bean Sauce, Somerfield*	½ Pack/175g	133	1.8	76	10.7	6.1	1	1.9
Black Bean Sauce, Takeaway, Iceland*	1 Pack/375g	345	11.2	92	8.6	7	3	1.5
Cabernet Sauvignon Wine, Finest, Tesco*	½ Pack/192g	213	6.1	111	14.7	5.6	3.2	0.6
Creamy Mushroom Sauce, Weight Watchers*	1 Pack/330g	343	9.6	104	7	12.5	2.9	0.6
Creamy Mustard Sauce, GFY, Asda*	1 Pack/400g	468	9.2	117	6	18	2.3	0.4
Creamy Tikka Style Sauce, Tesco*	1 Breast/190g	215	10.4	113	15.1	0.7	5.5	0.8
Gravy, Breast, Sainsbury's*	1 Box/200g	124	1	62	11.8	2.9	0.5	0.2
Hot Ginger Sauce with Thai Sticky Rice, Sainsbury's*	1 Pack/450g	603	20.7	134	6.8	16.3	4.6	0.5
Hunter's BBQ Sauce, Asda*	½ Pack /190g	348	14.1	183	19.1	10.3	7.4	0
Leek & Bacon Sauce, Chilled, Co-Op*	1 Pack/400g	460	20	115	15	2	5	0.2
Lemon & Garlic Marinade, Thighs, Go Cook, Asda*	½ Pack/265g	493	30.2	186	19.7	1.2	11.4	0.8
Lemon Sauce with Rice, Sainsbury's*	1 Pack/450g	513	6.8	114	8.1	17	1.5	0.7
Light Batter, Bites, Captain Birds Eye, Birds Eye*	1 Piece/15g	32	1.9	210	18.6	5.8	12.5	0.2
Madeira Sauce with Mushrooms, Finest, Tesco*	½ Pack/200g	210	8.3	105	13.8	3	4.2	1
Masala with Spiced Indian Lentils, M&S*	1 Pack/330g	297	8.2	90	10.3	6.1	2.5	5.9
Mexican Salsa, Tesco*	1 Pack/320g	368	8.6	115	19.5	3.1	2.7	0.6
Mexican Style Sauce, Tesco*	1 Serving/180g	128	1.4	71	13.3	2.6	0.8	0.7
Mushroom Sauce, 124, Oakhouse Foods Ltd*	1 Meal/380g	334	8	88	8.5	9.7	2.1	1.7
Oyster Sauce & Mushrooms, Tesco*	1 Pack/350g	252	5.6	72	8	6.3	1.6	0.7
Peanut Sauce, Cafe Classics, Lean Cuisine	1 Pack 9oz/255g	300	9	118	7.8	13.7	3.5	1.2
Red Wine Sauce, Breasts, Fresh Tastes, Asda*	½ Pack/190g	245	8	129	20.5	2.4	4.2	0.5
Reggae Reggae Sauce, Drumsticks, Levi Roots*	1 Serving/100g	165	7.3	165	21.5	3.4	7.3	0
Smoky Barbeque Sauce, Tesco*	1 Serving/185g	229	3.9	124	16.3	9.9	2.1	1
Smoky BBQ Marinade, Breast, Fillets, Mini, CBY, Asda*	3 Fillets/150g	144	1.5	96	18.5	3.3	1	0
Sticky Balsamic Glaze, Chargrilled, COU, M&S*	1 Pack/370g	296	2.2	80	7	11.2	0.6	1.3
Sweet Chilli Sauce, Breast, Fresh Tastes, Asda*	½ Pack/180g	288	9	160	18.4	10.3	5	0.5
Tomato & Basil Sauce, Breast Fillets, Morrisons*	½ Pack/171g	231	7.5	135	21.3	2.5	4.4	1.4
Tomato & Basil Sauce, Breast, GFY, Asda*	1 Pack/392g	447	13.3	114	12	9	3.4	1.5
Tomato & Herb Sauce, Breasts, Tesco*	½ Pack/172.5g	155	2.4	90	15	3.6	1.4	0.5
Tomato & Basil Sauce, Breast, Fresh Tastes, Asda*	½ Pack/130g	136	2.7	105	19.3	2.3	2.1	0.7
White Sauce, Canned, HL, Tesco*	½ Can/200g	180	5.8	90	14.3	1.3	2.9	5.4
White Wine & Tarragon Sauce, Breasts, Finest, Tesco*	½ Pack/200g	326	20.2	163	16.8	1.3	10.1	0

C

	Measure INFO/WEIGHT	per Measure KCAL	FAT	Nutrition Values per 100g / 100ml KCAL	PROT	CARB	FAT	FIBRE
CHICKEN IN								
White Wine & Tarragon Sauce, Waitrose*	½ Pack/225g	281	17.3	125	10.7	3.1	7.7	0.3
White Wine Sauce, Breasts, Tesco*	1 Serving/370g	388	14.1	105	16.9	0.8	3.8	0.6
Zesty Orange Sauce, Breast, Asda*	1 Serving/200g	326	14	163	16	9	7	0
CHICKEN KATSU								
Coconut, Everdine*	1 Serving/450g	585	28.4	130	9.1	7.2	6.3	4.4
Curry, City Kitchen, Tesco*	1 Pack/385g	465	13.2	121	6	16.3	3.4	1.3
CHICKEN LEMON								
Balls, Asda*	1 Ball/15g	42	2.6	279	14	19	17	1.6
Battered, Cantonese, Sainsbury's*	1 Pack/350g	560	19.6	160	10.7	16.6	5.6	0.9
Battered, Chinese Meal for Two, Tesco*	½ Serving/175g	294	13	168	6.6	18.8	7.4	2
Cantonese Style with Egg Fried Rice, Farmfoods*	1 Pack/324g	486	15.6	150	4.9	21.8	4.8	0.1
Cantonese, Sainsbury's*	½ Pack/140g	218	8.8	156	11	13.9	6.3	0.6
Chinese, Tesco*	1 Serving/350g	564	11.2	161	7	26	3.2	0.3
COU, M&S*	1 Pack/150g	150	1.4	100	17.9	5.6	0.9	0.8
Tesco*	½ Pack/175g	214	7.4	122	11	10.1	4.2	0.6
with Vegetable Rice, BGTY, Sainsbury's*	1 Pack/400g	428	6.4	107	6.5	16.8	1.6	0.8
CHICKEN MADEIRA								
with Mushroom Rice, Finest, Tesco*	1 Pack/413g	570	16.9	138	9.9	14.5	4.1	1.5
CHICKEN MOROCCAN								
Style with Spicy Cous Cous, BGTY, Sainsbury's*	1 Serving/225g	304	3.8	135	9.2	20.6	1.7	0
Style, Sainsbury's*	½ Pack/269g	334	7	124	14.7	10.4	2.6	3.1
with Bulgur Wheat, Good & Balanced, Asda*	1 Pack/375g	365	3.4	98	7.4	13.3	0.9	3.4
with Cous Cous & Fruity Sauce, BGTY, Sainsbury's*	1 Pack/400g	440	8	110	10	13.1	2	2.6
with Cous Cous, GFY, Asda*	1 Serving/450g	414	5.8	92	8	12	1.3	0.8
CHICKEN ORIENTAL								
with Noodles, SteamFresh, Birds Eye*	1 Pack/400g	336	8.8	84	7.1	9	2.2	0.3
CHICKEN PASANDA								
Sainsbury's*	1 Serving/200g	368	24.8	184	14.7	3.4	12.4	2.3
with Pilau Rice, HL, Tesco*	1 Pack/440g	466	11	106	5.7	15.2	2.5	0.9
CHICKEN PEPPERONATA								
M&S*	1 Pack/379g	258	5.7	68	6.1	6.5	1.5	1.8
CHICKEN PIRI PIRI								
& Rice, HE, Tesco*	1 Pack/395g	395	7.9	100	8.2	12	2	1.7
Breast, Fillets, Mini, Tesco*	½ Pack/100g	135	1.1	135	22.7	7.6	1.1	0
M&S*	1 Pack/300g	420	23.1	140	10	7.3	7.7	1.3
Sliced, Just Add, M&S*	½ Pack/60g	91	2.8	152	26.9	0.2	4.7	0
with Rice, BGTY, Sainsbury's*	1 Serving/399g	395	4.4	99	10.3	11.9	1.1	1.6
CHICKEN PROVENCALE								
M&S*	1 Pack/430g	366	11.6	85	13.2	2.3	2.7	0.6
CHICKEN STUFFED								
Breast with Mushrooms, HE, Tesco*	1 Serving/175g	152	3.2	87	16.3	1.5	1.8	0.2
with Moroccan Style Cous Cous, GFY, Asda*	½ Pack/180g	259	4.9	144	20	10	2.7	0
with Mushrooms, Finest, Tesco*	1 Serving/150g	177	7.6	118	15.9	2	5.1	0.6
CHICKEN SUPREME								
Breast, Sainsbury's*	1 Serving/187g	421	29.5	225	20.6	0.3	15.8	0.6
with Rice, Asda*	1 Pack/450g	616	31.5	137	15	3.4	7	1.1
with Rice, HE, Tesco*	1 Pack/400g	384	6.4	96	4.9	15.6	1.6	1.5
CHICKEN SZECHUAN								
Tesco*	1 Pack/350g	385	10.5	110	7.2	13.6	3	0.3
with Noodles, Sainsbury's*	1 Pack/450g	423	14	94	6	10.4	3.1	0.9
CHICKEN TANDOORI								
& Basmati Rice, Aromatic, Asda*	1 Pack/380g	399	8	105	7.5	12	2.1	3.7
& Spiced Rice, As Consumed, Eat Smart, Morrisons*	1 Pack/380g	416	4.8	113	7.8	16.1	1.3	2.8

	Measure INFO/WEIGHT	per Measure KCAL	FAT	Nutrition Values per 100g / 100ml KCAL	PROT	CARB	FAT	FIBRE
CHICKEN TANDOORI								
Fresh Tastes, Asda*	1 Pack/400g	356	5.6	89	6.4	12.7	1.4	2.1
Masala & Rice, HL, Tesco*	1 Serving/450g	410	7.6	91	6.6	12.9	1.7	0.6
Masala, Indian, Tesco*	1 Serving/350g	430	25.9	123	10.2	4	7.4	1.8
Masala, Sainsbury's*	1 Pack/400g	536	27.2	134	13.2	5	6.8	0.5
Royal, with Pilau Rice & Aloo Gobi, Co-Op*	1 Pack/451g	591	26.6	131	7.4	12	5.9	0.5
Sizzler, Sainsbury's*	1 Pack/400g	536	29.2	134	12.8	4.3	7.3	1.7
Sizzler, Tesco*	1 Serving/175g	243	11.6	139	10	10	6.6	1
Steam Meal, As Consumed, Simply Bistro, Aldi*	1 Pack/400g	317	7.5	80	5.5	9.3	1.9	2.1
with Rice, City Kitchen, Tesco*	1 Pack/385g	597	21.2	155	6.7	19.6	5.5	1.8
with Vegetable Pilau Rice, HL, Tesco*	1 Pack/347.8g	400	9	115	8.4	14.1	2.6	1.9
CHICKEN TERIYAKI								
& Noodles, Asda*	½ Pack/340g	445	8.8	131	9	18	2.6	0.9
Japanese with Ramen Noodles, Sainsbury's*	1 Pack/450g	482	9.4	107	6.5	15.5	2.1	0.8
Noodles, HL, Tesco*	1 Pack/367g	282	1.8	77	6.4	10.5	0.5	2.3
CHICKEN TIKKA								
& Cous Cous, Boots*	1 Pack/160g	307	17.6	192	6.2	17	11	1.3
& Lemon Rice, Deli Meal, M&S*	1 Pack/360g	342	7.2	95	9.8	10.2	2	0.7
& Coriander Rice, Weight Watchers*	1 Pack/400g	348	2.4	87	6.2	14.3	0.6	1.6
Creamy, Breast, Tesco*	1 Breast/190g	215	10.4	113	15.1	0.7	5.5	0.8
Masala, & Pilau Rice, Charlie Bigham's*	½ Pack/403g	657	38.3	163	5.9	14.2	9.5	0
Masala, with Rice, Weight Watchers*	1 Meal/320g	377	5.8	118	6.8	18.3	1.8	0.7
Takeaway	***1 Serving/350g***	***421***	***15***	***120***	***20.3***	***0***	***4.3***	***0.3***
with Basmati Rice, Weight Watchers*	1 Pack/380g	342	6.5	90	6.6	11.8	1.7	1.1
with Pilau Rice, GFY, Asda*	1 Pack/450g	382	2.7	85	7	13	0.6	1.8
CHICKEN WITH								
a Sea Salt & Black Pepper Crust, Breasts, Asda*	1 Serving/154g	186	4.3	121	19	5	2.8	0
a Sticky Honey & Chilli Sauce, Breast, Asda*	1 Serving/175g	247	5.6	141	20	8	3.2	0
Apricots & Almonds, HE, Tesco*	1 Pack/500g	465	9.5	93	11.8	7.3	1.9	0.5
Bacon & Leeks, GFY, Asda*	1 Pack/400g	328	8	82	13	3	2	0.6
Basil Pesto & Parmesan Crust, Breast, COOK!, M&S*	½ Pack/150g	240	11	160	20.9	1.8	7.3	0.8
Broccoli & Pesto Pasta, BGTY, Sainsbury's*	1 Pack/301g	328	5.1	109	10.3	13.2	1.7	2.5
Butternut Squash Rice, Reggae Reggae, Levi Roots*	1 Pack/450g	495	13.5	110	5.8	14	3	1.1
Caesar Melt & Prosciutto, Breast, M&S*	1 Pack/375g	488	18.8	130	19.6	1.3	5	1
Cheese Croutons & Onion, Asda*	1 Serving/200g	200	6.4	100	16	2	3.2	0.9
Cheese, Leek & Ham, Breast, Fresh Tastes, Asda*	1 Pack/430g	658	30.5	153	18.9	3.4	7.1	0.7
Chorizo & Tomato Sauce, Catalan, Charlie Bigham's*	1 Pack/479g	407	15.8	85	10.9	2.8	3.3	0.7
Chorizo & Manchego Cheese, Breasts, M&S*	½ Pack/178g	222	8.9	125	18.3	1.7	5	0.6
Chorizo & Patatas Bravas, COU, M&S*	1 Pack/400g	380	9.2	95	7.8	10.8	2.3	1.7
Coriander & Lime, Asda*	1 Serving/105g	122	0.9	116	24	2.9	0.9	0.2
Cous Cous, Harissa, PB, Waitrose*	1 Pack/400g	348	8	87	7.6	9.5	2	1.7
Cous Cous, Lemon & Herb, Finest, Tesco*	1 Pack/370g	492	18.5	133	10.5	11.5	5	0.9
Cranberry Stuffing, Breast, Finest, Tesco*	½ Pack/200g	252	4.8	126	16.2	9.9	2.4	0.9
Fresh Mango, Chilli & Coriander, British, COU, M&S*	1 Pack/168.8g	270	3.9	160	12.1	22.8	2.3	1.9
Fusilli & Courgette, Sainsbury's*	1 Pack/450g	675	28.8	150	8.6	14.6	6.4	0.5
Garlic & Herbs, Asda*	1 Slice/25g	28	0.4	114	23.9	1.1	1.5	0
Garlic & Chilli Balti, Tesco*	1 Pack/400g	320	7.6	80	11	4.4	1.9	0.8
Garlic Mushrooms, Asda*	1 Serving/320g	342	16	107	13.8	1.8	5	2.2
Garlic Mushrooms, Breast, Simply Cook, Tesco*	½ Pack/125g	170	6.6	136	22	0.1	5.3	0.1
Garlic Mushrooms, Breast, Tesco*	1 Breast/125g	149	5.9	119	19	0.2	4.7	0.1
Gravy & Stuffing, Breasts, Tesco*	½ Pack/173g	257	11.1	149	14.4	8.3	6.4	2.2
Honey & Ginger Sauce, 125, Oakhouse Foods Ltd*	1 Dinner/365g	339	8	93	8.7	9.8	2.2	1.2
Leek & Bacon, Creamy Sauce, Simply Bistro, Aldi*	1 Pack/400g	348	10.8	87	7.5	7.3	2.7	2.1
Leek & Bacon, M&S*	½ Pack/183g	239	12.8	131	15.3	1.2	7	0.9

	Measure INFO/WEIGHT	per Measure KCAL	FAT	Nutrition Values per 100g / 100ml KCAL	PROT	CARB	FAT	FIBRE
CHICKEN WITH								
Lemon Grass, Thai Greens & Baby Corn, Sainsbury's*	1 Serving/200g	196	6.8	98	10	6.9	3.4	1.4
Lime & Coriander, Easy, Waitrose*	½ Pack/168g	203	7.9	121	18.9	0.7	4.7	0.5
Lyonnaise Potatoes, M&S*	½ Pack/260g	286	8.1	110	12.6	8	3.1	0.9
Manchego & Sun Dried Tomato Filling, Tesco*	½ Pack/225g	325	10.5	144	24.3	1	4.7	0.5
Mango, Lime & Coriander, Asda*	1 Pack/400g	416	6	104	6.6	15.9	1.5	1.4
Mozzarella & Pancetta, Breast, Finest, Tesco*	½ Pack/225g	326	14	145	14.4	7.9	6.2	1.1
Mozzarella & Pesto Melt, Breasts, COOK!, M&S*	½ Pack/165g	206	10.2	125	16.4	1.3	6.2	0.7
Mushroom & Bacon, Fillets, M&S*	½ Pack/188g	225	11.2	120	15.5	0.5	6	1.7
Mushroom & Garlic Butter, Breasts, Sainsbury's*	½ Pack/195g	388	20.1	199	20	4.6	10.3	0.1
Mushroom Risotto, M&S*	1 Pack/400g	480	11.6	120	6.9	16.7	2.9	0.8
Mushrooms in Madeira Sauce, HE, Tesco*	½ Pack/200g	182	2	91	15	5.4	1	0.4
Pancakes & Plum Sauce, COU, M&S*	1 Pack/245g	257	5.6	105	7.9	12.7	2.3	0.3
Pasta, Chianti & Balsamic, BGTY, Sainsbury's*	1 Pack/400g	372	7.6	93	9.4	9.5	1.9	1.9
Plum Sauce, Battered, Tesco*	1 Serving/175g	324	10.2	185	6.7	26.5	5.8	0.8
Plum Tomatoes & Basil, Breast, Birds Eye*	1 Serving/172g	200	8.1	116	13.3	5	4.7	0.6
Pork Stuffing, Breast, Roast, M&S*	1 Serving/100g	165	6.5	165	24.1	3	6.5	0
Potato Wedges, Tomato & Basil, Weight Watchers*	1 Pack/330g	254	6.6	77	4.7	9.2	2	1.6
Rice 'n' Peas, Sainsbury's*	1 Pack/300g	489	18.3	163	12.5	14.4	6.1	2.1
Rice, Breast, Chargrilled, Spicy, Asda*	1 Pack/400g	372	2.4	93	6	16	0.6	1
Rice, Fiesta, Weight Watchers*	1 Pack/330g	307	6.6	93	6.1	12.8	2	0.4
Rice, Jamaican Jerk, Healthier Choice, Co-Op*	1 Pack/406g	365	9.3	90	7.8	9.8	2.3	3.4
Sage & Onion Stuffing, Breast, Roast, Sliced, M&S*	1 Slice/16.5g	27	1.1	165	24.1	3	6.5	0
Soured Cream, Cajun Spiced, Breast, COOK!, M&S*	½ Pack/200g	230	10.2	115	14.7	2.1	5.1	1.1
Soy & Ginger Noodles, Love Life, Waitrose*	1 Pot/360g	212	4.7	59	5	6.7	1.3	2.3
Spiced Butter, Jerk, Spicy, Half, Waitrose*	1 Pack/679g	1331	75.4	196	22.8	0.9	11.1	0.8
Spinach, Honey Mustard, American Style, Asda*	1 Serving/240g	394	24	164	14	4.4	10	0.3
Spirelli, Steam Meal, Tesco*	1 Serving/400g	400	10.8	100	6.6	12	2.7	1.2
Spring Vegetables, Chargrilled, COU, M&S*	1 Pack/414g	290	3.7	70	8.8	7.3	0.9	1.8
Stilton & Port Sauce, Breasts, Finest, Tesco*	1 Serving/400g	668	34.4	167	18.5	3.9	8.6	0.7
Stuffing, TTD, Sainsbury's*	1 Slice/34g	50	2	148	22.7	1.3	5.8	0.9
Sweet Chilli & Garlic, Chinese, Asda*	1 Serving/400g	436	2.4	109	8	18	0.6	2.1
Sweet Chilli Sauce & Egg Fried Rice, Tesco*	1 Pack/380g	494	10.3	130	7.5	18.2	2.7	1.3
Sweet Potato Mash, Jerk, Super Naturals, Sainsbury's*	1 Pack/400g	284	4.4	71	6.1	9.2	1.1	2.2
Tangy Lemon Sauce, Breasts, Just Cook, Sainsbury's*	1 Serving/164g	244	3	149	16.2	16.9	1.8	0.1
Vegetables, Curried, Plumrose*	1 Serving/196g	253	16.1	129	5.8	8	8.2	0
CHICORY								
Fresh, Raw, Average	*1 Head/150g*	*30*	*0.9*	*20*	*0.6*	*2.8*	*0.6*	*0.9*
CHILLI								
& Potato Wedges, Good Choice, Iceland*	1 Pack/400g	368	13.6	92	5.5	9.8	3.4	1.2
& Rice, Birds Eye*	1 Serving/285g	305	7.7	107	3.4	17.2	2.7	1
& Rice, GFY, Asda*	1 Pack/400g	352	1.6	88	5	16	0.4	1.8
& Wedges, BBQ, HL, Tesco*	1 Pack/420g	391	10.9	93	5.4	12.2	2.6	1.9
& Potato Wedges, Sainsbury's*	1 Pack/371g	393	15.2	106	7.2	10.1	4.1	2.2
& Rice, Morrisons*	1 Serving/500g	630	15.5	126	5.7	18.9	3.1	1.1
& Wedges, GFY, Asda*	1 Pack/400g	364	10	91	7	10.1	2.5	2.5
Beef & Mushrooms, GFY, Asda*	1 Pack/400g	364	6	91	9.1	10.2	1.5	1.2
Beef & Potato Crush, Weight Watchers*	1 Pack/400g	232	6	58	5	5.9	1.5	3.4
Beef & Rice Pot, Shapers, Boots*	1 Pot/301g	250	4.5	83	4	12	1.5	2.1
Beef with Rice, GFY, Asda*	1 Serving/402g	354	6	88	4.7	14	1.5	0.9
Beef with Rice, Sainsbury's*	1 Serving/300g	360	5.1	120	5.6	20.6	1.7	1.1
Beef, Asda*	½ Pack/200g	190	7.8	95	7	8	3.9	1.2
Beef, High Protein, Mexican Bean, Batchelors*	1 Pack/270g	228	4.1	84	4.7	11.3	1.5	3.4
Con Carne & Rice, Somerfield*	1 Pack/500g	490	5	98	5	18	1	0

C

CHILLI

INFO/WEIGHT	Measure	per Measure KCAL	FAT	Nutrition Values per 100g / 100ml KCAL	PROT	CARB	FAT	FIBRE
Con Carne & Rice, Everyday, Value, Tesco*	1 Pack/400g	455	11.1	115	5	15.5	2.8	3.3
Con Carne & Rice, Tex Mex, M Kitchen, Morrisons*	1 Pack/450g	580	22.9	129	0.5	14.9	5.1	0.5
Con Carne & Sweetcorn Mash, Fuller Longer, M&S*	1 Pack/400g	380	13.2	95	8.5	7.4	3.3	3.9
Con Carne with Rice, GFY, Asda*	1 Serving/400g	456	6.4	114	6	19	1.6	0.9
Con Carne with Rice, Healthy Choice, Asda*	1 Pack/400g	412	8.4	103	6	15	2.1	0.9
Con Carne with Rice, Morrisons*	1 Pack/400g	328	5.2	82	5.3	12.2	1.3	1.4
Con Carne with Rice, Organic, Sainsbury's*	1 Pack/400g	472	10.8	118	5	18.5	2.7	1.8
Con Carne, & Mexican Rice, Charlie Bigham's*	½ Pack/430g	563	22.8	131	6	14.7	5.3	0
Con Carne, & Rice, Fiesta, Aldi*	1 Pack/450g	648	24.3	144	6.7	16	5.4	2.3
Con Carne, 2 Minute Meals, Sainsbury's*	1 Pouch/200g	146	3.2	73	6	8.6	1.6	2.7
Con Carne, Asda*	1 Can/392g	376	13.7	96	7	9	3.5	0
Con Carne, Baked Bean, Heinz*	1 Can/390g	324	5.8	83	7	10.3	1.5	2.8
Con Carne, Beef, Look What We Found*	1 Pack/250g	243	9.5	97	7.5	6.2	3.8	4.1
Con Carne, Canned, El Tequito, Lidl*	1 Serving/320g	365	10.2	114	7.1	14	3.2	0.5
Con Carne, Canned, Morrisons*	1 Can/392g	368	11.8	94	8.8	8	3	2.4
Con Carne, Canned, Sainsbury's*	½ Can/200g	162	4.2	81	6.6	8.9	2.1	2.5
Con Carne, Canned, Tesco*	½ Can/200g	220	11.4	110	7.8	6.4	5.7	4.7
Con Carne, Classic, Canned, Stagg*	½ Can/200g	260	10	130	7	13	5	4.5
Con Carne, Cooked, BGTY, Sainsbury's*	1 Pack/400g	356	6.8	94	4.9	13.4	1.8	2.2
Con Carne, Diet Chef Ltd*	1 Pack/300g	333	13.5	111	7.3	10.4	4.5	2.1
Con Carne, Dynamite Hot, Stagg*	1 Serving/250g	310	15.5	124	7.6	9.6	6.2	2.5
Con Carne, From Restaurant, Average	*1 Serving/253g*	*256*	*8.3*	*101*	*9.7*	*8.7*	*3.3*	*0*
Con Carne, Frozen, Co-Op*	1 Pack/340g	306	3.4	90	6	15	1	1
Con Carne, Heston from Waitrose, Waitrose*	½ Pack/300g	429	27	143	8.4	5.9	9	2.3
Con Carne, Homepride*	1 Can/390g	234	2.3	60	2.5	11.2	0.6	0
Con Carne, M&S*	1 Pack/285g	285	10.5	100	8.7	7.4	3.7	2
Con Carne, Recipe Mix, Colman's*	1 Pack/50g	158	1.2	316	10.4	62.9	2.5	6.8
Con Carne, with Brown Rice, Everdine*	1 Meal/450g	459	18.4	102	7.2	6.4	4.1	5.2
Con Carne, with Long Grain Rice, COU, M&S*	1 Pack/400g	388	7.6	97	5	13.9	1.9	2.1
Con Carne, with Rice, BGTY, Sainsbury's*	1 Pack/400g	392	8.3	99	6.3	12.5	2.1	2.2
Con Carne, with Rice, Classic, Co-Op*	1 Pack/400g	464	13.6	116	5.9	14	3.4	2.7
Con Carne, with Rice, PB, Waitrose*	1 Pack/400g	404	7.2	101	5.8	15.3	1.8	1.7
Con Carne, with Rice, Weight Watchers*	1 Pack/300g	279	4.2	93	4.6	15.1	1.4	1.1
Con Veggie, Cook*	1 Portion/285g	194	4.3	68	5.9	7.8	1.5	0
Diced Beef,with Rice, 672, Wiltshire Farm Foods*	1 Portion/380g	328	9.2	86	5.5	10	2.4	1.6
Medium, Uncle Ben's*	1 Jar/500g	305	4	61	1.8	11.1	0.8	0
Mexican, Beanfeast, Batchelors*	1 Serving/65g	203	3.2	312	24.3	42.7	4.9	13.6
Minced Beef with Rice, Mini, CBY, Asda*	1 Pack/250g	308	9.8	123	5.3	15.8	3.9	1.7
Mixed Vegetable, Tesco*	1 Pack/400g	352	11.6	88	3.9	11	2.9	3.2
sin Carne, Bio, Reichenhof*	1 Portion/200g	132	0.8	66	4.9	8.9	0.4	0
Speckled Lentil, with Parisienne Potatoes, Everdine*	1 Serving/450g	450	14.4	100	2.9	12.7	3.2	4.5
Steak & Coriander Rice, Taste Mexico, M&S*	1 Pack/400g	532	15.2	133	7.1	16.4	3.8	2.4
Three Bean, & Cauliflower Rice, Goodlife*	1 Pack/400g	276	8	69	3.8	5.8	2	6.5
Three Bean, & Vegetable, Slimfree, Aldi*	1 Pack/500g	295	2.5	59	3.4	8.5	0.5	3.1
Three Bean, Diet Chef Ltd*	1 Pack/300g	195	2.7	65	4	10.3	0.9	3.6
Vegetable	*1oz/28g*	*16*	*0.2*	*57*	*3*	*10.8*	*0.6*	*2.6*
Vegetable & Rice, BGTY, Sainsbury's*	1 Pack/450g	410	5	91	3.5	16.7	1.1	3.5
Vegetable & Rice, HE, Tesco*	1 Pack/450g	392	5.4	87	2.8	16.1	1.2	1.5
Vegetable Garden, Stagg*	1 Can/400g	280	2	70	3.5	14	0.5	3
Vegetable, Canned, Heated, Asda*	½ Can/200g	158	1	79	3.2	14.1	0.5	2.5
Vegetable, Canned, Sainsbury's*	1 Can/400g	230	1.6	58	3.1	10.4	0.4	3.2
Vegetable, Diet Chef Ltd*	1 Pack/300g	258	4.8	86	3.4	14.5	1.6	4.4
Vegetable, Fast Diet Kitchen*	1 Pack/340g	194	1.4	57	3.6	12.2	0.4	4.8

C

	Measure INFO/WEIGHT	per Measure		Nutrition Values per 100g / 100ml				
		KCAL	FAT	KCAL	PROT	CARB	FAT	FIBRE
CHILLI								
Vegetable, Retail	*1oz/28g*	*20*	*0.6*	*70*	*4*	*9.4*	*2.1*	*0*
Vegetarian with Rice, Tesco*	1 Pack/500g	575	13	115	4	19	2.6	1.8
Vegetarian, Mexican, Chef's Selection, Quorn*	½ Pack/170g	143	4.3	84	6.6	6.5	2.5	4.5
Vegetarian, Soya Mince, & Rice, Waitrose*	1 Pack/402g	442	8.4	110	5.4	14.9	2.1	5.4
Vegetarian, Tesco*	1 Pack/400g	340	3.2	85	4.4	15	0.8	2.1
Vegetarian, with Rice, Ready Meal, Average	*1 Serving/400g*	*434*	*6*	*108*	*3.8*	*20*	*1.5*	*1.3*
CHILLI POWDER								
Average	*1 Tsp/4g*	*16*	*0.7*	*405*	*12.3*	*54.7*	*16.8*	*34.2*
CHIPS								
American Style, Oven, Co-Op*	1 Serving/150g	255	9	170	2	26	6	3
American Style, Thin, Oven, Tesco*	1 Serving/125g	210	8.1	168	2.7	24.6	6.5	2.1
Chip Shop, Fishnchickn*	1 Portion/311g	734	38.6	236	3.2	27.9	12.4	0
Chunky 11/5/17, M&S*	½ Pack/200g	292	7.6	146	2	24.7	3.8	2.6
Chunky Oven, Harry Ramsden's*	1 Serving/150g	184	5.4	123	2.8	19.9	3.6	1.6
Chunky, COU, M&S*	1 Serving/150g	158	2.4	105	2.1	20.5	1.6	2.3
Chunky, Crisp & Golden, Waitrose*	½ Pack/225g	259	7	115	2.1	17.7	3.1	3.9
Chunky, Fresh, Chilled, Finest, Tesco*	1 Pack/450g	608	18	135	2.1	22.3	4	2.7
Chunky, Gastropub, M&S*	1 Pack/400g	520	12.4	130	2.6	22.4	3.1	2.3
Chunky, Ready to Bake, M&S*	1 Serving/200g	310	8.4	155	2.2	26.8	4.2	2
Crinkle Cut, Frozen, Fried in Corn Oil	*1oz/28g*	*81*	*4.7*	*290*	*3.6*	*33.4*	*16.7*	*2.2*
Crinkle Cut, Oven Baked, Aunt Bessie's*	1 Serving/100g	206	9.2	206	2.9	28	9.2	3.2
Crinkle Cut, Oven, Asda*	1 Serving/100g	134	3.8	134	2	23	3.8	8
Family Fries, Oven, Tesco*	1 Serving/125g	164	4.6	131	2	22.4	3.7	1.8
Fine Cut, Frozen, Fried in Blended Oil	*1oz/28g*	*102*	*6*	*364*	*4.5*	*41.2*	*21.3*	*2.4*
Fine Cut, Frozen, Fried in Corn Oil	*1oz/28g*	*102*	*6*	*364*	*4.5*	*41.2*	*21.3*	*2.7*
Fried, Average	*1 Serving/130g*	*266*	*10.9*	*204*	*3.2*	*29.6*	*8.4*	*1.2*
Frozen, Crinkle Cut, Aunt Bessie's*	1 Serving/100g	163	7.3	163	3.1	21.3	7.3	2.2
Fry or Oven, Oven Cooked, Smart Price, Asda*	1 Serving/125g	192	4.3	153	2.1	26.9	3.4	3.3
Frying, Cooked in Sunflower Oil, Value, Tesco*	1 Portion/125g	172	4.9	138	2.5	23.1	3.9	1.6
Frying, Crinkle Cut, Tesco*	1 Serving/125g	161	4.1	129	2.6	22.2	3.3	1.9
Gourmet, Cornish Sea Salt, Oven Baked, McCain*	¼ Pack/100g	206	9.9	206	2	25.6	9.9	3
Homefries, Chunky, Weighed Baked, McCain*	1 Serving/100g	153	3.1	153	3.2	28	3.1	2.3
Homefries, Chunky, Weighed Frozen, McCain*	1 Serving/100g	123	2.5	123	2.5	22.6	2.5	1.6
Homefries, Crinkle Cut, Weighed Baked, McCain*	1 Serving/100g	176	5	176	2.6	30.1	5	2.3
Homefries, Crinkle Cut, Weighed Frozen, McCain*	1 Serving/100g	142	5.1	142	1.9	22.2	5.1	1.3
Homefries, Straight Cut, Weighed Baked, McCain*	1 Serving/100g	181	6.2	181	3.1	28.1	6.2	2.4
Homefries, Straight Cut, Weighed Frozen, McCain*	1 Serving/100g	134	4.6	134	2.2	21	4.6	1.7
Homemade, Fried in Blended Oil, Average	*1oz/28g*	*53*	*1.9*	*189*	*3.9*	*30.1*	*6.7*	*2.2*
Homemade, Fried in Corn Oil, Average	*1oz/28g*	*53*	*1.9*	*189*	*3.9*	*30.1*	*6.7*	*2.2*
Homemade, Fried in Dripping, Average	*1oz/28g*	*53*	*1.9*	*189*	*3.9*	*30.1*	*6.7*	*2.2*
Homestyle Oven, Sainsbury's*	1 Serving/125g	206	5.4	165	2.4	29.2	4.3	2.1
Homestyle, Frozen, Aunt Bessie's*	1 Serving/200g	292	8	146	2.4	24	4	1.7
Homestyle, Oven Cooked, Aunt Bessie's*	1 Serving/100g	191	7.8	191	3.1	27	7.8	2.9
Homestyle, Oven, Straight Cut , Tesco*	1 Serving/125g	251	10.6	201	3	26.2	8.5	3.5
Micro Chips, Crinkle Cut, Cooked, McCain*	1 Pack/100g	146	4	158	2.4	26	4.3	2.8
Micro Chips, Straight Cut, Cooked, McCain*	1 Pack/100g	163	4.8	163	2.3	27.7	4.8	2
Microwave, Cooked	*1oz/28g*	*62*	*2.7*	*221*	*3.6*	*32.1*	*9.6*	*2.9*
Oven, 5% Fat, Frozen, McCain*	1 Serving/200g	238	6	119	1.9	21	3	1.6
Oven, American Style, Champion*	1 Serving/200g	372	14.4	186	2.2	28.2	7.2	2
Oven, Best in the World, Iceland*	1 Serving/175g	332	11.7	190	3.4	28.9	6.7	3.5
Oven, Champion*	1 Pack/133g	210	6	158	2.5	27	4.5	0
Oven, Chunky, Extra Special, Asda*	1 Serving/125g	238	7	190	3.4	31.5	5.6	3.2
Oven, Cooked, Value, Tesco*	1 Serving/125g	308	9.8	246	4.5	39.5	7.8	2.9

CHIPS

	Measure INFO/WEIGHT	per Measure KCAL	FAT	Nutrition Values per 100g / 100ml KCAL	PROT	CARB	FAT	FIBRE
Oven, Crinkle Cut, Frozen, Essential, Waitrose*	1 Serving/165g	225	6.4	136	2.7	22.6	3.9	1.7
Oven, Crinkle Cut, Sainsbury's*	1 Serving/165g	297	9.1	180	3.3	29.5	5.5	2.4
Oven, Frozen, Baked	**1 Portion/80g**	**130**	**3.4**	**162**	**3.2**	**29.8**	**4.2**	**2**
Oven, Frozen, Basics, Sainsbury's*	1 Serving/165g	249	8.1	151	3	23.6	4.9	2.9
Oven, Frozen, BGTY, Sainsbury's*	1 Serving/165g	226	4.6	137	2.9	25	2.8	2.7
Oven, Frozen, Value, Tesco*	1 Serving/125g	189	5.7	151	2.8	24.7	4.6	1.9
Oven, Homefries, McCain*	1 Serving/100g	134	4.6	134	2.2	21	4.6	1.7
Oven, Morrisons*	1 Serving/100g	134	3.9	134	2.4	22.2	3.9	0
Oven, Original, McCain*	1 Serving/100g	158	3.8	158	2.5	28.5	3.8	2.3
Oven, Steak Cut, Asda*	1 Serving/100g	153	4.1	153	2	27	4.1	2.5
Oven, Steak Cut, Sainsbury's*	1 Serving/165g	266	7.8	161	2.6	27.1	4.7	2.8
Oven, Steak Cut, Waitrose*	1 Serving/165g	218	5.6	132	2.7	22.7	3.4	1.7
Oven, Steakhouse, Frozen, Tesco*	1 Serving/125g	165	4.2	132	2.7	22.7	3.4	1.7
Oven, Straight Cut, 5% Fat, Sainsbury's*	1 Serving/165g	280	8.1	170	3.4	28	4.9	2.5
Oven, Straight Cut, Asda*	1 Serving/100g	199	5	199	3.5	35	5	3
Oven, Straight Cut, BFY, Morrisons*	1 Serving/165g	249	5.8	151	2.8	27.1	3.5	2.1
Oven, Straight Cut, Reduced Fat, Tesco*	1 Serving/100g	127	3	127	2.3	22.7	3	2.1
Oven, Straight Cut, Waitrose*	1 Serving/165g	219	6.1	133	2	23	3.7	1.7
Oven, Sweet Potato, Cooked, Tesco*	¼ Pack/125g	180	7.1	145	2.5	18.2	5.7	3.7
Oven, Thick Cut, Frozen, Baked	**1oz/28g**	**44**	**1.2**	**157**	**3.2**	**27.9**	**4.4**	**1.8**
Oven, Thin & Crispy, Tesco*	1 Portion/100g	205	4.9	205	2.7	37.6	4.9	5.8
Oven, Thin Cut, American Style, Asda*	1 Serving/100g	240	10	240	3.4	34	10	3
Oven, Thin Fries, Morrisons*	1 Serving/100g	161	6.1	161	2.9	23.6	6.1	1.2
Potato, Lights, Reduced Fat, Lay's*	1 Serving/25g	118	5.5	470	7.5	60	22	5
Steak Cut, Frying, Asda*	1 Serving/97g	181	6.8	187	2.9	28	7	2.8
Steak Cut, Oven, Tesco*	1 Serving/165g	233	6.4	141	2	24.4	3.9	2
Steakhouse, Fry, Tesco*	1 Serving/125g	278	15.1	222	3.1	25.2	12.1	2
Straight Cut, Frozen, Fried in Blended Oil	**1oz/28g**	**76**	**3.8**	**273**	**4.1**	**36**	**13.5**	**2.4**
Straight Cut, Frozen, Fried in Corn Oil	**1oz/28g**	**76**	**3.8**	**273**	**4.1**	**36**	**13.5**	**2.4**
Straight Cut, Oven, BGTY, Sainsbury's*	1 Portion/165g	226	3.5	137	2.7	26.8	2.1	4.1
Thick Cut, Frozen, Fried in Corn Oil, Average	**1oz/28g**	**66**	**2.9**	**234**	**3.6**	**34**	**10.2**	**2.4**
Triple Cooked, Gastro, Frozen, McCain*	1 Serving/187g	379	22.2	203	1.9	21	11.9	2.2
Triple Cooked, Gastro, Oven Baked, McCain*	1 Serving/135g	379	20.5	281	2.9	31.6	15.2	3
Vegetable, Root, Ready to Roast, Tesco*	¼ Pack/125g	99	3.8	79	1.1	10.3	3	3.1
with Gravy, Mayflower*	1 Box/330g	403	19.2	122	1.8	15.8	5.8	1.4

CHIVES

	Measure INFO/WEIGHT	per Measure KCAL	FAT	Nutrition Values per 100g / 100ml KCAL	PROT	CARB	FAT	FIBRE
Fresh, Average	**1 Tsp/2g**	**0**	**0**	**23**	**2.8**	**1.7**	**0.6**	**1.9**

CHOC ICES

	Measure INFO/WEIGHT	per Measure KCAL	FAT	Nutrition Values per 100g / 100ml KCAL	PROT	CARB	FAT	FIBRE
Chocolate, Dark, Seriously Creamy, Waitrose*	1 Ice/82g	195	12.9	238	2.6	21.6	15.7	1.7
Chocolate, Real Milk, Sainsbury's*	1 Ice/48g	151	9.5	312	3.5	30.3	19.7	0.8
Dark, Sainsbury's*	1 Choc Ice/44g	156	4.7	354	0	0	10.6	0
Everyday, Value, Tesco*	1 Choc Ice/31g	95	6.3	300	2.3	26.7	19.9	1
Mini Mix, Eis Stern*	1 Ice/39g	129	8.9	334	4.2	29	23	0
Neapolitan Chocolate, Co-Op*	1 Ice/62g	120	8.2	194	2	16.9	13.2	0.4
Smart Price, Asda*	1 Ice/31g	81	5.9	262	2.8	20	19	0
White Chocolate, Sainsbury's*	1 Ice/48g	140	8.9	292	3.8	27.3	18.6	0.1

CHOCOLATE

	Measure INFO/WEIGHT	per Measure KCAL	FAT	Nutrition Values per 100g / 100ml KCAL	PROT	CARB	FAT	FIBRE
Advent Calendar, Dairy Milk, Cadbury*	.1 Chocolate/4.2g	22	1.3	525	7.5	56.6	30.1	0.7
Advent Calendar, Maltesers, Mars*	1 Chocolate/4g	21	1.2	537	6.8	57.9	30.9	0
Advent Calendar, Sainsbury's*	1 Chocolate/3.6g	20	1.2	557	7.2	52.7	34.3	2.1
Advent Calendar, The Snowman, M&S*	1 Chocolate/3.8g	21	1.2	550	6.6	60.4	31	0
Almond & Honey, Dairy Milk, Cadbury*	1 Sm Bar/54g	281	15.6	520	8	57.1	28.9	1
Alpine Milk , Milka*	1 Serving/25g	132	7.4	530	6.6	58.5	29.5	1.8

	Measure INFO/WEIGHT	per Measure KCAL	FAT	Nutrition Values per 100g / 100ml KCAL	PROT	CARB	FAT	FIBRE
CHOCOLATE								
Baking, Belgian, Milk for Cakes, Luxury, Sainsbury's*	1 Chunk/8g	44	2.7	556	7.6	56.5	33.3	1.5
Bar, Animal, Nestle*	1 Bar/19g	97	5	513	5.8	63.6	26.1	0
Bar, Apricot & Raisin, Thorntons*	1 Bar/40g	185	10.9	462	8	46	27.3	3.5
Bar, Bliss Truffle, Cadbury*	1 Bar/40g	226	14.9	565	6.6	48.8	37.3	2.8
Bar, Bliss, Hazelnut Truffle, Cadbury*	1 Serving/100g	565	37.9	565	7.2	47.7	37.9	2.6
Bar, Bliss, Toffee Flavour Truffle, Cadbury*	2 Chunks/23g	128	8.1	555	6.9	51.6	35.3	1.6
Bar, Cappuccino, Thorntons*	1 Bar/38g	201	13.2	529	5.2	49.7	34.7	0.5
Bar, Chocolate Cream, Fry's*	1 Piece/10g	42	1.3	415	2.8	70.8	13.2	1.2
Bar, Cookies & Cream, Hello, Lindt*	1 Square/10g	56	3.7	565	7	52	37	0
Bar, Dark Chocolate, Diabetic, Thorntons*	1 Bar/75g	345	26.8	460	5.4	28.5	35.8	8.1
Bar, Dark with Ginger, Thorntons*	1 Bar/90g	495	35.1	550	8	39	39	0
Bar, Dark, 60% Cocoa with Macadamia, Thorntons*	1 Bar/70g	183	12.8	523	6.5	42.3	36.5	12.6
Bar, Dark, Thorntons*	1 Sm Bar/48g	250	17.7	521	7.3	39.9	36.9	10.9
Bar, Deliciously, Free From, Sainsbury's*	1 Bar/35g	190	12.2	543	2.5	48.2	35	12.4
Bar, Extra Dark, 60% Cocoa, Lindor, Lindt*	1 Bar/150g	900	73.5	600	5	35	49	2
Bar, Free From, Asda*	1 Bar/35g	194	12.1	563	2.5	58	35	2.8
Bar, Hazel Nut & Cashew, Dairy Milk, Cadbury*	3 Chunks/18g	96	6	540	8.8	50.6	33.5	1.8
Bar, Jazz Orange, Thorntons*	1 Bar/56g	304	18.1	543	6.8	55.7	32.3	1.2
Bar, Milk, Thorntons*	1 Sm Bar/50g	269	16	538	7.5	54.8	32	1
Bar, Truffle, M&S*	1 Bar/35g	168	11.4	480	5.9	41.7	32.5	8.3
Bar, Truffle, Orange, M&S*	1 Bar/33g	177	10.5	535	6.6	55.6	31.9	1.4
Bar, Twisted, Creme Egg, Cadbury*	1 Bar/45g	210	9.4	465	5.2	64.6	20.8	0.5
Bar, Viennese, Continental, Thorntons*	1 Bar/38g	206	13	542	4.2	54	34.2	0.8
Bar, White, Thorntons*	1 Bar/50g	274	15.6	547	6.5	59.5	31.3	0
Bars, Alpini, Continental, Thorntons*	1 Bar/36g	192	11.4	538	6.9	55.3	32	2.7
Bars, Baby Ruth, Candy, Nestlé*	1 Bar/60g	296	14.1	494	6.7	63.9	23.5	1.7
Bars, Bubbles, Galaxy, Mars*	1 Bar/31g	172	10.6	555	6.5	54.7	34.2	1.5
Bars, Chocolate, Cherry, Lindt*	1 Bar/100g	470	22.8	470	4.5	61.7	22.8	0
Bars, Chocolate, Pistacho, Lindt*	1 Bar/100g	585	40.6	585	7.1	48.2	40.6	0
Bars, Chocolate, Strawberry, Lindt*	1 Bar/100g	470	22.8	470	4.5	61.6	22.8	0
Bars, Chocoletti, Stracciatella, Lindt*	1 Bar/5.5g	32	2.3	590	7.7	49	41	0
Bars, Milk Chocolate, Galaxy, Mars*	1 Bar/42g	229	13.6	546	6.7	56	32.4	1.5
Bars, Milk Chocolate, Gold, Lindt*	1 Bar/300g	1605	92.9	535	6.6	58.7	31	0
Bars, Milk Chocolate, Hazelnut, Gold, Lindt*	1 Bar/300g	1665	108.2	555	7.9	50.7	36.1	0
Bars, Milk Chocolate, Hazelnut, Lindt*	1 Bar/100g	570	38.8	570	8.5	47	38.8	0
Bars, Milk Chocolate, Lindt*	1 Bar/100g	535	31	535	6.6	57.6	31	0
Bars, Milk Chocolate, Raisin & Hazelnut, Lindt*	1 Bar/100g	530	31.6	530	3.1	54.7	31.6	0
Beans, Coffee, Dark, Solid, M&S*	1 Serving/10g	53	3.8	532	4.7	42.4	37.6	11.6
Bear, Lindt*	1 Bear/10.5g	60	3.6	572	7.5	57.7	34.6	0
Belgian Milk, TTD, Sainsbury's*	1 Piece/10g	55	3.5	549	9.6	48.3	35.3	2
Belgian, Kschocolat*	4 Pieces/40g	212	12.2	530	6	57.5	30.5	2.3
Belgian, Milk, Mini Eggs, M&S*	1 Egg/8g	43	2.5	535	7	55.8	31.7	2.7
Blueberry Intense, Excellence, Lindt*	1 Serving/40g	200	12.4	500	6	50	31	0
Bubbly Santa, M&S*	1 Santa/23g	124	7.3	540	7	55.8	31.7	2.7
Bubbly, Dairy Milk, Cadbury*	1 Bar/35g	185	10.5	525	7.7	56.9	29.7	0.7
Bunny, Easter, Mars*	1 Bunny/29g	155	9.2	535	6.2	56.2	31.7	0
Bunny, Lindt*	1 Bunny/10.5g	60	3.6	572	7.5	57.5	34.6	0
Buttons, Dairy Milk, Cadbury*	1 Pack/32g	170	9.7	525	7.7	56.7	29.9	0.7
Cappuccino, Nestle*	1 Serving/20g	109	6.6	545	6.1	56	32.9	0
Caramel, Chunk, Dairy Milk, Cadbury*	1 Chunk/33g	158	7.6	480	5	63	23	0
Caramel, Dairy Milk, Cadbury*	1 Bar/45g	215	10.4	480	4.9	62.8	23.2	0.4
Caramel, Irresistibly Smooth, Lindor, Lindt*	1 Bar/100g	625	48	625	4.7	43	48	0
Chips, Dark, The Pantry, Aldi*	1 Serving/25g	126	6.5	505	3.8	60	26	6.1

CHOCOLATE

	Measure INFO/WEIGHT	per Measure KCAL	FAT	Nutrition Values per 100g / 100ml KCAL	PROT	CARB	FAT	FIBRE
Chocolat Noir, Lindt*	1/6 Bar/17g	87	5.4	510	6	50	32	0
Chocolate Favourites, Tesco*	½ Box/227g	1015	43.6	447	4.2	64.3	19.2	0.3
Chomp, Cadbury*	1 Bar/24g	112	4.8	465	3.3	67.9	20	0.2
Christmas Tree Decoration, Average	**1 Chocolate/12g**	**63**	**3.6**	**522**	**7.6**	**56.4**	**29.9**	**0.4**
Christmas Tree Decoration, Cadbury*	1 Piece/12g	60	3.4	525	7.6	56.2	29.9	0
Chunk Bar, Dairy Milk, Cadbury*	1 Chunk/6.7g	35	2	525	7.5	57	29.8	0.1
Chunky Hazelnut Bar, M&S*	1 Bar/52g	293	19.4	563	8.8	48.1	37.3	1.7
Coco Mylk, Raw, Bar, Ombar*	1 Bar/35g	208	15.9	594	6.8	43.9	45.5	8
Coconut, White, Excellence, Lindt*	1 Square/10g	61	4.4	610	6	48	44	0
Coins, Marzipan, & Cherry , Favorina, Lidl*	1 Serving/30g	132	5.7	439	5.3	58	19	3.3
Coins, Marzipan, Plum, & Madeira, Favorina, Lidl*	1 Serving/30g	131	6	437	5.4	53	20	4.9
Coins, Milk, Sainsbury's*	1 Coin/5g	26	1.4	502	5.5	58.8	27.1	2.5
Cool & Delicious, Dairy Milk, Cadbury*	1 Bar/21g	110	6.3	525	7.6	56.1	30.1	0
Counters, Galaxy, Mars*	4 Counters/10g	53	2.9	529	6.8	59.4	29.1	1.4
Crispello Double Choc, Cadbury*	1 Piece/10g	55	3.5	560	7	51	36	1.9
Crispies, Chunk, Dairy Milk, Cadbury*	1 Chunk/31g	158	8.5	510	7.6	58.6	27.4	0
Crispies, Dairy Milk, Cadbury*	1 Bar/49g	250	13.4	510	7.6	58.6	27.4	0
Crispy, Sainsbury's*	4 Squares/19g	99	5.4	521	9.1	56.9	28.5	2.1
Dairy Milk with Oreo, Dairy Milk, Cadbury*	3 Chunks/15g	85	5.4	560	6.1	53.5	35.5	0.7
Dairy Milk, Cadbury*	1 Bar/45g	240	13.8	530	7.5	56.5	30.5	0.7
Dairy Milk, Toffee Popcorn, Dairy Milk, Cadbury*	1 Bar/150g	765	39.8	510	7	59.5	26.5	1.7
Dark + Nibs, Artisan, Raw, Raw Halo Ltd*	1 Bar/35g	212	17.6	606	8.3	29.4	50.4	0
Dark + Sweet Orange, Artisan, Raw, Raw Halo Ltd*	1 Bar/33g	199	16.4	602	7.8	31.3	49.7	0
Dark with Chilli, Thorntons*	4 Squares/20g	107	7.9	533	7.2	36.3	39.5	10.4
Dark, Finest, 85% Cocoa, Moser Roth, Aldi*	1 Bar/25g	152	12.8	608	11	18	51	15
Dark, 60%, Amazonas, Lidl*	1 Square/13g	75	5.2	574	5.7	44	40	7.5
Dark, 70% Cocoa Solids, Extra Fine, Lindt*	1 Square/10g	54	4.1	537	8	33	41	0
Dark, 70% Cocoa Solids, Organic, Green & Black's*	1 Sm Bar/35g	193	14.4	551	9.3	36	41.1	11.5
Dark, 70% Cocoa Solids, Organic, Morrisons*	½ Bar/50g	266	20.6	531	7.9	31.6	41.1	11
Dark, 70%, with Raspberries, Divine Chocolate*	1 Square/5g	29	2.2	584	6.7	32.2	45	11.3
Dark, 70%, Velvet, Green & Black's*	1 Piece/10g	62	4.9	619	6.1	33	49	9.7
Dark, 75% Cacao, Rausch*	1 Row/31.3g	163	12.9	522	8.8	28.5	41.1	15
Dark, 85% Cocoa, Excellence, Lindt*	1 Serving/40g	212	18.4	530	11	19	46	0
Dark, 85% Cocoa, TTD, Sainsbury's*	1 Serving/25g	142	12.8	569	9.7	17	51.4	14.1
Dark, 99% Cocoa, Excellence, Lindt*	1 Serving/25g	142	12.5	567	13	8	50	8
Dark, Assorted Collection, Velvet, Green & Black's*	1 Piece/10g	61	4.8	612	5.8	35	48	9.2
Dark, Belgian, Extra Special, Asda*	2 Squares/20g	102	8	508	11	26	40	16
Dark, Belgian, Luxury Continental, Sainsbury's*	1 Bar/100g	490	38.7	490	11.1	24.2	38.7	7.4
Dark, Belgian, No Added Sugar, Chocologic*	4 Pieces/13g	58	4.7	432	5.3	18.7	34.8	34.8
Dark, Bournville, Classic, Cadbury*	1 Bar/45g	238	13.5	530	3.8	59.5	29.9	5.5
Dark, Chilli, Excellence, Lindt*	1 Serving/40g	202	12.8	506	5.4	49	32	0
Dark, Classic, Bourneville, Cadbury*	4 Squares/24.8g	125	6.8	505	4.7	58.8	27.3	2
Dark, Co-Op*	1 Bar/50g	252	14.5	505	4	57	29	6
Dark, Continental, Luxury, Tesco*	1 Bar/100g	571	37.8	571	11.3	46.5	37.8	0.1
Dark, Fair Trade, Co-Op*	1 Bar/45g	214	13	475	4	49	29	6
Dark, Feuilles with Orange, Nestle*	1 Piece/8g	42	2.6	524	4.6	54.4	32	0
Dark, Goji, Cranberry & Linseed, M&S*	1 Bar/28g	172	11.7	614	12	41.4	41.7	12.6
Dark, Hazelnut Crisp, Mini Bar, Mister Choc, Lidl*	1 Mini Bar/18g	102	6.8	566	7.7	46.2	37.9	4.4
Dark, Luxury Continental, Sainsbury's*	½ Bar/50g	252	20	504	10.7	25.5	40	16.1
Dark, Mint, Intense, Lindt*	1 Square/10g	53	3.2	529	5	51	32	0
Dark, Orange & Almond, Moser Roth, Aldi*	1 Serving/25g	133	8	532	5.9	51	32	7.9
Dark, Plain, Average	**1oz/28g**	**143**	**7.8**	**510**	**5**	**63.5**	**28**	**2.5**
Dark, Plain, Rich, Co-Op*	1 Bar/200g	1010	58	505	4	57	29	6

CHOCOLATE

	Measure INFO/WEIGHT	per Measure KCAL	FAT	Nutrition Values per 100g / 100ml KCAL	PROT	CARB	FAT	FIBRE
Dark, Pure, Artisan, Raw, Raw Halo Ltd*	1 Bar/33g	201	16.9	610	7.7	30.1	51.1	0
Dark, Raw Organic, Loving Earth*	1 Serving/20g	99	7.9	495	9.3	46.4	39.5	0
Dark, Rich, Tesco*	1 Serving/20g	98	6.1	491	5.8	60	30.4	11.5
Dark, Simply, Lidl*	3 Squares/20g	98	5.6	491	4.6	51	28	8.1
Dark, Smooth, Bar, Galaxy, Mars*	1 Bar/125g	651	42	521	6.2	48	33.6	9.3
Dark, Smooth, No Added Sugar, Sainsbury's*	1 Piece/10g	53	4.2	529	8.2	34.3	42.2	11
Dark, Special, Hershey*	1 Pack/41g	180	12	439	4.9	61	29.3	7.3
Dark, Tiddly Pot, Hotel Chocolat*	1 Serving/58g	311	22.4	537	13.9	30.5	38.7	8.7
Dark, Whole Nut, Tesco*	1 Serving/13g	67	4.5	539	6.1	48.3	35.7	6.5
Dark, with Almonds, Green & Black's*	1 Row/18g	112	9	622	9.2	29	50	9.4
Dark, with Mint, Velvet, Green & Black's*	1 Row/18g	111	8.8	619	6.1	33	49	9.7
Dark, with Orange, 70% , Ecuador *	1 Square/13g	70	4.9	537	7.3	36	38	11
Dark, with Orange, Lidl*	1 Square/13g	67	4.7	537	7.3	36	38	11
Dark, with Salted Almonds, Benugo*	1 Bar/25g	138	9.2	550	6.1	43.7	37	7
Dark, with Salted Caramel, Velvet, Green & Black's*	1 Row/18g	108	8.1	600	5.2	39	45	8.2
Dark, with Sea Salt, Velvet, Green & Black's*	1 Row/18g	111	8.8	616	6.1	33	49	9.7
Diet, Ritter Sport*	1 Square/6g	25	1.8	412	6	44	30	0
Double Blend, Nestle*	1 Rectangle/11g	61	3.6	553	7.3	55.9	33	0
Dream with Real Strawberries, Cadbury*	1 Bar/45.0g	250	14.9	555	4.5	59.6	33.1	0
Drops, Plain, Asda*	1 Serving/100g	489	29	489	7	50	29	10
Drops, Plain, Sainsbury's*	1 Serving/125g	638	34.5	510	5.3	60.1	27.6	4
Drops, White for Cooking & Decorating, Sainsbury's*	1oz/28g	152	8.6	544	6.5	60.3	30.8	0
Egg n Spoon, Mousse Centre, Oreo Pieces, Cadbury*	1 Egg/34g	191	11.9	561	7.1	53	35	1.2
Egg, Caramel, Cadbury*	1 Egg/39g	187	9.5	480	4	60	24.5	0.4
Eggs, Milk, Raspberry, Favorina, Lidl*	1 Egg/19g	86	3.6	453	4.1	64.3	19.1	0
Elves, Magical, with Popping Candy, Cadbury*	1 Elf/15g	77	4.2	515	6.9	60	27.7	0
Espresso Coffee Kick, 5 Bars, M&S*	1 Bar/12g	77	5.5	644	5.5	46	46.2	11.3
Ferrero Rocher, Ferrero*	1 Chocolate/13g	75	5.3	603	8.2	44.4	42.7	0
Ferrero Rocher, Heart, Ferrero*	1 Chocolate/13g	75	5.3	603	8.2	44.4	42.7	0
Fingers, Milk, Mister Choc, Lidl*	1 Finger/18g	104	6.9	579	6.2	51.7	38.4	0.9
Football, Milk Chocolate, Thorntons*	1 Football/200g	1088	67	544	7.6	52.9	33.5	1
Freddo, Caramel, Dairy Milk, Cadbury*	1 Freddo/19g	93	4.7	490	5.5	60.5	24.8	0.5
Freddo, Dairy Milk, Cadbury*	1 Freddo/18g	95	5.4	530	7.5	57	29.8	0.7
Fruit & Nut, Belgian, Waitrose*	1 Serving/50g	254	14.6	508	8.6	54.6	29.2	3.4
Fruit & Nut, Dark, Tesco*	4 Squares/25g	124	7	494	5.8	54.8	27.9	6.5
Fruit & Nut, Dairyfine, Aldi*	4 Squares/25g	131	8	525	8.1	50	32	4.2
Galaxy, Crispy, Galaxy, Mars*	1 Portion/20.4g	111	6.6	546	6.4	56.7	32.2	0
Ginger, Traidcraft*	1 Bar/50g	212	7.4	424	3.9	68.2	14.8	0
Golden Biscuit Crunch, Dairy Milk, Cadbury*	4 Chunks /25g	135	8.2	545	6.2	55.5	33	0.8
Golf Balls, Milk Chocolate, Lindt*	1 Pack/110g	619	39.5	563	6.5	53.6	35.9	0
Hazelnut Crunch, Choceur, Aldi*	1 Serving/40g	226	14.4	564	9.2	49.7	36	2.4
Kinder Maxi, Ferrero*	1 Bar/21g	116	7.1	550	10	51	34	0
Kinder Surprise, Ferrero*	1 Egg/20g	110	7	550	10	50	35	0
Kinder, Bueno Bar, Milk, Ferrero*	1 Bar/21.5g	123	8	575	9.2	49.5	37.3	2
Kinder, Bueno, Bar, White, Ferrero*	1 Piece/19.5g	111	7	571	8.8	52.6	35.9	1
Kinder, Riegel, Ferrero*	1 Bar/21g	117	7.1	558	10	53	34	0
King Size, Dairy Milk, Cadbury*	1 Serving/85g	446	25.2	525	7.6	56.4	29.7	0
Kitten, Milk Chocolate, Lindt*	1 Kitten/10.5g	60	3.6	572	7.5	57.7	34.6	0
Lait Intense, Experiences, Cote D'or*	3 Squares/100g	575	40	575	7.2	44.5	40	5
Light & Whippy, Bite Sized, Sainsbury's*	1 Bar/15.0g	66	2.4	439	3.3	69.7	16.3	0.1
Little Bars, Dairy Milk, Cadbury*	1 Bar/20.8g	110	6.3	530	7.7	56.6	30.1	0.7
Macadamia Nut, Excellence, Lindt*	1 Bar/100g	560	37	560	7	51	37	0
Mandarin & Gubinge, Mylk, Loving Earth*	2 Squares/8g	55	4.4	621	4.6	42.7	50	0

CHOCOLATE

INFO/WEIGHT	Measure	per Measure		Nutrition Values per 100g / 100ml				
		KCAL	FAT	KCAL	PROT	CARB	FAT	FIBRE
Mars, Bites, Mars*	4 Bites/20g	90	3.3	449	4.1	70.2	16.6	0
Matchmakers, Mint, Nestle*	1 Stick/4g	20	0.8	477	4.3	69.7	20.1	0.9
Matchmakers, Yummy Honeycomb, Nestle*	4 Sticks/15g	72	3.1	495	3.7	70.6	21.3	2.4
Milk for Baking, Value, Tesco*	½ Bar/50g	265	14.5	530	6.7	60	29	2.2
Milk with Biscuit Pieces, Asda*	2 Squares/14g	73	4.1	521	8	57	29	1.9
Milk with Crisped Rice, Dubble*	1 Bar/40g	211	11.8	528	6.4	59.6	29.4	0
Milk with Honey & Almond Nougat, Swiss, Toblerone*	1 Piece/8g	42	2.4	525	5.4	59	29.5	2.2
Milk with Peanut Butter Filling, Ghirardelli*	1 Serving/45g	250	17	556	8.9	48.9	37.8	2.2
Milk with Raisins & Hazelnuts, Green & Black's*	1 Bar/100g	556	36.9	556	9.2	46.8	36.9	3.2
Milk with Whole Almonds, Organic, Green & Black's*	1 Bar/100g	578	42.2	578	11.8	37.7	42.2	5.2
Milk, Average	*1oz/28g*	*146*	*8.6*	*520*	*7.7*	*56.9*	*30.7*	*0.8*
Milk, Bars, M&S*	1 Bar/40g	214	12.8	535	7.8	54	32	1.9
Milk, Belgian, No Added Sugar, Chocologic*	4 Squares/13g	64	4.8	484	7.9	33.7	36.2	17
Milk, Biscuit Sticks, Mikado, Kraft*	1 Stick/2.3g	11	0.5	475	7.8	67	19.8	3.1
Milk, Bubbly, Swiss, M&S*	1 Serving/40g	218	13.7	545	8	52	34.3	2.5
Milk, Creamy, Organic, Green & Black's*	6 Pieces/20g	110	7	560	9.1	50.3	35.5	1.6
Milk, Extra Au Lait, Milch Extra, Lindt*	½ Bar/50g	268	15.5	535	6.5	57	31	0
Milk, Extra Creamy, Excellence, Lindt*	1 Bar/100g	560	37.1	560	6	51.1	37.1	0
Milk, Extra Fine, Swiss, M&S*	1 Serving/25g	141	9.2	565	7.2	50.9	36.7	2.3
Milk, Fair Trade, Tesco*	1 Serving/45g	236	13.3	524	7.6	56.7	29.6	2
Milk, Figures, Hollow, Dairyfine, Aldi*	1 Serving/11g	58	3.2	523	5.5	59.9	29	3.1
Milk, Giant Buttons, M&S*	1 Button/8g	44	2.7	550	7.1	52.3	34.2	0.4
Milk, Honey, Traidcraft*	1 Bar/50g	272	16.5	545	6	54	33	0
Milk, Italian, Low Sugar, Groder*	1 Serving/40g	199	14.6	498	6.9	51.2	36.5	1.9
Milk, Latte Macchiato, Mini Bar, Mister Choc, Lidl*	1 Mini Bar/18g	106	7.4	588	7.7	46.2	41.2	2.8
Milk, Lindor, Lindt*	1 Square/11g	68	5.2	615	4.7	43	47	0
Milk, Mini Bar, Mister Choc, Lidl*	1 Mini Bar/18g	103	6.6	571	7.1	51.1	36.8	2.8
Milk, Organic, Tesco*	1 Serving/25g	140	9.1	558	6.3	51.4	36.3	2.3
Milk, Ryelands*	4 Squares/29g	155	8.2	520	7.3	60.7	27.6	1.7
Milk, Sainsbury's*	4 Squares/25g	133	7.7	533	9.2	54.6	30.8	2.2
Milk, Salted Caramel, Godiva*	1 Square/10g	53	3	524	7.1	57	30	0
Milk, Salted Caramel, Thin, Organic, Green & Black's*	1 Square/12g	67	4.1	550	8.4	51.5	33.5	2.6
Milk, Santas, Tesco*	1 Bag/90g	433	21.8	481	4.5	61.4	24.2	1.4
Milk, Smart Price, Asda*	1 Square/6g	32	1.9	536	8	54	32	1.8
Milk, Strawberry Yogurt, Mini Bar, Mister Choc, Lidl*	1 Mini Bar/18g	102	6.5	566	6	52.8	36.3	2.8
Milk, Swiss, Diabetic with Fruit & Nuts, Boots*	½ Bar/21g	97	6.7	462	7	55	32	2.7
Milk, Swiss, Finest, Tesco*	2 Squares/20g	112	7	558	8.5	50.6	35.2	2.3
Milk, Tesco*	1 Serving/25g	133	7.7	533	9.5	54.7	30.7	2.2
Milk, Value, Tesco*	1/6 Bar/16g	83	4.5	520	6.8	60	28	2.3
Milk, Whole Nut, Tesco*	1 Serving/25g	129	8.4	517	8.7	53.4	33.8	9
Milk, Winnie the Pooh, Solid Shapes, M&S*	1 Chocolate/6g	32	1.9	540	8.1	54.1	32.4	1.3
Milky Bar, Giant Buttons, Mars*	1 Sweet/2g	11	0.6	546	7.5	57.7	31.6	0
Mini Bites, Chunky, Moments, Fox's*	1 Roll/20g	90	4.9	450	5.7	52.4	24.6	2.2
Mini Eggs, Cadbury*	1 Egg/3.1g	16	0.7	501	4.2	72	21	1.6
Mini Eggs, Caramel, Cadbury*	1 Mini Egg/11.3g	55	2.9	485	5.7	59	25.7	0.4
Mini Eggs, Daim, Cadbury*	1 Egg/11g	60	3.4	535	6.9	56.5	30.5	1.8
Mini Eggs, Golden, Galaxy *	½ Bag/40g	207	10.8	518	6.6	61.3	27	0
Mini Eggs, Lindor, Lindt*	3 Eggs/15g	92	6.8	611	5.4	45	45	0
Mini Eggs, Oreo, Cadbury*	1 Egg/10g	58	3.7	565	5.9	53.5	36	1.3
Mini, Toblerone*	1 Serving/6g	32	1.8	525	5.6	57.5	30	3.5
Mint Chips, Dairy Milk, Cadbury*	1 Bar/49g	247	12.8	505	6.6	61.6	26.1	0.6
Mint Creme, Sainsbury's*	1 Serving/20g	93	4.9	467	2.8	62.7	24.5	2.1
Mint Crisps, M&S*	1 Mint/8g	40	2.4	494	5.4	54.8	29.6	3.1

	Measure INFO/WEIGHT	per Measure KCAL	FAT	Nutrition Values per 100g / 100ml KCAL	PROT	CARB	FAT	FIBRE
CHOCOLATE								
Mint, Waves, Choceur, Aldi*	7 Waves/25g	129	7	516	6.4	56	28	6
Mistletoe Kisses, Mars*	1 Pack /42g	209	11.5	498	5.3	57	27.3	0
Mountain Bar with Orange, Swiss, M&S*	½ Bar/50g	268	16.4	535	8	52.2	32.8	3.2
Mountain Bar, Swiss, M&S*	1 Bar/100g	555	35.3	555	6.5	55.2	35.3	0.2
Mylk + Crispies, Artisan, Raw, Raw Halo Ltd*	1 Bar/33g	183	13.4	555	6.7	41.4	40.7	0
Mylk + Mint Crisp, Artisan, Raw, Raw Halo Ltd*	1 Bar/33g	187	13.9	567	7	41.5	42	0
Mylk + Salted Caramel, Artisan, Raw, Raw Halo Ltd*	1 Bar/32g	198	17.2	618	6.4	28.8	53.6	0
Mylk, Pure, Artisan, Raw, Raw Halo Ltd*	1 Bar/33g	205	17.8	621	6.4	29.1	53.8	0
Natural Orange, Excellence, Lindt*	1 Bar/100g	560	37	560	7	50	37	0
Natural Vanilla, Excellence, Lindt*	1 Bar/100g	590	40	590	6	51	40	0
Nibs, Raw, Cacao, Organic, Navitas Naturals*	1 Serving/28g	130	12	464	14.3	35.7	42.9	32.1
Noir, Special, Frey*	1 Bar/35g	197	15.8	562	8	30	45	0
NutRageous, Reese's, Hershey*	1 Bar/51g	260	16	510	11.8	54.9	31.4	3.9
Nuts About Caramel, Cadbury*	1 Bar/55g	272	15.1	495	5.8	56.6	27.4	0
Nutty Caramel, Dairy Milk, Cadbury*	4 Squares/28g	155	9.9	550	6.9	51	35	1.2
Nutty Nougat, Bite Sized, Sainsbury's*	1 Bar/23g	111	5.5	481	7.6	59	23.8	0.6
Oange, Crunchball, Terry's*	1 Segment/9g	45	2.4	520	6.9	59.8	28.1	2
Old Jamaica, Bournville, Cadbury*	4 Chunks/23g	107	5.4	465	4.2	59.6	23.4	2
Orange Cream, Cadbury*	1 Bar/51g	217	7.9	425	2.6	68.6	15.4	0
Orange Cream, Fry's*	1 Bar/50g	210	6.8	420	2.8	72.3	13.7	0
Orange, Bar, Terry's*	1 Bar/40g	210	11.7	530	7.3	58	29.5	2.1
Orange, Dark, Terry's*	1 Segment/9g	45	2.6	511	4.3	57	29.3	6.2
Orange, Fair Trade, Divine Foods*	4 Squares/17g	92	5.4	541	6.5	57.7	31.5	0
Orange, Milk, Mini Segments, Minis, Terry's*	1 Segment/4g	21	1.1	520	5.8	59.5	28	2.4
Orange, Milk, Terry's*	1 Orange/175g	910	49	520	5.8	59.5	28	2.4
Orange, Plain, Terry's*	1 Orange/175g	889	51.4	508	3.8	56.8	29.4	6.2
Orange, Sainsbury's*	4 Squares/19g	100	5.8	531	9.2	54.3	30.7	2.2
Orange, Segsations, Terry's*	1 Segsation/8g	43	2.3	520	6.9	58.5	28.5	2.8
Orange, White, Terry's*	1 Segment/11g	61	3.4	535	6.3	60.9	29.4	0
Oreo, Bar, Dairy Milk, Cadbury*	1 Bar/41g	226	13.7	550	6	55	33.5	1.6
Panna Cotta & Raspberry, M&S*	1 Bar/36g	190	12.1	528	4.7	51.4	33.6	0.3
Peanut Butter Cup, Big Cup, Reese's, Hershey*	1 Cup/39g	210	12	538	10.3	53.8	30.8	2.6
Peanut Butter Cup, Mini, Reeses, Hershey*	2 Mini Cups/7g	38	2.1	542	8.8	53.8	30.5	0
Peanut Butter Cup, Miniature, Reese's, Hershey*	1 Cup/8.8g	44	2.6	500	9.1	59.1	29.6	2.3
Peanut Butter Cup, Reese's, Hershey*	1 Cup/21g	105	6.5	500	11.9	57.1	31	5.9
Peanut Butter Cup, White, Mini, Reese's, Hershey*	5 Cups/39g	210	12	538	12.8	53.8	30.8	2.6
Peanut Butter Cups, Sugar Free, Reese's, Hershey*	1 Cup/11g	45	3.3	409	6.8	61.4	29.6	13.6
Peanut Caramel Crisp, Big Taste, Dairy Milk, Cadbury*	1 Chunk/12g	63	3.9	547	9.8	49	34	2.5
Peppermint Cream, Fry's*	1 Bar/51g	217	7.9	425	2.6	68.8	15.4	0
Peppermint Patty, Hershey*	3 Patties/41g	160	3	390	2.4	80.5	7.3	0
Peppermint, Ritter Sport*	1 Bar/100g	483	26	483	3	60	26	0
Plain with Hazelnuts, Tesco*	4 Squares/25g	135	8.9	539	6.1	48.3	35.7	6.5
Plain, 50% Cocoa Solids Minimum, Tesco*	4 Squares/22g	115	6.2	523	7.4	60	28.1	1.8
Plain, 72% Cocoa Solids, Finest, Tesco*	1 Square/10g	60	4.4	603	7.7	44	44	3.7
Plain, Belgian, Organic, Waitrose*	1 Bar/100g	505	37.6	505	9.6	32	37.6	5.6
Plain, Belgian, TTD, Sainsbury's*	1 Piece/10g	57	4.7	570	7	29.3	47.2	10.2
Plain, Continental, Waitrose*	1 Square/4g	23	1.8	558	7.7	32.9	44	5.9
Plain, Dark, Fruit & Nut, Rich, Sainsbury's*	4 Squares/25g	122	7	489	5.2	53.9	27.9	5.7
Plain, Fair Trade, Tesco*	1 Bar/40g	200	11.8	501	4.8	53.8	29.6	6.6
Plain, Whole Nut, Belgian, Waitrose*	4 Squares/25g	135	9.5	540	6.3	45.4	38	7.8
Plain, Wholenut, Sainsbury's*	1 Serving/25g	142	9	567	5.7	54.6	36.2	2.5
Planets, Mars*	1 Pack/37g	178	8.3	481	4.9	65.4	22.4	0
Praline, M&S*	1 Bar/34g	185	12	545	7.3	49.6	35.2	3.1

CHOCOLATE

	Measure INFO/WEIGHT	per Measure KCAL	FAT	Nutrition Values per 100g / 100ml KCAL	PROT	CARB	FAT	FIBRE
Probiotic, Bar, Ohso*	1 Bar/14g	72	5	514	5	47	36	15.5
Puddles, Hazelnut Flavour Filling, Dairy Milk, Cadbury*	¼ Bar/22.5g	114	6.2	505	6.3	57	27.5	0.9
Rafaello, Roche, Ferrero*	1 Sweet/10g	60	4.7	600	9.7	35.4	46.6	0
Reese's Pieces, Bite Size, Minis, Hershey*	11 Pieces/39g	200	12	513	7.7	59	30.8	2.6
Reese's, Fast Break, Candy Bar, Hershey*	1 Bar/56g	260	12	464	8.9	62.5	21.4	3.6
Reindeer, Lindt*	1 Reindeer/107g	588	35.3	550	7.2	55	33	0
Rocky Road, Clusters, Tesco*	1 Serving/32g	160	9.5	500	7.1	51	29.7	6.7
Salted Butterscotch, Milk, The Best, Morrisons*	2 Squares/20g	112	7.1	558	6.2	53.1	35.3	1.6
Shortcake, Snack Shots, Cadbury*	½ Bag/50g	260	14	520	5.8	60.4	27.9	2
Smooth Praline, Choceur, Aldi*	1 Square/5g	27	1.6	544	7.8	52	33	3.9
Snack Bar, Kinder*	1 Bar/21g	116	7.1	554	10	52	34	0
Snack Size, Dairy Milk, Cadbury*	1 Bar/30g	159	9	530	7.8	57.1	29.9	0
Snaps, Milk, Cadbury*	1 Snap/3g	15	0.8	505	6.3	60.5	27	1
Snickers, More Nuts, Snickers*	1 Bar/58g	299	17.3	515	10.1	52.8	29.8	0
Snowman, Mousse, Dairy Milk, Cadbury*	1 Snowman/29g	162	10.2	560	6.7	54.5	35	0.4
Speckled Eggs, M&S*	1 Egg/6g	25	1	440	6.6	63.1	18.2	1.5
Tabasco, Spicy, Tabasco*	1 Bar/28g	152	9.2	542	4.7	53.4	32.8	7.1
Tasters, Dairy Milk, Cadbury*	1 Bag/45g	238	13.7	530	7.6	56.4	30.5	0
Taz Chocolate Bar, Cadbury*	1 Bar/25g	121	6	485	4.8	62	24	0
Teddy Bear, Milk Chocolate, Thorntons*	1 Teddy/250g	1358	83.8	543	7.6	52.6	33.5	1
Tiffin, Limited Edition, Dairy Milk, Cadbury*	6 Chunks/24g	120	6	502	6.7	60	25	2.1
Toffee, Wholenut, Big Taste, Dairy Milk, Cadbury*	4 Chunks/33g	184	11.9	557	6.3	51	36	1.8
Toffifee, Storck*	1 Sweet/8g	43	2.4	516	5.9	58.5	28.7	0
Treatsize, Dairy Milk, Cadbury*	1 Bar/14g	73	4.2	525	7.5	57	29.8	0.7
Turkish Delight, Dairyfine, Aldi*	3 Squares/25g	119	6	475	3.4	62	24	0.5
Turkish Delight, Lge Bar, Dairy Milk, Cadbury*	1 Square/7.5g	35	1.6	470	5.6	63.2	21.4	0.5
Twirl, Bites, Cadbury*	1 Bite/2g	11	0.6	530	7.7	56.5	30.3	0.8
Ultimate, Bar, Waitrose*	1 Portion/60g	263	18.9	438	4.6	32.3	31.4	3.7
Wafer, Dairy Milk, Cadbury*	1 Bar/46g	235	12.9	510	7.7	57	28	0
Whips, Double Chocolate, M&S*	1 Whip/29g	140	7.3	485	6.6	57.8	25.3	1
White with Honey & Almond Nougat, Toblerone*	1 Serving/25g	132	7.2	530	6.2	60.5	29	0.2
White with Strawberries, Divine*	1 Piece/3g	16	0.9	534	7.6	59.9	29.3	0.1
White with Strawberry Pieces, Under 99 Cals, M&S*	1 Bar/16g	86	4.9	540	6.6	60.4	30.4	0.3
White, Average	*1oz/28g*	*148*	*8.7*	*529*	*8*	*58.3*	*30.9*	*0*
White, Creamy Vanilla, Green & Black's*	1 Sm Bar/35g	201	12.8	573	7.4	53.5	36.6	0.1
White, Creamy, Aldi*	1 Bar/40g	220	13.2	551	5.5	58	33	0
White, Creamy, Tesco*	1 Serving/25g	139	8.7	557	5.1	55.7	34.9	3.3
White, Crispy, Fair Trade, Co-Op*	½ Bar/50g	278	17.5	555	9	51	35	0.1
White, Nestle*	4 Pieces/40g	220	13	550	7.5	55	32.5	0
White, No Added Sugar, Belgian, Boots*	1 Serving/30g	146	10.8	488	6	47.8	36	7
White, Smart Price, Asda*	1 Serving/25g	137	8.2	549	7	56	33	0
White, Value, Tesco*	1 Serving/10g	55	3.1	548	4.7	62	31.2	0
Whole Nut, Dairy Milk, Cadbury*	1 Bar/49.1g	270	17.4	550	8.9	49.5	35.4	1.7
Whole Nut, Sainsbury's*	4 Chunks/25g	142	9.4	566	8.5	48.5	37.6	2.6
Whole Nut, Smart Price, Asda*	½ Bar/16g	92	6.2	562	8	47	38	3.3
Wildlife Bar, Cadbury*	1 Bar/21g	109	6.2	520	7.8	56.8	29.3	0
Wispa, Bitsa Wispa, Cadbury*	¼ Bag/43g	238	14.7	550	7.3	53	34	0.9
with Creme Egg, Dairy Milk, Cadbury*	1 Bar/45g	210	9.3	470	5.2	64.8	20.9	0.5
with Crunchie Bits, Dairy Milk, Cadbury*	1 Bar/200g	1000	48.8	500	6.2	63.3	24.4	0
with Shortcake Biscuit, Dairy Milk, Cadbury*	1 Square/6g	31	1.7	520	7.5	59	28	0

CHOCOLATE NUTS

	Measure INFO/WEIGHT	per Measure KCAL	FAT	Nutrition Values per 100g / 100ml KCAL	PROT	CARB	FAT	FIBRE
Peanuts, Assorted, Thorntons*	1 Bag/140g	785	57.1	561	13.8	34.8	40.8	3.6
Peanuts, Belgian Coated, M&S*	1 Serving/20g	109	7.6	545	14.7	35.6	38	5.8

	Measure INFO/WEIGHT	per Measure KCAL	FAT	Nutrition Values per 100g / 100ml KCAL	PROT	CARB	FAT	FIBRE
CHOCOLATE NUTS								
Peanuts, Milk, Tesco*	1 Bag/227g	1221	86	538	17.5	31.8	37.9	4.4
CHOCOLATE RAISINS								
Assorted, Thorntons*	1 Bag/140g	601	27.6	429	4.2	58.8	19.7	2.9
Californian, Belgian White Chocolate, M&S*	1 Pack/100g	450	20.9	450	4.3	60.6	20.9	0.8
Californian, Tesco*	½ Bag/57g	268	11.7	472	5.2	66.2	20.7	1.3
Co-Op*	½ Pack/50g	205	7.5	410	4	64	15	1
Milk Chocolate Coated, Average	*1 Serving/50g*	*207*	*7.7*	*415*	*4.4*	*64.6*	*15.4*	*2*
Milk, Asda*	1 Serving/28g	120	4.2	430	5.1	66.4	15.1	4.2
Milk, Tesco*	1 Lge Bag/227g	933	35	411	4.8	63.3	15.4	0.9
CHOCOLATE SPREAD								
& Caramel, CBY, Asda*	1 Serving/100g	564	34.7	564	2.5	60.1	34.7	0.8
Average	*1 Tsp/12g*	*68*	*4.5*	*569*	*4.1*	*57.1*	*37.6*	*0*
Hazelnut, Nutella, Ferrero*	1oz/28g	149	8.7	533	6.6	56.4	31	3.5
Hazelnut, Weight Watchers*	1 Serving/15g	50	1.8	333	4.7	45.3	12	12
Luxury, Atkins & Potts*	1 Tbsp/25g	115	7.1	459	6.3	46.6	28.3	2
Orange, Specially Selected, Aldi*	1 Tsp/3g	17	1	559	0.2	63	33	0.5
Snickers, Mars*	1 Serving/7g	38	2.6	548	8.7	43.3	37.8	0
with Nuts	*1 Tsp/12g*	*66*	*4*	*549*	*6.2*	*60.5*	*33*	*0.8*
CHOCOLATES								
All Gold, Dark, Terry's*	1 Serving/30g	152	8.7	505	4	57.5	29	4.3
All Gold, Milk, Terry's*	1 Serving/30g	158	9.2	525	4.8	58	30.5	1.5
Almond Marzipan, Milk Chocolate, Thorntons*	1 Chocolate/13g	60	2.9	464	6.6	59.4	22.6	5.6
Almond Mocca Mousse, Thorntons*	1 Chocolate/14g	76	5.3	543	8.5	40.7	37.9	2.9
Alpini, Thorntons*	1 Chocolate/13g	70	4.2	538	7	54.6	32.3	2.3
Assortment, Occasions, Tesco*	1 Chocolate/15g	70	3.1	470	4.6	65.8	20.9	0.5
Bites, Galaxy, Mars*	1 Pack/40g	197	9.7	492	5	63	24.2	0.8
Bittermint, Bendicks*	1 Mint/18g	80	3	440	4.3	68.9	16.3	2.4
Cafe Au Lait from Continental Selection, Thorntons*	1 Chocolate/16g	77	4	481	5.3	58.1	25	0.6
Cappuccino from Continental Selection, Thorntons*	1 Chocolate/13g	70	4.7	538	5.9	48.5	36.2	0.8
Caramels, Sainsbury's*	1 Sweet/11.6g	57	2.6	490	3.5	69	22.2	0.2
Celebrations, Mars*	1 Sweet/8g	40	2	497	5.6	61.2	25	1.7
Champagne Truffles, Milk, The Best, Morrisons*	1 Truffle/12g	57	2.9	479	5.2	57.9	24.8	1.4
Cherishes, Belgian, Hamlet *	2 Chocolates/24g	105	3.8	438	2.5	62.1	15.9	0
Coconut, Lindor, Lindt*	1 Ball/12.5g	79	6	632	5.4	42	48	0
Coffee Cream, Average	*1 Chocolate/12g*	*54*	*2*	*446*	*3.3*	*70.4*	*17*	*2.4*
Coffee Creme, Dark, Thorntons*	1 Chocolate/13g	52	1.4	400	3	71.5	10.8	0.8
Coffee Creme, Milk, Thorntons*	1 Chocolate/13g	52	1.3	400	2.8	74.6	10	0.8
Continental, Belgian, Thorntons*	1 Chocolate/13g	67	3.9	514	5.8	53.5	30.3	2.9
Continental, Thorntons*	1 Chocolate/15g	76	4.4	506	5.6	54.5	29.3	2.7
Country Caramel, Milk, Thorntons*	1 Chocolate/9g	45	2.4	500	4.6	62.2	26.7	0
Dairy Box, Milk, Nestle*	1 Piece/11g	50	2.1	456	4.4	65.9	19.4	0.7
Dark, Elegant, Elizabeth Shaw*	1 Chocolate/8g	38	1.8	469	2.9	62.5	23.1	0
Dark, Rose & Violet Creams	*1 Chocolate/13g*	*55*	*1.6*	*422*	*2.2*	*76.1*	*12.5*	*1.7*
Dark, Swiss Thins, Lindt*	1 Pack/125g	681	46.2	545	4.8	49.2	37	0
Eclipse, Truffle, Plain, Dark, Montezuma*	1 Truffle/16g	93	8.5	581	0.6	21.9	53.1	0
Filled, Average	*1 Chocolate/13g*	*58*	*2.8*	*447*	*4.9*	*62.9*	*21.3*	*1.3*
Fondant, Chocolate Coated, Usda Average*	1 Chocolate/11g	40	1	366	2.2	80.4	9.3	2.1
Heroes, Cadbury*	1 Sweet/8g	38	1.8	480	4.8	65.1	22.4	0.4
Italian Collection, Amaretto, M&S*	1 Chocolate/13g	60	3.1	480	4.4	59.7	25.1	2.3
Italian Collection, Favourites, M&S*	1 Chocolate/14g	74	4.7	530	5.7	50.4	33.7	1.6
Italian Collection, Panna Cotta, M&S*	1 Chocolate/13g	70	4.7	545	5.3	49.4	36.4	0.1
Lemon Selector In White Chocolate, Hotel Chocolat*	1 Sphere /5g	26	1.8	525	6	47.2	35.5	0
Liqueurs, Brandy, Asda*	1 Chocolate/8g	34	1.4	409	4	60	17	0.8

CHOCOLATES

INFO/WEIGHT	Measure	per Measure KCAL	FAT	Nutrition Values per 100g / 100ml KCAL	PROT	CARB	FAT	FIBRE
Liqueurs, Brandy, Favorina, Lidl*	1 Keg/12g	53	2.6	444	1.7	54.3	21.4	0
Liqueurs, Cherry, M&S*	1 Chocolate/12.6g	55	2.6	435	3.2	50.6	20.2	4.1
Liqueurs, Cherry, Mon Cheri, Ferrero*	1 Chocolate/11g	50	2.2	455	3	52.8	20.3	0
Liqueurs, Cognac Truffle, Thorntons*	1 Chocolate/14g	65	3.8	464	7.3	40	27.1	2.9
Liqueurs, Cointreau, Plain, Barrels	*1 Chocolate/10g*	*44*	*1.8*	*435*	*3.5*	*57*	*18*	*0*
Milk & White, Penguins, Cocoa Loco*	1 Chocolate/11g	63	4.1	572	6.5	52.3	37.2	0
Milk Tray, Cadbury*	1 Chocolate/9.4g	47	2.4	495	4.7	61.5	25.8	0.7
Milk, Mini Eggs, Green & Black's*	1 Mini Egg/7.5g	42	2.7	562	8.6	48.3	35.5	3.8
Milk, Swiss Thins, Lindt*	1 Pack/125g	688	43.3	550	5.8	53.6	34.6	0
Mini Eggs, Mix, Cadbury*	1 Pack/276g	1419	74.5	514	1.6	60	27	1.6
Mini Eggs, with Soft White Truffle Centre, M&S*	1 Egg/6g	33	2	550	6.5	56.3	33.9	1.4
Mint Creams, Dark, Smooth & Fragrant, Waitrose*	1 Sweet/10g	42	0.9	410	3	77.9	9.1	2.4
Mint Crisp, Bendicks*	1 Mint/8g	38	2.3	494	5.2	55	29.9	0
Mint Crisp, Dark, Elizabeth Shaw*	1 Chocolate/6g	27	1.2	458	1.9	68	20.7	0
Mint Crisp, Milk, Elizabeth Shaw*	1 Chocolate/6g	30	1.3	493	4	70.9	21.4	0
Mint Crisp, Thorntons*	1 Chocolate/7g	34	2.2	486	7.7	40	31.4	4.3
Mints, After Eight, Dark, Nestle*	1 Sweet/7g	32	0.9	461	5	63	12.9	2
Mints, After Eight, Orange, Nestle*	1 Sweet/7g	29	0.9	417	2.5	72.6	12.9	1.1
Mints, After Eight, Straws, Nestle*	1 Sweet/4.6g	24	1.4	526	5.1	56.6	31	4
Misshapes, Assorted, Cadbury*	1 Chocolate/8g	41	2.3	515	5.2	57.5	29.1	0
Moments, Thorntons*	1 Chocolate/7.2g	37	2	511	5.4	59.9	27.8	1.9
Neapolitans, No Added Sugar, Chocologic*	3 Chocolates/14g	66	5.1	472	8.8	27.8	36.2	22
Orange Cream, Average	*1 Chocolate/12g*	*53*	*2*	*440*	*3.2*	*69.3*	*16.7*	*0*
Orange Crisp, Elizabeth Shaw*	1 Chocolate/6g	29	1.3	478	2.9	68.2	21.5	0
Peppermint Cream, Average	*1 Chocolate/12g*	*50*	*1.4*	*418*	*1.9*	*76.4*	*11.4*	*1.6*
Praline, Coffee, Thorntons*	1 Chocolate/7g	37	2.4	529	7	47.1	34.3	2.9
Praline, Hazelnut, Thorntons*	1 Chocolate/5g	27	1.8	540	7	48	36	4
Praline, Marzipan, Thorntons*	1 Chocolate/14g	63	3	450	5.9	58.6	21.4	2.1
Praline, Roast Hazelnut, Thorntons*	1 Chocolate/13g	70	4.4	538	6	51.5	33.8	3.1
Quality Street, Nestle*	1 Sweet/9.4g	44	1.9	470	3.5	67.3	20.5	1.5
Roses, Cadbury*	1 Chocolate/8.5g	41	1.9	480	3.3	66	22.5	1.3
Sea Shells, Belgian, Guylian*	1 Shell/11.3g	62	3.8	550	7.6	52	34	0
Seashells, Belgian, Woolworths*	1 Box/63g	346	19.6	550	5.5	52.9	31.1	0
Seashells, Milk & White, Belgian, Waitrose*	1 Serving/15g	77	4.6	511	5	53.1	31	2.8
Stars, Mini Wishes, Truffle Centre, Cadbury*	1 Star/13g	70	4.1	540	6.9	55.6	31.8	1.3
Strawberries & Cream, Thorntons*	1 Chocolate/12g	64	3.9	533	5.1	54.2	32.5	0.8
Swiss Tradition, De Luxe, Lindt*	1 Pack/250g	1388	90.7	555	6.3	51.9	36.3	0
Swiss Tradition, Mixed, Lindt*	1 Pack/392g	2215	149.4	565	6.1	49.8	38.1	0
Truffle Balls, Swiss Milk Chocolate, Waitrose*	1 Chocolate/13g	78	5.8	621	4.1	47	46	1.4
Truffle Filled, Swiss, Balls, Finest, Tesco*	3 Balls/37g	240	19	640	5	40.7	50.8	1.5
Truffle Hearts, Baileys*	1 Chocolate/15g	76	4.3	506	5.2	52.6	28.9	1.3
Truffle, Amaretto, Thorntons*	1 Chocolate/14g	66	3.6	471	5.5	55	25.7	2.9
Truffle, Belgian, Flaked, Tesco*	1 Truffle/14g	80	5.4	575	4.4	52.7	38.5	2.3
Truffle, Brandy, Thorntons*	1 Chocolate/14g	68	3.8	486	6.1	52.1	27.1	0.7
Truffle, Caramel, Thorntons*	1 Chocolate/14g	67	3.6	479	4.2	57.9	25.7	2.1
Truffle, Champagne, Premier, Thorntons*	1 Chocolate/17g	88	5.6	518	6.9	45.3	32.9	2.4
Truffle, Cherry, Thorntons*	1 Chocolate/14g	58	3	414	4.2	50.7	21.4	1.4
Truffle, Continental Champagne, Thorntons*	1 Chocolate/16g	78	4.5	488	6.1	51.3	28	0.6
Truffle, Dark, Balls, Lindor, Lindt*	1 Ball/12g	76	6.2	630	3.4	38.5	51.4	0
Truffle, French Cocoa Dusted, Sainsbury's*	1 Truffle/10g	57	4.5	570	4	37	45	0
Truffle, Hazelnut, Balls, Lindor, Lindt*	1 Ball/12g	76	6.1	632	5	39.1	50.6	0
Truffle, Irish Milk Chocolate Cream, Elizabeth Shaw*	1 Chocolate/12g	57	2.7	477	3.9	63.4	22.8	0
Truffle, Lemon, White, Thorntons*	1 Chocolate/14g	63	3.5	450	4.6	64.3	25	0.7

	Measure INFO/WEIGHT	per Measure KCAL	FAT	Nutrition Values per 100g / 100ml KCAL	PROT	CARB	FAT	FIBRE
CHOCOLATES								
Truffle, Milk Chocolate, Balls, Lindor, Lindt*	1 Ball/12g	75	5.6	623	4.9	44	47	2.8
Truffle, Rum, Thorntons*	1 Chocolate/13g	63	3.2	485	4.8	58.5	24.6	4.8
Truffle, Selection, Tesco*	1 Chocolate/14g	75	4.2	539	5.1	62	29.8	0.5
Truffle, Seville, Thorntons*	1 Chocolate/14g	76	4.7	543	7.1	53.6	33.6	1.4
Truffle, Swiss, Somerfield*	1 Pack/125g	640	40	512	4	52	32	0
Truffle, Thorntons*	1 Chocolate/7g	33	1.9	471	6	48.6	27.1	1.4
Truffle, Vanilla, Thorntons*	1 Chocolate/13g	64	3.5	492	4.8	57.7	26.9	1.5
Truffle, Viennese, Dark, Thorntons*	1 Chocolate/10g	53	3.6	530	5.9	47	36	3
Truffle, Viennese, Milk, Thorntons*	1 Chocolate/10g	56	3.6	560	4.9	54	36	0
Truffle, White Chocolate, Balls, Lindor, Lindt*	1 Ball/12g	78	6.2	649	5.2	40.2	51.9	0
Truffles, Belgian Milk, Waitrose*	1 Truffle/14g	74	4.8	525	5.8	52.9	34.1	1.2
Truffles, Caramel Milk Chocolate, Aldi*	1 Truffle/12g	76	5.8	633	5.8	42.5	48.3	4.2
Truffles, Chocada, Blissed, Organic, Raw Health*	1 Pack/65g	232	11	357	7	48	17	12
Truffles, Mini Milk Chocolate Balls, Lindor, Lindt*	3 Balls/15g	90	7	600	6.7	40	46.7	0
Truffles, Rum, Average	**1 Truffle/11g**	**57**	**3.7**	**521**	**6.1**	**49.7**	**33.7**	**1.9**
Twilight, Dark with Mint, Terry's*	1 Chocolate/6g	33	1.9	530	3.1	59.5	30.5	4.2
Valentine, Thorntons*	1 Chocolate/11g	60	3.8	542	5.7	52	34.5	2.1
Winter Selection, Thorntons*	1 Chocolate/10g	51	3.1	506	6.2	51.3	30.6	3.8
CHOP SUEY								
Chicken with Noodles, Sainsbury's*	1 Pack/300g	300	7.5	100	5.7	13.6	2.5	1.2
Vegetable, M&S*	½ Pack/150g	90	6.1	60	2	3.1	4.1	2.9
CHOW MEIN								
Beef, Ready Meal, Average	**1 Serving/400g**	**422**	**12.2**	**106**	**6**	**13.4**	**3**	**1**
Beef, Sainsbury's*	1 Pack/450g	500	11.2	111	6.6	15.5	2.5	0.8
Cantonese Vegetable Stir Fry, Sainsbury's*	¼ Pack/100g	85	3.8	85	2.2	10.6	3.8	1.2
Chicken & Vegetable, Fuller Longer, M&S*	1 Pack/380g	266	4.9	70	6.3	8.7	1.3	2.1
Chicken, Chinese Takeaway, Sainsbury's*	1 Pack/316g	338	8.5	107	9.1	11.6	2.7	0.7
Chicken, Chinese Takeaway, Tesco*	1 Serving/350g	294	8.4	84	8.1	7.5	2.4	1.1
Chicken, Co-Op*	1 Pack/300g	270	9	90	8	9	3	0.9
Chicken, COU, M&S*	1 Pack/200g	170	5.4	85	5.9	9.5	2.7	1.4
Chicken, Less Than 3% Fat, BGTY, Sainsbury's*	1 Pack/400g	292	6.2	75	5.9	7.8	1.6	2.7
Chicken, Microwaved, Slimzone, Asda*	1 Pack/475g	342	3.3	72	7.4	8.4	0.7	1.5
Chicken, Morrisons*	1 Pack/400g	368	9.2	92	5.8	13	2.3	1.1
Chicken, Ready Meal, Average	**1 Serving/400g**	**375**	**9.4**	**94**	**6.5**	**11.5**	**2.4**	**1.2**
Chicken, Takeaway, Main, M&S*	1 Pack/400g	440	12	110	7.7	12.4	3	1.4
Pork, PB, Waitrose*	½ Pack/310g	332	2.8	107	7.6	17.2	0.9	1.6
Prawn, Takeaway, Chinese	**1 Portion/550g**	**792**	**60**	**144**	**5.6**	**6.1**	**10.9**	**2.8**
Special, COU, M&S*	1 Pack/400g	400	15.2	100	6.6	10.3	3.8	1.4
Special, Ready Meal, Average	**1 Serving/400g**	**383**	**9.7**	**96**	**6.5**	**12.1**	**2.4**	**1**
Vegetable, Ready Meal, Average	**1 Serving/400g**	**337**	**6.7**	**84**	**4.2**	**12.8**	**1.7**	**2**
Vesta*	1 Pack/433.3g	594	17.3	137	4.8	20.4	4	3.3
CHRISTMAS PUDDING								
Alcohol & Nut Free, Matthew Walker*	1 Pudding/100g	277	2.3	277	3.1	59.3	2.3	3.4
Alcohol Free, 450g, Sainsbury's*	1 Serving/114g	330	3.5	290	2.7	61.3	3.1	3.2
Average	**1oz/28g**	**81**	**2.7**	**291**	**4.6**	**49.5**	**9.7**	**1.3**
BGTY, Sainsbury's*	1 Serving/114g	302	2.8	266	2.8	58.2	2.5	4.6
Champagne, Luxury, Specially Selected, Aldi*	¼ Pudding/113g	346	8.4	306	3.5	54	7.4	5.1
Classic, Asda*	¼ Pudding/113g	362	6.2	319	2.7	63	5.5	3.4
Cognac Laced, 450g, TTD, Sainsbury's*	¼ Pudding/113g	341	10	303	2.8	51.3	8.9	3.1
Connoisseur, Holly Lane, Aldi*	1 Pudding/100g	303	4.9	303	2.3	61	4.9	3.6
Gluten & Wheat Free, Finest, Tesco*	1 Pudding/100g	305	7.1	305	3.3	55.1	7.1	3.7
Hidden Clementine, Heston, Waitrose*	1 Serving/114g	352	7.7	310	2.9	57.8	6.8	3.1
Hidden Clementine, Matured, Finest, Tesco*	¼ Pudding/113g	351	8.5	309	3	55.6	7.5	3.5

	Measure INFO/WEIGHT	per Measure KCAL	FAT	Nutrition Values per 100g / 100ml KCAL	PROT	CARB	FAT	FIBRE
CHRISTMAS PUDDING								
Individual, 6 Month Matured, Sainsbury's*	1 Pudding/100g	309	5.3	309	2.4	60.8	5.3	4
Light & Fruity, 450g, Sainsbury's*	¼ Pudding/113g	331	5.3	293	1.8	59.3	4.7	3.4
Luxury	*1 Serving/114g*	*416*	*18.8*	*365*	*2.5*	*48.6*	*16.4*	*1*
Luxury, Tesco*	¼ Pudding/114g	346	11	305	3.7	50.8	9.7	1.3
Matured, Finest, Tesco*	1 Serving/113g	340	8.3	300	3.2	54.1	7.3	2.5
Nut Free & Alcohol Free, Tesco*	1 Serving/114g	368	6.5	323	2.9	63.6	5.7	3
Pear & Calvados Pudding, Finest, Tesco*	1/8 Pudding/113g	330	5.7	291	3.3	56.8	5	2.9
Rich Fruit, Tesco*	1 Serving/114g	331	6.7	290	2.4	55	5.9	0
Sticky Toffee, Tesco*	¼ Pudding/114g	372	7.3	326	2.5	64.5	6.4	0.8
Ultimate, Finest, Tesco*	1 Serving/100g	285	7	285	3.7	51.6	7	4.7
Vintage, M&S*	1/8 Pudding/113g	335	6.4	295	2.6	59.8	5.6	1.4
CHUTNEY								
Albert's Victorian, Baxters*	1 Serving/25g	40	0.1	159	1.1	37.9	0.3	1.5
Apple & Pear, TTD, Sainsbury's*	1 Serving/20g	38	0.2	190	0.6	45.2	0.8	1.7
Apple & Walnut, Waitrose*	1 Serving/20g	49	0.5	243	12	53.8	2.6	3.8
Apricot, Sharwood's*	1 Tsp/16g	21	0	131	0.6	32	0.1	2.3
Bengal Spice Mango, Sharwood's*	1 Tsp/5g	12	0	236	0.5	58	0.2	1.2
Caramelised Onion, Sainsbury's*	1 Serving/25g	28	0.4	111	1.1	23.5	1.4	1.1
Caramelised Red Onion, Loyd Grossman*	1 Serving/10g	11	0	111	0.5	27.2	0	0.5
Cheese Board, Cottage Delight Ltd*	1 Tbsp/15g	42	0.5	277	1	46.6	3.1	0
Cranberry & Caramelised Red Onion, Baxters*	1 Serving/20g	31	0	154	0.3	38	0.1	0.3
Fruit, Spiced, Baxters*	1 Tsp/16g	23	0	143	6	34.8	0.1	0
Fruit, Traditional, M&S*	1oz/28g	43	0.1	155	0.9	37.2	0.3	1.7
Indian Appetisers, Pot, Waitrose*	1 Pot/158g	330	2.2	209	1.8	47.3	1.4	1.8
Lime & Chilli, Geeta's*	1 Serving/25g	69	0.4	277	2	64	1.4	1.9
Mango & Apple, Sharwood's*	1oz/28g	65	0	233	0.4	57.6	0.1	1.1
Mango & Ginger, Baxters*	1 Jar/320g	598	0.6	187	5	45.7	0.2	0.9
Mango & Chilli, Geeta's*	1 Serving/30g	74	0	246	0.5	60.7	0.1	0.2
Mango & Mint, Cofresh*	1 Tbsp/20g	31	0.1	155	1.7	36.4	0.3	2
Mango with Hint of Chilli & Ginger, Waitrose*	1 Serving/20g	52	0	259	0.5	64.2	0	0.7
Mango, Green Label, Sharwood's*	1 Tsp/10g	24	0	241	0.3	59.7	0.1	0.9
Mango, Hot & Spicy, Waitrose*	1 Serving/20g	46	0.1	230	0.6	51.6	0.3	1.8
Mango, Premium, Geeta's*	1 Serving/50g	126	0.1	253	0.8	62	0.2	0.8
Mango, Spicy, Sainsbury's*	1 Tbsp/15g	24	0.1	160	0.7	37	0.7	1.3
Mango, Sweet	*1 Tsp/16g*	*30*	*0*	*189*	*0.7*	*48.3*	*0.1*	*0*
Mango, Tesco*	1 Serving/20g	45	0	224	0.4	55.5	0.1	1.3
Mango, Waitrose*	1 Serving/20g	43	0.3	215	1	49	1.5	2
Mixed Fruit	*1 Tsp/16g*	*25*	*0*	*155*	*0.6*	*39.7*	*0*	*0*
Onion, Vitasia, Lidl*	1 Tbsp/15g	40	0.1	266	0.9	63.1	0.9	0
Peach, Spicy, Waitrose*	1 Serving/20g	43	0.3	215	1	49	1.5	1.5
Ploughman's Plum, The English Provender Co.*	1 Tsp/10g	16	0	160	1.3	38.1	0.2	1.6
Plum, Ploughman's, Tesco*	1 Tsp/5g	8	0	154	1	34.1	0.4	5.3
Red Onion & Sherry Vinegar, Sainsbury's*	1 Serving/10g	24	0.1	236	0.5	57.1	0.6	1.4
Spicy Fruit, Baxters*	1 Serving/15g	22	0	146	0.6	35.4	0.2	0
Spicy Onion, Organic, The English Provender Co.*	1 Serving/10g	24	0	245	1.2	59	0.5	3.5
Sticky Fig & Balsamic Chutney, M&S*	1 Servin/25g	57	0.3	228	1.6	49.8	1.3	5.4
Sweet Mango, Patak's*	1 Tbsp/15g	39	0	259	0.3	67.4	0.1	0.7
Sweet Tomato & Chilli, The English Provender Co.*	1 Tsp/10g	19	0	189	0.9	46	0.2	1.7
Tomato	*1 Tsp/16g*	*20*	*0*	*128*	*1.2*	*31*	*0.2*	*1.3*
Tomato & Chilli, Specially Selected, Aldi*	1 Tbsp/15g	21	0.1	138	12	32	0.5	1.3
Tomato & Red Pepper, Baxters*	1 Jar/312g	512	1.2	164	2	38	0.4	1.5
Tomato, Baxters*	1 Tsp/12g	18	0	152	1.1	35.9	0.4	1
Tomato, Waitrose*	1 Pot/100g	195	0.3	195	1.3	46.8	0.3	0

C

	Measure INFO/WEIGHT	per Measure KCAL	FAT	Nutrition Values per 100g / 100ml KCAL	PROT	CARB	FAT	FIBRE
CIDER								
Apple, Low Alcohol, Sainsbury's*	1 Glass/250ml	75	0.4	30	0.5	5.4	0.2	0
Basics, Sainsbury's*	1 Glass/250ml	200	0	80	0	0	0	0
Berry, Irish, Magner's*	1 Bottle/500ml	215	0	43	0	4.3	0	0
Cyder, Organic, Aspall*	1 Serving/200ml	120	0.2	60	0.1	3.1	0.1	0
Cyder, Perronelle's Blush, Aspall*	1 Serving/200ml	122	0.2	61	0.1	5.4	0.1	0.5
Cyder, Premier Cru, Aspall*	1 Serving/200ml	120	0	60	0	3.1	0	0
Cyder, Suffolk, Medium, Aspall*	1 Serving/200ml	134	0	67	0.1	4.4	0	0
Diamond White*	1fl oz/30ml	11	0	36	0	2.6	0	0
Dry, Average	*1 Pint/568ml*	*205*	*0*	*36*	*0*	*2.6*	*0*	*0*
Dry, French, So Good, Somerfield*	1 Bottle/500ml	150	0	30	0	0.3	0	0
Dry, Strongbow*	1 Bottle/375ml	161	0	43	0	3.4	0	0
Fruit, Mixed, Alcohol Free, Kopparberg*	1 Bottle/500ml	190	2.5	38	0.5	9.2	0.5	0
Gold, Thatchers*	1 Bottle/500ml	230	0	46	0	4.5	0	0
Light, Bulmers*	1 Can/500ml	140	0	28	0	0.8	0	0
Low Alcohol	*1 Pint/568ml*	*97*	*0*	*17*	*0*	*3.6*	*0*	*0*
Low Alcohol, M&S*	1 Serving/200ml	50	0	25	0	6.5	0	0
Low Alcohol, Sainsbury's*	1 Serving/200ml	62	0	31	0	6.4	0	0
Low Carb, Stowford*	1 Bottle/500ml	140	0	28	0	0.2	0	0
Magner's*	½ Pint/284ml	105	0	37	0	2	0	0
Medium Sweet, Somerfield*	1 Pint/568ml	233	0	41	0	5	0	0
Mulled, Waitrose*	½ Pint/284ml	145	0	51	0	0	0	0
Organic, Westons*	1 Serving/200ml	96	0	48	0	3.1	0	0
Original, Bulmers*	1 Serving/250ml	105	0	42	0	4	0	0
Original, Gaymers*	1 Bottle/330ml	148	0	45	0	4.7	0	0
Pear, Bulmers*	1 Serving/200ml	86	0	43	0	3.6	0	0
Pear, Gaymers*	1 Bottle/330ml	168	0	51	0	6.2	0	0
Pear, Magner's*	1 Bottle/568ml	179	0	32	0	0	0	0
Pear, Non Alcoholic, Kopparberg*	1 Bottle/500ml	170	0.5	34	0	8.4	0.1	0
Raspberry, Light, Kopparberg*	1 Can/250ml	85	1.2	34	0.5	2.6	0.5	0
Scrumpy, Average	*1 Serving/200ml*	*93*	*0*	*46*	*0*	*2.3*	*0*	*0*
Scrumpy, Westons*	1 Serving/200ml	94	0	47	0	1.8	0	0
Strawberry & Lime, Non Alcoholic, Kopparberg*	1 Bottle/500ml	205	2.5	41	0.5	10.1	0.5	0
Sweet, Average	*1 Pint/568ml*	*239*	*0*	*42*	*0*	*4.3*	*0*	*0*
Vintage	*1 Pint/568ml*	*574*	*0*	*101*	*0*	*7.3*	*0*	*0*
CINNAMON								
Ground, Average	*1 Tsp/3g*	*8*	*0.1*	*261*	*3.9*	*55.5*	*3.2*	*0*
CLAMS								
in Brine, Average	*1oz/28g*	*22*	*0.2*	*79*	*16*	*2.4*	*0.6*	*0*
Raw, Average	*20 Sm/180g*	*133*	*1.7*	*74*	*12.8*	*2.6*	*1*	*0*
CLEMENTINES								
Raw, Weighed with Peel, Average	*1 Med/61g*	*22*	*0.1*	*35*	*0.6*	*9*	*0.1*	*1.3*
Raw, Weighed without Peel, Average	*1 Med/46g*	*22*	*0.1*	*47*	*0.8*	*12*	*0.2*	*1.7*
COCKLES								
Boiled	*1 Cockle/4g*	*2*	*0*	*53*	*12*	*0*	*0.6*	*0*
Bottled in Vinegar, Drained	*1oz/28g*	*8*	*0.1*	*28*	*6.3*	*0*	*0.3*	*0*
in Parsley Oil, The Best, Morrisons*	½ Pack70g	91	5.2	129	9.6	5.9	7.4	0.4
COCKTAIL								
Alcoholic, Juice Based, Average	*1 Glass/200ml*	*464*	*29.2*	*232*	*6.4*	*18.7*	*14.6*	*1.4*
Bloody Mary, Average	*1 Glass/250ml*	*86*	*0*	*42*	*0*	*2.3*	*0*	*0.6*
Bucks Fizz, Premixed, M&S*	1 Glass/250ml	152	0	61	0	9	0	0
Cosmo, Skinny Brands*	1 Can/250ml	90	0.2	36	0	1.3	0.1	0
Cosmopolitan, Canned, M&S*	1 Serving/200ml	456	0	228	0	22	0	0
Daiquiri, Strawberry, Frozen, Average	*1 Glass/250ml*	*132*	*0*	*53*	*0*	*14.1*	*0*	*0*

	Measure INFO/WEIGHT	per Measure KCAL	FAT	Nutrition Values per 100g / 100ml KCAL	PROT	CARB	FAT	FIBRE
COCKTAIL								
Grenadine, Orange Juice, Pineapple Juice	*1 Serving/200ml*	*158*	*0.3*	*79*	*0.5*	*19.2*	*0.1*	*0.2*
Long Island Iced Tea, Average	*1 Glass/250ml*	*282*	*0*	*113*	*0*	*13.6*	*0*	*0*
Mai Tai, Average	*1 Serving/200ml*	*209*	*0.1*	*105*	*0.2*	*13.9*	*0.1*	*0.1*
Margarita, Skinny Brands*	1 Can/250ml	90	0.2	36	0	1	0.1	0
Mojito, Canned, My Cocktail, Manchester Drinks Co.*	1 Can/250ml	150	0	60	0	9.1	0	0
Mojito, Skinny Brands*	1 Can/250ml	90	0.2	36	0	1.1	0.1	0
Pina Colada	*1 Glass/250ml*	*592*	*20*	*237*	*1*	*28*	*8*	*0*
COCOA								
Nibs, Naturya*	1 Serving/10g	58	5	578	13	18.2	50.3	13.4
COCOA POWDER								
Cadbury*	1 Tbsp/16g	52	3.3	322	23.1	10.5	20.8	0
Dark, Fine, Dr Oetker*	3 Tbsp/25g	89	5.2	357	20	8.9	21	28
Dry, Unsweetened, Average	*1 Tbsp/5g*	*11*	*0.7*	*229*	*19.6*	*54.3*	*13.7*	*33.2*
Organic, Green & Black's*	1 Tsp/4g	16	0.8	405	22	19	21	27
COCONUT								
Chips, Caramel, Navitas Naturals*	1 Pack/57g	377	31.4	662	6.3	35	55	14
Creamed, Average	*1oz/28g*	*186*	*19.2*	*666*	*6*	*6.7*	*68.4*	*7*
Curls, Ape*	1 Pack/20g	108	7.8	540	6.9	28	39	22
Desiccated, Average	*1oz/28g*	*169*	*17.4*	*604*	*5.6*	*6.4*	*62*	*13.7*
Flaked, Neal's Yard*	1 Serving/30g	181	18.6	604	5.3	44.4	62	13.7
Flakes, Unsweetened, Dr Goerg*	1 Serving/100g	686	67	686	7	6	67	15.6
Fresh, Flesh Only, Average	*1oz/28g*	*69*	*7.1*	*246*	*2.2*	*2.6*	*25.2*	*5.1*
Ice, Average	*1oz/28g*	*104*	*3.6*	*371*	*1.7*	*66.7*	*12.7*	*2.6*
Water with Pineapple, Vita Coco*	1 Carton /330ml	82	0	25	0	6	0	0
Water, Vitasia, Lidl*	1 Can/330ml	63	0	19	0	4.2	0	0
COD								
Bake, with Crab & Potato, Finest, Tesco*	1 Pack/364g	312	10.9	86	6.9	7.3	3	1
Baked, Average	*1oz/28g*	*27*	*0.3*	*96*	*21.4*	*0*	*1.2*	*0*
Beer Battered, Crispy, Finest, Tesco*	1 Portion/250g	575	35	230	12	13.4	14	1.3
Bites & Chips, 573, Wiltshire Farm Foods*	1 Portion/310g	433	12.1	140	6.2	19	3.9	0
Dried, Salted, Average	*1oz/28g*	*82*	*0.7*	*290*	*62.8*	*0*	*2.4*	*0*
Dried, Salted, Boiled, Average	*1oz/28g*	*32*	*0.7*	*115*	*27*	*0*	*0.7*	*0*
Fillets with a Red Pepper Salsa, Love Life, Waitrose*	½ Pack/170g	92	1.5	54	9	2.5	0.9	0.5
Fillets, Battered, Average	*1 Fillet/125g*	*219*	*10.2*	*176*	*12.6*	*13*	*8.2*	*1*
Fillets, Breaded, Average	*1 Fillet/125g*	*258*	*12.2*	*206*	*13*	*16.7*	*9.8*	*1*
Fillets, Breaded, Chunky, Average	*1 Piece/135g*	*204*	*8*	*151*	*13.7*	*10.9*	*5.9*	*1.4*
Fillets, Breaded, Light, Healthy Range, Average	*1 Fillet/135g*	*209*	*6.9*	*154*	*13.6*	*13.3*	*5.1*	*1.2*
Fillets, Broccoli Mornay, Cooked, Ocean Trader*	½ Pack/155g	142	5.4	92	12	2.4	3.5	1.2
Fillets, Chunky, Average	*1 Fillet/198g*	*267*	*7.3*	*135*	*17.1*	*8.2*	*3.7*	*0.8*
Fillets, Mediterranean Herb Style, Tesco*	1 Serving/115g	163	11	142	13.8	0.1	9.6	0.1
Fillets, Skinless & Boneless, Raw, Average	*1 Fillet/140g*	*137*	*2.4*	*98*	*17.8*	*0*	*1.8*	*0.4*
Fillets, Smoked, Average	*1 Serving/150g*	*152*	*2.4*	*101*	*21.6*	*0*	*1.6*	*0*
Fillets, Tempura, Battered, Crispy, Gastro, Youngs*	1 Fillet/131g	252	12.1	192	12.9	14.1	9.2	0.8
Fillets, with Tomato & Basil Sauce, Simply Bake, Tesco*	1 Fillet/142g	170	8.1	120	15.2	1.8	5.7	0.1
Fillets, Beer Battered, Gastro, Youngs*	1 Fillet/119g	232	10.7	195	13.6	14.4	9	1.1
Loins, Average	*1 Serving/145g*	*116*	*1.2*	*80*	*17.9*	*0.1*	*0.8*	*0.2*
Loins, Beer Battered, TTD, Sainsbury's*	1 Fillet/93g	182	10.8	196	14.4	8.5	11.6	2.7
Mornay, Fillets, Sainsbury's*	1 Serving/153g	236	14.4	154	15.2	2.2	9.4	0.9
Mornay, Gratin, Cooked, Just Cook, Sainsbury's*	1 Pack/320g	518	32.2	185	13.3	6.9	11.5	0.5
Mornay, Nutritionally Balanced, M&S*	1 Pack/400g	320	10.4	80	6.8	7.2	2.6	1.6
Mornay, Sainsbury's*	1 Serving/180g	277	16.9	154	15.2	2.2	9.4	0.9
Mornay, with Mash & Peas, HL, Tesco*	1 Pack/327g	322	7.5	99	7.8	10.2	2.3	2.9
Poached, Average	*1oz/28g*	*26*	*0.3*	*94*	*20.9*	*0*	*1.1*	*0*

C

	Measure INFO/WEIGHT	per Measure KCAL	FAT	Nutrition Values per 100g / 100ml KCAL	PROT	CARB	FAT	FIBRE
COD								
Smoked, Raw, Average	*1oz/28g*	*22*	*0.2*	*78*	*18.1*	*0*	*0.6*	*0*
Steaks, Battered, Chip Shop Style, Average	*1 Serving/150g*	*321*	*18*	*214*	*12.5*	*14.3*	*12*	*1.1*
Steamed, Average	*1oz/28g*	*23*	*0.3*	*83*	*18.6*	*0*	*0.9*	*0*
Thai Green, Steamer, Cook In, Co-Op*	½ Pack/169g	149	4.7	88	13	2.4	2.8	0.9
COD & CHIPS								
& Peas, 240, Oakhouse Foods Ltd*	1 Meal/300g	510	18.6	170	6.4	22.3	6.2	2.2
Asda*	1 Serving/280g	450	14	161	8	21	5	1.1
Chunky, M&S*	1 Serving/340g	510	20.4	150	6.5	17.5	6	1.5
COD IN								
a Sweet Red Pepper Sauce, Fillets, GFY, Asda*	½ Pack/170g	143	2.7	84	15	2.3	1.6	0.1
Butter Sauce, Ross*	1 Serving/150g	126	5.8	84	9.1	3.2	3.9	0.1
Butter Sauce, Sainsbury's*	1 Serving/150g	198	13.5	132	10.6	2	9	0.1
Butter Sauce, Steaks, Birds Eye*	1 Pack/170g	185	9.4	109	9.8	5	5.5	0.1
Butter Sauce, Steaks, Frozen, Asda*	1 Pouch/152g	163	4	107	16	5	2.6	0.8
Butter Sauce, Steaks, Morrisons*	1 Steak/170g	153	5.6	90	10.9	4.1	3.3	0.4
Butter Sauce, Steaks, Youngs*	1 Pack/139g	107	3.2	77	9.7	4.1	2.3	0.4
Butter Sauce, Tesco*	1 Pack/150g	123	5.4	82	9.4	2.9	3.6	0.5
Cheese Sauce, BGTY, Sainsbury's*	1 Serving/170g	144	4.1	85	12.8	3.1	2.4	0
Cheese Sauce, Pre Packed, Average	*1 Serving/150g*	*136*	*4.4*	*90*	*11.8*	*4.2*	*3*	*0*
Cheese Sauce, Steaks, Birds Eye*	1 Pack/182g	175	6.4	96	10.9	5.2	3.5	0.1
Cheese Sauce, with Broccoli, Lidl*	½ Pack/155g	143	5.4	92	12	2.4	3.5	1.2
Mushroom Sauce, BGTY, Sainsbury's*	1 Serving/170g	112	2.9	66	9.9	2.8	1.7	0.1
Parsley Sauce, COU, M&S*	1 Pack/185g	130	4.6	70	10.6	1.4	2.5	0.6
Parsley Sauce, Frozen, M&S*	1 Pack/184g	156	7.2	85	11.1	1.9	3.9	1
Parsley Sauce, Portions, Ocean Trader*	1 Serving/120g	112	4.7	93	9.4	4	3.9	0.1
Parsley Sauce, Pre Packed, Average	*1 Serving/150g*	*123*	*4.7*	*82*	*10.1*	*3.3*	*3.1*	*0.5*
Parsley Sauce, Skinless & Boneless, Sainsbury's*	1 Portion/150g	162	9	108	11.3	2.2	6	0.5
Parsley Sauce, Steaks, Birds Eye*	1 Steak/172g	155	4.8	90	10.5	5.6	2.8	0.1
Red Pepper Sauce, SteamFresh, Birds Eye*	1 Serving/125g	115	2.4	92	14.4	4.7	1.9	0.3
COD MEDITERRANEAN								
Everdine*	1 Serving/450g	414	18	92	6.8	5.4	4	3.9
PB, Waitrose*	1 Serving/370g	255	3.7	69	13.1	1.9	1	1.2
Style, Fillets, GFY, Asda*	1 Pack/397g	274	9.9	69	9	2.5	2.5	0.9
COD WITH								
a Mediterranean Pepper Sauce, Fillets, Waitrose*	1 Pack/370g	240	4.8	65	12.2	1.1	1.3	0.9
a Thai Crust, PB, Waitrose*	1 Pack/280g	249	7	89	15.1	1.6	2.5	0.6
Fish Pesto, Fillets, COOK!, M&S*	½ Pack/165g	210	5.1	127	16.4	8.4	3.1	4.2
Parma Ham & Sardinian Chick Peas, M&S*	½ Pack/255g	268	12.5	105	9.8	5.3	4.9	0.5
Roasted Vegetables, M&S*	1 Serving/280g	238	10.6	85	8	4.9	3.8	1.7
Salsa & Rosemary Potatoes, BGTY, Sainsbury's*	1 Pack/450g	356	4	79	4.7	13.1	0.9	1.6
Sunblush Tomato Sauce, GFY, Asda*	½ Pack/177g	117	2.7	66	13	0.1	1.5	1
Sweet Chilli, COU, M&S*	1 Pack/400g	360	2	90	7.7	13.1	0.5	1.6
Tomato Sauce, Fillets, Asda*	1 Serving/181g	210	10.9	116	13	2.6	6	2.3
COFFEE								
& Chicory, Breakfast Drink, Ricore, Nestle*	1 Tsp/5g	7	0	141	2.7	9.1	0	45.3
Azera, Barista Style Instant, Nescafe*	1 Serving/200ml	2	0	1	0.1	0	0	0
Azera, Latte, To Go, Nescafe*	1 Serving/307ml	89	2.5	29	1	4.4	0.8	0.3
Black, Average	*1 Mug/270ml*	*5*	*0*	*2*	*0.2*	*0.3*	*0*	*0*
Cafe Caramel, Cafe Range, Nescafe*	1 Sachet/17g	72	2.4	423	9.2	64.6	14.1	1.3
Cafe Hazelnut, Nescafe*	1 Sachet/17g	73	2.4	428	9.3	66	14.1	0
Cafe Irish Cream, Cafe Range, Nescafe*	1 Sachet/23g	98	3.2	425	8.2	65.2	14.1	1.2
Cafe Latte, Dry, Douwe Egberts*	1 Serving/12g	58	2.6	480	10	60	22	0
Cafe Latte, Instant, Made Up, Maxwell House*	1 Serving/12.5g	53	1.7	424	6.4	68	13.6	0

COFFEE

INFO/WEIGHT	Measure	per Measure KCAL	FAT	Nutrition Values per 100g / 100ml KCAL	PROT	CARB	FAT	FIBRE
Cafe Latte, Vita Coco*	1 Carton/330g	132	3.3	40	1.7	6	1	0
Cafe Mocha, Cafe Range, Nescafe*	1 Sachet/22g	92	2.9	418	8.5	66.6	13.1	0
Cafe Vanilla, Latte, Cafe Range, Nescafe*	1 Sachet/18.5g	73	1.6	395	9.2	68.3	8.5	4.1
Cappuccino Ice, Made Up, Dolce Gusto, Nescafe*	1 Serving/240ml	111	2.8	46	1.8	7.2	1.2	0.2
Cappuccino, Cafe Mocha, Dry, Maxwell House*	1 Serving/23g	100	2.5	434	4.3	78.2	10.8	0
Cappuccino, Cafe Specials, Dry, M&S*	1 Serving/14g	55	1.6	395	14	59	11.5	0.7
Cappuccino, Cappio, Iced, Kenco*	1 Can/200ml	138	6	69	3	7	3	0
Cappuccino, Cappio, Kenco*	1 Sachet/18g	79	1.9	439	11.7	73.9	10.6	0.6
Cappuccino, Co-Op*	1 Serving/12.5g	55	2	440	16	64	16	8
Cappuccino, Decaff, Instant, Made Up, Nescafe*	1 Mug/200ml	68	2.3	34	1	5	1.2	0
Cappuccino, Decaff, Nescafe*	1 Sachet/16g	68	2.3	428	11.6	62.6	14.6	0
Cappuccino, Decaff, Unsweetened, Nescafe*	1 Sachet/16g	70	3.1	437	14.5	51.2	19.4	4.3
Cappuccino, Dreamy, Cafe, Options*	1 Serving/30g	77	5.1	256	12.9	58.1	16.9	0
Cappuccino, Dry, Maxwell House*	1 Mug/15g	52	1.4	350	12	64	9.6	0.4
Cappuccino, Dry, Waitrose*	1 Sachet/13g	58	2.3	439	15.1	56	17.2	4.4
Cappuccino, for Filter Systems, Kenco*	1 Sachet/6g	22	0.8	375	19	44	13.5	0
Cappuccino, Iced, Cowbelle, Aldi*	1 Serving/250ml	169	4.5	68	3.3	9.6	1.8	0.3
Cappuccino, Instant, Aldi*	1 Sachet/12.5g	49	1.7	393	12.5	55.1	13.6	0
Cappuccino, Instant, Asda*	1 Sachet/15g	60	2.3	399	13	53	15.2	0.9
Cappuccino, Instant, Kenco*	1 Sachet/20g	80	2.8	401	13.5	55.7	13.8	0
Cappuccino, Instant, Made Up, Maxwell House*	1 Serving/280g	123	5.3	44	0.6	5.8	1.9	0
Cappuccino, Instant, Unsweetened, Douwe Egberts*	1 Serving/12g	48	1.9	400	11	53	16	0
Cappuccino, Italian, Nescafe*	1 Cup/150ml	60	2.9	40	1.2	4.4	1.9	0
Cappuccino, Low Sugar, Tesco*	1 Serving/13g	55	2.6	425	18.4	43.3	19.8	0.4
Cappuccino, M&S*	1 Serving/164g	66	2.6	40	1.5	4.4	1.6	0
Cappuccino, Made Up, Dolce Gusto, Nescafe*	1 Serving/240ml	84	3.7	35	1.6	4	1.5	0.3
Cappuccino, Original Mugsticks, Maxwell House*	1 Serving/18g	73	2.8	406	14.4	52.8	15.6	0
Cappuccino, Original, Sachets, Nescafe*	1 Sachet/18g	80	3.1	444	11.7	60.3	17.4	0
Cappuccino, Sainsbury's*	1 Serving/12g	49	1.9	411	14.9	52.9	15.5	0.4
Cappuccino, Semi Skimmed Milk, Average	*1 Serving/200ml*	*63*	*2.3*	*31*	*2.2*	*3.2*	*1.2*	*0*
Cappuccino, Sweetened, Instant, Alcafe, Aldi*	1 Sachet/135ml	61	1.6	45	0.5	8.2	1.2	0.4
Cappuccino, to Go, Original, Nescafe*	1 Serving/19g	84	3.3	444	11.7	60.3	17.4	0
Cappuccino, Unsweetened Taste, Maxwell House*	1 Serving/15g	65	2.9	434	17.4	47.6	19.3	0.3
Cappuccino, Unsweetened, Cappio, Kenco*	1 Serving/18g	73	1.8	406	12.2	66.7	10	0.6
Cappuccino, Unsweetened, Gold, Nescafe*	1 Sachet/14g	55	1.8	392	12.9	52.5	13	5.7
Capuccino, Alcafe, Aldi*	1 Sachet/135ml	61	1.6	45	0.5	8.2	1.2	0.4
Chococino, Made up, Dolce Gusto, Nescafe*	1 Serving/210g	147	5.4	70	2.3	9.4	2.6	0.7
Columbian, Nescafe*	1 Serving/2g	2	0	111	16.7	11.1	0	5.6
Compliment*	1 Serving/14ml	20	1.8	143	1.4	6.4	12.9	0
Dandelion, Symingtons*	1 Tsp/6g	19	0	320	2.8	79.3	0	0
Espresso, Instant, Nescafe*	1 Tsp/1.8g	2	0	118	7.8	3.1	0.2	34.1
Espresso, Made Up, Dolce Gusto, Nescafe*	1 Serving/60ml	1	0.1	2	0.1	0	0.2	0.3
Frappe Iced, Nestle*	1 Sachet/24g	92	1	384	15	72	4	0.5
Gold Blend, Decafefinated, Nescafe*	1 Tsp/5g	3	0	63	7	9	0.2	27
Gold Blend, Nescafe*	1 Cup 200ml/5g	3	0	63	7	9	0.2	27
Green Mountain, Breakfast, Keurig*	1 Serving/227ml	0	0	0	0.1	0	0	0
Ice Mocha Drink, Nescafe, Nestle*	1 Bottle/280ml	160	3.4	57	1.1	10.5	1.2	0
Iced, Mocha, Jimmys Iced Coffee*	1 Carton/300g	138	3.6	46	2.3	6.6	1.2	0
Iced, Original, Jimmys Iced Coffee*	1 Carton/300ml	126	3	42	2	6.2	1	0
Iced, Skinny, Jimmys Iced Coffee*	1 Carton/330ml	106	0	32	2	6.3	0	0
Infusion, Avg with Semi-Skimmed Milk	*1 Cup/220ml*	*15*	*0.4*	*7*	*0.6*	*0.7*	*0.2*	*0*
Infusion, Avg with Single Cream	*1 Cup/220ml*	*31*	*2.6*	*14*	*0.4*	*0.3*	*1.2*	*0*
Instant, Alta Rica, Nescafe*	1 Tsp/1.8g	2	0	98	13.8	10	0.3	21

C

	Measure INFO/WEIGHT	per Measure		Nutrition Values per 100g / 100ml				
		KCAL	FAT	KCAL	PROT	CARB	FAT	FIBRE
COFFEE								
Instant, Decaffeinated, Nescafe*	1 Tsp/1.8g	2	0	101	14.9	10	0.2	8.4
Instant, Fine Blend, Nescafe*	1 Tsp/2g	1	0	63	7	9	0.2	27
Instant, Made with Skimmed Milk	***1 Serving/270ml***	***15***	***0***	***6***	***0.6***	***0.8***	***0***	***0***
Instant, Made with Water & Semi Skimmed Milk	***1 Serving/350ml***	***24***	***0.7***	***7***	***0.4***	***0.5***	***0.2***	***0***
Instant, Made with Water, & Whole Milk	***1 Cup/220ml***	***18***	***0.9***	***8***	***0.5***	***0.6***	***0.4***	***0***
Instant, Original, Nescafe*	1 Tsp/1.8g	1	0	63	7	9	0.2	27
Instant, with Skimmed Milk, Costa Rican, Kenco*	1 Mug/300ml	17	0.1	6	0.6	0.8	0	0
Irish Latte, Gold, Nescafe*	1 Mug/22g	90	2.2	411	8.3	70.6	9.9	2.6
Latte Macchiato, Made Up, Dolce Gusto, Nescafe*	1 Serving/220g	89	4.2	40	2	4.1	1.9	0.3
Latte, Cafe, M&S*	1 Serving/190g	142	5.3	75	4.3	8.3	2.8	0
Latte, Iced, M&S*	1 Bottle/300ml	186	3.6	62	2.9	9.8	1.2	0.5
Latte, Macchiato, Tassimo*	1 Cup/275ml	135	7.7	49	2.3	3.6	2.8	0
Latte, Nescafe*	1 Sachet/22g	110	6.3	498	14.5	45.7	28.5	0
Latte, No Sugar, In Cup, From Machine, Kenco*	1 Cup/4.2g	17	0.9	400	7.6	44	22	0
Latte, Skinny, Nescafe*	1 Sachet/20g	72	1.1	359	24.1	54.3	5.3	1.1
Mocha, Double Chocolate, Gold, Nescafe*	1 Sachet/23g	93	2.3	403	9.4	66.3	9.8	5.1
Mocha, Made Up, Dolce Gusto, Nescafe*	1 Serving/210g	117	5.1	56	2.4	6.1	2.4	0.6
Mocha, Sainsbury's*	1 Serving/22g	84	3	383	14	51	13.7	1.3
Mocha, Skinny, Nescafe*	1 Sachet/21g	77	0.7	367	13.6	70.3	3.5	4.3
Skinny Cappuccino, Made Up, Dolce Gusto, Nescafe*	1 Mug/15g	49	0.1	337	33.3	48.8	0.9	2.3
COFFEE SUBSTITUTE								
Bambu, Vogel*	1 Tsp/3g	10	0	320	3.5	75.3	0.5	0
COFFEE WHITENER								
Creamer, Hazelnut, Fat Free, Coffee Mate, Nestle*	1 Tbsp/15ml	25	0	167	0	33.3	0	0
Light, Asda*	1 Serving/3g	13	0.4	433	0.9	78	13	0
Light, Tesco*	1 Tsp/3g	13	0.4	429	0.9	77.7	12.7	0
Original, Coffee Mate, Nestle*	1 Tsp/3.5g	19	1.2	547	2.4	56.7	34.4	0
Tesco*	1 Tsp/3g	16	0.9	533	1.2	61.3	31.4	0
Virtually Fat Free, Coffee Mate, Nestle*	1 Tsp/5g	10	0.2	200	1	42	3	0
COGNAC								
40% Volume	***1 Pub Shot/35ml***	***78***	***0***	***222***	***0***	***0***	***0***	***0***
COLA								
Average	***1 Can/330ml***	***135***	***0***	***41***	***0***	***10.9***	***0***	***0***
Coke, Cherry, Coca-Cola*	1 Bottle/500ml	225	0	45	0	11.2	0	0
Coke, Cherry, Zero, Coca-Cola*	1 Can/330ml	1	0	0	0	0	0	0
Coke, Diet with Cherry, Coca-Cola*	1 Bottle/500ml	5	0	1	0	0	0	0
Coke, Diet, Caffeine Free, Coca-Cola*	1 Can/330ml	1	0	0	0	0.1	0	0
Coke, Vanilla, Coca-Cola*	1 Bottle/500ml	215	0	43	0	10.7	0	0
Coke, with Lemon, Diet, Coca-Cola*	1 Can/330ml	5	0	1	0	0	0	0
Coke, with Vanilla, Diet, Coca-Cola*	1 Glass/200ml	1	0	0	0	0.1	0	0
Curiosity, Fentiman's*	1 Bottle/275ml	129	0	47	0.1	11.6	0	0
Diet, Average	***1 Serving/200ml***	***1***	***0***	***1***	***0***	***0***	***0***	***0***
Pepsi Max, Ginger, Pepsi*	1 Can/250ml	1	0	0	0	0	0	0
Twist, Light, Pepsi*	1 Bottle/500ml	4	0	1	0	0.1	0	0
Zero, Caffeine Free, Coca-Cola*	1 Glass/200ml	0	0	0	0	0	0	0
Zero, Coca-Cola*	1 Can/330ml	2	0	0	0	0	0	0
COLESLAW								
Apple, Raisin & Walnut, TTD, Sainsbury's*	1 Serving/75g	212	19.6	283	2.3	8	26.2	2.8
Basics, Sainsbury's*	1 Serving/25g	27	2.4	107	1	3.7	9.8	1.6
Cheese, Deli Style, Waitrose*	¼ Tub/75g	247	24.3	330	3.8	5.1	32.5	0.9
Cheese, M&S*	1 Serving/57g	185	19.1	325	4.2	2	33.5	1.7
Cheese, Sainsbury's*	1 Serving/75g	184	16.8	246	3.8	6.5	22.4	1.4
Coronation, Sainsbury's*	¼ Pot/75g	145	11.6	193	1	11.4	15.5	1.9

	Measure INFO/WEIGHT	per Measure KCAL	FAT	Nutrition Values per 100g / 100ml KCAL	PROT	CARB	FAT	FIBRE
COLESLAW								
COU, M&S*	½ Pack/125g	75	3.4	60	1.3	7.4	2.7	1.7
Creamy, Asda*	1 Serving/25g	62	6	248	0.9	7	24	1.8
Creamy, GFY, Asda*	1 Serving/100g	163	14.9	163	0.7	6.5	14.9	0.8
Creamy, LC, Tesco*	1/3 Pot/100g	105	8.8	105	1.2	4.9	8.8	1.6
Creamy, Morrisons*	1 Serving/40g	111	11.1	277	1.1	5.5	27.7	1.3
Creamy, Tesco*	1 Serving/75g	142	13.4	190	1	5.5	17.8	1.5
Crunchy & Creamy, Aldi*	¼ Pack/75g	177	17.2	236	0.9	5.1	23	1.4
Deli Salad, Tesco*	1 Serving/50g	91	8.5	183	0.9	5.5	17.1	1.6
Deli Style, M&S*	1 Serving/50g	110	10.6	220	1	4.8	21.2	1.9
Essential, Waitrose*	1 Portion/125g	310	30.8	248	0.8	5.4	24.6	1.2
From Restaurant, Average	*3/4 Cup/99g*	*147*	*11*	*148*	*1.5*	*12.9*	*11.1*	*0*
Fruity, M&S*	1 Serving/63g	151	14.3	240	1.1	8.3	22.7	3.1
Half Fat, Waitrose*	1 Serving/100g	38	2.7	38	0.6	2.9	2.7	1.2
Iceland*	1 Serving/110g	112	8.2	102	0.7	7.8	7.5	1.6
Jalapeno, Sainsbury's*	1 Serving/75g	142	13.4	190	0.9	5.6	17.9	1.6
Light, Reduced Fat, Morrisons*	1 Serving/30g	38	3.1	125	0.8	7.4	10.2	0
Luxury, Asda*	1 Serving/50g	108	10.5	217	0.9	6	21	0
Luxury, Lidl*	1 Serving/50g	102	9.7	203	0.9	5.9	19.4	0
Luxury, Rich & Creamy, TTD, Sainsbury's*	1 Serving/50g	123	11.8	246	1.8	5.9	23.6	1.5
Piri Piri, Sainsbury's*	½ Tub/70g	113	9.9	162	1.1	6.6	14.2	1.8
Premium, Co-Op*	1 Serving/50g	160	17	320	1	3	34	2
Red, Tesco*	½ Pack/70g	53	1	76	1	13.5	1.5	2.4
Reduced Fat, Average	*1 Tbsp/20g*	*23*	*1.9*	*113*	*1*	*6.4*	*9.3*	*2*
Reduced Fat, Co-Op*	1 Serving/50g	45	3.5	90	0.9	6	7	2
Reduced Fat, Essential, Waitrose*	1/6 Tub/50g	65	5.1	130	1.2	8.3	10.2	1.6
Reduced Fat, M&S*	½ Tub/112.2g	230	22.4	205	1.1	5.4	20	2.8
TTD, Sainsbury's*	¼ Med Pot/75g	179	17.2	238	1.2	6	22.9	1.6
with Reduced Calorie Dressing, Retail	*1 Serving/40g*	*27*	*1.8*	*67*	*0.9*	*6.1*	*4.5*	*1.4*
COLEY								
Portions, Raw, Average	*1 Serving/92g*	*65*	*0.6*	*71*	*15.9*	*0*	*0.6*	*0*
Steamed, Average	*1oz/28g*	*29*	*0.4*	*105*	*23.3*	*0*	*1.3*	*0*
CONCHIGLIE								
Cooked, Average	*1 Serving/185g*	*247*	*1.6*	*134*	*4.8*	*26.6*	*0.8*	*0.6*
Cooked, Sainsbury's*	1 Serving/100g	160	0.6	160	4.4	33.6	0.6	1.4
Dry Weight, Average	*1 Serving/100g*	*352*	*1.7*	*352*	*12.5*	*71.6*	*1.7*	*2.6*
Shells, Dry, Average	*1 Serving/100g*	*346*	*1.5*	*346*	*12.3*	*70.4*	*1.5*	*3*
Whole Wheat, Dry Weight, Average	*1 Serving/75g*	*237*	*1.5*	*316*	*12.6*	*62*	*2*	*10.7*
CONCHIGLIONI								
Dry, Waitrose*	1 Serving/75g	256	1	341	12.5	69.8	1.3	3.7
CONSERVE								
Apricot, Average	*1 Tbsp/15g*	*37*	*0*	*244*	*0.5*	*59.3*	*0.2*	*1.5*
Apricot, Reduced Sugar, Streamline*	1 Tbsp/20g	37	0	184	0.5	45	0.2	0
Blackcurrant, Average	*1 Tbsp/15g*	*37*	*0*	*245*	*0.6*	*60*	*0.1*	*1.9*
Blueberry, M&S*	1 Tsp/8g	15	0	206	0.3	51.1	0.1	1.3
Hedgerow, TTD, Sainsbury's*	1 Tbsp/15g	41	0	276	0.5	68.2	0.1	0.5
Morello Cherry, Waitrose*	1 Tbsp/15g	39	0	258	0.4	64.2	0	1.4
Plum, TTD, Sainsbury's*	1 Tbsp/15g	44	0	295	0.3	73.1	0.1	0.5
Raspberry, Average	*1 Tbsp/15g*	*37*	*0.1*	*249*	*0.6*	*61*	*0.3*	*1.3*
Red Cherry, TTD, Sainsbury's*	1 Tbsp/15g	43	0	283	0.4	70.2	0.1	0.5
Rhubarb & Ginger, M&S*	1 Tbsp/15g	29	0	194	0.3	47.9	0.1	1
Strawberry, Average	*1 Tbsp/15g*	*37*	*0*	*250*	*0.4*	*61.6*	*0.1*	*0.5*
CONSOMME								
Average	*1oz/28g*	*3*	*0*	*12*	*2.9*	*0.1*	*0*	*0*

C

	Measure INFO/WEIGHT	per Measure KCAL	FAT	Nutrition Values per 100g / 100ml KCAL	PROT	CARB	FAT	FIBRE
CONSOMME								
Beef, Canned, Sainsbury's*	1 Can/415g	46	0	11	2	0.7	0	0
Beef, Luxury, with Sherry, Baxters*	1 Can/415g	62	0	15	2.7	1	0	0
COOKIES								
All Butter, Almond, Italian Style, M&S*	1 Cookie/23g	120	6.4	515	6.7	59.4	27.6	3.6
All Butter, Ginger Bread, M&S*	1 Cookie/23g	102	5	445	4.3	57.5	21.8	2.4
All Butter, Italian Style Sorrento Lemon, M&S*	1 Cookie/24g	120	6.4	500	4.9	60.4	26.7	2.1
All Butter, Melting Moment, M&S*	1 Cookie/23g	110	6.4	470	4.5	51.5	27.5	3.4
All Butter, Sultana, TTD, Sainsbury's*	1 Biscuit/17g	79	3.8	476	5.4	62.7	22.6	2
Almond, Ose*	1 Cookie/10g	46	1.4	456	8.4	74	14	0
Apple & Raisin, Go Ahead, McVitie's*	1 Cookie/15g	66	1.9	443	5.3	76.8	12.7	3.4
Apple Crumble, M&S*	1 Cookie/26g	90	0.5	345	4.6	76.8	2	2.9
Apple Pie, The Biscuit Collection*	1 Cookie/19g	90	4.2	474	3.9	65	22.1	0
Big Milk Chocolate Chunk, Cookie Coach*	1 Cookie/35g	174	8.8	497	6.2	61.4	25.1	0
Bites, Weight Watchers*	1 Pack/21g	97	4	464	5.8	67	19.2	4.3
Bounty, Mars*	1 Cookie/46g	215	9.6	468	5.7	63.4	20.9	0
Brazil Nut, Organic, Traidcraft*	1 Cookie/17g	91	5.4	547	5.8	57.7	32.6	2.1
Brazil Nut, Prewett's*	1 Cookie/50g	122	7.4	244	2.6	25.2	14.8	1
Butter & Sultana, Sainsbury's*	1 Cookie/13g	61	2.6	473	4.5	68.4	20.1	1.6
Cherry Bakewell, COU, M&S*	1 Cookie/25g	90	0.6	355	6	77.2	2.5	3.4
Chia & Coconut, with Afternoon Infusion, Graze*	1 Punnet/22g	118	6.9	528	5.8	53	31	5
Choc Chip & Coconut, Maryland*	1 Cookie/10g	55	2.5	512	5.1	62.9	23.7	0
Choc Chip & Hazelnut, Maryland*	1 Cookie/11g	55	2.7	513	6.3	65.3	25	0
Choc Chip 'n' Chunk, McVitie's*	1 Cookie/11g	55	2.9	498	5.8	59.2	26.4	3.5
Choc Chip, Bronte*	1 Cookie/16.7g	79	3.6	474	5.8	64	21.6	0
Choc Chip, Cadbury*	1 Cookie/11g	55	2.8	503	5.9	62.2	25.6	0
Choc Chip, Giant, Paterson's*	1 Cookie/60g	296	15.2	493	0.1	61.3	25.3	3.2
Choc Chip, Lyons*	1 Cookie/11.4g	57	2.7	499	5.2	68.3	23.4	1.7
Choc Chip, Mini, Good to Go, Waitrose*	1 Bag/25g	127	6.6	508	6	60.4	26.4	2.4
Choc Chip, Parkside*	1 Cookie/11.3g	56	2.7	495	5.3	64.5	23.7	0
Choc Chip, Reduced Fat, Maryland*	1 Cookie/10.7g	51	1.9	478	5.9	73	18	0
Choc Chip, Sainsbury's*	1 Cookie/10.8g	55	2.6	508	6.2	67	23.9	1.3
Choc Chunk & Hazelnut, Co-Op*	1 Cookie/17g	89	5.3	525	6	56	31	3
Choc Chunk, Fabulous Bakin' Boys*	1 Cookie/60g	270	12.6	450	5	59	21	3
Choc Chunk, Finest, Tesco*	1 Cookie/80g	355	14.1	445	5.7	65.3	17.7	1.8
Chocolate & Nut, Organic, Evernat*	1 Cookie/69g	337	15.6	489	7.2	64.1	22.6	0
Chocolate & Orange, COU, M&S*	1 Cookie/26g	90	0.7	350	5.7	77.2	2.6	3.2
Chocolate & Orange, Bites, Go Ahead, McVitie's*	1 Pack/23g	98	2.4	427	6.9	74.1	10.5	4
Chocolate Chip & Caramel, Bites, Maryland*	5 Biscuits/20g	103	5.3	513	5.7	61.8	26.4	3
Chocolate Chip & Hazelnut, Extra Special, Asda*	1 Cookie/25.2g	130	8.1	516	6	51	32	2.5
Chocolate Chip, Asda*	1 Cookie/12g	57	2.9	497	5	63	25	2.6
Chocolate Chip, Average	*1 Cookie/10g*	*49*	*2.5*	*489*	*5.5*	*64.1*	*24.7*	*2.9*
Chocolate Chip, BGTY, Sainsbury's*	1 Cookie/17g	72	2	428	4.5	75.6	11.9	2.5
Chocolate Chip, Chips Ahoy*	1 Cookie/11g	55	2.8	500	6	65	25	3
Chocolate Chip, Co-Op*	1 Cookie/11g	55	2.6	500	5	65	24	1
Chocolate Chip, Dough, Otis Spunkmeyer*	1 Cookie/38g	160	8	421	5.3	60.5	21	2.6
Chocolate Chip, GF, Organic, Dove's Farm*	1 Cookie/17g	77	3.1	451	4.3	66.9	18.5	0
Chocolate Chip, GFY, Asda*	1 Cookie/10g	48	2	463	5	68	19	3.5
Chocolate Chip, Gluten & Wheat Free, Lovemore*	1 Cookie/17g	81	4.5	483	3.8	57.8	26.8	3.5
Chocolate Chip, Handbaked, Border*	1 Cookie/15g	72	3.4	480	5.9	67.4	22.6	0
Chocolate Chip, Low Price, Sainsbury's*	1 Cookie/11g	54	2.3	500	7	70.1	21.3	2.5
Chocolate Chip, Lyons*	1 Cookie/12g	56	2.5	483	5.6	66.5	21.6	1.7
Chocolate Chip, M&S*	1 Cookie/12g	59	3	495	5.7	62.1	24.8	2.7
Chocolate Chip, Maryland*	1 Cookie/11g	53	2.5	487	5.4	63.8	22.6	3.5

	Measure INFO/WEIGHT	per Measure KCAL	FAT	Nutrition Values per 100g / 100ml KCAL	PROT	CARB	FAT	FIBRE
COOKIES								
Chocolate Chip, McVitie's*	1 Cookie/11g	54	2.8	496	5.8	60.2	25.8	3
Chocolate Chip, Mini, McVitie's*	1 Bag/40g	196	9.2	491	5.5	65.1	23.1	2.8
Chocolate Chip, Mini, Tesco*	1 Bag/30g	148	7.1	493	5.4	64.6	23.7	1.7
Chocolate Chip, Morrisons*	1 Cookie/10g	52	2.5	502	5	66.2	24.1	1.3
Chocolate Chip, Organic, Sainsbury's*	1 Cookie/17g	89	4.9	530	5	61.8	29.2	0.3
Chocolate Chip, Organic, Tesco*	1 Cookie/17g	88	4.7	520	4	63.3	27.4	2.8
Chocolate Chip, Tesco*	1 Cookie/11g	56	2.7	510	5.2	67.2	24.1	1.6
Chocolate Chip, Value, Tesco*	1 Cookie/11g	56	2.9	512	4.8	64.8	26	1.6
Chocolate Chip, Weight Watchers*	1 Cookie/11g	49	1.9	443	7.6	65.4	17.2	4.6
Chocolate Chunk & Hazelnut, Tesco*	1 Cookie/22g	118	6.7	538	6.2	60.2	30.3	1.9
Chocolate Chunk & Hazelnut, TTD, Sainsbury's*	1 Biscuit/17g	88	5.2	528	6.5	54.8	31.4	2.8
Chocolate Chunk & Orange, So Good, Somerfield*	1 Cookie/22g	117	6.5	525	5.3	60	29.3	1.8
Chocolate Chunk, All Butter, COU, M&S*	1 Cookie/23.9g	110	4.3	460	5.7	69.1	17.9	2.3
Chocolate Chunk, All Butter, M&S*	1 Cookie/24g	120	6	500	5.2	62.4	25.2	2.9
Chocolate Chunk, Cadbury*	1 Cookie/22g	119	6.9	540	6.5	58	31.2	0
Chocolate Chunk, Devondale*	1 Cookie/65g	308	16.3	474	4.6	59.2	25.1	2.8
Chocolate Fruit & Nut, Extra Special, Asda*	1 Cookie/25g	125	7.1	509	6	56	29	2
Chocolate Orange, Half Coated, Finest, Tesco*	1 Cookie/22g	107	5.6	488	4.9	59.6	25.5	1.2
Chocolate Thin Crisp, Simply Food, M&S*	1 Pack/23g	100	2	435	4.4	78.3	8.7	4.4
Chocolate, Belgian, Extra Special, Asda*	1 Cookie/26g	138	8	535	6	58	31	2
Chocolate, Milk, Free From, Tesco*	1 Cookie/20g	100	6.1	500	5.6	50.4	30.7	4.1
Chocolate, Quadruple, Sainsbury's*	1 Cookie/20g	117	6.6	585	6	66.5	33	1.5
Chocolate, Soft, American Style, Budgens*	1 Cookie/50g	216	9.3	431	5.1	60.8	18.6	2.2
Chocolate, Triple, Half Coated, Finest, Tesco*	1 Cookie/25g	131	7.3	525	5.7	58.7	29.3	2.3
Chunkie Extremely Chocolatey, Fox's*	1 Cookie/25.7g	130	6.8	506	6.2	61	26.3	2.6
Chunky Chocolate, Kate's Cakes Ltd*	1 Serving/100g	441	22	441	5.2	55.5	22	2.4
Cocoa, Organic, Bites, No Junk, Organix*	1 Bag/25g	105	3.2	421	7	69	13	5.5
Coconut & Raspberry, GF, Sainsbury's*	1 Cookie/20g	102	5.9	511	5.9	56	29.3	6.7
Coconut, Gluten-Free, Sainsbury's*	1 Cookie/20g	103	6.1	516	5.6	54.4	30.7	4.1
Cranberry & Orange, Finest, Tesco*	1 Cookie/25.5g	125	5.8	490	4.1	67.4	22.6	3.2
Cranberry & Orange, Go Ahead, McVitie's*	1 Cookie/17g	77	2.2	452	5.3	78	13.2	2.4
Crunchy Muesli, Mini, Shapers, Boots*	1 Pack/30g	134	4.5	448	6.7	71	15	1.8
Danish Butter, Tesco*	1 Cookie/26g	133	6.6	516	4.7	66.7	25.6	1.3
Dark Chocolate Chunk & Ginger, The Best, Morrisons*	1 Cookie/25g	126	6.4	503	4.6	63.7	25.5	2.8
Dark Treacle, Weight Watchers*	1 Cookie/11g	49	1.7	423	5.2	66.7	15.1	1.7
Double Choc Chip, Giant, Paterson's*	1 Cookie/60g	293	15.2	489	0.3	61.3	25.3	3.7
Double Choc Chip, Mini, M&S*	1 Cookie/22g	108	5.2	490	5.3	63.6	23.7	1.8
Double Choc Chip, Tesco*	1 Cookie/11g	55	2.7	500	4.2	65.3	24.7	3
Double Choc Chip, Weight Watchers*	1 Biscuit/11g	49	1.9	443	7.6	65.4	17.2	4.6
Double Choc, Maryland*	1 Cookie/10g	51	2.6	510	5.2	64.4	25.7	0
Double Chocolate & Nuts, Bens Cookie*	1 Cookie/85g	364	17.4	428	8.7	71.2	20.5	2.8
Double Chocolate & Walnut, Soft, Tesco*	1 Cookie/25g	116	6.4	463	5.8	52.1	25.7	4.7
Double Chocolate Chip, Co-Op*	1 Cookie/17g	87	4.6	510	5	63	27	2
Double Chocolate Chip, Organic, Waitrose*	1 Cookie/18g	96	5.6	535	5.1	58.6	31	1.9
Double Chocolate Chip, Somerfield*	1 Cookie/11g	56	2.8	513	5.2	64.9	25.8	1.3
Double Chocolate Chip, Traidcraft*	1 Cookie/22g	114	5.9	520	5.8	64.1	26.7	2.4
Double Chocolate Chip, Treat Yourself, Spar*	1 Cookie/20g	94	5	470	5.5	56	25	2.5
Double Fudge & Chocolate, Sugar Free, Murray*	1 Cookie/12g	47	2.3	400	5.7	65.7	20	5.7
Eton Mess, Finest, Tesco*	1 Cookie/66g	281	9.7	426	5.1	67.6	14.7	1.4
Farmbake, Arnotts*	1 Cookie/13g	61	2.4	470	5	68.4	18.7	0
Finest White Chocolate & Honeycomb, Bakery, Tesco*	1 Cookie/65g	289	11	445	5.5	67.1	17	0.9
Fortune, Average	*1 Cookie/8g*	*30*	*0.2*	*378*	*4.2*	*84*	*2.7*	*1.6*
Fruit & Oat, Soft, Diet Chef Ltd*	1 Cookie45g	198	9.1	440	4.8	61.9	20.2	4.3

	Measure INFO/WEIGHT	per Measure KCAL	FAT	Nutrition Values per 100g / 100ml KCAL	PROT	CARB	FAT	FIBRE
COOKIES								
Fruit, Giant, Cookie Coach*	1 Cookie/60g	280	13.2	466	4.9	62	22	0
Fruity Shrewsbury, Giant, Paterson's*	1 Cookie/60g	298	15.2	496	4.8	62.6	25.4	1.7
Fudge Brownie American Cream, Sainsbury's*	1 Cookie/12g	60	2.8	499	4.8	67.9	23.2	2.2
Fudge Brownie, Maryland*	1 Cookie/11g	56	2.8	510	5.8	63	25	0
Ginger & Brazil Nut, Organic, Dove's Farm*	1 Cookie/17g	79	3.5	464	5	65	20.5	4.8
Ginger & Choc Chip, BGTY, Sainsbury's*	1 Cookie/16.7g	69	3.2	415	5.8	55.3	19	12.1
Ginger, GF, Barkat*	1 Cookie/17g	85	4.4	501	3.2	63.8	25.9	0
Ginger, Low Fat, M&S*	1 Cookie/23g	82	1	358	5.1	74.9	4.3	2.4
Gman, Gingerbread, GF, Barkat*	2 Biscuits/34g	167	9.3	490	15.8	49.5	27.3	6
Hazelnut & Choc Chip 'n' Chunk, McVitie's*	1 Cookie/11g	55	3	505	6.1	57.8	27.7	3.5
Hazelnut, GF, Organic, Dove's Farm*	1 Cookie/17g	79	3.7	463	4.8	61.5	21.9	1.8
Honey, Lemon & Ginger, Nothing Naughty*	1 Cookie/60g	246	9	410	2.9	64.4	15	0
Jaffa, Tesco*	1 Cookie/42g	175	5.9	417	4.8	66.9	14	1.9
Lemon & Currant, Weight Watchers*	2 Cookies/19g	86	3.4	451	5.1	63.6	17.7	8.4
Lemon Meringue, COU, M&S*	1 Cookie/25g	89	0.6	355	5.6	77.6	2.6	3
Lemon Zest, GF, Organic, Dove's Farm*	1 Cookie/17g	80	3.1	473	3.3	73.7	18.3	0
Mango & Coconut, Tesco*	1 Cookie/20g	90	3.9	450	5.5	61	19.5	5.5
Milk Chocolate Chunk, Average	**1 Cookie/25g**	**129**	**6.9**	**515**	**6.6**	**60**	**27.6**	**1.6**
Milk Chocolate, Classic, Millie's Cookies*	1 Cookie/45g	190	10.2	422	5.1	49.3	22.7	1.3
Oat & Cranberry, BGTY, Sainsbury's*	1 Cookie/28g	126	5	449	6.8	65	18	5.1
Oat & Raisin, Health Matters*	1 Cookie/8g	33	0.7	414	7	76.6	8.8	3.3
Oat & Treacle, TTD, Sainsbury's*	1 Biscuit/25g	121	5.9	482	5.7	61.8	23.6	3.7
Oat & Fruit, Kate's Cakes Ltd*	1 Serving/100g	418	18.2	418	4.2	59.5	18.2	3
Oat & Raisin, GF, Prewett's*	1 Cookie18g	80	2.7	442	6.2	63	15	5.1
Oat & Sultana, Free From, Sainsbury's*	1 Cookie/19g	87	3.7	462	6.2	62.6	19.8	4.2
Oat, Giant Jumbo, Paterson's*	1 Cookie/60g	299	16.2	499	0.4	58.4	27	3.2
Oatflake & Honey, Organic, Sainsbury's*	1 Cookie/17g	82	3.6	480	6.3	66	21.2	2.6
Oatflake & Raisin, Waitrose*	1 Cookie/17g	80	3.8	469	5.8	61.7	22.1	4.7
Oatflake & Treacle, TTD, Sainsbury's*	1 Cookie/25g	122	5.9	490	5.7	61.8	23.6	3.7
Oaties, Grandma Wilds*	1 Cookie/50g	254	12.4	507	5.1	66	24.9	0
Oatmeal, Chocolate Chip, Chewy, Dad's*	1 Cookie/15g	70	3	467	6.7	66.7	20	3.3
Oreo, Mini, Oreo*	1 Pack/25g	120	4.8	480	4.8	70	19.2	2.4
Oreo, Nabisco*	1 Cookie/11g	52	2.3	471	5.9	70.6	20.6	2.9
Pecan & Maple, Mini, Bronte*	1 Pack/100g	509	27.3	509	5.4	60.3	27.3	1.6
Pineapple, Coconut & White Chocolate, M&S*	1 Cookie/23g	119	5.7	518	5.1	56.7	24.9	2.9
Quadruple Chocolate, TTD, Sainsbury's*	1 Biscuit/20g	104	5.7	518	6.2	59.8	28.2	1.6
Raisin & Cinnamon, Low Fat, M&S*	1 Cookie/22g	78	0.9	355	6.2	73	4.1	3.2
Red Velvet, Filled, Bakery, Tesco*	1 Cookie/42g	170	5.5	405	4.6	66.6	13.1	1.3
Rolo, Nestle*	1 Cookie/39g	178	7.4	456	5.4	64.8	19	2.2
Stem Ginger, Aldi*	1 Cookie/13g	58	2.4	463	3.6	68.5	19.4	0
Stem Ginger, All Butter, Deluxe, Lidl*	1 Biscuit/17g	80	3.6	468	5.1	62	21	5.4
Stem Ginger, Deluxe, Lidl*	1 Cookie/17g	80	3.6	468	5.1	62	21	5.4
Stem Ginger, Free From, Asda*	1 Biscuit/19g	89	3.6	467	3	69	19	4.1
Stem Ginger, Free From, Sainsbury's*	1 Cookie/17.1g	84	4.8	489	6.5	58	28	6.8
Stem Ginger, Kate's Cakes Ltd*	1 Serving/100g	376	11.7	376	5	62.7	11.7	1.7
Stem Ginger, Less Than 5% Fat, M&S*	1 Cookie/22g	79	0.9	360	6.2	73.9	4.3	3
Stem Ginger, Reduced Fat, Waitrose*	1 Cookie/16.7g	75	2.7	448	4.5	71	16.2	1.6
Stem Ginger, Tesco*	1 Cookie/20g	98	4.8	489	4.2	64	24	2
Stem Ginger, TTD, Sainsbury's*	1 Cookie/17g	79	3.7	476	5.2	64.3	22	2.3
Sultana, All Butter, Reduced Fat, M&S*	1 Cookie/17g	70	2.4	420	4.9	68.6	14.2	2.6
Sultana, Deluxe, Lidl*	1 Biscuit/17g	77	3.2	453	5.3	64.7	18.8	2.9
Sultana, Soft & Chewy, Sainsbury's*	1 Cookie/25g	104	3.5	414	4.4	67.8	13.9	2.5
Toffee Popcorn, Butter Buds*	1 Cookie/40g	184	7.6	459	4.2	66.8	19	1.4

	Measure INFO/WEIGHT	per Measure KCAL	FAT	Nutrition Values per 100g / 100ml KCAL	PROT	CARB	FAT	FIBRE
COOKIES								
Toffee, Weight Watchers*	2 Cookies/152g	686	27.4	451	6.8	61.7	18	7.5
Treacle & Oat, All Butter, Finest, Tesco*	1 Biscuit/20g	100	5	500	4.8	62.9	25	2.1
Triple Chocolate Chunk, Bakery, Finest, Tesco*	1 Cookie/80g	360	15.9	450	7.4	59.2	19.9	2.1
Triple Chocolate, TTD, Sainsbury's*	1 Cookie/72g	344	16.5	478	5.8	61.2	22.9	2
White Chocolate & Cranberry, Devondale*	1 Cookie/65g	300	15.3	462	4.7	60.7	23.5	2.1
White Chocolate & Raspberry, McVitie's*	1 Cookie/17g	87	4.4	512	4.7	64.1	25.9	1.8
White Chocolate & Cranberry, Kate's Cakes Ltd*	1 Serving/100g	389	13.4	389	4.7	62.3	13.4	2
White Chocolate & Raspberry, Finest, Tesco*	1 Cookie/76g	304	9.6	400	5.2	66.3	12.6	2.4
White Chocolate, Asda*	1 Cookie/54g	256	11.9	474	5	64	22	2.1
White Chocolate, Chunk, Average	*1 Cookie/25g*	*124*	*6.2*	*498*	*5.5*	*62.8*	*24.8*	*1*
White Chocolate, Maryland*	1 Cookie/10g	51	2.5	512	5.7	64	25	0
White Chocolate, TTD, Sainsbury's*	1 Cookie/25g	126	6.4	504	5.5	62.5	25.8	1.2
COQ AU VIN								
658, Oakhouse Foods Ltd*	1 Serving/400g	728	39.6	182	14	7.9	9.9	2.8
Diet Chef Ltd*	1 Pack/300g	285	13.2	95	7.7	6.1	4.4	2.2
Finest, Tesco*	1 Serving/273g	251	9.8	92	14.3	0.7	3.6	1.8
M&S*	1 Serving/295g	398	22.7	135	14.2	1.5	7.7	1
Oven Cooked, TTD, Sainsbury's*	½ Pack/244g	337	17.1	138	15.2	3.1	7	1.1
Sainsbury's*	1 Pack/400g	484	17.6	121	16.8	3.5	4.4	0.2
CORDIAL								
Apple & Mango, Hi Juice, As Prepared, Morrisons*	1 Serving/250ml	69	0	28	0	6.7	0	0.1
Blackcurrant, New Zealand Honey Co*	1 Serving/30ml	109	0.3	363	1	88	1	0
Cox's Apple & Plum, Diluted, Bottle Green*	1 Serving/10ml	3	0	29	0	7.2	0	0
Elderflower, Made Up, Bottle Green*	1 Glass/200ml	46	0	23	0	5.6	0	0
Elderflower, Undiluted, Waitrose*	1 Serving/20ml	22	0	110	0	27.5	0	0
Lemon & Lime, High Juice, M&S*	1 Glass/250ml	75	0	30	0	7	0	0
Lime Juice, Concentrated	*1 Serving/20ml*	*22*	*0*	*112*	*0.1*	*29.8*	*0*	*0*
Lime Juice, Diluted	*1 Glass/250ml*	*55*	*0*	*22*	*0*	*6*	*0*	*0*
Lime Juice, Waitrose*	1 Serving/20ml	21	0	104	10	23.7	0	0
Lime with Aromatic Bitters & Ginger, Sainsbury's*	1 Serving/40ml	12	0.1	29	0	6.9	0.3	0.3
Lime, Juice, Diluted, Rose's*	1 Serving/250ml	52	0	21	0	4.9	0	0
Lime, Sainsbury's*	1 Serving/50ml	14	0	27	0	6.2	0	0
Lime, Tesco*	1 Pint/74ml	8	0	11	0.2	0.5	0	0
Pomegranate & Elderflower, Bottle Green*	1 fl oz/30ml	9	0	30	0	7	0	0
CORIANDER								
Leaves, Dried, Average	*1oz/28g*	*78*	*1.3*	*279*	*21.8*	*41.7*	*4.8*	*0*
Leaves, Fresh, Average	*1 Bunch/20g*	*5*	*0.1*	*23*	*2.1*	*3.7*	*0.5*	*2.8*
Seeds, Ground, Schwartz*	1 Tsp/5g	22	0.9	446	14.2	54.9	18.8	0
CORN								
Baby, & Mange Tout, Eat Fresh, Tesco*	1 Serving/100g	31	0.2	31	2.9	3.3	0.2	2.1
Baby, Average	*1 Serving/80g*	*21*	*0.3*	*26*	*2.5*	*3.1*	*0.4*	*1.7*
Baby, Canned, Drained, Average	*1 Serving/80g*	*18*	*0.3*	*23*	*2.9*	*2*	*0.4*	*1.5*
Cobs, Boiled, Weighed with Cob, Average	*1 Ear/200g*	*78*	*1.7*	*39*	*1.5*	*6.8*	*0.8*	*0.8*
Cobs, with Butter, From Restaurant, Average	*1 Ear/146g*	*155*	*3.4*	*106*	*3.1*	*21.9*	*2.4*	*0*
Creamed Style, Green Giant*	1 Can/418g	238	2.1	57	1.2	11.9	0.5	3
CORN CAKES								
M&S*	½ Pack/85g	238	17	280	6.4	19.8	20	3.4
Organic, Kallo*	1 Cake/5g	16	0.2	340	12.7	74.3	4.1	11.2
Slightly Salted, Mrs Crimble's*	1 Pack/27.5g	104	0.9	380	7.9	80	3.4	5.4
Thick Slices, Orgran*	1 Cake/11g	42	0.4	385	13.2	79	3.7	14.2
with Chai Seeds, Kallo*	1 Cake/7g	27	0.2	389	8	81	2.4	0
CORN MEAL								
Yellow, Enriched & Degerminated, Dry, Quaker*	1 Tbsp/9g	30	0.2	333	7.4	77.8	1.8	7.4

	Measure INFO/WEIGHT	per Measure KCAL	FAT	Nutrition Values per 100g / 100ml KCAL	PROT	CARB	FAT	FIBRE
CORNED BEEF								
& Parsley Sauce, Mini, 279, Oakhouse Foods Ltd*	1 Serving/250g	343	17.3	137	8.9	10.6	6.9	0.4
Average	*1 Slice/35g*	*75*	*4.3*	*214*	*25.9*	*0.7*	*12.2*	*0*
Lean, Healthy Range, Average	*1 Slice/30g*	*57*	*2.6*	*191*	*27*	*1*	*8.7*	*0*
Sliced, Premium, Average	*1 Slice/31g*	*69*	*3.9*	*222*	*26.6*	*0.5*	*12.6*	*0*
CORNFLOUR								
Average	*1 Tsp/5g*	*18*	*0.1*	*355*	*0.6*	*86.9*	*1.2*	*0.1*
COULIS								
Passsion Fruit & Mango, TTD, Sainsbury's*	1 Tbs/15ml	23	0.1	155	1.2	34.7	1	0.9
Raspberry, TTD, Sainsbury's*	1 Tbsp/15ml	25	0.1	165	0.4	39.1	0.6	1.4
COURGETTE								
Baby, Raw, Average	*1 Courgette/29g*	*6*	*0.1*	*22*	*2*	*2*	*0.5*	*1.2*
Courgetti, Italian, Tomato, Pot, Bol*	1 Pot/380g	441	18.2	116	2.5	15	4.8	1.4
Fried, Average	*1oz/28g*	*18*	*1.3*	*63*	*2.6*	*2.6*	*4.8*	*1.2*
Raw, Average	*1 Courgette/224g*	*40*	*0.9*	*18*	*1.8*	*1.8*	*0.4*	*0.9*
Spaghetti, Waitrose*	½ Pack/80g	16	0.3	20	1.8	1.8	0.4	1.2
Stuffed, Round, Lovely Vegetables, M&S*	½ Pack/200g	110	2.6	55	1.8	7.7	1.3	1.8
COUS COUS								
& Chargrilled Vegetables, M&S*	1 Serving/200g	200	3	100	3.9	17.3	1.5	1.6
& Chickpeas, TTD, Sainsbury's*	¼ Pot/72g	121	6.8	167	4.7	15.8	9.4	1.4
& Wok Oriental, Findus*	½ Pack/300g	510	25.5	170	4.5	19	8.5	0
4 Grain, Unprepared, Artisan Grains*	1 Serving/100g	341	2.7	341	11.7	64.9	2.7	8
Cauliflower & Broccoli, Waitrose*	½ Pack/110g	43	1	39	4	2.4	0.9	2.8
Chargrilled Red & Yellow Pepper, Tesco*	1 Pack/200g	212	3.6	106	4.6	17.8	1.8	0.5
Chargrilled Vegetable, Morrisons*	1 Serving/225g	227	5.4	101	3.3	16.5	2.4	1.3
Chargrilled Vegetables & Olive Oil, Delphi*	½ Pot/75g	105	2.9	140	3.8	22.5	3.9	1.9
Citrus Kick, Cooked, Ainsley Harriott*	1 Serving/130g	182	1.6	140	4.3	27.9	1.2	2.4
Citrus Kick, Dry, Ainsley Harriott*	½ Sachet/50g	184	1.2	368	11.6	77	2.4	9.2
Cooked, Average	*1 Tbsp/15g*	*24*	*0.3*	*158*	*4.3*	*31.4*	*1.9*	*1.3*
Cooked, From Restaurant, Average	*1 Cup/157g*	*176*	*0.3*	*112*	*3.8*	*23.2*	*0.2*	*1.4*
Coriander & Lemon, Morrisons*	1 Serving/100g	159	3.4	159	4.4	27.7	3.4	1.4
Coriander & Lemon, As Consumed, Sainsbury's*	½ Pack/140g	195	1	139	4.8	27.5	0.7	1.9
Dry, Average	*1 Serving/50g*	*178*	*0.7*	*356*	*13.7*	*72.8*	*1.5*	*2.6*
Fruity, Sainsbury's*	1 Portion/100g	194	4.5	194	4.4	33.2	4.5	1.7
Garlic & Coriander, Dry, Waitrose*	1 Serving/70g	235	2.5	336	11.7	64.2	3.6	6.2
Giant, Tesco*	1 Pack/220g	350	14.4	160	4.1	20.7	6.6	1.2
Harissa Style Savoury, Sainsbury's*	1 Serving/260g	434	12	167	4.7	26.8	4.6	1.3
Hot & Spicy Flavour, Dry, Amazing Grains, Haldane's*	1 Serving/50g	182	2.1	365	12.5	67	4.2	3.1
Mediterranean Tomato, GFY, Asda*	½ Pack/141g	192	1.3	136	5	27	0.9	1.7
Mint & Coriander Flavour, Dry, Amazing Grains*	1 Sachet/99g	349	2.7	353	12.2	70	2.7	3.2
Moroccan Medley, Ainsley Harriott*	½ Sachet/130g	178	2	137	5.4	25.4	1.5	2.2
Moroccan Style, Break, GFY, Asda*	1 Pack/150.3g	215	2.7	143	5.6	26.1	1.8	1.8
Moroccan Style, Cooked, Sainsbury's*	½ Pack/140g	200	1.1	143	6.2	26.4	0.8	2.5
Moroccan Style, Finest, Tesco*	1 Tub/225g	292	5.6	130	4.3	22.6	2.5	3.7
Moroccan Style, Fruity, M&S*	1 Serving/200g	370	5.4	185	3.4	36.7	2.7	3.4
Moroccan Style, Spiced, Meadow Fresh, Lidl*	1 Pack/280g	456	14.8	163	3	25	5.3	1.6
Moroccan Style, TTD, Sainsbury's*	1 Pot/200g	364	7.2	182	4.4	30.3	3.6	5.5
Moroccan, Co-Op*	1 Pack/110g	155	1.8	141	4.8	26	1.6	1.6
Moroccan, Pot, Prepared, NutriPot*	1 Pot/322g	315	2.9	98	6.2	14.9	0.9	2.6
Mushroom, Prepared, without Oil or Butter, Tesco*	½ Pack/140g	194	1.3	139	4.3	27.7	0.9	1.4
Pearl, Cooked, Artisan Grains*	1 Serving/100g	114	0.5	114	3.8	23	0.5	0.9
Red Pepper & Chilli, Waitrose*	1 Pack/200g	344	13.8	172	4.5	23	6.9	1.3
Roasted Vegetable, Cooked, Ainsley Harriott*	1 Serving/130g	180	2	138	5.6	25.5	1.5	2.6
Roasted Vegetable, Dry, Ainsley Harriott*	½ Sachet/50g	180	2	360	14.6	66.4	4	6.8

	Measure INFO/WEIGHT	per Measure KCAL	per Measure FAT	Nutrition Values per 100g / 100ml KCAL	PROT	CARB	FAT	FIBRE

COUS COUS

	Measure INFO/WEIGHT	KCAL	FAT	KCAL	PROT	CARB	FAT	FIBRE
Roasted Vegetable, Snack Salad Pot, HL, Tesco*	1 Pack/60g	213	2.4	355	15.1	64.6	4	4.2
Roasted Vegetables, Waitrose*	1 Serving/200g	328	13.2	164	3.9	22	6.6	0.9
Spice Fusion, Lyttos*	1 Serving/100g	134	1.5	134	4.3	23.9	1.5	3.4
Spice Sensation, Batchelors*	1 Pack/120g	163	1.1	136	4.7	26.3	0.9	1.8
Spicy Vegetable, GFY, Asda*	½ Pack/55g	71	0.6	129	4.7	25	1.1	2
Spicy Vegetable, Morrisons*	1 Pack/110g	187	5.5	170	5.1	26.2	5	2.9
Sun Dried Tomato, Somerfield*	1 Jar/110g	176	5.5	160	3	25	5	0
Sundried Tomato, & Garlic, Newgate, Lidl*	1 Serving/135g	181	1.5	134	4.5	25.7	1.1	1.7
Sweet Vegetable, CBY, Asda*	1 Serving/100g	120	0	120	2.9	14.8	0	0
Tangy Tomato, Cooked, Ainsley Harriott*	1 Serving/133g	166	0.8	125	4.6	25.3	0.6	3.3
Tomato & Basil, Made Up, Tesco*	1 Serving/200g	348	16.6	174	3.9	21	8.3	3.4
Tomato & Mediterranean Herb, Made Up, Co-Op*	½ Pack/138g	189	1.5	137	5.3	26	1.1	1.6
Tomato & Onion, Dry Weight, Waitrose*	1 Pack/110g	376	4	342	12.6	64.9	3.6	5.1
Tricolour, Unprepared, Artisan Grains*	1 Serving/100g	350	1	350	14	67	1	5
Wholewheat, Tesco*	1 Serving/50g	178	1	355	12	72	2	5
with Sun Dried Tomato, CBY, Asda*	1 Pack/310g	515	12.1	166	4.6	26.2	3.9	4

CRAB

	Measure INFO/WEIGHT	KCAL	FAT	KCAL	PROT	CARB	FAT	FIBRE
Blue, Soft Shelled, Raw, Average	*1 Crab/84g*	*73*	*0.9*	*87*	*18.1*	*0*	*1.1*	*0*
Boiled, Meat Only, Average	*1 Tbsp/40g*	*51*	*2.2*	*128*	*19.5*	*0*	*5.5*	*0*
Brown, Cornish, Seafood & Eat It*	1 Pack/100g	171	10.7	171	17.9	1.9	10.7	0
Cocktail, Waitrose*	1 Serving/100g	217	17.6	217	10.8	3.8	17.6	0.4
Cornish 50/50, Seafood & Eat It*	1 Pot/100g	144	5.8	144	21.6	1.2	5.8	0.5
Cornish Potted, Seafood & Eat It*	1 Pack/100g	235	17.5	235	15	5.1	17.5	0.8
Dressed, Average	*1 Can/43g*	*66*	*3.4*	*154*	*16.8*	*4.1*	*7.9*	*0.2*
Meat in Brine, Average	*½ Can/60g*	*41*	*0.2*	*69*	*15.6*	*0.8*	*0.4*	*0.1*
Meat, Raw, Average	*1oz/28g*	*28*	*0.2*	*100*	*20.8*	*2.8*	*0.6*	*0*

CRAB CAKES

	Measure INFO/WEIGHT	KCAL	FAT	KCAL	PROT	CARB	FAT	FIBRE
Goan, M&S*	1 Pack/190g	228	7.6	120	8	12.9	4	1.8
Iceland*	1 Serving/18g	52	3.2	288	7.2	25.6	18	1.3
Shetland Isles, Dressed, TTD, Sainsbury's*	1 Cake/75g	130	8.3	174	12.4	6	11.1	0.5
Tesco*	1 Serving/130g	281	16	216	11	15.4	12.3	1.1
Thai, TTD, Sainsbury's*	½ Pack/106g	201	9.5	189	9.5	17.8	8.9	1.4

CRAB STICKS

	Measure INFO/WEIGHT	KCAL	FAT	KCAL	PROT	CARB	FAT	FIBRE
Average	*1 Stick/15g*	*14*	*0*	*94*	*9.1*	*13.9*	*0.3*	*0*

CRACKERBREAD

	Measure INFO/WEIGHT	KCAL	FAT	KCAL	PROT	CARB	FAT	FIBRE
Original, Ryvita*	1 Slice/5g	19	0.1	378	10.8	75	2.8	4.8
Wholegrain, Ryvita*	1 Slice/5.7g	20	0.2	360	12.4	68.7	3.9	9.8

CRACKERS

	Measure INFO/WEIGHT	KCAL	FAT	KCAL	PROT	CARB	FAT	FIBRE
Ancient Grains Crackers, Kirkland*	3 Crackers/18g	90	4	500	11.1	66.7	22.2	0
Bath Oliver, Jacob's*	1 Cracker/12g	52	1.6	432	9.6	67.6	13.7	2.6
Bean Mix, Habas Tapas, Graze*	1 Punnet/30g	131	3.8	438	11.7	68.9	12.8	1.5
Black Olive, M&S*	1 Cracker/4g	20	1	485	8.3	59.4	23.5	4.3
Black Pepper for Cheese, Ryvita*	1 Cracker/7g	27	0.2	384	13.2	72.9	2.9	6.8
Bran, Jacob's*	1 Cracker/7g	32	1.3	454	9.7	62.8	18.2	3.2
Brooklyn Bites, Graze*	1 Punnet/29g	157	11.3	541	4.1	33	39	4
Buckwheat & Chia, Rude Health*	1 Cracker/7g	29	0.7	388	14	56	8.8	15
Butter Puff, Sainsbury's*	1 Cracker/10g	54	2.7	523	10.4	60.7	26.5	2.5
Caramelised Onion, Ciabatta, Jacob's*	1 Cracker/10g	43	1	426	12.5	68.6	10.3	4.3
Carrot Crunch, Sweet & Smokey, Graze*	1 Punnet/28g	140	8.1	499	13	42	29	11
Charcoal, Wafer, Miller's Damsel*	1 Cracker/5g	21	0.7	420	13.8	59.5	13.9	0
Cheddar, & Black Pepper, Thins, Ryvita*	1 Thin/7g	30	0.7	422	17.5	63.8	10	3.3
Cheddar, Goldfish, Pepperidge Farm*	1 Pack/43g	200	7	465	11.6	65.1	16.3	2.3
Cheese & Onion, Crispy, Bites, Ritz*	1 Bag/23g	109	4.8	474	7	63	21	2.7

CRACKERS

INFO/WEIGHT	Measure	per Measure KCAL	FAT	Nutrition Values per 100g / 100ml KCAL	PROT	CARB	FAT	FIBRE
Cheese Bites, Sour Cream & Onion, Mrs Crimbles*	1 Pack/30g	125	4.6	416	15.9	54	15.2	2
Cheese Snack Mix, Christmas, M&S*	1 Serving/30g	133	4.2	442	9.9	67.2	14	4
Cheese Thins, Asda*	1 Cracker/4g	21	1.3	532	12	49	32	0
Cheese Thins, Cheddar, The Planet Snack Co*	1 Serving/30g	153	8.8	509	11.5	50.1	29.2	2.1
Cheese Thins, Co-Op*	1 Cracker/4g	21	1.3	530	12	49	32	3
Cheese Thins, Mini, Snack Rite*	1 Bag/30g	144	6.8	480	12.9	55.9	22.7	2.5
Cheese Thins, Waitrose*	1 Cracker/4g	21	1.2	545	11.9	52.6	31.9	2.5
Cheese, Cheddar, Crispies, TTD, Sainsbury's*	1 Thin/4g	21	1.5	576	14.2	39	40.4	2.2
Cheese, Mini, Heinz*	1 Pack/25g	108	3.6	433	9.4	68.6	14.6	0.6
Cheese, Mini, Shapers, Boots*	1 Serving/23g	97	3.2	421	9.4	65	14	4.6
Cheese, Oat Bakes, Nairn's*	1 Bag/30g	130	4.7	432	15	57.4	15.8	1.3
Cheese, Puff Pastry, Somerfield*	1 Cracker/4g	21	1.5	500	10.6	36.1	34.8	2.1
Cheese, Ritz*	1 Cracker/4g	17	0.9	486	10.1	55.9	24.7	2.2
Chives, Jacob's*	1 Cracker/6g	28	1	457	9.5	67.5	16.5	2.7
Choice Grain, Jacob's*	1 Cracker/7.5g	32	1.1	427	9	65.5	14.3	5.4
Corn Thins, 97% Fat Free, Real Foods*	1 Cracker/6g	23	0.2	378	10.2	81.7	3	8.6
Corn Thins, Real Foods*	1 Serving/6g	22	0.2	378	10.2	81.7	3	8.6
Cream Cheese & Onion Flavour, Bakefuls, Ritz*	1 Bag/23g	109	4.8	474	7	63	21	2.7
Cream, 45% Less Fat, Morrisons*	1 Cracker/8g	32	0.6	403	10.5	74.2	7.1	3.3
Cream, Aldi*	1 Cracker/8g	36	1.2	456	9.1	71.7	14.7	3
Cream, Asda*	1 Cracker/8g	35	1.2	443	10	67	15	0
Cream, Average	**1 Cracker/7g**	**31**	**1.1**	**440**	**9.5**	**68.3**	**16.3**	**2.2**
Cream, BFY, Morrisons*	1 Cracker/8g	32	0.6	406	10.9	74.4	7.2	2.8
Cream, BGTY, Sainsbury's*	1 Cracker/8g	32	0.6	400	10.9	71.7	7.7	3.1
Cream, Choice Grain, Jacob's*	1 Cracker/7g	30	0.9	400	9	64.5	11.8	7
Cream, Jacob's*	1 Cracker/8g	35	1.1	440	10	67.7	13.5	3.8
Cream, Light, Jacob's*	1 Cracker/8g	31	0.5	388	10.6	72.2	6.3	4.1
Cream, Lower Fat, Tesco*	1 Cracker/5g	20	0.3	393	11	72.4	6.6	3.1
Cream, Morrisons*	1 Cracker/8g	36	1.2	446	9.6	68.5	14.8	2.7
Cream, Reduced Fat, Tesco*	1 Cracker/8g	31	0.5	406	10.9	74.4	7.2	2.8
Cream, Roasted Onion, Jacob's*	1 Cracker/8g	35	1.2	441	10.2	66.8	14.8	2.9
Cream, Sainsbury's*	1 Cracker/8g	35	1.3	422	9.5	66.7	15.2	2.8
Cream, Sun Dried Tomato Flavour, Jacob's*	1 Cracker/8g	35	1.1	434	10.2	66.7	14	3
Cream, Tesco*	1 Cracker/7.7g	34	1.2	447	9	69	15	3
Crispy Cheese, M&S*	1 Cracker/4.3g	20	1	470	9.4	58.1	22.1	3
Crispy Chickpea, M&S*	¼ Pack/25g	99	1.4	396	17.6	67.8	5.5	2.5
Crispy, Salt & Vinegar Flavour, Walkers*	1 Serving/30g	130	4.5	434	6.9	66	15	3.6
Crunchy Grain, Breaks, Ritz*	5 Crackers/33g	143	5.8	440	8.6	60	18	3.3
Cruskits, Arnotts*	2 Cruskits/12g	40	0.2	331	9	63.7	1.5	0
El Picante, Graze*	1 Punnet/25g	126	6.7	506	15	49	27	6
Extra Wheatgerm, Hovis*	1 Serving/6g	27	1.1	447	10.2	60	18.5	4.4
Flamed Baked, Traditional English, Water, Rakusen's*	1 Cracker/20g	79	1.1	394	8.6	75.8	5.5	3.3
Flatbread, Multigrain, Jacob's*	1 Cracker/10g	42	0.7	411	11	73.8	6.8	5.3
Flax, Pumpkin, Organic, Raw Health*	1 Cracker/12g	64	5	533	19	8	42	21
Garden Herbs, Jacob's*	1 Cracker/6g	28	1	457	9.5	67.5	16.5	2.7
Garlic & Herb, Jacob's*	1 Cracker/10g	45	1.7	450	10	68.3	16.7	3.3
Garlic, CBY, Asda*	2 Biscuits/12g	58	2.6	483	7	63.3	21.5	4.2
Glutafin*	1 Serving/11g	52	2.2	470	2.4	70	20	0.7
Harvest Grain, Sainsbury's*	1 Cracker/6g	27	1.1	458	8.5	64.5	18.4	4.1
Herb & Onion, 99% Fat Free, Rakusen's*	1 Cracker/5g	18	0	360	9.1	82.6	1	3.9
Herb & Spice, Jacob's*	1 Cracker/6g	27	1	457	9.5	67.5	16.5	2.7
Herb & Onion, Trufree*	1 Cracker/6g	25	0.7	418	2.5	75	12	10
Herbs & Spice Selection, Jacob's*	1 Cracker/6g	27	0.9	451	9.5	68	15.7	2.7

CRACKERS

INFO/WEIGHT	Measure			Nutrition Values per 100g / 100ml				
		KCAL	FAT	KCAL	PROT	CARB	FAT	FIBRE
High Fibre, Dietary Specials*	1 Cracker/6g	23	0.6	391	2.1	60	11	17
Japanese Beef Teriyaki, Sensations, Walkers*	1 Serving/24g	118	6.3	490	1.4	62	26	3.5
Light & Crispy, Sainsbury's*	1 Cracker/11g	42	1.2	384	11.3	61	10.5	13
Lightly Salted, Crispy, Sainsbury's*	1 Cracker/5g	25	1.3	533	7.8	62.6	27.9	2.1
Lightly Salted, Italian, Jacob's*	1 Cracker/6g	26	0.8	429	10.3	67.6	13	2.9
Louisiana Wild Rice & Beans, Graze*	1 Pack/30g	136	5.7	454	17	49	19	8.8
Matzos, Flame Baked, Rakusen's*	1 Cracker/21g	75	0.2	357	10	79	1	4.3
Matzos, Tea, Flamed Baked, Round, Rakusen's*	1 Cracker/5g	19	0	382	9.9	85.7	0.8	3.7
Mediterranean Tomato & Herb, Oat Bakes, Nairn's*	1 Bag/30g	129	4.7	431	8.1	64.2	15.8	8.3
Mediterranean, Jacob's*	1 Cracker/6g	27	1	450	9.7	66.5	16.1	2.7
Melty, Sour Cream & Onion Flavour, Walkers*	1 Serving/30g	148	6.6	493	7.3	65	22	2.8
Melty, Sweet Chilli Flavour, Walkers*	1 Serving/30g	147	6.6	490	7.5	64	22	2.8
Mix, Yaki Soba, Graze*	1 Punnet/32g	159	9.3	498	24	36	29	6
Mixed Seed, Multi Grain, Asda*	1 Cracker/6g	28	1.1	445	11	62	17	4.4
Multi Seed, Thins, Ryvita*	1 Thin/9g	39	1.3	434	16.4	56.2	14.1	8.1
Multi-grain, Aldi, Savour Bakes, Aldi*	1 Cracker/5g	20	0.8	404	8.3	55	16.8	5.1
Multigrain, Corn Thins, Real Foods*	1 Cracker/6g	23	0.2	388	10.9	71	3.7	10.3
Multigrain, Morrisons*	10 Crackers/20g	76	2.2	379	8.8	61.3	11	5.1
Multigrain, Tesco*	1 Cracker/5g	24	1	477	8.8	60.8	20.8	5.7
Oat & Wheat, Weight Watchers*	4 Crackers/20g	74	0.5	370	10.5	75	2.5	4
Olive Oil & Oregano, Mediterreaneo, Jacob's*	1 Cracker/6g	25	0.7	412	12.4	65.5	11.2	6
Oriental, Asda*	1 Serving/30g	115	6	383	1.7	49	20	4.3
Original, Vita Wheat, Arnotts*	1 Cracker/20g	87	2.3	433	8.7	69.3	11.5	6.8
Passionately Pizza, Jacobites, Jacob's*	1 Pack/150g	708	38.1	472	5.7	55.3	25.4	1.7
Peanut, Wasabi, Graze*	1 Pack/26g	125	5.6	479	15.2	53.8	21.4	5.4
Pizza Flavour, Mini, Sainsbury's*	1 Serving/25g	113	4	454	7.6	68.7	15.9	2.7
Poppy & Sesame Seed, Sainsbury's*	1 Cracker/4g	21	1.1	530	9.6	58.9	28.4	3.4
Poppy Oat, Cracker Selection, TTD, Sainsbury's*	1 Cracker/4g	19	0.7	467	9.8	65	17.7	4.1
Ritz, Mini, Kraft*	1 Bag/25g	126	6	504	7.9	63	24	2
Ritz, Original, Jacob's*	1 Cracker/3.3g	17	1	509	6.9	55.6	28.8	2
Rosemary, CBY, Asda*	1 Cracker/6g	29	1.2	486	6.5	68.3	20.2	2.4
Rye Cakes, Lightly Salted, Ryvita*	1 Cake/6.3g	23	0.1	363	8.9	69.9	2	13.7
Rye Cakes, Multigrain, Ryvita*	1 Cake/6.5g	23	0.2	352	9.4	66.3	2.5	13.3
Rye, Organic, Dove's Farm*	1 Cracker/7g	28	1	393	7	58.4	14.6	8.7
Salada Original, Arnotts*	4 Crackers/16g	68	1.6	427	10.4	71.5	10	3.9
Salt & Black Pepper, Jacob's*	1 Cracker/6g	27	1	457	9.5	67.5	16.5	2.7
Salt & Black Pepper, Eat Well, M&S*	1 Pack/25g	106	3.7	422	9.6	62.9	14.7	5.1
Salt & Pepper, Sainsbury's*	1 Cracker/6g	27	1.2	485	7.3	64.5	21.3	3
Salted, Ritz, Nabisco*	1 Cracker/3.4g	17	0.9	493	7	57.5	26.1	2.9
Sea Salt & Vinegar Flavour, Bakefuls, Ritz*	1 Bag/23g	108	4.8	471	7	61	21	2.8
Seeds, & Sea Salt, Snacks, Finn Crisp*	1 Serving/30g	111	2.4	371	12	53	8.1	19
Selection, Finest, Tesco*	1 Serving/30g	136	4.3	452	9.6	71	14.4	0
Sesame & Poppy Thins, Tesco*	1 Cracker/4g	20	1	485	9.9	57.6	23.5	4.4
Smokehouse BBQ Crunch, Graze*	1 Box/31g	137	4.7	441	10	62	15	5.4
Sour Cream & Garlic, Crostini, Mix, Graze*	1 Punnet/25g	133	8	531	15	44	32	4
Spicy Indonesian Vegetable, Waitrose*	1 Pack/60g	295	16.3	492	1.2	60.6	27.2	2.2
Spicy, Trufree*	1 Cracker/6g	25	0.8	412	3.8	70	13	12.5
Sweet Chilli, Oat Bakes, Nairn's*	1 Bag/30g	128	4	426	8.1	68.4	13.3	7.2
Sweet Chilli, Thins, Ryvita*	1 Thin/8g	31	0.1	382	12	77.5	1.5	5.2
Sweet Chilli, Thins, Savours, Jacob's*	1 Cracker/4.4g	21	0.9	472	8	62.3	21.2	3.6
Table, Schar*	5 Crackers/30g	138	3	460	6.7	80	10	3.3
Tarallini with Fennel Seeds, Crosta & Mollica*	1 Cracker/4g	21	0.9	529	8.2	67.5	22	4.2
Thai Spiced, Blue Dragon*	10 Crackers/10g	54	3.1	536	1.5	61	31.2	2.1

	Measure INFO/WEIGHT	per Measure KCAL	FAT	KCAL	PROT	CARB	FAT	FIBRE
CRACKERS								
Thai Spicy Vegetable, Sainsbury's*	1 Pack/50g	231	10.4	462	7.2	61.5	20.8	2.6
The British Barbecue, Graze*	1 Punnet/25g	127	8	508	17.4	36.8	32.2	7.4
Tom Yum Yum, Graze*	1 Pack/23g	90	0.6	390	7.2	84.8	2.4	1.4
Tuc, Cheese Sandwich, Jacob's*	1 Cracker/13.6g	72	4.3	531	8.4	53.8	31.4	0
Tuc, Jacob's*	1 Cracker/5g	25	1.4	518	6.9	54.2	29.9	2.6
Tuc, Mini with Sesame Seeds, Jacob's*	1 Biscuit/2g	10	0.5	523	9.7	63.1	25.8	3.9
Unsalted, Tops, Premium Plus, Impress*	1 Cracker/3g	13	0.3	448	10.3	75.9	10.3	0
Wasabi, Vitasia, Lidl*	1 Serving/30g	167	9.9	557	3.6	61.3	32.9	0
Wasapeas, Graze*	1 Pack/32g	128	2.5	406	14.8	65.2	7.8	7.1
Waterthins, Wafers, Philemon*	1 Crackers/2g	7	0.1	392	10.6	77.9	3.6	5
Wheaten, M&S*	1 Cracker/4g	20	0.9	450	10.2	57	20.2	5
Whole Wheat, 100%, Oven Baked, Master Choice*	1 Cracker/4g	17	0.4	429	10	75	9.6	12.1
Wholemeal, Tesco*	1 Cracker/7g	29	1	414	9.4	60.6	14.9	10.4
Wholmeal, Organic, Nairn's*	1 Cracker/14g	58	2	413	9	61.4	14.6	8.7
CRANBERRIES								
& Blueberries, Delicious, Boots*	1 Pack/75g	220	1	293	0.7	70	1.3	9.1
& Raisins, Dried, Sweetened, Ocean Spray*	1 Serving/50g	163	0.2	326	0.1	80.3	0.5	4.6
Dried, Sweetened, Average	*1 Serving/10g*	*34*	*0.1*	*335*	*0.3*	*81.1*	*0.8*	*4.4*
Fresh, Raw, Average	*1oz/28g*	*4*	*0*	*15*	*0.4*	*3.4*	*0.1*	*3*
Frozen, Sainsbury's*	1 Portion/80g	18	0.1	22	0.4	3.4	0.1	3
CRAYFISH								
Raw	*1oz/28g*	*19*	*0.2*	*67*	*14.9*	*0*	*0.8*	*0*
Tails in Brine, Luxury, The Big Prawn Co*	½ Tub/90g	46	0.6	51	10.1	1	0.7	0
Tails, Chilli & Garlic, Asda*	1 Serving/140g	133	4.3	95	16	1.1	3.1	0.8
CREAM								
Aerosol, Average	*1oz/28g*	*87*	*8.7*	*309*	*1.8*	*6.2*	*30.9*	*0*
Aerosol, Reduced Fat, Average	*1 Serving/55ml*	*33*	*3*	*60*	*0.6*	*2*	*5.4*	*0*
Brandy, Extra Thick, TTD, Sainsbury's*	1 Serving/30ml	131	12.3	436	1.4	10.4	40.8	0.5
Brandy, Pourable with Remy Martin*, Finest, Tesco*	½ Pot/125ml	460	35.5	368	2.7	19.8	28.4	0
Brandy, Really Thick, Finest, Tesco*	½ Pot/125ml	579	49.5	463	1.3	19.7	39.6	0
Brandy, Really Thick, Tesco*	1 Pot/250ml	1162	98.2	465	1.4	21.3	39.3	0
Chantilly, TTD, Sainsbury's*	2 Tbsp/30g	136	14	455	1.4	6.9	46.8	0
Clotted, Fresh, Average	*1 Serving/28g*	*162*	*17.5*	*579*	*1.6*	*2.3*	*62.7*	*0*
Coconut, Soya, Cuisine, Alpro*	1 Tbsp/15g	15	1.3	100	1.2	2.3	8.8	0
Double, Average	*1 Tbsp/15ml*	*68*	*7.3*	*452*	*1.6*	*2.4*	*48.4*	*0*
Double, Brandy, Waitrose*	1 Serving/30ml	138	12.4	460	1.3	14.4	41.4	0
Double, Channel Island, Cointreau, Waitrose*	1 Serving/30ml	129	11.4	431	1.3	15.3	38.2	0
Double, Reduced Fat, Average	*1 Serving/30g*	*73*	*7*	*243*	*2.7*	*5.6*	*23.3*	*0.1*
Extra Thick, with Baileys, Baileys*	1 fl oz/30ml	129	11.6	431	1.5	13.4	38.6	0
Goat's, Double, St Helen's Farm*	1 Tbsp/15g	67	7.2	449	1.7	2.6	48	0
Half & Half, Dairyland*	2 Tbsp/30ml	40	3	133	3.3	6.7	10	0
Oat Alternative, Dairy Free, Oatly*	1 Carton/250ml	375	32.5	150	1	6	13	0.8
Remy Martin, Channel Island, Waitrose*	1 Serving/30ml	135	12.8	450	1.5	9.7	42.8	0
Single, Average	*1 Tbsp/15ml*	*28*	*2.7*	*188*	*2.6*	*3.9*	*18*	*0.1*
Single, Extra Thick, Average	*1 Serving/38ml*	*72*	*6.9*	*192*	*2.7*	*4.1*	*18.4*	*0*
Single, Soya, Fresh, Plant Based, Cuisine, Alpro*	1 Tbsp/15g	18	1.5	122	2	4.5	10.2	0.4
Single, Soya, UHT, Plant Based, Cuisine, Alpro*	1 Tbsp/15g	25	2.5	169	2	1.6	16.8	0.3
Soured, Fresh, Average	*1 Tsp/5ml*	*10*	*0.9*	*191*	*2.7*	*3.9*	*18.4*	*0*
Soured, Reduced Fat, Average	*1 Tsp/5ml*	*6*	*0.4*	*119*	*5.2*	*6.7*	*8.6*	*0.4*
Strawberry, Light, Real Dairy, Uht, Anchor*	1 Serving/12.5g	25	2.1	198	2.6	8.7	17	0
Thick, Sterilised, Average	*1 Tbsp/15ml*	*35*	*3.5*	*233*	*2.6*	*3.6*	*23.1*	*0*
Uht, Double, Average	*1 Tbsp/15g*	*41*	*3.9*	*274*	*2.2*	*7.4*	*26.3*	*0*
Uht, Reduced Fat, Average	*1 Serving/25ml*	*16*	*1.4*	*62*	*0.6*	*2.2*	*5.6*	*0*

	Measure INFO/WEIGHT	per Measure KCAL	FAT	Nutrition Values per 100g / 100ml KCAL	PROT	CARB	FAT	FIBRE
CREAM								
Uht, Single, Average	*1 Tbsp/15ml*	*29*	*2.8*	*194*	*2.6*	*4*	*18.8*	*0*
Whipping, Average	*1 Tbsp/15ml*	*52*	*5.5*	*348*	*2.1*	*3.2*	*36.4*	*0*
CREAM SODA								
American with Vanilla, Tesco*	1 Glass/313ml	75	0	24	0	5.9	0	0
Diet, Sainsbury's*	1 Serving/250ml	2	0	1	0	0	0	0
No Added Sugar, Sainsbury's*	1 Can/330ml	2	0.3	0	0.1	0.1	0.1	0.1
Shapers, Boots*	1 Bottle/300ml	3	0	1	0	0	0	0
Traditional Style, Tesco*	1 Can/330ml	139	0	42	0	10.4	0	0
CREME BRULEE								
Average	*1 Serving/100g*	*313*	*26*	*313*	*3.8*	*15.7*	*26*	*0.2*
Dine in Dessert, M&S*	1 Dessert/89g	186	13.1	210	4.9	14.2	14.8	0.5
Gastropub, M&S*	1 Brulee/83.8g	285	24.6	340	3.1	15.7	29.3	0.7
M&S*	1 Pot/100g	360	32.6	360	3.3	13	32.6	0
Nestle*	1 Serving/100g	305	25.6	305	4	14.6	25.6	0
Reduced Fat, M&S*	1 Serving/89g	186	13.1	210	4.9	14.2	14.8	0.5
Somerfield*	1 Pot/100g	316	27	316	4	15	27	0
CREME CARAMEL								
Asda*	1 Pot/100g	113	2.6	113	2.4	20	2.6	0
Average	*1 Serving/128g*	*140*	*2.8*	*109*	*3*	*20.6*	*2.2*	*0*
La Laitiere*	1 Pot/100g	135	4	135	5	20	4	0
Lidl*	1 Pot/89g	79	0.7	89	2.3	18.1	0.8	0.1
Tesco*	1 Pot/100g	115	1.6	115	2.8	21.8	1.6	0
CREME EGG								
Cadbury*	1 Egg/40g	177	6	440	3.2	73	15	0.4
Minis, Cadbury*	1 Egg/11.5g	50	1.9	435	4.2	67	16.5	0.5
CREME FRAICHE								
Average	*1 Pot/295g*	*1067*	*112.2*	*362*	*2.2*	*2.6*	*38*	*0*
Half Fat, Average	*1 Tbsp/15g*	*27*	*2.4*	*181*	*3.1*	*5.5*	*16.2*	*0*
Lemon & Rocket, Sainsbury's*	1 Serving/150g	188	17.2	125	2.2	3	11.5	0.5
Low Fat, Average	*1 Tbsp/30ml*	*43*	*3.6*	*143*	*3.3*	*5.6*	*12.1*	*0.1*
CREPES								
Chocolate Filled, Tesco*	1 Crepe/32g	140	5.8	438	5.9	62.5	18.1	1.6
Lobster, Finest, Tesco*	1 Serving/160g	250	10.2	156	10.7	14	6.4	1.2
Mushroom, M&S*	1 Pack/186g	195	4.5	105	5.7	17.1	2.4	2.5
CRISPBAKES								
Broccoli & Leek, Asda*	1 Bake/132.2g	263	13.2	199	6.3	21	10	2
Bubble & Squeak, M&S*	1 Bake/47g	79	4.1	170	2.7	19.6	8.8	1.5
Cheese & Onion, M&S*	1 Bake/114g	285	18.5	250	6.4	19.4	16.2	1.7
Cheese & Onion, Tesco*	1 Bake/109g	275	17.2	252	7.9	19.6	15.8	2.1
Cheese & Onion, Cooked, Dalepak*	1 Bake/86g	192	8.8	223	4.9	26.9	10.2	1.7
Cheese & Onion, Meat Free, Morrisons*	1 Crispbake/136g	282	13.8	207	1.5	23.5	10.1	4.9
Cheese & Onion, Ovenbaked, Iceland*	1 Crispbake/77g	145	5.3	189	4.8	25.9	6.9	2.3
Cheese, Spring Onion & Chive, Sainsbury's*	1 Bake/113.5g	287	16.8	253	7.1	24.5	14.8	1.7
Chicken & Mushroom, Sainsbury's*	1 Crispbake/85g	174	7.6	205	10.5	20.6	8.9	1.8
Dutch, Asda*	1 Bake/8g	31	0.3	388	14.7	74.9	3.3	4.2
Dutch, Co-Op*	1 Crispbake/10g	38	0.4	375	16	69.6	3.5	6.5
Dutch, HL, Tesco*	1 Bake/8g	30	0.2	385	14.7	74.9	2.7	4.2
Dutch, Sainsbury's*	1 Bake/10g	38	0.5	392	14.5	72.3	5	5.8
Mature Cheddar, Crispy Thins, TTD, Sainsbury's*	1 Thin/4g	21	1.5	581	14.2	38.3	40.6	2.8
Minced Beef, M&S*	1 Bake/113g	226	12.3	200	10	15.6	10.9	1.5
Roast Vegetable & Basil, Cauldron Foods*	1 Bake/115g	242	11	210	3.5	26	9.6	2.9
Vegetable, M&S*	1 Bake/114g	200	10.3	175	2.5	19.2	9	2.6
Vegetable, Sainsbury's*	1 Bake/114g	246	13	216	2	26.2	11.4	2

INFO/WEIGHT	Measure	per Measure		Nutrition Values per 100g / 100ml				
		KCAL	FAT	KCAL	PROT	CARB	FAT	FIBRE
CRISPBAKES								
Vegetarian, Salmon Style, & Dill, Quorn*	1 Crispbake/100g	182	6.6	182	7	22	6.6	3.5
CRISPBREAD								
3 Grain 3 Seed, Foodie Market, Aldi*	1 Crispbread/25g	109	4.2	436	15	52	17	8.8
3 Grain, Foodie Market, Aldi*	1 Crispbread/25g	113	4.7	461	15	49	19	10
3 Seed, Classic, Gourmet, Dr Karg*	1 Bread/25g	108	4.9	430	16.5	46.6	19.7	10.9
3 Seed, Organic, Gourmet	*1 Bread/25g*	*101*	*4.7*	*405*	*15.8*	*48.8*	*18.8*	*14.6*
Apple & Cinnamon, Ryvita*	1 Crispbread/15g	54	0.2	356	7.2	72.5	1.6	11.8
Chickpea, Mung Bean & Chive, Easy Bean*	1 Crispbread/22g	93	4.1	422	12.8	50.6	18.6	6.9
Corn Thins, Sesame, Real Foods*	1 Thin/6g	23	0.2	384	10.7	69.9	3.4	10.2
Corn, Orgran*	1 Bread/5g	18	0.1	360	7.5	83	1.8	3
Cracked Black Pepper, Thins, Ryvita*	1 Slice/10g	35	0.2	344	8.8	66.6	1.6	14.5
Cream Cheese & Chives, Minis, Ryvita*	1 Pack/30g	114	2.3	380	8.7	75.7	7.7	13
Crisp 'n' Light, Wasa*	1 Bread/7g	24	0.1	360	12	73	2.2	5.3
Dark Rye, Morrisons*	1 Bake/13g	39	0.4	300	11.5	61.5	3.1	16.9
Dark Rye, Ryvita*	1 Bread/10g	34	0.1	342	8.5	66.5	1.2	15.2
Fibre Plus, Wholegrain with Sesame, Wasa*	1 Bread/10g	35	0.7	350	13	47	7	24
Five Seed, Bites, Knacks, Peters Yard*	1 Portion/25g	99	2.3	397	14	69.6	9.2	10.3
Fruit Crunch, Ryvita*	1 Slice/15g	54	0.8	358	8.3	61.8	5.4	14.9
GF	*1 Serving/8g*	*25*	*0.1*	*331*	*6.4*	*72.9*	*1.5*	*0*
Hint of Chilli, Ryvita*	1 Slice/12g	42	0.2	349	8.6	66.6	1.9	16.8
Mini, Sesame & Linseed, Dr Karg*	1 Crispbread/3g	13	0.4	424	12.1	57.6	12.1	9.1
Mixed Grain, Jacobs*	1 Cracker/10g	41	1.3	436	9.1	66.7	13.9	4.2
Multigrain, Deli, Ryvita*	1 Slice/11g	41	0.8	370	11.2	56	7.2	18.3
Multigrain, Ryvita*	1 Slice/11g	41	0.8	370	11.2	56	7.2	18.3
Original Rye, Thin, Finn Crisp*	1 Slice/6g	22	0.2	339	10	59	2.6	20
Original Rye, Wasa*	1 Bread/11g	35	0.2	315	9	67	1.4	14
Original, Ryvita*	1 Bread/10g	35	0.2	350	8.5	66.9	1.7	16.5
Poppyseed, Wasa*	1 Bread/13g	46	1	350	13	56	8	14
Provita*	1 Bread/6g	26	0.6	416	12.5	68.4	9.9	0
Pumpkin Seeds & Oats, Rye, Deli, Ryvita*	1 Crispbread/12g	46	0.9	370	11.2	56	7.2	18.3
Pumpkin Seeds & Oats, Ryvita*	1 Slice/12.5g	46	0.9	370	11.2	56	7.2	18.3
Rice & Cracked Pepper, Orgran*	1 Bread/5g	18	0.1	388	8.4	81.9	1.8	2
Rice, Sakata*	1 Bread/25g	26	0.2	102	1.7	22	0.7	0.3
Roasted Onion, Organic, Dr Karg*	1 Bread/25g	98	3.7	390	15.8	48.5	14.8	12.9
Rosemary & Apricot, Toasts, M&S*	1 Toast/8g	34	1.4	434	12.3	54.3	17.8	3.7
Rounds, Multigrain, Finn Crisp*	1 Bread/12.5g	41	0.8	330	13	56	6	18
Rounds, Wholegrain Wheat, Finn Crisp*	1 Bread/12.5g	45	0.7	360	11	66	5.9	10
Rustikal, Wasa*	1 Crispbread/15g	51	0.2	340	9	6.4	1.5	16
Salt & Vinegar, Minis, Ryvita*	1 Pack/24g	90	1.9	376	8.2	74	7.8	11.4
Scan Bran, Slimming World*	1 Slice/10g	31	0.5	310	14.9	29	5.3	42.1
Seeded, Spelt, Organic, Dr Karg*	1 Bread/25g	108	4.5	430	17.2	44.4	18	11.2
Sesame & Rye, Tesco*	1 Biscuit/9g	34	0.8	385	12.5	55.6	8.7	17.2
Sesame, Ryvita*	1 Bread/10.1g	37	0.7	373	10.5	58.3	7	17.5
Sesame, Savour Bakes, Aldi*	1 Crispbread/9g	31	0.5	344	10	57.8	5.6	15.6
Snacks, Cheese, Onion & Chive Flavour, Quaker*	1 Pack/28g	118	2.5	420	8.3	76	9.1	2.4
Sour Cream & Onion, Mini, The Foodie Market, Aldi*	1/6 Pack/25g	107	3.8	427	14	54	15	7.9
Sourdough, Original, Peter's Yard*	1 Crispbread/10g	38	0.4	381	12.9	68.3	4.1	9.5
Spelt, Cheese, Sunflower Seeds, Organic, Dr Karg*	1 Bread/25g	103	4.5	411	19.2	42.8	18.1	10.4
Spelt, Muesli, Organic, Dr Karg*	1 Bread/25g	94	2.8	375	14.2	54.4	11.2	10.6
Sport, Wasa*	1 Bread/15g	46	0.2	310	9	64	1.5	16
Sunflower Seeds & Oats, Ryvita*	1 Bread/12g	46	1.1	384	9.7	58.4	9	15.3
Super Chia, GF, Semper*	1 Crispbread/14g	50	0.4	357	5.3	72	3.2	9.4
Sweet Chilli, Minis, Ryvita*	1 Pack/24g	90	1.8	376	8.5	75.9	7.4	10.3

INFO/WEIGHT	Measure	per Measure		Nutrition Values per 100g / 100ml				
		KCAL	FAT	KCAL	PROT	CARB	FAT	FIBRE
CRISPBREAD								
Sweet Onion, Ryvita*	1 Crispbread/12g	43	0.2	356	9	70.6	1.4	12.6
Sweet Onion, Wholegrain Rye, Deli, Ryvita*	1 Crispbread/10g	37	0.1	365	9	70.6	1.4	12.6
Thin Crisps, Original Taste, Finn Crisp*	1 Bread/6.3g	20	0.2	320	11	63	2.4	19
Toasted Corn, Orgran*	1 Crispbread/15g	55	0.2	367	6.7	75.5	1.4	1.9
Trufree*	1 Bread/6g	22	0.1	370	6	82	2	1
Wheat, Morrisons*	1 Crispbread/8g	28	0.3	377	11.5	73.1	3.4	4.2
Whole Grain, Crispy, Thin, Kavli*	3 Breads/15g	50	0.3	333	10	70	1.7	12.7
Wholegrain, Classic Three Seed, Organic, Dr Karg*	1 Bread/25g	101	4.5	405	15.8	44.8	18	14.6
Wholemeal Rye, Organic, Kallo*	1 Bread/10g	31	0.2	314	9.7	65	1.7	15.4
Wholemeal, Light, Allinson*	1 Bread/5g	17	0.1	349	11.7	69.7	2.6	11
Wholemeal, Organic, Allinson*	1 Bread/5g	17	0.1	336	14.2	66	1.7	12.2
Wholemeal, Rye with Milk, Grafschafter*	1 Bread/9.3g	29	0.1	316	11.4	64	1.6	15
CRISPS								
Aberdeen Angus, Aldi*	1 Serving/40g	208	11.6	519	5.1	59	29	2.5
Apple, Dried, Snapz*	1 Pack/15g	52	0	344	2	77	0	14.7
Apple, Eat Smart, Morrisons*	1 Pack/20g	68	0.1	338	1.9	75.3	0.7	11.4
Apple, Pure, Dusted with Cinnamon, Graze*	¼ Bag/13g	47	0	364	2	81	0	14
Apple, Thyme & Sage, M&S*	1 Bag/55g	253	13.4	460	5.5	55.3	24.3	6.1
Argentinean Flame Grilled Steak, Walkers*	1 Bag/35g	182	11.3	520	6.5	50.7	32.4	4.2
Bacon Crispies, Sainsbury's*	1 Bag/25g	117	5.7	468	19.9	45.8	22.8	4.8
Bacon Flavour Rashers, BGTY, Sainsbury's*	1 Pack/10g	34	0.2	340	10.8	70.3	1.6	3.5
Bacon Pillows, Light, Shapers, Boots*	1 Pack/12g	44	0.3	367	3.7	83	2.3	4
Bacon Rashers, Blazin, Tesco*	1 Bag/25g	121	6.6	485	16.5	45.7	26.3	3.8
Bacon Rashers, COU, M&S*	1 Pack/20g	72	0.6	360	9.4	77.5	2.9	3.5
Bacon Rashers, Iceland*	1 Bag/75g	330	13.2	440	8.3	61.9	17.6	2.9
Bacon Rashers, Snackrite, Aldi*	1 Bag/18g	89	4.3	496	5.6	63	24	1.7
Bacon Rice Bites, Asda*	1 Bag/30g	136	4.8	452	7	70	16	0.4
Bacon Sizzler, Ridge Cut, McCoys*	1 Bag/32g	165	9.7	516	7.1	53.6	30.3	3.9
Bacon, Shapers, Boots*	1 Bag/23g	99	3.4	431	8	66	15	3
Bacon, Sizzler, Ridged, Snackrite, Aldi*	1 Pack/30g	160	9.3	532	7.2	55	31	3.9
Bacon, Webs, Monster Munch*	1 Pack/15g	74	3.4	497	6.5	65.2	23.1	1.6
Baked Bean Flavour, Walkers*	1 Bag/35g	184	11.6	525	6.5	50	33	4
Baked, Average	**1 Bag/25g**	**93**	**1.5**	**374**	**6.5**	**73.5**	**5.9**	**5.8**
Baked, Ready Salted, Walkers*	1 Pack/37.5g	153	3	409	7	74.9	8	4.9
Baked, Sour Cream & Chive, Walkers*	1 Pack/37.5g	148	3.2	395	7	73	8.5	5
Barbecue Beef, Select, Tesco*	1 Pack/25g	134	8.7	536	6.4	49.2	34.8	4.4
Barbecue, Handcooked, Tesco*	1 Bag/40g	187	10	468	6.6	53.8	25.1	5.2
Barbecue, Savoury Snacks, Weight Watchers*	1 Pack/22g	81	1.9	366	18.6	61	8.7	6.1
Barbecue, Snack Rite*	1 Bag/25g	131	8.3	524	5.1	51.3	33.2	0
Barbecue, Sunseed Oil, Walkers*	1 Pack/32.5g	171	10.7	525	6.5	50	33	4
Barbeque Pop Outs, Passions, Aldi*	1 Pack/100g	422	13	422	5.8	69	13	3
BBQ Rib, Crusti Croc, Lidl*	1 Bag/25g	132	8.2	527	6.4	50	32.6	4
BBQ Rib, Sunseed, Walkers*	1 Bag/25g	131	8.2	525	6.5	50	33	4
Beautifully Barbecued, Cassava, GF, Hale & Hearty*	1 Bag/30g	143	6.9	478	3.3	66	23.1	6.6
Beef & Onion, Tayto*	1 Bag/35g	184	11.9	526	7.6	47.3	34	4.5
Beef & Horseradish, Hand Cooked , Deluxe, Lidl*	1 Pack/25g	121	6.8	484	7	50.5	27.1	5.1
Beef & Onion Flavour, Average	**1 Bag/25g**	**131**	**8.3**	**524**	**6.5**	**50**	**33.1**	**4.3**
Beef & Onion, Walkers*	1 Bag/32.5g	171	10.7	525	6.5	50	33	4
Beef & Red Wine, Specially Selected, Aldi*	1 Serving/25g	130	7.3	519	5.1	59	29	2.5
Beef, Discos, KP Snacks*	1 Pack/28g	145	8.2	518	5.1	58.7	29.3	2.4
Beef, Space Raiders, KP Snacks*	1 Pack/13g	64	2.9	495	6.5	65.3	22.8	1
Beef, Squares, Walkers*	1 Bag/25g	105	4.5	420	6	59	18	4.6
Beefy, Smiths, Walkers*	1 Bag/25g	133	9.2	531	4.3	45.2	37	0

C

	Measure INFO/WEIGHT	per Measure KCAL	per Measure FAT	Nutrition Values per 100g / 100ml KCAL	PROT	CARB	FAT	FIBRE

CRISPS

	Measure INFO/WEIGHT	KCAL	FAT	KCAL	PROT	CARB	FAT	FIBRE
Beetroot Chips, Crunchy, Apple Snapz*	1 Bag/20g	52	0.2	260	14.7	76	1	28
Beetroot Vinaigrette, Eat Well, M&S*	1 Pack/30g	92	0.1	306	13.6	51.4	0.2	21.9
Beetroot, Eat Smart, Morrisons*	1 Pack/20g	63	0.1	313	15.1	52	0.4	20.5
Beetroot, Seasoned In Salt, Glennans*	1 Bag/27g	130	8.9	480	8.2	36	32.8	13.2
Big Snak, Crisp 'n Tasty Potato Chips, Herrs*	1 Pack/43g	212	12.1	494	7.1	56.5	28.2	3.6
Buffalo Mozzarella & Herbs, Walkers*	1 Serving/35g	172	9.1	490	6.1	57	26	4.2
Buffalo Mozzarella Tomato & Basil, Kettle Chips*	1 Serving/50g	238	12.8	476	6.7	54.4	25.7	4.9
Bugles, Cheese Flavour, Walkers*	1 Pack/30g	158	8.8	525	7	56.9	29.3	3
Builders Breakfast, Walkers*	1 Sm Bag/25g	131	8.3	524	5.6	50.8	33.2	4
Butter & Chive, COU, M&S*	1 Bag/26g	95	0.5	365	7.7	77.3	1.9	4.6
Cajun Squirrel, Walkers*	1 Bag/25g	130	8.2	522	5.8	51.2	32.7	4.2
Canadian Ham Flavour, Seabrook*	1 Pack/30g	159	9.8	531	5.7	50.9	32.7	5.1
Carrot, Eat Smart, Morrisons*	1 Pack/200g	63	0.3	316	5.5	61.9	1.3	17.2
Chargrilled Chicken Crinkles, Shapers, Boots*	1 Bag/20g	96	4.8	482	6.6	60	24	4
Chargrilled Chicken, Ridge Cut, McCoys*	1 Pack/32g	167	10	521	7	52.9	31.3	4
Chargrilled Chicken, Ridged, Snackrite, Aldi*	1 Pack/30g	157	9	524	6.5	54	30	4
Chargrilled Steak, Max, Walkers*	1 Bag/55g	289	18.2	525	6.5	50	33	4
Cheddar & Red Onion Chutney, Sensations, Walkers*	1 Bag/40g	198	11.2	495	6.5	54	28	4.5
Cheddar & Spring Onion, 35% Less Fat, Sainsbury's*	1 Pack/20g	93	4.2	463	6.3	62.4	20.9	0.9
Cheddar & Onion, Crinkles, Walkers*	1 Pack/28g	150	9.3	538	6	51.5	33.3	3.5
Cheddar & Onion, Ridge Cut, McCoys*	1 Bag/32g	165	9.8	516	7	53.2	30.6	3.9
Cheddar & Sour Cream, Extra Crunchy, Walkers*	1 Serving/30g	143	6.8	476	6.6	59.1	22.6	4.7
Cheddar Cheese & Bacon, Temptingly, Walkers*	1 Pack/32g	169	10	520	6.2	52.3	30.9	4.2
Cheese & Onion Rings, Crunchy, Shapers, Boots*	1 Bag/15g	56	0.4	374	5.9	81	2.9	2
Cheese & Onion, 30% Less Fat, Sainsbury's*	1 Pack/25g	115	5.4	459	7.5	58.1	21.8	5.4
Cheese & Onion, BGTY, Sainsbury's*	1 Bag/25g	120	6.2	479	7	57	24.8	5.7
Cheese & Onion, Crinkle Cut, Low Fat, Waitrose*	1 Bag/25g	122	5.8	490	7.7	62.6	23.2	4.7
Cheese & Onion, Flavour Crinkles, Shapers, Boots*	1 Bag/20g	96	4.8	482	6.6	60	24	4
Cheese & Onion, GFY, Asda*	1 Pack/26g	122	5.7	470	7	61	22	4.2
Cheese & Onion, KP Snacks*	1 Bag/25g	134	8.7	534	6.6	48.7	34.8	4.8
Cheese & Onion, M&S*	1 Bag/25g	134	8.9	535	5.5	48.8	35.5	5
Cheese & Onion, Max, Walkers*	1 Pack/50g	262	16	525	6.8	52	32	5.2
Cheese & Onion, Organic, Tesco*	1 Bag/25g	128	8.2	514	5.2	49.9	32.6	7
Cheese & Onion, Potato Heads, Walkers*	1 Pack/23g	108	5.3	470	6	60	23	5.5
Cheese & Onion, Sainsbury's*	1 Bag/25g	132	8.7	527	4.6	48.8	34.8	3.9
Cheese & Onion, Snack Rite*	1 Pack/25g	132	8.4	527	5.3	51.3	33.4	0
Cheese & Onion, Sprinters*	1 Bag/25g	137	9.2	549	5.4	49.4	36.6	0
Cheese & Onion, Squares, Walkers*	1 Bag/25g	108	4.5	430	6.5	61	18	5.5
Cheese & Onion, Value, Tesco*	1 Bag/20g	108	7.2	541	6	48.3	36	4.8
Cheese & Chives, Walkers*	1 Bag/32.5g	172	10.7	530	6.5	50	33	4.1
Cheese & Onion Flavour, Asda*	1 Bag/25g	130	7.8	519	5.6	53.6	31.4	3.7
Cheese & Onion, Baked, Walkers*	1 Bag/25g	104	2.1	418	6.5	75.5	8.5	4.8
Cheese & Onion, Crinkle, Seabrook*	1 Pack/32g	170	10.5	536	5.9	51.1	33.1	5.2
Cheese & Onion, Discos, KP Snacks*	1 Pack/28g	146	8.2	520	5.1	59.1	29.3	2.5
Cheese & Onion, Golden Wonder*	1 Bag/25g	129	7.9	516	5.8	52.4	31.5	3.8
Cheese & Onion, Hand Cooked, Ten Acre*	1 Bag/40g	201	11.5	503	6.6	51.8	28.7	6.2
Cheese & Onion, Lights, Walkers*	1 Bag/24g	113	5	470	7.5	62	21	5
Cheese & Onion, Oven Baked, Asda*	1 Bag/25g	95	2	380	5.1	72	8	3.3
Cheese & Onion, Oven Baked, Tesco*	1 Bag/25g	102	1.6	410	5.3	74.7	6.6	7.7
Cheese & Onion, Pom Bear, Intersnack Ltd*	1 Bag/19g	95	5.3	498	3.8	58.1	27.8	3.2
Cheese & Onion, Sunseed Oil, Walkers*	1 Bag/32.5g	171	10.7	525	7	50	33	4
Cheese & Onion, Tesco*	1 Pack/25g	135	8	535	5.4	54.8	31.8	3.2
Cheese & Red Onion, Extra Crunchy, Walkers*	1 Serving/30g	140	6.3	468	6.8	60.6	20.9	4.9

CRISPS

INFO/WEIGHT	Measure		Nutrition Values per 100g / 100ml				
	KCAL	FAT	KCAL	PROT	CARB	FAT	FIBRE
Cheese Bites, Weight Watchers*	1 Pack/18g	73	1	406	13.9	71.1	5.6	2.2
Cheese Curls, Morrisons*	1 Bag/17g	95	6.1	557	3.1	54.8	35.6	2.6
Cheese Curls, Shapers, Boots*	1 Pack/14g	68	3.8	489	4.5	57	27	2.7
Cheese Curls, Sprinters*	1 Bag/14g	68	3.8	483	4.1	56.4	26.8	0
Cheese Curls, Tesco*	1 Bag/14.4g	75	4.5	520	4.5	54.4	31.1	1.9
Cheese Curls, Weight Watchers*	1 Pack/20g	78	1.7	392	5	73.8	8.6	3.4
Cheese Heads, Walkers*	1 Bag/27g	128	6	475	10.8	58	22.3	2.8
Cheese Moments, Smiths*	1 Pack/28g	148	9.2	530	8	50	33	2
Cheese Puffs, Weight Watchers*	1 Pack/18g	80	1.9	444	7.8	77.2	10.6	3.3
Cheese Tasters, M&S*	1 Sm Bag/30g	154	8.8	515	8.1	55	29.3	1.7
Cheese Twirls, Boulevard, Simply Delicious*	1 Pack/25g	138	8.8	550	12.1	46.7	35	0
Cheese, Curls, Asda*	1 Bag/16g	87	5.3	541	3.6	57	33	1.7
Cheese, Space Raiders, KP Snacks*	1 Bag/16g	76	3.5	473	7.1	61.6	22	3.1
Cheeses with Onion, Soulmates, Kettle Chips*	1 Pack/40g	195	11.6	488	7.7	50.2	29	5.4
Cheesy Curls, Bobby's*	1 Bag/40g	225	14.8	563	7.6	50.1	36.9	0
Cheesy Curls, Tesco*	1 Pack/17g	90	5.4	530	3.5	56	32	1.9
Cheesy Puffs, Co-Op*	1 Bag/60g	321	20.4	535	3	54	34	2
Chicken & Thyme, Oven Roasted, Tesco*	1 Pack/150g	728	40.5	485	6.5	54	27	4.5
Chicken, Firecracker, McCoys*	1 Bag/35g	177	10.3	506	6.2	54	29.5	4
Chilli & Lemon, Walkers*	1 Pack/25g	131	8.2	525	6.3	51	33	3.8
Chilli & Lemon, Houmous Chips, Eat Real*	1 Serving/28g	126	4.8	449	6.5	68.4	17	4.5
Chilli & Lemon, Lentil Chips, Eat Real*	1 Serrving/28g	130	5.4	466	9.3	66	19.5	3.2
Chilli & Lime, Quinoa Chips, Eat Real*	1 Pack/30g	165	8.7	549	7	66.2	28.9	2.5
Chinese Sizzling Beef, McCoys*	1 Bag/35g	178	10.6	506	6.9	51.8	30.2	4
Chinese Spare Rib, Walkers*	1 Bag/25g	131	8.2	525	6.5	50	33	4
Cider Vinegar & Sea Salt, Tyrrells*	1 Pack/40g	192	9.8	481	7.2	60.1	24.6	2.4
Cool Cheese Curly, Tesco*	1 Bag/14g	71	4.5	510	4.5	51	32	2.6
Corn Chips, Fritos*	1 Pack/42.5g	240	15	565	4.7	56.5	35.3	0
Corn Snacks, Crispy, Bugles*	1 Bag/20g	102	5.6	508	4.8	60.7	28	1.4
Coronation Chicken, Walkers*	1 Bag/25g	131	8.2	525	6.5	50	33	4
Cream Cheese & Chive, Waffles, Spar*	1 Pack/27g	132	6.8	488	4.2	60.7	25.3	1.3
Cream Cheese & Onion, Crisp & Thin, Ritz*	1 Serving/30g	135	4.8	450	5.7	68	16	5.1
Creamy Dill, Houmous Chips, Eat Real*	1 Serving/28g	126	4.8	449	6.5	68.4	17	4.5
Creamy Dill, Lentil Chips, Eat Real*	1 Serving/28g	130	5.4	466	9.3	66	19.5	3.2
Crinkle Cut, Lower Fat, No Added Salt, Waitrose*	1 Bag/40g	193	10	483	6.5	58	25	3.9
Crispy Duck & Hoisin, Walkers*	1 Bag/25g	131	8.2	523	5.8	51.5	32.6	4
Crunchy Sticks, Ready Salted, M&S*	1 Pack/75g	398	24.8	530	5.6	52.2	33	3.8
Crunchy Sticks, Ready Salted, Tesco*	1 Serving/25g	119	5.9	475	5.6	60.3	23.5	3
Crunchy Sticks, Salt & Vinegar, Sainsbury's*	1 Bag/25g	118	6.1	474	5.9	58	24.3	2.4
Crunchy Sticks, Salt & Vinegar, Tesco*	1 Serving/25g	118	6.1	470	6.9	55.7	24.4	2.7
Crunchy Sticks, Salt & Vinegar, Value, Tesco*	1 Bag/22g	113	5.9	512	5.7	62.1	26.8	0.7
Crushed Natural Sea Salt, Darling Spuds*	1 Bag/40g	195	12	488	5.6	53.4	30	4.5
Curls, Cheesy, Asda*	1 Pack/17g	87	4.9	511	3.8	59.7	28.6	1.7
Double Gloucester & Red Onion, Kettle Chips*	1 Serving/40g	188	9.9	471	6.6	55.5	24.7	4.8
English Roast Beef & Yorkshire Pudding, Walkers*	1 Bag/34.5g	180	11.3	522	6.6	50.4	32.7	4
Extra Crunchy, Salt & Malt Vinegar, Walkers*	1 Pack/30g	139	6.2	463	6.6	59.9	20.8	4.8
Far Out Fajita, Chickpea Puffs, Organic, Hippeas*	1 Bag/22g	91	4	414	13.2	49.6	18.2	7.7
Flame Grilled Steak, Extra Crunchy, Walkers*	1 Bag /150g	702	31.6	468	6.9	60	21.1	5
Flame Grilled Steak, Ridge Cut, McCoys*	1 Bag/47g	250	14.7	526	6.9	53	31	3.9
Flamed Grilled Steak, Deep Ridge, Walkers*	1 Pack/28g	144	8.4	515	6.4	52.6	30.1	4.3
Flamed Grilled Steak, Max, Walkers*	1 Pack/50g	266	16.4	533	6.5	51.6	32.8	2.8
Four Cheese & Red Onion, Sensations, Walkers*	1 Bag/40g	194	10.8	485	6.5	54	27	4.5
Gammon & Mustard, Hand Cooked, Deluxe, Lidl*	1 Pack/25g	122	6.8	487	6	52.6	27	4.9

CRISPS

INFO/WEIGHT	per Measure KCAL	FAT	KCAL	PROT	CARB	FAT	FIBRE
Garlic & Herbs Creme Fraiche, Kettle Chips*							
1 Bag/50g	248	14.2	497	6	54.7	28.3	4.2
Greek Kebab, Mediterranean, Walkers*							
1 Pack/25g	128	8.2	510	6	49	33	4.5
Guinness, Burts*							
1 Bag/40g	206	11.5	514	5.1	58.6	28.8	2.5
Ham & English Mustard Flavour, Real*							
1 Bag/35g	176	9.9	502	6.2	53.9	28.2	4.2
Ham & Mustard, Salty Dog*							
1 Pack/40g	192	10.8	480	7.5	54.5	27.1	4.2
Hand Cooked, Honey Roast Ham, Finest, Tesco*							
1 Serving/25g	130	7.3	515	5.1	58.6	28.8	2.5
Honey & BBQ, Wholgrain, Snacks, M&S*							
1 Serving/30g	146	7.5	485	7.8	57.6	24.9	5.2
Honey Roasted Ham, Sensations, Walkers*							
1 Bag/40g	196	10.8	490	6.5	55	27	4
Hoops, Ready Salted, Weight Watchers*							
1 Bag/20g	73	0.3	365	3.4	82.7	1.4	4.1
Hot & Spicy Salami, Tesco*							
1 Bag/50g	216	18	431	26.2	0.7	35.9	0
Hot & Spicy, Quinoa Chips, Eat Real*							
1 Serving/30g	159	8.6	531	7.1	62.3	28.7	2.4
Hot Jalapeño Chilli, Hand Cooked, Finest, Tesco*							
1 Serving/25g	130	7.2	519	5.1	58.6	28.8	2.5
Jalapeno & Cheddar, Quinoa & Puffs, Eat Real*							
1 Serving/28g	130	6.9	465	4.6	52.9	24.7	2.8
Jalapeno Peppers, Fire Roasted, Darling Spuds*							
1 Pack/40g	191	11.4	478	6.3	53.4	28.5	4.5
Kale, Tomato, Spinach & Potato, Chips, Eat Real*							
1 Serving/28g	143	8.1	510	4.4	60.1	28.8	3.6
Lamb & Mint, Slow Roasted, Sensations, Walkers*							
1 Bag/35g	170	9.4	485	6.5	54	27	4.5
Lant Chips, Ikea*							
1 Serving/25g	126	6.9	505	8.3	55.9	27.6	4.5
Lentil Curls, Sour Cream, & Chive, Tesco*							
1 Pack/20g	90	3.1	448	11.3	64.1	15.6	3.3
Lentil Tubes, Smokey Bacon, M&S*							
1 Pack/22g	87	1.8	394	11.4	67.3	8	3.7
Lightly Salted, Baked, COU, M&S*							
1 Bag/25g	88	0.6	350	8.5	76.4	2.3	5.7
Lightly Salted, Crinkle Cut, Low Fat, Waitrose*							
1 Pack/35g	163	8	466	5.2	60.1	22.8	5.1
Lightly Salted, Deluxe, Lidl*							
1 Pack/25g	123	6.4	492	6.3	56	25.8	5.1
Lightly Salted, Handcooked, Finest, Tesco*							
1 Bag/40g	206	11.5	515	5.1	58.6	28.8	2.5
Lightly Salted, Kettle Chips*							
1 Serving/50g	256	15	513	5.8	51.5	30.1	6.5
Lightly Salted, Low Fat, Waitrose*							
1 Bag/25g	125	6.2	500	7.5	61.3	25	4.8
Lightly Salted, Potato Bakes, Weight Watchers*							
1 Pack/20g	78	1.8	392	5	72	9	5
Lightly Salted, Thicker Cut, Tear 'n' Share, Walkers*							
1 Serving/30g	142	6.5	473	6.8	59.8	21.8	5
Lightly Sea Salted, Hand Cooked, English, Tyrrells*							
1 Pack/25g	125	6.4	501	5.9	49	25.4	5.3
Lightly Sea Salted, Jonathan Crisp*							
1 Bag/35g	176	10.2	503	6.5	52	29	5.4
Lightly Sea Salted, Potato Chips, Hand Fried, Burts*							
¼ Bag/50g	252	13.8	504	6.4	57.4	27.7	0
Lightly Sea Salted, Potato Chips, Tyrrells*							
1 Pack/150g	740	38.1	493	7.7	58.9	25.4	2.6
Lincolnshire Sausage, Tyrrells*							
1 Pack/100g	530	28.2	530	8.6	60.8	28.2	3
Mango Chilli, Kettle Chips*							
1 Serving/40g	190	9.6	475	6.3	53.9	24	6.1
Marmite, Sunseed, Walkers*							
1 Bag/32.5g	168	9.9	517	7.3	51.1	30.5	4.3
Mature Cheddar & Chive, Kettle Chips*							
1 Serving/50g	239	12.7	478	8.1	54.4	25.4	5
Mature Cheddar & Shallot, Temptations, Tesco*							
1/6 Bag/25g	131	8.6	524	6.6	47.4	34.2	4.4
Mature Cheddar & Chive, Tyrrells*							
1 Serving/30g	134	6.9	447	6.9	53.7	23.1	2.4
Mature Cheddar & Onion, Deep Ridge, Walkers*							
1 Pack/28g	145	8.6	518	6.4	51.8	30.7	4.3
Mature Cheddar & Red Onion, Deluxe, Lidl*							
1 Pack/25g	121	6.2	483	7.4	54.6	25	5
Mature Cheddar & Red Onion, Finest, Tesco*							
1 Bag/40g	208	8.3	519	5.1	58.6	20.8	2.5
Mature Cheddar, Hand Fried, Potato Chips, Burts*							
1 Serving/40g	202	11.1	504	6.4	57.4	27.7	0
Mature Cheese & Chives, Potato Chips, Tyrrells*							
1 Bag/50g	261	14	522	6.1	56.5	27.9	0
Mexican Chilli, Ridge Cut, McCoys*							
1 Bag/32g	164	9.8	514	6.9	53	30.5	4.5
Mexican Lime with a Hint of Chilli, Kettle Chips*							
1 Serving/50g	242	13.8	484	5	54.1	27.5	5.4
Mixed Pepper Flavour Burst, M&S*							
1 Bag/55g	286	18.4	520	6	50.1	33.5	4
Mozzarella, & Pesto, Lentil, Curls, Bites, Kettle*							
1 Pack/22g	97	3.1	439	12.9	62.8	14.3	3.9
Munchies, Cheese Fix, Snack Mix, Rold Gold*							
1 Serving/28g	140	7	500	7.1	64.3	25	3.6
Mystery Meaty Flavour B, Walkers*							
1 Pack/25g	132	8.1	527	5.9	51.2	32.3	4.1
Naked, Tyrrells*							
1 Pack/150g	680	36.8	453	5.6	50.8	24.5	0
New York Cheddar, Kettle Chips*							
1 Bag/50g	242	13.4	483	6.7	53.9	26.7	4.5
Olive Oil, Mozzarella & Oregano, Walkers*							
1 Serving/30g	152	8.7	505	6.5	54	29	4
Onion Rings, Corn Snacks, Average							
1 Bag/25g	*122*	*6.1*	*486*	*5.8*	*60.9*	*24.2*	*2.7*
Onion Rings, M&S*							
1 Pack/40g	186	8.6	465	5.2	62.1	21.5	4.3

CRISPS	Measure INFO/WEIGHT	per Measure KCAL	FAT	Nutrition Values per 100g / 100ml KCAL	PROT	CARB	FAT	FIBRE
Onion Rings, Pickled, HE, Tesco*	1 Pack/15g	51	0.3	340	6.2	74.7	1.8	6.5
Onion Rings, Tayto*	1 Pack/17g	82	4.1	484	3	63.4	24	2.4
Onion Rings, Tesco*	1 Serving/30g	148	7.6	495	8.4	57.8	25.5	2.5
Oriental Ribs, Ridge Cut, McCoys*	1 Pack/50g	256	15	511	7.3	52.7	30.1	4.2
Paprika Flavour, Corn Snacks, Shapers, Boots*	1 Pack/13g	64	3.5	494	8.7	54	27	2.2
Paprika, Max, Walkers*	1 Bag/50g	260	16	520	6.5	52	31.9	5.1
Parsnip, Passions, Snack Rite*	1 Serving/25g	124	9.4	494	4.5	34.5	37.6	18.8
Pastrami & Cheese, Crinkle, M&S*	1 Bag/25g	120	5.9	485	6.5	61	24	3.5
Pea & Pinto Bean, Sticks, Off The Eaten Path*	1 Bag/23g	102	3.9	443	9.6	59	17	7.9
Pepper Power, Chickpea Puffs, Organic, Hippeas*	1 Pack/22g	90	4	409	12.7	49.6	18.2	7.3
Pickled Onion Flavour Rings, BGTY, Sainsbury's*	1 Serving/10g	34	0.2	345	5	81.7	1.5	3.7
Pickled Onion Rings, COU, M&S*	1 Bag/20g	69	0.3	345	5	81.7	1.5	3.7
Pickled Onion, Beastie Bites, Asda*	1 Bag/20g	100	5.2	498	6	60	26	0
Pickled Onion, Golden Wonder*	1 Bag/25g	131	8.5	524	5.6	49	34	2
Pickled Onion, Space Raiders, KP Snacks*	1 Bag/13g	64	2.9	495	6.5	65.3	22.8	1
Pickled Onion, Stompers, Morrisons*	1 Pack/25g	129	7.9	518	6.1	52.2	31.6	1.3
Pickled Onion, Sunseed, Walkers*	1 Bag/32.5g	171	10.7	525	6.5	50	33	4
Plain, Quinoa Chips, Eat Real*	1 Serving/30g	159	8.6	531	7.1	62.3	28.7	2.4
Pom Bear, Zoo, Really Cheesy, Potato Snack	*1 Bag/19g*	*100*	*5.8*	*525*	*3.6*	*57*	*30.7*	*3.1*
Potato	*1oz/28g*	*148*	*9.6*	*530*	*5.7*	*53.3*	*34.2*	*5.3*
Potato Chips, Anglesey Sea Salt, Red Sky*	1 Serving/40g	185	8.7	463	6.8	59.8	21.8	5
Potato Rings, Ready Salted, M&S*	1 Serving/75g	375	21.1	500	3.5	58.9	28.1	2.6
Potato Rings, Ready Salted, Sainsbury's*	1 Serving/50g	257	14.2	514	3.2	61.5	28.4	1.8
Potato Squares, Ready Salted, Sainsbury's*	1 Bag/50g	192	8	384	6.5	53.8	15.9	7.8
Potato Thins, Lightly Salted, LC, Tesco*	1 Pack/20g	72	0.4	360	5.1	79.5	2	4.2
Potato Twirls, Sainsbury's*	1 Serving/50g	218	7.3	435	3	72.8	14.6	3.1
Potato Zoo, Crispy Potato Animals, Kids, Tesco*	1 Bag/30g	57	1.9	190	2.5	24.5	6.3	2.1
Potato, Baked, COU, M&S*	1 Bag/25g	88	0.6	350	8.5	76.4	2.3	5.7
Potato, Cheddar & Onion, Hand Cooked, Aldi*	1 Pack/150g	753	41.8	502	7.7	54.9	27.9	4
Potato, Low Fat	*1oz/28g*	*128*	*6*	*458*	*6.6*	*63.5*	*21.5*	*5.9*
Potato, Tyrrells*	1 Pack/261g	1362	72.8	522	6.1	56.5	27.9	0
Prawn Cocktail Flavour, Seabrook*	1 Bag/30g	163	10.1	544	5.7	49.2	33.7	4.5
Prawn Cocktail, 30% Less Fat, Sainsbury's*	1 Pack/25g	118	5.9	470	6.3	58.9	23.6	5.7
Prawn Cocktail, Boots*	1 Pack/21g	99	4.6	470	6.8	60	22	4.3
Prawn Cocktail, Crusti Croc, Lidl*	1 Pack/25g	136	8.2	546	5.3	55.1	33	3.9
Prawn Cocktail, Golden Wonder*	1 Bag/25g	131	7.7	521	5.3	53.9	30.8	3.5
Prawn Cocktail, Lites, Advantage, Tayto*	1 Pack/21g	96	4.1	455	5.3	65.1	19.3	3.8
Prawn Cocktail, Lites, Shapers, Boots*	1 Bag/21g	92	3.8	438	5.1	64	18	4.1
Prawn Cocktail, Snack Rite*	1 Bag/25g	129	8.3	516	5	49.2	33.2	0
Prawn Cocktail, Snaktastic, Lidl*	1 Pack/25g	134	8	535	5.9	54	32	3.5
Prawn Cocktail, Spirals, Shapers, Boots*	1 Bag/15g	73	3.8	489	3.3	61	25	3
Prawn Cocktail, Sunseed Oil, Walkers*	1 Bag/32.5g	171	10.7	525	6.5	50	33	4
Prawn Cocktail, Tayto*	1 Bag/35g	185	12.3	526	7.5	46.6	35	4.5
Prawn Crackers, Tesco*	1 Bag/60g	316	17.5	527	3.2	62.8	29.2	0.8
Prawn, Spirals, Shapers, Boots*	1 Pack/100g	468	22	468	3.1	64	22	2.8
Pretzel, Salted, Original, Pretzel Crisps*	1 Serving/28g	100	0	357	7.1	85.7	0	3.6
Ready Salted, 30% Less Fat, Sainsbury's*	1 Serving/25g	122	5.6	486	7.3	63.7	22.4	8.2
Ready Salted, Average	*1 Bag/25g*	*127*	*7.4*	*508*	*6.1*	*53.4*	*29.7*	*4*
Ready Salted, BGTY, Sainsbury's*	1 Bag/25g	122	6.6	486	6.8	55.7	26.2	6.6
Ready Salted, Co-Op*	1 Bag/25g	131	8.5	525	6	51	34	3
Ready Salted, Deep Ridge, Walkers*	1 Pack/28g	148	9	529	6.4	51.1	32.1	4.6
Ready Salted, Everyday Value, Tesco*	1 Pack/18g	100	6.1	535	5	52.8	32.7	3.8
Ready Salted, GFY, Asda*	1 Bag/23g	109	5.3	475	7	60	23	4.3

CRISPS

INFO/WEIGHT	Measure	per Measure		Nutrition Values per 100g / 100ml				
		KCAL	FAT	KCAL	PROT	CARB	FAT	FIBRE
Ready Salted, Golden Wonder*	1 Bag/25g	135	8.8	539	5.5	49.9	35.3	2
Ready Salted, KP Snacks*	1 Bag/24g	131	8.8	545	5.6	47.9	36.8	4.9
Ready Salted, Lidl*	1 Bag/25g	138	9.2	554	4.9	50.3	37	0
Ready Salted, Lower Fat, Asda*	1 Bag/25g	120	6.2	481	6	58	25	4.8
Ready Salted, M&S*	1 Bag/25g	136	9.2	545	5.6	47.8	36.6	4.9
Ready Salted, Morrisons*	1 Bag/25g	134	8.7	536	4.9	50.9	34.8	4.3
Ready Salted, Oven Baked, Asda*	1 Bag/25g	95	1.9	379	4.4	73.1	7.7	2.6
Ready Salted, Oven Baked, Tesco*	1 Bag/25g	95	1.9	380	4.4	73.1	7.7	8.4
Ready Salted, Potato Chips, Sainsbury's*	¼ Pack/33g	174	10.9	526	5.6	51.7	33	3.8
Ready Salted, Potato Chips, Tesco*	1 Bag/25g	132	8.2	526	5.6	51.7	33	3.8
Ready Salted, Reduced Fat, Tesco*	1 Pack/25g	114	6.2	456	6.3	52	24.7	5.9
Ready Salted, Ridge Cut, McCoys*	1 Bag/32g	168	10.2	524	6.6	52.6	31.9	4.1
Ready Salted, Sainsbury's*	1 Bag/25g	132	8.1	530	5	52.5	32.5	3.7
Ready Salted, Smart Price, Asda*	1 Bag/18g	96	5.9	531	5	52.6	32.6	3.8
Ready Salted, Squares, M&S*	1 Bag/35g	150	6.3	430	6.8	63.5	18.1	3.9
Ready Salted, Squares, Walkers*	1 Pack/25g	109	4.8	435	6.5	60	19	6
Ready Salted, Sunseed Oil, Walkers*	1 Bag/32.5g	175	11.1	537	5.9	49.7	34.1	4.2
Ready Salted, Tesco*	1 Bag/25g	140	8.5	545	5	55.4	33.2	1.8
Ready Salted, Value, Morrisons*	1 Pack/18g	95	6	528	6.7	50	33.3	0.6
Red Leicester & Spring Onion, Handcooked, M&S*	1 Pack/40g	194	10.6	485	6.8	55	26.4	5.1
Reggae Reggae, Grove Cut, Levi Roots*	1 Pack/40g	200	11.5	500	5.1	58.6	28.8	2.5
Ridge, Thick & Chunky, Ready Salted, Eastmans*	1 Pack/30g	155	9.2	515	5.9	53.5	30.6	4.1
Roast Beef & Mustard, Thick Cut, Brannigans*	1 Bag/40g	203	12	507	7.6	51.7	30	3.7
Roast Beef & Horseradish, Tyrrells*	¼ Pack/38g	165	10.1	439	5.3	41.7	26.9	4.7
Roast Beef, KP Snacks*	1 Bag/25g	134	8.8	534	6.6	47.5	35.3	4.7
Roast Chicken & Sage Flavour, M&S*	1 Bag/25g	135	8.6	540	5.9	50.6	34.6	4.6
Roast Chicken Flavour	**1 Bag/25g**	**130**	**7.7**	**519**	**5.2**	**53.5**	**30.8**	**3.7**
Roast Chicken Flavour, Average	**1 Bag/25g**	**132**	**8.6**	**528**	**6.1**	**48.8**	**34.2**	**3.9**
Roast Chicken Flavour, Crinkle, Weight Watchers*	1 Pack/16g	76	3.3	475	5.6	63.1	20.6	6.2
Roast Chicken, 30% Less Fat, Sainsbury's*	1 Pack/25g	115	5.5	460	7.4	58.3	21.9	5.2
Roast Chicken, Golden Wonder*	1 Bag/25g	130	8.4	522	6.2	48.6	33.6	2
Roast Chicken, Select, Tesco*	1 Bag/25g	134	8.8	536	6.6	48.6	35	4.4
Roast Chicken, Snack Rite*	1 Bag/25g	132	8.3	526	5.3	51.3	33.3	0
Roast Chicken, Sunseed Oil, Walkers*	1 Bag/32.5g	171	10.7	525	6.5	50	33	4
Roast Ham & Mustard, Ridge Cut, McCoys*	1 Bag/32g	166	9.8	518	7.1	53.5	30.6	3.9
Roast Pork & Apple Sauce, Select, Tesco*	1 Bag/25g	136	8.8	544	6.5	50	35.3	3.7
Roasted Peanut Puffs, Ellert*	1 Serving/25g	125	6	500	13	56	24	4.1
Salsa with Mesquite, Kettle Chips*	1 Serving/50g	231	12.1	462	5.8	55.2	24.2	5.7
Salt & Balsamic Vinegar, PB, Waitrose*	1 Bag/20g	69	0.5	347	4.2	76.4	2.7	5.2
Salt & Black Pepper, Handcooked, M&S*	1 Bag/40g	180	9.2	450	5.7	55	22.9	5.2
Salt & Malt Vinegar Flavour, Sainsbury's*	1 Bag/25g	134	8.8	538	4.9	50.3	35.2	2.3
Salt & Vinegar Flavour, Asda*	1 Bag/25g	130	8.5	522	6	48	34	4.2
Salt & Vinegar Flavour, Half Fat, M&S*	1 Bag/40g	168	6.8	420	5.8	61	17	7.7
Salt & Vinegar Flavour, Sprinters*	1 Bag/25g	133	8.8	532	4.8	49.1	35.2	0
Salt & Vinegar Fries, COU, M&S*	1 Bag/25g	85	0.4	340	5	80	1.6	4
Salt & Vinegar, 30% Less Fat, Sainsbury's*	1 Bag/25g	114	5.4	458	7.2	58.3	21.8	5.1
Salt & Vinegar, Crinkle, M&S*	1 Pack/25g	120	5.9	485	6.5	61	24	3.5
Salt & Vinegar, Crinkles, Shapers, Boots*	1 Pack/20g	96	4.8	482	6.6	60	24	4
Salt & Vinegar, Everyday, Co-Op*	1 Bag/17g	77	3.4	455	6	62	20	2
Salt & Vinegar, GFY, Asda*	1 Bag/26g	120	5.7	466	6	61	22	4.1
Salt & Vinegar, Golden Lights, Golden Wonder*	1 Bag/21g	94	3.9	446	4.2	65.7	18.5	3.7
Salt & Vinegar, Golden Wonder*	1 Bag/25g	130	8.5	522	5.4	48.5	34	2
Salt & Vinegar, Lights, Walkers*	1 Bag/28g	133	6.2	475	7	62	22	4.5

CRISPS

INFO/WEIGHT	Measure		Nutrition Values per 100g / 100ml				
	KCAL	FAT	KCAL	PROT	CARB	FAT	FIBRE
Salt & Vinegar, Lower Fat, Asda*	1 Bag/25g	120	6.2	481	5	58	25	4.8
Salt & Vinegar, M&S*	1 Bag/25g	131	8.6	525	5.4	48.8	34.5	4.6
Salt & Vinegar, Morrisons*	1 Bag/25g	129	7.8	515	4.9	53.9	31.1	3.6
Salt & Vinegar, Rough Cuts, Tayto*	1 Bag/30g	152	9.2	506	4.6	56.8	30.8	0
Salt & Vinegar, Sainsbury's*	1 Bag/25g	130	8.8	522	4.1	46.9	35.3	3.9
Salt & Vinegar, Select, Tesco*	1 Bag/25g	132	8.7	529	5.9	47.8	34.9	4.3
Salt & Vinegar, Snack Rite*	1 Bag/25g	127	8.2	508	4.7	48.1	33	0
Salt & Vinegar, Tayto*	1 Bag/35g	184	11.9	526	7.6	47.3	34	4.5
Salt & Vinegar, Waitrose*	1 Pack/25g	132	8.4	529	6.3	50.5	33.8	4.4
Salt & Malt Vinegar, Deep Ridge, Walkers*	1 Pack/28g	143	8.6	511	6.1	50.7	30.7	4.3
Salt & Malt Vinegar, Hunky Dorys*	1 Serving/25g	132	7.9	527	5.1	54.7	31.4	0
Salt & Malt Vinegar, Ridge Cut, McCoys*	1 Bag/32g	169	9.9	529	6.5	54	31	3.9
Salt & Shake, Walkers*	1 Pack/24g	128	7.8	533	6.2	52.2	32.3	4.4
Salt & Vinegar Chiplets, M&S*	1 Pack/50g	220	9.4	440	5.7	61.3	18.9	4.7
Salt & Vinegar in Sunflower Oil, Sainsbury's*	1 Serving/25g	131	8.4	524	5.2	49.7	33.8	3.7
Salt & Vinegar, Average	*1 Bag/25g*	*130*	*8.2*	*519*	*5.5*	*50.3*	*32.9*	*3.4*
Salt & Vinegar, Baked, Walkers*	1 Pack/37.5g	150	3	400	6	73.5	8.1	4.6
Salt & Vinegar, Crinkle Cut, Reduced Fat, Lidl*	1 Pack/25g	116	5.2	464	6.7	60.6	20.8	3.6
Salt & Vinegar, Crinkle Cut, Seabrook*	1 Pack/25g	126	7.2	502	5.9	52.9	28.7	3.9
Salt & Vinegar, Crispy Discs, Shapers, Boots*	1 Bag/21g	92	4	439	4.8	63	19	4.9
Salt & Vinegar, Discos, KP Snacks*	1 Bag/28g	145	8.3	517	4.7	58.3	29.5	2.3
Salt & Vinegar, Distinctively, Walkers*	1 Pack/32.5g	169	10	519	5.9	52.6	30.8	4.2
Salt & Vinegar, Everyday Value, Tesco*	1 Bag/18g	95	5.7	530	5	54.1	31.7	3.7
Salt & Vinegar, Odd Bites, Savoury Bakes, Aldi*	1 Bag/25g	115	4	459	8.6	69	16	3.4
Salt & Vinegar, Oven Baked, Asda*	1 Bag/25g	95	2	380	5.1	72	8	2.9
Salt & Vinegar, Pom Bear, Intersnack Ltd*	1 Pack/25g	124	6.8	494	3	58.8	27.4	2.7
Salt & Vinegar, Potato Bakes, Weight Watchers*	1 Bag/20g	81	1.8	404	5.3	76	8.8	2.3
Salt & Vinegar, Space Raiders, KP Snacks*	1 Bag/17g	81	3.8	478	6.9	61.7	22.6	2.2
Salt & Vinegar, Spirals, Shapers, Boots*	1 Pack/15g	73	3.8	486	3	61	25	3.4
Salt & Vinegar, Squares, Walkers*	1 Bag/27.5g	122	5	443	6.5	61	18	5.5
Salt & Vinegar, Sunseed Oil, Walkers*	1 Bag/32.5g	171	10.7	525	6.5	50	33	4
Salt & Vinegar, Thick Ridged, Snackrite, Aldi*	1 Bag/30g	159	9.3	529	5.8	55	31	3.4
Salt Your Own, Excluding Salt, Aldi*	1 Pack/24.3g	130	8.1	536	6	52.6	33.5	4.5
Salt Your Own, Sainsbury's*	1 Pack/24.4g	127	7.9	520	5	52.2	32.3	3.7
Salt Your Own, Snackrite, Aldi*	1 Pack/24.3g	130	8.1	536	6	52.6	33.5	4.5
Salt, & Vinegar, Snaktastic, Lidl*	1 Pack/25g	130	7.8	520	5.6	52	31.2	3.6
Sausage & Tomato Flavour, Golden Wonder*	1 Bag/35g	174	10.6	505	6.1	51.3	30.6	4.5
Scampi, Smiths, Walkers*	1 Bag/27g	134	7	496	13	52.5	26	0
Sea Sal & Vinegar, Crisp & Thin, Ritz*	1 Serving/30g	134	4.8	445	5.6	67	16	5.3
Sea Salt & Malt Vinegar, Handcooked, Real *	1 Bag/35g	179	10.2	512	5.6	54.6	29.2	4.2
Sea Salt & Black Pepper, GFY, Asda*	1 Bag/100g	476	24	476	6	59	24	6
Sea Salt & Black Pepper, Highlander*	1 Serving/25g	141	9.6	564	5.6	44	38.4	4.8
Sea Salt & Black Pepper, Shapers, Boots*	1 Bag/20g	96	4.8	482	6.6	60	24	4
Sea Salt & Cider Vinegar, TTD, Sainsbury's*	1/3 Pack/50g	245	14.3	489	5.5	52.7	28.5	6.1
Sea Salt & Cracked Black Pepper, Lights, Walkers*	1 Bag/24g	115	5.3	480	7	63	22	5
Sea Salt & Malt Vinegar, Sensations, Walkers*	1 Bag/40g	194	10.8	485	6.5	54	27	4.5
Sea Salt & Balsamic Vinegar, Delux, Lidl*	1 Pack/25g	121	6.3	484	6	56.8	25.2	4.4
Sea Salt & Balsamic Vinegar, Handcooked, M&S*	1 Bag/40g	208	12.1	521	6.7	52.8	30.4	4.6
Sea Salt & Balsamic Vinegar, Kettle Chips*	1 Bag/40g	201	11.4	502	5.4	53	28.4	6.1
Sea Salt & Black Pepper, Tyrrells*	¼ Pack/38g	182	9.3	480	7.3	59.9	24.5	2.4
Sea Salt & Black Peppercorn, Delux, Lidl*	1 Pack/25g	123	6.1	492	6.4	57.2	24.4	4.8
Sea Salt & Crushed Black Peppercorn, Deluxe, Lidl*	1 Pack/25g	120	6.1	481	6.2	57	24.3	4.9
Sea Salt & Indian Black Pepper, Pipers Crisps*	1 Pack/40g	195	11.6	487	6.6	49.9	29	0

CRISPS

INFO/WEIGHT	Measure	per Measure		Nutrition Values per 100g / 100ml				
		KCAL	FAT	KCAL	PROT	CARB	FAT	FIBRE
Sea Salt, Golden Lights, Golden Wonder*	1 Bag/21g	94	3.9	448	3.9	66.4	18.5	4.4
Sea Salt, Gourmet, TTD, Sainsbury's*	1/3 Pack/50g	249	15	498	5.7	51.4	30	6.4
Sea Salt, Handcooked, Extra Special, Asda*	1 Pack/31g	149	7.8	477	7	56	25	4.1
Sea Salt, Houmous Chips, Eat Real*	1 Serving/28g	126	4.8	449	6.5	68.4	17	4.5
Sea Salt, Lentil Chips, Eat Real*	1 Serving/28g	130	5.4	466	9.3	66	19.5	3.2
Sea Salt, Potato, Mackies*	1 Pack/40g	200	10.8	499	7.4	55	27	4.5
Sea Salt, Ridge Crisps, Morrisons*	1 Serving/25g	126	6.6	504	6.5	58.8	26.3	2.9
Sea Salted, Crinkle Cut, Seabrook *	1 Bag/32g	165	10	517	5.7	53.7	31.1	0
Sea Salted, Furrows, Tyrells *	1 Serving/30g	143	7.2	476	6.2	59.9	23.9	0
Shells, Prawn Cocktail, Asda*	1 Bag/18g	90	5.3	501	4.6	54.9	29.2	6.2
Simply Salted, Extra Crunchy, Walkers*	1 Bag/30g	142	6.5	473	6.8	59.8	21.8	5
Simply Salted, Lights, Walkers*	1 Bag/24g	113	5.3	470	7	61	22	5
Sizzling Beef, Spice, McCoys*	1 Bag/35g	175	10.4	501	6.4	51.7	29.8	4
Sizzling King Prawn, Ridge Cut, McCoys*	1 Pack/50g	259	15.2	518	6.6	54.7	30.3	4
Slightly Salted, Lay's*	1 Serving/30g	153	9.3	510	6.1	49	31.1	5
Smoked Ham & Pickle, Thick Cut, Brannigans*	1 Bag/40g	203	11.9	507	7	52.8	29.8	3.8
Smokey Bacon Potato Hoops, COU, M&S*	1 Pack/16g	58	0.4	360	5.6	78.7	2.7	4.5
Smokey Bacon, Budgens*	1 Bag/25g	130	8.2	519	6.2	49.3	33	4.8
Smokey Bacon, Crinkle, Shapers, Boots*	1 Pack/20g	96	4.8	482	6.6	60	24	4
Smokey Bacon, Select, Tesco*	1 Bag/25g	134	8.7	536	6.4	49	34.9	4.3
Smoky Bacon Flavour, Average	*1 Bag/25g*	*132*	*8.4*	*527*	*6.2*	*49.7*	*33.7*	*3.2*
Smoky Bacon, BGTY, Sainsbury's*	1 Bag/25g	118	5.9	472	6.5	58.5	23.6	5.7
Smoky Bacon, Golden Wonder*	1 Bag/25g	131	8.4	523	5.9	49.1	33.7	2
Smoky Bacon, Snack Rite*	1 Bag/25g	131	8.3	525	5.5	51.2	33.1	0
Smoky Bacon, Sunseed Oil, Walkers*	1 Bag/34.5g	183	11.4	530	6.5	51	33	4
Smoky Bacon, Tayto*	1 Bag/35g	184	11.9	526	7.6	47.3	34	4.5
Snax, Tayto*	1 Pack/17g	82	3.7	483	2.4	70	21.5	1.6
Sour Cream & Chive Crispy Discs, Shapers, Boots*	1 Bag/21g	94	4	448	5.7	61.9	19	4.3
Sour Cream & Chive, Crinkle, Reduced Fat, M&S*	1 Bag/40g	178	8.2	445	5.6	58.8	20.6	5.6
Sour Cream & Chive, Lights, Walkers*	1 Bag/24g	114	5.3	475	7.5	62	22	5
Sour Cream & Chive, PB, Waitrose*	1 Pack/20g	69	0.5	347	4.4	76.3	2.7	5.2
Sour Cream & Chilli Lentil Curls, M&S*	1 Pack/60g	243	5.2	405	13.6	65.3	8.7	4.3
Sour Cream & Chive Flavour, Average	*1 Bag/25g*	*127*	*7.7*	*508*	*6.8*	*50.7*	*30.9*	*4.6*
Sour Cream & Chives, Quinoa Chips, Eat Real*	1 Pack/30g	165	8.6	550	8	66.4	28.8	2.5
Spiced Chilli, McCoys*	1 Bag/35g	175	10.1	500	6.1	54.2	28.8	4.2
Spicy Chilli, Sunseed, Walkers*	1 Pack/34.5g	183	11.4	530	6.5	51	33	4
Spring Onion Flavour, Tayto*	1 Bag/35g	184	11.9	526	7.6	47.3	34	4.5
Steak & Onion, Walkers*	1 Pack/32.5g	169	10.7	520	6.5	49	33	4
Sun Bites, Honey Glazed Barbecue, Walkers*	1 Pack/25g	123	6.1	493	6.5	58.7	24.4	6.1
Sunbites, Cheddar & Caramelised Onion, Walkers*	1 Bag/25g	120	5.4	480	7.6	60.8	21.6	6.4
Sweet & Smokin', Hippeas*	1 Pack/22g	91	4	414	12.7	50.4	18.2	7.3
Sweet Chill, Mexican, Phileas Fogg*	1 Bag/38g	193	11	507	6.7	54.8	29	4.2
Sweet Chilli & Red Pepper, Potato Chips, Tyrrells*	¼ Pack/37.4g	180	9.2	481	7.9	59.7	24.5	2.4
Sweet Chilli & Red Peppers, Fusion, Tayto*	1 Bag/28g	140	8.3	500	4.9	52.2	29.8	4.6
Sweet Chilli Chicken, Extra Crunchy, Walkers*	1 Bag/30g	143	6.8	477	6.5	59.9	22.5	4.8
Sweet Chilli Flavour, Average	*1 Bag/25g*	*115*	*5.6*	*461*	*5.1*	*59.9*	*22.6*	*4.6*
Sweet Chilli, Baked Potato, COU, M&S*	1 Bag/26g	91	0.7	350	7.6	73.9	2.8	8.5
Sweet Chilli, Cracker, Special K, Kellogg's*	21 Crisps/23g	94	2.1	409	5	73	9	8
Sweet Chilli, Crinkle Cut, Weight Watchers*	1 Sm Bag/20g	94	4.1	470	5.6	62.9	20.6	5.8
Sweet Chilli, Hand Cooked, Asda*	1 Pack/25g	120	7.1	479	5.7	54.5	28.3	4.5
Sweet Chilli, Lentil, Curls, Bites, Kettle Chips*	1 Pack/22g	94	2.6	428	13.2	65	11.9	4
Sweet Chilli, Thicker Cut, Tear 'n' Share, Walkers*	1 Serving/30g	141	6.3	469	6.8	60.5	21.1	4.8
Sweet Potato, Lightly Salted, Baked, Kettle Chips*	1 Serving/20g	82	2.7	409	6.3	60	13.4	11.6

	Measure INFO/WEIGHT	per Measure KCAL	FAT	Nutrition Values per 100g / 100ml KCAL	PROT	CARB	FAT	FIBRE
CRISPS								
Sweet Red Chilli, Crisp & Thin, Ritz*	1 Serving/30g	135	4.8	450	6.1	68	16	5.3
T Bone Steak, Bubble Chips, Roysters*	1 Pack/28g	151	8.9	540	5.5	55	32	2.6
Tangy Sweet Chilli, Delight Bites, Snackrite, Aldi*	1 Pack/25g	111	4.2	445	6.6	66	17	2.3
Tangy Toms, Red Mill*	1 Bag/15g	76	4.1	507	6	60	27.3	0.7
Tasty Thai Sweet Chilli Flavour, CBY, Asda*	1 Serving/25g	126	6.7	505	5.9	59	27	3.5
Thai Bites, Mild, Jacob's*	1 Bag/25g	93	0.8	373	6.9	79	3.3	1
Thai Curry & Coriander, Tyrrells*	1 Pack/50g	261	14	522	6.1	56.5	27.9	5.4
Thai Sweet Chicken, Ridge Cut, McCoys*	1 Bag/50g	257	15	514	7	54	30	4.1
Thai Sweet Chilli Flavour, Velvet Crunch, King*	1 Pack/20g	81	1.9	404	1.6	77.5	9.7	2
Thai Sweet Chilli, Lentil Waves, Burts*	1 Pack/20g	91	3.3	453	11.7	62.6	16.3	4.9
Thai Sweet Chilli, Sensations, Walkers*	1 Bag/40g	194	10.4	485	6	57	26	4.2
Tomato & Herb, Shapers, Boots*	1 Bag/20g	94	4.2	468	3.7	66	21	3.9
Tomato & Basil, Houmous Chips, Eat Real*	1 Serving/28g	126	4.8	449	6.5	68.4	17	4.5
Tomato & Basil, Lentil Chips, Eat Real*	1 Serving/28g	130	5.4	466	9.3	66	19.5	3.2
Tomato & Herbs, Baked Fusions, Snacks, Walkers*	1 Pack/22g	95	3	433	6.7	68.3	13.5	6.4
Tomato Ketchup Flavour, Golden Wonder*	1 Bag/25g	135	8	521	5.1	54	30.8	3.6
Tomato Ketchup Flavour, Seabrook*	1 Pack/25g	124	6.8	497	5.9	55.5	27.1	0
Tortillas, Nacho Cheese Flavour, Weight Watchers*	1 Pack/18g	78	2.9	433	6.1	66.7	16.1	3.9
Traditional, Hand Cooked, Finest, Tesco*	1 Bag/150g	708	39.2	472	6.4	52.9	26.1	5.1
Twirls, Prawn Cocktail, Bobby's*	1 Pack/26g	116	4.8	445	3.4	65.9	18.6	0
Twirls, Salt & Vinegar, Co-Op*	1 Bag/40g	170	8	425	5	57.5	20	5
Twirls, Salt & Vinegar, Sainsbury's*	½ Bag/40g	167	5.6	418	3	70.1	14	3
Twirls, Salt & Vinegar, Tesco*	1 Bag/80g	349	14	436	3.9	65.8	17.5	2.4
Unsalted, Seabrook*	1 Bag/30g	163	10.7	544	5.7	47.9	35.8	4.1
Vegetable, Average	***1 Bag/25g***	***118***	***7.4***	***470***	***4.1***	***46.5***	***29.6***	***12.1***
Vegetable, Crunchy, Asda*	½ Bag/50g	251	12	502	1.4	70	24	6
Vegetable, Finest, Tesco*	1 Serving/50g	203	12.8	406	5	39	25.5	14.6
Vegetable, Pan Fried, Glennans*	1 Bag/20g	98	6.7	490	5	42.5	33.5	11
Vegetable, TTD, Sainsbury's*	½ Pack/52g	254	17.9	490	4.8	39.9	34.5	12.8
Vegetable, Waitrose*	1 Pack/100g	490	35.2	490	4.7	38.5	35.2	13
Veggie & Kale, Straws, Eat Real*	1 Bag/22g	109	5.6	497	3.1	65.1	25.5	2.8
Waffles, Bacon Flavour, BGTY, Sainsbury's*	1 Serving/12g	41	0.2	345	6.4	79.7	1.4	2.9
Wheat Crunchies, Golden Wonder*	1 Pack/35g	172	8.7	491	11.1	55.9	24.8	0
Wheat Crunchies, Salt & Vinegar, Golden Wonder*	1 Bag/34g	165	8.5	484	10.5	54.5	24.9	2.8
White Cheddar, Quinoa & Kale Puffs, Eat Real*	1 Serving/28g	130	6.9	465	2.7	53.6	24.7	5
White Cheddar, Quinoa Puffs, Eat Real*	1 Serving/28g	130	6.9	465	5	53.6	24.7	2.7
Wild Paprika Flavour, Croky*	1 Pack/45g	234	13	521	6	58	29	0
Worcester Sauce Flavour, Hunky Dorys*	1 Bag/45g	211	12.9	469	6.3	49.3	28.7	0
Worcester Sauce, Sunseed Oil, Walkers*	1 Bag/32.5g	168	9.9	516	6.2	52	30.5	4.3
CRISPY PANCAKE								
Beef Bolognese, Findus*	1 Pancake/65g	104	2.6	160	6.5	25	4	1
Chicken, Bacon & Sweetcorn, Findus*	1 Pancake/63g	101	2.5	160	5.5	26	4	1.1
Minced Beef, As Consumed, Findus*	1 Pancake/115g	90	1.4	78	2.9	12.8	1.2	0.9
Three Cheeses, As Consumed, Findus*	2 Pancakes/107g	183	3.6	171	6.5	28	3.4	1.4
CROISSANT								
All Butter, Bakers Selection, Asda*	1 Croissant/40g	164	8.4	412	6.9	48	21	1.9
All Butter, BGTY, Sainsbury's*	1 Croissant/44g	151	6.5	343	9.3	42.7	14.8	1.8
All Butter, Budgens*	1 Croissant/45g	185	11.1	412	7.9	39.7	24.6	3.3
All Butter, Finest, Tesco*	1 Croissant/77g	328	18.2	426	8.6	44.9	23.6	1.9
All Butter, M&S*	1 Croissant/54g	222	12.8	415	7.4	45.2	23.8	1.6
All Butter, Mini, Sainsbury's*	1 Croissant/30g	126	7	420	8.1	42.9	23.4	2.6
All Butter, Mini, Tesco*	1 Croissant/35g	150	8.2	430	9.3	45.2	23.5	2
All Butter, Reduced Fat, Tesco*	1 Croissant/52g	164	5.5	315	7.5	47.4	10.6	1.8

	Measure INFO/WEIGHT	per Measure KCAL	FAT	Nutrition Values per 100g / 100ml KCAL	PROT	CARB	FAT	FIBRE

CROISSANT

	Measure INFO/WEIGHT	KCAL	FAT	KCAL	PROT	CARB	FAT	FIBRE
All Butter, Sainsbury's*	1 Croissant/44g	188	10.8	428	9.2	42.6	24.5	1.2
All Butter, Tesco*	1 Croissant/48g	192	10.4	400	8.5	41.7	21.6	2.6
Asda*	1 Croissant/47g	190	9.9	405	9	45	21	0
Average	*1 Croissant/50g*	*180*	*10.2*	*360*	*8.3*	*38.3*	*20.3*	*1.6*
Belgian Dark Chocolate Orange, Finest, Tesco*	1 Croissant/95g	348	18.1	367	6.5	41.3	19.1	1.8
Butter, Charentes, Waitrose*	1 Croissant/68g	289	17.2	426	8	40.5	25.3	2.1
Butter, GFY, Asda*	1 Croissant/44g	153	7	352	6	46	16	2
Butter, Morrisons*	1 Croissant/44g	196	12.5	446	9.3	38.2	28.4	2
Butter, Part Baked, De Graaf*	1 Croissant/45g	170	8.4	378	7.3	45.2	18.7	0
Cheese & Ham, Delice de France*	1 Serving/91g	225	12.3	247	7	24.4	13.5	2.5
Cheese & Ham, Mini, Waitrose*	1 Croissant/16.7g	64	4.1	383	13.2	28.1	24.6	3
Continental, Mini, CBY, Asda*	1 Croissant/35g	150	8.9	427	9.2	40.6	25.3	1.6
Creme Patissiere & Raisins, Mini Chinois, Aldi*	1 Chinois/50g	133	3.4	266	0	20.2	6.8	0
Egg, Cheese & Tomato	1 Pack/149g	434	25.1	291	9	20.8	16.8	1.6
Flaky Pastry with a Plain Chocolate Filling, Tesco*	1 Croissant/78g	318	19	408	6.5	41	24.3	2
French Butter, Bon Appetit, Aldi*	1 Croissant/40g	171	9.2	428	7	47.2	23	2.2
French Butter, You Count, Love Life, Waitrose*	1 Croissant/44g	168	7.4	382	9.8	46.4	16.8	3.1
Hazlenut, Waitrose*	1 Croissant/95g	466	29.9	490	8.3	41.6	31.5	3.6
Low Fat, M&S*	1 Croissant/49g	195	7.8	398	9.8	52.9	15.9	1.8
Mini, Lidl*	1 Croissant/30g	112	5	373	7.8	48	16.6	0
Organic, Tesco*	1 Croissant/45g	195	11.6	433	8.2	42	25.8	2.2
Ready to Bake, Frozen, Chateau Blanc*	1 Croissant/65g	226	11.1	347	7.2	40	17	2.9
Reduced Fat, Asda*	1 Croissant/44g	159	6.5	361	9.7	47.2	14.8	2
Reduced Fat, Sainsbury's*	1 Croissant/44g	173	7.7	393	9.8	49.2	17.5	2.2
TTD, Sainsbury's*	1 Croissant/70g	289	16.1	413	8.1	43.4	23	2.5
Wholesome, Sainsbury's*	1 Croissant/44g	192	12.1	436	8.8	38.3	27.5	4
with Egg & Cheese, From Restaurant, Average	*1 Croissant/127g*	*368*	*24.7*	*290*	*10.1*	*19.1*	*19.4*	*0*
with Egg, Cheese & Ham from Restaurant, Average	*1 Croissant/152g*	*474*	*33.6*	*312*	*12.4*	*15.9*	*22.1*	*0*

CROQUETTES

	Measure INFO/WEIGHT	KCAL	FAT	KCAL	PROT	CARB	FAT	FIBRE
Cheesy, Morrisons*	1 Croquette/42g	117	5.5	278	7	32.9	13	0.6
Morrisons*	1 Serving/150g	231	8.1	154	3.3	23.1	5.4	1.1
Potato & Parsnip, Finest, Tesco*	2 Croquettes/74g	155	7.3	210	6	23.2	9.9	3.9
Potato, Asda*	3 Croquettes/81g	144	5.7	177	2	26.5	7	2.2
Potato, Birds Eye*	1 Croquette/29g	44	1.7	152	2.6	22.6	5.7	1.2
Potato, Chunky, Aunt Bessie's*	1 Serving/41g	62	2.5	152	2.3	23.9	6.1	1.8
Potato, Cooked, Sainsbury's*	2 Croquettes73g	157	7.6	214	2.9	26	10.3	2.6
Potato, Fried in Blended Oil, Average	*1 Croquette/80g*	*171*	*10.5*	*214*	*3.7*	*21.6*	*13.1*	*1.3*
Potato, M&S*	1 Croquette/41g	68	3.6	165	2.4	19.3	8.8	2.2
Potato, Waitrose*	1 Croquette/30g	47	2.4	157	3	17.9	8.1	1.5
Serrano Ham & Manchego, World Cafe, Waitrose*	½ Pack/78g	238	14	305	8.4	26.1	18	2.6
Vegetable, Sainsbury's*	1 Serving/175g	392	20.8	224	5.8	23.3	11.9	2.2

CROSTINI

	Measure INFO/WEIGHT	KCAL	FAT	KCAL	PROT	CARB	FAT	FIBRE
with Goats Cheese & Red Onion Chutney, Waitrose*	1 Crostini/17g	47	1.3	274	9.1	33.5	7.8	3.1
with Oregano, Crosta & Mollica*	1 Pack/150g	726	21.2	484	11.7	74.2	14.1	6.4

CROUTONS

	Measure INFO/WEIGHT	KCAL	FAT	KCAL	PROT	CARB	FAT	FIBRE
Fresh, M&S*	1 Serving/10g	53	3.3	530	11.4	50	32.8	3.2
Garlic, Waitrose*	1 Serving/40g	209	12	522	10.8	52.1	30	2.7
Herb, Sainsbury's*	1 Serving/15g	64	1.7	429	13.4	68.2	11.4	2.8
La Rochelle*	1 Bag/70g	400	28	572	7	49	40	0
Lightly Sea Salted, Asda*	1 Serving/20g	83	1.9	414	12.9	69.7	9.3	4.3
Prepacked, Average	*1 Serving/15g*	*74*	*3.6*	*495*	*10.8*	*58.7*	*24*	*2.6*
Sun Dried Tomato, Sainsbury's*	¼ Pack/15g	75	3.8	497	11.7	55.2	25.5	2.5

	Measure INFO/WEIGHT	per Measure KCAL	FAT	Nutrition Values per 100g / 100ml KCAL	PROT	CARB	FAT	FIBRE
CRUDITES								
Platter, Sainsbury's*	1 Pack/275g	96	0.8	35	1.4	6.6	0.3	1.6
Selection, Prepared, M&S*	1 Serving/250g	75	1	30	1.4	5.8	0.4	2
Vegetable Sticks, Average	*1 Serving/100g*	*24*	*0.2*	*24*	*0.7*	*4.5*	*0.2*	*1.9*
CRUMBLE								
Almond & Apricot, Devondale*	1 Cake/80g	314	13.2	392	3.6	57	16.5	9.8
Apple & Blackberry, Asda*	1 Serving/175g	427	15.8	244	2.7	38	9	1.2
Apple & Blackberry, Budgens*	1 Serving/240g	821	31.2	342	3.7	54	13	0.6
Apple & Blackberry, M&S*	1 Serving/135g	398	15.1	295	3.5	44.9	11.2	1.6
Apple & Blackberry, Sainsbury's*	1 Serving/110g	232	6.2	211	3	37.1	5.6	2.1
Apple & Custard, Asda*	1 Serving/125g	250	8.8	200	2.3	32	7	0
Apple & Toffee, Weight Watchers*	1 Pot/98g	190	4.5	194	1.6	36.6	4.6	0
Apple & Blackberry with Custard, Somerfield*	1 Serving/120g	324	15	270	2.3	36.3	12.5	1.1
Apple & Blackberry, Tesco*	1/6 Pie/90g	286	11.7	318	3	45.8	13	2.8
Apple with Custard, Green's*	1 Serving/79g	171	5.3	216	1.9	37	6.7	1.2
Apple with Custard, Individual, Sainsbury's*	1 Pudding/120g	286	13.9	238	2	31.4	11.6	2.4
Apple with Sultanas, Weight Watchers*	1 Dessert/110g	196	4.3	178	1.4	34.2	3.9	1.3
Apple, Average	*1 Serving/240g*	*497*	*12*	*207*	*0.9*	*40.5*	*5*	*1.1*
Apple, Basics, Sainsbury's*	¼ Crumble/125g	235	4.9	188	1.7	36.5	3.9	1.2
Apple, Co-Op*	¼ Crumble/110g	270	7.7	245	2	43	7	2
Apple, Fresh, Chilled, Tesco*	¼ Pack/150g	368	13.4	245	2.8	38	8.9	1.4
Apple, Frozen, Tesco*	¼ Pack/150g	345	16.3	230	2.1	30.7	10.9	3.9
Apple, Sainsbury's*	1 Crumble/565g	1034	32.8	183	2.3	30.5	5.8	2.9
Apple, Sara Lee*	1 Serving/200g	606	18	303	2.3	53.3	9	1.2
Apple, Somerfield*	1 Serving/195g	454	16.4	233	2.5	36.8	8.4	1.1
Apple, Waitrose*	1 Serving/125g	310	2.9	248	2.2	54.5	2.3	1.2
Blackcurrant & Apple, Devondale*	1 Cake/80g	314	13.2	393	3.6	57	16.5	9.8
Bramley Apple & Blackberry, BGTY, Sainsbury's*	1 Crumble/120g	217	3.2	181	1.7	35.8	2.7	2.2
Bramley Apple, Blackberry & Plum, Finest, Tesco*	½ Pack/175g	396	14.9	226	2.6	33.5	8.5	2.6
Bramley Apple, CBY, Asda*	1 Serving/100g	257	8.4	257	2.5	41.8	8.4	2.3
Bramley Apple, Favourites, M&S*	1 Serving/140g	390	13.8	279	4.6	43.2	9.9	1.2
Bramley Apple, M&S*	1 Serving/149g	387	13.7	260	4.3	40.3	9.2	1.1
Bramley Apple, Tesco*	1/3 Pack/155g	378	14.9	244	2.8	36.7	9.6	1.8
Crumble, Bramley Apple, 2 Pots, Sainsbury's*	1 Pot/116g	303	9.5	261	2.6	43.2	8.2	2.1
Fruit	*1 Portion/170g*	*337*	*11.7*	*198*	*2*	*34*	*6.9*	*1.7*
Fruit with Custard	*1 Serving/270g*	*463*	*17.6*	*171*	*2.4*	*27*	*6.5*	*1.3*
Fruit, Wholemeal	*1oz/28g*	*54*	*2*	*193*	*2.6*	*31.7*	*7.1*	*2.7*
Gooseberry, M&S*	1 Serving/133g	379	14.2	285	3.5	43.3	10.7	1.7
Plum & Cherry, 775, Wiltshire Farm Foods*	1 Serving/120g	248	7.4	194	2.3	34	5.8	0
Pork & Apple, Mini, 282, Oakhouse Foods Ltd*	1 Serving/250g	420	23.3	168	9	12.5	9.3	0.6
Rhubarb with Custard, Sainsbury's*	1 Serving/120g	288	13.9	240	2.4	31.4	11.6	2.3
Rhubarb, Asda*	½ Crumble/200g	460	24	230	2.4	28	12	5
Rhubarb, Average	*1 Portion/150g*	*330*	*11.1*	*220*	*2.7*	*35.5*	*7.4*	*1.9*
Rhubarb, Devondale*	1 Cake/80g	316	13.2	395	3.5	57	16.5	9
Rhubarb, M&S*	1 Serving/133g	366	13.2	275	3.4	42.6	9.9	1.4
Rhubarb, Sainsbury's*	1 Serving/50g	112	2.8	224	3.1	40.4	5.6	1.8
Rhubarb, Tesco*	1/6 Crumble/117g	228	9.7	195	2.8	27.3	8.3	1.7
Toffee Apple, As Consumed, Morrisons*	¼ Crumble/122g	326	11.4	267	1.9	42.9	9.3	2
CRUMBLE MIX								
Luxury, Tesco*	¼ Pack/55g	243	9	441	5.7	67.9	16.3	3.2
Topping, Morrisons*	1 Serving/40g	179	6.6	448	5.4	69.5	16.5	2.8
Topping, Sainsbury's*	1 Serving/47g	188	9.2	401	5.9	50.3	19.6	5.3
CRUMPETS								
Asda*	1 Crumpet/45g	85	0.4	188	6	39	0.9	2.1

C

C

	Measure INFO/WEIGHT	per Measure KCAL	FAT	Nutrition Values per 100g / 100ml KCAL	PROT	CARB	FAT	FIBRE
CRUMPETS								
Bakers Selection, Asda*	1 Crumpet/50g	106	0.6	211	6.7	42	1.2	2.7
Buttermilk, TTD, Sainsbury's*	1 Crumpet/52g	102	0.6	195	6.5	38.5	1.1	2.6
Co-Op*	1 Crumpet/40g	70	0.3	175	7	35	0.7	2
Essential, Waitrose*	1 Crumpet/52g	94	0.6	182	6.5	35.1	1.1	2.6
Everyday, Value, Tesco*	1 Crumpet/40g	75	0.4	190	6	37.5	0.9	2.9
Fruit from Bakery, Tesco*	1 Crumpet/73g	161	1.7	220	6.2	43.2	2.3	1.1
Gluten, Wheat & Milk Free, Free From, Livwell*	1 Crumpet/55g	83	1.7	151	3.6	26.9	3.1	2
Golden Sun, Lidl*	1 Crumpet/43g	83	0.7	193	7.8	37.1	1.6	1.6
Kwik Save*	1 Crumpet/41g	79	0.4	192	5.9	39.9	1	2.5
Less Than 2% Fat, M&S*	1 Crumpet/61g	116	0.8	190	8	36.9	1.3	2.1
Morning Fresh*	1 Crumpet/20g	36	0.3	180	7.3	34.8	1.3	5.2
Morrisons*	1 Crumpet/40g	90	0.2	225	7.8	47.2	0.5	3.2
Mother's Pride*	1 Crumpet/43g	80	0.4	185	5.6	38.3	1	2.3
PB, Waitrose*	1 Crumpet/55g	94	0.2	171	6.1	36.1	0.3	4.4
Premium, Sainsbury's*	1 Crumpet/50g	96	0.7	191	6.1	38.6	1.4	1.7
Rowan Hill Bakery, Lidl*	1 Crumpet/44g	78	0.5	178	5.5	34.5	1.2	0
Smart Price, Asda*	1 Crumpet/35.6g	67	0.3	188	6	39	0.9	2.1
Somerfield*	1 Crumpet/41.1g	79	0.4	192	5.9	39.9	1	2.5
Square, Tesco*	1 Crumpet/60g	101	0.5	168	6.3	33.8	0.8	2.7
Thins , Kingsmill*	1 Thin/27g	54	0.3	199	6.9	39.3	1.1	2.3
Toasted, Average	*1 Crumpet/40g*	*80*	*0.4*	*199*	*6.7*	*43.4*	*1*	*2*
Toasted, Tesco*	1 Crumpet/65g	120	0.6	185	5.2	37.9	0.9	3.7
Village Bakery, Aldi*	1 Crumpet/46g	86	0.5	187	5.7	38	1	2.8
Waitrose*	1 Crumpet/62g	116	0.7	188	6.3	37.9	1.2	2.1
Warburton's*	1 Crumpet/55g	98	0.4	178	5.6	36.1	0.7	2.3
CRUNCHIE								
Blast, Cadbury*	1 Serving/42g	199	8.3	480	4.7	69.6	20.1	0.7
Cadbury*	1 Bar/40g	185	7.5	465	4	69.5	18.9	0.5
Nuggets, Cadbury*	1 Bag/125g	569	20.5	455	3.8	73.1	16.4	0
Treat Size, Cadbury*	1 Bar/17g	80	3.1	470	4	71.5	18.4	0
CUCUMBER								
Average	*1 Serving/80g*	*8*	*0.1*	*10*	*0.7*	*1.5*	*0.1*	*0.6*
Baby, Pickled, Always Fresh*	1 Serving/30g	14	0.1	47	2	8	0.3	0
Crunchies with a Yoghurt & Mint Dip, Shapers, Boots*	1 Serving/110g	35	1	32	2.1	3.7	0.9	0.8
Juiced, Average*	1 Serving/100g	9	0.1	9	0.4	2.5	0.1	0.1
CUMIN								
Seeds, Whole, Average	*1 Tsp/2g*	*8*	*0.5*	*375*	*17.8*	*44.2*	*22.7*	*10.5*
CUPCAKES								
Assorted, Sainsbury's*	1 Cake/38g	130	2.3	341	2.2	69.3	6.1	0.4
Carrot, Average	*1 Cake/40g*	*157*	*8.6*	*392*	*3.6*	*45.4*	*21.6*	*0.6*
Chocolate, Average	*1 Cake/40g*	*159*	*6.4*	*398*	*3.5*	*59.9*	*16*	*1.2*
Chocolate, BGTY, Sainsbury's*	1 Cake/38g	121	1.7	318	2.5	66.5	4.6	0.8
Chocolate, COU, M&S*	1 Cake/45g	130	1.3	290	4.6	62.2	2.8	4.3
Chocolate, Fabulous Bakin' Boys*	1 Cupcake/34g	152	8.1	448	4	54	24	1
Chocolate, Lyons*	1 Cake/39g	125	1.8	321	2.4	67.5	4.6	0.8
Chocolate, Mini, Weight Watchers*	1 Cupcake/20g	87	4.3	426	6.1	52	21.1	1.8
Cookies & Cream, Secret Chocolate Centre, Tesco*	1 Cupcake/69g	335	20	485	2.7	52.2	29	1
Iced Cupcake, Gluten & Wheat Free, Lovemore*	1 Cake/33g	138	6.3	418	2.1	54.5	19	0.4
Jam Splatter, Tesco*	1 Cake/47g	221	10.2	470	2.3	65.6	21.8	0.5
Lemon, Average	*1 Cake/40g*	*184*	*10.1*	*461*	*3*	*55.5*	*25.3*	*1.1*
Lemon, COU, M&S*	1 Cupcake/43g	130	0.9	305	3.3	68.1	2.1	2
Lemon, Healthy Option, Average	*1 Cake/40g*	*131*	*1.5*	*328*	*2.7*	*68.9*	*3.7*	*5.2*
Lemon, Mini, Weight Watchers*	1 Cupcake/16.8g	56	0.8	333	2.4	63.3	4.9	12.1

	Measure INFO/WEIGHT	per Measure KCAL	per Measure FAT	Nutrition Values per 100g / 100ml KCAL	PROT	CARB	FAT	FIBRE
CUPCAKES								
Pink, M&S*	1 Cupcake/39g	160	3.3	410	2.5	81.3	8.5	0.6
Toffee, Thorntons*	1 Cupcake/80g	330	16	412	2.4	56	20	0
CURACAO								
Average	*1 Pub Shot/35ml*	*109*	*0*	*311*	*0*	*28.3*	*0*	*0*
CURLY WURLY								
Cadbury*	1 Bar/26g	115	4.5	442	3.5	69.2	17.3	0.8
Squirlies, Cadbury*	1 Squirl/3g	13	0.5	442	3.5	69.2	17.3	0.8
CURRANTS								
Average	*1oz/28g*	*75*	*0.1*	*267*	*2.3*	*67.8*	*0.4*	*1.9*
CURRY								
& Chips, Curry Sauce, Chipped Potatoes, Kershaws*	1 Serving/330g	391	8.2	118	10	14	2.5	2
Aubergine	*1oz/28g*	*33*	*2.8*	*118*	*1.4*	*6.2*	*10.1*	*1.5*
Aubergine, Masala, TTD, Sainsbury's*	½ Pack/115g	135	11.4	117	2.9	4.1	9.9	5.8
Beef, Sainsbury's*	1 Serving/400g	552	32.8	138	10.7	5.4	8.2	0.9
Beef, Thai, Finest, Tesco*	1 Serving/500g	770	29	154	9	16.5	5.8	1.2
Beef, with Rice, Iceland*,	1 Pack/400g	404	6.8	101	6.7	14.7	1.7	1
Beef, with Rice, Morrisons*	1 Serving/400g	480	20	120	6	12.6	5	0.6
Blackeye Bean, Gujerati	*1oz/28g*	*36*	*1.2*	*127*	*7.2*	*16.1*	*4.4*	*2.8*
Cabbage	*1oz/28g*	*23*	*1.4*	*82*	*1.9*	*8.1*	*5*	*2.1*
Cauliflower & Potato	*1oz/28g*	*17*	*0.7*	*59*	*3.4*	*6.6*	*2.4*	*1.8*
Cauliflower, & Chickpea, Lovely Vegetables, M&S*	1 Serving/390g	351	13.6	90	2.9	11.2	3.5	3.7
Chick Pea, Whole, Average	*1oz/28g*	*50*	*2.1*	*179*	*9.6*	*21.3*	*7.5*	*4.5*
Chick Pea, Whole, Basic, Average	*1oz/28g*	*30*	*1*	*108*	*6*	*14.2*	*3.6*	*3.3*
Chicken, Chinese with Rice, Ready Meal, Average	*1 Serving/450g*	*490*	*11.5*	*109*	*7.2*	*14.1*	*2.6*	*1.3*
Chicken, Chinese, Morrisons*	1 Pack/340g	347	15.6	102	10.3	5	4.6	0.8
Chicken, Chinese, Sharwoods*	1 Pack/375g	420	10.1	112	5	16.1	2.7	1.5
Chicken, Green Thai Style & Sticky Rice, Asda*	1 Pack/450g	585	10.8	130	7	20	2.4	0.1
Chicken, Green Thai, Balanced for You, M&S*	1 Pack/395g	383	5.9	97	7.8	12.7	1.5	1
Chicken, Green Thai, Charlie Bigham's*	½ Pack/300g	342	21	114	8.7	4.8	7	0
Chicken, Hot, Can, Tesco*	1 Can/418g	514	26.3	123	9.7	6.9	6.3	0.9
Chicken, Kashmiri, Waitrose*	1 Serving/400g	640	36.4	160	14.5	5	9.1	0.6
Chicken, Malaysian, Finest, Tesco*	1 Pack/375g	375	8.3	100	7.4	12.2	2.2	0.8
Chicken, Mild, Canned, Bilash, Aldi*	½ Can/200g	180	7.6	90	9.5	4.5	3.8	0.7
Chicken, Mild, Tinned, Sainsbury's*	1 Serving/200g	214	7	107	12.7	6.1	3.5	1.1
Chicken, Piri Piri, & Cajun Rice, Asda*	1 Pack/380g	410	8.7	108	6.7	14	2.3	2.6
Chicken, Thai, Green, & Jasmine Rice, Ready Meal	*1 Serving/450g*	*520*	*17.2*	*116*	*7.7*	*12.6*	*3.8*	*1.1*
Chicken, Thai, Green, No Rice, Average	*1 Serving/200g*	*174*	*7*	*87*	*8.2*	*5*	*3.5*	*1.4*
Chicken, Thai, Red, & Jasmine Rice, Ready Meal	*1 Serving/450g*	*500*	*15.3*	*111*	*7.5*	*12.6*	*3.4*	*1*
Chicken, Thai, Red, & Rice, Ready Meal, Healthy	*1 Serving/400g*	*400*	*7.8*	*100*	*6.4*	*14*	*2*	*1*
Chicken, Thai, Red, & Sticky Rice, Ready Meal	*1 Serving/450g*	*527*	*15.7*	*117*	*6.7*	*14.2*	*3.5*	*1.7*
Chicken, Thai, Red, No Rice, Average	*1 Serving/200g*	*194*	*6.9*	*97*	*7.2*	*9*	*3.4*	*1.4*
Chicken, with Rice, Average	*1 Serving/400g*	*465*	*11*	*116*	*5.1*	*17.8*	*2.8*	*0.8*
Chicken, with Rice, Fresh, Co-Op*	1 Pack/300g	270	9	90	3	13	3	1
Chicken, with Rice, Fruity, HL, Tesco*	1 Pack/450g	495	5.4	110	6.5	18.2	1.2	1.2
Chicken, with Rice, Ready Meal, Average	*1 Serving/400g*	*446*	*10.5*	*112*	*5.2*	*16.8*	*2.6*	*1*
Chicken, Yellow Thai Style, HL, Tesco*	1 Pack/450g	504	12.2	112	9.3	12.6	2.7	0.5
Courgette, & Potato	*1oz/28g*	*24*	*1.5*	*86*	*1.9*	*8.7*	*5.2*	*1.2*
Dudhi, Kofta	*1oz/28g*	*32*	*2.1*	*113*	*2.6*	*9.4*	*7.4*	*2.8*
Fish, & Vegetable, Bangladeshi, Average	*1oz/28g*	*33*	*2.4*	*117*	*9.1*	*1.4*	*8.4*	*0.5*
Fish, Bangladeshi, Average	*1oz/28g*	*35*	*2.2*	*124*	*12.2*	*1.5*	*7.9*	*0.3*
Fish, Red Thai, Waitrose*	1 Pack/500g	275	11	55	5.2	3.7	2.2	1
Jamaican Jerk, Veg Pot, Vegan, Bol*	1 Pot/345g	310	3.8	90	4	14.1	1.1	3.9
Lamb, & Potato, 385, Wiltshire Farm Foods*	1 Serving/210g	334	23	159	8.9	6.2	11	1.7

C

	Measure INFO/WEIGHT	per Measure KCAL	FAT	Nutrition Values per 100g / 100ml KCAL	PROT	CARB	FAT	FIBRE
CURRY								
Lamb, Aromatic, Balanced for You, M&S*	1 Pack/380g	388	9.1	102	9	9.2	2.4	3.7
Lamb, Hot, M&S*	½ Can/213.3g	320	19.6	150	14.9	6	9.2	2.3
Mushroom, & Pea, Masala, Indian, Sainsbury's*	1 Pack/300g	264	14.7	88	3.3	5.2	4.9	5.1
Paneer, & Parsnip, Everdine*	1 Serving/450g	567	22.9	126	5.3	12.8	5.1	3.9
Paneer, & Sweet Potato, Kofte Biryani, Everdine*	1 Serving/450g	562	22.1	125	3.8	13.1	4.9	6.7
Potato & Pea	*1oz/28g*	*26*	*1.1*	*92*	*2.9*	*13*	*3.8*	*2.4*
Prawn & Mushroom	*1oz/28g*	*47*	*4*	*168*	*7.3*	*2.5*	*14.4*	*1*
Prawn, Coconut & Lime, King, Sainsbury's*	½ Pack/351g	207	8.8	59	3.7	5.4	2.5	1
Prawn, Goan, King, M&S*	1 Pack/400g	680	44.4	170	5.1	11.6	11.1	1.5
Prawn, Malay, King, Waitrose*	1 Pack/350g	364	19.2	104	6.6	7.1	5.5	0.9
Prawn, Red Thai, King, City Kitchen, Tesco*	1 Pack/385g	460	14.4	119	4.5	16.7	3.7	1
Prawn, Red Thai, Sainsbury's*	1 Pack/300g	546	39.6	182	6.3	9.4	13.2	1.7
Prawn, Takeaway, Average	*1 Serving/350g*	*410*	*29.8*	*117*	*8.2*	*2.2*	*8.5*	*2*
Prawn, with Rice, Frozen, Sainsbury's*	1 Pack/400g	552	7.6	138	3.9	26.4	1.9	2.1
Red Kidney Bean, Punjabi	*1oz/28g*	*30*	*1.6*	*106*	*4.7*	*10.1*	*5.6*	*3.8*
Red Thai, Vegetarian, Tesco*	1 Pack/429ml	588	21.9	137	5.4	17.3	5.1	1.6
Salmon, Green, Waitrose*	1 Pack/401g	581	40.5	145	9.1	4.5	10.1	2.7
Sambhar Mix, Lentil & Vegetable, Fudco*	1 Box/100g	354	13.2	354	13.6	45.3	13.2	9.6
Sri Lankan Sambar, Pot, Bol*	1 Pot/345g	310	8.6	90	5.3	9.4	2.5	4.4
Sri Lankan Veg, Weight Watchers*	1 Pack/380g	171	6.1	45	1.5	5.2	1.6	2
Sweet Potato, Slimfree, Aldi*	½ Pack/275g	138	1.6	50	2.3	6.5	0.6	4.8
Thai, Coconut, Veg Pot, Vegan, Bol*	1 Pot/345g	266	6.6	77	1.8	12.3	1.9	1.8
Vegetable, & Chickpea, Cook*	1 Serving/330g	224	6.3	68	3.2	7.9	1.9	3.3
Vegetable, Asda*	1 Pack/350g	329	21	94	1.9	8	6	1.9
Vegetable, Canned, Sainsbury's*	½ Can/200g	200	12.2	100	1.4	9.8	6.1	1.8
Vegetable, Canned, Tesco*	1 Can/400g	308	11.2	77	2	9.7	2.8	2.4
Vegetable, Diet Chef Ltd*	1 Pack/300g	153	3.6	51	2	8	1.2	2.1
Vegetable, Frozen, Mixed Vegetables, Average	*1oz/28g*	*25*	*1.7*	*88*	*2.5*	*6.9*	*6.1*	*0*
Vegetable, in Sweet Sauce, Average	*1 Serving/330g*	*162*	*6.9*	*49*	*1.4*	*6.7*	*2.1*	*1.3*
Vegetable, Indian Meal for One, Tesco*	1 Serving/200g	218	14.4	109	2	9	7.2	1.2
Vegetable, Indian, Canned, Tesco*	1 Can/400g	320	18	80	2	6.7	4.5	1.1
Vegetable, Indian, Sainsbury's*	½ Pack/200g	206	14.6	103	2.5	6.8	7.3	4.6
Vegetable, Indian, Tesco*	1 Serving/225g	257	17.8	114	2.1	8.6	7.9	1.6
Vegetable, LC, Tesco*	1 Pack/350g	350	4.2	100	2.3	19.4	1.2	1.5
Vegetable, Medium, Tesco*	1 Pack/350g	326	21.7	93	2.3	7.1	6.2	1.9
Vegetable, Mixed, Organic, Pure & Pronto*	1 Pack/400g	368	11.6	92	4.2	12.4	2.9	4.8
Vegetable, Pakistani, Average	*1oz/28g*	*17*	*0.7*	*60*	*2.2*	*8.7*	*2.6*	*2.2*
Vegetable, Sabzi Tarkari, Patak's*	1 Pack/400g	500	31.2	125	2.5	11.1	7.8	2.2
Vegetable, South Indian, Weight Watchers*	1 Pack/400g	256	7.6	64	2.7	7.9	1.9	2.4
Vegetable, Takeaway, Average	*1 Serving/330g*	*346*	*24.4*	*105*	*2.5*	*7.6*	*7.4*	*0*
Vegetable, with Rice, Healthy Range, Average	*1 Serving/400g*	*351*	*4.6*	*88*	*2.3*	*16.8*	*1.1*	*1.9*
Vegetable, with Rice, Ready Meal, Average	*1 Serving/400g*	*408*	*12*	*102*	*3.3*	*16.4*	*3*	*0*
Vegetable, with Yoghurt, Average	*1oz/28g*	*17*	*1.1*	*62*	*2.6*	*4.6*	*4.1*	*1.4*
Vegetable, Yellow Thai, Sainsbury's*	1 Pack/400g	624	48.8	156	2.2	9.4	12.2	1.1
CURRY LEAVES								
Fresh	*1oz/28g*	*23*	*0.3*	*81*	*6.6*	*11*	*1.1*	*0*
CURRY PASTE								
Balti, Sharwood's*	¼ Pack/72.5g	328	28.7	453	5	19.2	39.6	3.1
Balti, Tomato & Coriander, Original, Patak's*	1 Tbsp/15g	58	5.1	388	4	14.6	34	3.7
Green Thai, Average	*1 Tsp/5g*	*6*	*0.4*	*128*	*2.1*	*11.7*	*7.9*	*3.1*
Jalfrezi, Patak's*	1 Serving/30g	96	8.1	320	3.7	14.2	26.9	5.6
Korma, Asda*	1 Tube/100g	338	23.5	338	5.1	26.6	23.5	1.2
Madras, Cumin & Chilli, Hot, Patak's*	¼ Jar/70g	202	18.1	289	4.7	7.6	25.9	10.8

	Measure INFO/WEIGHT	per Measure KCAL	FAT	Nutrition Values per 100g / 100ml KCAL	PROT	CARB	FAT	FIBRE
CURRY PASTE								
Medium, Asda*	1 Tsp/5g	18	1.6	364	5	14	32	5
Mild, Coriander & Cumin, Original, Patak's*	1 Serving/35g	99	8.6	283	4.8	9.1	24.6	10.7
Red, Thai, Average	*1 Tsp/5g*	*7*	*0.5*	*132*	*2.3*	*9.5*	*9.1*	*3*
Rogan Josh, Tomato & Paprika, Patak's*	1 Serving/30g	119	11	397	4.1	12.7	36.7	5.9
Tandoori, Tamarind & Ginger, Patak's*	1 Serving/30g	33	0.5	110	3.1	20.4	1.8	2.6
Tikka Masala, Coriander & Lemon, Medium, Patak's*	1 Serving/30g	111	9.5	369	3.8	16.9	31.8	2.9
Tikka Masala, Spice, Patak's*	1 Tbsp/15g	46	3.4	305	3.4	17.8	22.8	5.6
Tikka, Asda*	½ Tube/50g	118	8.5	235	4.5	16.1	17	1.6
Tom Yum, Thai Taste*	1 Tsp/13g	35	2	269	5.4	30.8	15.4	7.7
Yellow Thai, Tesco*	1 Tbsp/15g	15	0.6	100	1.9	13.6	4.1	4.9
Yellow, Thai, Barts*	1 Serving/30g	84	3.8	281	2.7	30.4	12.8	8.3
CURRY POWDER								
Average	*1 Tsp/2g*	*6*	*0.3*	*325*	*12.7*	*41.8*	*13.8*	*0*
CUSTARD								
Banana Flavour, Ambrosia*	1 Sm Pot/135g	139	3.9	103	2.9	16.1	2.9	0
Banana Flavour, Pot, Average	*1 Pot/135g*	*138*	*3.9*	*102*	*2.9*	*16*	*2.9*	*0*
Canned, Essential, Waitrose*	¼ Can/100g	101	3.2	101	2.7	15.3	3.2	0
Chocolate Flavour, Ambrosia*	1 Pot/150g	177	4.4	118	3	20	2.9	0.7
Chocolate Flavour, Pot, Average	*1 Pot/125g*	*138*	*3.4*	*111*	*3.1*	*18.2*	*2.7*	*0.6*
Instant, Just Add Water, Made Up, Weight Watchers*	1 Serving/145g	93	0.6	64	1.2	13.9	0.4	0.9
Instant, Mix, As Sold, Smart Price, Asda*	1 Pack/70g	204	2.7	291	2.6	61.3	3.9	0
Low Fat, Average	*1/3 Pot/141g*	*116*	*1.6*	*82*	*2.9*	*15*	*1.2*	*0*
Powder	*1 Tsp/5g*	*18*	*0*	*354*	*0.6*	*92*	*0.7*	*0.1*
Ready to Eat, Chocolate, Tesco*	1 Pot/150g	150	3.4	100	3.2	16.2	2.3	0.3
Ready to Eat. Low Fat, Pot, Tesco*	1 Pot/150g	132	2	88	3.2	15.9	1.3	0
Ready To Serve, Aldi*	¼ Pot/125g	152	7.2	122	2.7	15	5.8	0
Ready to Serve, Average	*1 Serving/50g*	*59*	*2.3*	*118*	*3.3*	*16.1*	*4.6*	*0.2*
Ready to Serve, Canned, Everyday Value, Tesco*	½ Can/192g	133	1.3	69	2.8	12.9	0.7	0
Salted Caramel Flavour, Morrisons*	½ Pot/150g	167	4.8	111	2.9	17.4	3.2	0.5
Soya, Vanilla, Dairy Free, Deliciously, Alpro*	1 Tbsp/15g	12	0.3	81	3	13.3	1.8	0.5
Toffee Flavour, Ambrosia*	1 Pot/150g	156	4.2	104	2.8	17	2.8	0
Vanilla Bean, Dollop*	1 Dollop/100g	127	3	127	20.2	27.7	3	0
Vanilla Flavour, Pot, Average	*1 Pot/125g*	*128*	*3.5*	*102*	*2.8*	*16.4*	*2.8*	*0*
Vanilla with Apple Crunch, Ambrosia*	1 Pack/193g	276	8.7	143	3.4	22.4	4.5	0.8
Vanilla, Low Fat, Fresh, Waitrose*	1/5 Pot/100g	104	2.4	104	3.5	17.1	2.4	0
Vanilla, TTD, Sainsbury's*	1 Pot/150g	312	23.2	208	2.5	14.7	15.5	0.1
CUSTARD APPLE								
Cherimoya, Weighed without Skin & Seeds, Average	*1 Serving/312g*	*234*	*2.1*	*75*	*1.6*	*17.7*	*0.7*	*3*
CUTLETS								
Nut, Goodlife*	1 Cutlet/88g	283	19.4	322	9.1	21.8	22	3.4
Nut, Meat Free, Tesco*	1 Cutlet/70g	240	16.2	340	8	22.7	23	3.8
Nut, Retail, Fried in Vegetable Oil, Average	*1 Cutlet/90g*	*260*	*20.1*	*289*	*4.8*	*18.7*	*22.3*	*1.7*
Nut, Retail, Grilled, Average	*1 Cutlet/90g*	*191*	*11.7*	*212*	*5.1*	*19.9*	*13*	*1.8*
Vegetable & Nut, Asda*	1 Cutlet/88g	296	20.3	335	10	22	23	4.6
CUTTLEFISH								
Raw	*1oz/28g*	*16*	*0.2*	*56*	*12.7*	*0*	*0.6*	*0*

	Measure INFO/WEIGHT	per Measure KCAL	FAT	Nutrition Values per 100g / 100ml KCAL	PROT	CARB	FAT	FIBRE
DAB								
Raw	*1oz/28g*	*21*	*0.3*	*74*	*15.7*	*0*	*1.2*	*0*
DAIM								
Mondelez*	1 Bar/28g	148	8.7	530	2.9	59	31	1.2
DAIRYLEA DUNKERS								
with Jumbo Tubes, Kraft*	1 Pack/42.5g	108	5.1	255	9.1	27	12	0.9
with Ritz Crackers, Dairylea, Kraft*	1 Tub/46g	118	5.5	258	9.6	26	12	2.2
DAMSONS								
Raw, Weighed with Stones, Average	*1oz/28g*	*9*	*0*	*31*	*0.4*	*7.7*	*0*	*1.4*
Raw, Weighed without Stones, Average	*1oz/28g*	*11*	*0*	*38*	*0.5*	*9.6*	*0*	*1.8*
DANDELION & BURDOCK								
Barr*	1 Bottle/250ml	40	0	16	0	4	0	0
Fermented, Botanical, Fentiman's*	1 Bottle/275ml	130	0	47	0	11.6	0	0
Original, Ben Shaws*	1 Can/440ml	128	0	29	0	7	0	0
Slightly Sparkling, Fentiman's*	1 Serving/200ml	98	0	49	0	11.7	0	0
Sparkling, Diet, Morrisons*	1 Glass/200ml	2	0	1	0	0.3	0	0
DANISH PASTRY								
Apple & Cinnamon, Danish Twist, Entenmann's*	1 Serving/52g	150	1	288	5.6	62	1.9	1.5
Apple & Sultana, Tesco*	1 Pastry/72g	293	16.4	407	5.4	45	22.8	1.4
Apple Danish, Bakery, Waitrose*	1 Pastry/123g	400	22.2	325	5.1	35.7	18	2.4
Apple, Fresh Cream, Sainsbury's*	1 Pastry/67g	248	14.6	368	3.1	40.2	21.6	0.4
Apple, Iceland*	¼ Pastry/95g	223	5	235	5.3	41.5	5.3	2.3
Average	*1 Pastry/110g*	*411*	*19.4*	*374*	*5.8*	*51.3*	*17.6*	*1.6*
Cherry & Custard, Bar, Tesco*	1 Bar/350g	910	49	260	3.5	29.9	14	7.7
Custard, Bar, Sara Lee*	¼ Bar/100g	228	6.4	228	6.6	36.1	6.4	0.8
Fruit Bears Claw , Waitrose*	1 Pastry/97g	339	15.8	349	4.6	45	16.3	2
Fruit Filled, Average	*1 Pastry/94g*	*335*	*15.9*	*356*	*5.1*	*47.9*	*17*	*0*
Pecan & Maple Plait, M&S*	1 Serving/85g	394	26.3	464	5.9	40.5	31	4.1
Raspberry Trifle Crown, Bakery, Tesco*	1 Pastry/90g	321	19	356	6.1	34.3	21.1	2.3
Toasted Pecan, Danish Twist, Entenmann's*	1 Slice/48g	171	7.6	351	7	47.2	15.6	1.4
DATES								
Dried, Average	*1 Date/5g*	*13*	*0*	*266*	*2.8*	*64.1*	*0.4*	*4.1*
Dried, Medjool, Average	*1 Date/20g*	*56*	*0.1*	*279*	*2.2*	*69.3*	*0.3*	*4.3*
Fresh, Raw, Yellow, Average	*1 Date/20g*	*21*	*0*	*107*	*1.3*	*27.1*	*0.1*	*1.5*
Medjool, Stuffed with Walnuts, Tesco*	2 Dates/40g	98	2.3	245	4.4	44	5.7	3.4
Milk Chocolate Coated, Julian Graves*	1 Pack/200g	768	22.6	384	4.5	66	11.3	2.6
DELI FILLER								
Cheese & Onion, Essential, Waitrose*	1 Pot/170g	692	64.8	407	10.8	4.5	38.1	1.5
Cheese & Onion, Sainsbury's*	1 Pack/170g	673	62.7	396	10.8	4.8	36.9	0.9
Chicken & Bacon, Co-Op*	1 Pack/200g	420	29.6	210	17.6	1	14.8	2.6
Chicken, Caesar Style, Sainsbury's*	1 Pack/80g	212	18.2	265	14	1	22.7	2.6
King Prawn & Avocado, M&S*	1 Pack/170g	425	38.8	250	9.5	1.4	22.8	0.5
Prawn & Mayonnaise, M&S*	1 Serving/60g	150	13.8	250	11.3	1	23	0.5
Prawn Cocktail, Eat Well, M&S*	½ Pot/85g	119	7.3	140	9.1	6.4	8.6	0.6
Smoked Salmon & Soft Cheese, M&S*	1 Serving/85g	207	17.3	244	11.7	3.3	20.4	0.5
Tuna & Sweetcorn, BGTY, Sainsbury's*	1 Serving/50g	64	2.6	128	12.6	7.2	5.1	1.2
DELIGHT								
Butterscotch Flavour, No Added Sugar, Tesco*	1 Pack/49g	225	10	460	4.8	63.3	20.5	0
Chocolate Flavour, Dry, Tesco*	1 Pack/49g	220	9	450	6.2	64.2	18.4	2.3
Vanilla, No Added Sugar, Dry, Tesco*	1 Pack/49g	51	1.8	105	3.4	13.7	3.7	0.1
DESSERT								
After Dark, Black Forest, Gateaux, Gu*	1 Pot/85g	258	18.5	303	3	24.7	21.8	1.3
After Eight, Dark Chocolate & Mint, Nestle*	1 Pot/70g	125	4.9	178	4.2	25.3	7	0
Apple Crumble, Sainsbury's*	1 Pot/136g	291	10.5	214	3.2	33	7.7	2.7

DESSERT

INFO/WEIGHT	Measure		per Measure		Nutrition Values per 100g / 100ml				
			KCAL	FAT	KCAL	PROT	CARB	FAT	FIBRE
Banana Split	**1 Serving/175g**		**368**	**25.5**	**210**	**2.2**	**18**	**14.6**	**0.2**
Banoffee Layered, Sainsbury's*	1 Pot/115g		270	14.7	235	2.2	27.8	12.8	1
Banoffee, Frozen, HL, Tesco*	1 Serving/60g		92	1.6	153	2.5	29.9	2.6	0.6
Banoffee, Sainsbury's*	1 Pot/140g		360	19.1	257	2.7	30.9	13.6	1.3
Banoffee, Weight Watchers*	1 Dessert/81g		170	3.6	210	4.9	37.7	4.4	1.4
Billionaire Bullion Bar, M&S*	1 Dessert/80g		353	22.5	441	5.4	41.2	28.1	0.7
Black Cherry, Dragana, Waitrose*	1 Pot/125g		236	11.4	189	2.1	24.7	9.1	0.5
Black Forest, LC, Tesco*	1 Pot/145g		188	2.3	130	3.2	25.8	1.6	0.9
Black Forest, Somerfield*	1 Pot/100g		275	11.5	275	4.8	37.6	11.5	2.5
Black Forest, Tesco*	1 Pot/100g		287	14.4	287	3.5	35.8	14.4	2.4
Blueberry Muffin, Tesco*	1 Pot/91g		265	18.7	291	2	24.5	20.6	3
Butterscotch Flavour Whip, Co-Op*	1 Pack/64g		241	0.1	377	0.6	93.4	0.1	0
Buttons, Milk Chocolate, Cadbury*	1 Pot/100g		280	14.9	280	6.2	30.8	14.9	0
Cafe Mocha, COU, M&S*	1 Dessert/115g		155	3.1	135	5.5	21.8	2.7	1
Cappuccino, Italian, Co-Op*	1 Pack/90g		256	10.8	285	5	39	12	0.1
Caramel Crunch, Weight Watchers*	1 Serving/89g		174	2.6	196	4.6	37.9	2.9	1.7
Caramel Flavour, Soya, Dairy Free, Organic, Provamel*	1 Pot/125g		125	2.2	100	3	17.8	1.8	0.5
Caramel, Delights, Shape, Danone*	1 Pot/110g		109	2.5	99	3.3	16.3	2.3	0.1
Caramel, Pots Of Joy, Dairy Milk, Cadbury*	1 Pot/70g		150	7.3	215	2.5	27.1	10.5	0.1
Caramel, Soya, Creamy, Sweet, Alpro*	1 Pot/125g		106	2.2	85	3.2	13.7	1.8	0.5
Charlotte, Strawberry & Raspberry, COU, M&S*	1 Pot/110g		153	1.2	139	2.1	29.7	1.1	1.1
Cheeky & Saucy Little Pots Au Chocolat, Gu*	1 Pot/45g		199	16.6	443	3.3	24.1	36.9	2.3
Chocolate Fudge, Pot, Fabulous, Thorntons*	1 Pot /65g		168	10.4	258	5.5	22.7	16	0
Chocolate Banoffee, Gu*	1 Pot/85g		325	21.5	382	3.9	35	25.3	1
Chocolate Brownie, M&S*	¼ Pack/144g		610	39.5	425	4.7	39.6	27.5	1
Chocolate Buttons, Cadbury*	1 Pack/100g		275	14.5	275	5	30.5	14.5	0
Chocolate Creme, King Frais, Lidl*	1 Pot/125g		131	3.6	105	2.6	17	2.9	0
Chocolate Duetto, Weight Watchers*	1 Pot/85g		99	2.4	117	4.4	18.4	2.8	0
Chocolate Flavour, Soya, Dairy Free, Organic, Provamel*	1 Pot/125g		111	3	89	3	13.6	2.4	1
Chocolate Fudge Brownie, Tesco*	1 Pot/125g		374	16.6	299	4.6	40.2	13.3	1.3
Chocolate Hazelnut, Charolait, Aldi*	1 Serving/200g		270	11	135	3.3	18.1	5.5	0
Chocolate Hazelnut, Alpro*	1 Dessert/125g		98	2.9	78	2.6	11.2	2.3	1.1
Chocolate Honeycomb Crisp, COU, M&S*	1 Serving/71g		110	2.1	155	4.6	27.6	2.9	1
Chocolate Marshmallow, Weight Watchers*	1 Serving/50g		97	2.4	194	3.2	34.5	4.7	1.3
Chocolate Mint Torte, Weight Watchers*	1 Dessert/88g		174	4.1	198	4.7	34.3	4.7	5.2
Chocolate Mousse Cake, Weight Watchers*	1 Dessert/75g		148	2.2	198	5.9	37.1	2.9	1
Chocolate Muffin, LC, Tesco*	1 Pot/107.7g		140	2.4	130	4.3	22.6	2.2	1.3
Chocolate Muffin, Skinny, Low Fat, COU, M&S*	1 Pot/110g		154	3.1	140	5.2	23.5	2.8	0.5
Chocolate Muffin, Tesco*	1 Serving/104g		354	21.2	340	3.5	35.5	20.4	2.1
Chocolate Muffin, Waitrose*	1 Serving/110g		138	3	126	5.2	20	2.7	0.4
Chocolate Orange, Pots of Joy, Terry's*	1 Pot/70g		150	7.3	215	3.7	26	10.5	0.1
Chocolate Toffee, Weight Watchers*	1 Dessert/89g		177	4	197	4.3	34.9	4.5	2.2
Chocolate, Dark, Soya, Alpro*	1 Pot/125g		118	2.9	94	3	14.7	2.3	1.4
Chocolate, Delights, Shape, Danone*	1 Pot/110g		109	2.4	99	3.3	16.3	2.2	0.6
Chocolate, Everyday Value, Tesco*	1 Pot/100g		121	4	121	2.7	18.4	4	0.4
Chocolate, Frappe, Skinny, COU, M&S*	1 Pot/100g		116	2.6	116	6.2	16.9	2.6	0.5
Chocolate, Soya, Silky Smooth, Alpro*	1 Pot/125g		104	2.4	83	3	13	1.9	1.1
Chocolate, Weight Watchers*	1 Serving/82g		145	2.5	177	5.2	32.3	3	2.9
Crazy Chocolate Overload, M&S*	1 Pot/120g		402	27	335	3.1	30	22.5	0.5
Creme Au Chocolat, Bonne Maman*	1 Pot/100g		182	9.4	182	5	19	9.4	0
Creme Caramel, Sainsbury's*	1 Pot/100g		116	1.6	116	2.6	22.9	1.6	0
Custard with Caramel, Layers, Ambrosia*	1 Pot/161g		183	4.7	114	2.5	19.6	2.9	0
Double Chocolate Brownie, Weight Watchers*	1 Pot/86g		167	3.3	194	5.1	33.7	3.8	2.4

D

	Measure INFO/WEIGHT	per Measure KCAL	FAT	Nutrition Values per 100g / 100ml KCAL	PROT	CARB	FAT	FIBRE
DESSERT								
Double Chocolate Fudge, M&S*	1 Pot/119g	387	25.5	325	3	30.6	21.4	1.6
Dreamy Vanilla, BGTY, Sainsbury's*	1 Serving/58g	146	8.2	252	3.5	27.6	14.2	5.3
Egg Custard, King Frais, Lidl*	1 Dessert/100g	161	7.9	161	4.5	18	7.9	0
Fudge, Cadbury*	1 Pot/90g	216	11.2	240	4.1	28.5	12.4	0
Fudge, Pot, Fabulous, Thortons*	1 Pot/65g	177	10.8	272	4.9	25.8	16.6	0
Galaxy, Mars*	1 Pot/75g	166	9.2	221	4.9	22.7	12.3	0
Gulabjam Indian, Waitrose*	1 Pot/180g	479	15.5	266	4.8	42.9	8.6	0.6
Hot Chocolate & Raspberry Truffle Bakes, M&S*	1 Truffle/92g	363	15.5	395	3.2	30.9	16.9	2
Jaffa Cake, COU, M&S*	1 Serving/120g	138	3.1	115	2.4	20.1	2.6	1
Jaffa, COU, M&S*	1 Pot/107g	155	4.3	145	3.7	23.3	4	0.5
Key Lime Pie	**1 Serving/125g**	**431**	**25**	**344**	**4.1**	**37.9**	**20**	**1.4**
Lemon & Sultana Sponge, COU, M&S*	1 Pot/130g	169	1.6	130	2.8	26.5	1.2	0.5
Lemon & Raspberry Semifreddo, Waitrose*	1 Slice/63g	193	12.3	305	1.9	30.4	19.4	0.5
Lemon Meringue, Weight Watchers*	1 Pot/85g	161	0.4	189	2.4	43.1	0.5	0.6
Lemon Mousse Cake, Weight Watchers*	1 Serving/90g	130	2.4	144	3.2	26.7	2.7	0.5
Lemon, Sainsbury's*	1 Pot/115g	136	1.7	118	2.8	23.2	1.5	0.9
Lemoncello, Italian, Co-Op*	1 Pot/90g	266	14.4	295	3	34	16	0.1
Little Choc Pots, The Coconut Collaborative*	1 Pot/45g	105	6.5	234	2.2	23	14.4	1.5
Mandarin, COU, M&S*	1 Serving/150g	195	5.7	130	1	22	3.8	0.1
Millionaire's Shortbread, M&S*	1 Dessert/120g	440	27.8	365	3.2	35.5	23.1	1
Millionaires Shortbread, Tesco*	1 Serving/81g	321	21.7	397	2.8	35.7	26.8	0.7
Mint Chocolate Top, Weight Watchers*	1 Pot/75g	160	6.9	214	4	31.4	9.2	3.5
Mississippi Mud Pie	**1 Serving/125g**	**480**	**32**	**384**	**5.3**	**33.1**	**25.6**	**1.8**
Mix, Chocolate, Basics, Sainsbury's*	1 Serving/100g	92	3.3	92	4	11.5	3.3	0.5
Pineapple & Passionfruit, M&S*	1 Pot/100g	130	3.8	130	0.8	21.7	3.8	0.3
Pots Of Joy , Dairy Milk, Cadbury*	1 Pot /70g	158	8.2	225	4.2	25.6	11.7	0.1
Raspberry & Chardonnay, COU, M&S*	1 Serving/135g	155	0.7	115	1.6	25.5	0.5	2.7
Raspberry & Blackcurrant, Afternoon, Mini Pots, Fru, Gu*	1 Pot/50g	145	11.1	290	1.2	22.5	22.2	0.6
Raspberry Flavour Whip, Co-Op*	1 Whip/64g	241	0.1	377	1.2	92.5	0.2	0
Raspberry Frappe, Skinny, COU, M&S*	1 Pot/94g	114	2.1	121	3.1	22	2.2	0.5
Raspberry Royale, Essential, Waitrose*	1 Pot/150g	216	10.6	144	1.1	18.9	7.1	0.5
Rich Chocolate, Weight Watchers*	1 Pot/70g	62	1.7	89	3.5	13.4	2.4	1.4
Rocky Road, Sainsbury's*	1 Pot/110g	328	21.6	298	3.6	26.8	19.6	2.1
Rolo, Nestle*	1 Pot/70g	170	8.3	243	3.3	30.8	11.9	0.5
Semifreddo, Chocolate & Caramel, Waitrose*	1 Slice/64g	217	12.3	342	3.4	37.4	19.4	2.1
Skinny Dippers, Minis, Skinny Cow*	1 Lolly/40ml	65	2	162	3.4	24.3	5	3.3
Skinny Lemon Muffin, COU, M&S*	1 Pot/105g	144	2.6	137	3.5	24.7	2.5	0.6
Snowy Delight, Pots Of Joy , Dairy Milk, Cadbury*	1 Pot/70g	156	7	223	4.8	28.5	10	0.5
Strawberry & Rhubarb, COU, M&S*	1 Pot/110g	104	0.8	95	1.5	20.1	0.7	0.9
Strawberry Flavour with Cream, Somerfield*	1 Pot/100g	119	5	119	2	16	5	0
Strawberry Flavour, Smart Price, Asda*	1 Pot/115g	113	2.6	98	2.4	17	2.3	0
Strawberry Mousse Cake, Weight Watchers*	1 Serving/90g	124	2.4	138	3	25.5	2.7	0.5
Tart, Millionaire, Tesco*	1 Pot/105g	420	26.3	405	3.5	38.7	25.4	1.6
Tiramisu	**1 Serving/150g**	**420**	**20.8**	**280**	**4.4**	**34**	**13.9**	**0.8**
Toffee & Vanilla, Weight Watchers*	1 Pot/67g	107	0.5	159	3.1	34.8	0.8	3.9
Toffee Banana Crunch, Farmfoods*	1/6 Dessert/82g	219	9.3	267	2.6	38.5	11.4	0.7
Toffee Fudge , Pot, Fabulous, Thorntons*	1 Pot/65g	178	10.5	274	4.8	27.3	16.1	0
Toffee with Biscuit Pieces, Iced, Weight Watchers*	1 Pot/57g	93	2.7	163	2.7	26.2	4.8	0.2
Toffee with Biscuit Pieces, Weight Watchers*	1 Pot/57g	93	2.7	163	2.7	26.2	4.8	0.2
Trifle, Chocolate, Cadbury*	1 Pot /90g	234	13.8	260	4.8	22.5	15.3	0
Triple Chocolate Layered, BGTY, Sainsbury's*	1 Pot/105g	147	2.9	140	4.2	24.4	2.8	0.5
Triple Chocolate, Delice, Sainsbury's*	1 Serving/105g	399	27.4	380	3.8	32.4	26.1	0.7
Vanilla & Caramel, Little Desserts, Petits Filous, Yoplait*	1 Pot/50g	75	2.6	150	4.7	21	5.3	0.2

D

INFO/WEIGHT	Measure	KCAL	FAT	KCAL	PROT	CARB	FAT	FIBRE
				Nutrition Values per 100g / 100ml				

DESSERT

	Measure INFO/WEIGHT	per Measure KCAL	FAT	KCAL	PROT	CARB	FAT	FIBRE
Vanilla & Chocolate Twist, Desira, Aldi*	1 Pack/150g	182	7.2	121	0	15	4.8	0
Vanilla Choc Fudge, Non Dairy Soya, Frozen, Tofutti*	1 Tub/500ml	825	45	165	1.6	20	9	0.4
Vanilla Creamed Rice, Weight Watchers*	1 Pot/130g	112	0.6	86	3.2	16.9	0.5	0.4
Vanilla Creme, With Raspberries, Bonne Maman*	1 Pot/90g	158	9	175	1.7	19	10	1.1
Vanilla Flavour, Soya, Dairy Free, Organic, Provamel*	1 Pot/125g	105	2.2	84	3.2	13.4	1.8	0.5
Vanilla Supreme, Sainsbury's*	1 Pot/95g	116	3.8	122	3	18	4	0
Vanilla with Strawberries Swirl, Weight Watchers*	1 Pot/57g	46	1.3	81	1.5	13.3	2.2	0.2
Vanilla, Frozen, BGTY, Sainsbury's*	1 Serving/75g	89	2.2	119	3	19.9	3	3.7
Vanilla, Frozen, GFY, Asda*	1 Serving/52g	72	2.3	139	2.7	22	4.5	0
Vanilla, Soya, Heavenly Velvet, Alpro*	1 Pot/125g	106	2.4	85	3.2	13.6	1.9	0.5
White Buttons, Pots of Joy, Cadbury*	1 Pot /70g	158	6.6	225	4.8	30.4	9.4	0
White Chocolate, Delights, Shape, Danone*	1 pot/110g	109	2.6	99	3.5	15.9	2.4	0.1
Zabaglione	*1 Serving/100g*	*278*	*18.3*	*278*	*3.6*	*24.3*	*18.3*	*2.3*

DHAL

	Measure INFO/WEIGHT	per Measure KCAL	FAT	KCAL	PROT	CARB	FAT	FIBRE
Black Gram, Average	*1oz/28g*	*21*	*1*	*74*	*4.2*	*7*	*3.4*	*1.7*
Chick Pea	*1oz/28g*	*42*	*1.7*	*149*	*7.4*	*17.7*	*6.1*	*3.8*
Chick Pea, Canned, Asda*	½ Can/194g	198	6.2	102	4.3	14	3.2	2.9
Chick Pea, Sainsbury's*	½ Can/200g	432	18.2	216	10.8	22.7	9.1	7.1
Chickpea, Mazadar*	1 Tin/400g	360	11.2	90	4.5	11.6	2.8	4.5
Lentil, Patak's*	1 Can/283g	156	2.8	55	2.8	9.3	1	1
Lentil, Red Masoor & Tomato with Butter, Average	*1oz/28g*	*26*	*1.4*	*94*	*4*	*9.7*	*4.9*	*0.9*
Lentil, Red Masoor & Vegetable, Average	*1oz/28g*	*31*	*1.1*	*110*	*5.8*	*14.7*	*3.8*	*1.8*
Lentil, Red Masoor with Vegetable Oil, Average	*1oz/28g*	*48*	*2.2*	*172*	*7.6*	*19.2*	*7.9*	*1.8*
Lentil, Red Masoor, Punjabi, Average	*1oz/28g*	*39*	*1.3*	*139*	*7.2*	*19.2*	*4.6*	*2*
Lentil, Red Masoorl & Mung Bean, Average	*1oz/28g*	*32*	*1.9*	*114*	*4.8*	*9.9*	*6.7*	*1.6*
Lentil, Red, WTF, Sainsbury's*	½ Pack/273g	254	4.1	93	5.5	14.4	1.5	1.4
Lentil, Tesco*	1 Serving/200g	248	13.2	124	5.1	10.6	6.6	2.5
Makhani, Curry Collection, Veetee*	1 Pack/300g	306	17.4	102	4.2	11.1	5.8	2.8
Mung Bean, Bengali	*1oz/28g*	*20*	*0.9*	*73*	*4.2*	*7.4*	*3.3*	*1.7*
Mung Beans, Dried, Boiled in Unsalted Water	*1oz/28g*	*26*	*0.1*	*92*	*7.8*	*15.3*	*0.4*	*0*
Split Peas, Yellow, Chana, Asda*	1 Serving/275g	300	19.2	109	2.6	9	7	1.8
Sri Lankan Vegetable, Gym Bowl, Pod Foods*	1 Bowl/324g	311	16.8	96	3.4	9.5	5.2	2.9
Tadkha, Rich & Golden, Waitrose*	½ Pack/150g	172	8.3	114	6	10.9	5.5	5.5
Tarka, Asda*	½ Pack/150g	216	12	144	6	12	8	6
Tarka, M&S*	1 Serving/250g	235	8.8	94	4.3	9.4	3.5	3.7
Vegetable, with Lentil, Slimming World*	1 Pack/550g	242	2.8	44	2.5	5.8	0.5	2.9

DHANSAK

	Measure INFO/WEIGHT	per Measure KCAL	FAT	KCAL	PROT	CARB	FAT	FIBRE
Chicken with Bagara Rice, Waitrose*	1 Pack/450g	549	8.1	122	8.2	18.2	1.8	1.2
Vegetable, Curry, Microwaved, Slimzone, Asda*	1 Portion/459g	225	2.3	49	2.5	7.7	0.5	2.6
Vegetable, Sainsbury's*	1 Serving/200g	148	5.6	74	3.1	8.9	2.8	2.8

DILL

	Measure INFO/WEIGHT	per Measure KCAL	FAT	KCAL	PROT	CARB	FAT	FIBRE
Dried, Average	*1 Tsp/1g*	*3*	*0*	*253*	*19.9*	*42.2*	*4.4*	*13.6*
Fresh, Average	*1 Tbsp/3g*	*1*	*0*	*25*	*3.7*	*0.9*	*0.8*	*2.5*

DIP

	Measure INFO/WEIGHT	per Measure KCAL	FAT	KCAL	PROT	CARB	FAT	FIBRE
Aubergine, Fresh, Waitrose*	1 Serving/85g	159	12.8	187	2.5	10.5	15	1.7
Baba Ganoush, Sabra*	1 Serving/75g	188	17.6	251	3.9	4.4	23.5	0
Beetroot & Sesame, Sainsbury's*	¼ Pot/45g	65	3.7	145	4.2	11.8	8.3	3.1
Blue Cheese, Fresh, Sainsbury's*	1/5 Pot/34g	115	11.7	337	3.6	3.1	34.5	0.1
Cajun Red Pepper, Sainsbury's*	1 Serving/50g	25	0.9	50	1.4	7	1.8	1.4
Cheddar & Spring Onion, M&S*	1 Pack/125g	581	60.4	465	3.6	4.7	48.3	0.5
Cheese & Chive, 50% Less Fat, Asda*	1 Pot/125g	261	21.5	209	4.5	9	17.2	0
Cheese & Chive, 50% Less Fat, Morrisons*	1 Serving/50g	86	6.4	172	8.8	5.2	12.7	0.2
Cheese & Chive, Asda*	1 Serving/43g	190	19.6	447	4.9	3.4	46	0

D

DIP

INFO/WEIGHT	Measure	per Measure		Nutrition Values per 100g / 100ml				
		KCAL	FAT	KCAL	PROT	CARB	FAT	FIBRE
Cheese & Chive, Tesco*	¼ Pack/50g	268	27.6	535	4.3	4.3	55.1	0.1
Chilli Cheese, Asda*	1 Serving/50g	131	11	262	8	8	22	1.1
Chilli, M&S*	1 Pot/35g	103	0.1	295	0.4	73.2	0.2	0.4
Endamame & Pea, Waitrose*	¼ Pot/51g	85	5.9	166	6.3	8	11.6	2
Feta Cheese, Fresh, Tesco*	1oz/28g	81	7.1	288	6.8	7.9	25.5	0.7
Frijolemole, Cannellini Bean & Chick Pea, Waitrose*	¼ Pot/50g	104	7.6	208	4.3	12.2	15.2	2.6
Garlic & Herb, Big Dipper, Morrisons*	¼ Pot/75g	278	28.1	370	1.3	6.9	37.5	0.4
Garlic & Herb, Reduced Fat, M&S*	1 Serving/10g	10	0.4	95	6	8.1	4	0.5
Garlic & Herb, Tesco*	¼ Pack/43g	257	27.8	604	0.9	3.2	65.4	0.3
Garlic & Herb	*1 Serving/100g*	*584*	*62.4*	*584*	*1.4*	*4.1*	*62.4*	*0.2*
Garlic Butter, for Dough Balls, Pizza Express*	½ Pot/8g	54	5.8	673	1.3	5.2	71.9	0.6
Garlic, Olive Oil & Butter, Pizza Express*	½ Pot/17g	106	11.5	621	1.5	2.8	67.4	0.5
Hot Salsa, Doritos, Walkers*	1 Jar/300g	99	0.3	33	1.1	6.4	0.1	0.9
Houmous, Black Olive, Wild Garden*	2 Tbsp/30g	35	2	117	6.7	13.3	6.7	3.3
Houmous, Red Pepper, Wild Garden*	2 Tbsp/30g	35	2	117	6.7	13.3	6.7	3.3
Houmous, Roasted Garlic, Wild Garden*	2 Tbsp/30g	35	2	117	6.7	13.3	6.7	3.3
Houmous, Sun Dried Tomato, Wild Garden*	2 Tbsp/30g	35	2	117	6.7	13.3	6.7	3.3
Houmous, Traditional, Wild Garden*	2 Tbsp/30g	35	2	117	6.7	13.3	6.7	4.3
Indian Snack Selection, Vitasia, Lidl*	1 Serving/70g	122	7	175	1	19.7	10	1.2
Jalapeno & Lime Hummus, with Coriander, Lisa's*	1 Serving/20g	47	2.8	235	7.3	21.5	13.9	6.9
Jalapeno, Greek Yoghurt, Skotidakis*	1 Tbsp/15g	25	1.8	167	6.7	13.3	11.7	0
Mature Cheddar Cheese & Chive, Fresh, Waitrose*	½ Pot/85g	393	40.5	462	5.8	2.4	47.7	1.7
Mexican Bean, Doritos, Walkers*	1 Tbsp/20g	18	0.7	89	2.7	12.1	3.3	2.4
Mild Salsa, Doritos, Walkers*	1 Tbsp/30g	9	0.1	30	0.8	6	0.3	1.5
Nacho Cheese, Average	*1 Serving/50g*	*175*	*17.2*	*350*	*6.3*	*3.4*	*34.4*	*0.9*
Nacho Cheese, Doritos, Walkers*	1 Serving/40g	92	8.1	231	3.4	8.5	20.2	0.6
Nacho Cheese, Primula*	1 Serving/57g	144	14.2	253	2.7	3.6	24.9	2.1
Nacho Cheese, Sainsbury's*	1 Serving/50g	244	25.1	487	4.8	3.9	50.2	0
Nacho Cheese, Tex-Mex Multipack Selection, Tesco*	1 Tub/125g	619	62	495	5.9	5.8	49.6	0
Onion & Garlic, Classic, Tesco*	1 Serving/30g	133	13.9	442	1.7	4.6	46.3	0.2
Onion & Garlic, GFY, Asda*	1/5 Pot/34g	56	4.8	166	2.1	8	14	0.2
Onion & Garlic, HE, Tesco*	1 Pot/170g	345	29.9	203	3.3	7.9	17.6	0.1
Onion & Garlic, Average	*1 Tbsp/15g*	*62*	*6.4*	*410*	*1.7*	*4.8*	*42.7*	*0.4*
Onion & Garlic, HL, Tesco*	1 Serving/43g	80	7.2	188	2.5	6.3	17	0.1
Pea, Yogurt & Mint, Sainsbury's*	¼ Pack/50g	119	10.8	238	3.4	7.5	21.6	2.1
Peanut, Satay Selection, Occasions, Sainsbury's*	1 Serving/2g	4	0.2	186	7.1	13.8	11.4	1.1
Pecorino, Basil & Pine Nut, Fresh, Waitrose*	½ Pot/85g	338	33.7	398	5.1	5.1	39.7	0
Red Pepper, Sainsbury's*	1 Pot/100g	103	4	103	2.3	14.6	4	0
Roast Onion, Garlic & Rocket, Reduced Fat, Waitrose*	1 Serving/25g	50	4.7	202	2.7	5.4	18.8	1.5
Salsa Mild, Asda*	1 Portion/100g	47	0.3	47	1.4	8.7	0.3	1.8
Salsa, Chunky Tomato, Tesco*	1 Pot/170g	68	2.2	40	1.1	5.9	1.3	1.1
Salsa, Chunky, Fresh, Sainsbury's*	1 Serving/100g	51	1.7	51	1.1	7.8	1.7	1.2
Smoked Salmon & Dill, Fresh, Waitrose*	½ Pot/85g	373	38	439	5.1	4.1	44.7	0.1
Smoky Red Pepper, Gazpacho, Graze*	1 Punnet/22.5g	54	1.3	242	5.7	40.1	5.9	3.7
Sour Cream & Chive, Doritos, Walkers*	1 Tbsp/20g	52	4.9	258	1.9	6.9	24.7	1.9
Sour Cream & Chive, Fresh, Tesco*	½ Pot/75g	305	31.8	407	2.1	4.1	42.4	0
Sour Cream & Chive, Half Fat, Waitrose*	½ Pot/85g	133	9.9	157	5.5	7.6	11.6	0.1
Sour Cream & Chive, Sainsbury's*	1 Serving/50g	141	13.8	282	3.1	5.4	27.5	0.1
Sour Cream & Chives, Mexican Style, Morrisons*	¼ Pack/25g	68	7	274	2.2	3.4	27.9	0.4
Sour Cream & Chive, Average	*1 Tbsp/15g*	*48*	*4.8*	*317*	*3.2*	*4*	*32*	*0.3*
Sour Cream & Chive, M&S*	½ Pack/57g	218	22.5	383	2.2	4.9	39.4	0.1
Sour Cream & Chive, Primula*	1 Serving/57g	169	17.4	297	4.3	1.3	30.5	1
Sour Cream, Tesco*	1 Serving/38g	111	11.2	297	3.4	3.9	29.8	0.2

	Measure INFO/WEIGHT	per Measure		Nutrition Values per 100g / 100ml				
		KCAL	FAT	KCAL	PROT	CARB	FAT	FIBRE
DIP								
Soured Cream & Chive, BGTY, Sainsbury's*	1 Serving/170g	253	17.5	149	4.2	9.9	10.3	0.1
Soured Cream & Chive, Classic, Tesco*	1 Serving/25g	81	8.4	323	1.7	3.2	33.7	0.2
Soured Cream & Chive, HL, Tesco*	1 Serving/31g	45	3.3	145	3.8	7.5	10.6	0.2
Soured Cream & Chive, Morrisons*	1 Serving/100g	317	32.6	317	2.6	3.3	32.6	0
Soured Cream & Chive, LC, Tesco*	¼ Pot/50g	65	4.5	130	4.3	7.4	9	0.1
Spiced Mango, Ginger & Chilli Salsa, Weight Watchers*	1 Serving/56g	48	0.1	85	1	19.9	0.2	2.6
Spicy Moroccan, BGTY, Sainsbury's*	½ Pot/85g	56	1.7	66	2.1	10	2	1.7
Sweet Chilli Mango, Encona*	1 Tbsp/15ml	22	0.1	148	0.4	35.4	0.6	0
Sweet Chilli, Chinese Snack Selection, Morrisons*	½ Pot/20g	64	0	320	0.1	79.4	0.2	0.6
Thai Sweet Chilli, Primula*	1 Serving/57g	126	0.1	221	0.6	54.4	0.1	0.3
Thousand Island, HL, Tesco*	1 Serving/31g	57	4.6	183	2.5	9.6	14.9	0.3
Thousand Island, M&S*	1oz/28g	69	6.2	245	2.1	9.4	22.2	0.7
Tortilla Chips, Cool Flavour, Big, Morrisons*	½ Pack/100g	453	22	453	6.4	57.4	22	8.1
Yoghurt & Cucumber Mint, Tesco*	1oz/28g	34	2	121	7	7.2	7.1	0.6
DIP & DIPPERS								
Blueberry Toasts, & White Chocolate Dip, Graze*	1 Punnet/25g	130	6.8	519	5.7	62	27	3.2
Boston Baguettes, Graze*	1 Pack/31g	84	2.1	274	5.9	45.7	6.9	2.1
Cranberry & Hazelnut Toasts, Deep Cocoa Dip, Graze*	1 Punnet/28g	139	7.3	497	6.3	60	26	4.8
Korai Chutney, Graze*	1 Punnet/24g	69	0.5	286	3	65	2	2
My Thai, Graze*	1 Punnet/25g	84	1.2	336	2.4	70.2	4.7	0.4
Oatbakes with Caramelised Onion Marmalade, Graze*	1 Serving/36g	111	4	309	8	42	11	6
Pretzel, & Chocolate, Retail, Graze*	1 Punnet/29g	142	6.4	488	9	61	22	3.9
Summer Berry Compote, Wholemeal Shortbread, Graze*	1 Punnet/34g	128	6.2	377	4	50.1	18.3	2.8
DOLMADES								
Stffed Vine Leaves, Delphi*	½ Pack/75g	120	9	160	2.2	16	12	1.1
Stuffed with Rice, M&S*	1 Leaf/38g	40	1.6	105	2.6	14.2	4.1	1.2
DOPIAZA								
Chicken, M&S*	1 Pack/350g	402	21.4	115	11.5	3.7	6.1	2.5
Chicken, with Pilau Rice, Tesco*	1 Pack/400g	424	15.2	106	5.7	12.3	3.8	1.5
Mushroom, Retail	*1oz/28g*	*19*	*1.6*	*69*	*1.3*	*3.7*	*5.7*	*1.1*
Mushroom, Waitrose*	½ Pack/150g	81	4.6	54	2.2	4.3	3.1	2.3
DORITOS								
Cheesy 3d's, Doritos, Walkers*	1 Pack/20g	89	3.2	445	7	68	16	3
Chilli Heatwave, Walkers*	1 Bag/30g	148	7.6	495	6.3	57.3	25.3	6.7
Cool Original, Walkers*	1 Bag/40g	200	10.8	500	7.5	58	27	3
Cool Spice 3ds, Walkers*	1 Bag/24g	108	4.3	450	8	64	18	4.4
Dippas, Hint of Lime, Walkers*	1 Bag/35g	173	8.8	495	7	60	25	3.5
Lighly Salted, Corn Chips, Doritos*	1 Bag/30g	149	7.1	497	6.9	62.9	23.6	3.3
Tangy Cheese, Walkers*	1 Bag/40g	200	10.8	500	7	57	27	3
DOUBLE DECKER								
Cadbury*	1 Bar/54.5g	251	10.3	460	4.4	68.4	18.9	0.6
Snack Size, Cadbury*	1 Bar/36g	165	7.4	465	4.8	64.5	20.9	0
with Nuts, Cadbury*	1 Bar/60g	291	14.7	485	7.9	58.6	24.5	0
DOUGH BALLS								
Garlic & Herb, Asda*	4 Balls/48g	173	8.5	361	9.2	40.9	17.8	3.6
Garlic, Tesco*	1 Serving/10g	40	2.3	400	7	40	23	1
Garlic, Waitrose*	1 Ball/11g	38	1.8	347	8.5	41.4	16.4	3.3
Original, Plain as Sold, Supermarket, Pizza Express*	1 Ball/11g	34	0.3	311	10.8	59	3	2.5
Sainsbury's*	1 Ball/12g	41	2.1	343	8.4	38.7	17.2	2.2
with Garlic & Herb Butter (Cooked with Dip), Sainsbury's*	½ Pack/100g	362	14.8	362	9.6	47.7	14.8	2.9
with Garlic & Herb Butter, Aldi*	1 Ball/12g	45	2.2	365	7.7	46.7	18.2	1.8
DOUGHNUTS								
Chocolate , Cadbury*	1 Doughnut/74g	332	19.2	449	6.2	46.8	25.9	2.3

D

DOUGHNUTS

INFO/WEIGHT	Measure	per Measure KCAL	FAT	Nutrition Values per 100g / 100ml KCAL	PROT	CARB	FAT	FIBRE
Chocolate Iced, Ring, Bakery, Tesco*	1 Doughnut/59g	249	13.8	423	5.9	46.4	23.4	1.4
Chocolate Orange, Filled, Krispy Kreme*	1 Doughnut/93g	357	17.1	384	5.7	47.6	18.4	2.8
Cream & Jam, Tesco*	1 Doughnut/90g	288	14.1	320	5.4	39.4	15.7	2
Custard Filled, Average	*1 Doughnut/75g*	*268*	*14.2*	*358*	*6.2*	*43.3*	*19*	*0*
Custard, Sainsbury's*	1 Doughnut/70g	172	7.5	246	5.1	32.3	10.7	2.3
Custard, Tesco*	1 Doughnut/70g	204	8.2	292	5.2	40.3	11.8	1.7
Glazed, Bakery, Tesco*	1 Doughnut/52g	202	10.1	389	6.5	45.9	19.5	2
Jam Filled, Average	*1 Doughnut/75g*	*252*	*10.9*	*336*	*5.7*	*48.8*	*14.5*	*0*
Jam, American Style, Sainsbury's*	1 Doughnut/65g	220	20.6	339	4.9	49.6	31.8	3.5
Jam, Bakery, Tesco*	1 Doughnut/70g	225	7.6	321	5.6	49.2	10.9	2
Jam, M&S*	1 Doughnut/49g	141	2	287	5	57.6	4	1.3
Jam, Mini, Somerfield*	1 Doughnut/45g	138	4	307	6.4	50.1	9	1.4
Lemon Meringue, Krispy Kreme*	1 Doughnut/84g	346	20.3	410	8	40	24	1.8
Mini, Ring, Bites, Sugar Coated, Simply Doughnuts*	1 Ring/12g	57	3.5	474	6.9	43	29	0
Mini, Sainsbury's*	1 Doughnut/14g	53	2.7	379	5.2	47.9	18.9	2.1
Nutty Chocolatta , Krispy Kreme*	1 Doughnut/87g	379	20.9	436	6.7	46.9	24.1	2.2
Oreo, CSM, UK LTD*	1 Doughnut/72g	326	19.5	453	5	46.8	27	1.1
Plain, Ring, Average	*1 Doughnut/60g*	*238*	*13*	*397*	*6.1*	*47.2*	*21.7*	*0*
Raspberry Jam, Sainsbury's*	1 Doughnut/58g	203	8.9	350	5.5	46.4	15.3	2.3
Reese's Peanut Butter, Krispy Kreme*	1 Doughnut/93g	377	21.3	405	8.3	40.2	22.9	2.6
Ring, Iced, Average	*1 Doughnut/70g*	*268*	*12.2*	*383*	*4.8*	*55.1*	*17.5*	*0*
Ring, Sugar, Tesco*	1 Doughnut/56g	217	13.5	388	5.7	34.8	24.2	4.2
Selection, Bakers Selection, Asda*	1 Doughnut/75g	273	17.9	365	4.5	32	24	1.4
Strawberry Iced, Ring, Bakery, Tesco*	1 Doughnut/58g	248	14.3	428	5.4	45.3	24.7	1.4
Strawberry Iced, Ring, Mini, Bakery, Tesco*	1 Doughnut/15g	62	3.1	415	4.9	51.5	20.8	1.3
White Iced, Bakery, Sainsbury's*	1 Doughnut/55g	214	10.1	389	6.5	48.9	18.4	1.1
Yum Yums, Glazed, Sweet, Waitrose*	1 Doughnut/45g	172	10	382	4	41.6	22.2	2
Yum Yums, M&S*	1 Doughnut/37g	155	8.9	420	4.9	45.7	23.9	1.6

DOVER SOLE

INFO/WEIGHT	Measure	per Measure KCAL	FAT	Nutrition Values per 100g / 100ml KCAL	PROT	CARB	FAT	FIBRE
Fillet, Raw, Average	*1oz/28g*	*25*	*0.5*	*89*	*18.1*	*0*	*1.8*	*0*

DR PEPPER*

INFO/WEIGHT	Measure	per Measure KCAL	FAT	Nutrition Values per 100g / 100ml KCAL	PROT	CARB	FAT	FIBRE
Coca-Cola*	1 Bottle/500ml	145	0	29	0	7.2	0	0
Zero, Coca-Cola*	1 Can/330ml	2	0	0	0	0	0	0

DRAGON FRUIT

INFO/WEIGHT	Measure	per Measure KCAL	FAT	Nutrition Values per 100g / 100ml KCAL	PROT	CARB	FAT	FIBRE
Raw, Edible Portion, Average	*1 Serving/100g*	*41*	*0.5*	*41*	*0.7*	*9.6*	*0.5*	*3.6*

DRAMBUIE

INFO/WEIGHT	Measure	per Measure KCAL	FAT	Nutrition Values per 100g / 100ml KCAL	PROT	CARB	FAT	FIBRE
39% Volume	*1 Pub Shot/35ml*	*125*	*0*	*358*	*0*	*23*	*0*	*0*

DREAM TOPPING

INFO/WEIGHT	Measure	per Measure KCAL	FAT	Nutrition Values per 100g / 100ml KCAL	PROT	CARB	FAT	FIBRE
Dry, Bird's*	1oz/28g	193	16.4	690	6.7	32.5	58.5	0.5
Sugar Free, Dry, Bird's*	1oz/28g	195	16.9	695	7.3	30.5	60.5	0.5

DRESSING

INFO/WEIGHT	Measure	per Measure KCAL	FAT	Nutrition Values per 100g / 100ml KCAL	PROT	CARB	FAT	FIBRE
French Style, BGTY, Sainsbury's*	1 Tbsp/15ml	11	0.4	76	0.7	12.6	2.5	0.5
Aioli, Deli Style, Light, Praise*	1 Tbsp/20ml	76	7.1	380	5	15.5	35.5	0
Balsamic Bliss, Ainsley Harriott*	1 Tbsp/15g	41	3.2	272	0.8	19.3	21.1	0
Balsamic Glaze, Odysea *	1 Tsp/5ml	9	0	171	0.5	40	0	0
Balsamic Vinegar, Asda*	1 Pack/44ml	121	11.9	275	0.9	7	27	0
Balsamic Vinegar, Light, Kraft*	1 Serving/15ml	15	0.9	100	0.3	9.6	6.3	0.5
Balsamic Vinegar, Morrisons*	1 Serving/15ml	17	0.2	111	0.1	22.9	1.6	0.1
Balsamic with Olive Oil, Pizza Express*	1 Serving/10g	42	4.1	421	0.3	10.3	41.2	0
Balsamic, Fig Glaze, Tesco*	1 Tbsp/15ml	31	0	208	1.4	47.9	0	0
Balsamic, LC, Tesco*	1 Tbsp/14g	12	0.2	85	0.3	16.7	1.5	0.2
Balsamic, M&S*	1 Tbsp/15g	74	7.2	490	0.3	9.7	48	0.5
Balsamic, New, Sainsbury's*	1 Tbsp/15g	58	5.2	389	0.6	18.3	34.8	0.8

DRESSING

INFO/WEIGHT	Measure	per Measure KCAL	FAT	Nutrition Values per 100g / 100ml KCAL	PROT	CARB	FAT	FIBRE
Balsamic, Oak Aged, TTD, Sainsbury's*	1 Tbsp/15ml	54	4.8	338	0.5	16.3	30	0.5
Balsamic, Sweet, BGTY, Sainsbury's*	1 Tsp/5g	3	0	61	0.5	13.6	0.5	0.5
Balsamic, Sweet, Finest, Tesco*	1 Serving/10ml	16	0	155	0.4	36.9	0.1	0.4
Balsamic, Vinaigrette, Newman's Own*	1 Tbsp/15ml	56	5.7	372	0.1	7.2	38.2	0.5
Balsamic, Weight Watchers*	1 Serving/15ml	12	0.3	81	0.1	16	1.8	0.5
Blue Cheese, British, Specially Selected, Aldi*	1 Tbsp/15ml	60	6	403	2	9.3	40	0.9
Blue Cheese, Hellmann's*	1 Tbsp/15g	69	7.1	459	0.7	6.3	47.2	1.1
Blue Cheese, Salad, Waitrose*	1 Serving/50g	265	25.2	530	2.1	17.3	50.3	4.1
Caesar Style, GFY, Asda*	1 Sachet/44ml	34	1	77	5	9	2.3	0
Caesar, 95% Fat Free, Tesco*	1 Tsp/6g	5	0.2	88	4.1	8.9	3.7	0.3
Caesar, Asiago, Briannas*	1 Tbsp/15ml	70	7.5	467	3.3	3.3	50	0
Caesar, Chilled, Reduced Fat, Tesco*	1 Tsp/5ml	13	1.2	252	6.5	3.1	23.7	0.1
Caesar, Classic, Sainsbury's*	1 Tsp/5ml	22	2.3	442	2.7	4.6	45.9	0.5
Caesar, Fat Free, Average	*1 Tsp/5g*	*4*	*0.2*	*84*	*4.6*	*11*	*4.1*	*0.2*
Caesar, Finest, Tesco*	1 Tbsp/15ml	72	7.6	477	1.9	2.8	50.9	0.2
Caesar, Fresh, Asda*	1 Dtsp/10ml	45	4.8	454	2.4	3.2	48	0
Caesar, Hellmann's*	1 Tsp/6g	30	3.1	499	2.5	4.5	51.7	0.3
Caesar, LC, Tesco*	1 Serving/15g	9	0.2	60	1.5	9.5	1.5	0.5
Caesar, Less Than 3% Fat, BGTY, Sainsbury's*	1 Serving/20g	10	0.4	48	0.8	7	1.9	0.3
Caesar, Low Fat, Average	*1 Tsp/5g*	*4*	*0.1*	*77*	*2.3*	*11.1*	*2.6*	*0.2*
Caesar, Mary Berry*	1 Serving/100g	573	56.9	573	2.4	12.8	56.9	0.1
Caesar, Original, Cardini's*	1 Serving/10g	56	6	555	2.3	1.5	60	0.2
Caesar, Tesco*	1 Tbsp/15ml	65	6.8	435	0.9	5.4	45.1	0.3
Caesar, Waitrose*	1 Serving/15ml	72	7.6	479	4.5	0.9	50.8	0.2
Classic French, Fresh, M&S*	1 Serving/10ml	52	5.3	515	0.6	8.2	53.1	0.2
Cream Cheese & Chive, Creamy Ranch, Kraft*	1 Serving/15ml	31	2.6	205	1.2	11	17	0
Creamy Ranch, 95% Fat Free, Kraft*	1 Tsp/6ml	7	0.3	111	1.4	14.5	5	0.3
Creme Fraiche, Salad, Kraft*	1 Tbsp/15ml	12	0.4	78	0.8	12.5	2.5	0
Dijon Honey Mustard, Briannas*	1 Tbsp/15ml	65	6	433	0	20	40	0
Fat Free, Vinegar & Oil Based, Average	*1 Tsp/5g*	*2*	*0*	*37*	*0.4*	*7.9*	*0.2*	*0.4*
French Salad, M&S*	1 Serving/25ml	156	16.8	625	0.5	3.8	67.3	0.1
French, Batts, Lidl*	2 Tbsp/30ml	95	8.7	317	1.7	12	29	0
French, Chilled, Tesco*	1 Tbsp/15ml	63	5.9	421	1.1	15.1	39.6	0
French, Classic, Sainsbury's*	1 Tbsp/15ml	71	7.4	473	1	5.7	49.6	0.5
French, Classics, M&S*	1 Tbsp/15ml	77	8	516	0.6	8.2	53.1	0.2
French, Finest, Tesco*	1 Tbsp/15g	56	5.8	370	0.4	5.1	38.7	1
French, Fresh, Organic, Sainsbury's*	1 Tbsp/15ml	45	4.6	301	0.4	5.5	31	0.4
French, Fresh, Sainsbury's*	1 Tbsp/15ml	64	6.7	429	0.6	6.6	44.6	0.6
French, LC, Tesco*	1 Tbsp/16g	8	0.3	50	0.8	7.6	1.6	1.1
French, Less Than 3% Fat, M&S*	1 Tbsp/15ml	10	0.4	68	0.7	11.5	2.6	0.7
French, Reduced Fat, M&S*	1 Tbsp/15g	10	0.4	70	0.7	11.5	2.8	0.7
French, Sainsbury's*	1 Tbsp/15ml	33	2.9	219	0.6	9.8	19.1	0.5
French, Tesco*	1 Serving/25ml	110	11.2	441	0.7	7.2	44.9	0.2
French, Virtually Fat Free, Aldi*	1 Serving/10g	3	0	33	0.9	6.7	0.3	1.1
Garlic & Herb, Reduced Calorie, Hellmann's*	1 Tbsp/15ml	35	2.9	232	0.6	12.8	19.3	0.4
Garlic & Herb, Tesco*	1 Tbsp/15g	32	3	210	0.9	5.8	20.2	0.8
Ginger & Toasted Sesame, Naturally Righteous *	1 Serving/15ml	66	6.3	440	2.7	16	42	0
Honey & Mustard, BGTY, Sainsbury's*	1 Tbsp/20g	14	0.1	71	0.4	16.1	0.5	0.2
Honey & Mustard, Finest, Tesco*	1 Serving/25ml	72	5.6	288	1.7	19.6	22.5	0.7
Honey & Mustard, Fresh, M&S*	1 Serving/10ml	43	4.2	430	1.7	9.7	42.4	0.5
Honey & Mustard, Hellmann's*	1 Serving/15ml	27	0.2	182	0.7	13.7	1.6	0.3
Honey & Mustard, LC, Tesco*	1 Tbsp/13.8g	9	0.2	65	1.3	11.6	1.1	0.6
Honey & Mustard, M&S*	1 Tbsp/15ml	64	6.4	427	1.7	9.7	42.4	0.6

D

	Measure INFO/WEIGHT	per Measure KCAL	FAT	Nutrition Values per 100g / 100ml KCAL	PROT	CARB	FAT	FIBRE
DRESSING								
Honey & Mustard, Sainsbury's*	1 Serving/10ml	37	3.3	366	1	15.4	33	0.1
Honey & Mustard, Tesco*	1 Tbsp/15ml	33	2.3	220	0.8	18.8	15.2	2.5
Honey, Orange & Mustard, BGTY, Sainsbury's*	1 Tbsp/15ml	16	0.4	105	1.8	18.6	2.5	1.8
Italian Balsamic, Loyd Grossman*	1 Serving/10g	36	3.4	357	0.9	13.1	33.5	0.1
Italian, Salad, Essential, Waitrose*	1 Serving/15ml	62	6	414	0.3	12	40.4	0.5
Lemon & Cracked Black Pepper, GFY, Asda*	1 Tbsp/15g	9	0	57	0.2	14	0	0.3
Lemongrass, Ginger & Lime, Waitrose*	1 Serving/5ml	27	2.9	544	1.2	5.6	57.3	0.5
Oil & Lemon	**1 Tbsp/15g**	**97**	**10.6**	**647**	**0.3**	**2.8**	**70.6**	**0**
Olive Oil & Balsamic Vinegar, Sainsbury's*	1 Serving/25ml	104	10.4	415	0.9	9.4	41.8	0.2
Passion Fruit & Mango, HE, Tesco*	1 Tbsp/15ml	25	0.3	169	0.6	36.7	2.2	0.4
Raspberry, & Balsamic, with Rosemary, Suzanne's*	1 Tbsp/15ml	22	0	148	1	48.1	0.1	0.5
Salad, Honey & Mustard, Light, Kraft*	1 Tbsp/15ml	19	0.7	126	1.2	19	4.6	1.1
Salad, Italian, Newman's Own*	1 Tbsp/15g	82	9	545	0.2	1	59.8	0
Salad, Mary Berry*	1 Serving/15g	77	6.6	513	0.8	28.5	44	0.1
Salad, Raspberry Balsamic, GFY, Asda*	1 Tbsp/15ml	6	0.1	40	0.7	9.3	0.7	1.3
Sauce, Dressing, Finest, Tesco*	1 Serving/30ml	108	11.1	360	3.5	2.9	37.1	0.9
Thousand Island	**1 Tsp/6g**	**19**	**1.8**	**323**	**1.1**	**12.5**	**30.2**	**0.4**
Thousand Island, BGTY, Sainsbury's*	1 Serving/20g	19	1.4	95	0.4	7.3	7.2	0.5
Thousand Island, Eat Smart, Morrisons*	1 Tbsp/15ml	38	3.2	253	0	0	21.3	0
Thousand Island, Hellmann's*	1 Tbsp/15ml	36	3	238	1	14	20	0
Thousand Island, Reduced Calorie	**1 Tsp/6g**	**12**	**0.9**	**195**	**0.7**	**14.7**	**15.2**	**0**
Thousand Island, Tesco*	1 Tbsp/15g	55	4.7	360	1.1	19.5	30.5	0.3
Thousand Island, Walden Farms*	2 Tbsps/30ml	3	0	9	0	4.3	0	1
Tomato & Red Pepper, BGTY, Sainsbury's*	1 Serving/50ml	42	2.2	83	1.1	10	4.3	0.6
True Blue Cheese, Briannas*	2 Tbsp/30ml	120	11	400	3.3	16.7	36.7	0
Whole Grain Dijon Mustard & Honey, Loyd Grossman*	1oz/28g	93	8.9	331	1.2	9.9	31.8	1.3
Yoghurt & Mint, HE, Tesco*	1 Tbsp/15g	20	0.4	135	1.5	26.2	2.7	0
Yoghurt & Mint, HL, Tesco*	1 Serving/50g	31	1.2	62	4.1	6.9	2.5	0.2
Yoghurt & Mint, PB, Waitrose*	1 Serving/100ml	130	2.6	130	4.6	22.1	2.6	0.7
Yoghurt & Mint, Crucials*	1 Tbsp/15g	58	5.9	387	1.4	6.2	39.5	0.4
DRIED FRUIT								
Apples & Sultanas, The Foodie Market, Aldi*	1 Pack/30g	86	0.2	287	2.1	67	0.5	4.3
Apricots, Soft, Alesto, Lidl*	1 Serving/30g	69	0.2	230	1.3	51.1	0.7	6.7
Banana, Bites, Kiddylicious, Babylicious*	1 Serving/15g	74	4	493	1.7	65.1	26.8	6.6
Banana, Raw, Terrafertil*	1 Banana/25g	70	0.2	282	4	56.5	0.6	17.5
Beach Bum, Graze*	1 Pack/28g	93	4.2	332	4	46	15	9
Dragons Nest, Kids, Graze*	1 Punnet/33g	119	3.3	362	3	68	10	4
Figgy Pop, Graze*	1 Pack/40g	100	0.4	251	2.5	61.6	1.1	0
Goji Berry, Graze*	1 Pack/45g	234	17.3	521	17.1	28.4	38.4	0
Honey Coated Banana Chips, Whitworths*	1 Serving/25g	132	7.8	526	1	59.9	31.4	1.7
Mixed, Value, Tesco*	1 Serving/25g	71	0.2	285	2.1	67.5	0.7	2.3
Pineapple, Sweetened, Whitworths*	1 Bag/35g	122	0.1	350	0.4	86.3	0.2	0.5
Prunes, Juicy, Whitworths*	1 Pack/500g	740	2	148	2.5	34	0.4	5.7
Raisin & Chocolate, Shot, Whitworths*	1 Pack/25g	91	2.3	364	4	63.2	9.2	5.6
Strawberry, Banana & Cherry, Sunshine Mix, Graze*	1 Pack/50g	78	0.2	157	9.7	37.2	0.4	0
Trail Mix, Kick Start, Wholefoods, Asda*	1 Serving/50g	194	10.2	387	10.9	40	20.4	10.7
DRIED FRUIT MIX								
5 Fruits, Ready to Eat, Sundora*	½ Pack/100g	233	0.4	233	1.6	58.4	0.4	6.8
Agadoo, Pineapple, Jumbo & Green Raisins, Graze*	1 Pack/40g	110	0.4	275	2.1	69	0.9	0
Apple Strudel, Graze*	1 Pack/40g	99	0.3	247	2.2	58.7	0.7	5.9
Asda*	1 Serving/50g	152	0.2	305	2	74	0.5	0.6
Average	**1 Tbsp/25g**	**67**	**0.1**	**268**	**2.3**	**68.1**	**0.4**	**2.2**
Berry, Love Life, Waitrose*	1 Serving/30g	89	0.3	296	1.9	70	0.9	3

	Measure INFO/WEIGHT	per Measure		Nutrition Values per 100g / 100ml				
		KCAL	FAT	KCAL	PROT	CARB	FAT	FIBRE
DRIED FRUIT MIX								
Berry, Whole Foods, Tesco*	1 Serving/25g	66	0.2	265	3.3	60	0.7	7.5
Dates, Raisins & Apricots, Wholefoods, Tesco*	1 Serving/20g	52	0.1	260	3.1	59	0.4	4
Eden, Graze*	1 Punnet /25g	69	0.2	275	2	63.7	1	8.1
Exotic Mix, Sundora*	1 Sm Pack/50g	138	1.4	276	2.3	60.6	2.7	3.8
Fruit & Oat Bites, Mixed Berry, Planet Lunch*	1 Bar/20g	53	0.6	265	3.9	56	2.8	8
Garden of England, Graze*	1 Punnet/25g	70	0.2	280	1	71.2	0.7	5.6
Little Figgy Went to Market, Graze*	1 Punnet/36g	97	0.3	272	2	66	0.9	7
Luxury, Co-Op*	1 Serving/40g	114	0.2	285	2	68	0.6	4
Pear Tatin, Graze*	1 Punnet/35g	143	6.3	408	7	57.2	18.1	5.9
Raisins & Berries, Tesco*	1 Pot/60g	200	0.3	334	2.2	78.2	0.5	3.8
Raisins Mix, Wholesome, Love Life, Waitrose*	1 Serving/30g	88	0.3	293	2.1	69	0.9	3.7
Scandinavian Forest, Graze*	1 Punnet/28g	79	0.2	282	2	71	0.6	8
Scrumptious Blueberry Swirl, Graze*	1 Punnet/40g	155	3.2	392	1.2	76	8	3
Sultanas Raisins & Cranberries, Dunnes*	1 Handful/15g	47	0.1	315	2	80.2	0.9	4.7
Sultanas, Currants, Raisins & Citrus Peel, Asda*	1 Serving/100g	283	0.5	283	2.6	67	0.5	1.7
Taste of Hawaii, Extra Special, Asda*	1 Serving/100g	314	0.8	314	1.7	75	0.8	4.4
Tesco*	1 Tbsp/25g	71	0.1	284	2.3	67.9	0.4	2.2
Traditional, Bake With, Whitworths*	1 Serving/30g	84	0.2	279	2.1	64.7	0.8	2.2
Tropical Sundae, Graze*	1 Punnet/29g	86	0.3	299	2.7	72.7	1	8.5
Vine Fruit, Wholesome, Waitrose*	1 Serving/30g	87	0.1	289	2.1	69.3	0.4	5.3
Wholefoods, Tesco*	1 Serving/25g	79	0.2	315	1.6	73.6	0.9	3
DRIFTER								
Nestle*	1 Finger/20g	99	4.3	484	4.1	68.9	20.9	1.2
DRINKING CHOCOLATE								
Made Up with Semi-Skimmed Milk, Average	*1 Mug/227ml*	*129*	*4.3*	*57*	*3.5*	*7*	*1.9*	*0.2*
Made Up with Skimmed Milk, Average	*1 Mug/227ml*	*100*	*1.1*	*44*	*3.5*	*7*	*0.5*	*0*
Made Up with Whole Milk, Average	*1 Mug/227ml*	*173*	*9.5*	*76*	*3.4*	*6.8*	*4.2*	*0.2*
Powder, Made Up with Skimmed Milk	*1 Mug/227ml*	*134*	*1.4*	*59*	*3.5*	*10.8*	*0.6*	*0*
Powder, Made Up with Whole Milk	*1 Mug/227ml*	*204*	*9.3*	*90*	*3.4*	*10.6*	*4.1*	*0*
DRIPPING								
Beef	*1oz/28g*	*249*	*27.7*	*891*	*0*	*0*	*99*	*0*
DUCK								
Breast, Meat Only, Cooked, Average	*1oz/28g*	*48*	*2*	*172*	*25.3*	*1.8*	*7*	*0*
Breast, Meat Only, Raw, Average	*1 Serving/160g*	*206*	*6.8*	*128*	*22.6*	*0*	*4.2*	*0.2*
Breast, Roast, & Blueberries, Everdine*	1 Serving/450g	436	18.4	97	6	7.7	4.1	2.9
Leg, Meat & Skin, Average	*1oz/28g*	*80*	*5.6*	*286*	*17.2*	*0.5*	*20*	*0.4*
Raw, Meat Only, Weighed with Fat, Skin & Bone	*1 Serving/100g*	*38*	*1.8*	*38*	*5.5*	*0*	*1.8*	*0*
Raw, Meat, Fat & Skin	*1oz/28g*	*109*	*10.4*	*388*	*13.1*	*0*	*37.3*	*0*
Roast, Duckling, Half, Irish, Crispy, Deluxe, Lidl*	1 Serving/50g	172	12.4	343	13.1	17.4	24.7	0
Roasted, Meat Only, Weighed with Fat, Skin & Bone	*1 Serving/100g*	*41*	*2.2*	*41*	*5.3*	*0*	*2.2*	*0*
Roasted, Meat, Fat & Skin	*1oz/28g*	*118*	*10.7*	*423*	*20*	*0*	*38.1*	*0*
DUCK &								
Plum Sauce, Roasted, Sainsbury's*	½ Pack/150g	174	3.8	116	6.9	16	2.5	1.8
DUCK AROMATIC								
Crispy, Asda*	1/3 Pack/166g	469	24.9	283	19	18	15	0.8
Crispy, Half Duck & Pancakes, M&S*	½ Pack/311g	590	26.7	190	13.9	14	8.6	2.1
Crispy, Half with Hoisin Sauce & 12 Pancakes, Tesco*	1/6 Pack/70g	162	7.4	232	18.3	15.9	10.6	1.1
Crispy, Quarter with Hoisin Sauce & 6 Pancakes, Tesco*	1/6 Pack/40g	100	4.2	250	12.3	25.3	10.6	2
Crispy, Somerfield*	1 Serving/265g	782	49	295	18.1	14	18.5	0.7
Crispy, Whole with Hoisin Sauce & 18 Pancakes, Tesco*	1/9 Pack/100g	280	17.2	280	18.9	12	17.2	0.4
with a Plum Sauce, Finest, Tesco*	1 Serving/250g	400	14	160	16.1	11.3	5.6	4.6
with Plum Sauce, Tesco*	½ Pack/250g	350	11.5	140	9.3	15.2	4.6	0.3

D

	Measure INFO/WEIGHT	per Measure KCAL	FAT	Nutrition Values per 100g / 100ml KCAL	PROT	CARB	FAT	FIBRE
DUCK CANTONESE								
Style, Roast, Tesco*	1 Pack/300g	375	6.9	125	8.2	17.9	2.3	0.5
DUCK IN								
a Plum Sauce, Crispy, M&S*	1 Pack/325g	569	31.2	175	10.7	11.2	9.6	0.9
Chinese Barbecue, Wings, Sainsbury's*	1 Serving/175g	430	25	246	19.4	9.7	14.3	0
Filo Pastry, Christmas Trees, Iceland*	1 Tree/24g	63	2.4	267	9.6	32.8	10	3.6
Orange Sauce, Breast, Simply, Gressingham Foods*	½ Pack/175g	254	11.9	145	15.9	5.1	6.8	0.4
Orange Sauce, Roast, a L'Orange, M&S*	½ Pack/259g	482	26.9	186	16.2	6.5	10.4	0.8
DUCK PEKING								
Crispy, Aromatic, Sainsbury's*	½ Pack/300g	1236	110.7	412	19.5	0.6	36.9	0.1
DUCK WITH								
Port & Orange Sauce, Legs, Slow Cooked, M&S*	½ Pack/158g	284	14.7	180	20.8	3.2	9.3	0.9
Noodles, Shanghai Roast, Sainsbury's*	1 Pack/450g	580	17.1	129	5.6	18	3.8	1.2
Pancakes & Hoisin Sauce, M&S*	1 Pack/80g	136	3.2	170	13	19.9	4	0.9
DUMPLINGS								
Average	*1oz/28g*	*58*	*3.3*	*208*	*2.8*	*24.5*	*11.7*	*0.9*
Dim Sum, Assorted Stuffing, Steamed, Restaurant	*1 Serving/100g*	*230*	*8.2*	*230*	*7.9*	*32*	*8.2*	*3*
Dim Sum, Chicken, Asian Fusion, Waitrose*	1 Dumpling/20g	30	0.4	152	9.5	22.8	2.2	1.4
Dim Sum, Chicken, Steamed, Restaurant	*1 Serving/100g*	*230*	*5.9*	*230*	*7.5*	*37*	*5.9*	*2.1*
Dim Sum, Chinese, Deep Fried, Restaurant	*1 Serving/100g*	*430*	*23*	*430*	*4.9*	*50*	*23*	*1.8*
Dim Sum, From Restaurant, Average	*1 Piece/12g*	*50*	*2.4*	*433*	*28.9*	*31.3*	*20.4*	*0*
Dim Sum, Meat Dumpling, Deep Fried, Restaurant	*1 Serving/100g*	*340*	*16*	*340*	*4.9*	*43*	*16*	*1*
Dim Sum, Pork, Restaurant, Average	*1 Serving/100g*	*270*	*7.3*	*270*	*7.3*	*43*	*7.3*	*1.6*
Dim Sum, Prawn, Steamed, Eat Well, M&S*	1 Dim Sum/20g	28	0.2	138	6.7	25.1	1.1	0.6
Dim Sum, Steamed, Prawn, M&S*	6 Dim Sum/120g	222	3.2	185	1.1	39	2.7	1.5
Dim Sum, Vegetable & Meat, Pan Fried, Restaurant	*1 Serving/100g*	*280*	*13*	*280*	*6.4*	*34*	*13*	*3.7*
Dim Sum, Vegetable & Meat, Steamed, Restaurant	*1 Serving/100g*	*240*	*7.9*	*240*	*5.9*	*37*	*7.9*	*2.5*
Dim Sum, Wonton, Deep Fried, Restaurant	*1 Serving/100g*	*430*	*29*	*430*	*9.7*	*32*	*29*	*1.2*
Gyozas, Chicken, Microwaved, Iceland*	1 Gyozas/18g	31	0.5	176	8.3	28	2.7	3.3
Homestyle, Baked Weight, Frozen, Aunt Bessie's*	1 Dumpling/49g	188	8.6	384	9.7	44.4	17.6	2.8
Mix, Cooked as Directed, Aunt Bessie's*	2 Dumplings/53g	126	4.9	238	4.5	33	9.2	2.4
Pork & Garlic Chive, Waitrose*	1 Pack/115g	215	8.1	187	9.4	20.4	7	1.1
Prawn Sui Mai, Selection, M&S*	6 Sui Mai/120g	143	0.8	119	9.4	13.3	0.7	1.5
Prawn, Siu Mai, Chinese, M&S*	8 Dumplings/170g	170	2.9	100	7.8	13.1	1.7	1.3
Vegetable, Steamed, Bibigo*	1 Dumpling/28g	29	1.9	103	6.9	18.5	6.7	1.4

	Measure INFO/WEIGHT	per Measure KCAL	FAT	Nutrition Values per 100g / 100ml KCAL	PROT	CARB	FAT	FIBRE
EASTER EGG								
After Eight Giant Chocolate Egg, Nestle*	¼ Egg Shell/50g	274	16.9	547	5.5	51.8	33.8	7.1
Buttons, Chocolate Egg Shell Only, Cadbury*	1 Med Egg/162g	859	48.6	530	7.5	56.8	30	0.7
Caramel, Chocolate Egg Shell Only, Cadbury*	1 Lge Egg/343g	1801	102.9	525	7.5	56.8	30	0.7
Chick, Dairy Milk, Chocolate Egg Shell Only, Cadbury*	1 Egg/167g	877	50.1	525	7.5	56.8	30	0.7
Chocolate Egg Shell Only, Dairy Milk, Cadbury*	1 Med Egg/178g	943	53.4	530	7.5	56.8	30	0.7
Chocolate Orange, Terry's*	1 Egg/120g	636	36.6	530	7.4	57	30.5	2.4
Creme Egg, Chocolate Egg Shell Only, Cadbury*	1 Egg/178g	943	53.4	530	7.5	56.8	30	0.7
Crunchie, Cadbury*	1 Med Egg/167g	885	50.1	530	7.5	56.8	30	0.7
Dark Chocolate, 70%, Green & Black's*	1 Med Egg/165g	960	69.5	580	9.1	36.5	42	10
Disney, Nestle*	1 Egg/65g	342	18.9	526	6.3	59.7	29.1	0.6
Flake, Chocolate Egg Shell Only, Cadbury*	1 Med Shell/153g	811	46.7	530	7.6	56.5	30.5	0.7
Galaxy Ripple Indulgence, with Chocolate Egg, Mars*	1 Egg Shell/198g	1047	57.2	529	7	59.2	28.9	1.6
Kit Kat, Chunky, Nestle*	1 Med Egg/235g	1248	67.2	531	5.3	62.3	28.6	1.7
Milk Chocolate, Nestle*	½ Egg/42g	205	9.7	489	5	65.2	23.1	0.5
Milk Chocolate, Swiss, Hollow, M&S*	1 Egg/18g	100	6.3	555	6.7	53.2	34.8	2.5
Milky Bar, Nestle*	1 Egg/40g	182	6.9	454	4.2	70.8	17.2	0
Roses, Chocolate Egg Shell Only, Cadbury*	1 Egg/200g	1060	60	530	7.5	56.8	30	0.7
Smarties, Nestle*	1 Med Egg/258g	1367	74	530	5.3	62.2	28.7	1.7
Twirl, Chocolate Egg Shell Only, Cadbury*	1 Lge Egg/325g	1722	97.5	530	7.5	56.8	30	0.7
White Chocolate, Thorntons*	1 Egg/360g	1958	109.1	544	5.5	62.2	30.3	2.1
Wispa, Chocolate Egg Shell Only, Cadbury*	1 Lg Egg/313g	1643	93.9	525	7.5	56.8	30	0.7
ECLAIR								
Chocolate, 25% Less Fat, Sainsbury's*	1 Eclair/58g	171	9.3	295	6.8	31.1	16	1.2
Chocolate, Asda*	1 Eclair/33g	144	11	436	6.7	27.3	33.3	4.8
Chocolate, Belgian, Fresh Cream, Tesco*	1 Eclair/61g	233	15.4	382	7.3	30.6	25.3	1
Chocolate, Fresh Cream, M&S*	1 Eclair/43.6g	170	12.2	390	6.3	28.4	27.9	2
Chocolate, Fresh Cream, Sainsbury's*	1 Eclair/59g	212	13.9	360	4.2	32.7	23.6	0.5
Chocolate, Frozen, Morrisons*	1 Eclair/31g	116	9.6	374	5	18.8	31	1.3
Chocolate, Mini, Iceland*	1 Eclair/12g	49	3.6	418	5.3	29.3	30.8	1
EEL								
Cooked or Smoked, Dry Heat, Average	**1 Serving/100g**	**236**	**15**	**236**	**23.6**	**0**	**15**	**0**
Jellied, Average	**1oz/28g**	**26**	**1.9**	**93**	**8**	**0**	**6.7**	**0**
Raw, Average	**1oz/28g**	**32**	**2.1**	**113**	**11.1**	**0**	**7.6**	**0**
EGG SUBSTITUTE								
Vegan Egg, Follow Your Heart*	1 Serving/10g	40	1.7	401	5	0	17	40
EGGS								
Araucana, Bluebell, Free Range, Finest, Tesco*	1 Egg/50g	66	4.5	131	12.6	0.1	9	0
Dried, White, Average	**1 Tbsp/14g**	**41**	**0**	**295**	**73.8**	**0**	**0**	**0**
Dried, Whole, Average	**1oz/28g**	**159**	**11.6**	**568**	**48.4**	**0**	**41.6**	**0**
Duck, Boiled & Salted, Weight with Shell	**1 Egg/75g**	**148**	**11.6**	**198**	**14.6**	**0**	**15.5**	**0**
Duck, Whole, Raw, Weight with Shell	**1 Egg/75g**	**122**	**8.8**	**163**	**14.3**	**0**	**11.8**	**0**
Free Range, Large, Weight with Shell	**1 Egg/68g**	**97**	**6.8**	**143**	**12.6**	**0.8**	**9.9**	**0**
Fried in Veg Oil, Average	**1 Med/60g**	**107**	**8.3**	**179**	**13.6**	**0.7**	**13.9**	**0**
Fried, without Fat, Average	**1 Med/60g**	**104**	**7.6**	**174**	**15**	**0.7**	**12.7**	**0**
Goose, Whole, Fresh, Raw, Weight with Shell	**1 Egg/144g**	**232**	**16.6**	**161**	**12.1**	**1.2**	**11.5**	**0**
Large, Weight with Shell	**1 Egg/68g**	**97**	**6.8**	**143**	**12.6**	**0.8**	**9.9**	**0**
Medium, Boiled, Weight with Shell	**1 Egg/60g**	**86**	**6**	**143**	**12.6**	**0.8**	**9.9**	**0**
Medium, Weight with Shell	**1 Egg/58g**	**83**	**5.8**	**143**	**12.6**	**0.8**	**9.9**	**0**
Poached, Weight with Shell	**1 Med/58g**	**83**	**5.8**	**143**	**12.6**	**0.8**	**9.9**	**0**
Quail, Whole, Raw, Weight with Shell	**1 Egg/13g**	**20**	**1.4**	**151**	**12.9**	**0.4**	**11.1**	**0**
Savoury, Bites, Mini, Sainsbury's*	1 Egg/12g	35	2.2	288	9.4	21.7	17.8	1.6
Savoury, Mini, Tesco*	1 Egg/20g	55	3.5	274	9.2	20.2	17.4	2.3
Savoury, Vegetarian, Mini, Quorn*	1 Egg/20g	51	2.3	257	15	21	11.5	4.6

E

	Measure INFO/WEIGHT	per Measure KCAL	FAT	Nutrition Values per 100g / 100ml KCAL	PROT	CARB	FAT	FIBRE
EGGS								
Scotch, Asda*	1 Egg/114g	286	19.2	251	11.2	13.7	16.8	1.4
Scotch, Cumberland, Waitrose*	1 Egg/114g	243	14.3	214	13	12.1	12.6	1.6
Scotch, Finest, Tesco*	1 Egg/114g	280	20.1	247	11.6	10.4	17.7	1.1
Scotch, Free Range, Sainsbury's*	1 Egg/112.7g	284	19	252	12.4	12.5	16.9	2.5
Scotch, Lincolnshire, M&S*	1 Egg/114g	306	21.1	268	12	12.8	18.5	1.2
Scotch, Morrisons*	1 Egg/114g	286	19.1	251	11.2	13.7	16.8	1.4
Scotch, Retail	*1 Egg/120g*	*301*	*20.5*	*251*	*12*	*13.1*	*17.1*	*0*
Scrambled with Milk, Average	*1 Serving/100g*	*257*	*23.4*	*257*	*10.9*	*0.7*	*23.4*	*0*
Scrambled, Average	*1 Serving/100g*	*160*	*11.6*	*160*	*13.8*	*0*	*11.6*	*0*
Turkey, Whole, Raw, Weight with Shell	*1 Egg/79g*	*135*	*9.6*	*171*	*13.7*	*1.2*	*12.2*	*0*
Very Large, Average, Weight with Shell	*1 Egg/78g*	*112*	*7.8*	*143*	*12.6*	*0.8*	*9.9*	*0*
White, Free Range, Liquid, Two Chicks*	3 Tbsp/45g	23	0	50	10.5	1	0	0
Whites Only, Raw, Average	*1 Lg Egg/33g*	*12*	*0*	*36*	*9*	*0*	*0*	*0*
Yolks, Raw	*1 Yolk/14g*	*47*	*4.3*	*339*	*16.1*	*0*	*30.5*	*0*
ELICHE								
Dry Weight, Buitoni*	1 Serving/80g	282	1.5	352	11.2	72.6	1.9	0
ELK								
Raw, Meat only	*1 Serving/100g*	*111*	*1.4*	*111*	*23*	*0*	*1.4*	*0*
Roasted, Meat only	*1 Serving/100g*	*146*	*1.9*	*146*	*30.2*	*0*	*1.9*	*0*
ENCHILADAS								
3 Bean, Ready Meal, Average	*1 Pack/400g*	*505*	*16.6*	*126*	*4.4*	*16.9*	*4.2*	*3.2*
Beef, LC, Tesco*	1 Pack/400g	440	11.2	110	5.4	13.4	2.8	3.1
Chicken, American, HL, Tesco*	1 Serving/240g	353	4.3	147	10.4	22.5	1.8	1.2
Chicken, Asda*	1 Serving/500g	690	30	138	10	17	6	1
Chicken, Average	*1 Serving/295g*	*483*	*18.8*	*164*	*11.6*	*16*	*6.4*	*1.7*
Chicken, Diner Specials, M&S*	½ Pack/227g	340	12	150	9.9	15.4	5.3	2
Chicken, in a Spicy Salsa & Bean Sauce, Asda*	½ Pack/212g	373	17	176	10	16	8	0
Chicken, PB, Waitrose*	1 Pack/450g	482	14.4	107	6.9	12.7	3.2	1.1
Chicken, Suiza, Smart Ones, Weight Watchers*	1 Pack/255g	290	5	114	4.3	18	2	1.2
Spicy, Three Bean, Cooked, CBY, Asda*	1 Pack/400g	466	15.9	117	4.4	13.7	4	4.1
Vegetable, & Bean, Eat Smart, Morrisons*	1 Pack/380g	475	9.9	125	4.7	20.7	2.6	3.2
Vegetable, Morrisons*	1 Pack/400g	468	18.4	117	4.5	14.4	4.6	1.8
with Cheese & Beef, From Restaurant	*1 Serving/295g*	*496*	*27.1*	*168*	*6.2*	*15.9*	*9.2*	*0*
with Cheese, From Restaurant	*1 Serving/163g*	*319*	*18.8*	*196*	*5.9*	*17.5*	*11.6*	*0*
ENDIVE								
Raw	*1oz/28g*	*2*	*0*	*8*	*1.1*	*0.6*	*0.1*	*1.3*
ENERGY DRINK								
Average	*1 Can/250ml*	*118*	*0*	*47*	*0*	*11.4*	*0*	*0*
Blue Bolt, Sainsbury's*	1 Can/250ml	124	0	49	0	11.3	0	0
Cherry, Lucozade*	1 Bottle/500ml	345	0	69	0	17.1	0	0
Citrus Blast, Soft Drink, Mountain Dew, Britvic*	1 Bottle/500ml	240	0	48	0	13	0	0
Citrus, Isotonic, Umbro*	1 Bottle/500ml	139	0	28	0	6.5	0	0
Isostar Sport, Isostar*	1 Glass/250ml	74	0	30	0	7	0	0
Juiced Berry, Relentless*	1 Can/500g	230	0	46	0	10.7	0	0
Juiced Orange & Tropical Fruit, Relentless*	1 Can/500ml	220	0	44	0	10.7	0	0
KX, Sugar Free, Diet, Tesco*	1 Can/250ml	5	0	2	0	0	0	0
KX, Sugar Free, Tesco*	1 Can/250ml	8	0	3	0	0	0	0
Lemon, Active Sport, Tesco*	1 Bottle/500ml	135	0	27	0	6.5	0	0
Libertus, Blue, Sugar Free, Relentless*	1 Can/500ml	20	0	4	0	0	0	0
Monster*	1 Can/500ml	240	0	48	0	12	0	0
Orange, Active Sport, Tesco*	1 Bottle/500ml	135	0	27	0	6.5	0	0
Original, Rockstar*	1 Can/500ml	290	0	60	0.4	13.6	0	0
Powerade, Aqua+*	1 Bottle/500ml	80	0	16	0	3.7	0	0

	Measure INFO/WEIGHT	per Measure KCAL	FAT	Nutrition Values per 100g / 100ml KCAL	PROT	CARB	FAT	FIBRE
ENERGY DRINK								
Red Devil, Britvic*	1 Can/250ml	160	0	64	0.4	15.1	0	0
Red Rooster, Hi Energy Mixer, Cott Beverages Ltd*	1 Can/250ml	112	0	45	0.6	10.3	0	0
Red Thunder, Diet, Low Calorie, Aldi*	1 Can/250ml	5	0	2	0.1	0	0	0
Relentless, Original, Relentless*	1 Can/500ml	230	0	46	0	10.4	0	0
Relentless, Sugar Free, Coca-Cola*	1 Can/500ml	20	0	4	0	0	0	0
Revive, Cranberry with Acai, Light Sparkling, Lucozade*	1 Bottle/380ml	50	0	13	0	2.8	0	0
Simulation, Emerge, Aldi*	1 Can/105g	44	0.1	42	0	10	0.1	0.1
SoBe, Appleberry Burst, Britvic*	1 Can/250ml	135	0	54	0.4	12	0	0
Sparkling Orange, Dual Energy, Powerade*	1 Bottle/500ml	225	0	45	0	10.5	0	0
Sugar Free, Boost Drinks Ltd*	1 Can/250ml	5	0	2	0	0	0	0
Sugar Free, Diet, Mountain Dew, Britvic*	1 Can/440ml	3	0	1	0	0	0	0
Tropical, Emerge, Cott Beverages Ltd*	1 Can/250ml	115	0	46	0	10.7	0	0
Ultra Citron, Zero Calorie, Monster*	1 Can/500ml	9	0	2	0	1	0	0
Ultra Red, Zero Sugar Plus Calorie, Monster*	1 Can/500ml	15	0	3	0	0.9	0	0
Ultra, Zero Calorie, Monster*	1 Can/500ml	10	0	2	0	0.9	0	0
V, Frucor Beverages*	1 Can/250ml	112	0	45	0	11.2	0	0
ESCALOPE								
Vegetarian, Garlic & Herb, Quorn*	1 Escalope/140g	293	16.5	209	8.9	16.9	11.8	3.8
Vegetarian, Garlic & Mushroom, Creamy, Quorn*	1 Escalope/120g	291	15	243	10.5	20.5	12.5	3
Vegetarian, Gruyere Cheese, Quorn*	1 Escalope/110g	267	15.4	243	10	18	14	2.6
Vegetarian, Korma, Quorn*	1 Escalope/120g	270	15.6	225	7	20	13	3
Vegetarian, Lemon & Black Pepper, Quorn*	1 Escalope/110g	256	12.9	233	9.6	20.5	11.7	2.1
Vegetarian, Mozzarella & Pesto, Quorn*	1 Escalope/120g	271	15.6	226	10	15	13	4.5
Vegetarian, Turkey Style, Sage & Onion, Quorn*	1 Escalope/100g	188	9.8	188	10	15	9.8	4.5

E

	Measure INFO/WEIGHT	per Measure KCAL	FAT	Nutrition Values per 100g / 100ml KCAL	PROT	CARB	FAT	FIBRE
FAGGOTS								
British Pork with Streaky Bacon, Essential, Waitrose*	2 Faggots/128g	255	14.5	199	16.7	7.5	11.3	0.9
Mushy Peas & Mash, Sainsbury's*	1 Pack/450g	576	19.4	128	6	16.3	4.3	1.6
Pork, West Country Sauce, Six Pack, Cooked, Mr Brains*	2 Faggots/134g	170	8.8	127	5.5	10.9	6.6	1
FAJITA								
Beef, GFY, Asda*	½ Pack/208g	354	9.8	170	11	21	4.7	1.6
Chicken, Average	**1 Serving/240g**	**357**	**12.8**	**149**	**10.2**	**15**	**5.4**	**2.3**
Chicken, BGTY, Sainsbury's*	1 Pack/172g	256	4.3	149	10.8	20.9	2.5	1.7
Chicken, Co-Op*	1 Serving/230g	391	16.1	170	11	15	7	3
Chicken, COU, M&S*	1 Pack/230g	288	5.3	125	10	16.5	2.3	1.5
Chicken, M&S*	1 Pack/230g	345	12.2	150	8.6	17.7	5.3	1
Chicken, Mexican, No Mayo, Foo-Go*	1 Pack/198g	360	11.1	182	9.6	23.3	5.6	2.4
Chicken, Sainsbury's*	½ Pack/275g	396	14.6	144	9.5	14.5	5.3	1.9
Chicken, Salt Balanced, COU, M&S*	1 Pack/230g	253	5.3	110	9.5	13.2	2.3	1.7
Chicken, Tesco*	½ Pack /275g	382	14.3	139	9.2	13.9	5.2	1.9
Crispy Chicken, Old El Paso*	1 Fajita/70g	183	5.4	263	7.6	41	7.8	1.8
Gammon Steaks, Tesco*	1 Serving/250g	368	15.5	147	17.5	5.3	6.2	0
Meal Kit, Tesco*	1 Serving/100g	210	3.4	210	6.1	38.2	3.4	2.1
Mexican Style, Meal Kit, Made Up, CBY, Asda*	¼ Pack/120g	280	6.6	234	6	39	5.5	2.3
Mini Chicken, Tesco*	1 Fajita/18g	37	1.1	205	8.7	27.8	6.3	3.4
Sizzling Fajita Kit, Smoky BBQ, As Sold, Old El Paso*	1 Fajita/63g	141	2.3	224	6.8	40	3.7	1.8
Smoky Chicken, Everdine*	1 Serving/450g	585	15.3	130	9.1	14.3	3.4	3.1
Vegetable	**1 Serving/275g**	**472**	**14.9**	**172**	**4.9**	**25.6**	**5.4**	**1.9**
Vegetable, Tesco*	1 Fajita/112g	133	5.6	119	4.2	14.3	5	1.1
Vegetarian, Meal Kit, Quorn*	½ Pack/214g	268	5.4	125	7	18.5	2.5	3.5
Vegetarian, Strips, Cooked, Quorn*	½ Pack/70g	81	1.1	115	14.8	9.3	1.6	2.4
FALAFEL								
& Feta, Snack pot, Lovely Vegetables, M&S*	1 Pack/300g	270	13.2	90	4.4	8.5	4.4	5.2
& Houmous, Snack Pot, Tesco*	1 Pack/106g	354	26.2	324	8.4	14.5	24	8.4
12 pack, Sainsbury's*	1 Falafel/17g	44	2.5	259	7.3	20.6	14.8	7.2
Asda*	½ Pack/50g	140	9.6	281	8.3	18.9	19.1	8.2
Authentic Mediterranean, Great Food*	1 Falafel/22g	56	2.6	253	9.1	29.9	11.7	4.1
Balls, Meat Free, Meat Free, Tesco*	3 Balls/67g	135	5.3	205	7.1	21.7	8.1	6.3
Fried in Vegetable Oil, Average	**1 Falafel/25g**	**45**	**2.8**	**179**	**6.4**	**15.6**	**11.2**	**3.4**
Gourmet, Meat Free, Vegideli, The Redwood Co*	1 Patty/16.7g	26	1.4	159	6.1	20.5	8.5	8.1
Herby & Aromatic, Waitrose*	2 Falafels/38g	85	3.4	224	8.5	23.3	8.9	8.4
Mini, M&S*	1 Falafel/14g	43	2.5	310	7.9	28.1	18.4	2.6
Mini, Sainsbury's*	1 Serving/168g	499	29.6	297	8	26.8	17.6	3.2
Mix, Asda*	1 Pack/120g	313	15	261	6.4	30.8	12.5	2.6
Mix, Authentic, Al'fez*	1 Serving/100g	235	13.8	235	7.1	26.3	13.8	8.8
Mix, Lebanese Style, Al'fez*	½ Pack/200g	470	27.6	235	7.1	26.3	13.8	0
Mix, Organic, Quick & Easy, Hale & Hearty*	1 Pack/200g	646	11	323	19.2	43.8	5.5	10.7
Moroccan Chicken & Butternut Squash, Asda*	1 Pack/400g	428	12	107	8.9	9.2	3	3.7
Organic, Cauldron Foods*	1 Falafel/25g	51	2.4	203	8.4	20.3	9.8	7.2
Original, Mediterranean, Great Food*	1 Falafel/22g	69	4	316	9.2	32	18.3	6.6
Shawarma, Everdine*	1 Serving/450g	590	18.4	131	4.5	16.7	4.1	5
Sweet Potato, Meat Free, Vegan, Tesco*	3 Falafels/62g	123	6.2	199	4.2	18.1	10	9.6
Vegetarian, Organic, Waitrose*	1 Felafel/25g	55	2.6	220	8	23.3	10.5	7.6
FANTA								
Fruit Twist, Coca-Cola*	1 Serving/250ml	132	0	53	0	13	0	0
Icy Lemon, Coca-Cola*	1 Can/330ml	112	0	34	0	8.3	0	0
Icy Lemon, Zero, Coca-Cola*	1 Can/330ml	7	0	2	0	0.2	0	0
Lemon, Coca-Cola*	1 Can/330ml	165	0	50	0	12	0	0
Light, Coca-Cola*	1 Glass/250ml	5	0	2	0	0.5	0	0

F

	Measure INFO/WEIGHT	per Measure KCAL	FAT	Nutrition Values per 100g / 100ml KCAL	PROT	CARB	FAT	FIBRE
FANTA								
Orange, Coca-Cola*	1 Glass/250ml	75	0	30	0	7.1	0	0
Orange, Zero, Coca-Cola*	1 Can/330ml	11	0	3	0	0.5	0	0
Peach, Singapore, Coca-Cola*	1 Bottle/500ml	230	0	46	0	11	0	0
Red Fruits, Coca-Cola*	1 Serving/100ml	37	0	37	0	9	0	0
Summer Fruits, Z, Coca-Cola*	1fl oz/30ml	1	0	3	0	0.6	0	0
FARFALLE								
Bows, Dry, Average	***1 Serving/75g***	***265***	***1.4***	***353***	***11.4***	***72.6***	***1.9***	***1.9***
Salmon, Hot Smoked, Slimming World*	1 Pack/550g	605	12.1	110	6	15.3	2.2	2.4
FAT								
Duck, Sainsbury's*	1 Serving/15g	135	15	900	0.5	0.5	100	0.5
Goose, Sainsbury's*	1 Serving/15g	135	14.9	897	0.5	0.7	99.3	0.5
Vegetable, Pure, Trex*	1 Tbsp/12g	108	12	900	0	0	100	0
FENNEL								
Florence, Boiled in Salted Water	***1oz/28g***	***3***	***0.1***	***11***	***0.9***	***1.5***	***0.2***	***2.3***
Florence, Raw, Unprepared, Average	***1 Bulb/250g***	***24***	***0.4***	***10***	***0.7***	***1.4***	***0.2***	***1.9***
Florence, Steamed	***1 Serving/80g***	***9***	***0.2***	***11***	***9***	***1.5***	***0.2***	***2.3***
FENUGREEK								
Leaves, Raw, Fresh, Average	***1 Serving/80g***	***28***	***0.2***	***35***	***4.6***	***4.8***	***0.2***	***1.1***
FETTUCCINE								
Chicken & Roasted Pepper, Love Life, Waitrose*	1 Pack/375g	329	5.7	92	6.3	12.1	1.6	1.9
Chicken, Cajun Spiced, COU, M&S*	1 Pack/400g	400	8	100	8	12.3	2	1.3
Dry Weight, Buitoni*	1 Serving/90g	326	1.5	362	12.2	74.4	1.7	0
Edamame & Mung Bean, Explore Asian*	¼ Pack/50g	168	2.1	335	47.2	16.8	4.2	20.6
Slim Pasta, Eat Water*	½ Pack/100g	9	0	9	0.2	0	0	4
with Tomato & Mushroom, Easy Cook, Napolina*	1 Pack/120g	461	8.6	384	11.8	67.9	7.2	0
FIG ROLLS								
Asda*	1 Biscuit/19g	71	1.7	372	4.8	68	9	0
Bolands*	1 Biscuit/17g	63	1.4	372	4.1	68.3	8	5
Go Ahead, McVitie's*	1 Biscuit/15g	55	0.7	365	4.2	76.8	4.6	2.9
Jacob's*	1 Biscuit/17g	66	1.5	386	3.4	72.2	8.6	3
Sainsbury's*	1 Biscuit/19g	67	1.6	360	4.3	64.5	8.7	3.4
Vitalinea, Jacob's*	1 Biscuit/18g	61	1	339	3.7	68.2	5.8	3.8
FIGS								
Almond Stuffed, Kounos*	3 Figs/34g	99	22.2	291	2.2	63.9	65.3	0.2
Dried, Average	***1 Fig/14g***	***32***	***0.1***	***232***	***3.6***	***53.2***	***1.1***	***8.6***
Raw, Fresh, Average	***1 Fig/35g***	***16***	***0.1***	***45***	***1.3***	***9.8***	***0.2***	***1.5***
FISH								
Balls, Gefilte, M&S*	1 Pack/200g	280	7.8	140	14.1	11.9	3.9	1
Char, Arctic, Whole, Raw	***1 Serving/100g***	***137***	***6***	***137***	***20.8***	***0***	***6***	***0***
Chargrills, Sun Ripened Tomato, Basil, Birds Eye*	1 Chargrill/162g	123	2.6	76	14	1.5	1.6	0.5
Fillet, Battered Or Breaded, & Fried, From Restaurant	***1 Portion/256g***	***594***	***31.5***	***232***	***14.7***	***17***	***12.3***	***0.5***
Fillets in Parsley Sauce, Light & Easy, Youngs*	1 Pack/224g	139	4.3	62	8.4	2.8	1.9	1.4
Fillets, Dinner, Meal for One, Youngs*	1 Pack/378g	340	11	90	6	9.1	2.9	1.5
Fillets, Lemon & Pepper, Youngs*	1 Fillet/130g	283	16.7	218	10.3	15.3	12.9	4.3
Fillets, Lime & Chilli, Fish Fusions, Birds Eye*	1 Portion/160g	270	10.1	169	15	12.9	6.3	0.5
Garlic & Herb, Inspirations, Birds Eye*	½ Pack/160g	254	9.8	159	14	11.8	6.1	0.4
Goujons, Asda*	1 Serving/125g	240	8	192	12.8	20.8	6.4	0.2
Grouper	***1 Serving/100g***	***92***	***1***	***92***	***19.4***	***0***	***1***	***0***
Medley, SteamFresh, Birds Eye*	1 Bag/170g	170	6.3	100	13	2.3	3.7	0.1
Melts with Tomato & Mozzarella Filling, Birds Eye*	1 Fillet/100g	255	15	255	13	17	15	0.6
Pie Mix, Ocado*	1 Pack/320g	410	18.2	128	19	0	5.7	0
Pie Mix, Seasonal, Sainsbury's*	1 Pack/320g	480	28.2	150	17.7	0	8.8	0
Pouting, Fillets, Tesco*	1 Serving/100g	85	0.3	85	19.7	0.3	0.3	0

F

	Measure INFO/WEIGHT	per Measure KCAL	FAT	Nutrition Values per 100g / 100ml KCAL	PROT	CARB	FAT	FIBRE
FISH								
River Cobbler, Smoked, Tesco*	1 Fillet /165g	124	3.5	75	13.9	0	2.1	1.5
River Cobbler, Value, Tesco*	½ Pack/133g	133	5.3	100	15.1	0.1	4	0.1
Salted, Chinese, Steamed	*1oz/28g*	*43*	*0.6*	*155*	*33.9*	*0*	*2.2*	*0*
Sticks, Crunchy, Mrs. Paul's*	6 Sticks/95g	220	10	232	11.6	21	10.5	0
White, Smoked, Average	*1 Serving/100g*	*108*	*0.9*	*108*	*23.4*	*0*	*0.9*	*0*
FISH & CHIPS								
Breaded, Budgens*	1 Pack/340g	544	18	160	8.6	19.3	5.3	1.5
Co-Op*	1 Pack/250g	388	15	155	6	18	6	2
Mini Meal, 093, Wiltshire Farm Foods*	1 Serving/185g	255	8.3	138	6.9	17.7	4.5	2.8
Quinoa Coated, Everdine*	1 Serving/450g	405	16.2	90	6.9	5.7	3.6	3.6
Takeaway or Fast Food, Average	*1 Serving/469g*	*998*	*115.6*	*213*	*17.7*	*45.7*	*24.6*	*2.6*
Tesco*	1 Serving/300g	489	18.6	163	5.5	21.2	6.2	1.6
with Mushy Peas, Kershaws*	1 Pack/315g	450	18.3	143	6.4	16.4	5.8	1.6
FISH CAKES								
Breaded, Sainsbury's*	1 Cake/42g	75	3.4	179	10	16.2	8.1	0.7
Bubbly Batter, Youngs*	1 Cake/44g	109	6.7	247	7.1	20.5	15.1	1.4
Cod & Parsley, Waitrose*	1 Cake/85g	147	6.5	173	9.2	16.9	7.6	1.1
Cod & Pollock, Breaded, Youngs*	2 Cakes/98g	165	7.1	168	7.3	18.1	7.2	1.1
Cod & Prawn, Red Thai, Ovenbaked, Extra Special, Asda*	1 Cake/147g	258	8.6	176	9.5	20	5.9	2.3
Cod Fillet, & Sweet Potato, Finest, Tesco*	1 Cake/136g	202	6.4	149	8.4	17.1	4.7	2.3
Cod in Crunch Crumb, Birds Eye*	1 Cake/49.5g	93	4.3	187	11.4	16	8.6	1
Cod Mornay, Easy to Cook, Waitrose*	1 Cake/149g	234	9.1	157	10.5	15	6.1	1.4
Cod, As Consumed, Morrisons*	1 Cake/130g	221	9	170	9.5	17.2	6.9	0.8
Cod, Baked, (2 Pack), Tesco*	1 Cake/135g	255	9.9	189	9.1	21.1	7.3	3.2
Cod, Birds Eye*	1 Cake/51g	93	4.4	182	10	16	8.7	1.1
Cod, Breaded, Lighthouse Bay, Lidl*	1 Cake/132g	224	8.4	170	9.7	17.5	6.4	1.6
Cod, Chunky, Breaded, Chilled, Youngs*	1 Cake/90g	192	11.5	213	9.5	14.9	12.8	1.2
Cod, Fresh, Asda*	1 Cake/75g	164	8.2	219	7	23	11	1.6
Cod, Homemade, Average	*1 Cake/50g*	*120*	*8.3*	*241*	*9.3*	*14.4*	*16.6*	*0.7*
Cod, M&S*	1 Cake/85g	153	7.8	180	8.9	15.4	9.2	1.3
Cod, with Davidstow Cheddar, Aldi*	1 Cake/136g	252	12.1	185	6.3	19	8.9	1.3
Fried in Blended Oil	*1 Cake/50g*	*109*	*6.7*	*218*	*8.6*	*16.8*	*13.4*	*0*
Frozen, Average	*1 Cake/85g*	*112*	*3.3*	*132*	*8.6*	*16.7*	*3.9*	*0*
Haddock in Breadcrumbs, Sainsbury's*	1 Cake/88g	158	6.2	179	10.8	18.2	7	1.4
Haddock, & Vintage Cheddar, Smoked, Saucy Fish Co*	1 Cake/135g	220	7.6	163	9.7	18	5.6	0.9
Haddock, Sainsbury's*	1 Cake/135g	253	10	188	10.8	18.7	7.4	1.5
Haddock, Smoked, Breaded, Asda*	1 Cake/90g	202	11.7	225	9	18	13	1.6
Haddock, Smoked, Extra Special, Asda*	1 Cake/115g	218	10.9	190	12.8	13.2	9.5	1.3
Haddock, Smoked, M&S*	1 Cake/85g	153	8	180	10.6	13.4	9.4	2.6
Prawn, Thai Inspired, Finest, Tesco*	1 Cake/135g	196	6.8	145	9.5	14.6	5	1.8
Prawn, Thai Style, Finest, Tesco*	1 Cake/145g	305	13.5	210	6.7	24.2	9.3	1
Salmon & Dill, Waitrose*	1 Cake/85g	206	11.9	242	11.5	17.5	14	1.8
Salmon & Hollandaise Sauce, Saucy Fish Co*	1 Cake/135g	270	13	200	9.2	19.2	9.6	1.4
Salmon & Watercress, Aldi*	1 Cake/139g	316	18.1	227	10	17	13	0.5
Salmon Fillet & Spinach, Finest, Tesco*	1 Cake/133g	267	10.5	201	12.7	19.2	7.9	1
Salmon, & Broccoli, Morrisons*	1 Cake/110g	211	10.3	191	9	16.7	9.3	2.2
Salmon, Asda*	1 Cake/86g	215	12	250	8	23	14	1.4
Salmon, Coated in a Light & Crispy Breadcrumb, Tesco*	1 Cake/90g	212	10.8	235	9.7	21	12	1.2
Salmon, Ginger & Chilli, Sainsbury's*	1 Cake/150g	332	17	221	11.1	17.7	11.3	2.3
Salmon, Homemade, Average	*1 Cake/50g*	*136*	*9.8*	*273*	*10.4*	*14.4*	*19.7*	*0.7*
Salmon, M&S*	1 Cake/86g	180	10.9	210	9.1	15.1	12.7	1.7
Salmon, Melting Middle, Lochmuir, M&S*	1 Pack/290g	551	30.4	190	9.1	14.3	10.5	1.5

	Measure INFO/WEIGHT	per Measure KCAL	FAT	Nutrition Values per 100g / 100ml KCAL	PROT	CARB	FAT	FIBRE
FISH CAKES								
Salmon, Morrisons*	1 Cake/90g	241	11.8	268	10.1	27.6	13.1	1.5
Salmon, Sainsbury's*	1 Cake/88g	171	7.6	194	12.6	16.5	8.6	1.6
Salmon, Spinach & Sicilian Lemon, Finest, Tesco*	1 Cake/145g	290	16.2	200	9.9	14.3	11.2	1.4
Salmon, Tesco*	1 Cake/90g	239	13.5	266	11.4	21.3	15	0
Smart Price, Asda*	1 Cake/42g	78	3.3	188	7	22	8	0.9
Thai, Frozen, Sainsbury's*	1 Cake/15g	28	1.1	187	21.3	9.3	7.3	0.7
Thai, Oriental Selection, Waitrose*	1 Cake/11g	18	0.3	161	17.8	15.8	3	1.5
Tuna, Lime & Coriander, BGTY, Sainsbury's*	1 Cake/91g	200	10.7	220	10.7	17.7	11.8	2.6
Tuna, Sainsbury's*	1 Cake/90g	183	7.5	203	13.7	18.4	8.3	2.1
Value, Tesco*	1 Cake/42g	88	4.8	210	8.2	19.5	11.5	1.1
FISH FINGERS								
Chip Shop, Youngs*	1 Finger/30g	75	4.9	251	9.3	16.6	16.4	1.2
Chunky, Cooked, Tesco*	2 Fingers/98g	230	10	235	13.2	21.6	10.2	1.3
Cod, 100% Cod Fillet, Tesco*	1 Finger/30g	53	2.2	177	12.4	14.9	7.5	1.4
Cod, Fillets, Asda*	1 Finger/31g	66	3.1	214	13	18	10	0
Cod, Fillets, Chunky, M&S*	1 Finger/40g	70	2.4	175	12	17.2	6	1
Cod, Fillets, Essential, Waitrose*	1 Finger/28g	57	2.2	205	13.6	19.1	8	1.1
Cod, Fillets, Waitrose*	1 Finger/30g	55	2.2	183	11.9	16.9	7.5	0.7
Cod, Fried in Blended Oil, Average	*1 Finger/28g*	*67*	*3.9*	*238*	*13.2*	*15.5*	*14.1*	*0.6*
Cod, Frozen, Average	*1 Finger/28g*	*48*	*2.2*	*170*	*11.6*	*14.2*	*7.8*	*0.6*
Cod, Grilled, Average	*1 Finger/28g*	*56*	*2.5*	*200*	*14.3*	*16.6*	*8.9*	*0.7*
Cod, Morrisons*	1 Finger/30g	54	2.2	180	11.7	16.4	7.5	1.1
Cod, Sainsbury's*	1 Finger/28g	53	2.1	190	12.5	17.7	7.7	1
Cod, Youngs*	1 Finger/24g	50	2	209	13.3	19.8	8.3	0.8
Economy, Sainsbury's*	1 Finger/26g	51	2.2	198	12.6	17.7	8.5	1.3
Fishless, Vegan, Quorn*	1 Finger/20g	37	1.4	187	4.4	24.1	7.1	4.7
Free From, Sainsbury's*	1 Finger/30g	56	2.3	188	11.4	18	7.8	0.7
Haddock in Crispy Batter, Birds Eye*	1 Finger/30g	56	2.3	188	14.3	15.1	7.8	0.7
Haddock in Crunchy Crumb, Morrisons*	1 Finger/30g	57	2.4	190	13.1	16.3	8	1.1
Haddock, Fillets, Asda*	1 Finger/30g	62	2.7	205	14	17	9	0
Iceland*	1 Finger/23g	44	2	192	11.5	17.3	8.5	1.3
in Batter, Crispy, Jumbo, Morrisons*	1 Finger/71g	146	8.9	205	11.3	12.2	12.5	0.6
Omega 3, Grilled, Tesco*	3 Fingers/71g	150	6.8	210	12.4	17.8	9.5	1.3
Plaice, Cider Battered, M&S*	½ Pack/140g	372	24.6	266	12.3	14.1	17.6	1.2
Pollock, Sainsbury's*	3 Fingers/85g	160	6.7	188	13	15.9	7.9	0.8
Salmon, Birds Eye*	1 Finger/28g	63	2.7	225	13.2	21.7	9.5	0.9
FISH IN								
Butter Sauce, Steaks, Ross*	1 Serving/140g	111	4	84	10.6	3.6	3	0.3
Butter Sauce, Steaks, Youngs*	1 Steak/140g	102	2.9	73	9.6	3.7	2.1	0.5
Parsley Sauce, Steaks, Ross*	1 Serving/150g	123	5.6	82	9.1	3.1	3.7	0.1
FIVE SPICE								
Powder, Sharwood's*	1 Tsp/2g	3	0.2	172	12.2	11.6	8.6	23.4
FLAKE								
Dipped, Cadbury*	1 Bar/41g	215	12.5	530	7.6	56.1	30.8	0.8
Luxury, Cadbury*	1 Bar/45g	240	13.6	533	7.3	57.8	30.2	0
Praline, Cadbury*	1 Bar/38g	201	12.9	535	7.7	49.5	34.3	0
FLAN								
Cauliflower, Cheese & Broccoli, Hot, Sainsbury's*	¼ Flan/100g	303	19.8	303	6.4	24.7	19.8	1.2
Cheese & Potato, Hot, Tesco*	¼ Flan/100g	282	19.7	282	6	20	19.7	2.3
Chicken & Smoked Bacon, Hot, Sainsbury's*	¼ Flan/100g	293	18.5	293	10.2	21.5	18.5	1.2
Mediterranean Vegetable, Co-Op*	¼ Flan/88g	188	10.5	215	4	22	12	3
Pastry with Fruit	*1oz/28g*	*33*	*1.2*	*118*	*1.4*	*19.3*	*4.4*	*0.7*
Sponge with Fruit	*1oz/28g*	*31*	*0.4*	*112*	*2.8*	*23.3*	*1.5*	*0.6*

F

FLAN CASE

	Measure INFO/WEIGHT	per Measure KCAL	FAT	Nutrition Values per 100g / 100ml KCAL	PROT	CARB	FAT	FIBRE
Sponge, Average	**1oz/28g**	**90**	**1.5**	**320**	**7**	**62.5**	**5.4**	**0.7**
FLAPJACK								
Lemon Curd, Graze*	1 Punnet/53g	248	12.7	468	6	60	24	6
7 Fruits, Graze*	1 Punnet/55g	223	10.5	406	5.1	54.9	19.1	4.3
All Butter, Sainsbury's*	1 Flapjack/35g	156	8	446	5.7	54.5	22.8	2.7
All Butter, Squares, M&S*	1 Flapjack/34g	150	7.2	441	6.2	56.2	21.2	4.4
All Butter, Topped with Caramel, Spar*	1 Bar/65g	292	12.9	449	5	60.5	19.9	3.8
Apple & Raspberry, Fox's*	1 Flapjack/26g	105	5	403	4.8	52.5	19.4	3.7
Apple & Cinnamon, Graze*	1 Punnet/52g	236	12	453	5	54	23	5
Apricot & Raisin, Waitrose*	1 Flapjack/38g	143	4.2	376	4.7	64.3	11.1	5.8
Average	**1 Sm/50g**	**242**	**13.3**	**484**	**4.5**	**60.4**	**26.6**	**2.7**
Cappuccino, Blackfriars*	1 Flapjack/110g	481	27.5	437	5	61	25	0
Caramel Bake, The Handmade Flapjack Company*	1 Flapjack/90g	375	13	417	6	65.6	14.5	0
Cherry & Coconut, Blackfriars*	1 Flapjack/110g	490	23.1	445	5	58	21	0
Cherry & Sultana, Cookie Coach*	1 Pack/90g	373	15.6	414	6.2	58.2	17.3	0
Cherry Bakewell, Iced, Devondale*	1 Flapjack/95g	432	21.9	455	3.7	54	23.1	2.6
Chocolate Chip, Boots*	1 Flapjack/75g	313	11.2	417	5.6	65	15	3.5
Chocolate Chip, Devondale*	1 Flapjack/95g	434	24.7	457	4.3	49	26	3.6
Chocolate Dipped, M&S*	1 Flapjack/96g	442	21.5	460	6.1	61.3	22.4	3
Chocolate Special, The Handmade Flapjack Company*	1 Flapjack/90g	392	17.8	436	5.7	58.7	19.8	0
Chunky Chocolate, M&S*	1 FlapJack/80g	348	15.1	435	5.8	59.9	18.9	2.2
Co-Op*	1 Flapjack/38g	175	9.4	465	5	54	25	4
Cranberry, Apple & Raisin, LC, Tesco*	1 Flapjack/30g	98	1.7	325	5.7	63.1	5.6	5.7
Dark Chocolate, Delectable , Thomas J Fudge*	1 Flapjack/36g	171	7.4	476	5.5	64.9	20.6	0
Golden Oaty, Fingers, Fabulous Bakin' Boys*	1 Finger/28g	130	6.8	464	4.5	60.2	24.3	3.1
Hobnobs, Milk Chocolate, McVitie's*	1 Flapjack/35g	155	6	443	5.8	64.2	17.2	4.2
Jaffa Cake, Graze*	1 Punnet/53g	242	12.7	457	6	53	24	5
Lemon Drizzle, Graze*	1 Punnet/53g	248	12.7	468	5.9	54	24	5.8
M&S*	1 Flapjack/53g	228	10.1	430	6	59.1	19	3.5
Mince Pie, Graze*	1 Punnet/52g	234	10.9	450	4.9	63	21	6.3
Mini, Sainsbury's*	1 Slice/15g	65	2.9	431	5.6	59.3	19	2.7
Mixed Fruit, Fabulous Bakin' Boys*	1 Serving/90g	350	9.4	389	5.5	71	10.5	4
Oat, GF, Hale & Hearty*	1 Cake/36g	165	9.1	457	6.8	55.1	25.2	8.9
Raspberry Preserve, The Handmade Flapjack Company*	1 Flapjack/90g	310	2.1	345	6.4	74.4	2.4	0
Summer Berry, Graze*	1 Punnet/52g	230	10.9	442	5	56	21	5
Toffee, Finest, Tesco*	1 Flapjack/35g	156	6.7	446	4.9	63.6	19.1	1.3
FLATBREAD								
BBQ Chicken, Improved, Shapers, Boots*	1 Pack/165g	268	3.8	162	10	25	2.3	1.2
BBQ Style Chicken, Shapers, Boots*	1 Serving/108g	187	5	173	10	23	4.6	2.8
Cajun Style Chicken, GFY, Asda*	1 Wrap/176g	231	2.1	131	9	21	1.2	0.9
Chargrilled Chicken, COU, M&S*	1 Pack/163g	245	3.1	150	10.8	23	1.9	5.2
Cheddar, & Tomato, Cooked, Sainsbury's*	¼ Pack/56g	153	3.8	284	11.6	42.4	7	2.2
Cheese, & Tomato, Tesco*	¼ Pack/54g	160	3.5	295	11.6	45.7	6.4	1.9
Chicken Tikka, Shapers, Boots*	1 Pack/1734g	303	5.7	175	11	25	3.3	1.8
Chicken, & Mango Salad, Sainsbury's*	1 Pack/100g	251	2.5	251	16.9	40.4	2.5	2.5
Chicken, Cajun, Greggs*	1 Pack/173g	309	6.2	179	9.8	26	3.6	0
Chicken, Peri Peri, Hot, Greggs*	1 Pack/148g	308	7.3	208	14	27	4.9	0
Chicken, Tikka, BGTY, Sainsbury's*	1 Flatbread/186g	292	4.5	157	11.6	20.5	2.4	3.5
Chicken, with Mango Salsa, Jerk Style, Chargrilled, M&S*	1 Flatbread/200g	300	7.6	150	12.5	15.4	3.8	2.6
Falafel, Greggs*	1 Pack/165g	361	9.1	219	5.9	35	5.5	0
Feta Cheese, COU, M&S*	1 Pack/180g	225	4	125	6.3	20.6	2.2	1.9
Goats Cheese, Butternut Squash, & Beetroot, Tesco*	1 Pack/164g	378	13.6	231	5.9	31.8	8.3	2.6
Greek Feta Salad, Boots*	1 Pack/158g	241	5.7	153	6.4	24	3.6	1.2

	Measure INFO/WEIGHT	per Measure KCAL	FAT	Nutrition Values per 100g / 100ml KCAL	PROT	CARB	FAT	FIBRE

FLATBREAD

	Measure INFO/WEIGHT	KCAL	FAT	KCAL	PROT	CARB	FAT	FIBRE
Harissa Chicken, & Roasted Vegetable, M&S*	1 Pack/186g	342	4.8	184	10.7	19.7	2.6	0
Italian Chicken, Improved, Shapers, Boots*	1 Pack/151g	263	6.8	174	11	22	4.5	1.8
King Prawn, Tikka, Waitrose*	1 Pack/165g	257	3.3	156	9.4	25.1	2	1.5
Mature Cheddar, & Garlic, Finest, Tesco*	¼ Flatbread/66g	188	6.3	285	7.2	41.8	9.6	2.6
Mexican, Chicken, Stonebaked, Finest, Tesco*	1 Pack/155g	280	5.1	180	11.7	25.1	3.3	1.6
Moroccan Chicken, Shapers, Boots*	1 Pack/164g	289	2.1	176	9.8	30	1.3	2.2
Multiseed, Spelt, Suzie's*	1 Portion/100g	364	6	364	10.6	66.9	6	3.3
Noccelara Olive Fougasse, Waitrose*	½ Pack/120.8g	331	8.4	331	0	52.3	8.4	3.1
Plain, Thins, Deli Kitchen*	1 Flatbread/35g	103	1.9	295	8.5	51.4	5.3	4.1
Pork, Bramley Apple, & Stuffing, Tesco Finest*	1 Pack/201g	385	4.8	192	8.1	33.8	2.4	1.9
Red Pepper, & Mozzarella, Morrisons*	¼ Pack/65g	148	2.6	226	10.1	36.4	3.9	2.7
Smoked Ham, & Emmental, Fold, Delicious, Boots*	1 Fold/165g	394	16.5	239	12	24	10	3.6
Spiced Chicken, & Mango, Love Life, Waitrose*	1 Pack/174g	298	4.7	171	9.7	26.1	2.7	1.9
Spicy Chicken, Shapers, Boots*	1 Pack/181g	292	4.5	161	11	23	2.5	0
Spicy Mexican, Shapers, Boots*	1 Pack/190g	296	7.6	156	7	23	4	3.7
Sticky BBQ Style Chicken, Shapers, Boots*	1 Pack/158g	274	7.3	173	10	23	4.6	2.8

FLAXSEED

	Measure INFO/WEIGHT	KCAL	FAT	KCAL	PROT	CARB	FAT	FIBRE
Milled, Organic, Linwoods*	2 Dtsp/30g	152	12	508	22.1	3	40	23.7
Organic, Premium Ground, Prewett's*	1 Tbsp/15g	73	6	489	24	2	40	23
with Bio Cultures & Vitamin D, Linwoods*	2 Tbsps/30g	144	11	481	17.9	6	36.6	28.4

FLOUR

	Measure INFO/WEIGHT	KCAL	FAT	KCAL	PROT	CARB	FAT	FIBRE
Arrowroot, Average	*1oz/28g*	*100*	*0*	*357*	*0.3*	*88.2*	*0.1*	*3.4*
Bread, White, Strong, Average	*1oz/28g*	*94*	*0.4*	*336*	*11.8*	*68.4*	*1.5*	*3.4*
Brown, Chapati, Average	*1 Tbsp/20g*	*67*	*0.2*	*333*	*11.5*	*73.7*	*1.2*	*0*
Brown, Wheat	*1oz/28g*	*90*	*0.5*	*323*	*12.6*	*68.5*	*1.8*	*6.4*
Chakki Wheat Atta, Whole Wheat, Pillsbury*	1 Portion/30g	98	0.5	327	12	65	1.7	0
Chick Pea	*1oz/28g*	*88*	*1.5*	*313*	*19.7*	*49.6*	*5.4*	*10.7*
Coconut, Average	*1 Serving/100g*	*344*	*13.6*	*344*	*18.2*	*15.4*	*13.6*	*43.8*
Millet	*1oz/28g*	*99*	*0.5*	*354*	*5.8*	*75.4*	*1.7*	*0*
Millet, GF, Bob's Red Mill*	1 Serving/30g	111	1.5	370	10	77	5	7
Peanut, Protein Plus*	¼ Cup/30g	110	4	367	53.3	26.7	13.3	13.3
Plain, Average	*1oz/28g*	*98*	*0.4*	*349*	*10.3*	*73.8*	*1.5*	*2.2*
Potato	*1oz/28g*	*92*	*0.3*	*328*	*9.1*	*75.6*	*0.9*	*5.7*
Rice	*1 Tsp/5g*	*18*	*0*	*366*	*6.4*	*80.1*	*0.8*	*2*
Soya, Low Fat, Average	*1oz/28g*	*99*	*2*	*352*	*45.3*	*28.2*	*7.2*	*13.5*
Speciality GF, Dove's Farm*	1 Serving/100g	353	1.8	353	4.7	85.2	1.8	2.7
Spelt, Average	*1 Serving/57g*	*216*	*1.7*	*381*	*14.3*	*74.5*	*3*	*6.4*
White, Average	*1oz/28g*	*89*	*0.3*	*319*	*9.8*	*66.8*	*1*	*2.9*
White, Chapati, Average	*1 Tbsp/20g*	*67*	*0.1*	*335*	*9.8*	*77.6*	*0.5*	*0*
White, Self Raising, Average	*1oz/28g*	*94*	*0.4*	*336*	*9.9*	*71.8*	*1.3*	*2.9*
White, Self Raising, Gluten & Wheat Free, Dove's Farm*	1 Serving/100g	344	1	344	5.5	78.1	1	1.4
Wholemeal, Average	*1oz/28g*	*87*	*0.6*	*312*	*12.6*	*61.9*	*2.2*	*9*

FLYTE

	Measure INFO/WEIGHT	KCAL	FAT	KCAL	PROT	CARB	FAT	FIBRE
Mars*	1 Bar/23g	99	3.2	441	3.4	74.8	14.2	0
Snacksize, Mars*	1 Bar/23g	98	3.3	436	3.8	72.5	14.5	0

FOOL

	Measure INFO/WEIGHT	KCAL	FAT	KCAL	PROT	CARB	FAT	FIBRE
Apricot, Fruit, Tesco*	1 Pot/113g	200	12.7	177	2.6	16.4	11.2	0.3
Apricot, Somerfield*	1 Pot/114g	201	13	177	2.5	16	11.4	0.4
Fruit, Average	*1 Pot/120g*	*196*	*11.2*	*163*	*1*	*20.2*	*9.3*	*1.2*
Gooseberry, BFY, Morrisons*	1 Pot/114g	99	3.9	87	3.4	10.7	3.4	0.4
Gooseberry, Fabulously Fruity, Sainsbury's*	1 Pot/113g	197	11.6	173	2.7	17.1	10.2	1.2
Gooseberry, Fruit, Co-Op*	1 Pot/114g	211	11.4	185	3	22	10	1
Gooseberry, Fruit, Somerfield*	1 Pot/114g	215	12.5	189	3	19	11	0

F

	Measure INFO/WEIGHT	per Measure KCAL	FAT	Nutrition Values per 100g / 100ml KCAL	PROT	CARB	FAT	FIBRE
FOOL								
Gooseberry, Tesco*	1 Pot/112g	225	14.1	200	3	17.8	12.5	0.7
Lemon, Fruit, BGTY, Sainsbury's*	1 Pot/113g	94	3.8	83	3.4	9.7	3.4	0.3
Lemon, Signature, Morrisons*	1 Pot/114g	213	11.8	187	3	20	10.4	0.5
Raspberry, Fruit, Tesco*	1 Pot/113g	234	12.8	207	2.6	23.6	11.3	0.3
Rhubarb, Fruit, Somerfield*	1 Pot/114g	201	12.5	176	3	16	11	0
Rhubarb, Fruit, Waitrose*	1 Pot/114g	182	12.9	160	2.7	11.9	11.3	0.3
Rhubarb, Timberly, Fabulously Fruity, Sainsbury's*	1 Pot/113g	167	11.7	147	2.4	10.9	10.3	0.5
Strawberry, Fruit, BGTY, Sainsbury's*	1 Pot/120g	100	3.1	83	3.7	11.1	2.6	0.8
Strawberry, Fruit, Co-Op*	1 Pot/114g	188	10.3	165	2	18	9	0.8
FRANKFURTERS								
Average	*1 Frankfurter/42g*	*123*	*11.2*	*292*	*12*	*1.3*	*26.6*	*0*
Vegetarian, Quorn*	1 Frankfurter/45g	92	6.3	205	13.5	4.5	14	3.5
Vegetarian, Tivall*	1 Sausage/30g	73	4.8	244	18	7	16	3
FRAZZLES								
Bacon, Smith's, Walkers*	1 Bag/23g	113	5.3	488	7.5	62	23	1.3
FREEKEH								
Greenwheat, Cooked, Artisan Grains*	1 Serving/100g	165	2	165	8.8	30.2	2	5.2
Wholegrain, Unprepared, Artisan Grains*	1 Serving/100g	347	4.3	347	18.5	63.5	4.3	10.9
FRENCH FRIES								
Cheese & Onion, Walkers*	1 Pack/22g	95	3.5	430	5	66	16	5
Ready Salted, Walkers*	1 Bag/21g	91	3.4	434	5	65	16	5
Salt & Vinegar, Walkers*	1 Bag/22g	95	3.5	430	5	66	16	5
Seasoned, Frozen, Ovenbaked, Asda*	1/6 Pack/125g	286	10.9	229	3.1	33	8.7	3
Worcester Sauce, Walkers*	1 Bag/22g	96	3.5	435	5	65	16	5
FRENCH TOAST								
Asda*	1 Toast/8g	30	0.4	381	10	74	5	4
Morrisons*	1 Toast/8g	31	0.5	393	11	72.5	6.6	3
Sainsbury's*	1 Toast/8g	31	0.5	382	10	72	6.6	5
Tesco*	1 Toast/9g	37	1	440	7.8	74.5	11.7	2.8
FRIES								
Chips, From Restaurant, Average	*1 Serving/105g*	*294*	*16.3*	*280*	*3.3*	*34*	*15.5*	*2.1*
Curly, Cajun, Weighed Frozen, McCain*	1 Portion/100g	156	8.7	156	1.6	17.7	8.7	1.8
Curly, Ovenbaked, Iceland*	1 Serving/100g	253	12.1	253	3.5	30.8	12.1	3.5
Curly, Southern Style, Tesco*	1 Serving/50g	124	3.6	248	3.8	41.7	7.3	3.8
Extra Chunky, Oven Baked, Homefries, McCain*	1 Serving/200g	306	6.2	153	3.2	28	3.1	2.3
Skin on, Ovenbaked, Iceland*	1/10 Bag/100g	204	6.9	204	3.3	30.6	6.9	3.2
Sweet Potato, Crispy, McCain*	1 Serving/125g	170	5.7	136	1.6	20.4	4.6	3.5
Sweet Potato, Iceland*	1 Serving/125g	252	9.9	202	1.9	28.4	7.9	4.7
Sweet Potato, Oven Baked, CBY, Asda*	1 Serving/125g	188	6.5	150	5.6	19	5.2	2.4
Sweet Potato, Prefried & Frozen, Cooked, Sainsbury's*	1 Serving/125g	297	14.7	237	2.4	28.3	11.7	4.6
Sweet Potato, Ready to Roast, Cooked, Sainsbury's*	½ Pack/116g	201	8.3	174	2.1	23.7	7.2	3.2
Sweet Potato, Slims Kitchen *	1 Bowl/340g	578	25.5	170	1.5	22	7.5	0
FRISPS								
Tangy Salt & Vinegar, KP Snacks*	1 Bag/30g	160	10	532	5	52.6	33.5	2.9
Tasty Cheese & Onion, KP Snacks*	1 Bag/28g	150	9.4	537	5.5	53.2	33.6	3.2
FRITTATA								
Spinach & Courgette, Meat Free, Tesco*	1 Frittata/120g	199	12.8	166	5.8	10.2	10.7	2.9
Vegetable, CBY, Asda*	1 Frittatas/150g	183	7.8	122	6.2	12.1	5.2	1
FROMAGE FRAIS								
0% Fat, Vitalinea, Danone*	1 Tbsp/28g	14	0	50	7.4	4.7	0.1	0
Apricot, Summer Fruit, Layered, Weight Watchers*	1 Pot/100g	46	0.1	46	5.4	5.8	0.1	0.2
Blackberry, Berry Fruits, Layered, Weight Watchers*	1 Pot/100g	49	0.2	49	5.5	5.7	0.2	0.4
Cherry, 0% Fat, Vitalinea, Danone*	1 Serving/150g	88	0.2	59	6.1	8	0.2	1.6

F

Measure INFO/WEIGHT	per Measure KCAL	FAT	Nutrition Values per 100g / 100ml KCAL	PROT	CARB	FAT	FIBRE

FROMAGE FRAIS

	Measure INFO/WEIGHT	KCAL	FAT	KCAL	PROT	CARB	FAT	FIBRE
Fabby, Loved By Kids, M&S*	1 Pot/43g	45	1.6	105	6.2	12.3	3.7	0
Fat Free, Average	*1 Pot/60g*	*35*	*0.1*	*58*	*7.7*	*6.8*	*0.2*	*0*
Forest Fruit, Layered, Weight Watchers*	1 Pot/100g	47	0.2	47	5.5	5.7	0.2	0.4
Kids, Yeo Valley*	1 Serving/90g	111	4.8	123	6.6	12.6	5.3	0
Munch Bunch, Nestle*	1 Pot/42g	44	1.3	105	6.7	12.6	3	0
Peach, BGTY, Sainsbury's*	1 Pot/100g	53	0.2	53	7.2	5.5	0.2	0.5
Peach, Summer Fruit, Layered, Weight Watchers*	1 Pot/100g	46	0.1	46	5	8	0.1	0.4
Plain, Average	*1oz/28g*	*32*	*2*	*113*	*6.8*	*5.7*	*7.1*	*0*
Raspberry, Berry Fruits, Layered, Weight Watchers*	1 Pot/100g	47	0.2	47	5.5	5.7	0.2	0.4
Raspberry, Little Stars, Muller*	1 Pot/60g	66	2.4	110	5	12.7	4	0.4
Raspberry, Organic, Yeo Valley*	1 Pot/100g	127	6.5	127	6.1	11.1	6.5	0.4
Raspberry, Value, Tesco*	1 Serving/60g	56	0.8	93	7.2	13.5	1.3	0
Strawberry Cheesecake, Dessert Selection, Sainsbury's*	1 Pot/90g	95	2.2	106	5.8	15.3	2.5	0.1
Strawberry Tart, Sainsbury's*	1 Pot/100g	54	0.2	54	7.6	5.5	0.2	1.1
Strawberry, 99.9% Fat Free, Onken*	1 Serving/50g	46	0	91	6.9	15.3	0.1	0
Strawberry, GFY, Asda*	1 Pot/100g	58	0.2	58	6	8	0.2	0
Strawberry, HE, Tesco*	1 Pot/100g	54	0.2	54	6.2	6.8	0.2	0.1
Strawberry, Langley Farm*	1 Pot/125g	189	9.8	151	7	13.3	7.8	0
Strawberry, Organic, Yeo Valley*	1 Pot/90g	116	5.4	129	6.3	12.5	6	0.2
Strawberry, Petits Filous, Yoplait*	1 Pot/50g	52	1.4	104	6.7	12.6	2.9	0.2
Strawberry, Thomas the Tank Engine, Yoplait*	1 Pot/50g	50	0.6	101	6.8	15.4	1.3	0
Strawberry, Value, Tesco*	1 Pot/60g	55	0.8	92	7.2	13	1.3	0
Toffee & Pecan Pie, Smooth & Creamy, Tesco*	1 Pot/100g	148	6.8	148	6.9	14.8	6.8	0.2
Vanilla, Danone*	1 Serving/200g	274	8.2	137	5.3	19.6	4.1	0
Wildlife, Strawberry, Raspberry Or Peach, Yoplait*	1 Pot/50g	46	0.6	93	7.1	13.2	1.3	0.2
with Fruit, Average	*1 Avg Pot/90g*	*74*	*2.2*	*83*	*6.1*	*9*	*2.5*	*0.8*
with Fruit, Healthy Range, Average	*1 Avg Pot/90g*	*40*	*0.1*	*45*	*5.8*	*5.1*	*0.2*	*0.3*

FROZEN YOGHURT

	Measure INFO/WEIGHT	KCAL	FAT	KCAL	PROT	CARB	FAT	FIBRE
Belgian Chocolate, Calorie Controlled, Love Life, Waitrose*	1/5 Pot/100g	89	1.7	89	4.3	14	1.7	0.3
Black Cherry, M&S*	1 Pot/125g	164	1.4	131	3.1	27.1	1.1	0.5
Cherry Garcia, Low Fat, Ben & Jerry's*	1 Serving/100g	143	2.4	143	3	26	2.4	1
Chocmoo, Yoomoo*	1 Serving/100g	142	1.7	142	3.5	26	1.7	4.1
Chocolate, Average	*1 Portion/100g*	*120*	*1.9*	*120*	*4.3*	*22*	*1.9*	*2.1*
Chocolate, Pinkberry*	1 Sm Pot/140g	168	2.1	120	5	23	1.5	2
Chocolate, Snog*	1 Serving/100g	109	1.6	109	4.5	19.9	1.6	1.7
Coconut, Pinkberry*	1 Sm Pot/140g	196	0	140	4	30	0	0
Frae*	1 Sm/83ml	56	0	67	2.4	12	0	0
Green Tea, Pinkberry*	1 Sm Pot/100g	110	0	110	4	25	0	0
Mango, Pinkberry*	1 Sm Cup/140g	140	0	100	3	23	0	0
Mango, Snowconut, The Coconut Collaborative*	1 Serving/200ml	372	15	186	1.8	21	7.5	1
Nakedmoo, Yoomoo*	1 Serving/125g	168	2	134	3.3	24.5	1.6	4.1
Natural, Average	*1 Portion/100g*	*101*	*0.8*	*101*	*3.8*	*19.9*	*0.8*	*0.9*
Original, Pinkberry*	1 Sm Pot/140g	140	0	100	3	21	0	0
Passionfruit, Pinkberry*	1 Sm Pot/140g	140	0	100	3	22	0	0
Peanut Butter, Pinkberry*	1 Sm Pot/140g	238	9.8	170	7	23	7	1
Phish Food, Lower Fat, Ben & Jerry's*	½ Pot/211g	464	10.6	220	4	40	5	1.5
Pomegranate, Pinkberry*	1 Sm Pot/140g	168	0	120	3	26	0	0
Pumpkin, Pinkberry*	1 Sm Pot/140g	154	0	110	3	23	0	0
Raspberry Snowconut, The Coconut Collaborative*	1 Serving/200ml	378	15	189	1.8	21.2	7.5	1.2
Raspberry, Handmade Farmhouse, Sainsbury's*	1 Serving/100g	132	3.8	132	2.7	21.8	3.8	2.2
Salted Caramel, Pinkberry*	1 Sm Pot/140g	168	0	120	4	26	0	0
Strawberry Cheesecake, Low Fat, Ben & Jerry's*	1 Serving/100g	170	3	170	4	31	3	1
Strawberry, Average	*1 Portion/100g*	*114*	*2.2*	*114*	*2.6*	*21.2*	*2.2*	*0.5*

F

	Measure INFO/WEIGHT	per Measure KCAL	FAT	Nutrition Values per 100g / 100ml KCAL	PROT	CARB	FAT	FIBRE
FROZEN YOGHURT								
Strawberry, Tesco*	1 Pot/60g	82	1.3	136	2.6	26.5	2.2	0.8
Strawbmoo, Yoomoo*	1 Serving/100g	133	1.5	133	3.2	24.7	1.5	4.1
Tropicoolmoo, Yoomoo*	1 Pot/92g	134	1.2	146	2.9	28.9	1.3	3.6
Vanilla, Less Than 5% Fat, Tesco*	1 Pot/120g	179	2.9	149	8.1	23.8	2.4	0.7
FRUIT								
5 a Day Selection, Waitrose*	1 Pack/400g	224	0.8	56	0.7	12.2	0.2	1.3
Apple & Pear, Snack Pack, Great Stuff, Asda*	1 Pack/80g	42	0.1	52	0.4	11	0.1	2.6
Apple, Pineapple & Grape, Ready to Eat, Sainsbury's*	1 Pack/180g	94	0.2	52	0.5	8.3	0.1	1.3
Apples & Grape, Snack Pack, Goodness for Kids, Tesco*	1 Pack/80g	44	0.1	55	0.4	12.3	0.1	2.6
Baked, Nibbles, Cherry Berry, We Are Bear*	1 Pack/30g	87	0	290	1.2	76	0.2	10.3
Baked, Nibbles, Mango Pineapple, We Are Bear*	1 Bag/30g	85	0	285	1.4	73	0.2	11
Berry Medley, Freshly Prepared, M&S*	1 Pack/180g	90	0.4	50	0.7	10.9	0.2	2.9
Black Forest, Frozen, Tesco*	1 Serving/80g	37	0	46	0.8	10.5	0	1.8
Cempedak	*1 Serving/100g*	*116*	*0.4*	*116*	*3*	*28.6*	*0.4*	*0*
Citrus Selection, Fresh, Sainsbury's*	1 Pack/240g	79	0.2	33	0.9	7.1	0.1	1.6
Fabulous Fruity Fingers, Melon & Mango, M&S*	1 Pack/240g	96	0.5	40	0.6	8.2	0.2	1
Fingers, Melon & Pineapple, Sainsbury's*	1 Pack/240g	74	0.2	31	0.5	6.5	0.1	0.8
Grapefruit & Orange Segments, Breakfast, Del Monte*	1 Can/411g	193	0.4	47	1	10.2	0.1	1
Melon & Grape Munchies, Eat Well, M&S*	½ Pack/200g	70	0.2	35	0.5	8.3	0.1	0.7
Melon & Grape Pot, Co-Op*	1 Pot/130g	39	0.1	30	0.6	6.9	0.1	0.7
Melon & Grape, Sainsbury's*	½ Pack/200g	66	0.2	33	0.5	7.1	0.1	0.7
Melon & Grape, Snack Pack, Goodness for Kids, Tesco*	1 Pack/90g	34	0	38	0.5	9	0	0.7
Melon & Grapes, Morrisons*	1 Pack/360g	112	0.4	31	0.6	6.4	0.1	0.8
Melon, Kiwi Fruit & Strawberries, Fresh Tastes, Asda*	1 Pack/240g	96	0.5	40	0.8	7.7	0.2	2.1
Melon, Kiwi, & Strawberry, Fully Prepared, Sainsbury's*	1 Pack/245g	74	0.5	30	0.8	6.3	0.2	1.3
Melon, Pineapple & Mango Fingers, Good to Go, Waitrose*	1 Pot/160g	82	0.3	51	0.7	11.6	0.2	1.2
Melon, Wedges, Snack Pack, Goodness for Kids, Tesco*	1 Pack/90g	17	0.1	19	0.4	4.1	0.1	0.6
Mixed, Fresh, 5 a Day, Tesco*	1 Pack/400g	136	0.8	34	0.8	7.4	0.2	1.4
Mixed, Fresh, Tesco*	1 Pack/200g	70	0.4	35	0.8	7.4	0.1	1.4
Mixed, Pieces, in Orange Jelly, Fruitini, Del Monte*	1 Can/140g	94	0.1	67	0.3	15.8	0.1	0
Mixed, Tropical, Fruit Express, Del Monte*	1 Pot/185g	89	0.2	48	0.2	11.2	0.1	1.2
Mixed, Vine, Crazy Jack*	1 Serving/10g	31	0	309	2.8	74	0.3	4.7
Orchard, Frozen, British, Delicious & Colourful, Waitrose*	½ Pack/150g	60	0.2	40	0.6	7.7	0.1	2.7
Peach Pieces in Fruit Juice, Tesco*	1 Pot/125g	60	0	48	0.4	11.7	0	1
Peach, Slices, Frozen, Sainsbury's*	1 Serving/80g	30	0	37	1	7.6	0	1.5
Pieces, Mixed in Fruit Juice, Fruitini, Del Monte*	1 Serving/120g	61	0.1	51	0.4	12	0.1	0.5
Pineapple & Mango Tango; Eat Well, M&S*	1 Pack/200g	100	0.8	50	1	22.2	0.4	2.6
Pineapple Fingers, Snack Pack, Goodness for Kids, Tesco*	1 Pack/70g	31	0.1	44	0.4	10.1	0.2	2
Pineapple Pot, CBY, Asda*	1 Pot/200g	106	0	53	0.4	12.5	0	0.7
Pineapple, Grape & Kiwi, Asda*	1 Serving/200g	98	0.6	49	0.6	11	0.3	1.7
Pineapple, Grape & Kiwi, Fresh Tastes, Asda*	1 Pack/200g	106	0.6	53	0.6	11	0.3	1.8
Pineapple, Mango & Nectarine, Fresh Tastes, Asda*	1 Pack/240g	127	0.5	53	0.8	11	0.2	2.1
Pink Lady Apple & Grape, Snack Pack, On The Go, Tesco*	1 Pack/80g	44	0.1	55	0.3	12.3	0.1	2.6
Rolls, Peach, Yo Yo, Bear*	1 Roll/10g	28	0	275	1.4	72	0.2	10
Snack Pack, Fresh, Sainsbury's*	1 Serving/120g	54	0.1	45	0.1	11	0.1	1.3
Snack, Sweet Grape, Shapers, Boots*	1 Pack/80g	53	0.1	66	0.4	15	0.1	1
Strawberries, Apple & Grapes, Fresh Tastes, Asda*	1 Pot/190g	91	0.2	48	0.5	10.6	0.1	0
Summer Berries, M&S*	1 Pack/160g	80	0.3	50	0.7	10	0.2	3
Tayberry	*1 Serving/100g*	*25*	*0*	*25*	*1.2*	*12*	*0*	*7*
Tropical in Juice, Dole*	1 Pot/113g	59	0	52	0.3	14.2	0	1.8
Tropical Shaker with Coulis, Morrisons*	1 Pot/250g	168	1	67	0.8	14.6	0.4	0.9
Tutti Frutti Collection, Freshly Prepared, Tesco*	1 Pack/200g	86	0.4	43	0.6	9.1	0.2	1.4

F

FRUIT & NUT MIX	Measure INFO/WEIGHT	per Measure KCAL	FAT	Nutrition Values per 100g / 100ml KCAL	PROT	CARB	FAT	FIBRE
FRUIT & NUT MIX								
Billionaire's Shortbread, Graze*	1 Punnet/41g	192	10.2	469	8	53	25	5
Bounty Hunter, Graze*	1 Punnet/31g	147	8.3	474	4	54.4	26.8	5.6
Cacao & Orange, with Dates & Raw Almonds, Graze*	1 Punnet/43g	174	8.1	406	8.7	55	19	9.2
Cherry Fudge Sundae, Graze*	1 Punnet/45g	186	8.1	414	7.2	56	18	4.9
Daily Vigour Mix, Waitrose*	1 Pack/50g	265	18.8	530	14.6	30	37.6	6.4
Dried, Selection, Wholesome, Love Life, Waitrose*	1 Serving/30g	144	9.6	479	9.8	38	32	4.4
Eleanor's Apple Crumble, Graze*	1 Pack/32g	115	4	356	6.4	62	12.5	8
Flapjack, Fruit & Seed, Graze*	1 Punnet/53g	226	11.1	426	6	54	21	5
Honeycomb Crunch, Graze*	1 Punnet/40g	181	9.7	446	9	50	24	4
Jaffa Cake, Graze*	1 Punnet/44g	208	13.7	472	7	43	31	6
Jam Doughnut, Graze*	1 Punnet/31g	131	4.7	422	7	65	15	6
Marvellous Macaroon, Graze*	1 Punnet/28g	157	10.9	562	11	41	39	6
Nuts & Raisins, Mixed, Natural, Love Life, Waitrose*	1 Serving/50g	258	16.4	515	16.5	38.4	32.8	7.2
Salted Caramel, Nibbles, N'akd*	1 Bag/40g	138	4.7	345	6.6	56.1	11.8	3.3
Seed, Cashew & Blueberry Mix, Love Life, Waitrose*	1 Serving/103g	142	8.1	472	13.9	40.8	26.8	5.9
Strawberry Milkshake, Graze*	1 Pack/39g	148	3.9	380	2	72	10	2
Trail Mix, Average	*1oz/28g*	*121*	*8*	*432*	*9.1*	*37.2*	*28.5*	*4.3*
Tropical Praline, Graze*	1 Punnet/35g	121	4.2	347	4.2	59.2	12.1	2
Unsalted, Tesco*	1 Serving/25g	112	4.6	449	12.6	58.1	18.5	12.2
Walnut & Vanilla Truffle, Graze*	1 Punnet/38g	187	12.1	496	10	43.9	32.2	6
White Chocolate & Raspberry Cheesecake, Graze*	1 Punnet/39g	204	13.7	524	7.5	44.7	35.1	4.5
FRUIT & NUTS								
Cocoa & Raspberry, Posh Bits, Nak'd*	1 Serving/35g	134	3.9	384	8	59	11.1	8
Cocoa Mandarin, Posh Bits, Nak'd*	1 Serving/35g	131	3.8	373	7.6	57	10.9	8.7
Dried, Date & Toasted Almond, Shots, Whitworths*	1 Pack/25g	94	3.4	377	9.1	52.3	13.6	4.5
FRUIT COCKTAIL								
Fresh & Ready, Sainsbury's*	1 Pack/300g	117	0.3	39	0.6	9	0.1	1.2
in Apple Juice, Asda*	1/3 Can/80g	40	0.1	50	0.3	12	0.1	1.6
in Fruit Juice, Heinz*	1 Pot/125g	78	0	62	0.5	15	0	1
in Fruit Juice, Sainsbury's*	1 Serving/198g	97	0.2	49	0.3	11.9	0.1	1.3
in Fruit Juice, Waitrose*	1 Can/142g	71	0	50	0.4	12	0	1
in Juice, Del Monte*	1 Can/415g	203	0.4	49	0.4	11.2	0.1	0
in Light Syrup, Princes*	1 Serving/206g	64	0	31	0.4	7.3	0	1
in Light Syrup, Sainsbury's*	½ Can/125g	72	0.1	58	0.4	14	0.1	1.3
in Light Syrup, Valfrutta*	1 Serving/206g	95	0	46	0.2	11.4	0	1.5
in Syrup, Morrisons*	½ Can/205g	129	0.2	63	0.3	14.9	0.1	0
in Syrup, Smart Price, Asda*	1 Can/411g	173	0.4	42	0.3	10	0.1	1.6
Tropical, Canned, Asda*	½ Can/200g	120	0	60	0	15	0	1.6
FRUIT COMPOTE								
& Vanilla Sponge, Weight Watchers*	1 Pack/140g	202	2.9	144	2.2	29	2.1	1.8
Apple, Strawberry & Blackberry, Organic, Yeo Valley*	½ Pot/112g	73	0.1	65	0.5	15.5	0.1	1.9
Apricot & Prune, Yeo Valley*	1 Pot/225g	207	0.2	92	0.6	22.3	0.1	1.6
HE, Tesco*	1 Pot/140g	113	0.3	81	0.9	19.1	0.2	1.6
Orchard Fruits, GFY, Asda*	1 Pot/180g	113	0.2	63	0.5	15	0.1	0
Spiced, Tesco*	1 Serving/112g	122	0.6	109	1.7	24.4	0.5	3.1
Strawberry & Raspberry, M&S*	1 Serving/80g	72	0.1	90	0.7	23.5	0.1	2.3
Summerfruit, M&S*	¼ Pot/125g	119	0.8	95	0.9	22.7	0.6	0.8
FRUIT DRINK								
Gazpacho, Spirit of Summer, M&S*	1 Serving/150ml	39	0.2	26	0.8	5.1	0.1	0.7
Lemon & Lime, Diet, Carbonated, M&S*	1 Glass/250ml	5	0	2	0	0.2	0	0
Multivitamin, Rejuvenation, Active Life, Purdy's*	1 Bottle/330ml	125	0	38	0	9.5	0	0
Pineapple, Sparkling, KA, Barr's*	1 Can/330ml	168	0	51	0	12.5	0	0

F

	Measure INFO/WEIGHT	per Measure KCAL	FAT	Nutrition Values per 100g / 100ml KCAL	PROT	CARB	FAT	FIBRE
FRUIT DRINK								
Refresco LÃfmon, La Casera*	1 Serving/200ml	2	0	1	0	0	0	0
Sparkling Pink Grapefruit, Shapers, Boots*	1 Serving/200ml	6	0	3	0	0.3	0	0
FRUIT FLAKES								
Blackcurrant with Yoghurt Coating, Fruit Bowl*	1 Bag/21g	95	4	453	1.3	69	19	3.9
Raspberry with Yoghurt Coating, Fruit Bowl*	1 Serving/21g	95	4	453	1.3	69	19	3.9
Strawberry with Yoghurt Coating, Fruit Bowl*	1 Serving/21g	95	4	453	1.3	69	19	3.9
FRUIT GUMS								
Fruit Salad, Tesco*	6 Sweets/30g	100	0.2	335	8.3	73.4	0.5	0.3
Rowntree's*	1 Tube/49.4g	170	0.1	344	4.8	81.3	0.2	0
Sugar Free, Sainsbury's*	1 Serving/30g	63	0.1	209	7.7	71.3	0.2	0.1
FRUIT MEDLEY								
Citrus, Somerfield*	1 Serving/81g	25	0.1	31	0.6	6.9	0.1	0.4
Dried, Tropical, Soft, Love Life, Waitrose*	1 Serving/30g	86	0	288	0.2	70.6	0	2.5
Exotic, Co-Op*	1 Serving/120g	54	0.2	45	0.6	10	0.2	0
Fresh, Tesco*	1 Pack/200g	86	0.2	43	0.4	10	0.1	1.1
in Fresh Orange Juice, Co-Op*	1 Serving/140g	49	0	35	0.5	9	0	0
Mango, Melon, Kiwi & Blueberry, Fresh, M&S*	1 Pack/260g	104	0.8	40	0.7	9.1	0.3	1.6
Mixed, Fruit Harvest, Whitworths*	1 Pack/50g	166	0.4	331	1.8	79.4	0.7	4.8
Nectarine, Mango & Blueberry, Fresh, M&S*	1 Pack/245g	122	0.5	50	1	11.1	0.2	2.1
Pineapple, Papaya & Mango, Waitrose*	1 Pack/550g	297	0.6	54	0.6	12.8	0.1	1.1
Raisin, Fruit Harvest, Whitworths*	1 Pack/50g	158	0.6	315	1.8	74.4	1.3	4.3
Shapers, Boots*	1 Pack/140g	55	0.3	39	0.7	8.6	0.2	1
FRUIT MIX								
Apple Cosmo, Graze*	1 Punnet/34g	100	0.2	292	1.5	69.8	0.7	4.6
Apple, & Strawberry, Pot, Market Street , Morrisons*	1 Serving/125g	61	0.6	49	0.6	9.8	0.5	1.2
Apricot, Torte, Graze*	1 Pack/45g	151	3.6	335	3.3	63	8	4
Banana, Coconut & Mango, Dried, Graze*	1 Punnet/45g	144	3.7	320	18.7	57.1	8.2	0
Berry, Sainsbury's*	1 Serving/20g	64	0.4	319	1	78.1	1.9	5.5
Date To Remember, Graze*	1 Punnet/40g	131	1.8	327	3.3	68.3	4.4	6.3
Fig Roll, Graze*	1 Punnet/35g	110	0.6	313	1.6	23.1	1.7	2
Forest Fruit, Dried, Graze*	1 Pack/50g	160	0.4	319	1.8	76	0.8	0
Juicy Orange Raisins, Graze*	1 Pack/40g	110	0.4	275	2.1	69	0.9	0
Love Mix, Graze*	1 Pack/40g	99	0.4	245	4	58	0.9	5.9
Luxury, Sainsbury's*	1 Serving/30g	78	0.2	261	1.8	62.3	0.5	2.7
Melon, Strawberry & Grape, Sainsbury's*	1 Pack/180g	58	0.4	32	0.5	7	0.2	0.4
Muffin, Dried, Graze*	1 Box/60g	221	6.8	368	1.7	65.8	11.3	1.7
Nectarine, Raspberry & Blueberry, Seasonal, M&S*	1 Pack/160g	72	0.3	45	1.3	8.3	0.2	2.7
Pineapple, Kiwi, Mango & Blueberry, Waitrose*	1 Pack/330g	208	1	63	0.7	14.5	0.3	1.9
Pineapple, Melon, Mango, Tesco*	1 Pack/440g	242	0.9	55	1.1	11.4	0.2	1.3
Plum, Pomegranate, & Blueberry, Market Street, Morrisons*	1 Serving/80g	38	0.1	47	0.6	10	0.1	1.8
Pumpkin Pie, Graze*	1 Pack/65g	274	11.2	422	11.4	48.2	17.2	0
Red, Frozen, Crops*	3 Tbsp/80g	28	0.1	35	1	5.2	0.1	4.6
Sour Mango Tangtastic, Graze*	1 Pack/34g	110	0.2	323	1.3	79.8	0.6	2
Summer Fruits, British, Frozen, Waitrose*	1 Pack/380g	99	0.8	26	1	5.2	0.2	5.5
Summer Fruits, Frozen, Asda*	1 Serving/100g	28	0	28	0.9	6	0	2.5
Summer Fruits, Frozen, Four Seasons*	1/5 Pack/100g	53	1	53	1.1	6.5	1	7.3
Summer Fruits, Frozen, Sainsbury's*	1 Serving/80g	43	0.1	54	0.9	6.9	0.1	2
Summer Fruits, in Syrup, Sainsbury's*	1 Pudding/289g	188	0.3	65	0.5	15.6	0.1	1.2
Summer Fruits, Sainsbury's*	1 Serving/80g	26	0	32	0.9	7.4	0	2.4
Summer Pudding, Graze*	1 Punnet/32g	109	0.4	342	1.6	81.2	1.2	4.2
Super Wholefood with Blueberries & Mango, M&S*	1 Pack/215g	260	7.7	121	4.4	17	3.6	8.7
Tropical, Fresh, Waitrose*	1 Pack/240g	122	0.5	51	0.6	11.6	0.2	1.9
Tutti Frutti, Graze*	1 Punnet/41g	120	0.4	292	1.9	72.3	0.9	4

	Measure INFO/WEIGHT	per Measure KCAL	per Measure FAT	Nutrition Values per 100g / 100ml KCAL	PROT	CARB	FAT	FIBRE
FRUIT MIX								
with Cherry in Juice, Drained, Dole*	1 Pouch/220g	119	0.2	54	0.4	12.2	0.1	1.7
FRUIT PUREE								
Apple & Blueberry, Organic, Clearspring*	1 Tub/100g	76	0.3	76	0.4	17.8	0.3	0
Apple & Blueberry, Organix*	1 Pot/100g	54	0.6	54	0.4	11.6	0.6	2.5
Apple & Peach, Organix*	1 Pot/100g	49	0.3	49	0.6	11	0.3	2.1
Apple, Kale & Mango, Twist, Organic, Happy Squeeze*	1 Pouch/60g	40	0	67	0	15.6	0	1.1
Banana, Apple & Apricot, Organix*	1 Pot/100g	68	0.4	68	0.8	15.4	0.4	2
FRUIT SALAD								
Apple, Orange, Pineapple & Grape, Morrisons*	1 Serving/64g	40	0.1	62	0.8	13.1	0.1	2.6
Apple, Pineapple & Grape, Sweet & Tangy, Sainsbury's*	1 Pack/180g	70	0.2	39	0.5	8.3	0.1	1.3
Autumn, Fresh, M&S*	½ Pack/160g	64	0.2	40	0.7	9.4	0.1	2.9
Berry, Asda*	1 Pack/250g	122	0.2	49	0.6	10.9	0.1	0
Berry, Seasonal, Asda*	1 Pack/300g	93	0.3	31	0.6	7	0.1	2.1
Chunky in Fruit Juice, Canned, John West*	1 Can/411g	193	0.8	47	0.4	11	0.2	0.8
Citrus, Fresh, M&S*	½ Pack/225g	79	0.2	35	0.9	7.7	0.1	1.5
Classic, Co-Op*	1 Box/285g	142	0.3	50	0.6	11	0.1	2.3
Classic, Fresh, Prepared, Sainsbury's*	1 Pack/320g	157	0.3	49	0.6	10.3	0.1	2
Classic, M&S*	1 Pack/369g	166	1.1	45	0.6	9.1	0.3	1.7
Classic, Ocado*	1 Pack/265g	130	0.3	49	0.7	12.1	0.1	1.2
Dried, M&S*	½ Pack/125g	269	0.5	215	1.8	51.4	0.4	5.9
Exotic with Melon, Mango, Kiwi Fruit & Grapes, Asda*	1 Pot/300g	141	0.9	47	0.6	10.5	0.3	1.4
Exotic, Fresh, Tesco*	1 Serving/225g	86	0.4	38	0.7	8.4	0.2	1.5
Exotic, Fully Prepared, Sainsbury's*	1 Serving/200g	74	0.4	37	0.6	8.3	0.2	1.3
Exotic, Morrisons*	1 Serving/150g	78	0.3	52	0.6	12.2	0.2	0
Exotic, Waitrose*	1 Pack/300g	126	0.6	42	0.6	9.5	0.2	1.1
Fresh for You, Tesco*	1 Pack/160g	59	0.3	37	0.6	8.2	0.2	1.1
Fresh, Morrisons*	1 Tub/350g	150	0.4	43	0.7	9.9	0.1	0
Fresh, Tesco*	1 Pack/200g	84	0.4	42	0.7	9.3	0.2	1.5
Fresh, Washed, Ready to Eat, Tesco*	1 Pack/200g	92	0.2	46	0.7	10.6	0.1	1.6
Freshly Prepared, M&S*	1 Pack/350g	140	0.7	40	0.5	9.3	0.2	1
Fruit Crunch, Salad Bowl, M&S*	½ Pack/120g	174	4.1	145	3.1	25.5	3.4	0.6
Golden, Fresh, Asda*	1 Pot/147g	69	0.1	47	0.6	11	0.1	1.6
Grapefruit & Orange, Fresh, M&S*	1 Serving/250g	88	0.2	35	0.9	7.4	0.1	1.6
Green, M&S*	1 Pack/400g	200	0.8	50	0.6	10.9	0.2	1.2
Homemade, Unsweetened, Average	*1 Serving/140g*	*77*	*0.1*	*55*	*0.7*	*13.8*	*0.1*	*1.5*
Juicy Melon, Pineapple & Grapes, Asda*	1 Pot/300g	111	0.3	37	0.5	8.4	0.1	0.9
Kiwi, Pineapple & Grape, Fresh Tastes, Asda*	1 Pack/200g	106	0.6	53	0.6	11	0.3	1.8
Layered, Tropical Rainbow, Freshly Prepared, M&S*	1 Pack/375g	206	1.1	55	0.7	12.6	0.3	1.7
Mango, Kiwi, Blueberry & Pomegranate, Fresh, M&S*	1 Pack/350g	210	1	60	0.9	13.4	0.3	2.4
Mediterranean Style, Budgens*	1 Serving/250g	95	0.5	38	0.6	8.5	0.2	0.8
Melon & Red Grape, Freshly Prepared, M&S*	1 Pack/450g	158	0.4	35	0.5	8.4	0.1	0.7
Melon & Mango, Shapers, Boots*	1 Pack/80g	29	0.1	36	0.6	7.8	0.1	1.2
Melon, Grape, Kiwi, Strawberry, & Pomegranate, Tesco*	1 Pot/375g	172	0.8	46	0.8	9.6	0.2	1.2
Melon, Kiwi, Grapes & Pomegranate Seeds, Morrisons*	1 Pack/400g	152	1.2	38	0.7	8.2	0.3	1.2
Melon, Kiwi, Strawberry, WTF, Sainsbury's*	1 Pack/245g	74	0.5	30	0.8	6.3	0.2	1.3
Melon, Pineapple & Grapes, Fresh, Tesco*	1 Pack/300g	120	0.3	40	0.5	9.2	0.1	1
Mixed, Average	*1 Bowl/100g*	*42*	*0.2*	*42*	*0.6*	*9.4*	*0.2*	*1.5*
Mixed, Food to Go, M&S*	1 Pack/400g	400	1.2	100	0.9	23.3	0.3	2.8
Mixed, Fresh, Sainsbury's*	1 Pack/200g	84	0.4	42	0.7	9.4	0.2	1.9
Mixed, Tesco*	1 Pack/225g	86	0.4	38	0.7	8.3	0.2	1.3
Nectarine, Melon, Strawberry, & Blueberry, Morrisons*	1 Pot/230g	78	0.5	34	0.9	6.7	0.2	1.1
Oranges, Apple, Pineapple & Grapes, Fresh, Asda*	1 Pack/260g	120	0.3	46	0.6	10.5	0.1	2.1
Pineapple, Apple & Strawberries, Tesco*	1 Pack/190g	80	0.2	42	0.4	9.8	0.1	1.4

F

	Measure INFO/WEIGHT	per Measure KCAL	FAT	Nutrition Values per 100g / 100ml KCAL	PROT	CARB	FAT	FIBRE
FRUIT SALAD								
Pineapple, Apple, Melon & Grape, Shapers, Boots*	1 Serving/100g	49	0.1	49	0.4	10.5	0.1	1.2
Pineapple, Mango & Passion Fruit, Prepared, M&S*	1 Pack/400g	200	0.8	50	0.7	10.8	0.2	1.8
Pineapple, Mango, Apple & Grape, Waitrose*	1 Pack/300g	186	0.6	62	0.5	14.7	0.2	1.7
Pineapple, Melon & Grape, Eat Well, M&S*	1 Pot/120g	52	0.1	43	0.5	9.3	0.1	1.4
Pineapple, Melon, Kiwi & Blueberry, Shapers, Boots*	1 Pack/179g	75	0.4	42	0.6	8.7	0.2	1.4
Pineapple, Strawberry, Grape & Carrot, M&S*	1 Pack/240g	101	1	42	0.6	8.3	0.4	1.4
Plum, Blackberries, & Fig, Tesco*	1 Pot/260g	109	0.5	42	0.8	8.2	0.2	2.5
Plum, Blackberry, Seasonal Opal Apple, Tesco*	1 Pack/105g	51	0.3	49	0.6	9.8	0.3	2.1
Rainbow Layers, Tesco*	1 Pack/270g	122	0.5	45	0.5	9.8	0.2	1.1
Rainbow, Asda*	1 Pack/350g	140	1	40	0.6	8.8	0.3	1.4
Rainbow, Fresh, Tesco*	1 Tub/270g	105	0.5	39	0.5	8.8	0.2	0.9
Seasonal Melon & Grapes, Asda*	½ Pack/200g	66	1	33	0.5	7.5	0.5	0.4
Seasonal, Fresh, Asda*	1 Pack/125g	55	0.1	44	0.5	10.4	0.1	1.2
Seasonal, M&S*	1 Serving/200g	100	0.4	50	0.5	11.8	0.2	2.1
Sharing, Fresh Tastes, Asda*	1 Pack/450g	220	0.9	49	0.4	10.4	0.2	0
Strawberry & Blueberry, Asda*	1 Pack/240g	86	0.2	36	0.9	7	0.1	1.5
Summer, Red, Fresh, M&S*	1 Pack/400g	160	0.8	40	0	10	0.2	1.2
Summer, Sainsbury's*	1 Pack/240g	84	0.5	35	0.7	7.8	0.2	1.3
Sunshine, Fresh, M&S*	1 Serving/200g	70	0.2	35	0	8.3	0.1	1.3
Tropical in Light Syrup, Passion Fruit Juice, Tesco*	½ Can/216g	130	0.2	60	0.3	14.1	0.1	1.1
Tropical Mix, Tesco*	½ Pack/140g	71	0.3	51	0.5	11	0.2	1.5
Tropical, Fresh, Asda*	1 Pack/400g	164	0.8	41	0.7	9	0.2	1.8
Tropical, Fruit Snacks, Frozen, Sainsbury's*	1 Serving/175g	79	0.2	45	0.7	10.4	0.1	1.6
Tropical, Tropical Harvest*	1 Serving/100g	52	0	52	0.3	12.8	0	1.4
Virgin Trains*	1 Serving/140g	56	0.1	40	0.4	10	0.1	0.8
FRUIT SHOOT								
Apple & Blackcurrant, Robinson's*	1 Bottle/200ml	10	0	5	0.1	0.8	0	0
Apple, Low Sugar, Robinson's*	1 Bottle/200ml	14	0	7	0	1.2	0	0
FRUIT SPREAD								
Apricot, Pure, Organic, Whole Earth*	1 Serving/20g	33	0.1	167	0.8	40	0.4	0.9
Blackcurrant, Carb Check, Heinz*	1 Tbsp/15g	8	0	54	0.5	12.8	0.1	2.7
Cherries & Berries, Organic, Meridian Foods*	1 Tbsp/15g	16	0	109	0.5	26	0.3	1.1
Cherry & Berry, Meridian Foods*	1 Serving/10g	14	0.1	138	0.7	33.7	0.6	3.2
Raspberry & Cranberry, No Added Sugar, Superjam*	1 Spread/10g	22	0	216	2.1	47	0.3	0
Raspberry, Weight Watchers*	1 Tsp/6g	7	0	111	0.4	27.1	0.1	0.9
Seville Orange, Weight Watchers*	1 Tsp/15g	17	0	111	0.2	27.5	0	0.3
FU YUNG								
Chicken, Chinese Takeaway, Tesco*	1 Pack/350g	315	3.5	90	5.6	14.5	1	0.8
Egg, Average	***1oz/28g***	***67***	***5.8***	***239***	***9.9***	***2.2***	***20.6***	***1.3***
FUDGE								
All Butter, Finest, Tesco*	1 Sweet/10g	43	1.4	429	1.3	73.4	14.5	0
Butter Tablet, Thorntons*	1oz/28g	116	3.1	414	0.9	77.6	11.1	0
Butter, Milk, Thorntons*	1 Sweet/13g	60	2.5	462	3.7	68.5	19.2	0
Cadbury*	1 Bar/25g	118	4	445	2.5	74.5	15	0.5
Chocolate, Average	***1 Sweet/30g***	***132***	***4.1***	***441***	***3.3***	***81.1***	***13.7***	***0***
Chocolate, Thorntons*	1 Bag/100g	459	19.1	459	3.1	69	19.1	0.6
Chunks for Baking	***1 Serving/100g***	***428***	***12.2***	***428***	***1.7***	***77.2***	***12.2***	***0.6***
Clotted Cream, Sainsbury's*	1 Sweet/8g	35	0.9	430	1.9	81.5	10.7	0.7
Dairy, Co-Op*	1 Sweet/9g	39	1.2	430	2	76	13	0
Salted Caramel, Fudgelicious, Ryedale Farm*	1 Piece/9g	43	1.8	473	2.1	72	20	0
Vanilla, Bar, M&S*	1 Bar/43g	205	10	476	3.7	63	23.3	0.4
Vanilla, Julian Graves*	1 Serving/10g	41	1	407	1	78.9	9.7	0
Vanilla, Thorntons*	1 Bag/100g	465	21.9	465	1.8	65.9	21.9	0

	Measure INFO/WEIGHT	per Measure KCAL	FAT	Nutrition Values per 100g / 100ml KCAL	PROT	CARB	FAT	FIBRE
FUSILLI								
Brown Rice, Fusilli, GF, Dove's Farm*	1 Serving/30g	101	0.4	338	7.9	70.3	1.5	4.1
Cooked, Average	*1 Serving/210g*	*248*	*1.4*	*118*	*4.2*	*23.8*	*0.6*	*1.2*
Dry, Average	*1 Serving/90g*	*316*	*1.4*	*352*	*12.3*	*72*	*1.6*	*2.2*
Fresh, Cooked, Average	*1 Serving/200g*	*329*	*3.6*	*164*	*6.4*	*30.6*	*1.8*	*1.8*
Fresh, Dry, Average	*1 Serving/75g*	*208*	*2*	*277*	*10.9*	*53.4*	*2.7*	*2.1*
Fusilloni, TTD, Sainsbury's*	1 Serving/90g	321	1.5	357	12.3	73.1	1.7	2.5
Green Pea & Quinoa, Pasta, GF, Dry, Clearspring*	1 Serving/80g	277	2	346	21	56	2.5	7.2
Green Pea, Organic, Uncooked, Napolina*	1 Serving/75g	99	0.1	132	9.2	20.4	0.1	6.9
Red Lentil, Dry, Cook Italian*	1 Serving/80g	283	1.6	354	23	58	2	6
Tricolore, Dry, Average	*1 Serving/75g*	*264*	*1.3*	*351*	*12.2*	*71.8*	*1.7*	*2.7*
Whole Wheat, Dry Weight, Average	*1 Serving/90g*	*290*	*2.1*	*322*	*13.1*	*62.3*	*2.3*	*9*
Wholegrain Spelt, Cooked, Sainsbury's*	1 Serving/75g	120	0.8	160	6.2	30.3	1	2.6
FYBOGEL								
Lemon, Reckitt Benckiser*	1 Serving/4.3g	4	0	95	2.4	11.3	1.1	64.8
Orange, Reckitt Benckiser*	1 Serving/4.3g	5	0	106	2.4	12.7	1.1	64.4

F

	Measure INFO/WEIGHT	per Measure KCAL	FAT	Nutrition Values per 100g / 100ml KCAL	PROT	CARB	FAT	FIBRE
GALANGAL								
Raw, Root, Average	*100g*	*71*	*0.6*	*71*	*1.2*	*15.3*	*0.6*	*2.4*
GALAXY								
Amicelli, Mars*	1 Serving/13g	66	3.5	507	6.2	59.7	27.1	0
Bubbles Filled, Chocolate Egg, Galaxy, Mars*	1 Egg/28g	155	9.5	555	6.5	54.7	34.1	1.5
Caramel Crunch, Promises, Mars*	1 Bar/100g	540	31.8	540	6.1	57.5	31.8	0
Caramel, Mars*	1 Bar/49g	254	13	518	5.8	64.2	26.4	0
Cookie Crumble, Mars*	1 Bar/114g	627	37.6	550	6.2	56	33	1.9
Fruit & Hazelnut, Milk, Mars*	1 Bar/47g	235	13.2	501	7.1	55.2	28	0
Hazelnut, Mars*	1 Piece/6g	37	2.5	582	7.8	49.4	39.2	0
Hazelnut, Roast, Promises, Mars*	1 Bar/100g	544	32.9	544	6.4	55.6	32.9	0
Swirls, Mars*	1 Bag/150g	747	39.8	498	4.9	60.2	26.5	0
GAMMON								
Breaded, Average	*1oz/28g*	*34*	*0.9*	*120*	*22.5*	*1*	*3*	*0*
Dry Cured, Ready to Roast, M&S*	½ Joint/255g	255	3.8	100	20.5	0.5	1.5	0.5
Grills, Grilled, Savers, Morrisons*	1 Grill/97g	135	4.5	139	24.2	0	4.6	0
Honey & Mustard, Average	*½ Pack/190g*	*294*	*13.5*	*155*	*19.1*	*3.6*	*7.1*	*0.1*
Joint, Boiled, Average	*1 Serving/60g*	*122*	*7.4*	*204*	*23.3*	*0*	*12.3*	*0*
Joint, Honey Glaze, Just Cook, Sainsbury's*	1/3 Pack/123g	242	12.8	197	23.4	2.1	10.4	0
Joint, Raw, Average	*1 Serving/100g*	*138*	*7.5*	*138*	*17.5*	*0*	*7.5*	*0*
Joint, Smoked, As Sold, Woodside Farms, Tesco*	1 Portion/150g	243	15.6	162	16.8	0.2	10.4	0
Joint, Unsmoked, Ovenbaked, Butchers Selection, Asda*	1 Serving/150g	178	6.1	119	20	0.5	4.1	0
Steak, Freshcure, Aldi*	1 Steak/88g	141	6.6	160	23	0.5	7.5	0.5
Steak, Umsmoked, As Prepared, Waitrose*	1 Serving/200g	358	21.4	179	20.4	0.1	10.7	0.1
Steaks, Cooked, Average	*1 Steak/97g*	*157*	*7.1*	*161*	*23.3*	*0.4*	*7.4*	*0*
Steaks, Healthy Range, Average	*1 Serving/110g*	*107*	*3.5*	*97*	*18*	*0.4*	*3.2*	*0.2*
Steaks, Honey Roast, Average	*1 Steak/100g*	*142*	*5.3*	*142*	*21.5*	*2.3*	*5.3*	*0*
Steaks, Smoked, Average	*1 Steak/110g*	*150*	*5.5*	*137*	*22.7*	*0.1*	*5*	*0.1*
Steaks, with Pineapple & Mango Salsa, Easy, Waitrose*	1 Steak/163g	239	11.6	146	14.1	6.5	7.1	0.5
GAMMON &								
Cheese, Ovenbaked, CBY, Asda*	½ Pack/182g	253	9.8	139	17.8	4.5	5.4	0.5
Parsley Sauce, Steak, Tesco*	½ Pack/140g	217	7.3	155	23.7	2.9	5.2	0.5
GARAM MASALA								
Dry, Ground, Average	*1 Tbsp/15g*	*57*	*2.3*	*379*	*15.6*	*45.2*	*15.1*	*0*
GARLIC								
Black	*1 Clove/5g*	*13*	*0*	*264*	*13.3*	*53.3*	*0*	*20*
Pickled, Bevellini*	1 Serving/12g	5	0	42	2.5	0.8	0.1	0
Powder, Average	*1 Tsp/3g*	*7*	*0*	*246*	*18.7*	*42.7*	*1.2*	*9.9*
Raw, Average	*1 Clove/3g*	*3*	*0*	*98*	*7.9*	*16.3*	*0.6*	*2.1*
Spice Blend, Gourmet Garden*	1 Squeeze/10ml	32	2.4	210	4.5	10.8	16.2	10.3
Very Lazy, The English Provender Co.*	1 Tsp/3g	3	0	111	6	20.9	0.4	3
Wild	*1 Clove/3g*	*1*	*0*	*23*	*2.8*	*1.7*	*0.6*	*1.9*
GARLIC PUREE								
Average	*1 Tbsp/18g*	*68*	*6*	*380*	*3.5*	*16.9*	*33.6*	*0*
in Vegetable Oil, GIA*	1 Tsp/5g	12	0.9	248	3.6	18.8	17.7	0
with Tomato, GIA*	10g	7	0.1	70	5.1	0.5	1.2	0
GATEAU								
Black Forest, 500g Size, Tesco*	1 Cake/500g	1125	55	225	4	27.1	11	1.8
Black Forest, Dome, Tesco*	1 Dome/600g	1626	68.4	271	4	37.4	11.4	1.6
Black Forest, Mini, Tesco*	1 Serving/55g	136	5.1	247	5.7	35.3	9.2	1
Black Forest, Sara Lee*	1 Serving/80g	221	9.8	276	3.6	37.9	12.3	1.2
Chocolate Layer, M&S*	1 Serving/86g	278	15.7	323	4.2	35.9	18.3	0.9
Chocolate, Swirl, Tesco*	1 Serving/83g	230	13.3	277	3.8	29.3	16	0.2
Double Chocolate, Frozen, Tesco*	1/5 Gateau/70g	119	4.7	265	5	35.8	10.4	4

G

	Measure INFO/WEIGHT	per Measure KCAL	FAT	Nutrition Values per 100g / 100ml KCAL	PROT	CARB	FAT	FIBRE
GATEAU								
Double Strawberry, Sara Lee*	1/8 Cake/199g	533	24.3	268	3.2	36.2	12.2	0.6
Ice Cream, Chocolate & Vanilla, Iceland*	1 Serving/130g	252	12.2	194	3.3	24.1	9.4	0.6
Orange & Lemon, Iceland*	1 Serving/90g	220	9.9	245	2.6	33.8	11	0.3
Strawberry, Co-Op*	1 Serving/77g	222	12.9	288	5.1	29.2	16.7	1
Strawberry, Frozen, Tesco*	1/5 Gateau/75g	155	6.3	205	2.8	28.8	8.3	0.9
Swiss, Cadbury*	1/6 Gateau/60g	228	10.1	380	5.2	52	16.8	0.9
Triple Chocolate, Heinz*	¼ Cake/85g	209	9.5	245	5.1	31.2	11.1	2.4
GELATINE								
Average	*1 Tsp/3g*	*10*	*0*	*338*	*84.4*	*0*	*0*	*0*
GHEE								
Butter	*1oz/28g*	*251*	*27.9*	*898*	*0*	*0*	*99.8*	*0*
Vegetable	*1oz/28g*	*251*	*27.8*	*895*	*0*	*0*	*99.4*	*0*
GHERKINS								
Pickled, Average	*1 Gherkin/36g*	*4*	*0*	*12*	*0.8*	*2.1*	*0.1*	*1*
GIN								
& Diet Tonic, Can, Greenalls*	1 Can/250ml	95	0	38	0	0	0	0
& Tonic, Canned, Ready to Drink, M&S*	1 Can/250ml	175	0.8	70	0.2	5.6	0.3	0.1
37.5% Volume	*1 Pub Shot/35ml*	*72*	*0*	*207*	*0*	*0*	*0*	*0*
40% Volume	*1 Pub Shot/35ml*	*78*	*0*	*224*	*0*	*0*	*0*	*0*
Gordons & Bitter Lemon, Canned, Gordons*	1 Can/250ml	170	0	68	0	7.1	0	0
Gordons & Schweppes Slimline Tonic, Canned, Diageo*	1 Can/250ml	75	0	30	0	0	0	0
Gordons & Schweppes Tonic, Canned, Diageo*	1 Can/250ml	152	0	61	0	6.2	0	0
GINGER								
& Garlic, Minced, Nishaan*	1 Tsp/10g	6	0	59	2.4	10.5	0.3	2.4
Chopped, Frozen	*1 Serving/4g*	*2*	*0*	*51*	*1.8*	*8.1*	*0.8*	*2*
Chunks, Crystallised, Julian Graves*	1 Serving/10g	28	0	283	0.2	70.1	0.2	1.5
Crystalised, Graze*	1 Pack/25g	61	0.1	243	2.9	58	0.3	0
Ground, Average	*1 Tsp/2g*	*5*	*0.1*	*258*	*7.4*	*60*	*3.3*	*0*
Paste, Very Lazy, The English Provender Co.*	1 Pack/75g	14	0.2	19	0.8	2.4	0.2	0
Root, Raw, Pared, Average	*1 Tsp/2g*	*2*	*0*	*81*	*1.8*	*18*	*0.8*	*2*
Root, Raw, Unprepared, Average	*1 Tsp/2g*	*1*	*0*	*74*	*1.7*	*16.3*	*0.7*	*1.8*
Stem in Sugar Syrup, Sainsbury's*	1oz/28g	76	0	271	0.2	67.3	0.1	1.4
Very Lazy, The English Provender Co.*	1 Tsp/5g	3	0	52	0.7	10.9	0.8	0.8
GINGER ALE								
1870, Siver Spring*	1 Serving/100ml	18	0	18	0	4.2	0	0
American, Finest, Tesco*	1 Serving/150ml	68	0	45	0	11	0	0
American, Low Calorie, Tesco*	1fl oz/30ml	0	0	1	0	0	0	0
American, Tesco*	1 Glass/250ml	58	0	23	0	5.5	0	0
Dry	*1 Glass/250ml*	*38*	*0*	*15*	*0*	*3.9*	*0*	*0*
Dry, Sainsbury's*	1 Glass/250ml	95	0.2	38	0.1	9.1	0.1	0.1
GINGER BEER								
Alcoholic, Crabbies*	1 Bottle/500ml	254	0	51	0	7.1	0	0
Asda*	1 Can/330ml	144	0	44	0	10.9	0	0
Classic, Schweppes*	1 Can/330ml	115	0	35	0	8.4	0	0
D & G Old Jamaican*	1 Can/330ml	211	0	64	0	16	0	0
Diet, Crabbies*	1 Bottle/700ml	7	0	1	0	0	0	0
Fiery, Canned, Waitrose*	1 Can/330ml	178	0	54	0	13.3	0	0
Fiery, Low Calorie, Waitrose*	1 Can/330ml	3	0	1	0.1	0	0	0
Fiery, Root, Cawston Press*	1 Can/330ml	109	0	33	0.1	7.5	0	0
Light, Waitrose*	1 Glass/250ml	2	0.2	1	0	0	0.1	0.1
No Added Sugar, Aldi*	1 Glass/250ml	5	0	2	0	0	0	0
No Added Sugar, Canned, Tesco*	1 Can/330ml	3	0.3	1	0	0.1	0.1	0.1
Sainsbury's*	1 Can/330ml	69	0	21	0	5.1	0	0

G

	Measure INFO/WEIGHT	per Measure KCAL	FAT	Nutrition Values per 100g / 100ml KCAL	PROT	CARB	FAT	FIBRE
GINGER BEER								
Scottish Raspberry, John Crabbie & Co*	1 Serving/200ml	64	0	32	0	7.9	0	0
Sparkling, Organic, Whole Earth*	1 Can/330ml	116	0	35	0	8.2	0	0
Tesco*	1 Serving/200ml	70	0.2	35	0.1	8.2	0.1	0
Traditional, Fentiman's*	1 Bottle/275ml	130	0	47	0	11.3	0	0
GINGER WINE								
Green Ginger Wine & Scots Whisky, Crabbies*	1 Glass/125ml	192	0	153	14.3	14.3	0	0
Green, Crabbies*	1 Serving/125ml	202	0	162	0	21.8	0	0
GINGERBREAD								
Average	*1oz/28g*	*106*	*3.5*	*379*	*5.7*	*64.7*	*12.6*	*1.2*
GLYCERINE								
Average	*1 Tsp/5ml*	*22*	*0*	*440*	*0*	*100*	*0*	*0*
GNOCCHI								
Carrot & Swede, Tesco*	¼ Pack/100g	51	1.1	51	3.3	5.6	1.1	2.8
Di Patate, Italfresco*	½ Pack/200g	296	0.4	148	3.3	33.2	0.2	0
Fresh, Cooked, Essential, Waitrose*	¼ Pack/134g	242	0.5	181	4.7	39	0.4	1
Fresh, Italian, Chilled, Sainsbury's*	¼ Pack/125g	190	0.4	152	3.8	33.6	0.3	1.4
Fresh, Raw, Essential, Waitrose*	¼ Pack/125g	225	0.5	180	4.7	39	0.4	1
Fresh, Tesco*	½ Pack/200g	230	0.2	115	2.5	25.1	0.1	2
Potato, Cooked, Average	*1 Serving/150g*	*200*	*0*	*133*	*0*	*33.2*	*0*	*0*
GNOCCHI								
Potato, Fresh, Dell'ugo*	¼ Pack/87g	124	0.3	142	4	30.2	0.4	1
Potato, with Steamed Greens, Everdine*	1 Serving/450g	342	11.2	76	3.2	8.8	2.5	2.8
GOAT								
Meat, Uncooked	*1 Portion/100g*	*109*	*2.3*	*109*	*20*	*0*	*2.3*	*0*
GOJI BERRIES								
Average	*1 Serving/100g*	*287*	*0.7*	*287*	*6.6*	*65.1*	*0.7*	*6.8*
GOOSE								
Leg with Skin, Fire Roasted	*1 Leg/174g*	*482*	*29.8*	*277*	*28.8*	*0*	*17.1*	*0*
Meat & Skin, Roasted	*½ Goose/774g*	*2361*	*169.5*	*305*	*25.2*	*0*	*21.9*	*0*
Meat, Fat & Skin, Raw	*1oz/28g*	*101*	*9.2*	*361*	*16.5*	*0*	*32.8*	*0*
Meat, Raw	*1 Portion/185g*	*298*	*13*	*161*	*23*	*0*	*7*	*0*
Meat, Roasted	*1 Portion/143g*	*340*	*18.6*	*238*	*29*	*0*	*13*	*0*
GOOSEBERRIES								
Dessert, Raw, Tops & Tails Removed	*1oz/28g*	*11*	*0.1*	*40*	*0.7*	*9.2*	*0.3*	*2.4*
Stewed with Sugar	*25g*	*14*	*0.1*	*54*	*0.7*	*12.9*	*0.3*	*4.2*
Stewed without Sugar	*25g*	*4*	*0.1*	*16*	*0.9*	*2.5*	*0.3*	*4.4*
GOULASH								
Beef with Tagliatelle, COU, M&S*	1 Pack/360g	414	8.3	115	8.5	14.5	2.3	1
Beef, Average	*1 Serving/300g*	*310*	*9.5*	*103*	*8.1*	*10.4*	*3.2*	*0.9*
Beef, Finest, Tesco*	½ Pack/300g	297	9.3	99	11.6	6.2	3.1	0.6
Beef, Weight Watchers*	1 Pack/330g	241	5.6	73	4.8	9.5	1.7	0.6
GRAPEFRUIT								
in Juice, Canned, Average	*1/3 Can/179g*	*82*	*0.1*	*46*	*0.5*	*10.6*	*0*	*0.4*
in Syrup, Average	*1oz/28g*	*19*	*0*	*69*	*0.5*	*16.8*	*0.1*	*0.5*
Raw, Flesh Only, Average	*½ Fruit/160g*	*48*	*0.2*	*30*	*0.8*	*6.8*	*0.1*	*1.3*
Raw, Weighed with Skin & Seeds, Average	*1 Lge/340g*	*54*	*0.2*	*16*	*0.3*	*4*	*0*	*0.6*
Ruby Red in Juice, Average	*1 Serving/135g*	*54*	*0.1*	*40*	*0.6*	*9.4*	*0*	*0.5*
GRAPES								
Cotton Candy, 1, Waitrose*	1 Serving/80g	53	0.1	66	0.4	15.4	0.1	0.9
Cotton Candy, Black, Seedless, Finest, Tesco*	1 Portion/80g	53	0.1	66	0.4	15.4	0.1	0.7
Green, Average	*1 Grape/5g*	*3*	*0*	*62*	*0.4*	*15.2*	*0.1*	*0.7*
Red & Green Selection, Average	*1 Grape/5g*	*3*	*0*	*62*	*0.4*	*15.2*	*0.1*	*0.8*

G

	Measure INFO/WEIGHT	per Measure KCAL	FAT	Nutrition Values per 100g / 100ml KCAL	PROT	CARB	FAT	FIBRE
GRAPES								
Red, Average	*1 Grape/5g*	*3*	*0*	*65*	*0.4*	*15.8*	*0.1*	*0.6*
Sable, 1, Waitrose*	1 Pack/400g	264	0.4	66	0.4	15.4	0.1	0.9
Sable, Finest, Tesco*	1 Serving/80g	53	0.1	66	0.4	15.4	0.1	0.7
GRAPPA								
Average	*1 Serving/30ml*	*85*	*0*	*283*	*0*	*6.7*	*0*	*0*
GRATIN								
Cauliflower, Findus*	1 Pack/400g	340	20	85	3.5	7	5	0
Cheesy Potato, Ovenbaked, Asda*	½ Pack/200g	179	8	90	1.7	11	4	1.4
Crab & Lobster Mac & Cheese, Iceland*	1 Pot/100g	148	7.1	155	7.4	14	7.4	1.5
Dauphinoise, Budgens*	½ Pack/218g	277	15.7	127	3	12.5	7.2	2.5
Leek & Carrot, Findus*	1 Pack/400g	440	26	110	3.5	9.5	6.5	0
Potato, & Spinach, M&S*	1 Serving/225g	259	16	115	2.9	9.1	7.1	1.3
Potato, Creamy, M&S*	½ Pack/225g	360	25	160	2.2	11.9	11.1	0.9
Potato, HL, Tesco*	1 Serving/225g	169	5	75	2.3	11.4	2.2	0.6
Potato, On The Side, M Kitchen, Morrisons*	½ Pack/200g	241	12.5	120	3.1	12.4	6.2	1.3
Potato, Sainsbury's*	½ Pack/225g	448	34	199	4.4	11.4	15.1	1
Potato, Somerfield*	½ Pack/225g	356	27	158	2	11	12	0
Root Vegetable, Finest, Tesco*	½ Pack/214g	365	23.9	171	2.4	14	11.2	2
Smoked Haddock, Rarebit, Iceland*	½ Pack/100g	174	11.2	184	14.6	4.1	11.8	1.4
Vegetable, Somerfield*	1 Pack/300g	417	39	139	1	5	13	0
GRAVY								
Beef with Winter Berry & Shallot, Made Up, Oxo*	1 Serving/105ml	24	0.3	23	0.6	4.3	0.3	0.1
Beef, Aunt Bessie's*	1 Serving/100g	73	5.3	73	1	5.3	5.3	0.5
Beef, Favourite, Granules, Made Up, Bisto*	1 Serving/50ml	13	0.5	26	0	4.2	1	0
Beef, Free From, Sainsbury's*	½ Pack/151g	47	1.5	31	1.5	4.1	1	0.2
Beef, Fresh, Sainsbury's*	1 Serving/83ml	47	2.7	56	2.4	4.5	3.2	0.6
Beef, Heat & Serve, Morrisons*	1 Serving/150g	27	0.4	18	0.3	3.9	0.3	0.5
Beef, Roast, Traditional, Finest, Tesco*	¼ Pot/125g	68	3	54	2.4	5.5	2.4	0.3
Caramelised Onion, Made Up, Bisto*	1 Serving/70ml	20	0.3	29	0.1	6.1	0.4	0.1
Chicken, Finest, Tesco*	¼ Pouch/88ml	38	1.1	43	2.3	5.6	1.3	0
Chicken, Granules For, Dry Weight, Bisto*	1 Serving/20g	80	3.2	400	1.9	62.5	15.8	0.2
Favourite, Granules, Made Up, Bisto*	1 Serving/50ml	15	0.6	30	0.2	4.4	1.2	0
for Chicken & Turkey, Christmas, TTD, Sainsbury's*	¼ Pot/112g	66	1.7	59	6.9	4.2	1.5	0.5
Fresh, Somerfield*	1 Pack/300g	69	3	23	0	4	1	0
Granules for Chicken, Made Up, Smart Price, Asda*	1 Serving/100ml	34	2.3	34	0.2	3	2.3	0.1
Granules for Meat, Made Up, Asda*	1 Serving/100ml	38	2.4	38	0.6	4	2.4	0.1
Granules for Meat, Made Up, Sainsbury's*	1 Serving/100ml	37	2.4	37	0.4	3.5	2.4	0.1
Granules for Vegetarian Dishes, Dry Weight, Bisto*	1 Serving/28g	100	3.7	356	2.7	56	13.3	4.5
Granules, Beef, Dry, Tesco*	1 Serving/6g	29	2.1	480	5.5	36.4	34.7	1.5
Granules, Beef, Made Up, Tesco*	1 Serving/140ml	48	3.6	35	0.3	2.6	2.5	0.1
Granules, Chicken & Hint of Sage & Onion, Oxo*	1 Serving/30g	95	1.8	316	11.1	54.2	6.1	0.7
Granules, Chicken, Dry, Average	*1 Tsp/4g*	*17*	*0.9*	*428*	*4.5*	*49.4*	*23.6*	*1.2*
Granules, Chicken, Dry, Oxo*	1oz/28g	83	1.4	296	11.1	54.2	4.9	0.7
Granules, Chicken, Made Up, Oxo*	1fl oz/30ml	5	0.1	18	0.7	3.3	0.3	0
Granules, Dry, Bisto*	1 Serving/10g	38	1.6	384	3.1	56.4	16.2	1.5
Granules, Dry, Value, Tesco*	1oz/28g	111	5.2	397	3.2	54.4	18.5	1
Granules, for Chicken, Made Up, Average	*1 Serving/50ml*	*15*	*0.8*	*30*	*0.4*	*3.6*	*1.5*	*0.1*
Granules, for Vegetarian Dishes, Made Up, Sainsbury's*	1 Serving/50ml	16	1.1	32	0.2	2.8	2.2	0.8
Granules, Instant, Made Up	*1oz/28g*	*10*	*0.7*	*34*	*0.3*	*3*	*2.4*	*0*
Granules, Lamb, Dry, Average	*1 Tsp/4g*	*14*	*0.3*	*344*	*10.8*	*56.2*	*8.4*	*2.8*
Granules, Made Up, Oxo*	1 Serving/150ml	28	0.4	19	0.6	3.4	0.3	0
Granules, Vegetable, Dry, Oxo*	1oz/28g	88	1.4	316	8.4	59.5	4.9	0.9
Granules, Vegetable, Dry, Tesco*	½ Pint/20g	94	6.7	470	3.8	38.5	33.4	3.7

G

	Measure INFO/WEIGHT	per Measure KCAL	FAT	Nutrition Values per 100g / 100ml KCAL	PROT	CARB	FAT	FIBRE
GRAVY								
Instant, Made Up, BGTY, Sainsbury's*	1fl oz/30ml	10	0	32	0.3	7.4	0.1	0.1
Lamb, Granules, As Prepared, Best, Bisto*	1 Serving/50ml	13	0.5	26	1	5.4	1	1
Meat, Granules, As Consumed, Quixo, Aldi*	1 Serving/70ml	24	1.6	34	0.5	3.1	2.3	0.5
Onion, Fresh, Asda*	1/6 Pot/77g	30	1.6	39	1.7	3.3	2.1	0.4
Onion, Fresh, Somerfield*	1 Pack/300g	195	12	65	1	7	4	0
Onion, Granules For, Dry Weight, Bisto*	4 Tsp/20g	78	2.9	391	2.4	62.3	14.7	2.3
Onion, Granules, Made Up, Bisto*	1 Serving/50ml	14	0.3	28	0.2	5.6	0.6	0
Onion, Rich, M&S*	½ Pack/150g	60	1.8	40	2	5.9	1.2	0.3
Pork, Best, Made Up, Bisto*	1 Serving/50ml	14	0.2	28	0.6	5.8	0.4	0
Powder, GF, Dry, Allergycare*	1 Tbsp/10g	26	0	260	0.3	63.8	0.4	0
Powder, Made Up, Sainsbury's*	1 Serving/100ml	15	0.1	15	0.4	3.2	0.1	0.1
Powder, Vegetarian, Organic, Marigold*	1 Serving/22g	79	1.7	361	10.6	61.5	7.7	1.3
Roast Beef, Best in Glass Jar, Made Up, Bisto*	1 Serving/70ml	21	0.3	30	0.3	6.1	0.4	0
Roast Lamb, Bisto*	1 Serving/20g	60	0.9	302	3.4	62.3	4.3	0
Roast Onion, Classic, Dry, Schwartz*	1 Pack/27g	85	1.1	315	8.8	61	4	4.6
Roast Pork & Sage, Classic, Dry, Schwartz*	1 Pack/25g	88	1.4	354	11.8	63.8	5.8	0
Roast Pork, Best, in Glass Jar, Dry Weight, Bisto*	4 Tsp/20g	63	0.9	314	4.3	64.1	4.5	0
Turkey, Finest, Tesco*	¼ Pouch/88ml	49	1.4	56	3.9	6.4	1.6	0
Turkey, Granules For, Dry Weight, Bisto*	4 Tsp/20g	75	3.1	377	2.4	57.2	15.5	1
Turkey, Rich, Ready to Heat, Schwartz*	1 Pack/200g	62	2.4	31	1.9	3.1	1.2	0.5
Vegetable, Granules For, Dry Weight, Bisto*	1 Tsp/4g	15	0.5	380	2.1	63	13.3	4.5
Vegetable, Granules For, Made Up, Bisto*	1 Serving/50ml	14	0.2	28	0.2	5.6	0.4	0.2
GRITS								
Hominy, White, Enriched, Old Fashioned, Quaker*	¼ Cup/41g	140	0.5	341	7.3	78	1.2	4.9
GROUSE								
Meat Only, Roasted	*1oz/28g*	*36*	*0.6*	*128*	*27.6*	*0*	*2*	*0*
GUACAMOLE								
Average	*1 Tbsp/17g*	*33*	*3.3*	*194*	*1.6*	*3.4*	*19.2*	*2.4*
Avocado, Reduced Fat, The Fresh Dip Company*	1 Serving/113g	128	9.8	113	2.5	6.1	8.7	2.3
Chunky, M&S*	1 Pot/170g	221	19.2	130	1.5	5.1	11.3	1.7
Fresh, Sainsbury's*	1oz/28g	59	5.7	212	1.5	4.2	20.2	3.7
Reduced Fat Average	*1 Serving/100g*	*129*	*10.8*	*129*	*2.4*	*5.2*	*10.8*	*3*
Reduced Fat, Dip, BGTY, Sainsbury's*	¼ Pot/42.5g	62	5.7	146	1.3	2.9	13.5	4
Style, Topping, Dip, Discovery*	1 Seving/37g	29	2.1	79	1.2	6	5.6	1.2
GUAVA								
Canned in Syrup	*1oz/28g*	*17*	*0*	*60*	*0.4*	*15.7*	*0*	*3*
Raw, Flesh Only, Average	*1 Fruit/55g*	*37*	*0.6*	*68*	*3*	*14*	*1*	*5*
GUINEA FOWL								
Boned & Stuffed, Fresh, Fayrefield Foods*	1 Serving/325g	650	39.3	200	19.1	3.3	12.1	0.5
Fresh, Free Range, Waitrose*	1 Portion/193g	258	11.9	134	19.5	0	6.2	0.3
GUMS								
American Hard, Sainsbury's*	1 Sweet/6g	22	0	360	0.1	90	0.1	0
American Hard, Tesco*	1 Serving/200g	646	0	323	0	80.8	0	0
Milk Bottles, Bassett's*	1 Pack/25g	88	0.4	353	6.2	78.3	1.6	0
Milk Bottles, Milk Flavour, Asda*	1 Pack/100g	369	2.3	369	7	80	2.3	0.4

INFO/WEIGHT	Measure			Nutrition Values per 100g / 100ml				
		KCAL	FAT	KCAL	PROT	CARB	FAT	FIBRE
HADDOCK								
Fillets, Battered, Average	*1oz/28g*	*64*	*3.4*	*228*	*13.4*	*16.3*	*12.2*	*1.1*
Fillets, in Breadcrumbs, Average	*1 Fillet/125g*	*253*	*12.4*	*203*	*13.5*	*14.9*	*9.9*	*1.2*
Fillets, in Lemon & Chive Butter Sauce, Birds Eye*	1 Portion/148g	190	11.3	128	14.6	0.4	7.6	0
Fillets, in Seeded Breadcrumbs, Waitrose*	1 Fillet/121g	278	12.8	230	15.6	16.8	10.6	2.5
Fillets, Raw, Average	*1 Fillet/140g*	*111*	*1.2*	*79*	*17.7*	*0.2*	*0.8*	*0*
Fillets, Seeded, Crunchy & Flavoursome, Waitrose*	1 Fillet/109g	259	12.8	238	15.6	16.3	11.7	2.2
Fillets, Seeded, Super, Loved by Us, Co-Op*	1 Portion/150g	265	13.3	177	14	9.5	8.9	1.8
Fillets, Smoked, Cooked, Average	*1 Pack/300g*	*337*	*7.7*	*112*	*21.9*	*0.4*	*2.6*	*0.1*
Fillets, Smoked, in Mustard & Dill, The Saucy Fish Co.*	2 Fillets/270g	262	9.7	97	15.5	0.1	3.6	0
Fillets, Smoked, Raw, Average	*1 Pack/227g*	*190*	*1*	*84*	*19.9*	*0.1*	*0.4*	*0.2*
Fillets, with Lemon & Chive Sauce, Inspirations, Birds Eye*	1 Fillet/148g	200	11.8	135	15.4	0.3	8	0.1
Flour, Fried in Blended Oil	*1oz/28g*	*39*	*1.1*	*138*	*21.1*	*4.5*	*4.1*	*0.2*
Goujons, Batter, Crispy, M&S*	1 Serving/100g	250	14.1	250	11.7	18.5	14.1	0.8
Mornay, COU, M&S*	½ Pack/190g	162	3.8	85	14.5	2.6	2	0.6
Smoked, Ocean Trader, Lidl*	1 Portion/100g	96	0.2	96	23.2	0.1	0.2	0.5
HAGGIS								
Hall's*	1 Haggis/454g	1053	64.5	232	9.7	15.1	14.2	2.5
Traditional, Average	*1 Serving/454g*	*1119*	*66.5*	*246*	*12.4*	*17.2*	*14.6*	*1*
Traditional, Macsween*	1 Haggis/454g	1149	70.8	253	11.1	19.1	15.6	2.1
Vegetarian, Macsween*	1/3 Pack/151g	412	24.6	273	6	22.9	16.3	0
Vegetarian, Simon Howie*	1/3 Pack/151g	305	14.6	202	11.8	17.6	9.7	0
HAKE								
Fillets, in Breadcrumbs, Average	*1oz/28g*	*66*	*3.7*	*234*	*12.9*	*16*	*13.4*	*1*
Goujons, Average	*1 Serving/150g*	*345*	*17.8*	*230*	*12.4*	*18.6*	*11.9*	*1.3*
Raw, Average	*1oz/28g*	*28*	*0.6*	*100*	*20.1*	*0*	*2.2*	*0*
with Tomato & Basil Sauce, Vegetable Selection, Tesco*	1 Pack/450g	248	5.8	55	4.3	6.7	1.3	1.5
HALIBUT								
Cooked, Dry Heat, Average	*1oz/28g*	*38*	*1.1*	*135*	*24.6*	*0.4*	*4*	*0*
Raw	*1oz/28g*	*28*	*0.5*	*101*	*21.1*	*0*	*1.9*	*0*
with Roasted Pepper Sauce, Fillets, M&S*	1 Serving/145g	218	14.4	150	12.7	2.4	9.9	0.6
HALVA								
Average	*1oz/28g*	*107*	*3.7*	*381*	*1.8*	*68*	*13.2*	*0*
HAM								
Applewood Smoked, Average	*1 Slice/28g*	*31*	*0.8*	*112*	*21.2*	*0.6*	*2.8*	*0.2*
Baked, Average	*1 Slice/74g*	*98*	*3.7*	*133*	*21*	*1*	*5*	*0*
Beechwood Smoked, Morrisons*	1 Slice/20g	32	1.8	160	19.5	0.5	9	0
Black Forest, Slices, Dulano, Lidl*	1 Slice/11g	26	1.6	240	25	1	15	0.5
Boiled, Average	*1 Pack/113g*	*154*	*6.5*	*136*	*20.6*	*0.6*	*5.8*	*0*
Breaded, Average	*1 Slice/37g*	*57*	*2.3*	*155*	*23.1*	*1.8*	*6.3*	*1.6*
Breaded, Dry Cured, Average	*1 Slice/33g*	*47*	*1.8*	*142*	*22.2*	*1.4*	*5.4*	*0*
Brunswick, Average	*1 Slice/20g*	*32*	*1.8*	*160*	*19.5*	*0.6*	*8.8*	*0*
Cooked, Sliced, Average	*1 Slice/17g*	*18*	*0.5*	*109*	*19*	*1*	*3.2*	*0.1*
Crumbed, Sliced, Average	*1 Slice/28g*	*33*	*0.9*	*117*	*21.5*	*0.9*	*3.1*	*0*
Danish, Average	*1 Slice/11g*	*14*	*0.6*	*125*	*18.4*	*1*	*5.4*	*0*
Danish, Lean, Average	*1 Slice/15g*	*14*	*0.3*	*92*	*17.8*	*1*	*1.8*	*0*
Dry Cured, Average	*1 Slice/18g*	*26*	*1*	*144*	*22.4*	*1*	*5.6*	*0.2*
Extra Lean, Average	*1 Slice/11g*	*10*	*0.2*	*90*	*18*	*1.4*	*1.4*	*0*
Gammon, Breaded, Average	*1 Serving/25g*	*31*	*0.8*	*122*	*22*	*1.5*	*3.1*	*0*
Gammon, Dry Cured, Sliced, Average	*1 Slice/33g*	*43*	*1.4*	*131*	*22.9*	*0.4*	*4.2*	*0*
Gammon, Honey Roast, Average	*1 Serving/60g*	*81*	*2.8*	*134*	*22.4*	*0.4*	*4.8*	*0*
Gammon, Smoked, Average	*1 Slice/43g*	*59*	*2.1*	*137*	*22.3*	*0.7*	*4.9*	*0.2*
German Black Forest, Average	*½ Pack/35g*	*93*	*6*	*267*	*27.2*	*1.3*	*17*	*0.5*
Hock, Cooked, Shredded, Sainsbury's*	½ Pack50g	69	1.6	138	26.3	0.7	3.3	0

H

	Measure INFO/WEIGHT	per Measure KCAL	FAT	Nutrition Values per 100g / 100ml KCAL	PROT	CARB	FAT	FIBRE
HAM								
Hock, Pulled, M&S*	1 Pack/100g	165	6.5	165	26.5	0.1	6.5	0.1
Hock, with Apple Sauce, Slow Cooked, M&S*	1 Hock/167g	321	7.2	192	23.2	14.9	4.3	0.5
Honey & Mustard, Average	*1oz/28g*	*39*	*1.2*	*140*	*20.8*	*4.6*	*4.3*	*0*
Honey Roast, Average	*1 Slice/20g*	*25*	*0.8*	*123*	*20.3*	*1.6*	*3.8*	*0.1*
Honey Roast, Dry Cured, Average	*1 Slice/33g*	*46*	*1.5*	*140*	*22.7*	*2.3*	*4.4*	*0.2*
Honey Roast, Lean, Average	*1 Serving/25g*	*28*	*0.8*	*111*	*18.2*	*2.7*	*3.1*	*0*
Honey Roast, Wafer Thin, Average	*1 Slice/10g*	*11*	*0.3*	*113*	*17.4*	*3.7*	*3.2*	*0.3*
Honey Roast, Wafer Thin, Premium, Average	*1 Slice/10g*	*15*	*0.6*	*149*	*22*	*1.6*	*6*	*0*
Jamon, Iberico de Bellota, Hand Carved, 1, Waitrose*	¼ Pack/16g	56	3.9	344	31.5	0.7	23.7	0.9
Joint, Cured, Roasted, Average	*1 Serving/100g*	*138*	*5.2*	*138*	*21.7*	*1*	*5.2*	*0.1*
Joint, Roast, Christmas, Tesco*	1/6 Joint/167g	225	10.8	135	17.9	1.1	6.5	0
Lean, Average	*1 Slice/18g*	*19*	*0.4*	*104*	*19.5*	*1.1*	*2.4*	*0.3*
Oak Smoked, Average	*1 Slice/20g*	*26*	*0.9*	*130*	*21*	*1*	*4.7*	*0.3*
Parma, Average	*1 Slice/10g*	*21*	*1.1*	*213*	*29.3*	*0*	*10.6*	*0*
Parma, Premium, Average	*1 Slice/14g*	*36*	*2.3*	*258*	*27.9*	*0.3*	*16.1*	*0*
Peppered, Average	*1 Slice/12g*	*13*	*0.3*	*110*	*18.5*	*2*	*2.7*	*0*
Peppered, Dry Cured, Average	*1 Slice/31g*	*43*	*1.5*	*140*	*23.1*	*1.3*	*4.7*	*0.2*
Prosciutto, Average	*1 Slice/12g*	*27*	*1.5*	*226*	*28.7*	*0*	*12.4*	*0.4*
Serrano, Average	*1 Slice/20g*	*46*	*2.4*	*230*	*30.5*	*0.4*	*11.8*	*0*
Smoked, Average	*1 Slice/18g*	*21*	*0.7*	*117*	*19.7*	*0.9*	*3.7*	*0*
Smoked, Dry Cured, Average	*1 Slice/28g*	*38*	*1.2*	*137*	*23*	*1.4*	*4.4*	*0.2*
Smoked, Wafer Thin, Average	*1 Serving/40g*	*41*	*1.2*	*102*	*17.7*	*1.2*	*2.9*	*0.2*
Thick Cut, Average	*1 Slice/74g*	*94*	*2.9*	*127*	*22.4*	*0.6*	*3.9*	*0.1*
Tinned, Average	*½ Can/100g*	*136*	*8.8*	*136*	*12.2*	*2*	*8.8*	*0*
Tinned, Lean, Average	*½ Can/100g*	*94*	*2.3*	*94*	*18.1*	*0.2*	*2.3*	*0.4*
Vegetarian, Slices, Deli, Wafer Thin, Deli, Quorn*	1/3 Pack/60g	66	1.3	110	16	6.5	2.2	5.8
Vegetarian, Slices, Quorn*	¼ Pack/25g	30	0.5	122	16	6.5	2.2	5.8
Wafer Thin, Average	*1 Slice/10g*	*10*	*0.3*	*101*	*17.9*	*1.4*	*2.6*	*0.1*
Wiltshire, Average	*1oz/28g*	*41*	*1.7*	*148*	*23.1*	*0*	*6*	*0*
Wiltshire, Breaded, Average	*1oz/28g*	*41*	*1.4*	*145*	*23.9*	*1*	*5*	*0*
HARE								
Raw, Lean Only, Average	*1oz/28g*	*35*	*1*	*125*	*23.5*	*0.2*	*3.5*	*0*
Stewed, Lean Only, Average	*1oz/28g*	*48*	*1.5*	*170*	*29.5*	*0.2*	*5.5*	*0*
HARIBO*								
American Hard Gums, Haribo*	1 Pack/175g	630	3.3	360	0.3	85.5	1.9	0.2
Cola Bottles, Fizzy, Haribo*	1 Pack/175g	595	0.4	340	6.3	78.3	0.2	0.3
Cola Bottles, Haribo*	1 Pack/16g	56	0	348	7.7	78.9	0.2	0.3
Dolly Mixtures, Haribo*	1 Pack/175g	719	8.4	411	1.8	90.2	4.8	0.2
Fantasy Mix, Haribo*	1 Pack/100g	344	0.2	344	6.6	79	0.2	0.3
Gold Bears, Haribo*	1 Pack/100g	348	0.2	348	7.7	78.9	0.2	0.3
Happy Cherries, Haribo*	1 Serving/40g	139	0.1	348	7.7	78.9	0.2	0.3
Horror Mix, Haribo*	1 Pack/100g	344	0.2	344	6.6	79	0.2	0.3
Jelly Babies, Haribo*	1oz/28g	97	0.1	348	4.5	82.1	0.2	0.5
Jelly Beans, Haribo*	1 Pack/100g	379	0.2	379	0.6	93.8	0.2	0.1
Kiddies Super Mix, Haribo*	1 Pack/100g	344	0.2	344	6.6	79	0.2	0.3
Liquorice Favourites, Haribo*	1 Serving/40g	143	1.2	357	2.8	78.8	3	2.3
Liquorice with Stevia, Stevi-Lakritz, Haribo*	¼ Bag/25g	46	0	185	8.1	16	0.1	48.6
Magic Mix, Haribo*	1oz/28g	102	0.5	366	5.4	82	1.9	0.3
Maoam Stripes, Haribo*	1 Chew/7g	27	0.4	384	1.2	81.7	6.1	0.3
Mega Roulette, Haribo*	1oz/28g	97	0.1	348	7.7	78.9	0.2	0.3
Milky Mix, Haribo*	1 Pack/175g	607	0.4	347	7.1	79.6	0.2	0.4
Mint Imperials, Haribo*	1 Pack/175g	695	0.9	397	0.4	98.8	0.5	0.1
Pontefract Cakes, Haribo*	1 Serving/40g	118	0.1	296	5.3	68.2	0.2	0.5

H

	INFO/WEIGHT	KCAL	FAT	KCAL	PROT	CARB	FAT	FIBRE
HARIBO*								
Snakes, Haribo*	1 Snake/8g	28	0	348	7.7	78.9	0.2	0.3
Starmix, Haribo*	1 Pack/100g	344	0.2	344	6.6	79	0.2	0.3
Tangfastics, Haribo*	1 Pack/100g	359	2.3	359	6.3	78.3	2.3	0.5
Tropifruit, Haribo*	1oz/28g	97	0.1	348	4.5	82.1	0.2	0.5
HARISSA PASTE								
Average	*1 Tsp/5g*	*6*	*0.3*	*123*	*2.9*	*12.9*	*6.7*	*2.8*
Barts*	1 Tbsp/15g	11	0.3	76	4	10.7	1.9	0
Easy, M&S*	1 Tbsp/15g	16	0.8	105	2.5	11.2	5.5	4.4
HASH								
Corned Beef, Asda*	1 Pack/400g	416	14.4	104	6	12	3.6	1.1
Corned Beef, M&S*	½ Pack/321g	385	20.2	120	8.1	7.4	6.3	1.3
Steak, in London Porter Gravy, British, TTD, Sainsbury's*	1 Pack/400g	408	13.6	102	8.5	8.5	3.4	1.4
Steak, Potato & Onion, Gastropub, M&S*	1 Meal/370g	399	14.8	108	9	8.1	4	1.7
HASH BROWNS								
Homestyle, Aunt Bessie's*	2 Pieces/98g	182	9.2	186	1.6	23	9.4	1.9
Oven Baked, Weighed Cooked, McCain*	1 Piece/37.5g	80	4.3	214	2.1	25.7	11.4	2.2
Oven Baked, Weighed Frozen, McCain*	1 Piece/40g	75	4.1	187	1.7	21.8	10.3	2.1
Potatoes, From Restaurant, Average	*1 Portion/150g*	*489*	*32.5*	*326*	*2.6*	*32.1*	*21.6*	*2.7*
Uncooked, Average	*1 Piece/45g*	*78*	*3.7*	*173*	*2*	*22.5*	*8.3*	*1.9*
HAZELNUTS								
Blanched, Average	*1 Serving/25g*	*164*	*15.9*	*656*	*15.4*	*5.8*	*63.5*	*6.5*
Chopped, Average	*1 Serving/10g*	*67*	*6.4*	*666*	*16.8*	*5.6*	*64*	*6.6*
Roasted, Graze*	1 Pack/26g	173	16.9	665	14	6.1	65	0
Whole, Average	*10 Whole/10g*	*66*	*6.4*	*655*	*15.4*	*5.8*	*63.5*	*6.5*
HEART								
Lambs, Average	*1 Heart/75g*	*92*	*4.5*	*122*	*16*	*1*	*6*	*0*
Ox, Raw	*1oz/28g*	*23*	*0.8*	*82*	*14.4*	*0*	*2.8*	*0*
Ox, Stewed	*1oz/28g*	*44*	*1.4*	*157*	*27.8*	*0*	*5.1*	*0*
HERMESETAS								
Powdered, Hermes*	1 Tsp/0.8g	3	0	387	1	96.8	0	0
The Classic Sweetener, Hermes*	1 Tablet/0.5g	0	0	294	14.2	59.3	0	0
HERRING								
Canned in Tomato Sauce, Average	*1oz/28g*	*57*	*4.3*	*204*	*11.9*	*4.1*	*15.5*	*0.1*
Dried, Salted, Average	*1oz/28g*	*47*	*2.1*	*168*	*25.3*	*0*	*7.4*	*0*
Fillets in Mustard & Dill Sauce, John West*	1 Can/190g	332	26.6	175	9.4	2.9	14	0.1
Fillets in Olive Oil, Succulent, Princes*	1 Serving/50g	108	7.5	215	20	0	15	0
Fillets, Raw, Average	*1 Herring/100g*	*139*	*9.4*	*139*	*13.8*	*0*	*9.4*	*0*
Fillets, Smoked, & Peppered, Sainsbury's*	½ Pack/80g	163	8.7	204	22.8	3.5	10.9	0
Grilled, Average	*1oz/28g*	*51*	*3.1*	*181*	*20.1*	*0*	*11.2*	*0*
in Dill Marinade, Drained, Elsinore*	1 Jar/140g	336	15.4	240	9.8	27	11	0
Pickled in Mustard Sauce, Abba*	1 Serving/58g	150	10.9	260	7	16	19	0
Pickled, Average	*1oz/28g*	*42*	*2.9*	*149*	*8.1*	*5.5*	*10.3*	*0*
Rollmops, with Onion, Asda*	1 Rollmop/65g	89	3.1	137	13.2	10.3	4.8	0.8
Smoked, Pepper in Oil, GlyngÃƒ¸re*	1 Can/130g	338	24.7	260	21	0	19	0
Whole, Raw, Average	*1 Serving/100g*	*95*	*6.6*	*95*	*8.9*	*0*	*6.6*	*0*
HOKI								
Grilled	*1oz/28g*	*34*	*0.8*	*121*	*24.1*	*0*	*2.7*	*0*
Raw	*1oz/28g*	*24*	*0.5*	*85*	*16.9*	*0*	*1.9*	*0*
HONEY								
Acacia Blossom, Sainsbury's*	1 Serving/24g	81	0	339	0.1	84.7	0.1	0.3
Acacia, Tesco*	1 Tsp/4g	12	0	307	0.4	76.4	0	0
Clear, Basics, Sainsbury's*	1 Tsp/15g	46	0	307	0.4	76.4	0.1	0
Clear, Everyday Essentials, Aldi*	1 Serving/10g	33	0	328	0.5	81	0.5	0.5

H

	Measure INFO/WEIGHT	per Measure KCAL	FAT	Nutrition Values per 100g / 100ml KCAL	PROT	CARB	FAT	FIBRE
HONEY								
Clear, Runny, Sainsbury's*	1 Serving/15g	51	0	339	0.1	84.7	0.1	0.3
Clear, Value, Tesco*	1 Serving/27g	86	0	320	1	78	0	0
Clear, with a Hint of Cinnamon, Rowse*	1 Tbsp/15g	49	0.1	329	0.5	81.5	0.5	0.5
Greek, Waitrose*	1 Tsp/6g	18	0	307	0.4	76.4	0	0
Pure, Clear, Average	*1 Tbsp/20g*	*63*	*0*	*315*	*0.5*	*78.5*	*0*	*0*
Pure, Set, Average	*1 Tbsp/20g*	*62*	*0*	*312*	*0.4*	*77.6*	*0*	*0*
Raw, British Wildflower, Hilltop*	1 Tsp/5g	17	0	333	0.2	83.1	0.2	0
Runny, Organic, Ocado *	1 Tsp/15g	49	0	324	0	81	0	0
Scottish Heather, Waitrose*	1 Serving/20g	61	0	307	0.4	76.4	0	0
Spanish Orange Blossom, Sainsbury's*	1 Tbsp/15g	51	0	339	0.1	84.7	0	0.3
HONEYCOMB								
Natural, Epicure*	1 Serving/100g	290	4.6	290	0.4	74.4	4.6	0
HOOCH*								
Vodka, Calculated Estimate, Hooch*	1 Bottle/330ml	145	0	44	0.3	5.1	0	0
HORLICKS								
Malted Drink, Chocolate, Extra Light, Dry Weight, Horlicks*	1 Serving/32g	95	2.5	296	9.2	47	7.8	17.3
Malted Drink, Extra Light, Instant, Dry Weight, Horlicks*	1 Serving/11g	35	0.7	319	8.4	57.4	6.2	10.5
Malted Drink, Light, Dry Weight, Horlicks*	1 Serving/32g	116	1.2	364	14.8	72.2	3.8	1.9
Malted Drink, Light, Made Up, Horlicks*	1 Mug/200ml	116	1.2	58	2.4	11.6	0.6	0.3
Powder, Made Up with Semi-Skimmed Milk	*1 Mug/227ml*	*184*	*4.3*	*81*	*4.3*	*12.9*	*1.9*	*0*
Powder, Made Up with Whole Milk	*1 Mug/227ml*	*225*	*8.9*	*99*	*4.2*	*12.7*	*3.9*	*0*
HORSERADISH								
Prepared, Average	*1 Tsp/5g*	*1*	*0*	*28*	*2*	*5*	*0.1*	*2.8*
HOT CHOCOLATE								
Belgian Choc & Butterscotch, Made Up, Options*	1 Sachet/11g	39	0.9	353	2.7	52	8.1	8.5
Belgian Choc, Options*	1 Sachet/11g	40	0.8	365	8.9	59	7.3	0
Cadbury*	1 Serving/12g	44	0.7	370	6.3	73.3	5.9	0
Caramel, Whittards of Chelsea*	1 Serving/20g	71	1.5	355	7.5	64.5	7.5	13
Choc Mint, Highlights, Made Up, Cadbury*	1 Serving/200ml	40	1.4	20	1	2.5	0.7	0.3
Choca Mocha Drink, Options, Ovaltine*	1 Sachet/11g	39	1.3	359	14.1	50.1	11.4	7
Chocolate Au Lait, Options, Ovaltine*	1 Sachet/10g	36	1	355	11.8	54.5	10	7.3
Cocoa, Lidl*	1 Serving/20g	77	1.2	386	6.1	74.1	6.2	0
Dairy Fudge, Highlights, Dry Weight, Cadbury*	1 Serving/11g	38	1.2	347	16	41	11	9.7
Dairy Fudge, Highlights, Made Up, Cadbury*	1 Serving/200ml	40	1	20	1	2.7	0.5	0.2
Dark, Bournville, Highlights, Made Up, Cadbury*	1 Serving/200ml	35	0.9	18	1.2	2	0.4	0
Dreamy Caramel, Options, Ovaltine*	1 Sachet/11g	39	0.9	354	12.3	48.5	7.8	0
Drink, Organic, Green & Black's*	1 Tsp/5g	20	0.4	395	8.6	67	7.5	12
Fairtrade, Whittards of Chelsea*	4 Tsp/20g	68	0.8	342	7.8	69	3.9	10.9
From Coffee Shop, Waitrose*	1 Serving/298ml	217	5.9	73	3.6	10.9	2	0
Galaxy, Mars*	1 Sachet/25g	97	1.9	386	4.8	71.9	7.7	4.7
Highlights, Instant, Dry Weight, Cadbury*	1 Sachet/11g	42	1.4	380	16.8	46.9	13.1	3.4
Highlights, Instant, Made Up, Cadbury*	1 Cup/200ml	40	1.4	20	1	2.5	0.7	0.3
Instant Break, Cadbury*	1 Sachet/28g	119	3.9	425	10.9	64.2	14	0
Instant, Highlights, Cadbury*	1 Sachet/22g	80	2.8	364	17.3	44.6	12.7	0
Instant, Tesco*	1 Serving/32g	155	10.3	485	10.5	38.1	32.3	5
Low Calorie, Dry Weight, As Sold, Average	*1 Sachet/11g*	*41*	*1.2*	*374*	*14.6*	*50*	*10.7*	*11.1*
Luxury, Skinny, Whittards of Chelsea*	1 Serving/28g	92	0.8	328	12.9	67.1	2.8	13.5
Made Up, Tassimo, Suchard*	1 Serving/280ml	88	2.4	31	0.3	5.5	0.9	0.2
Maltesers, Malt Drink, Instant, Made Up, Mars*	1 Serving/220ml	104	3	47	0.9	7.7	1.4	0
Mint Madness, Belgian, Options, Ovaltine*	1 Sachet/11g	38	0.8	348	12.3	49.2	6.9	20
Mint, Highlights, Cadbury*	1 Serving/200ml	40	1.4	20	1	2.5	0.7	0
Outrageous Orange, Options, Ovaltine*	1 Serving/11g	38	0.8	348	12.3	49.3	6.9	20
Tempting Toffee, Options, Ovaltine*	1 Sachet/11g	43	1	391	13.6	66.4	9.1	0

H

	Measure INFO/WEIGHT	per Measure KCAL	FAT	Nutrition Values per 100g / 100ml KCAL	PROT	CARB	FAT	FIBRE
HOT CHOCOLATE								
Velvet, Cadbury*	1 Serving/28g	136	6.9	487	8.6	57.8	24.6	2
Wicked White, Options, Ovaltine*	1 Sachet/11g	44	1.1	398	10.5	64.6	10	3.7
Wispa, Hot Frothy, Cadbury*	1 Sachet/27g	107	1.4	395	11	74	5.3	2.9
HOT DOG								
Plain, From Restaurant, Average	*1 Sandwich/98g*	*242*	*14.5*	*247*	*10.6*	*18.4*	*14.8*	*0*
Sausage, American Style, Average	*1 Sausage/75g*	*180*	*14.3*	*241*	*11.6*	*6.2*	*19*	*0*
Sausage, Average	*1 Sausage/23g*	*40*	*3*	*175*	*10.8*	*4.3*	*12.8*	*0.3*
Vegetarian, Meat Free, Sainsbury's*	1 Sausage/30g	71	4.5	237	18	7.6	15	1
Vegetarian, Tesco*	1 Sausage/30g	66	4.5	220	18	2.7	15	2
HOT POT								
Beef, Classic, 800g, Asda*	1 Serving/400g	400	20.8	100	5.7	7.1	5.2	1.2
Beef, Healthy Options, Birds Eye*	1 Pack/350g	294	7	84	4.5	12	2	1.2
Beef, Minced, Sainsbury's*	1 Pack/450g	464	22.1	103	5.3	9.5	4.9	2.2
Beef, Ross*	1 Pack/310g	255	11.2	82	2.2	9.4	3.6	1.5
Beef, Weight Watchers*	1 Pack/320g	231	7.7	72	3.6	8.4	2.4	1.6
Chicken & Mushroom, HL, Tesco*	1 Serving/450g	369	6.8	82	6.3	11.8	1.5	0.5
Chicken, Chunky, Weight Watchers*	1 Pack/320g	275	9	86	4.7	10.4	2.8	0.6
Chicken, Co-Op*	1 Pack/340g	289	10.2	85	6	9	3	0.7
Chicken, GFY, Asda*	1 Serving/400g	256	5.2	64	4.8	8.2	1.3	1.4
Chicken, Good Choice, Iceland*	1 Pack/400g	276	5.2	69	5	9.3	1.3	1
Chicken, LC, Tesco*	1 Pack/361g	250	4.6	70	5.1	9.1	1.3	1.5
Chicken, LC, Tesco*	1 Pack/363g	272	5.4	75	4.9	8.7	1.5	1.4
Chicken, Sainsbury's*	1 Pack/400g	340	11	85	5.2	9.8	2.8	1.3
Chicken, Weight Watchers*	1 Pack/320g	296	6.7	93	6.3	11.8	2.1	1.1
Corned Beef, 876, Oakhouse Foods Ltd*	1 Serving/340g	370	13.6	109	6	13.1	4	0.8
Lamb & Vegetable, Asda*	1 Pot/500g	240	2	48	4	7	0.4	0
Lamb Shank, Extra Special, Asda*	1 Pack/450g	508	20.2	113	10.2	7.8	4.5	1.3
Lamb, & Vegetable, Sliced, 035, Wiltshire Farm Foods*	1 Meal/179g	234	12.4	131	7	9.9	6.9	0
Lamb, British, Little Dish*	1 Pack/200g	206	7	103	5.1	11.8	3.5	2.1
Lamb, Classic, CBY, Asda*	1 Pack/399g	323	13.6	81	3.9	8.1	3.4	1.2
Lamb, Classic, Tesco*	1 Pack/335g	429	18.1	128	5.1	13.7	5.4	1.9
Lamb, Cumbrian, Look What We Found*	1 Pack/300g	276	5.4	92	8.9	10.1	1.8	3
Lamb, Diet Chef Ltd*	1 Pack/300g	276	5.4	92	8.9	10.1	1.8	3
Lamb, Minced, Classic Kitchen, Tesco*	1 Pack/450g	374	11.2	83	4.6	10	2.5	0.9
Lamb, Minced, Morrison*	1 Pack/400g	376	11.6	94	4.1	11.7	2.9	2.2
Lamb, Minced, New Zealand, Sainsbury's*	1 Pack/450g	580	30.2	129	7.3	8.2	6.7	3.6
Lamb, Mini, Classics, Asda*	1 Pack/300g	223	10.5	74	5.3	5.4	3.5	3.3
Lamb, Organic, Great Stuff, Asda*	1 Pack/300g	327	10.2	109	8	11.6	3.4	1.1
Lancashire, 305, Oakhouse Foods Ltd*	1 Serving/400g	344	14	86	5.6	7.4	3.5	1.1
Lancashire, Asda*	1 Pack/401g	269	5.2	67	3.8	10	1.3	0.9
Lancashire, M&S*	1 Pack/454g	431	15	95	10.1	6.7	3.3	1
Lancashire, Tesco*	½ Pack/225g	205	7	91	6	9.7	3.1	0.5
Lancashire, with Sliced Potatoes, Cooked, Aldi*	1 Pot/450g	460	17	108	7.3	9.3	4	2.7
Liver & Bacon, Tesco*	1 Pack/550g	693	31.4	126	6.4	12.3	5.7	1.5
Minced Beef & Vegetable, COU, M&S*	1 Pack/400g	380	6.8	95	10.3	9	1.7	2.4
Minced Beef, Bisto*	1 Pack/375g	363	13.5	97	4.1	11.3	3.6	1.4
Minced Beef, Classic, Asda*	1 Pack/400g	424	18.4	106	6.8	8.7	4.6	1.1
Minced Beef, Frozen, Tesco*	1 Pack/450g	338	11.2	75	4	9.1	2.5	1.4
Minced Beef, Iceland*	1 Pack/500g	505	15.5	101	5.5	12.7	3.1	1.3
Minced Lamb & Vegetable, COU, M&S*	1 Pack/400g	340	10.8	85	5.7	12.5	2.7	1.8
Potato, Slim & Save*	1 Pack/40g	147	2.2	368	36	26.6	5.5	11.3
Sausage with Baked Beans, Heinz*	1 Can/340g	354	10.9	104	4.6	14.3	3.2	2.4
Sausage, Aunt Bessie's*	¼ Pack/200g	212	9.2	106	3.6	12.6	4.6	1.9

H

	Measure INFO/WEIGHT	per Measure		Nutrition Values per 100g / 100ml				
		KCAL	FAT	KCAL	PROT	CARB	FAT	FIBRE

HOT POT

Sausage, Smart Price, Asda*	1 Pack/300g	239	7	80	3.7	11	2.3	0.4
Vegetable, Ready Meal, Average	*1 Serving/400g*	*261*	*7.4*	*65*	*1.9*	*10.7*	*1.9*	*1.9*
Vegetable, Weight Watchers*	1 Pack/335g	228	6.4	68	2.6	9.9	1.9	1.5
Vegetarian Sausage & Vegetable, Linda McCartney*	1 Pot/400g	516	20.4	129	6.4	15.7	5.1	2.3
Vegetarian, Quorn*	1 Pack/400g	252	8	63	3.3	8	2	1.9

HOUMOUS

Avocado, Fresh, San Amvrosia*	1 Serving/50g	172	16	344	5.4	8.5	32.1	2.5
Beetroot, Cannellini Bean, & Mint, HL, Tesco*	¼ Tub/45g	82	5.1	183	5.9	11.2	11.3	6.5
Broad Bean, Asparagus & Mint, Tesco*	¼ Pot/42g	120	9.7	285	7.1	9.7	23	3.7
Caramelised Onion, Tesco*	¼ Pack/50g	125	9.7	250	5.5	13	19.4	4.2
Caramelised Onion, The Deli, Aldi*	½ Pack/42g	94	5.9	224	7.4	15	14	4.1
Chargrilled Red Pepper & Chilli, 30% Less Fat, Asda*	1 Serving/50g	116	8.2	233	7.5	11.5	16.4	4.9
Extra Chick Peas, with Pine Nuts, & Olive Oil, Yarden*	1 Serving/30g	106	9.3	353	6.5	12	31	0
Jalapeno, Asda*	1 Serving/50g	166	14.5	331	7	10.6	29	4.5
Jalapeno, Sainsbury's*	¼ Pot/50g	148	13.4	296	6.4	7.2	26.8	5.7
Jalapeno, Tesco*	½ Pot/100g	360	31.1	360	7.5	11.4	31.1	3.9
Lemon & Coriander, Sainsbury's*	¼ Tub/50g	146	12.6	291	7	9.1	25.1	6
Lemon & Coriander, GFY, Asda*	1 Serving/50g	130	9.9	259	8.3	12	19.8	5.1
Lemon & Coriander, M&S*	½ Pack/100g	296	24.5	296	6.5	9.1	24.5	6.3
Lemon & Coriander, Tesco*	¼ Pack/45g	127	10.3	278	6.4	9.8	22.5	5.7
Moroccan Style, Sainsbury's*	¼ Pot/50g	114	9.8	227	5.5	7.3	19.5	6.6
Moroccan with Coriander & Spices, Tesco*	¼ Pot/50g	131	9.9	262	9.4	11.6	19.8	5.2
Moroccan, Tesco*	¼ Pot/50g	144	12.8	289	6.8	8.1	25.5	7.3
Red Pepper, Meadow Fresh, Lidl*	1 Serving/50g	158	12.9	307	7.1	11	25	5
Red Pepper, Reduced Fat, Tesco*	¼ Pot/45g	99	6.2	218	8.5	13.3	13.6	4.5
Reduced Fat, Average	*1 Tbsp/30g*	*72*	*5*	*241*	*9.2*	*13.3*	*16.8*	*3.6*
Reduced Fat, Moroccan Style, Topped, M&S*	1 Tub/170g	374	26	220	6.6	13.2	15.3	9.2
Reduced Fat, with Crunchy Carrot Sticks, M&S*	1 Pack/130g	157	9.9	121	3.3	7.8	7.6	3.9
Roasted Red Pepper, Sainsbury's*	½ Pot/100g	317	27.2	317	6.2	9	27.2	5.7
Smoked, Chilli Harissa, Moorish*	1 Pot/150g	432	34	288	7.2	11.9	22.7	3.5
Smoked, Moorish*	1 Pack/150g	448	36.3	299	7.1	11.5	24.2	3.4
Sweet Chilli, Tesco*	¼ Pot/50g	120	8.4	240	6.9	15.2	16.7	5.4
Three Bean, Reduced Fat, BGTY, Sainsbury's*	¼ Tub/50g	92	6	183	7.3	11.4	12	6
with Extra Virgin Olive Oil, Tesco*	1 Pack/190g	564	46.2	297	7.9	11.7	24.3	5.1

HULA HOOPS

BBQ Beef, 55% Less Saturated Fat, KP Snacks*	1 Pack/34g	172	9	505	3.7	61.8	26.4	2.2
BBQ Beef, Big Hoops, Hula Hoops*	1 Pack/50g	250	12	499	3.8	65	24	2.8
Beef Puft, Hula Hoops*	1 Pack/15g	72	3	478	9	64	20	4
Cheese & Onion 55% Less Saturated Fat, KP Snacks*	1 Bag/34g	175	9.7	515	3.6	61	28.5	1.9
Cheese, Puft, KP Snacks*	1 Pack/28g	132	5.6	471	8.8	61	20	4.1
Minis, Original, KP Snacks*	1 Tub/140g	752	48.7	537	3	52.9	34.8	1.7
Original, 55% Less Saturated Fat, KP Snacks*	1 Bag/34g	172	8.8	507	3.3	63	26	2.2
Ready Salted, Puft, KP Snacks*	1 Pack/15g	72	3.2	482	8.3	64	21	4
Salt & Vinegar, 50% Less Saturated Fat, KP Snacks*	1 Pack/25g	128	7	510	3.1	60.9	28.2	1.8
Salt & Vinegar, Puft, KP Snacks*	1 Pack/15g	72	3	478	8.1	63	20	3.9

H

ICE CREAM

	Measure INFO/WEIGHT	per Measure KCAL	FAT	Nutrition Values per 100g / 100ml KCAL	PROT	CARB	FAT	FIBRE
Praline, Carte d'Or*	1 Serving/100g	225	11	225	4	27	11	0
After Dinner, Mint, Dairy, Asda*	1 Serving/100g	182	8	182	3.4	24	8	0.4
Baked Alaska, Ben & Jerry's*	1 Serving/100g	260	15	260	4	29	15	0.1
Bananas Foster, Haagen-Dazs*	1 Serving/125ml	260	15	208	3.2	22.4	12	0
Banoffee Fudge, Sainsbury's*	1/8 Pot/67g	119	4	178	2.8	28.7	5.9	0.2
Banoffee, Haagen-Dazs*	1 Serving/120ml	274	15.6	228	4	23	13	0
Bar, Belgian Chocolate & Vanilla, Giant, M&S*	1 Bar/120g	384	26.3	320	3.5	27.7	21.9	0.1
Belgian Chocolate, Haagen-Dazs*	1 Sm Tub/78g	249	16.2	318	4.6	28.4	20.7	0
Belgian Milk Chocolate, Tesco*	1 Lolly/85g	255	15.5	300	3.9	29.8	18.2	0.7
Berry Neighbourly, Ben & Jerry's*	1 Scoop/44g	123	7	279	3.5	29	16	0
Blondie Brownie, Ben & Jerry's*	1 Scoop/43g	109	6	253	4.2	29	14	0
Blueberry, Gelateria, Carte d'Or*	2 Scoops/56g	110	4.1	190	28	31	7	0
Bob Marleys One Love, Ben & Jerry's*	1 Scoop/45g	123	6.3	273	3.2	33	14	0
Bounty, Mini Bar, Mars*	1 Bar/25ml	72	4.8	288	4.5	24.8	19	1
Caffe Latte, The Best, Morrisons*	1/5 Tub/100ml	144	6.6	144	2.9	18	6.6	0.4
Cappuccino, Thorntons*	1oz/28g	61	3.6	218	4.4	20.7	12.9	0
Caramel Craze, Organic, Tesco*	1 Serving/100g	253	15.3	253	3.3	25.5	15.3	0
Caramel, Chew Chew, Ben & Jerry's*	1 Scoop/45g	122	6.8	270	3.5	28	15	0
Caramel, with Caramel Pieces, Carte d'Or*	1 Serving/100g	230	7.4	230	2.9	38	7.4	0
Caramella, Sundae, Tesco*	1 Sundae/80g	165	5.5	205	2.2	32.9	6.8	1.9
Caramella, Tesco*	1 Serving/51g	120	5.5	235	2.6	32	10.7	1.1
Cheeky Choc, Brownie, Skinny Cow*	1 Tub/500ml	590	5.5	118	3	23.9	1.1	4.1
Cheesecake Brownie, Ben & Jerry's*	1 Serving 100g	260	16	260	4	26	16	0
Choc Chip, Cookie Dough, Haagen-Dazs*	1oz/28g	74	4.7	266	3.8	24.9	16.9	0
Chocolate & Orange, Organic, Green & Black's*	1 Serving/100g	248	14.1	248	5	25.3	14.1	0.1
Chocolate Brownie with Walnuts, Haagen-Dazs*	1 Cup/101g	223	16.4	221	4.4	21	16.2	0
Chocolate Chip, Baskin Robbins*	1 Serving/75g	170	10	227	4	24	13.3	0
Chocolate Flavour, Average	**1 Serving/70g**	**149**	**7.9**	**212**	**4.1**	**23.7**	**11.3**	**0.6**
Chocolate Flavour, Soft Scoop, Sainsbury's*	1 Serving/70g	122	5.2	174	3.1	23.6	7.5	0.3
Chocolate Honeycomb, Co-Op*	¼ Pot/81g	186	10.5	230	4	26	13	0.3
Chocolate Ripple, PB, Waitrose*	1 Serving/125ml	205	3.1	164	4.8	30.5	2.5	4.1
Chocolate Trio, Thorntons*	1 Bar/100g	310	20.6	310	3.3	28	20.6	1.8
Chocolate with Chocolate Chips, Milfina*	1oz/28g	66	3.5	235	3.8	26.7	12.5	0.8
Chocolate, Caramel, Cookie Dough, Topped, Ben & Jerry's	1 Scoop/45g	137	7.6	305	3.9	33	17	0
Chocolate, Fudge, Brownie, Ben & Jerry's*	1 Scoop/41.5g	102	5.4	245	4.2	29	13	0
Chocolate, Fudge, Brownie, Non-Dairy, Ben & Jerry's*	1 Scoop/39.5g	88	4.3	222	2.9	26	11	0
Chocolate, Gelatelli, Lidl*	1 Portion/50g	126	6.8	251	3.8	27.3	13.6	2.1
Chocolate, Haagen-Dazs*	1 Serving/120ml	269	18	224	4	19	15	0
Chocolate, Heavenly, Non Dairy, Swedish Glace, Wall's*	1 Serving/100g	206	11	206	3.3	23	11	0
Chocolate, Inspiration, Gelateria, Carte d'Or*	1 Serving/100g	210	9	210	3.5	28	9	0
Chocolate, on Stick, Chocolate Covered, Green & Black's*	1 Stick/100g	214	13.6	214	3.7	19.3	13.6	2.1
Chocolate, Organic, Green & Black's*	1 Serving/125g	310	17.6	248	5	25.3	14.1	1.1
Chocolate, Organic, M&S*	1oz/28g	71	4.5	255	5	24	16	1.5
Chocolate, Santo Domingo, 1, Waitrose*	1 Serving/66g	220	16.4	333	4.5	22.8	24.8	0.5
Chocolate, Soft Scoop, Asda*	1 Scoop/47g	84	3.8	179	3.7	23	8	0
Chocolate, Soft Scoop, Tesco*	1 Serving/50g	93	4	186	3.2	25.1	8.1	0.3
Chocolate, Swirl Pot, Skinny Cow*	1 Pot/100ml	98	0.6	98	2.9	20.2	0.6	2.7
Chocolatino, Sundae, Tesco*	1 Tub/80g	160	5.9	200	4.4	29	7.4	2.4
Chunky Monkey, Non-Dairy, Ben & Jerry's*	1 Scoop/41.5g	109	5.8	262	2.4	30	14	0
Clotted Cream, Cornish, Kelly's Of Cornwall*	1 Serving/125g	282	18.6	226	2.9	20.1	14.9	0.1
Coconut, Alpro*	1 Serving/100g	167	8.2	167	0.2	16.1	8.2	12.5
Coconut, Carte d'Or*	1 Serving/100ml	125	7.1	125	1.8	14	7.1	0.5
Coffee Coffee Chip, Baskin Robbins*	1 Scoop/112g	264	15	236	3.8	25	13.4	0

ICE CREAM

	Measure INFO/WEIGHT	per Measure KCAL	FAT	Nutrition Values per 100g / 100ml KCAL	PROT	CARB	FAT	FIBRE
Coffee, Finest, Tesco*	¼ Pot/93g	236	14.9	254	4.9	22.5	16	0
Coffee, Haagen-Dazs*	1 Serving/120ml	271	18.4	226	4.1	17.9	15.3	0
Coffee, Waitrose*	¼ Tub/125ml	292	16.4	234	3.6	25.4	13.1	0
Cookie Dough, Ben & Jerry's*	1 Scoop/42.5g	115	6.4	270	4	30	15	0
Cookie Dough, S'wich Up, Ben & Jerry's*	1 Scoop/40.5g	117	6.5	290	4.2	31	16	0
Cookie Dough, Tesco*	1 Serving/125g	301	14.2	241	3.3	31	11.4	0.6
Cookies & Cream, Haagen-Dazs*	1 Sm Tub/100ml	226	14.7	226	4	19.5	14.7	0
Cream Di Frutta, Noblissima, Lidl*	1 Scoop/50g	89	2.4	178	2.2	29.9	4.7	0
Crunchie, Blast, Cadbury*	1 Lolly/100ml	230	13.9	230	2.8	23.1	13.9	0.1
Dairy Cornish, Tesco*	1 Serving/49g	112	6	228	3.2	24.7	12.3	0.1
Dairy Milk, Orange, Cadbury*	1 Serving/120ml	259	13.9	216	3.5	26	11.6	0
Dairy, Flavoured	*1oz/28g*	*50*	*2.2*	*179*	*3.5*	*24.7*	*8*	*0*
Double Chocolate, Nestle*	1 Serving/78g	248	14.3	320	4.8	33.7	18.4	0
Dulce De Leche, Bar, Haagen-Dazs*	1 Bar/105g	370	24	352	3.8	32.3	22.9	0
Eton Mess, Gelateria, Carte d'Or*	1 Serving/100g	181	5.8	181	2.2	30	5.8	0
Exotic, Solero, Wall's*	1 Lolly/68g	98	2.1	144	1.7	27	3.1	0
Fig & Orange Blossom Honey, Waitrose*	1 Serving/100g	219	11.8	219	3.9	24.3	11.8	0.4
Fruit & Fresh Tropical, Carte d'Or*	1 Serving/83g	154	7.1	185	2.5	24.5	8.5	0
Galaxy, Mars*	1 Bar/60ml	203	13.4	339	4.7	29.7	22.4	0
Gelato, Vanilla	*1 Serving/100g*	*162*	*7.2*	*162*	*2.4*	*22.6*	*7.2*	*0.3*
Gingerbread, Specially Selected, Aldi*	1 Scoop/64g	169	8.3	264	4	33	13	0.6
Gold Digger Dynamite, Chokablok*	¼ Tub/125ml	288	14	230	3.2	28.2	11.2	0.9
Greek Yoghurt & Honey, Carte d'Or*	1 Serving/55g	114	4.8	207	2.7	29	8.8	0
Half Baked, Ben & Jerry's*	1 Scoop/41g	107	5.3	262	4.1	32	13	0
Hazelnut Chocolate, Alpro*	1 Serving/100g	177	9.4	177	0.8	17.2	9.4	8.6
Home Sweet Honeycomb, Ben & Jerry's*	1 Scoop/43g	114	6.4	266	3.8	30	15	0
Honeycomb & Caramel, Dairy, Sainsbury's*	2 Scoops/76g	180	8	236	3.2	32	10.5	0.6
Honeycomb Harvest, Mackies*	1 Serving/100g	209	10	209	4	25	10	0
Hunky Punky Chocolate, Dairy Free, Booja-Booja*	1 Tub/500ml	685	35	137	3.3	17	7	0
Jam Roly Poly & Custard, Aunt Bessie's*	1 Scoop/50g	92	4.1	185	4	23	8.3	0.1
Karamel Sutra, Ben & Jerry's*	1 Scoop/43g	112	6	260	4	27	14	0
Knickerbocker Glory	*1oz/28g*	*31*	*1.4*	*112*	*1.5*	*16.4*	*5*	*0.2*
Lavazza, Carte d'Or*	1 Serving/55g	120	5.4	218	3.5	29	9.9	0
Lemon Cream, Dairy, Sainsbury's*	1 Serving/100g	199	9.3	199	3	25.9	9.3	0.1
Lemon Curd Swirl, Duchy Originals*	¼ Pot/101g	247	14.2	245	3.7	25.8	14.1	0
Lemon Meringue Bar, Heston from Waitrose, Waitrose*	1 Serving/60g	108	2.8	181	1.8	32	4.7	1.5
Lemon Meringue Pie, Aunt Bessie's*	1 Serving/50g	101	4.6	202	3.6	26	9.1	0.1
Lemon, Haagen-Dazs*	1 Serving/120ml	144	0.2	120	0.3	29.3	0.2	0
Light Chocolate Ices, Co-Op*	1 Ice/62g	121	8.1	195	2	18	13	0.5
Log, Mint Chocolate, Sainsbury's*	1 Serving/51g	100	5.1	197	3	23.8	10	0.2
Luscious Mint Choc Chip, Morrisons*	1 Serving/50g	99	5.2	198	2.9	23.1	10.5	0.7
Lychee Cream & Ginger, Haagen-Dazs*	1 Serving/120ml	258	12.7	215	3.6	26.1	10.6	0
Macadamia Nut, Baskin Robbins*	1 Serving/113g	270	18	239	4.4	22.1	15.9	0.9
Mango, 98% Fat Free, Bulla*	1 Serving/70g	94	1.1	134	4.2	25.4	1.6	0
Maple & Walnut, American, Sainsbury's*	1/8 Pot/68g	121	4.9	179	3.1	25.6	7.2	0.2
Mince Pie, Farmhouse Dairy, TTD, Sainsbury's*	¼ Pot/100g	272	14.9	272	4.5	29.3	14.9	1.3
Mince Pie, Finest, Tesco*	¼ Pack/188g	476	22.1	254	3.9	33	11.8	1.1
Mini Mix, Chocolate Coated, Gelatelli, Lidl*	1 Lolly/36g	123	7.8	342	3.9	32	21.8	1.2
Mini Mix, Sorbet Coated, Gelatelli, Lidl*	1 Lolly/40g	64	2.4	160	1.7	24.7	5.9	0
Mini Sticks, Milk Chocolate, Weight Watchers*	1 Mini Stick/45ml	96	5	213	2.7	25.8	11.1	0.7
Mint & Chocolate Flavour, Average	*1 Serving/70g*	*129*	*6.3*	*184*	*3*	*22.6*	*9*	*1.2*
Mint & Chocolate, Sainsbury's*	1 Serving/71g	137	6.7	192	3.4	23.5	9.4	0.4
Mint Choc Chip Soft Scoop, Asda*	1 Serving/46g	86	4.1	189	2.9	24	9	0.3

ICE CREAM

INFO/WEIGHT	Measure			Nutrition Values per 100g / 100ml				
		KCAL	FAT	KCAL	PROT	CARB	FAT	FIBRE
Mint Chocolate Chip, Baskin Robbins*	1 Scoop/113g	270	16	239	4.4	24.8	14.2	0.9
Mint Crunch, Dairy Milk, Cadbury*	1 Serving/60ml	162	13.3	270	3	29	22.2	0
Mint Ripple, Good Choice, Iceland*	1 Scoop/50g	58	1	117	3	21.7	2.1	0.1
Mint, Majestic Luxury, Iceland*	1 Serving/80g	269	14.6	337	3.8	39.3	18.3	1.3
Mint, Viennetta, Wall's*	1 Serving/50g	125	8	250	2.5	25	16	0
Minter Wonderland, Ben & Jerry's*	1 Scoop/44g	117	7.5	266	4	24	17	0
Mocha Coffee Indulgence, Sainsbury's*	¼ Pot/82g	178	10.6	217	3.2	22.1	12.9	0.1
Monster Mint, Sainsbury's*	1/8 Pot/67g	121	4.6	180	3	26.3	6.9	0.3
My Carte D'or, Chocolate, Carte d'Or*	1 Tub/200ml	220	11	110	1.8	12.5	5.5	0.4
Neapolitan, Average	**1 Serving/70g**	**111**	**4.6**	**158**	**3.1**	**21.9**	**6.5**	**0.6**
Neapolitan, Brick, Tesco*	1 Serving/50g	82	3.4	163	3.3	21.9	6.9	0.4
Neapolitan, Iceland*	1oz/28g	46	2.1	164	3	21.3	7.4	0
Neapolitan, Lidl*	1 Serving/48g	108	4.8	226	4.3	29.5	10	0
Neapolitan, Soft Scoop, Asda*	1 Scoop/47g	82	3.8	175	2.8	23	8	0.2
Neapolitan, Soft Scoop, M&S*	1/8 Tub/62.5g	100	4.6	160	2.7	21.3	7.4	0.3
Neapolitan, Soft Scoop, Sainsbury's*	1 Serving/75g	124	5.2	165	2.8	22.8	6.9	0.2
Neopolitian, Soft Scoop, Tesco*	1 Serving/43g	70	3	163	3.3	21.9	6.9	0.4
Non-Dairy, Reduced Calorie	**1oz/28g**	**33**	**1.7**	**119**	**3.4**	**13.7**	**6**	**0**
Organic, Madagascan Vanilla, Yeo Valley*	1 Serving/40ml	45	2.5	112	2.4	11.4	6.3	0.1
Panna Cotta, & Raspberry Swirl, Haagen-Dazs*	1 Serving/120ml	250	14.9	208	3.2	21	12.4	0
Peanut Butter Cup, Ben & Jerry's*	1 Scoop/43g	138	9	320	7	25	21	0
Peanut Butter, & Cookies, Non-Dairy, Ben & Jerry's*	1 Scoop/40.5g	113	6.5	280	4.3	29	16	0
Phish Food, Ben & Jerry's*	1 Scoop/43g	116	5.2	270	3.5	36	12	0
Pistachio, Haagen-Dazs*	1 Serving/120ml	276	18.8	230	4.4	17.7	15.7	0
Pistachio, Joe Deluccis Gelato*	1 Scoop/70g	148	6.6	211	2.4	28	9.4	0
Pistachio, Seriously Nutty, Waitrose*	1 fl oz/30ml	48	3.2	161	3.2	12.6	10.8	0.3
Praline, Green & Black's*	1 Sm Pot/100g	191	10.8	191	3.5	20	10.8	0.9
Pralines & Cream, Haagen-Dazs*	1 Sm Tub/78g	213	12.9	272	3.9	27.2	16.5	0
Protein, Banoffee, WheyHey*	1 Pot/150ml	149	4.4	99	13.4	7.8	2.9	0
Protein, Chocolate, WheyHey*	1 Pot/150ml	154	4.3	103	14	8	2.9	0
Protein, Chocolate, WheyHey*	1 Tub/100ml	85	3.5	85	8	8.5	3.5	0.7
Protein, Vanilla, WheyHey*	1 Pot/150ml	149	4.4	99	13.4	7.8	2.9	0
Raspberries, Clotted Cream, Waitrose*	1 Tub/500ml	790	39.5	158	2.9	18.9	7.9	0.1
Raspberry Ripple & Shortbread, Gelato, Pizza Express*	1 Serving/125g	322	18.9	257	3.8	26.9	15.1	0.5
Raspberry Ripple Brick, Tesco*	1 Serving/48g	71	2.9	148	2.6	20.8	6	0.2
Raspberry Ripple, Average	**1 Serving/70g**	**93**	**3.3**	**134**	**1.9**	**20.8**	**4.7**	**0.1**
Raspberry Ripple, Dairy, Waitrose*	1 Serving/186ml	195	10	105	1.9	12.3	5.4	0
Raspberry Ripple, Soft Scoop, Asda*	1 Scoop/46g	78	3.2	170	2.5	24	7	0.3
Raspberry Ripple, Soft Scoop, Sainsbury's*	1 Serving/75g	128	5.2	170	2.6	24.2	7	0.3
Raspberry Ripple, Soft Scoop, Tesco*	1 Scoop/25g	39	1.5	157	2.5	23	6.1	0.2
Raspberry, Delightful, Non Dairy, Swedish Glace, Wall's*	1 Serving/100g	211	9.4	211	2.6	29	9.4	0
Raspberry, Easy Serve, Co-Op*	1oz/28g	43	1.7	152	2.5	22.3	5.9	0
Really Creamy Chocolate, Asda*	1 Serving/100g	227	11	227	4.1	28	11	0.4
Really Creamy Toffee, Asda*	1 Serving/120ml	146	6	122	1.8	17.5	5	0.1
Red Berries, Solero, Wall's*	1 Lolly/75g	111	2	148	1.4	29	2.7	0
Rhubarb Crumble, Aunt Bessie's*	1 Serving/50g	96	4.4	192	3.8	25	8.7	0.2
Rocky Road, M&S*	1 Tub/500g	1475	88.5	295	4.2	29.5	17.7	1.2
Rocky Road, Sainsbury's*	1/8 Pot/67g	137	4.9	205	3.8	30.9	7.3	1
Rum & Raisin, Haagen-Dazs*	1 Serving/120ml	264	17.6	220	3.4	18.6	14.7	0
Rum & Raisin, TTD, Sainsbury's*	¼ Pot/100g	220	10.4	220	3.8	27.7	10.4	1
Run & Raisin, with West Indies Rum, Carte d'Or*	1 Serving/100g	201	7.5	201	2.6	25	7.5	0
Salted Caramel, Brownie, Topped, Ben & Jerry's*	1 Scoop/44.5g	134	8	301	4.2	30	18	0
Salted Caramel, The Best, Morrisons*	1 Serving/100ml	188	11.5	188	2.8	17.9	11.5	0.5

ICE CREAM

INFO/WEIGHT	Measure	per Measure KCAL	FAT	Nutrition Values per 100g / 100ml KCAL	PROT	CARB	FAT	FIBRE
Screwball, Asda*	1 Screwball/60g	122	6	203	3.3	25	10	1.5
Screwball, Farmfoods*	1 Lolly/72ml	127	4.4	177	3.3	27.1	6.1	0
Screwball, Tesco*	1 Screwball/61g	116	5.2	190	2.9	25.2	8.6	0.3
Smarties Ice Cream Pot, Nestle*	1 Pot/69g	151	5.7	218	4.4	33.6	8.2	0
Smarties, Nestle*	1 Serving/50g	125	6	250	3.6	32.3	11.9	0.2
Sofa So Good , Ben & Jerry's*	1 Scoop/42.5g	110	5.5	259	4	31	13	0
Spagnola, Carte d'Or*	1 Serving/100g	187	5.7	187	2	32	5.7	0
Speculoos? Specu-Love, Ben & Jerry's*	1 Scoop/41.5g	129	8.3	310	3.8	28	20	0
Stem Ginger with Belgian Chocolate, Waitrose*	1 Lolly/110g	255	14.4	232	2.9	25.5	13.1	1.7
Sticky Toffee, Cream O' Galloway*	1 Serving/30g	80	4.4	266	4.7	28.7	14.7	0
Strawberry & Cream, Mivvi, Nestle*	1 Serving/60g	118	4.6	196	2.6	29.4	7.6	0.2
Strawberry Cheesecake, Ben & Jerry's*	1 Serving 100g	240	14	240	3	27	14	0
Strawberry Cheesecake, Co-Op*	1/6 Pot/86g	163	6	190	3	29	7	0.2
Strawberry Cheesecake, Haagen-Dazs*	¼ Tub/125ml	295	17	236	3.3	25.1	13.6	0.3
Strawberry, Majestic, Luxury, Iceland*	1 Lolly/100g	281	18.6	281	2.7	25.8	18.6	0.1
Strawberry, Soft Scoop, Tesco*	1 Serving/45.8g	78	3.4	170	2.8	23.1	7.4	0.1
Strawberry, Swirled, Topped, Ben & Jerry's*	1 Scoop/43g	126	7.3	294	3.5	32	17	0
Strawberry, Viennetta, Wall's*	1 Serving/50g	120	7	240	2.5	24	14	0
Strawberry, Weight Watchers*	1 Pot/57g	81	2.2	142	2.5	23.4	3.9	0.2
Taste of Carrot Cake, Iced Dessert, Perfect World*	1 Tub/120ml	170	12	142	3.1	14	10	2.6
Taste Sensation, Mascarpone Forest Fruits, Aldi*	1 Pot/73.3g	159	7.4	217	1.8	29.6	10.1	0.6
Tiramisu, Haagen-Dazs*	1 Serving/120ml	303	19.6	253	3.8	22.7	16.3	0
Toffee & Biscuit, Weight Watchers*	1 Pot/100ml	93	2.7	93	1.5	14.9	2.7	0.1
Toffee & Honeycomb Sundaes, Weight Watchers*	1 Pot/98g	119	1.8	122	1.7	18.1	1.8	5.9
Toffee & Vanilla, Sainsbury's*	1 Serving/71g	146	6.8	205	3.1	26.7	9.5	0.1
Toffee Fudge, Soft Scoop, Asda*	1 Serving/50g	92	3.5	185	2.6	28	7	0
Toffee Vanilla, HE, Tesco*	1 Serving/73g	106	1.8	145	2.5	28.1	2.5	0.5
Triple Chocolate, Brownie, Skinny Cow*	1 Ice Cream/65g	93	1.7	144	3.5	24.1	2.6	5.3
Triple Chocolate, Carte d'Or*	1 Serving/58g	122	5.7	210	3.7	27	9.8	0
Triple Chocolate, Dairy, Morrisons*	1 Serving/100g	233	10.8	233	3.8	30	10.8	0.4
Vanilla & Cinnamon, Finest, Tesco*	1 Serving/50g	114	7.4	229	3.9	20.2	14.7	0.4
Vanilla & Cinnamon, Spar*	1 Serving/120g	247	10.3	206	3.8	28	8.6	0
Vanilla Bean, Light, Deluxe, Lidl*	1 Serving/64g	110	2.5	172	4.7	26.6	3.9	0
Vanilla Bean, Purbeck*	1 Serving/100g	198	11.5	198	4.8	18.7	11.5	0
Vanilla Caramel Brownie, Haagen-Dazs*	1 Serving/150g	410	24.8	273	4.5	26.8	16.5	0
Vanilla Chocolate, Taste Sensation, Frosty's, Aldi*	1 Pot/73.3g	164	7	224	2.1	32.4	9.6	0.7
Vanilla Flavour, Soft Scoop, Sainsbury's*	1 Serving/71g	96	3.9	136	2.9	18.8	5.5	0.2
Vanilla Florentine, Specially Selected, Aldi*	1 Scoop/62g	148	7.4	238	4.4	28	12	0.7
Vanilla with Strawberry Swirl, Mini Tub, Weight Watchers*	1 Mini Tub/57.0g	81	2.2	142	2.5	23.4	3.9	0.2
Vanilla, & Chocolate, Viennetta, Wall's*	1 Serving/100ml	125	7	250	2.5	27	14	0
Vanilla, Alpro*	1 Serving/100g	166	8	166	2.3	16.4	8	9.8
Vanilla, Ben & Jerry's*	1 Mini Tub/112g	258	16.8	230	4	20	15	0.1
Vanilla, COU, M&S*	¼ Pot/79g	111	2.2	140	1.7	25.9	2.8	0.8
Vanilla, Criminally Creamy, Co-Op*	1oz/28g	60	4.2	215	3	18	15	0.1
Vanilla, Dairy Milk, Cadbury*	1 Serving/120g	259	13.9	216	3.5	26	11.6	0.1
Vanilla, Dairy, Average	*1 Scoop/40g*	*80*	*4.4*	*201*	*3.5*	*23.6*	*11*	*0.7*
Vanilla, Dairy, Finest, Tesco*	1 Serving/92g	227	16	247	4.5	18	17.4	0.3
Vanilla, Dairy, Organic, Yeo Valley*	1 Serving/100g	206	11.2	206	4.9	21.3	11.2	0
Vanilla, Easy Serve, Co-Op*	1oz/28g	39	2	140	3	18	7	0.2
Vanilla, Haagen-Dazs*	1oz/28g	70	4.8	250	4.5	19.7	17.1	0
Vanilla, Light Soft Scoop, 25% Less Fat, Morrisons*	1 Scoop/50g	75	2.5	150	2.9	23.2	5	0.2
Vanilla, Light, Soft Scoop, Wall's*	1 Serving/100g	139	5.9	139	3	17	5.9	0
Vanilla, Low Fat, Average	*1 Scoop/50g*	*59*	*1.7*	*118*	*2.3*	*19.4*	*3.4*	*0.6*

ICE CREAM	Measure INFO/WEIGHT	per Measure KCAL	FAT	Nutrition Values per 100g / 100ml KCAL	PROT	CARB	FAT	FIBRE
Vanilla, Low Fat, Weight Watchers*	1 Scoop/125ml	75	2.1	60	1.1	9.7	1.7	0.1
Vanilla, Mackies*	1 Serving/100g	193	11	193	4	18	11	0
Vanilla, Madagascan, Carte d'Or*	1 Serving/100g	197	7.4	197	2.6	30	7.4	0
Vanilla, Madagascan, Light, 4.5% Fat, Carte d'Or*	1 Serving/100g	140	4.5	140	2.1	21	4.5	4
Vanilla, Made with Madagascan Vanilla, Sainsbury's*	1 Serving/56g	101	4	181	3	25.6	7.2	0.6
Vanilla, Non-Dairy, Average	*1 Serving/60g*	*107*	*5.2*	*178*	*3.2*	*23.1*	*8.7*	*0*
Vanilla, Organic, Sainsbury's*	1 Serving/85g	176	10.2	207	4.3	20.5	12	0.1
Vanilla, Organic, Waitrose*	1 Serving/125g	178	11.2	142	2.7	12.4	9	0
Vanilla, Pecan, Haagen-Dazs*	1 Serving/120ml	316	23.5	263	4.3	17.1	19.6	0
Vanilla, Really Creamy, Asda*	1 Serving/50g	98	5	196	3.5	23	10	0.1
Vanilla, Smart Price, Asda*	1 Scoop/40g	55	2.4	137	2.8	19	6	0.2
Vanilla, Smooth, Soy, Non Dairy, Swedish Glace, Wall's*	1 Serving/100g	210	11	210	3	24	11	0
Vanilla, Soft Scoop, BGTY, Sainsbury's*	1 Serving/75g	88	1.3	117	3.1	22.2	1.7	0.2
Vanilla, Soft Scoop, Tesco*	1oz/28g	46	2	164	3.1	21.8	7.1	0.1
Vanilla, Soft Scoop, Value, Tesco*	1 Scoop/41.6g	57	2.4	137	2.8	18.7	5.7	0.2
Vanilla, Soft Scoop, Wall's*	1 Serving/100g	187	9.1	187	3	23	9.1	0
Vanilla, Toffee Crunch, Ben & Jerry's*	1 Tub/407g	1099	65.1	270	4	29	16	0.5
Vanilla, TTD, Sainsbury's*	¼ Pot/100g	246	16.9	246	5.2	18.2	16.9	0
Vanilla, Waitrose*	1 Serving/100ml	156	10.8	156	2.6	12	10.8	0
Venezuelan Chocolate, Truly Irresistible, Co-Op*	1 Serving/100g	329	21	329	4.5	30	21	0.5
Walnut & Maple, Waitrose*	1 Serving/60g	68	2.3	114	1.8	18.2	3.8	0
What-a-lotta Chocolate, Ben & Jerry's*	1 Scoop/41g	123	7.4	300	4.3	30	18	0
with Cherry Sauce, Tesco*	1 Serving/58g	121	3.2	210	2.8	37	5.6	0.2
with Raspberry Sauce, Movenpick*	1 Serving/50g	130	7	260	4	27	14	0.2
Zesty Lemon Meringue, COU, M&S*	¼ Pot/73g	120	1.8	165	2.6	33	2.5	0.5
ICE CREAM BAR								
Bailey's, Haagen-Dazs*	1oz/28g	86	5.9	307	4.1	24.8	21.2	0
Bounty, 100 Ml Bar, Mars*	1 Bar/100ml	278	18.5	278	3.4	24.7	18.5	0.7
Chocolate Covered	*1 Bar/40g*	*128*	*9.3*	*320*	*5*	*24*	*23.3*	*0*
Crunchie, Cadbury*	1 Bar/60ml	165	9.7	275	3	29.5	16.2	0.5
Dairy Milk, Caramel, Cadbury*	1 Bar/60ml	175	10.3	290	3.6	30.2	17.1	0
Dairy Milk, Fruit & Nut, Cadbury*	1 Bar/90ml	243	15.3	270	3.5	26.1	17	0
Dairy Milk, Lolly, Cadbury*	1 Lolly/100g	235	15	235	3	25.1	15	0
Dream, Cadbury*	1 Serving/118g	260	14	220	3.6	26	11.9	0
Galaxy, Mars*	1 Bar/54g	184	12.2	341	3.8	30.7	22.5	0.6
Lion, Nestle*	1 Bar/45g	166	9.9	370	4.2	39.1	21.9	1
Maltesers, Mars*	1 Bar/45ml	113	7	252	2.9	25	15.6	0.7
Mars, Mars*	1 Bar/65g	182	10.5	280	3.4	29.7	16.2	0.8
Snickers, Mars*	1 Bar/53ml	179	10.4	337	6.5	33.2	19.6	0
Toffee Crunch, English, Weight Watchers*	1 Bar/40g	110	6	275	2.5	32.5	15	5
Twix, Mars*	1 Serving/43ml	128	7.3	301	4	32	17.1	1.2
Vanilla & Raspberry, Weight Watchers*	1 Serving/100g	81	0.3	81	2	23	0.3	0
Yorkie, Nestle*	1 Bar	144	8.7	359	4.8	36.5	21.6	0
ICE CREAM CONE								
Average	*1 Cone/75g*	*140*	*6.4*	*186*	*3.5*	*25.5*	*8.5*	*0*
Choc Chip with Hazelnut, Flirt, Cornetto, Wall's*	1 Cone/70g	223	11.2	320	4	40	16	0
Chocolate & Nut, Co-Op*	1 Cone/110g	307	17	279	3.9	31	15.5	0.6
Chocolate & Vanilla, Good Choice, Iceland*	1 Cone/110ml	161	7.2	146	2.7	22.9	6.5	0.8
Chocolate & Vanilla, M&S*	1oz/28g	83	4.8	295	4.2	31.8	17	0.7
Chocolate, & Caramel, Crunch, Cornetto, Wall's*	1 Cornetto/75g	247	15	329	3.6	34	20	0
Chocolate, M&S*	1oz/28g	94	6.4	335	4	28	23	2.3
Chocolate, Mini, Cornetto, Wall's*	1 Cone/36g	110	5.9	300	3.5	34	16	2
Chocolate, Vanilla & Hazelnut, Sainsbury's*	1 Cone/62g	190	10.5	306	4.5	33.9	16.9	0.6

	Measure INFO/WEIGHT	per Measure KCAL	FAT	Nutrition Values per 100g / 100ml KCAL	PROT	CARB	FAT	FIBRE
ICE CREAM CONE								
Cornet, Wafer Cone, Askeys*	1 Cone/4g	13	0.1	376	10.7	77.6	2.5	0
Cornetto, GFY, Asda*	1 Cone/67g	162	6	241	3	37	9	0.1
Cornetto, Wall's*	1 Cone/75g	195	9.7	260	3.7	34.5	12.9	0
Cup Cornet, Wafer Cone, Askeys*	1 Cone/4g	13	0.1	376	10.7	77.6	2.5	0
Dairy Milk Buttons, Cadbury*	1 Cone/100ml	204	10.4	204	0	24.6	10.4	0.6
Flake 99, Cadbury*	1 Cone/125ml	244	12.5	195	2.6	23.2	10	0
Mint Choc Chip, Iceland*	1 Cone/72g	210	9.4	292	3.3	40.4	13	1
Mint, Cornetto, Wall's*	1 Cornetto/60g	169	8.4	282	3.4	37	14	0
Peanut Butter, Giannis, Aldi*	1 Cone/72g	230	11.5	320	4.7	39	16	1.6
Peanut Butter, Love, Cornetto, Wall's*	1 Cornetto/75g	245	15	326	3.3	33	20	0
Salted Butter Caramel, Gelatelli*	1 Cone/76g	216	8.1	284	3.6	43.4	10.6	0
Strawberry & Vanilla, Iceland*	1 Serving/70g	182	7.6	260	3.3	37.5	10.8	0.7
Strawberry & Vanilla, Tesco*	1 Cone/70g	194	9.4	277	3	35.9	13.5	0.3
Strawberry, Cornetto, Wall's*	1 Cornetto/75g	198	8.2	264	2.1	40	11	0
Toffee & Vanilla, Giannis, Aldi*	1 Cone/71g	195	7.1	275	4.5	42	10	0.6
Vanilla, & Chocolate, Classico, Cornetto, Wall's*	1 Cornetto/75g	233	12.7	311	3.3	36	17	0
ICE CREAM ROLL								
Arctic, Average	*1 Serving/70g*	*140*	*4.6*	*200*	*4.1*	*33.3*	*6.6*	*0*
Tesco*	¼ Roll/57g	131	4.9	230	3.7	34.5	8.6	0.4
ICE CREAM SANDWICH								
'Wich, Ben & Jerry's*	1 Pack/117g	398	19.9	340	4	44	17	1
Chocolate, Skinny Cow*	1 Portion/36g	101	2.8	280	6	46	7.9	2.9
Mint, Skinny Cow*	1 Sandwich/71g	140	2	197	4.2	39.4	2.8	1.4
Neapolitan, Gelatelli, Lidl*	1 Sandwich/106g	233	9.5	220	4.9	29	9	1.9
Vanilla, Skinny Cow*	1 Portion/36g	100	3	277	5.4	45.1	8.2	2.1
ICE CREAM STICK								
Belgian Milk Chocolate Ices , Waitrose*	1 Bar/62g	208	12.7	338	4	33.5	20.6	1.6
Chocolate Cookies, Haagen-Dazs*	1 Stick/43g	162	10.9	376	4.9	31.8	25.4	0
Chocolate, Feast, Wall's*	1 Lolly/70g	245	16.1	350	3.6	31	23	0
Chocolate, Mini Milk, Wall's*	1 Lolly/23g	32	0.7	138	4.4	22	3.2	0
Mint Double Chocolate, Skinny Cow*	1 Stick/110ml	94	1.8	85	2.7	15.1	1.6	2.4
Strawberry, Mini Milk, Wall's*	1 Lolly/23g	31	0.7	133	3.9	22	3	0
Strawberry, Refreshing, Non Dairy, Swedish Glace, Wall's*	1 Lolly/37g	117	7.8	317	2.3	29	21	0
Vanilla, Mini Milk, Wall's*	1 Lolly/23g	30	0.7	130	3.9	22	3.1	0
ICE LOLLY								
Assorted, De Roma*	1 Lolly/55ml	48	0.2	87	0.2	20.9	0.4	0.2
Assorted, Farmfoods*	1 Lolly/56ml	35	0	62	0	15.6	0	0
Assorted, Iceland*	1 Lolly/51g	33	0	65	0	16.2	0	0
Baby, Tesco*	1 Lolly/32g	26	0	80	0.1	20	0	0.1
Berry Burst, Sainsbury's*	1 Serving/90ml	93	1.6	103	1.1	20.8	1.8	0.7
Blackcurrant Split, Iceland*	1 Lolly/75g	61	2.4	81	1.1	12	3.2	0.1
Blackcurrant, Dairy Split, Sainsbury's*	1 Lolly/73ml	88	2.6	121	1.8	20.4	3.6	0.1
Blackcurrant, Ribena*	1 Lolly/35ml	25	0	68	0	16.4	0	0
Bubblegum, Calippo, Wall's*	1 Calippo/106g	90	0.5	85	0.5	21	0.5	0
Cherry Tango, Liquid Ice, Britvic*	1 Lolly/65ml	84	0.1	129	0.1	31	0.1	0.2
Choc & Almond, Mini, Tesco*	1 Lolly/31g	103	7.4	331	4.4	24.8	23.8	0.9
Choc Lime Split, Morrisons*	1 Lolly/73ml	120	6.1	164	1.6	20.4	8.4	0.1
Chocolate Wonderpops, Sainsbury's*	1 Lolly/43g	118	8.3	276	2.6	21.8	19.4	0.7
Chocolate, Plain, Mini, Tesco*	1 Lolly/31g	94	6.6	304	3.1	24.8	21.4	1.2
Cider Refresher, Treats*	1 Lolly/70ml	54	0	77	0	19.2	0	0
Cola Lickers, Farmfoods*	1 Lolly/56ml	38	0	68	0	17	0	0
Exotic Fruit, Ice Cream, Gelatelli, Lidl*	1 Lolly/110g	148	2.8	135	1.8	25.6	2.5	0
Exotic Fruit, Mini, HL, Tesco*	1 Lolly/31g	41	0.6	131	1	26.4	2	1

ICE LOLLY

INFO/WEIGHT	Measure KCAL	FAT	per Measure KCAL	PROT	CARB	FAT	FIBRE

	Measure INFO/WEIGHT	per Measure		Nutrition Values per 100g / 100ml				
		KCAL	FAT	KCAL	PROT	CARB	FAT	FIBRE
Fab, Nestle*	1 Lolly/64g	90	3.2	141	0.5	23.4	5	0.4
Fab, Orange, Nestle*	1 Lolly/58g	81	2.7	140	0.6	24	4.7	0
Fruit Assorted, Basics, Somerfield*	1 Lolly/56ml	32	0	58	0	15	0	0
Fruit Flavour, Assorted, Basics, Sainsbury's*	1 Lolly/50g	33	0	66	0	16.5	0	0
Fruit Fusion, Mini, Farmfoods*	1 Lolly/45ml	36	0	79	0.2	19.2	0.1	0.2
Fruit Ices, Made with Orange Juice, Del Monte*	1 Lolly/75ml	79	0	105	0.5	25.7	0	0
Fruit Luxury, Mini, Co-Op*	1 Lolly/45g	58	2.7	130	2	18	6	0.2
Fruit Pastilles, Rowntree's*	1 Lolly/65ml	61	0	94	0.2	23.2	0	0
Fruit Split, Asda*	1 Lolly/74g	85	2.7	115	1.7	19	3.6	0
Fruit Split, Assorted, Co-Op*	1 Lolly/73g	80	2.2	110	1	20	3	0.1
Fruit Split, BFY, Morrisons*	1 Lolly/73g	50	0.5	69	1.6	13.9	0.7	0.1
Fruit Split, Waitrose*	1 Lolly/73g	91	2.6	124	2.5	21.7	3.6	0.4
Fruit Splits, Assorted, Somerfield*	1 Lolly/73ml	74	2.2	102	0	18	3	0
Fruit Splits, Treats*	1 Lolly/75ml	77	3.1	103	1.4	17.6	4.1	0
Fruit, Assorted, Waitrose*	1 Lolly/73g	59	0	81	0	20	0	0.1
Fruits of the Forest, Ice Cream, Gelatelli, Lidl*	1 Lolly/110g	145	2.8	132	1.9	24.5	2.5	0
Fruity 'n' Freezy, Asda*	1 Lolly/30ml	24	0	80	0.1	20	0	0
Ice Burst, Aldi*	1 Lolly/60g	67	1.1	112	0.5	24	1.8	0.5
Ice Lolly, Twister, Choc, Wall's*	1 Mini Lolly/27g	40	1.6	150	3.5	22	6	0.9
Icicles, All Flavours, Freezepops, Calypso*	1 Lolly/50ml	1	0	1	0	0.3	0	0
Kiwi Burst, Pineapple Sorbet in Kiwi Ice, Sainsbury's*	1 Serving/90ml	76	0.1	84	0.1	20.7	0.1	0.4
Lemon & Lime, Mini Bar, M&S*	1 Lolly/50g	48	0	95	0.1	23.6	0.1	0.2
Lemon & Lime, Rocket Split, De Roma*	1 Lolly/60ml	65	2.6	108	1	16	4.3	0.2
Lemon & Blackcurrant, Twister, Wall's*	1 Lolly/71g	68	0.4	96	0.7	21	0.6	0
Lemon & Lime, Mini, Calippo, Wall's*	1 Mini/78g	70	0.4	90	0.5	21	0.5	0
Lemon & Lime, Mini, Lemon Core, Twister, Wall's*	1 Mini/39g	42	0.5	107	0.6	22	1.2	0
Lemon & Lime, Mini, Strawberry Core, Twister, Wall's*	1 Mini/39g	41	0.5	105	0.6	22	1.2	0
Lemon & Lime, Twister, Wall's*	1 Lolly/71g	76	0.9	107	0.5	22	1.2	0
Lemon Sorbet, Mercadona*	1 Lolly/63g	38	0.2	61	0.5	32.4	0.3	8
Lemonade & Cola, Morrisons*	1 Lolly/55ml	36	0	65	0	16.2	0	0
Lemonade Flavour, R White*	1 Lolly/75ml	56	1.1	75	0.5	15.1	1.5	0.1
Lemonade Sparkle, Wall's*	1 Lolly/55ml	40	0	73	0	18.2	0	0
Mango & Passion Fruit Bursts, Sainsbury's*	1 Lolly/89ml	75	0.1	84	0.2	20.4	0.1	0
Mango & Passion Fruit Smoothie, Waitrose*	1 Lolly/73g	60	0.3	82	0.7	18.9	0.4	0.7
Milk, Blue Parrot Cafe, Sainsbury's*	1 Lolly/30ml	34	1	113	2.7	18	3.3	0.3
Mint Chocolate, Tesco*	1 Lolly/70g	234	13.9	334	3.6	35.4	19.8	1.2
Morrisons*	1 Lolly/100g	30	0	30	0	7.4	0	0
No Added Sugar, Tesco*	1 Lolly/32g	26	0	80	0.1	20	0	0.1
Nobbly Bobbly, Nestle*	1 Lolly/70ml	219	11.6	312	2.9	38.1	16.5	0.6
Orange & Lemon Splits, Farmfoods*	1 Lolly/56ml	69	2.4	124	1.6	19.8	4.3	0.2
Orange 'n' Cream, Tropicana*	1 Lolly/65g	83	2.9	129	1.4	20.5	4.5	0.3
Orange Juice, Asda*	1 Lolly/70g	58	0	83	0.7	20	0	0
Orange Juice, Bar, M&S*	1 Lolly/75g	64	0	86	0.5	21	0	0.1
Orange Juice, Co-Op*	1 Lolly/73g	51	0.1	70	0.4	17	0.1	0.1
Orange Juice, Freshly Squeezed, Finest, Tesco*	1 Lolly/80ml	89	0	111	0.7	27	0	0
Orange Juice, Freshly Squeezed, Waitrose*	1 Lolly/73g	88	0.1	120	0.6	29.7	0.1	0
Orange Juice, Morrisons*	1 Lolly/55ml	46	0	84	0	20	0	0
Orange, Average	**1 Lolly/72g**	**66**	**0**	**92**	**0.4**	**22.4**	**0**	**0.1**
Orange, Calippo, Wall's*	1 Calippo/105g	100	0.5	95	0.5	23	0.5	0
Orange, Lidl*	1 Lolly/50g	50	0	100	0.5	24.4	0	0
Orange, Mini, Calippo, Wall's*	1 Mini/79g	75	0.4	95	0.5	23	0.5	0
Orange, Real Fruit Juice, Sainsbury's*	1 Lolly/73ml	49	0.1	67	0.2	16.5	0.1	0.1
Orange, Real Juice, Sainsbury's*	1 Lolly/72ml	63	0.1	88	0.7	21	0.1	0.1

I

	Measure INFO/WEIGHT	per Measure		Nutrition Values per 100g / 100ml				
		KCAL	FAT	KCAL	PROT	CARB	FAT	FIBRE

ICE LOLLY

	Measure INFO/WEIGHT	KCAL	FAT	KCAL	PROT	CARB	FAT	FIBRE
Orange, Real Juice, Tesco*	1 Lolly/32g	25	0	78	0.6	18.7	0	0.3
Orange, Tesco*	1 Lolly/77g	53	0	68	0.2	16.8	0	0.3
Orange, Water, Iceland*	1 Lolly/75g	74	0	98	0.2	24.4	0	0.2
Pineapple & Coconut Colada, Waitrose*	1 Lolly/73ml	79	1.5	108	1	21	2.1	0.6
Pineapple, Dairy Split, Sainsbury's*	1 Lolly/72ml	84	2.6	116	1.8	19	3.6	0.1
Pineapple, Real Fruit Juice, Sainsbury's*	1 Lolly/73ml	55	0.1	76	0.1	19	0.1	0.1
Pop Up, CBY, Asda*	1 Lolly/80ml	65	0	81	0	20.1	0	0.3
Raspberry & Apple, Sainsbury's*	1 Lolly/57ml	39	0.1	68	0.1	17.1	0.1	0.1
Raspberry, Real Fruit Juice, Sainsbury's*	1 Lolly/72g	62	0.1	86	0.3	21	0.1	0.1
Raspberry, Smoothie, Iced, Del Monte*	1 Lolly/90ml	84	0	94	0.3	22.8	0	0.8
Real Fruit Juice, Rocket, Blue Parrot Cafe, Sainsbury's*	1 Lolly/58ml	45	0	77	0.2	19.1	0	0.1
Real Fruit, Dairy Split, Sainsbury's*	1 Lolly/73ml	100	3.1	137	2.1	22.8	4.2	0.1
Refresher, Fruit Flavour, Bassett's*	1 Lolly/45g	56	0.7	125	1.6	26	1.6	0.3
Rocket, Co-Op*	1 Lolly/60g	42	0	70	0	17	0	0
Rocket, Essential, Waitrose*	1 Lolly/58ml	42	0.1	72	0.4	16.8	0.2	0.7
Rocket, Sainsbury's*	1 Lolly/60g	50	0.3	83	0.5	19.9	0.5	0.5
Rolo, Nestle*	1 Lolly/75ml	243	14.1	324	3.8	36.5	18.8	0
Salted Caramel, Tesco*	1 Lolly/70g	227	12.5	324	3.6	36.7	17.9	1.1
Scooby Doo, Freezepops, Calypso*	1 Lolly/45ml	13	0	28	0	7	0	0
Scottish Raspberry, The Best, Morrisons*	1 Lolly/73ml	63	0.1	86	0.5	20.3	0.2	0.6
Seriously Fruity, Mango Sorbet, Waitrose*	1 Lolly/100ml	79	0.3	79	0.8	18.4	0.3	0.5
Skinny Dippers Minis, Caramel & Chocolate, Skinny Cow*	1 Lolly/38ml	62	1.9	162	3.4	24.3	5	3.3
Spotty Dotty, Sainsbury's*	1 Lolly/47g	111	6.5	236	1.8	25.5	13.8	1.3
Sprinkle Tops, Sainsbury's*	1 Lolly/40g	51	1.2	126	0.2	24.8	2.9	0.1
Strawberries & Cream, Cadbury*	1 Lolly/100ml	225	11.7	225	2.9	27	11.7	0
Strawberries 'n' Cream, Tropicana*	1 Lolly/50g	58	0.6	117	1.6	25	1.2	0
Strawberry & Banana, Smoothies, Sainsbury's*	1 Lolly/60g	100	3.2	166	1.5	28	5.3	0.2
Strawberry & Vanilla, 99% Fat Free, So-Lo, Iceland*	1 Lolly/92g	98	0.4	107	2.3	23.5	0.4	2.2
Strawberry Lemon, Shots, Calippo, Wall's*	1 Pack/81g	25	1	31	0.5	4.8	1.3	0
Strawberry Split, Average	*1 Lolly/72g*	*78*	*2.3*	*108*	*1.5*	*18.5*	*3.2*	*0.2*
Strawberry Split, Co-Op*	1 Lolly/71ml	75	2.1	105	1	17	3	0.1
Strawberry, Blackcurrant & Vanilla, Mini, Twister, Wall's*	1 Lolly/50ml	38	0.3	77	0.7	16	0.7	0
Strawberry, Dairy Split, Sainsbury's*	1 Lolly/73ml	86	2.6	118	1.7	19.8	3.6	0.1
Strawberry, Fruit Split, Iceland*	1 Lolly/73g	77	2.4	105	0.9	17.8	3.3	0.5
Strawberry, Orange & Pineapple, Rocket, Iceland*	1 Lolly/47g	38	0	81	0	20.2	0	0.1
Tip Top, Calypso*	1 Lolly/20ml	6	0	30	0.1	7.1	0.1	0
Traffic Light, Co-Op*	1 Lolly/52g	55	0.4	105	0.4	25	0.8	0
Tropical Fruit Sorbet, Waitrose*	1 Lolly/110g	90	2.2	82	1.5	14.5	2	0.2
Tropical Fruit, Starburst, Mars*	1 Lolly/93ml	94	0.1	101	0.3	24.8	0.1	0
Tropical, Mmmm, Tesco*	1 Lolly/73g	109	3.1	150	1.2	26.6	4.3	0.4
Whirlz, Giannis, Aldi*	1 Lolly/50g	49	0.9	98	0	17.4	1.8	0
Wonka Super Sour Tastic, Nestle*	1 Lolly/60ml	84	2.2	140	0	26.1	3.6	0
Zoom, Nestle*	1 Lolly/58ml	54	0.4	93	0.9	20.6	0.7	0

INDIAN MEAL

	Measure INFO/WEIGHT	KCAL	FAT	KCAL	PROT	CARB	FAT	FIBRE
Banquet for One, COU, M&S*	1 Pack/500g	400	6	80	6.7	10.2	1.2	3.1
for One, Asda*	1 Pack/550g	834	25.3	152	6.7	20.9	4.6	1.4
for One, Vegetarian, Asda*	1 Pack/499g	789	44.9	158	3.2	16	9	1.4
for Two, Hot, Takeaway, Tesco*	1 Pack/825g	1215	60.6	147	6.6	13.6	7.4	1.9
for Two, Menu, Tesco*	1 Serving/537g	811	34.4	151	6.3	17	6.4	0.8
Takeaway for One, Heated, HL, Tesco*	1 Pack/400g	410	6.4	103	7.2	14	1.6	2.1

IRN BRU

	Measure INFO/WEIGHT	KCAL	FAT	KCAL	PROT	CARB	FAT	FIBRE
Diet, Sugar Free, Barr's*	1 Can/330ml	2	0	1	0.5	0	0	0
Original, Barr's*	1 Bottle/500ml	214	0	43	0	10.5	0	0

	Measure INFO/WEIGHT	per Measure KCAL	FAT	Nutrition Values per 100g / 100ml KCAL	PROT	CARB	FAT	FIBRE
IRN BRU								
Xtra, Barr's*	1 Serving/250ml	2	0	1	0.5	0	0	0

I

	Measure INFO/WEIGHT	per Measure KCAL	FAT	Nutrition Values per 100g / 100ml KCAL	PROT	CARB	FAT	FIBRE
JACKFRUIT								
Raw, Average, Flesh Only	**1 Portion/162g**	**155**	**0.5**	**95**	**1.5**	**24.4**	**0.3**	**1.6**
JALFREZI								
Chicken, & Rice, Serves 1, Tesco*	1 Serving/475g	589	38	124	7.4	5.7	8	1.6
Chicken, & Coriander Rice, TTD, Sainsbury's*	1 Pack/473g	501	15.1	106	6.2	13.2	3.2	3.1
Chicken, & Pilau Rice, Sainsbury's*	1 Pack/500g	600	20.5	120	6.9	13.9	4.1	1.5
Chicken, & Pilau Rice, Takeaway, Asda*	1 Pack/557.7g	792	23.4	142	7	19	4.2	1.3
Chicken, , Slimzone, Asda*	1 Pack/467g	336	4.2	72	11	4.1	0.9	1.6
Chicken, Asda*	1 Pack/340g	415	20.4	122	10	7	6	1.6
Chicken, Canned, Tesco*	½ Can/200g	190	6.8	95	10.8	4.1	3.4	1.4
Chicken, Chef Select, Lidl*	1 Pack/367g	455	7.7	124	6.6	18.8	2.1	1.9
Chicken, Diet Chef Ltd*	1 Pack/300g	285	5.7	95	10.5	9	1.9	2.2
Chicken, Finest, Tesco*	1 Pack/350g	402	16.4	115	10.4	6.9	4.7	1.2
Chicken, GFY, Asda*	1 Pack/350g	238	3.2	68	9	6	0.9	1.8
Chicken, Hot & Spicy, Sainsbury's*	½ Pack/200g	228	11.4	114	12.8	2.9	5.7	1
Chicken, Indian Takeaway, Tesco*	1 Serving/350g	245	8.7	70	7.4	4.3	2.5	1.8
Chicken, Medium, GFY, Asda*	1 Pack/644g	972	27.7	151	6	22	4.3	0.9
Chicken, Specially Selected, Aldi*	1 Pack/350g	406	17.2	116	13	3.8	4.9	1.7
Chicken, Thali, Meal for One, M&S*	1 Pack/500g	680	28.5	136	7	12.7	5.7	3.1
Chicken, with Basmati Rice, Weight Watchers*	1 Pack/330g	238	1.6	72	5	11.8	0.5	0.5
Chicken, with Lemon Pilau Rice, Finest, Tesco*	1 Pack/493g	665	21.7	135	6.9	16.4	4.4	1.8
Chicken, with Pilau Basmati Rice, Frozen, Patak's*	1 Pack/400g	556	18.4	139	9.8	14.7	4.6	0.9
Chicken, with Pilau Rice, Charlie Bigham's*	½ Pack/424g	488	21.2	115	5.4	12.7	5	0
Chicken, with Pilau Rice, Cooked, CBY, Asda*	1 Pack/450g	682	15.4	151	8.1	21.5	3.4	1.2
Chicken, with Pilau Rice, GFY, Asda*	1 Pack/446g	495	11.1	111	8	14	2.5	1.2
Chicken, with Pilau Rice, Indian Cuisine, Aldi*	1 Pack/450g	673	21.3	158	8.7	18	5	3.3
Chicken, with Pilau Rice, Tesco*	1 Pack/460g	506	17.5	110	5.3	13.6	3.8	0.9
Chicken, with Rice, Morrisons*	1 Pack/400g	564	20.8	141	7.7	15.9	5.2	1.4
Chicken, with Rice, Ready Meal	**1 Serving/450g**	**557**	**18.9**	**124**	**6.9**	**14.5**	**4.2**	**1.5**
Chicken, with Rice, Ready Meal, Healthy Range	**1 Serving/400g**	**363**	**5.7**	**91**	**7.1**	**12.3**	**1.4**	**1.4**
Chicken, with Rice, Tesco*	1 Pack/550g	732	26.4	133	6.1	13.4	4.8	1
Meal for One, M&S*	1 Serving/500g	700	35	140	6.1	13.4	7	3
Vegetable, Eastern Indian, Sainsbury's*	1 Pack/400g	208	13.6	52	3.4	2	3.4	1.7
Vegetable, Indian, Sainsbury's*	½ Pack/200g	156	9	78	2	5.3	4.5	4.2
Vegetable, Waitrose*	1 Pack/400g	256	16	64	2.2	4.7	4	3.7
JAM								
Apricot, Average	**1 Tbsp/15g**	**37**	**0**	**248**	**0.2**	**61.6**	**0**	**1.5**
Apricot, Reduced Sugar, Average	**1 Serving/20g**	**37**	**0.1**	**186**	**0.4**	**46**	**0.3**	**0.4**
Black Cherry, Average	**1 Tsp/5g**	**12**	**0**	**247**	**0.4**	**61.2**	**0.3**	**0.4**
Blackberry, Extra Special, Asda*	1 Tbsp/15g	29	0.1	190	0.9	45	0.7	0
Blackcurrant, Average	**1 Tbsp/15g**	**38**	**0**	**250**	**0.2**	**62.3**	**0**	**1**
Blackcurrant, Reduced Sugar, Average	**1 Tsp/6g**	**10**	**0**	**178**	**0.4**	**44.4**	**0.2**	**1**
Blueberry, Best, Hartley's*	1 Tsp/20g	49	0	244	0.3	60.6	0.1	0
Damson, Extra Fruit, Best, Hartley's*	1 Tsp/5g	12	0	244	0.2	60.8	0	0
Fig	**1 Tsp/15g**	**36**	**0**	**242**	**0.5**	**60**	**0**	**0**
Golden Peach, Rhapsodie De Fruit, St Dalfour*	1 Tsp/10g	23	0	227	0.5	56	0.1	1.3
Kiwi & Gooseberry, 66% Fruit, Asda*	1 Serving/30g	56	0.2	187	0.5	45	0.5	0
Mixed Fruit, Average	**1 Tbsp/15g**	**38**	**0**	**252**	**0.3**	**63.5**	**0**	**0.5**
Peach, Pure, Summerland Sweets*	1 Tsp/5g	25	0	500	0	130	0	0
Plum, Tesco*	1 Serving/50g	130	0	261	0.2	64.4	0	0.6
Raspberry, Average	**1 Tbsp/15g**	**36**	**0**	**239**	**0.6**	**58.6**	**0.1**	**0.9**
Raspberry, Reduced Sugar, Average	**1 Tsp/6g**	**10**	**0**	**160**	**0.5**	**39.3**	**0.2**	**0.6**
Raspberry, Seedless, Average	**1 Tsp/10g**	**26**	**0**	**257**	**0.4**	**63.6**	**0**	**0.3**
Rhubarb & Ginger, Baxters*	1 Tsp/15g	40	0	264	0.4	65	0.1	0.8

J

	Measure INFO/WEIGHT	per Measure		Nutrition Values per 100g / 100ml				
		KCAL	FAT	KCAL	PROT	CARB	FAT	FIBRE
JAM								
Strawberry & Redcurrant, Reduced Sugar, Streamline*	1 Tbsp/15g	29	0	192	0.4	46.8	0.3	0
Strawberry, Average	*1 Tsp/10g*	*24*	*0*	*243*	*0.3*	*60.2*	*0.1*	*0.7*
Strawberry, Reduced Sugar, Average	*1 Tbsp/15g*	*28*	*0*	*187*	*0.4*	*45.8*	*0.3*	*0.2*
Wild Blackberry Jelly, Baxters*	1 Tsp/15g	32	0	210	0	53	0	1.2
JAMBALAYA								
American Style, Tesco*	1 Serving/275g	432	19.2	157	7.7	16	7	0.5
Cajun Chicken, Cooked, BGTY, Sainsbury's*	1 Pack/400g	392	6.5	103	6.6	14.6	1.7	1.6
Chicken & Prawn, World Cafe, Waitrose*	1 Pack/350g	413	12.2	118	5.3	15.3	3.5	2.3
COU, M&S*	1 Pack/400g	340	8	85	6.5	10.8	2	0.9
Ready Meal, Average	*1 Pack/450g*	*569*	*18.2*	*126*	*6.4*	*15.7*	*4*	*1.3*
JELLY								
Apple & Watermelon, Low Calorie, Hartley's*	1 Serving/175g	5	0	3	0	0.3	0	0.3
Apple, No Added Sugar, Hartley's*	1 Pot/115g	7	0.3	6	0	1.1	0.3	0
Blackberry, Unprepared, Morrisons*	1 Serving/20g	52	0	261	0.3	65	0	0
Blackcurrant & Tahitian Vanilla, M&S*	¼ Pack/143g	77	0.4	54	0.3	12.1	0.3	0.6
Blackcurrant, Made Up, Rowntree's*	¼ Jelly/140ml	100	0.1	71	1.4	16.4	0.1	0
Blackcurrant, Made Up, Sainsbury's*	¼ Jelly/150g	98	0	65	1.2	15.1	0	0
Blackcurrant, Sugar Free, Unprepared, Rowntree's*	1 Pack/24g	73	0	305	50	25	0	25
Blackcurrant, Tesco*	1 Serving/100g	84	0.1	84	0.2	20.5	0.1	0.4
Bramble, Tesco*	1 Serving/100g	257	0.1	257	0.3	63.7	0.1	1.3
Cherry Flavoured, Waitrose*	1 Pot/175g	87	0.5	50	0.3	11.3	0.3	0.2
Cloudy Lemonade, Pot, Hartley's*	1 Pot/183g	11	0.9	6	0.5	0.9	0.5	0
Crystals, Orange, Sugar Free, Bird's*	1 Sachet/12g	39	0.1	335	62.5	6.4	0.9	0
Crystals, Strawberry, Made Up, Tesco*	1 Serving/145g	9	0	6	1.3	0.3	0	0
Exotic Fruit, M&S*	1 Pot/175g	140	0.4	80	0.1	18.9	0.2	0.9
Fresh Fruit, M&S*	1 Pot/175g	131	0.2	75	0.2	18.4	0.1	0.3
Fruitini, Del Monte*	1 Serving/120g	78	0.1	65	0.3	15.3	0.1	0.5
Lime Flavour, Cubes, Hartley's*	1 Cube/12g	36	0	296	5.1	68.9	0	0
Lime, Made Up, Rowntree's*	¼ Jelly/140ml	100	0.1	71	1.4	16.4	0.1	0
Lime, Unprepared, Co-Op*	1 Pack/135g	397	0.1	294	5.5	68.1	0	1
Made Up with Water, Average	*1oz/28g*	*17*	*0*	*61*	*1.2*	*15.1*	*0*	*0*
Mandarin & Pineapple, Sainsbury's*	1 Pot/125g	95	0.1	76	0.2	18.9	0.1	1.2
Mixed Berry, WT5, Sainsbury's*	1 Serving/160g	112	0.3	70	0.7	16.3	0.2	1.5
Orange, Sugar Free, Crystals, Dry Weight, Hartley's*	1 Pack/26g	66	0	254	57.4	6.1	0	0
Orange, Sugar Free, Made Up, Hartley's*	1 Serving/140ml	9	0	6	1.3	0.3	0	0
Orange, Sugar Free, Rowntree's*	1 Serving/140ml	8	0	6	1.4	0.1	0	0
Orange, Sugar Free, Unprepared, Asda*	1 Serving/12g	36	0	303	63.6	12	0.1	0.2
Orange, Unprepared, Rowntree's*	1 Square/11g	33	0	296	4.4	69.6	0	0
Peach Melba, Eat Well, M&S*	1 Pot/175g	114	0.4	65	0.2	15.9	0.2	0.2
Raspberry & Elderflower, Seriously Fruity, Waitrose*	1/6 Pack/103g	71	0.3	69	2.3	13.9	0.3	0.5
Raspberry Flavour, Sugar Free, Made Up, Rowntree's*	1 Serving/140ml	9	0	6	1.4	0.1	0	0
Raspberry Flavour, Tesco*	1 Serving/34g	22	0	64	1	15	0	0.1
Raspberry Glitter, Made Up, Hartley's*	1 Serving/150g	94	0	63	0	15.4	0	0
Raspberry, Crystals, Vegetarian, Just Wholefoods*	1 Pack/85g	293	0	345	0.5	85.7	0	0
Raspberry, Individual Pot, Waitrose*	1 Pot/175g	92	1.2	53	0.3	10.7	0.7	1.1
Raspberry, Unprepared, Rowntree's*	1 Serving/135g	405	0.5	300	5.6	67.3	0.4	0
Redcurrant, Average	*1oz/28g*	*70*	*0*	*250*	*0.2*	*64.4*	*0*	*0*
Strawberry & Raspberry, Sainsbury's*	½ Pot/280g	230	0	82	0.2	20.2	0	1.2
Strawberry Flavour, Sugar Free, Made Up, Rowntree's*	1 Serving/140ml	10	0	7	1.5	0.1	0	0
Strawberry, Glitter, Made Up, Hartley's*	1 Serving/150g	94	0	63	0	15.4	0	0
Strawberry, Sugar Free, Crystals, Dry Weight, Hartley's*	1 Sachet/26g	73	0	280	56.8	13.1	0	0
Strawberry, Unprepared, Co-Op*	1 Pack/135g	402	0.1	298	5.5	69.1	0	0
Sugar Free, Dry, Tesco*	1 Pack/12.5g	36	0	285	55.4	15.6	0	0.2

J

	Measure INFO/WEIGHT	per Measure KCAL	FAT	Nutrition Values per 100g / 100ml KCAL	PROT	CARB	FAT	FIBRE
JELLY BABIES								
Bassett's*	1 Sweet/6g	20	0	335	3.5	79.7	0	0
M&S*	1 Pack/125g	418	0	334	5.2	78	0	0
Mini, Rowntree's*	1 Sm Bag/35g	128	0	366	4.6	86.9	0	0
JELLY BEANS								
Asda*	1 Bag/100g	364	0.4	364	0.1	90	0.4	0.2
Average	*1 Serving/100g*	*365*	*0.1*	*365*	*0.1*	*91.2*	*0.1*	*0.1*
Jelly Belly*	35 Beans/40g	140	0	350	0	90	0	0
Rowntree's*	1 Pack/35g	128	0	367	0	91.8	0	0
JERKY								
Beef, BBQ Flavour, Kings*	1 Bag/40g	116	1.9	291	36.3	26.2	4.9	1.3
Beef, Honey BBQ, Wild West*	1 Pack/50g	150	2.4	300	34.2	29.9	4.8	0.5
Beef, Peppered, Jack Link's*	1 Serving/28g	80	0.5	286	53.6	14.3	1.8	0
Beef, with Tomato Relish, Graze*	1 Pack/36g	91	1	253	22.2	30.6	2.8	2.5
JUICE								
Apple & Cranberry, Average	*1 Glass/250ml*	*114*	*0*	*46*	*0.1*	*10.2*	*0*	*0*
Apple & Elderflower, Copella*	1 Glass/250ml	108	0.2	43	0.4	10.2	0.1	0
Apple & Mango, Average	*1 Glass/200ml*	*108*	*0.1*	*54*	*0.3*	*12.6*	*0*	*0.1*
Apple & Orange, Fresh Up*	1 Serving/250ml	105	0	42	0	10.3	0	0
Apple & Raspberry, Average	*1 Serving/200ml*	*89*	*0.1*	*44*	*0.4*	*10.2*	*0*	*0.2*
Apple & Cherry, Sainsbury's*	1 Serving/200ml	96	0	48	0.3	10.8	0	0.8
Apple & Mango, 100% Pressed, Tesco*	1 Glass/150ml	72	0	48	0.4	10.7	0	0.9
Apple & Mango, Pressed, Waitrose*	1 Glass/100ml	54	0	54	0.3	12.6	0	0
Apple & Raspberry, Tropicana*	1 Glass/150ml	72	0	48	0.2	10.5	0	0.9
Apple & Rhubarb, Caxton Vale*	1 Glass/250ml	115	1	46	0.2	9.7	0.4	0
Apple & Rhubarb, Pressed, Cawston Press*	1 Serving/200ml	92	0.8	46	0.2	9.7	0.4	0
Apple, Cloudy, Pressed, Copella*	1 Glass/100ml	46	0	46	0.2	10.7	0	0.7
Apple, Concentrate, Average	*1 Tbsp/15ml*	*45*	*0*	*302*	*0*	*73.6*	*0.2*	*0*
Apple, Peach & Pear, Innocent*	1 Serving/100ml	45	0.1	45	0.4	10	0.1	1.4
Apple, Pure, Average	*1 Glass/250ml*	*116*	*0.1*	*47*	*0.1*	*11.2*	*0*	*0*
Apple, Pure, Organic, Average	*1 Serving/200ml*	*92*	*0.1*	*46*	*0*	*11.2*	*0*	*0*
Apple, Pure, Value, Tesco*	1 Glass/200ml	94	0	47	0.1	11.4	0	0
Beetroot, Apple, & Rhubarb, Morrisons*	1 Glass/150ml	68	0.2	45	0.7	9.9	0.1	0.7
Breakfast, Ruby, Tropicana*	1 Glass/200ml	90	0	45	0.8	9.7	0	0.7
Carrot, Average	*1 Glass/200ml*	*48*	*0.2*	*24*	*0.5*	*5.7*	*0.1*	*0*
Carrot, Orange, & Apple, Cold Pressed, B Fresh *	1 Bottle/250ml	65	0	26	0	6.2	0	0
Chia Watermelon & Pomegranate, WOW, Planet Organic*	1 Bottle/250ml	122	3.8	49	2.3	5.6	1.5	2.2
Clementine, 100% Pure Squeezed, Tesco*	1 Serving/150ml	71	0	48	0.4	10.7	0	0.2
Clementine, Morrisons*	1 Serving/100ml	48	0.1	48	0.5	10.9	0.1	0.1
Cranberry, Average	*1 Bottle/250ml*	*139*	*0.2*	*56*	*0.1*	*13.4*	*0.1*	*0.3*
Cranberry, No Added Sugar, Average	*1 Glass/200ml*	*11*	*0.1*	*6*	*0.1*	*0.8*	*0*	*0*
Exotic Fruit, Pure, Del Monte*	1 Glass/200ml	96	0	48	0.3	11.3	0	0
Exotic Fruit, Waitrose*	1 Glass/175ml	88	0	50	0.4	11.6	0	0
Froot Refresh, Orange & Passion Fruit, Minute Maid*	1 Bottle/330ml	79	0	24	0	6	0	0
Fruit, Tropical in Sparkling Spring Water, Light, Rio*	1 Can/330ml	17	0	5	0.1	1.1	0	0
Fruit, Tropical, Pure Premium, Tropicana*	1 Glass/200ml	98	0	49	0.5	11	0	0.8
Grape, Purple, Welch's*	1 Serving/200ml	136	0	68	0.1	16.5	0	0
Grape, Red, Average	*1 Serving/100ml*	*62*	*0*	*62*	*0.2*	*15.2*	*0*	*0*
Grape, White, Average	*1 Can/160ml*	*95*	*0.1*	*60*	*0.2*	*14.3*	*0.1*	*0.1*
Grapefruit, Pink, Average	*1 Glass/200ml*	*81*	*0.1*	*40*	*0.6*	*9*	*0*	*0.2*
Grapefruit, Pure, Average	*1 Glass/200ml*	*77*	*0.2*	*38*	*0.5*	*8.5*	*0.1*	*0.1*
Lemon, Fresh, Average	*1 Lemon/35.5ml*	*2*	*0*	*7*	*0.3*	*1.6*	*0*	*0.1*
Lemon, from Concentrate	*5ml*	*1*	*0*	*28*	*0.4*	*6.5*	*0*	*0*
Lime, Fresh, Average	*1 Tsp/5ml*	*0*	*0*	*9*	*0.4*	*1.6*	*0.1*	*0.1*

JUICE

	Measure INFO/WEIGHT	KCAL	FAT	KCAL	PROT	CARB	FAT	FIBRE
Mandarin Orange, Tropicana*	1 Serving/200ml	94	0	47	0.6	10	0	0.8
Mango Veggie, Naked Juice Co*	1 Serving/240ml	150	1	62	1.2	15.8	0.4	2.1
Mango, Peach, Papaya, Pure, Premium, Tropicana*	1 Glass/200ml	88	0	44	0.5	9.8	0	0.1
Mango, Pure, Canned	*1 Glass/250ml*	*98*	*0.5*	*39*	*0.1*	*9.8*	*0.2*	*0*
Multivitamin, Fruit, Vitafit, Lidl*	1 Carton/250ml	135	0.2	54	0.3	12.5	0.1	0.5
Orange & Kiwi Fruit, Tropicana*	1 Serving/175ml	90	0	51	0.5	12	0	0
Orange & Pineapple, Average	*1 Glass/120ml*	*56*	*0.6*	*46*	*0.4*	*10.5*	*0.5*	*0.5*
Orange & Raspberry, Average	*1fl oz/30ml*	*15*	*0*	*50*	*0.6*	*11.4*	*0.1*	*0.2*
Orange & Banana, Pure, Average	*1 Glass/150ml*	*79*	*0.1*	*53*	*0.7*	*12.1*	*0.1*	*0.2*
Orange & Grapefruit, Average	*1 Glass/200ml*	*84*	*0.2*	*42*	*0.8*	*9.2*	*0.1*	*0.4*
Orange & Lime, Tropicana*	1 Serving/250ml	115	0	46	1.1	9.4	0	0.6
Orange & Mango, Average	*1 Bottle/375ml*	*176*	*0.4*	*47*	*0.5*	*10.7*	*0.1*	*0.2*
Orange & Passionfruit, Tropicana*	1 Serving/200ml	94	0	47	0.8	10	0	0.7
Orange & Raspberry, Tropicana*	1 Bottle/330ml	139	0	42	0.4	9	0	0.8
Orange 100% from Concentrate, Farmfoods*	1 Serving/200ml	84	0.2	42	0.6	9.1	0.1	0.1
Orange with Bits, Freshly Squeezed, TTD, Sainsbury's*	1 Serving/249g	132	0	53	0.7	11.4	0	0.2
Orange with Bits, Innocent*	1 Glass/250ml	120	0	48	0.8	10.9	0	0.3
Orange with Bits, Not From Concentrate, Tesco*	1 Glass/250ml	110	0	44	0.4	10.6	0	0
Orange, Apple & Mango, Calypso*	1 Carton/200ml	92	0.4	46	0	11	0.2	0.1
Orange, Carrot & Passionfruit, Morrisons*	1 Glass/250ml	88	0.2	35	0.6	7.5	0.1	0.9
Orange, Freshly Squeezed, Average	*1 Serving/200ml*	*66*	*0*	*33*	*0.6*	*8.1*	*0*	*1*
Orange, Freshly Squeezed, with Bits, 1, Waitrose*	¼ Bottle/250ml	108	0.2	43	0.7	9.5	0.1	0.5
Orange, Mango & Passionfruit, Pure Squeezed, Waitrose*	1 Serving/250ml	130	0.8	52	0.6	10.9	0.3	0.3
Orange, Pure from Concentrate, Carton, Value, Tesco*	1 Serving/250ml	115	0	46	0.5	10.4	0	0
Orange, Pure Premium, Smooth, No Bits, Tropicana*	1 Glass/200ml	96	0	48	0.8	10	0	0.4
Orange, Pure with Bits, Average	*1 Glass/200ml*	*90*	*0.1*	*45*	*0.6*	*10.2*	*0.1*	*0.1*
Orange, Pure, Smooth, Average	*1 Glass/200ml*	*88*	*0.1*	*44*	*0.7*	*9.8*	*0*	*0.2*
Orange, Pure, Smooth, From Concentrate, Sainsbury's*	1 Serving/200ml	84	0.2	42	0.5	9.1	0.1	0.1
Orange, Pure, Tesco*	1 Glass/200ml	94	0	47	0.5	10.5	0	0
Orange, Red, Average	*1 Glass/250ml*	*115*	*0.1*	*46*	*0.4*	*10.7*	*0*	*0.2*
Orange, Smooth, Freshly Squeezed, TTD, Sainsbury's*	1 Serving/249g	132	0	53	0.7	11.4	0	0.2
Orange, Smooth, Innocent*	1 Serving/200ml	76	0	38	0.7	8.2	0	0
Orange, Sparkling, 55, Britvic*	1 Bottle/275ml	135	0.3	49	0.3	11.3	0.1	0.1
Orange, Vitafit*	1 Glass/200ml	78	0.2	39	0.7	8.3	0.1	0.7
Passion Fruit, Average	*1 Glass/200ml*	*94*	*0.2*	*47*	*0.8*	*10.7*	*0.1*	*0*
Pineapple, Average	*1 Glass/200ml*	*100*	*0.1*	*50*	*0.3*	*11.7*	*0.1*	*0.2*
Pomegranate, Grape & Apple, Tropicana*	1 Bottle/330ml	211	0	64	0.2	15.5	0	0.6
Pomegranate, Pomegreat*	1 Glass/200ml	88	0	44	0.1	11.1	0	0
Pomegranate, Pure, Organic, Biona*	1 Portion/100g	74	0.6	74	0.7	16.7	0.6	0.4
Prune, Average	*1 Serving/200ml*	*123*	*0.1*	*61*	*0.6*	*15.3*	*0.1*	*1.8*
Sweet Carrot & Orange, Shapers, Boots*	1 Serving/250ml	100	0.4	40	0.9	8.8	0.2	0.4
Tomato from Concentrate, Sainsbury's*	1 Glass/250ml	40	0.2	16	0.7	2.7	0.1	0.7
Tomato, Average	*1 Glass/200ml*	*40*	*0.1*	*20*	*0.8*	*4*	*0*	*0.4*
Tomato, Tangy, Princes*	1 Serving/200ml	34	0	17	0.8	3.1	0	0.6
Tomato, Vitafit, Lidl*	1 Serving/250ml	47	0.5	19	0.8	2.9	0.2	0.7
Tropical made from Concentrate, Sainsbury's*	1 Glass/250ml	120	0.2	48	0.5	10.7	0.1	0.1
Tropical, Pure, Sainsbury's*	1 Glass/200ml	104	0.2	52	0.5	12	0.1	0.1
Turmeric Booster, Cold Pressed, Moju*	1 Shot/60ml	22	0.1	36	0.8	7.5	0.1	0
V Fusion, Passion Fruit, Mango & Carrot, V8*	1 Serving/150ml	72	0	48	0.3	11.8	0	0.4
V Fusion, Raspberry & Beetroot, V8*	1 Serving/150ml	68	0	45	0.3	10.8	0	0.3
Vegetable, Organic, Evernat*	1 Glass/200ml	36	0.2	18	0.9	3.5	0.1	0.2
Vegetable, Organic, James White*	1 Sm Glass/100g	22	0.2	22	0.6	4.4	0.2	0
Vegetable, Original, V8*	1 Glass/150ml	26	0.2	17	0.9	2.8	0.1	0.9

J

	Measure INFO/WEIGHT	per Measure KCAL	FAT	Nutrition Values per 100g / 100ml KCAL	PROT	CARB	FAT	FIBRE
JUICE								
Watermelon, Mello Drinks*	1 Bottle/250ml	100	0.2	40	1	8.5	0.1	0.7
White Apple & Ginger, James White*	1 Glass/250ml	122	0	49	0.1	11.8	0	0
White Grape, Raspberry & Blackcurrant, Asda*	1 Serving/200ml	120	0.2	60	0.4	13.8	0.1	0.1
JUICE DRINK								
Aloe Vera, OKF*	1 Bottle/500ml	175	0	35	0	9	0	0
Apple & Blueberry, The Feel Good Drinks Co*	1 Serving/375ml	163	0.4	44	0.1	10.6	0.1	0
Apple & Elderflower, Tesco*	1 Serving/200ml	76	0	38	0	9.4	0	0
Apple & Raspberry, Sainsbury's*	1 Serving/200ml	112	0.2	56	0.1	13.8	0.1	0.1
Apple & Strawberry, Sainsbury's*	1 Serving/250ml	13	0.1	5	0	1	0	0
Apple & Mango, CBY, Asda*	1 Carton/250ml	115	0	46	0	11	0	0
Apple & Pomegranate, Sparkling Water, Sainsbury's*	1 Serving/200ml	4	0	2	0	0.3	0	0
Apple & Raspberry, Light, Just Drink, Don Simon*	1 Glass/250ml	50	0	20	0.1	6.1	0	0.3
Apple & Raspberry, Tesco*	1 Serving/300ml	138	0	46	0.1	11.2	0	0
Apple Lemonade, Cawston Press*	1 Glass/200g	106	0.2	53	0.2	11.9	0.1	0
Apple, Cranberry, & Blueberry, Waitrose*	1 Serving/150ml	75	0	50	0.1	11.9	0	0.1
Apple, No Added Sugar, Asda*	1 Glass/200ml	10	0	5	0	1	0	0
Apple, No Added Sugar, LC, Tesco*	1 Glass/250ml	12	0	5	0	0.9	0	0
Apple, Plum & Pear, Pure Pressed, CBY, Asda*	1 Glass/200ml	92	0	46	0.4	10.5	0	0.2
Berry & Elderberry, Fusion, Oasis*	1 Bottle/375ml	11	0	3	0	0.4	0	0
Blackcurrant & Apple, Oasis*	1 Serving/500ml	90	0	18	0	4.1	0	0
Blackcurrant, 45% High, No Added Sugar, Asda*	1 Serving/25ml	2	0	7	0	1.4	0	0
Blackcurrant, Extra Light, Ribena*	1 Serving/200ml	8	0	4	0	0.5	0	0
Blackcurrant, Pouch, Sun Shots, Aldi*	1 Pouch/200ml	10	0.5	5	0.2	1.1	0.2	0.2
Blueberry, BGTY, Sainsbury's*	1 Serving/250ml	15	0	6	0.1	1	0	0
Cherry & Cinnamon Presse, CBY, Asda*	1 Can/250ml	95	1.3	37	0.5	9.2	0.5	0.5
Cherry, No Added Sugar, Sainsbury's*	1 Carton/250ml	25	0.1	10	0.2	1.9	0	0
Cranberry & Blackberry, Ocean Spray*	1 Glass/250ml	120	0.2	48	0.1	11.3	0.1	0.2
Cranberry & Blackcurrant, Ocean Spray*	1 Bottle/500ml	265	0	53	0.2	12.7	0	0
Cranberry & Orange, HE, Tesco*	1 Glass/200ml	10	0	5	0	0.8	0	0
Cranberry & Raspberry, BGTY, Sainsbury's*	1 Glass/250ml	10	0.2	4	0.1	0.7	0.1	0.1
Cranberry & Raspberry, Sainsbury's*	1 Serving/250ml	105	0	42	0.1	9.9	0	0
Cranberry & Raspberry, Tesco*	1 Serving/200ml	96	0	48	0	11.6	0	0
Cranberry & Mango, Light, Ocean Spray*	1 Glass/250ml	22	0	9	0	2	0	0.1
Cranberry & Pomegranate, Ocean Spray*	1 Glass/250ml	120	0	48	0	11.5	0	0
Cranberry & Raspberry, No Add Sugar, LC, Tesco*	1 Serving/250ml	12	0	5	0	0.8	0	0
Cranberry & Raspberry, Ocean Spray*	1 Glass/200ml	96	0	48	0	11.6	0	0
Cranberry & Raspberry, with Spring Water, Zeo*	1 Serving/275ml	33	0	12	0	2.6	0	0
Cranberry Blend, Ocean Spray*	1 Glass/250ml	148	0	59	0.1	13.9	0	0
Cranberry, Asda*	1 Serving/200ml	40	0	20	0	4.5	0	0
Cranberry, Classic, Ocean Spray*	1 Bottle/500ml	245	0.5	49	0.1	11.7	0.1	0.1
Cranberry, Grape & Apple, Ocean Spray*	1 Glass/200ml	108	0	54	0.1	12.9	0	0
Cranberry, Light, Classic, Ocean Spray*	1 Glass/200ml	16	0	8	0	1.4	0	0
Cranberry, McEnnedy, Lidl*	1 Glass/200ml	98	0	49	0	11.7	0	0
Cranberry, Morrisons*	1 Glass/200ml	92	0	46	0	11.6	0	0
Cranberry, No Added Sugar, BGTY, Sainsbury's*	1 Glass/200ml	4	0	2	0	0.3	0	0
Cranberry, No Added Sugar, HL, Tesco*	1 Glass/200ml	8	0	4	0	1.1	0	0
Cranberry, Organic, Sainsbury's*	1 Serving/200ml	100	0	50	0	11.9	0	0
Cranberry, Original, Concentrated, Ocean Spray*	1 Serving/15ml	27	0	183	0.2	44.1	0	0
Cranberry, Solevita*	1 Serving/200ml	98	0	49	0.5	11.7	0	0
Cranberry, Tesco*	1 Serving/250ml	127	0	51	0.1	12.2	0	0
Cranberry, Waitrose*	1 Serving/250ml	145	0	58	0.1	13.9	0	0.1
Exotic, Tesco*	1 Serving/250ml	128	0	51	0.1	12.3	0	0
Forest Fruits, Asda*	1 Serving/200ml	88	0	44	0.3	10.9	0	0.3

J

JUICE DRINK

INFO/WEIGHT	Measure per Measure KCAL	FAT	Nutrition Values per 100g / 100ml KCAL	PROT	CARB	FAT	FIBRE
Fruit Cocktail, Sainsbury's*	1 Glass/200ml	90	0	45	0.2	10.6	0	0.1
Fruit Shoot, My-5, Apple & Pear, Robinson's*	1 Bottle/200ml	78	0.2	39	0.2	8.9	0.1	0
Grape & Elderflower, White, Sparkling, Shloer*	1 Glass/200ml	74	0	37	0	9.2	0	0
Grape, Apple & Raspberry, Co-Op*	1 Serving/150ml	75	0	50	0.4	12	0	0.1
Grape, Apple & Raspberry, Asda*	1 Glass/200ml	82	1	41	0.5	9.8	0.5	0.5
Grape, Red, Sparkling, Shloer*	1 Glass/200ml	84	0	42	0	10.4	0	0
Grape, White, Sparkling, Light, Shloer*	1 Glass/125ml	28	0	22	0.7	5.3	0	0
Grape, White, Sparkling, Shloer*	1 Serving/120ml	59	0	49	0	11.6	0	0
Guava Exotic, Rubicon*	1 Carton/288ml	150	0.3	52	0.2	12.9	0.1	0
J20, Apple & Mango, Britvic*	1 Bottle/275ml	83	0	30	0.1	6.8	0	0.2
J20, Apple & Raspberry, Britvic*	1 Bottle/275ml	88	0	32	0.1	7.3	0	0.3
J20, Orange & Passion Fruit, Britvic*	1 Bottle/275ml	88	0	32	0.3	7.2	0	0.2
J2O, Apple & Blueberry, Britvic*	1 Bottle/275g	124	0	45	0.1	11	0	0.2
J2O, Apple & Watermelon, Sparkling, Spritz, Britvic*	1 Serving/250ml	58	0	23	0	5.4	0	0
J2O, Glitterberry, Britvic*	1 Bottle/275ml	110	0	40	0.2	9.4	0	0
Lemon & Lime, Light, Oasis*	1 Bottle/250ml	6	0	3	0	0.2	0	0
Lemon, Cloudy, Lightly Carbonated, Zeo*	1 Serving/275ml	28	0	10	0.1	2.3	0	0
Lemon, The Feel Good Drinks Co*	1 Bottle/171ml	78	0.2	46	0.1	10.8	0.1	0
Lemonade, Asda*	1 Glass/200ml	88	0	44	0.1	11	0	0
Lychee, Sparkling, Rubicon*	1 Can/330g	182	0	55	0	13.6	0	0
Mango & Passionfruit, Shot, Big Shotz*	1 Shot/120ml	67	0.5	56	0	12.1	0.4	3.4
Mango Madness, Snapple*	1 Bottle/227ml	104	0	46	0	12	0	0
Mango, & Earl Grey Tea, Rio Doro, Aldi*	1 Bottle/ 330ml	3	0.3	1	0.1	0.3	0.1	0.1
Mango, Rubicon*	1 Serving/100ml	54	0.1	54	0.1	13.1	0.1	0
Mango, Sparkling, Rubicon*	1 Can/330ml	172	0	52	0	12.8	0	0
Mixed Berry Crush, Sparkling, CBY, Asda*	1 Glass/250ml	8	0	3	0	0.5	0	0
Mulled Lemonade, Sainsbury's*	1 Serving/150ml	67	0.8	44	0.5	10.8	0.5	0.5
Netar Multifruit, Light, Linessa, Lidl*	1 Glass /200ml	54	0.1	27	0.3	5.8	0.1	0
Orange & Lime, Refresh'd, Robinson's*	1 Bottle/500ml	55	0	11	0	2.2	0	0
Orange & Lime, Sparkling, Innocent*	1 Can/330ml	93	0	28	0.6	6.5	0	0
Orange & Mango, Spring Water, Sparkling, Rubicon*	1 Bottle/500ml	15	0	3	0	0.5	0	0
Orange, Caprisun*	1 Pouch/200ml	89	0	45	0	10.8	0	0
Orange, Carrot & Lemon, Pago*	1 Serving/200g	90	0.2	45	0.2	10.5	0.1	0
Orange, Diluted, Mi Wadi*	1 Serving/250ml	26	0	10	0	2.3	0	0
Orange, Fruitish, Spar*	1 Carton/330ml	13	0.3	4	0.1	0.8	0.1	0
Orange, HE, Tesco*	1 Glass/200ml	56	0.2	28	0.3	6.1	0.1	0
Orange, Juice Burst, Purity Soft Drinks Co*	1 Bottle/500ml	220	0	44	1	10.2	0	0
Orange, Mango & Lime, Fruit Crush, Shapers, Boots*	1 Bottle/330ml	150	0.6	45	0.4	10.6	0.2	0.4
Orange, Morrisons*	1 Serving/250ml	12	0.2	5	0.1	0.9	0.1	0.1
Orange, Sainsbury's*	1 Serving/250ml	18	0.2	7	0.1	1.4	0.1	0.1
Orange, Value, Tesco*	1 Glass/250ml	32	0	13	0	3.3	0	0
Orange, Zero, Vive, Aldi*	1 Serving/200g	2	1	1	0.5	0.5	0.5	0.5
Passion Fruit, Exotic, Rubicon*	1 Serving/200ml	110	0	55	0.1	13.6	0	0
Peach & Passionfruit Fruit, Sunmagic*	1 Serving/330ml	172	0	52	0.3	13	0	0.1
Peach & Apricot, Sparkling, J2O Spritz, Britvic*	1 Serving/250ml	52	0	21	0	4.9	0	0
Peach & Grapefruit, Lightly Carbonated, Zeo*	1 Serving/275ml	30	0	11	0	2.3	0	0
Peach, Passion Fruit, Extra Light, Oasis*	1 Bottle/500ml	18	0	4	0	0.6	0	0
Pear & Raspberry, Sparkling, J2O Spritz, Britvic*	1 Serving/250ml	55	0	22	0	5.2	0	0
Pear, Partially Made with Concentrate, Tesco*	1 Glass/200ml	110	0	55	0	12.4	0	0.2
Pineapple & Grapefruit, Shapers, Boots*	1 Bottle/500ml	10	0.5	2	0.1	0.2	0.1	0
Pink Cranberry Lemonade, Diet, Sparkling, M&S*	1 Bottle/500ml	15	0.5	3	0.1	0.5	0.1	0.1
Pink Grapefruit, Juice Burst, Purity Soft Drinks Co*	1 Bottle/500ml	210	0	42	0.4	10	0	0
Pink Guava, & Yuzu, Presse, Sparkling, M&S*	1 Serving/200ml	84	0.2	42	0.1	9.1	0.1	0.4

J

	Measure INFO/WEIGHT	per Measure KCAL	per Measure FAT	Nutrition Values per 100g / 100ml KCAL	PROT	CARB	FAT	FIBRE
JUICE DRINK								
Pomegranate & Raspberry, Still, Shapers, Boots*	1 Bottle/500ml	45	0	9	0	2	0	0
Pomegranate, Rubicon*	1 Can/330ml	108	0	54	0	13.5	0	0
Purple Grape & Mango, Welch's*	1 Glass/200ml	54	0	27	0	6.1	0	0.2
Raspberry & Pear, Tesco*	1 Serving/250ml	118	0	47	0	11.3	0	0
Raspberry, Ribena*	1 Bottle/500ml	215	0	43	0	10.4	0	0
Sicilian Lemon & Garden Mint, Presse, Finest, Tesco*	1 Serving/250ml	50	0	20	0	5	0	0
Spirit, Lemon & Grapefruit, Tropicana*	1 Bottle/400ml	184	0	46	0.3	10.4	0	0.6
Summer Fruits, Fresh, Tesco*	1 Glass/250ml	112	0.2	45	0.1	10.8	0.1	0.3
Summer Fruits, Oasis*	1 Bottle/500ml	90	0	18	0	4.2	0	0
Tropical Fruit, Tesco*	1 Glass/250ml	118	0	47	0	11.4	0	0
Tropical Fruit, Waitrose*	1 Glass/250ml	118	0	47	0.2	11.2	0	0
Tropical, Be Light, Aldi*	1 Glass/250ml	62	0.2	25	0.2	5.4	0.1	0.2
Tropical, No Added Sugar, Tesco*	1 Carton/250ml	12	0	5	0	1.1	0	0
White Cranberry & Lychee, Ocean Spray*	1 Glass/200ml	86	0	43	0	11.5	0	0
White Grape & Peach, Sainsbury's*	1 Glass/250ml	95	0.2	38	0.2	9	0.1	0.1
White Grape, Raspberry & Cranberry, Sparkling, Shloer*	1 Serving/250ml	117	0	47	0	11	0	0

J

	Measure INFO/WEIGHT	per Measure KCAL	per Measure FAT	Nutrition Values per 100g / 100ml KCAL	PROT	CARB	FAT	FIBRE
KALE								
Cavolo Nero, Boiled, Growers Selection, Asda*	½ Pack/150g	45	1.7	30	2.4	1	1.1	2.8
Curly, Boiled in Salted Water, Average	*1 Serving/60g*	*14*	*0.7*	*24*	*2.4*	*1*	*1.1*	*2.8*
Curly, Raw, Average	*1 Serving/90g*	*25*	*1.2*	*28*	*2.9*	*1.2*	*1.4*	*2.6*
Kalettes, Sprouts, Sweet Nutty & Versatile, Waitrose*	1 Serving/80g	41	1.1	51	3.5	4.1	1.4	4.1
Sprouts, Kalettes, Staples*	½ Bag/100g	53	1.5	53	3	5.2	1.5	3.5
KANGAROO								
Raw, Average	*1 Serving/200g*	*196*	*2*	*98*	*22*	*1*	*1*	*0*
KARELA								
Frozen, Shana*	1 Serving/80g	14	0.1	18	1.4	1.3	0.1	0
KEBAB								
BBQ Pork, Sainsbury's*	1 Serving/90g	65	2.2	72	11	1.4	2.4	0.9
Beef & Pepper, Kofta, Waitrose*	1 Kebab/138g	223	13.9	162	14.8	2.9	10.1	0.6
Beef, Kofta, Uncooked, Tesco*	1 Kebab/72.5g	163	12.5	225	14	3.2	17.3	1.2
Chicken & Pineapple, Caribbean Style, Iceland*	1 Kebab/44g	41	0.6	93	11.6	8.7	1.4	1.4
Chicken, & Chorizo, Waitrose*	1 Kebab/70g	135	8.2	195	20.4	1.3	11.8	1.1
Chicken, Breast, Moroccan Style, Sainsburys*	4 Kebabs/133g	170	2.5	128	26.8	0.9	1.9	0.5
Chicken, Mini Fillet, Ginger, Lime & Coriander, Waitrose*	1 Kebab/13g	22	0.5	172	32.3	2.1	3.8	0.1
Chicken, Mini Fillets, M&S*	1 Serving/150g	210	8.7	140	20.2	2	5.8	0.3
Chicken, Shish in Pitta Bread with Salad	*1 Kebab/250g*	*388*	*10.2*	*155*	*13.5*	*17.2*	*4.1*	*1*
Chicken, Shish, Meat Only, Average	*1 Kebab/250g*	*312*	*5.2*	*125*	*25.7*	*0.9*	*2.1*	*0.1*
Chicken, Thigh, Sticky Barbecue, M&S*	1 Kebab/100g	160	7.5	160	15.6	7.4	7.5	0.8
Chicken, Tikka, Oakhurst, Aldi*	1 Kebab/59g	52	0.7	88	14	5.1	1.2	0.5
Doner, in Pitta, with Salad, Average	*1 Serving/400g*	*1020*	*64.8*	*255*	*14.2*	*14*	*16.2*	*0.8*
Lamb & Chicken, Seekh, Indian Kitchen, Heated, Tesco*	½ Pack/64g	145	7.9	226	15.4	11.8	12.3	3.4
Lamb Shami with a Mint Raita Dip, M&S*	½ Pack/90g	189	12.1	210	12.8	9.7	13.4	3.5
Lamb with Mint, Tesco*	1 Serving/80g	192	13.4	240	16	5.5	16.7	0.4
Lamb, Kofta, Citrus Tikka, Sainsbury's*	1 Kebab/84g	199	11.6	235	18.1	9.8	13.7	2.6
Lamb, Kofta, Indian Style, Waitrose*	1 Kebab/125g	266	19.8	213	12.3	5.5	15.8	1.6
Lamb, Minted, Ashfield Farm, Aldi*	1 Kebab/54g	137	9.2	254	18.5	5.7	17	0
Lamb, Minted, Shish, As prepared, Waitrose*	1 Kebab/57g	123	7.3	217	17.2	7.9	12.9	0.1
Lamb, Shish, Sainsbury's*	1 Kebab/85g	178	11.3	210	19.7	2.8	13.3	0.7
Shish with Onions & Peppers	*1oz/28g*	*59*	*4.5*	*212*	*12.9*	*3.9*	*16.2*	*1.2*
KEDGEREE								
Average	*1oz/28g*	*48*	*2.4*	*171*	*15.9*	*7.8*	*8.7*	*0.1*
COU, M&S*	1 Pack/370g	388	8.1	105	7.6	13.7	2.2	2.1
Smoked Haddock, Big Dish, M&S*	1 Pack/450g	585	22.5	130	8.5	13	5	1.9
KETCHUP								
Barbeque, Asda*	1 Tbsp/15g	20	0	136	0.9	33	0	0
BBQ, Heinz*	1 Serving/10g	14	0	137	1.3	31.3	0.3	0.3
Chilli, Smoked, Gran Luchito*	1 Tsp/5g	18	0	358	1.8	18.4	0.9	0
Tomato, Average	*1 Tsp/5g*	*6*	*0*	*120*	*1.5*	*28.1*	*0.2*	*0.8*
Tomato, Batts, Lidl*	1 Tbsp/20g	20	0	99	1.5	21	0.1	2
Tomato, Everyday Value, Tesco*	1 Tbsp/15ml	21	0	140	0.9	32.6	0.2	0.5
Tomato, Morrisons*	1 Serving/15g	16	0	110	1.6	24	0.2	1.6
Tomato, Reduced Sugar, Average	*1 Tbsp/10g*	*9*	*0.1*	*87*	*2*	*16.9*	*1.2*	*0.9*
KIDNEY								
Lamb, Fried, Average	*1oz/28g*	*53*	*2.9*	*188*	*23.7*	*0*	*10.3*	*0*
Lamb, Raw, Average	*1oz/28g*	*25*	*0.7*	*91*	*17*	*0*	*2.6*	*0*
Ox, Raw	*1oz/28g*	*22*	*0.5*	*77*	*15.1*	*0*	*1.8*	*0*
Ox, Stewed	*1oz/28g*	*39*	*1.2*	*138*	*24.5*	*0*	*4.4*	*0*
Pig, Fried	*1oz/28g*	*57*	*2.7*	*202*	*29.2*	*0*	*9.5*	*0*
Pig, Raw	*1oz/28g*	*22*	*0.7*	*77*	*14*	*0*	*2.4*	*0*
Pig, Stewed	*1oz/28g*	*43*	*1.7*	*153*	*24.4*	*0*	*6.1*	*0*

K

	Measure INFO/WEIGHT	per Measure KCAL	FAT	Nutrition Values per 100g / 100ml KCAL	PROT	CARB	FAT	FIBRE
KIDNEY								
Veal, Raw, Average	**1 Serving/100g**	**99**	**3.1**	**99**	**15.8**	**0.8**	**3.1**	**0**
KIEV								
Chicken, Cooked, M Kitchen, Fresh Ideas, Morrisons*	1 Kiev/188g	371	13.5	198	18.5	14.4	7.2	0.7
Chicken, COU, M&S*	1 Kiev/150g	188	2.7	125	15.8	10.8	1.8	0.5
Chicken, Creamy Peppercorn, Tesco*	1 Kiev/132g	290	17.3	220	13.1	12.1	13.1	0.6
Chicken, Finest, Tesco*	1 Kiev/217g	380	12.8	175	21.9	8.3	5.9	0.5
Chicken, Garlic & Parsley Butter, Breaded, Waitrose*	1 Kiev/156g	375	21.3	241	17.5	11.1	13.7	1.4
Chicken, Garlic & Herb Sauce, Inspirations, Birds Eye*	1 Breast/125g	305	16.5	244	12.2	18.8	13.2	0.7
Chicken, Garlic & Herb, Frozen, Birds Eye*	1 Piece/91g	240	11.9	264	15.3	20.6	13.1	1
Chicken, Garlic & Herb, Reduced Fat, Sainsbury's*	1 Kiev/142g	317	18	223	15.1	12.7	12.7	0.6
Chicken, Garlic & Herb, Sainsbury's*	1 Kiev/134g	319	19.6	239	15	11.7	14.7	1.3
Chicken, Garlic & Parsley, BGTY, Sainsbury's*	1 Kiev/126.2g	289	15.3	229	14	15.9	12.1	1.1
Chicken, Garlic & Parsley, Sainsbury's*	1 Kiev/120g	365	25.6	304	11.1	17.1	21.3	0.8
Chicken, Garlic Butter, CBY, Asda*	1 Kiev/130g	359	25.7	276	12.4	11.9	19.8	0.5
Chicken, Garlic Butter, Frozen , Tesco*	1 Kiev/126g	340	22.6	270	13.1	14	17.9	0
Chicken, Garlic Butter, HL, Tesco*	1 Kiev/143g	285	16.4	200	14.3	9.9	11.5	0.6
Chicken, Garlic, Ashfield Farm, Aldi*	1 Kiev/131g	363	25.9	277	9.5	13.8	19.8	2.9
Chicken, Garlic, M&S*	1 Kiev/150g	370	24.8	247	15.6	8.2	16.5	2.9
Chicken, Garlic, Whole Breast, Asda*	1 Pack/290g	638	38	220	15.2	10.4	13.1	0
Chicken, Ham, & Cheese, Tesco*	1 Serving/143g	307	18.6	215	14.4	9.3	13	1.3
Chicken, with Cheese & Ham Sauce, Birds Eye*	1 Breast/124g	294	14.9	237	13	19	12	0.7
Chicken, with Wild Garlic Cornish Butter, Gastropub, M&S*	1 Kiev/225g	493	32.2	219	17.3	5	14.3	0.6
Mushroom & Spinach, Good Life*	1 Kiev/125g	290	14	232	6.4	24.5	11.2	3.7
Vegetarian, Chicken Style, Cheesy, Garlic, Tesco*	1 Kiev/113g	262	12.5	232	14.9	17	11.1	2.5
Vegetarian, Mini, Quorn*	1 Kiev/20g	41	2.2	207	14	13	11	6.5
Vegetarian, Vegetable, M&S*	1 Kiev/155g	287	16	185	3.5	18.2	10.3	2.9
KIPPER								
Baked, Average	**1oz/28g**	**57**	**3.2**	**205**	**25.5**	**0**	**11.4**	**0**
Fillets in Brine, John West*	1 Can/140g	269	16.8	192	21	0	12	0
Fillets in Sunflower Oil, John West*	1 Can/140g	321	23.8	229	19	0	17	0
Fillets, Raw, Average	**1 Serving/200g**	**384**	**29.1**	**192**	**14.5**	**0**	**14.6**	**0**
Fillets, Smoked with Butter, Scottish, Boil in Bag, Tesco*	1 Serving/100g	225	17.2	225	17	0	17.2	0
Fillets, Smoked, TTD, Sainsbury's*	1 Serving/100g	255	19.4	255	20.1	0.1	19.4	0
Grilled, Average	**1oz/28g**	**71**	**5.4**	**255**	**20.1**	**0**	**19.4**	**0**
Smoked, Average	**1 Serving/150g**	**322**	**23**	**214**	**18.9**	**0**	**15.4**	**0**
Whole, with Bone, Grilled, Average	**1 Serving/100g**	**161**	**12.2**	**161**	**12.7**	**0**	**12.2**	**0**
KIT KAT								
2 Finger, Dark, Nestle*	2 Fingers/21g	107	5.4	510	5.4	62.2	25.5	5.4
2 Finger, Nestle*	2 Fingers/21g	107	5.3	512	6	63.5	25.5	2.1
4 Finger, Nestle*	4 Fingers/42g	208	10.2	502	6.7	62.7	24.5	2.1
Caramac, 4 Finger, Nestle*	4 Fingers/49g	259	14.1	532	5.9	61.9	29	0.6
Chunky, Caramel, Nestle*	1 Bar/48g	259	15.3	539	5.2	58.6	31.8	0
Chunky, Double Caramel, Nestle*	½ Bar/21g	109	5.8	520	6.5	61	27.6	1
Chunky, Nestle*	1 Bar/48g	248	12.6	516	5.9	62.5	26.3	2.1
Chunky, Orange, Nestle*	1 Bar/48g	247	12.5	515	5.8	62	26.1	0
Chunky, Peanut, Nestle*	1 Bar/50g	268	15.8	537	8.4	54.9	31.5	0
Chunky, Snack Size, Nestle*	1 Bar/26g	133	7.1	513	6.6	60.4	27.2	1.1
Cookies & Cream, 2 Finger, Nestle*	1 Bar/21g	107	5.2	510	6.3	64	25	1.4
Cookies & Cream, Snap & Share, Nestle*	1 Row/16g	81	4.2	522	7.2	61.5	26.9	1.5
Editions, Mango & Passionfruit, Nestle*	1 Bar/45g	225	10.5	499	4.7	69	23.4	0
Editions, Seville Orange, Nestle*	1 Bar/45g	223	10.4	496	4.6	69.3	23	0.8
Kubes, Nestle*	1 Pack/50g	258	13.8	515	5.9	60.9	27.5	1
Low Carb, 2 Finger, Nestle*	2 Fingers/21g	92	6.6	438	9.2	28.3	31.3	1.3

K

	Measure INFO/WEIGHT	per Measure KCAL	FAT	Nutrition Values per 100g / 100ml KCAL	PROT	CARB	FAT	FIBRE
KIT KAT								
Low Carb, 4 Finger, Nestle*	1 Finger/11g	46	3.3	438	9.2	28.3	31.3	1.3
Mini, Nestle*	1 Bar/15g	75	3.9	502	7.5	59.4	26	0
Mint, 4 Finger, Nestle*	4 Fingers/48g	244	12.7	508	6	61.5	26.4	1.1
Orange, 2 Finger, Nestle*	2 Fingers/21g	107	5.6	507	5.5	61.7	26.5	0
Peanut Butter, Bites, Nestle*	4 Pieces/23g	120	6.1	521	5.7	63.5	26.7	1.8
Senses, Nestle*	1 Bar/31g	165	9.5	531	7.5	56.3	30.7	0
White, Chunky, Nestle*	1 Bar/53g	276	14.6	521	8.3	60.3	27.5	0.7
KIWI BERRY								
Tesco*	1 Serving/80g	70	0.5	87	1.2	17.6	0.6	3.2
KIWI FRUIT								
Fresh, Raw, Flesh & Seeds, Average	*1 Kiwi/60g*	*29*	*0.3*	*49*	*1.1*	*10.6*	*0.5*	*1.9*
Weighed with Skin, Average	*1 Kiwi/60g*	*25*	*0.3*	*42*	*0.9*	*9.1*	*0.4*	*1.6*
KOHLRABI								
Boiled in Salted Water	*1oz/28g*	*5*	*0.1*	*18*	*1.2*	*3.1*	*0.2*	*1.9*
Raw	*1oz/28g*	*5*	*0*	*16*	*1.1*	*2.6*	*0.1*	*1.5*
KORMA								
Chicken, & Basmati Rice, Tesco*	1 Pot/350g	588	32.6	168	4.3	16.9	9.3	2.3
Chicken, & Pilau Rice, Morrisons*	1 Pack/450g	889	48.2	198	9.4	15.9	10.7	1.4
Chicken, & Pilau Rice, Tesco*	1 Serving/460g	722	45.1	157	5.6	11.5	9.8	1.3
Chicken, & Rice, 95% Fat Free, Birds Eye*	1 Pack/370g	444	7	120	6.2	19.6	1.9	1.1
Chicken, & Rice, Everyday, Value, Tesco*	1 Pack/400g	625	28.9	160	7.3	13.8	7.4	2.6
Chicken, & White Rice, BGTY, Frozen, Sainsbury's*	1 Pack/375g	341	3.8	91	5.6	14.9	1	0.5
Chicken, & Pilau Rice, Charlie Bigham's*	½ Pack/405g	624	34	154	6.4	14	8.4	0
Chicken, & Rice, Indian Meal for Two, Sainsbury's*	1 Pack/500g	785	40.5	157	6.8	14.3	8.1	3.1
Chicken, CBY, Asda*	1 Pack/316g	518	34.8	164	11	4.2	11	1.8
Chicken, Indian Meal for 2, Finest, Tesco*	½ Pack/200g	348	24	174	10.3	6.2	12	2.5
Chicken, Indian Takeaway for One, Sainsbury's*	1 Serving/300g	498	30.9	166	13	5.3	10.3	1.6
Chicken, Indian Takeaway, Iceland*	1 Pack/400g	656	44	164	11.8	4.5	11	1.4
Chicken, Indian, Takeaway, Tesco*	½ Pack/175g	222	13.5	127	9	5.5	7.7	1.8
Chicken, Indian, Waitrose*	½ Pack/175g	280	17.5	160	12.4	4.7	10	1.2
Chicken, Morrisons*	1 Pack/350g	707	46.6	202	13.6	7	13.3	0.7
Chicken, with Peshwari Coriander Rice, Finest, Tesco*	1 Pack/550g	908	48.4	165	7.5	13.9	8.8	0.9
Chicken, with Pilau Rice, Co-Op*	1 Pack/450g	783	44.6	174	7.4	13	9.9	1.8
Chicken, with Pilau Rice, PB, Waitrose*	1 Pack/400g	452	6.8	113	8.9	15.4	1.7	1.3
Chicken, with Rice, Ready Meal	*1 Pack/400g*	*740*	*34.7*	*185*	*8.4*	*18.1*	*8.7*	*1.7*
Chicken, with Rice, Ready Meal, Healthy Range	*1 Serving/400g*	*450*	*8.2*	*112*	*7.3*	*16.1*	*2.1*	*1.2*
Vegetable, Ready to Cook, Fresh, Sainsbury's*	½ Pack/255g	263	17.3	103	2.8	7.7	6.8	2.1
Vegetable, Takeaway or Restaurant	*1 Serving/300g*	*336*	*13.5*	*112*	*3.4*	*15.4*	*4.5*	*2.6*
KRISPROLLS								
Cracked Wheat, Original, Pagen*	1 Krisproll/12.5g	48	0.9	380	12	67	7	9
Golden, Swedish Toasts, Pagen*	1 Krisproll/12g	48	1	400	11	69	8.5	5
Organic, Bio, Pagen*	1 Krisproll/12g	46	0.8	380	12	67	7	8
Swedish Toasts, Wholegrain, Pagen*	1 Toast/13g	51	0.8	390	11	67	6.5	8.5
KULFI								
Average	*1oz/28g*	*119*	*11.2*	*424*	*5.4*	*11.8*	*39.9*	*0.6*
KUMQUATS								
Raw	*1oz/28g*	*12*	*0.1*	*43*	*0.9*	*9.3*	*0.5*	*3.8*
KUNG PO								
Chicken, Sainsbury's*	½ Pack/175g	131	4.4	75	9.2	4	2.5	1
Chicken, Waitrose*	1 Pack/350g	318	3.9	91	8.2	12.1	1.1	1.2

K

	Measure INFO/WEIGHT	per Measure KCAL	FAT	Nutrition Values per 100g / 100ml KCAL	PROT	CARB	FAT	FIBRE
LAGER								
Alcohol Free, Becks*	1 Serving/275ml	55	0	20	0.7	5	0	0
Alcohol Free, Heineken*	1 Can/330ml	69	0	21	0	4.8	0	0
Amstel, Heineken*	1 Pint/568ml	227	0	40	0.5	3	0	0
Average	*½ Pint/284ml*	*117*	*0*	*41*	*0.3*	*3.1*	*0*	*0*
Basics, Sainsbury's*	1 Can/440g	71	0	16	0	1	0	0
Becks*	1 Can/275ml	113	0	41	0	3	0	0
Blanc, Kronenbourg*	½ pt/284ml	119	0	42	0	3.3	0	0
Boston, Samuel Adams*	1 Bottle/355ml	160	0	45	0	0	0	0
Bottled, Brahma*	1 Bottle/330ml	125	0	38	0	0	0	0
Budweiser, 66, Anheuser-Busch*	1 Bottle/330ml	102	0	31	0	0	0	0
C2, Carling*	½ Pint/284ml	80	0	28	0	3.5	0	0
Can, Carlsberg*	1 Can/440ml	141	0	32	0	2	0	0
Draught, Carling*	1 Pint/568ml	189	0	33	0	1.4	0	0
Export, Carlsberg*	1 Can/440ml	185	0	42	0.4	2.8	0	0.4
Export, Foster's*	1 Pint/568ml	210	0	37	0	2.2	0	0
Foster's*	1 Pint/568ml	193	0	34	0	3.1	0	0
German, Low Alcohol, Sainsbury's*	1 Bottle/330ml	92	0.3	28	0.4	5.9	0.1	0.1
Gold, Foster's, Heineken*	1 Can/440ml	145	0	33	0.3	1.2	0	0
Grolsch*	1 Sm Can/330ml	145	0	44	0	2.2	0	0
Heineken v 5, Heineken*	1 Pint/568ml	256	0	45	0.5	3	0	0
Heineken*, 5%, Heineken*	1 Bottle/250ml	110	0	44	0.4	3.4	0	0
Innis & Gunn*	1 Bottle/330ml	132	0	40	0.3	3.5	0	0
Kaliber, Guinness*	1 Can/440ml	110	0	25	0.2	6	0	0
KÃf¶lsch, FrÃf¼h*	1 Glass/200ml	112	0	56	0.5	4	0	0
Light, Coors*	1 Pint/568ml	170	0	30	0.3	1.5	0	0
Light, Corona*	1 Bottle/330ml	105	0	32	1.5	0	0	0
Lite, Carlsberg*	1 Bottle/330ml	89	0	27	0.1	0.5	0	0
Low Alcohol	*1 Can/440ml*	*44*	*0*	*10*	*0.2*	*1.5*	*0*	*0*
Organic, Tesco*	1 Bottle/500ml	215	0	43	0.2	3.5	0	0
Pils, Holsten*	1 Can/440ml	167	0	38	0.3	2.4	0	0
Pilsner, Efes*	1 Can/500ml	226	0	45	0	7.6	0	0
Pilsner, Premium, Bavaria*	1 Bottle/330ml	142	0	43	0.4	3.5	0	0
Polish, Tyskie*	1 Can/549ml	236	0	43	0	0	0	0
Premier, Kronenbourg*	½ Pint/284ml	136	0	48	0	0	0	0
Premium	*1 Can/440ml*	*260*	*0*	*59*	*0.3*	*2.4*	*0*	*0*
Premium, French, Biere Speciale, Tesco*	1 Serving/250ml	105	0	42	0.3	3.3	0	0
Premium, Light, Amstel*	1 Can/355ml	95	0	27	0	1.4	0	0
Premium, San Miguel*	1 Bottle/330ml	148	0	45	0.3	3.7	0	0
Premium, Tesco*	1 Can/440ml	145	0	33	0.3	4	0	0
Shandy, Traditional Style, Asda*	1 Serving/200ml	44	0	22	0	4.6	0	0
Skinny Brands*	1 Bottle/330ml	89	0.3	27	0	0.9	0.1	0
Stella Artois*	1 Can/550ml	220	0	40	0.4	3.1	0	0
Tuborg Green, Carlsberg*	1 Serving/200ml	78	0	39	0.5	2.5	0	0
Vier, Becks*	1 Bottle/275ml	110	0	40	0	3	0	0
LAKSA								
Chicken & Coconut Noodle, Cooked, Tesco*	1 Pack/351g	321	10.6	91	7.1	8.4	3	1.2
Chicken & Prawn, Asian, Waitrose*	1 Pack/380g	505	19.8	133	4.6	15.7	5.2	2.3
Chicken, COU, M&S*	1 Pack/450g	360	9.9	80	7.5	7	2.2	1.1
Thai Noodle, with Chicken, M&S*	1 Pack/400g	460	21.6	115	7	9.8	5.4	1.1
LAMB								
Breast, Lean, Roasted, Average	*1 Serving/100g*	*273*	*18.5*	*273*	*26.7*	*0*	*18.5*	*0*
Chops, Average	*1 Chop/82g*	*190*	*13.4*	*231*	*20.6*	*0.4*	*16.4*	*0*
Chops, Minted, Average	*1 Chop/100g*	*260*	*15.1*	*260*	*25.9*	*5.1*	*15.1*	*0.3*

L

	Measure INFO/WEIGHT	per Measure KCAL	FAT	Nutrition Values per 100g / 100ml KCAL	PROT	CARB	FAT	FIBRE
LAMB								
Cutlets, Neck, Raw, Lean & Fat, Weighed with Bone	1 Pack 210g	359	31.7	171	8.8	0	15.1	0
Diced, From Supermarket, Healthy Range, Average	½ Pack/200g	277	8.9	138	24.6	0.1	4.5	0
Grill Steak, Average	1oz/28g	70	4.7	250	20.2	4.4	16.9	0.4
Grill Steak, Prime, Average	1 Steak/63g	197	16.1	312	18.5	2	25.5	0.1
Leg, Joint, Raw, Average	1 Joint/510g	858	45.5	168	20.9	1.4	8.9	0.2
Leg, Roasted, Lean & Fat, Average	1oz/28g	66	3.8	237	28.6	0	13.6	0
Leg, Roasted, Lean, Average	1oz/28g	58	2.7	206	29.9	0	9.6	0
Loin, Chop, Grilled, Lean & Fat, Weighed with Bone	1 Serving/100g	193	14	193	16.8	0	14	0
Loin, Chops, Raw, Lean & Fat, Weighed with Bone	1 Serving/100g	216	17.9	216	13.7	0	17.9	0
Mince, Average	1oz/28g	58	4.2	207	17.6	0.5	14.8	0
Mince, Extra Lean, Sainsbury's*	1 Serving/225g	324	11.9	144	24.1	0	5.3	0.1
Mince, Lean, Raw, Tesco*	1 Pack/400g	860	63.6	215	17.6	0	15.9	0
Neck Fillet, Lean, Raw	1 Serving/100g	232	17.6	232	18.4	0	17.6	0
Rack, Raw, Lean & Fat	1oz/28g	79	6.7	283	17.3	0	23.8	0
Rack, Raw, Lean Only, Weighed with Bone	1oz/28g	21	1.1	73	8.6	0	4	0
Rack, Roasted, Lean	1oz/28g	63	3.6	225	27.1	0	13	0
Rack, Roasted, Lean & Fat	1oz/28g	102	8.4	363	23	0	30.1	0
Shank, in Mint Gravy, Simply Heat, Tesco*	1 Shank/332g	551	29.2	166	17.5	4	8.8	0.5
Shank, Just Cook, Sainsbury's*	1 Shank/225g	394	18.7	175	22.9	1.8	8.3	0
Shank, Mediterranean, Finest, Tesco*	1 Serving/404g	671	35.6	166	15	6.6	8.8	2
Shank, Shoulder, Fresh, British, Value, Tesco*	1 Shank/220g	242	5.3	110	22.1	0	2.4	0
Shoulder, Cooked, Lean & Fat	1oz/28g	84	6.3	301	24.4	0	22.5	0
Shoulder, Fillet, Average	1oz/28g	66	5.1	235	17.6	0	18.3	0
Shoulder, Raw, Average	1oz/28g	70	5.7	248	16.8	0	20.2	0
Shoulder, Roasted, Whole, Lean	1oz/28g	61	3.4	218	27.2	0	12.1	0
Sliced, in Rich Mint Gravy, Iceland*	½ Pack/150g	164	6.9	109	11.9	4.5	4.6	0.6
Steak, Leg, Raw, Average	1 Steak/150g	169	5.5	112	20	0	3.6	0
Steak, Minted, Average	1 Steak/125g	212	9	170	22.7	3.4	7.2	0.9
Steak, Raw, Average	1 Steak/140g	190	7.6	136	21.7	0.2	5.4	0
Stewing, Raw, Lean & Fat	1oz/28g	57	3.5	203	22.5	0	12.6	0
Stewing, Stewed, Lean	1oz/28g	67	4.1	240	26.6	0	14.8	0
Stewing, Stewed, Lean & Fat	1oz/28g	78	5.6	279	24.4	0	20.1	0
Trimmed Fat, Raw, Average	1 Serving/100g	518	51.6	518	13.3	0	51.6	0
LAMB IN								
Garlic & Rosemary Gravy, Shank, Asda*	1 Shank/280g	451	23.2	161	19.8	1.7	8.3	0.5
Rich Minted Gravy, Shank, Morrisons*	1 Pack/400g	612	26.4	153	18.8	5.2	6.6	0
LAMB MOROCCAN								
with Cous Cous, PB, Waitrose*	1 Pack/400g	390	5.2	98	7.7	13.6	1.3	2.2
LAMB WITH								
Carrot & Swede Mash, Braised, Eat Smart, Morrisons*	1 Pack/400g	304	9.2	76	5.2	8.2	2.3	1.5
Chunky Vegetables, Shanks, Braised, M&S*	½ Pack/425g	808	38.2	190	24.7	2	9	0.7
Gravy, Joint, Tesco*	1 Serving/225g	277	13	123	14.9	2.8	5.8	0
Honey Roast Vegetables, Extra Special, Asda*	1 Pack/400g	400	14.8	100	9.9	6.7	3.7	2.5
Mango & Mint, Shoulder Chops, Waitrose*	1 Chop/250g	555	40.5	222	16.7	2.3	16.2	0.5
Mash, Braised, Tesco*	1 Serving/450g	413	12.2	92	6.1	10.7	2.7	0.8
Mint Butter, Leg Steaks, Waitrose*	1 Serving/155g	270	16.3	174	19.6	0.4	10.5	0
Mint Glaze & Redcurrant Sauce, Steaks, Leg, Asda*	½ Pack/145g	247	8.7	170	18	11	6	0.5
Mint Gravy, Leg Chops, Tesco*	1 Serving/175g	214	9.8	122	15	3.2	5.6	1.7
Mint, Leg Chops, Morrisons*	2 Chops/350g	858	45.2	245	29.4	2.4	12.9	0.9
Redcurrant & Rosemary Sauce, Chops, Leg, Tesco*	1 Pack/325g	604	36.1	186	17.6	4	11.1	0.5
Roasted Vegetables, Shank, M&S*	½ Pack/420g	660	30.6	157	14.9	8.3	7.3	0.7
Rosemary Gravy, Shank, Sainsbury's*	1 Serving/200g	204	8.2	102	13.2	3.1	4.1	0.3
Sweet Mint Dressing, Joint, Tesco*	1 Serving/50g	96	5.9	193	19.9	1.8	11.8	0.6

L

INFO/WEIGHT	Measure	per Measure KCAL	FAT	Nutrition Values per 100g / 100ml KCAL	PROT	CARB	FAT	FIBRE

LARD

	Measure INFO/WEIGHT	per Measure KCAL	FAT	KCAL	PROT	CARB	FAT	FIBRE
Average	*1oz/28g*	*249*	*27.7*	*891*	*0*	*0*	*99*	*0*

LASAGNE

Al Forno, Beef, with a Chianti Classico Ragu, M&S*	1 Pack/400g	640	38	160	8.2	10.7	9.5	2.8
Al Forno, Heated, Finest, Tesco*	1 Pack/385g	608	29.2	158	9.8	11.8	7.6	1.5
Al Forno, TTD, Sainsbury's*	1 Pack/383g	571	30.3	149	8.6	10.9	7.9	2.1
Asda*	1 Pack/398g	502	23.9	126	7.3	10.6	6	1.1
Basics, Sainsbury's*	1 Pack/300g	330	12.9	110	4.8	13.1	4.3	1.2
Beef & Chunky Vegetable, HL, Tesco*	1 Pack/340g	354	9.5	104	5.9	13.8	2.8	1.2
Beef, al Forno, Cooked, 1, Waitrose*	1 Pack/400g	663	34.7	170	9.5	12.2	8.9	1.7
Beef, BGTY, Sainsbury's*	1 Pack/390g	376	8.5	102	6.2	13.2	2.3	1.7
Beef, Calorie Controlled, As Prepared, Love Life, Waitrose*	1 Pack/400g	341	7.1	91	6.7	10.6	1.9	2.4
Beef, Cooked, Italian, Sainsbury's*	1 Serving/375g	555	32.2	148	7.8	6.8	8.6	6.7
Beef, Frozen, Co-Op*	1 Pack/340g	388	15.6	114	7.5	10.7	4.6	1.4
Beef, Frozen, Eat Smart, Morrisons*	1 Pack/380g	331	10.3	87	6.1	9.5	2.7	1.3
Beef, Frozen, Tesco*	1 Pack/450g	608	25.2	135	7.5	12.6	5.6	0.8
Beef, Italian, Classic, Tesco*	1 Pack/600g	948	51	158	7.5	12.7	8.5	0.5
Beef, Less Than 3% Fat, Frozen, GFY, Asda*	1 Pack/400g	369	10	92	7.3	8.9	2.5	2.5
Beef, Little Dish*	1 Pack/200g	349	20.8	174	9.3	10.7	10.4	0.8
Beef, Ready Meal, Average	*1 Serving/400g*	*553*	*24*	*138*	*8.2*	*12.7*	*6*	*1.4*
Beef, Ready Meals, Waitrose*	1 Pack/400g	444	20.5	111	5.8	10.4	5.1	0.8
BFY, Morrisons*	1 Pack/350g	340	14	97	7.1	8.6	4	0.2
Bolognese, Lidl*	1 Serving/200g	336	18	168	8	13.7	9	0
Charlie Bigham's*	½ Pack/344g	557	29.2	162	8.5	11.3	8.5	0.7
Chicken, Italian, Sainsbury's*	1 Pack/450g	549	18.9	122	8.4	12.6	4.2	0.5
Creamy Ricotta & Vegetable, HL, Tesco*	1 Pack/384g	407	10.8	106	5.5	14.6	2.8	3.6
Extra Special, Asda*	½ Pack/291g	416	20.4	143	7	13	7	0.3
Family, Big Value Pack, Iceland*	¼ Pack/237g	322	14	136	5	15.9	5.9	1.4
Family, M&S*	¼ Pack/225g	281	14	125	10.3	6.9	6.2	1.1
GFY, Asda*	1 Pack/410g	344	8.2	84	5.5	11	2	0.3
Mediterranean Vegetable, COU, M&S*	1 Pack/360g	306	9.7	85	3.4	11.5	2.7	1.4
Mushroom & Spinach, Waitrose*	1 Pack/400g	373	14	93	3.1	12.3	3.5	1.3
Primana, Aldi*	1 Serving/250g	422	22.5	169	8	14	9	0
Roasted Vegetable, M&S*	1 Pack/400g	440	20.4	110	3.4	12.8	5.1	1.7
Sheets, Boiled, Average	*1 Sheet/20g*	*20*	*0.1*	*100*	*3*	*22*	*0.6*	*0.9*
Sheets, Dry, Average	*1 Sheet/20g*	*70*	*0.3*	*349*	*11.9*	*72.1*	*1.5*	*2.9*
Spinach & Ricotta, Finest, Tesco*	1 Pack/350g	584	37.1	167	6.1	11.7	10.6	1.2
Vegetable, BGTY, Sainsbury's*	1 Pack/385g	339	7.7	88	3.5	13.9	2	2.3
Vegetable, Healthy Range, Average	*1 Serving/400g*	*318*	*8.2*	*80*	*3.5*	*11.8*	*2.1*	*1.5*
Vegetable, Ready Meal, Average	*1 Serving/400g*	*408*	*17.6*	*102*	*4.1*	*12.4*	*4.4*	*1*
Vegetarian, Butternut Squash, Ovenbaked, Asda*	1 Pack/400g	376	13.1	92	2.4	13	3.2	0.6
Vegetarian, Frozen or Chilled, Quorn*	1 Pack/300g	303	8.1	101	4.8	12.5	2.7	1.6
Vegetarian, Linda McCartney*	1 Pack/360g	451	20.2	125	6.3	12.4	5.6	1.4
Vegetarian, Meat Substitute, Ready Meal, Average	*1 Serving/400g*	*468*	*20.8*	*117*	*5.3*	*12.2*	*5.2*	*1.6*
Vegetarian, Tesco*	1 Pack/450g	630	34.6	140	6	11.6	7.7	1.6
Vegetarian, Vegetable, Meat Free, Tesco*	1 Pack/353g	290	8.1	82	3.4	11.3	2.3	1.4

LAVERBREAD

Average	*1oz/28g*	*15*	*1*	*52*	*3.2*	*1.6*	*3.7*	*0*

LEEKS

Boiled, Average	*1oz/28g*	*6*	*0.2*	*21*	*1.2*	*2.6*	*0.7*	*1.7*
Creamed, Frozen, Waitrose*	1 Serving/225g	115	5.4	51	1.8	5.5	2.4	0
Raw, Unprepared, Average	*1 Leek/166g*	*37*	*0.8*	*22*	*1.6*	*2.9*	*0.5*	*2.2*

LEMON

Fresh, Raw, Average	*1 Slice/5g*	*1*	*0*	*18*	*0.9*	*2.9*	*0.3*	*2.1*

L

	Measure INFO/WEIGHT	per Measure KCAL	FAT	Nutrition Values per 100g / 100ml KCAL	PROT	CARB	FAT	FIBRE
LEMON								
Peel, Raw, Average	*1 Tbsp/6g*	*3*	*0*	*47*	*1.5*	*16*	*0.3*	*10.6*
LEMON CURD								
Average	*1 Tbsp/15g*	*44*	*0.7*	*294*	*0.7*	*62.9*	*4.7*	*0.1*
Grandessa, Aldi*	1 Tbsp/15g	45	0.6	300	0.8	64	4.3	0.6
Luxury, Average	*1 Tsp/7g*	*23*	*0.6*	*326*	*2.8*	*59.7*	*8.4*	*0.1*
Sainsbury's*	1 Portion/20g	51	1	254	0.7	51.3	4.8	1.3
LEMON GRASS								
Easy, Asda*	1 Tsp/10g	5	0.1	52	0.4	7.4	1.2	5.2
Stalks, Tesco*	1 Stalk/13g	12	0.1	99	1.8	25.3	0.5	0
LEMON SOLE								
Fillets, Raw, Average	*1 Serving/220g*	*177*	*2.8*	*81*	*17*	*0.2*	*1.3*	*0.3*
Goujons, Average	*1 Serving/150g*	*359*	*18.3*	*239*	*13.9*	*18.5*	*12.2*	*1*
Grilled, Average	*1oz/28g*	*27*	*0.5*	*97*	*20.2*	*0*	*1.7*	*0*
in Breadcrumbs, Average	*1 Fillet/142g*	*322*	*17.4*	*228*	*13.7*	*15.7*	*12.3*	*1*
in White Wine & Herb Butter, Fillets, M&S*	1 Pack/220g	385	27.7	175	15.1	0.1	12.6	0
Steamed, Average	*1oz/28g*	*25*	*0.3*	*91*	*20.6*	*0*	*0.9*	*0*
LEMONADE								
7 Up, Zero, Britvic*	1 Can/330ml	6	0	2	0.1	0.1	0	0
7-Up, Light, Britvic*	1 Can/330ml	4	0	1	0.1	0.2	0	0
Asda*	1 Glass/250ml	82	0	33	0	8	0	0
Average	*1 Glass/250ml*	*52*	*0.2*	*21*	*0.1*	*5*	*0.1*	*0.1*
Cloudy, Diet, Sainsbury's*	1 Can/330ml	7	0.3	2	0.1	0.2	0.1	0.3
Cloudy, Diet, Sparkling, M&S*	1 Serving/250ml	8	0.2	3	0.1	0.1	0.1	0.1
Cloudy, Diet, Tesco*	1 Serving/200ml	6	0	3	0	0.8	0	0
Cloudy, Gastropub, M&S*	1 Bottle/500ml	25	0	5	0	0	0	0
Cloudy, Sainsbury's*	1 Glass/250ml	118	0.2	47	0.1	12	0.1	0.1
Cloudy, Shapers, Boots*	1 Bottle/500ml	15	0	3	0	0.3	0	0
Cloudy, Sparkling, Shapers, Boots*	1 Bottle/500ml	15	0.5	3	0.1	0.3	0.1	0.2
Cloudy, Waitrose*	1 Glass/250ml	125	0	50	0	12.2	0	0
Diet with Black Cherry Flavouring, CBY, Asda*	1 Serving/250ml	5	0	2	0	0	0	0
Diet, Average	*1 Glass/250ml*	*4*	*0.1*	*2*	*0.1*	*0.2*	*0*	*0*
Diet, Premium, Tesco*	1 Glass/250ml	8	0	3	0	0.4	0	0
Diet, Toppers, Aldi*	1 Glass/100ml	1	0	1	0	0	0	0
Diet, Traditional Style, Tesco*	1 Glass/200ml	6	0	3	0	0.8	0	0
Low Calorie, Smart Price, Asda*	1 Glass/250ml	1	0	0	0	0.1	0	0
Pink, Still, Pure Premium, Tropicana*	1 Serving/200ml	90	0	45	0.2	10	0	0.7
Pink, Zero Calories, Lucozade*	1 Bottle/380ml	8	0	2	0.1	0.1	0	0
Pure Premium, Still, Tropicana*	1 Glass/200ml	86	2	43	0.2	9.5	1	0.7
R White*	1 Glass/250ml	65	0	26	0.1	6.2	0	0
Sainsbury's*	1 Glass/250ml	52	0.2	21	0.1	4.9	0.1	0.1
Schweppes*	1 Glass/250ml	45	0	18	0	4.2	0	0
Sicilian, Sainsbury's*	1 Glass/200ml	98	0.2	49	0.1	11.5	0.1	0.1
Sicilian, The Best, Morrisons*	1 Serving/150ml	52	0.2	34	0.1	7.9	0.1	0.5
Sparkling with Spanish Lemon Juice, Waitrose*	1 Glass/250ml	85	0	34	0	8.3	0	0
Sparkling, Co-Op*	1 Can/330ml	25	0	8	0	1.5	0	0
Sparkling, Morrisons*	1 Glass/250ml	63	0	25	0	6.1	0	0
Still, Freshly Squeezed, M&S*	½ Bottle/250ml	100	0.5	40	0.1	9	0.2	0.5
Still, Raspberry, M&S*	1 Glass/250ml	112	0	45	0.2	10.3	0	0.1
Sugar Free, Everyday Value, Tesco*	1 Glass/250ml	1	0	0	0	0	0	0
Tesco*	1 Glass/200ml	30	0	15	0	3.6	0	0
Traditional Style, Tesco*	1 Glass/200ml	100	0	50	0	12.3	0	0
TTD, Sainsbury's*	1 Serving/248g	159	0	64	0.1	14.8	0	0.2
Victorian, Fentiman's*	1 Bottle/275ml	130	0	47	0	11.3	0	0

L

	Measure INFO/WEIGHT	per Measure KCAL	FAT	Nutrition Values per 100g / 100ml KCAL	PROT	CARB	FAT	FIBRE
LEMSIP								
Beechams*	1 Sachet/2.9g	11	0	387	0	100	0	0
LENTILS								
Black Beluga, Ready to Eat, Merchant Gourmet*	1 Serving/62.5g	92	0.8	147	10.9	20.5	1.2	5.2
Brown, in Water, Drained, Canned, Cooks & Co*	½ Can/120g	65	0.4	54	4	6.8	0.3	4
Green & Brown, Dried, Boiled in Salted Water, Average	*1 Tbsp/30g*	*32*	*0.2*	*105*	*8.8*	*16.9*	*0.7*	*3.8*
Green or Brown in Water, Tinned, Average	*½ Can/132g*	*131*	*0.8*	*99*	*8.1*	*15.4*	*0.6*	*3.8*
Green or Brown, Dried, Average	*1 Serving/50g*	*150*	*0.8*	*301*	*22.8*	*49.8*	*1.5*	*9.6*
Puy, Green, Dry, Average	*1 Serving/100g*	*306*	*1.4*	*306*	*24.7*	*49.5*	*1.4*	*10.3*
Red, Boiled in Unsalted Water, Average	*1oz/28g*	*28*	*0.1*	*102*	*7.6*	*17.5*	*0.4*	*2.6*
Red, Dried, Average	*1oz/28g*	*88*	*0.4*	*315*	*23.8*	*53.8*	*1.3*	*4.9*
Red, Split, Wholefoods, Tesco*	1 Serving/100g	335	1.3	335	23.8	56.3	1.3	4.9
LETTUCE								
Average, Raw	*½ Cup/28g*	*4*	*0.1*	*13*	*1*	*1.7*	*0.3*	*1.1*
Cos, Sweet, Baby, Somerfield*	1 Pack/600g	90	3	15	0.8	1.7	0.5	0.9
Crest, Sainsbury's*	1 Serving/80g	11	0.4	14	0.8	1.7	0.5	0
Curly Leaf, Sainsbury's*	1 Serving/80g	11	0.4	14	0.8	1.7	0.5	0
Iceberg, Average	*1 Serving/80g*	*10*	*0.2*	*13*	*0.8*	*1.8*	*0.3*	*0.4*
Lamb's, Average	*1 Serving/80g*	*12*	*0.2*	*14*	*1.4*	*1.6*	*0.2*	*1*
Leafy, Tesco*	1 Serving/80g	11	0.3	14	1.2	1.5	0.4	1.9
Little Gem, Average	*1 Lettuce/90g*	*14*	*0.4*	*15*	*0.8*	*1.8*	*0.5*	*0.7*
Radicchio, Red, Raw, Average	*1 Head/220g*	*29*	*0.2*	*13*	*1.4*	*1.6*	*0.1*	*3*
Red Gem, Tesco*	½ Lettuce/45g	7	0.2	15	0.8	1.7	0.5	0.9
Romaine, Average	*1 Serving/80g*	*12*	*0.4*	*15*	*0.9*	*1.7*	*0.5*	*0.7*
Romaine, Hearts, Average	*1 Serving/80g*	*12*	*0.4*	*16*	*0.9*	*1.7*	*0.6*	*1*
Romaine, Sweet, Average	*1 Serving/80g*	*12*	*0.4*	*16*	*0.9*	*1.6*	*0.6*	*0.8*
Round, Average	*1 Serving/80g*	*10*	*0.2*	*13*	*1.4*	*2.2*	*0.2*	*1.1*
Sweet Gem, TTD, Sainsbury's*	1 Serving/100g	15	0.5	15	0.8	1.7	0.5	0.9
LILT								
Fruit Crush, Coca-Cola*	1 Can/330ml	66	0	20	0	4.6	0	0
Fruit Crush, Zero, Coca-Cola*	1 Can/330ml	12	0	4	0	0.3	0	0
Z, Coca-Cola*	1 Can/330ml	10	0	3	0	0.4	0	0
LIME								
Peel, Raw	*1 Tbsp/6g*	*3*	*0*	*47*	*1.5*	*16*	*0.3*	*10.6*
Raw, Flesh Only, Average	*1 Lime/71g*	*18*	*0.1*	*25*	*0.6*	*8.8*	*0.2*	*2.4*
Raw, Weighed with Peel & Seeds, Average	*1 Lime/85g*	*21*	*0.1*	*25*	*0.6*	*8.9*	*0.2*	*2.4*
LINGUINE								
Cooked	*1 Serving/100g*	*133*	*0.7*	*133*	*5.1*	*26.3*	*0.7*	*1.1*
Crab, Rocket & Chilli, Italian, Heated, Finest, Tesco*	1 Pack/325g	659	37.3	203	5.8	18.2	11.5	1.6
Dry, Average	*1 Serving/100g*	*352*	*2.2*	*352*	*13.1*	*70*	*2.2*	*2.8*
Fresh, Dry, Average	*1 Pack/250g*	*681*	*6.5*	*272*	*12.3*	*51.7*	*2.6*	*4*
King Prawn, Asda*	1 Pack/400g	380	10.4	95	6.4	11.5	2.6	1.5
King Prawn, COU, M&S*	1 Meal/360g	400	9	111	5.9	16.4	2.5	0.8
King Prawn, FreshTastes, Asda*	1 Serving/356g	338	9.3	95	6.4	11.5	2.6	1.5
King Prawn, Sundried Tomato & Chilli, City Kitchen, Tesco*	1 Pack/385g	424	16.2	110	4	13.5	4.2	1.4
Prawn, in a White Wine Sauce, Microwaved, HL, Tesco*	1 Pack/350g	410	7	117	5.6	18.5	2	1.4
Smoked Salmon, Sainsbury's*	1 Serving/400g	586	28.8	146	6.2	14.2	7.2	1.2
with Chicken & Basil Dressing, HL, Tesco*	1 Pack/359g	503	15.4	140	8.6	16.6	4.3	2.2
with Mushrooms, Vegelicious, Tesco*	1 Bowl/380g	399	12.5	105	4.3	13.7	3.3	2
with Scallops, Pancetta & Peas, Spirit of Summer, M&S*	1 Pack/380g	528	14.8	139	6.7	18.4	3.9	1.7
LINSEEDS								
Average	*1 Tsp/5g*	*23*	*1.7*	*464*	*21.7*	*18.5*	*33.5*	*26.3*
LION BAR								
Mini, Nestle*	1 Bar/16g	80	3.6	486	4.6	67.7	21.7	0

L

	Measure INFO/WEIGHT	KCAL	FAT	KCAL	PROT	CARB	FAT	FIBRE
LION BAR								
Nestle*	1 Bar/52g	248	11.2	478	6.5	64.6	21.6	0
Peanut, Nestle*	1 Bar/40g	195	10	488	8.1	57.1	25	2.3
LIQUEURS								
Amaretto, Average	*1 Pub Shot/25ml*	*97*	*0*	*388*	*0*	*60*	*0*	*0*
Aperol, Cocktail Mixer, Aperol*	1 Serving/150ml	142	0	95	0	6.7	0	0
Chambord*	1 Serving/35ml	79	0	225	0	29.3	0	0
Cherry, Choceur, Aldi*	1 Chocolate/13g	58	2.7	450	3.9	51	21	3.4
Cointreau, Specialite De France	*1 Serving/37ml*	*80*	*0*	*215*	*0*	*8.5*	*0*	*0*
Cream, Average	*1 Shot/25ml*	*81*	*4*	*325*	*0*	*22.8*	*16.1*	*0*
Grand Marnier*	1 Pub Shot/35ml	94	0	268	0	22.9	0	0
High Strength, Average	*1 Shot/25ml*	*78*	*0*	*314*	*0*	*24.4*	*0*	*0*
Kirsch, Average	*1 Shot/25ml*	*67*	*0*	*267*	*0*	*20*	*0*	*0*
Marula Fruit & Cream Cocktail, Amarula*	1 fl oz/30ml	103	0	343	0	36.7	0	0
LIQUORICE								
Allsorts, Average	*1 Sm Bag/56g*	*195*	*2.9*	*349*	*3.7*	*76.7*	*5.2*	*2*
Allsorts, Bassett's*	1 Pack/225g	855	11	380	5.6	77.8	4.9	1.6
Assorted, Filled, Panda*	1 Sweet/4g	15	0.4	385	3.7	68	11	0
Catherine Wheels, Barratt*	1 Wheel/22g	65	0.1	290	3.8	67.2	0.3	0.7
Catherine Wheels, Sainsbury's*	1 Wheel/17g	49	0.1	286	3.8	67.2	0.3	0.7
Log, Raspberry, Choc, RJ's Licorice Ltd*	1 Log/45.1g	178	4.5	395	3.9	74	10	0.9
Organic, Laidback Liquorice*	1 Bar/28g	90	0.3	320	4.7	75	1	3
Panda*	1 Bar/32g	109	0.2	340	3.8	78	0.5	0
Red, Fresh, 98% Fat Free, RJ's Licorice Ltd*	1oz/28g	96	0.5	342	3	75	1.7	0
Shapes, Average	*1oz/28g*	*78*	*0.4*	*278*	*5.5*	*65*	*1.4*	*1.9*
Soft Eating, Australia, Darrell Lea*	1 Piece/20g	68	0.4	338	2.8	76.1	1.9	0
Torpedos, Panda*	1 Serving/25g	92	0	366	1.9	88	0.2	1.4
LIVER								
& Sausages, 152, Oakhouse Foods Ltd*	1 Meal/400g	528	22	132	11.4	9.4	5.5	1
Calves with Fresh Sage Butter, M&S*	1 Serving/117g	210	12.5	180	12.8	10.1	10.7	1.5
Calves, Fried	*1oz/28g*	*49*	*2.7*	*176*	*22.3*	*0*	*9.6*	*0*
Calves, Raw	*1oz/28g*	*29*	*1*	*104*	*18.3*	*0*	*3.4*	*0*
Chicken, Cooked, Simmered, Average	*1 Serving/100g*	*167*	*6.5*	*167*	*24.5*	*0.9*	*6.5*	*0*
Chicken, Fried, Average	*1oz/28g*	*47*	*2.5*	*169*	*22.1*	*0*	*8.9*	*0*
Chicken, Raw, Average	*1oz/28g*	*26*	*0.6*	*92*	*17.7*	*0*	*2.3*	*0*
Lamb's, Braised, Average	*1 Serving/100g*	*220*	*8.8*	*220*	*30.6*	*2.5*	*8.8*	*0*
Lamb's, Fried, Average	*1oz/28g*	*66*	*3.6*	*237*	*30.1*	*0*	*12.9*	*0*
Lamb's, Raw, Average	*1 Serving/125g*	*171*	*7.8*	*137*	*20.3*	*0*	*6.2*	*0*
Ox, Raw	*1oz/28g*	*43*	*2.2*	*155*	*21.1*	*0*	*7.8*	*0*
Ox, Stewed	*1oz/28g*	*55*	*2.7*	*198*	*24.8*	*3.6*	*9.5*	*0*
Pig's, Raw	*1oz/28g*	*32*	*0.9*	*113*	*21.3*	*0*	*3.1*	*0*
Pig's, Stewed	*1 Serving/70g*	*132*	*5.7*	*189*	*25.6*	*3.6*	*8.1*	*0*
Veal, Deluxe, Lidl*	1 Slice/150g	188	5.2	125	19.6	3.8	3.5	0
LIVER & BACON								
& Onions, Cook*	1 Portion/280g	372	21.3	133	11.8	4.3	7.6	0.5
Meal for One, M&S*	1 Pack/452g	430	16.7	95	7	8	3.7	1.2
with Fresh Mashed Potato, Waitrose*	1 Pack/400g	416	17.2	104	7.3	9	4.3	1.3
with Mash, Cooked, British Classics, Tesco*	1 Pack/450g	562	20.2	125	11.9	7.6	4.5	1
LIVER & ONIONS								
Finest, Tesco*	½ Pack/225g	349	18.7	155	15.6	3.7	8.3	1.6
LIVER SAUSAGE								
Average	*1 Slice/10g*	*22*	*1.5*	*216*	*15.3*	*4.4*	*15.2*	*0.2*
LLAMA								
Steak, Average	*1 Steak/150g*	*158*	*2*	*105*	*23*	*0.2*	*1.3*	*0*

L

	Measure INFO/WEIGHT	per Measure KCAL	FAT	Nutrition Values per 100g / 100ml KCAL	PROT	CARB	FAT	FIBRE
LOBSTER								
Boiled, Average	*1oz/28g*	*29*	*0.4*	*103*	*22.1*	*0*	*1.6*	*0*
Dressed, Canned, John West*	1 Can/43g	45	2.1	105	13	2	5	0
Raw, Average	*1 Serving/100g*	*92*	*1.4*	*92*	*18.7*	*0.3*	*1.4*	*0*
Tail, Main, Waitrose*	1 Serving/100g	58	0.2	58	14.1	0	0.2	0
Thermidor, Finest, Tesco*	½ Pack/140g	381	25.2	272	15.3	12.1	18	1
Thermidor, M&S*	1 Serving/140g	287	19.2	205	10.7	9.7	13.7	0
LOGANBERRIES								
Raw	*1oz/28g*	*5*	*0*	*17*	*1.1*	*3.4*	*0*	*2.5*
LOLLIPOPS								
Assorted, Co-Op*	1 Lolly/10g	40	0	400	0	97	0	0
Chupa Chups*	1 Lolly/18g	44	0.2	247	0	96.5	1.3	0
Cremosa, Sugar Free, Chupa Chups*	1 Lolly/10g	28	0.5	275	0.2	92.5	5.4	0
Drumsticks, Swizzels*	1 Lolly/12g	50	0.7	413	0.4	87.9	6.1	0
Refreshers, Bassett's*	1 Lolly/6g	25	0	417	0	108.3	0	0
LOQUATS								
Raw	*1oz/28g*	*5*	*0*	*18*	*0.4*	*4*	*0.1*	*0*
LOZENGES								
Blackcurrant Flavour, Fishermans Friend, Lofthouses*	1 Lozenge/1g	3	0	251	0.1	97.2	1.3	0
Original Extra Strong, Fishermans Friend, Lofthouses*	1 Lozenge/1g	4	0	382	0.3	94.9	0	0.5
Original, Victory V*	1 Lozenge/3g	9	0	350	0	91	0	0
LUCOZADE								
Caribbean Crush, Energy, Lucozade*	1 Bottle/380ml	217	0	57	0	13.9	0	0
Energy, Original, GlaxoSmithKline UK Limited*	1 Bottle/380ml	266	0	70	0	17.2	0	0
Orange Energy Drink, GlaxoSmithKline UK Limited*	1 Bottle/500ml	350	0	70	0	17.2	0	0
Orange, Sport Lite, GlaxoSmithKline UK Limited*	1 Serving/500g	50	0	10	0	2	0	0
Raspberry Sport Body Fuel, GlaxoSmithKline UK Limited*	1 Bottle/500ml	140	0	28	0	6.4	0	0
Summer Berries, Sport, Lite, GlaxoSmithKline UK Limited*	1 Serving/200ml	20	0	10	0	2	0	0
Tropical, GlaxoSmithKline UK Limited*	1 Bottle/380ml	266	0	70	0	17.2	0	0
Zero Calories, Lucozade*	1 Serving/250ml	10	0	4	0.1	0.5	0	0
LUNCHEON MEAT								
Pork, Average	*1oz/28g*	*81*	*6.8*	*288*	*13.3*	*4*	*24.3*	*0*
LYCHEES								
Fresh, Raw, Flesh Only	*1oz/28g*	*16*	*0*	*58*	*0.9*	*14.3*	*0.1*	*0.7*
in Juice, Amoy*	1oz/28g	13	0	46	0.4	10.9	0	0
in Syrup, Average	*1oz/28g*	*19*	*0*	*69*	*0.4*	*17.7*	*0*	*0.4*
Raw, Weighed with Skin & Stone	*1oz/28g*	*6*	*0*	*22*	*0.3*	*5.5*	*0.1*	*0.2*

L

	Measure INFO/WEIGHT	per Measure KCAL	FAT	Nutrition Values per 100g / 100ml KCAL	PROT	CARB	FAT	FIBRE
M&M'S								
Crispy, Mars*	1 Serving/36g	179	8.8	498	4.1	63.9	24.4	2.7
Mars*	1 Pack/45g	218	9.7	485	5	68	21.5	0
Mini, Mars*	1 Sm Pack/36g	176	8.4	489	6.3	63.6	23.2	0
Peanut Butter, Mars*	1 Pack/46g	240	14	520	8.7	56.3	30.3	2.2
Peanut, Mars*	1 Pack/45g	228	11.4	506	9.4	60.1	25.4	2.7
MACADAMIA NUTS								
Plain, Average	*1 Pack/100g*	*750*	*77.6*	*750*	*7.9*	*4.8*	*77.6*	*5.3*
Roasted, Salted, Average	*6 Nuts/10g*	*75*	*7.8*	*748*	*7.9*	*4.8*	*77.6*	*5.3*
MACARONI								
Dry, Average	*1oz/28g*	*99*	*0.5*	*354*	*11.9*	*73.5*	*1.7*	*2.6*
MACARONI CHEESE								
& Spinach, TTD, Sainsbury's*	1 Pack/500g	1025	57.5	205	6.5	18.9	11.5	1.3
Canned	*1oz/28g*	*39*	*1.8*	*138*	*4.5*	*16.4*	*6.5*	*0.4*
Canned, Sainsbury's*	1 Can/400g	480	24	120	4.4	12	6	0.3
Charlie Bigham's*	½ Pack/335g	771	36.9	230	10.5	21.8	11	0.2
Creamy, Weight Watchers*	1 Pack/360g	344	9.7	96	4.4	12.9	2.7	1
Italian, Cooked, Morrisons*	1 Pack/400g	651	28.7	170	6.9	18.1	7.5	1
Italian, Tesco*	1 Pack/420g	830	40.7	198	9.2	18.2	9.7	1.2
Lobster & Orkney Crab, Gastropub, M&S*	1 Pack/370g	666	32.2	180	7.6	17.5	8.7	0.7
M&S*	1 Pack/400g	700	28.4	175	7	20.9	7.1	0.9
Newgate, Lidl*	½ Can/205g	181	8.2	88	2.5	10.2	4	0.8
Pasta, Italian Kitchen, Tesco*	1 Pack/450g	801	36	178	7.1	18.3	8	2.3
Prawn & Crab, Balanced for You, M&S*	1 Meal/350g	399	9.8	114	7.7	14	2.8	0.8
Ready Meal, Average	*1 Serving/400g*	*580*	*25.5*	*145*	*6*	*15.8*	*6.4*	*1*
Rice Mac, GF, Dairy Free, Amy's Kitchen*	1 Pack/227	581	24.7	228	3.5	32	9.7	1.3
Waitrose*	1 Pack/350g	466	32.9	133	6.8	5.2	9.4	0
with Bacon, 287, Oakhouse Foods Ltd*	1 Serving/370g	873	57	236	11.9	12	15.4	0.4
MACAROONS								
Coconut, Sainsbury's*	1 Macaroon/33g	146	6.1	441	4.7	63.7	18.6	0.8
Coconut, Tesco*	1 Macaroon/33g	140	6.1	425	4.4	59	18.6	5.7
French, Average	*1 Serving/60g*	*225*	*11*	*375*	*6.7*	*46.7*	*18.3*	*3.3*
MACKEREL								
Atlantic, Raw, Average	*1 Fillet/75g*	*154*	*10.4*	*205*	*18.6*	*0*	*13.9*	*0*
Fillets, in a Hot Chilli Dressing, Princes*	1 Pack/125g	370	33.8	296	13.3	0	27	0
Fillets, in Brine, Average	*1 Can/88g*	*206*	*15.3*	*234*	*19.4*	*0*	*17.4*	*0*
Fillets, in Curry Sauce, John West*	1 Can/125g	275	20.8	220	14.2	3.5	16.6	0.2
Fillets, in Hot Smoked Peppered, Asda*	1 Fillet/100g	341	28	341	19	3.3	28	0.6
Fillets, in Mustard Sauce, Average	*1 Can/125g*	*274*	*19.4*	*219*	*14.1*	*5.4*	*15.5*	*0*
Fillets, in Olive Oil, Average	*1 Serving/50g*	*149*	*12.2*	*298*	*18.5*	*1*	*24.4*	*0*
Fillets, in Spicy Tomato Sauce, Average	*1oz/28g*	*56*	*3.9*	*199*	*14.3*	*3.8*	*14*	*0*
Fillets, in Sunflower Oil, Average	*1 Can/94g*	*262*	*20.6*	*279*	*20.2*	*0.2*	*21.9*	*0.2*
Fillets, in Teriyaki Sauce, Boneless & Skinless, Tesco*	1 Can/125g	320	20.3	255	12.6	13.4	16.2	2
Fillets, in Tomato Sauce, Average	*1 Can/125g*	*251*	*18.3*	*200*	*14.3*	*2.7*	*14.7*	*0*
Fillets, Lemon & Parsley, Smoked, Fishmonger, Aldi*	1 Pack/200g	658	53	329	19.6	2.9	26.5	0
Fillets, Mexican, Canned, Princes*	1 Can/125g	241	13.8	193	11.4	11.8	11	0.5
Fillets, Smoked, Average	*1 Fillet/75g*	*251*	*21.1*	*334*	*19.7*	*0.5*	*28.2*	*0.3*
Fried in Blended Oil	*1oz/28g*	*76*	*5.5*	*272*	*24*	*0*	*19.5*	*0*
Grilled	*1oz/28g*	*67*	*4.8*	*239*	*20.8*	*0*	*17.3*	*0*
King, Raw	*1 Fillet/198g*	*208*	*4*	*105*	*20.3*	*0*	*2*	*0*
Raw with Skin, Weighed with Bone, Average	*1oz/28g*	*64*	*4.7*	*227*	*18.9*	*0*	*16.8*	*0*
Smoked, Peppered, Average	*1oz/28g*	*87*	*7*	*310*	*20.4*	*0.3*	*25.2*	*0.2*
Whole, Raw, Average	*1 Serving/100g*	*156*	*11.4*	*156*	*13.3*	*0*	*11.4*	*0*

M

M

MADRAS

INFO/WEIGHT	Measure	per Measure		Nutrition Values per 100g / 100ml				
		KCAL	FAT	KCAL	PROT	CARB	FAT	FIBRE
Beef, Indian, Takeaway, CBY, Asda*	½ Pack/200g	246	14.2	123	8.9	4.7	7.1	2.5
Beef, Tesco*	1 Pack/460g	616	37.7	134	10.6	4.5	8.2	1.2
Chicken, & Pilau Rice, Somerfield*	1 Pack/340g	496	23.8	146	7	14	7	0
Chicken, Sainsbury's*	1 Pack/400g	468	27.2	117	11.7	2.2	6.8	2.8
Chicken, Waitrose*	1 Pack/400g	672	42	168	14.6	3.7	10.5	1.8

MAGNUM

INFO/WEIGHT	Measure	KCAL	FAT	KCAL	PROT	CARB	FAT	FIBRE
Almond, Mini, Wall's*	1 Mini/50g	176	11.5	352	5.1	32	23	0
Almond, Wall's*	1 Magnum/73g	243	14.6	332	4.8	32	20	0
Bites, After Dinner Classic, Wall's*	1 Bite/29g	102	6.9	353	4	30	24	0
Caramel, Double, Mini, Wall's*	1 Mini/50g	174	10	348	3.2	37	20	0
Caramel, Double, Wall's*	1 Magnum/73g	246	14.6	338	3.2	36	20	0
Chocolate, Double, Mini, Wall's*	1 Mini/50g	182	11.5	365	4	33	23	0
Chocolate, Double, Wall's*	1 Magnum/69g	248	15.9	359	4.1	33	23	0
Classic, Mini, Wall's*	1 Mini/50g	168	11	336	3.7	31	22	0
Classic, Wall's*	1 Magnum/79g	244	15	309	3.6	29	19	1.2
Dark, Mini, Wall's*	1 Mini/50g	165	11	329	3.8	29	22	0
Double Coconut, Wall's*	1 Magnumg/73g	239	14.6	328	3.8	32	20	0
Espresso, Black, Mini, Wall's*	1 Mini/50g	159	10.5	317	3.7	29	21	0
Espresso, Black, Wall's*	1 Magnum/82g	237	15.6	289	3.4	27	19	0
Honeycomb, Wall's*	1 Magnum/78g	240	13.2	308	3.6	35	17	0
Mint, Mini, Wall's*	1 Mini/50g	165	10.5	330	4.2	30	21	0
Mint, Wall's*	1 Magnum/78g	244	14	313	3.1	33	18	0
Peanut Butter, Double, Mini, Wall's*	1 Mini/50g	173	11	346	4.3	32	22	0
Peanut Butter, Double, Wall's*	1 Magnum/73g	245	15.3	336	4.2	32	21	0
Pistachio, Wall's*	1 Magnum/75g	250	15.8	333	4.2	30	21	0
Raspberry, Pink, Mini, Wall's*	1 Mini/50g	166	11.5	332	2.9	31	23	0
Raspberry, Pink, Wall's*	1 Magnum/73g	239	15.3	328	2.9	30	21	0
Strawberry, & White, Wall's*	1 Magnum/88g	250	13.2	284	3	34	15	0
White, Mini, Wall's*	1 Mini/50g	167	10	333	3.7	35	20	0
White, Wall's*	1 Magnum/79g	239	14.2	303	3.5	33	18	0

MAKHANI

INFO/WEIGHT	Measure	KCAL	FAT	KCAL	PROT	CARB	FAT	FIBRE
Chicken, Sainsbury's*	½ Pack/199g	313	21.3	157	12.2	2.9	10.7	2.5
Chicken, Tikka, & Pilau Rice, BGTY, Sainsbury's*	1 Pack/400g	448	4	112	8.3	17.5	1	1.9
Chicken, Tikka, Waitrose*	1 Pack/400g	560	30.4	140	14	3.8	7.6	2.1
Prawn, King, Curry, M&S*	1 Pack/400g	732	51.6	183	8	8.1	12.9	1
Prawn, King, Finest, Tesco*	1 Pack/350g	514	38.8	147	6	6	11.1	1.3

MALTESERS

INFO/WEIGHT	Measure	KCAL	FAT	KCAL	PROT	CARB	FAT	FIBRE
MaltEaster, Chocolate Bunny, Mars*	1 Bunny/29g	156	9	539	6.9	57.6	31	1.2
Mars*	1 Reg Bag/37g	187	9.3	505	8	61.8	25	0.9
Mini Bunnies, Mars*	1 Bunny/12g	64	3.6	534	8	53.5	30.2	0
White Chocolate, Mars*	1 Pack/37g	186	9.4	504	7.9	61	25.4	0

MANDARIN ORANGES

INFO/WEIGHT	Measure	KCAL	FAT	KCAL	PROT	CARB	FAT	FIBRE
in Juice, Average	*1oz/28g*	*11*	*0*	*39*	*0.7*	*9*	*0*	*0.5*
in Light Syrup, Average	*1 Can/298g*	*201*	*0.1*	*68*	*0.6*	*16*	*0*	*0.1*
Weighed with Peel, Average	*1 Sm/50g*	*14*	*0*	*27*	*0.7*	*6.2*	*0.1*	*0.9*

MANGE TOUT

INFO/WEIGHT	Measure	KCAL	FAT	KCAL	PROT	CARB	FAT	FIBRE
& Sugar Snap Peas, Tesco*	1 Pack/150g	102	0.6	68	7	9.2	0.4	3.8
Boiled in Salted Water	*1oz/28g*	*7*	*0*	*26*	*3.2*	*3.3*	*0.1*	*2.2*
Raw, Average	*1 Serving/80g*	*25*	*0.2*	*31*	*3.5*	*4*	*0.2*	*1.1*
Stir-Fried in Blended Oil	*1oz/28g*	*20*	*1.3*	*71*	*3.8*	*3.5*	*4.8*	*2.4*

MANGO

INFO/WEIGHT	Measure	KCAL	FAT	KCAL	PROT	CARB	FAT	FIBRE
& Lime, Co-Op*	1 Pot/90g	51	0.4	57	0.7	12	0.5	1.6
& Pineapple, Fingers, Tesco*	1 Pack/80g	43	0.2	54	0.6	11.7	0.2	1.5

INFO/WEIGHT	Measure		per Measure		Nutrition Values per 100g / 100ml				
			KCAL	FAT	KCAL	PROT	CARB	FAT	FIBRE
MANGO									
Dried, Average	1 Serving/50g		174	0.5	347	1.4	83.1	1	4.9
in Syrup, Average	1oz/28g		22	0	80	0.3	20.5	0	0.9
Ripe, Raw, Weighed with Skin & Stone, Average	1 Mango/225g		60	0.2	27	0.3	6.5	0.1	1.2
Ripe, Raw, without Peel & Stone, Flesh Only, Average	1 Mango/207g		118	0.4	57	0.7	14.1	0.2	2.6
MANGOSTEEN									
Raw, Fresh, Average*	1 Serving/80g		50	0.5	63	0.6	15.6	0.6	5.1
MARINADE									
Barbeque, Sticky, Sainsbury's*	¼ Jar/77g		112	2.8	145	0.8	26.7	3.6	1
BBQ, Sticky, Newman's Own*	1/3 Jar/83ml		139	0.7	167	0.9	39	0.8	2.5
Cajun Spice, The English Provender Co.*	1 Serving/50g		94	6.7	187	1.3	15.3	13.4	1.6
Coat 'n Cook, Medium, Nando's*	1 Sachet/120g		94	5.4	78	1.1	9.6	4.5	2.8
Hickory Dickory Smokey, Ainsley Harriott*	1 Pot/300ml		360	0.3	120	0.6	28.1	0.1	0
Hot & Spicy Barbecue, M&S*	1 Serving/18g		23	0.1	130	1	31.1	0.3	0.8
Sticky Barbecue, Tesco*	¼ Jar/69.6g		80	0.1	115	0.7	26.7	0.2	0.6
Tandoori, Spice, Patak's*	1 Tbsp/15g		15	0.4	99	3.5	10.1	2.7	5.9
Tequila Chilli Lime, M&S*	1 Serving/75ml		116	1.2	155	0.6	34	1.6	0.5
Texan, Hickory Style, BBQ, Quick, Batts, Lidl*	1 Serving/16g		29	0.1	181	1.2	42.5	0.6	3.1
MARJORAM									
Dried	1 Tsp/1g		2	0	271	12.7	42.5	7	0
MARLIN									
Steaks, Chargrilled, Sainsbury's*	1 Steak/240g		367	14.6	153	23.6	0.8	6.1	0.6
MARMALADE									
3 Fruit, Thick Cut, Waitrose*	1 Tsp/15g		39	0	262	0.4	64.8	0.1	0.7
Blood Orange, TTD, Sainsbury's*	1 Tbsp/15g		40	0	264	0.3	65.7	0	0.8
Lemon & Lime, Average	1 Tbsp/20g		53	0	267	0.2	66.4	0.1	0.4
Lemon with Shred, Average	1 Serving/20g		50	0	248	0.2	61.6	0	0.6
Lime with Shred, Average	1 Tbsp/15g		39	0	261	0.2	65	0.1	0.4
Onion, Organic, Duchy Originals*	1 Serving/40g		103	1	257	1	57.8	2.4	2.6
Orange & Ginger, Average	1 Tbsp/15g		40	0	264	0.2	65.7	0.1	0.3
Orange & Tangerine, Tiptree, Wilkin & Sons*	1 Tsp/15g		40	0	268	0	67	0	0
Orange Shred, Med Cut, Tesco*	1 Serving/15g		39	0	260	0.3	64.7	0	0.5
Orange with Shred, Average	1 Tsp/5g		13	0	263	0.2	65.2	0	0.3
Orange, Fine Shred, Bonne Maman*	1 Tsp/5g		12	0	238	0.3	59	0.1	0.6
Orange, Reduced Sugar, Average	1 Tbsp/15g		26	0	170	0.4	42	0.1	0.6
Orange, Reduced Sugar, Thin Cut, Streamline*	1 Serving/10g		18	0	178	0.5	43	0.3	0
Orange, Shredless, Average	1 Tsp/10g		26	0	261	0.2	65	0	0.1
Orange, with Stem Ginger, Mrs Bridges*	1 Tbsp/15g		41	0	273	0	67.6	0	0
Three Fruit, Finest, Tesco*	1 Serving/15g		39	0	262	0.5	63.6	0.2	1.6
Three Fruits, Fresh Fruit, Sainsbury's*	1 Tsp/15g		38	0	250	0	61.3	0	0
MARMITE*									
XO, Marmite*	1 Serving/4g		10	0	250	37.5	25	0.2	0.2
Yeast Extract with Gold Coloured Flecks, Marmite*	1 Serving/4g		10	0	250	39	24	0.1	3.5
Yeast Extract, Marmite*	1 Tsp/9g		22	0	250	39	24	0.1	3.5
MARROW									
Boiled, Average	1oz/28g		3	0.1	9	0.4	1.6	0.2	0.6
Raw	1oz/28g		2	0	6	0.3	1.2	0.1	0.3
MARS									
Bar, 5 Little Ones, Mars*	1 Piece/8g		38	1.5	477	4.5	73.6	18.3	0
Bar, Duo, Mars*	1 Bar/42g		191	7.6	450	4.4	67.5	18	1.2
Bar, Funsize, Mars*	1 Bar/18g		80	3	446	3.5	70.1	16.8	1.1
Bar, Mars*	1 Std Bar/51g		229	8.7	449	4	69	17	1
Bar, Medium, 58g, Mars*	1 Bar/58g		263	10.5	453	4.6	67.9	18.1	0
Bar, Minis, Mars*	1 Bar/18g		80	11.6	444	3.3	0	64.4	1.1

M

	Measure INFO/WEIGHT	per Measure KCAL	FAT	Nutrition Values per 100g / 100ml KCAL	PROT	CARB	FAT	FIBRE
MARS								
Choc Brownie, Bar, Mars*	1 Bar/51g	231	9.4	452	4.6	66	18.3	0
Triple Choc, Bar, Limited Edition, Mars*	1 Bar/52g	233	9	448	4.5	67.7	17.3	2
MARSHMALLOWS								
Average	*1 Mallow/5g*	*16*	*0*	*327*	*3.9*	*83.1*	*0*	*0*
Chocolate Mallows, Cadbury*	1 Mallow/13g	56	2.2	435	4.7	64.7	17.4	0.8
Dark Chocolate Covered, Mister Choc, Lidl*	1 Mallow/25g	95	2.5	380	4	68	10	0
Fat Free, Tesco*	1 Mallow/7g	24	0	339	3.4	80.8	0.2	0.5
Haribo*	1 Mallow/5g	16	0	330	3	80	0	0
No Added Sugar, Sainsbury's*	1 Mallow/2.4g	5	0	206	3.3	77	0.1	0
Pascall*	1 Mallow/5g	15	0	335	2.6	80	0	0
Pink & White, Co-Op*	1 Mallow/7g	24	0	340	3	82	0	0
Princess*	1 Mallow/5g	16	0	314	3.4	80	0	0
Raspberry & Cream, Sainsbury's*	1 Mallow/7g	23	0	330	4.1	78.5	0	0.5
Sainsbury's*	1 Mallow/7g	23	0	330	4.1	78.5	0	0.5
MARZIPAN								
Bar, Chocolate, Plain, Thorntons*	1 Bar/46g	206	8	448	5.2	69.1	17.4	2
Dark Chocolate, Thorntons*	1 Serving/46g	207	8	451	5.2	69.4	17.4	2.1
Plain, Average	*1oz/28g*	*115*	*4*	*412*	*5.8*	*67.5*	*14.2*	*1.7*
MASALA								
Mixed Vegetable, M&S*	½ Pack/200g	170	9	85	2.3	7.4	4.5	2.9
Prawn Mango, Waitrose*	½ Pack/175g	175	11.2	100	5.8	4.3	6.4	1.3
Vegetable, Waitrose*	1 Serving/400g	288	19.2	72	2.2	4.9	4.8	2.5
Vegetable, with Cauliflower Rice, Goodlife*	1 Pack/400g	296	14	74	2.9	5.5	3.5	4.2
MAYONNAISE								
Aioli, Finest, Tesco*	1 Tsp/5g	20	2.1	408	0.8	8.5	41.2	0
Average	*1 Tsp/5g*	*35*	*3.8*	*690*	*0.9*	*1.6*	*75.5*	*0*
Beolive Roasted Garlic Flavour, Vandemooetele*	1 Serving/15ml	46	4.2	305	1.3	11.3	28.2	0
Branston, with a Twist of Pesto, Crosse & Blackwell*	1 Tbsp/30ml	124	11.6	412	1.2	14.1	38.6	0.2
Extra Light, Average	*1 Tbsp/33g*	*34*	*2*	*102*	*0.7*	*10.5*	*6.2*	*0.8*
French, Light, Sainsbury's*	1 Serving/15ml	46	4.7	307	0.4	6.1	31.1	0.2
French, Mustardy, Tracklements*	1 Tbsp/15g	111	12.2	739	2.1	0.4	81	0.4
Garlic & Herb, M&S*	1 Tsp/6g	43	4.6	712	3.4	2.4	76.9	0.9
Garlic & Herb, Reduced Calorie, Hellmann's*	1 Serving/25ml	58	4.8	233	0.7	13.1	19.3	0.4
Garlic, Organic, Simply Delicious*	1 Tbsp/15ml	100	10.9	670	1.6	3	72.7	0.1
Garlic, Retail, Average	*1 Tsp/11g*	*44*	*4.4*	*403*	*1.2*	*8.6*	*40.3*	*0*
Garlic, Waitrose*	1 Tsp/6g	21	2.1	346	0.6	8.6	34.3	0
Lemon, Waitrose*	1 Tsp/8ml	56	6.1	694	1.2	1.3	76	5.4
Light Dijon, Benedicta*	1 Tbsp/15g	44	4.4	292	0.7	6.7	29.2	0
Reduced Calorie, Average	*1 Tsp/6g*	*18*	*1.7*	*301*	*0.7*	*8.9*	*29*	*0.1*
Smoked Chilli, Gran Luchito*	1 Tsp/5g	42	4.1	838	0.4	3.1	81.1	0
with a Spark of Chilli, Hellmann's*	1 Tbsp/15ml	41	4	276	0.8	7.5	27	0.3
with Dijon Mustard, Hellmann's*	1 Tbsp/15ml	32	3	210	2.9	5.1	19.7	0
MEAL REPLACEMENT								
Banana Flavour Shake, Celebrity Slim*	1 Sachet/55g	214	2.4	389	34.5	51.5	4.4	0.6
Bars, Crispy Caramel Flavour, Slim & Save*	1 Bar/45g	169	5.3	377	26.7	37.5	11.8	6.9
Breakfast Shake, Banana, Be Fast*	1 Bottle/250ml	200	3.8	80	3.4	12	1.5	2.4
Breakfast Shake, Chocolate, Be Fast*	1 Bottle/250ml	200	3.8	80	3.3	12	1.5	2.5
Breakfast Shake, Strawberry, Be Fast*	1 Bottle/250ml	200	3.8	80	3.4	12	1.5	2.4
Breakfast Shake, Vanilla, Be Fast*	1 Bottle/250ml	190	3.8	76	3.6	10.9	1.5	2.6
Caramel Flavour Shake, Celebrity Slim*	1 Pack/55g	212	2.4	385	34.2	50.9	4.4	0.6
Chocolate Flavour Shake, Celebrity Slim*	1 Sachet/55g	211	2.5	383	34	49.1	4.6	2.2
Chocolate, Slender Shake, Boots*	1 Serving/30g	116	2.1	385	15	60	7	11
Chocolate, Weight Loss Shake, As Consumed, Yokobe*	1 Serving/300ml	302	7.2	101	9.6	9.4	2.4	1.4

	Measure INFO/WEIGHT	per Measure KCAL	per Measure FAT	Nutrition Values per 100g / 100ml KCAL	PROT	CARB	FAT	FIBRE
MEAL REPLACEMENT								
Nutra Cookies, Chocolate Chip, Visalus Sciences*	1 Cookie/40g	170	7	425	22.5	45	17.5	10
Nutra Cookies, Peanut Butter, Visalus Sciences*	1 Cookie/40g	185	9	463	25	40	22.5	10
Scrambled Eggs, Slim & Save*	1 Pack/40g	196	10.5	491	39.4	16.6	26.3	5
Shake Mix, Made with Water, Visalus Sciences*	1 Serving/31g	115	3	371	38.7	32.3	9.7	16.1
Shake, Chocolate, Advantage, Atkins*	1 Serving/34g	121	4.2	361	49	8.1	12.5	15.5
Shake, Chocolate, Ready to Drink, Advantage, Atkins*	1 Carton/330ml	172	9.2	52	6	0.6	2.8	1.2
Shake, Herbalife*	1 Serving/250ml	245	6.4	98	10	8.8	2.6	1
Shake, Vanilla, Ready to Drink, Advantage, Atkins*	1 Carton/330ml	175	8.9	53	6.2	0.6	2.7	0.9
Strawberry Flavour Shake, Celebrity Slim*	1 Sachet/55g	214	2.4	389	34.4	51.6	4.4	0.6
Strawberry, High Protein, Energy Meal, Spiru-tein*	1 Serving/34g	99	0	291	41.2	32.4	0	2.9
Strawberry, Slender Shake, Boots*	1 Serving/30g	115	1.9	383	15	61	6.3	11
Strawberry, Weight Loss Shake, As Consumed, Yokobe*	1 Serving/300ml	302	7.2	101	9.4	9.6	2.4	1.2
Ultra Slim, Ready to Drink, Strawberry, Tesco*	1 Carton/330ml	231	3	70	4.2	10.5	0.9	1.5
Ultra Slim, Ready to Drink, Vanilla, Tesco*	1 Carton/330ml	224	3	68	4.2	10.5	0.9	1.5
Ultra-Slim, Ready to Drink, Chocolate, Tesco*	1 Carton/330ml	214	3.6	65	4	9.8	1.1	1.3
Vanilla Bean Sundae, Protein Shake, Skinnygirl*	1 Bottle/340ml	80	1.5	24	3.5	1.5	0.4	0.3
Vanilla Flavour Shake, Celebrity Slim*	1 Sachet/55g	215	2.4	391	34.2	52	4.4	0.6
Vanilla Flavoured, Shake, Mealpak, All About Weight*	1 Shake/32g	120	3.3	375	37.5	30.6	10.3	8.1
MEAT LOAF								
Beef & Pork, Co-Op*	¼ Loaf/114g	314	25.1	275	13	7	22	1
Iceland*	1 Serving/150g	332	23.6	221	10.8	9.3	15.7	0.9
Pork, in Onion Gravy, 561, Wiltshire Farm Foods*	1 Portion/390g	328	18	84	3.9	6.3	4.6	0
Turkey & Bacon, Tesco*	1 Serving/225g	400	22.3	178	14.7	7.4	9.9	1.1
MEATBALLS								
& Pasta, Sainsbury's*	1 Serving/300g	333	9.3	111	5.3	15.5	3.1	1.9
Aberdeen Angus in Sauce, PB, Waitrose*	½ Pack/240g	228	7.2	95	10.5	6.5	3	1.1
Aberdeen Angus, Fresh, Chilled, Waitrose*	1 Meatball/36g	92	7.1	256	18	1.5	19.8	0
Al Forno, Charlie Bigham's*	½ Pack/324g	532	32.4	164	7	11.5	10	1.1
Beef, & Pork, TTD, Sainsbury's*	3 Meatballs/40g	111	8.6	278	19.5	1.1	21.4	1.2
Beef, Aberdeen Angus, 12 Pack, Waitrose*	1 Meatball/36g	93	7.1	259	18	2.3	19.8	0.1
Beef, Aberdeen Angus, with Tomato Sauce, Tesco*	½ Pack/250g	362	19.5	145	10.7	7.1	7.8	1.2
Beef, As Sold, Tesco*	1 Meatball/28g	78	6.2	277	16.6	2.3	22.3	0.9
Beef, Ashfield Farm, Aldi*	1 Meatball/20g	45	2.7	232	23	3.9	14	0.5
Beef, British with Italian Herbs, Finest, Tesco*	1oz/28g	63	4.7	225	15.4	2.1	16.8	1.7
Beef, Italian Style, As Consumed, Morrisons*	3 Meatballs/104g	235	14.7	226	19.7	4.5	14.1	0.9
Beef, Mini, Oven Cooked, Finest, Tesco*	5 Meatballs/72g	149	8.2	207	21.8	4	11.4	0.8
Beef, Sainsbury's*	1 Meatball/24g	59	4	251	19.6	4.8	16.9	0.5
Beef, Skinny, Mini, 24, M&S*	½ Pack/120g	132	2.9	110	17.9	4.3	2.4	0.5
Beef, TTD, Sainsbury's*	1 Meatball/35g	73	5.2	208	16.7	1.5	15	0.1
Chicken in Tomato Sauce, Average	*1 Can/392g*	*580*	*32.9*	*148*	*7.7*	*10.4*	*8.4*	*0*
Chicken, Italia, Baked, Heck*	1 Ball/28g	30	0.7	106	18.7	1.5	2.3	0
in Gravy, Campbell's*	½ Can/205g	164	5.3	80	5.6	8.6	2.6	0
in Tomato Sauce, Canned, Average	*1 Can/410g*	*387*	*15.1*	*94*	*5.6*	*9.8*	*3.7*	*0*
Italian Pork, Al Forno, Sainsbury's*	1 Pack/450g	644	23.8	143	6.1	17.6	5.3	1.4
Lamb, Asda*	1 Pack/340g	928	71.4	273	16	5.1	21	0.6
Pork & Beef, Swedish Style, Tesco*	1 Meatball/14g	34	2.5	245	14.3	6.5	17.7	2
Pork & Chorizo with Paprika Potatoes, Finest, Tesco*	½ Pack/425g	527	25.9	124	7.5	9.8	6.1	2.8
Pork, & Herb, Finest, Tesco*	6 Balls/168g	356	26.7	212	16	1	15.9	0.7
Pork, Alpenmark, Aldi*	1 Meatball/30g	78	5.7	259	12	7.3	19	3.6
Pork, British, Simply, M&S*	½ Pack/180g	396	27.2	220	17	4.3	15.1	0.5
Pork, Duchy Originals, Waitrose*	5 Meatballs/68g	184	12.6	270	21.7	4	18.6	0
Pork, Mini, Richmond*	5 Meatballs/50g	128	8	255	14	13	16	14
Spaghetti, Tesco*	1 Pack/385g	377	16	98	5.4	9.8	4.2	1.2

M

	Measure INFO/WEIGHT	per Measure KCAL	FAT	Nutrition Values per 100g / 100ml KCAL	PROT	CARB	FAT	FIBRE
MEATBALLS								
Spanish, with Patatas Bravas, TTD, Sainsbury's*	1 Pack/391g	543	30.1	139	9.6	6.7	7.7	2.6
Swedish, Average	*¼ Pack/88g*	*198*	*13.8*	*224*	*14*	*7.4*	*15.7*	*1.3*
Turkey, GFY, Asda*	½ Pack/330g	333	12.2	101	10	7	3.7	0
Turkey, Marinara, Frozen, Microwaved, Slimzone, Asda*	1 Pack/500g	448	4.1	99	7.1	14	0.9	2.6
Veal, with Parmesan, Mini, British, Waitrose*	½ Pack/110g	235	13.2	214	22.9	2.8	12	1.4
Vegetarian, Super Greens Balls, as Sold, Heck*	1 Ball/28g	41	0.8	146	5.4	25.1	3	5.8
Venison, Uncooked, Tesco*	1 Ball/30g	62	3.7	205	17.8	5.4	12.3	0.5
MEDLAR								
Raw, Flesh Only	*1 Fruit/28g*	*11*	*0.1*	*40*	*0.5*	*10.6*	*0.4*	*10*
MELBA TOAST								
Asda*	1 Slice/3.3g	13	0.2	395	12	76	4.8	4.6
Average	*1 Serving/3g*	*13*	*0.2*	*396*	*12*	*76*	*4.9*	*4.6*
Buitoni*	1 Serving/33g	130	1.6	395	12.1	75.5	4.9	4.6
Dutch, LC, Tesco*	1 Pack/20g	75	0.5	375	13.1	75	2.4	4.6
NUME, Morrisons*	6 Slices/20g	77	0.5	384	11.8	76.9	2.4	3.9
Original, Van Der Meulen*	1 Slice/3g	12	0.1	399	12.8	80.5	2.9	3.9
Thinly Sliced Toasted Wheat Bread, Sainsbury's*	1 Slice/3g	12	0.1	374	13.1	75.1	2.4	4.6
MELON								
Cantaloupe, Flesh Only, Average	*½ Melon/255g*	*87*	*0.5*	*34*	*0.8*	*8.2*	*0.2*	*0.9*
Cantaloupe, Weighed with Rind, Average	*1 Wedge/100g*	*18*	*0.2*	*18*	*0.4*	*4.2*	*0.2*	*0.4*
Galia	*1 Serving/240g*	*60*	*0.1*	*25*	*0.8*	*5.8*	*0*	*0.2*
Honeydew, Raw, Flesh Only, Average	*1oz/28g*	*8*	*0*	*30*	*0.7*	*7*	*0.1*	*0.5*
Medley, Pre Packed, Average	*1 Pack/240g*	*66*	*0.3*	*27*	*0.6*	*6*	*0.1*	*0.5*
Orange Melon, Purely, M&S*	1 Pack/500g	110	0.5	22	0.6	4.2	0.1	0.8
Piel de Sapo, Waitrose*	1 Pack/200g	80	0.4	40	0.8	8.2	0.2	0.9
MERINGUE								
Average	*1 Meringue/8g*	*30*	*0*	*379*	*5.3*	*95.4*	*0*	*0*
Bombe, Raspberry & Vanilla, M&S*	1 Bombe/100g	155	1.8	155	3.4	33.3	1.8	2.6
Chocolate, Waitrose*	1 Meringue/77g	341	11.3	444	2.6	75.3	14.7	0.5
Coffee Fresh Cream, Asda*	1 Meringue/28g	109	4.7	396	3.8	57	17	0.3
Cream, Fresh, Sainsbury's*	1 Meringue/35g	142	5.1	407	3.5	65.4	14.6	0.5
Cream, M&S*	1 Meringue/34.1g	145	7.6	425	4.1	52.6	22.2	1.4
Mini, M&S*	1 Meringue/3.8g	15	0	395	6.1	91.6	0	0.2
Nests, Average	*1 Nest/16g*	*63*	*0*	*397*	*4.8*	*93.3*	*0.1*	*0.1*
Nests, M&S*	1 Nest/12g	47	0	390	6.1	91.6	0	0
Nests, Mini, Tesco*	1 Nest/4.9g	19	0	386	4.8	91.2	0.2	0
Nests, Sainsbury's*	1 Nest/13.3g	52	0	392	4.2	93.6	0.1	0.1
Raspberry, M&S*	1 Serving/105g	215	13.8	205	1.8	20.6	13.1	3.1
Strawberry, Mini, Extra Special, Asda*	1 Meringue/4g	15	0	387	5	91	0.3	0.5
Toffee Cream, Tesco*	1 Meringue/30g	114	5	380	4.2	52.9	16.5	0
MIDGET GEMS								
M&S*	1 Bag/113g	367	0.1	325	6.3	75.1	0.1	0
Smart Price, Asda*	1 Pack/178g	586	0.2	329	6	76	0.1	0
MILK								
Almond, & Rice, Almond Dream*	1 Glass/95ml	36	1.2	38	0.6	5.2	1.3	0.4
Almond, Dark Chocolate, Alpro*	1 Serving/200ml	94	2.6	47	0.8	7.6	1.3	0.8
Almond, Original, Alpro*	1 Serving/200ml	48	2.2	24	0.5	3	1.1	0.2
Almond, Original, Fresh, Alpro*	1 Serving/200ml	48	22	24	0.5	3	11	0.2
Almond, Unsweetened, Breeze, Blue Diamond*	1 Serving/250ml	35	3	14	0.5	0.4	1.2	0.3
Almond, Unsweetened, Roasted, Alpro*	1 Serving/200ml	26	2.2	13	0.4	0	1.1	0.4
Almond, Unsweetened, Roasted, Fresh, Alpro*	1 Serving/200ml	26	2.2	13	0.4	0	1.1	0.4
Almond, Unsweetened, Unroasted, Alpro*	1 Serving/200ml	26	2.6	13	0.5	0	1.3	0.2
Alternative, Original, Good Hemp*	1 Glass/250ml	90	6	36	1.3	2.2	2.4	0.2

MILK

	Measure INFO/WEIGHT	per Measure KCAL	FAT	Nutrition Values per 100g / 100ml KCAL	PROT	CARB	FAT	FIBRE
Camel, 100% Raw, Fresh, Desert Farms*	100ml	53	3.5	53	3.4	3.4	3.5	0
Coconut, & Almond, Fresh, Alpro*	1 Serving/200ml	48	2.6	24	0.3	2.6	1.3	0
Coconut, Average	*1 Can/400ml*	*698*	*69.7*	*174*	*1.4*	*2.9*	*17.4*	*2.9*
Coconut, Canned, Pride*	½ Can/200ml	284	30	142	1	1.6	15	0
Coconut, Canned, Tesco*	¼ Can/100ml	151	15	151	0.9	3.2	15	0
Coconut, Chocolate, Alpro*	1 Serving/200ml	82	2.2	41	0.4	7	1.1	0
Coconut, Half Fat, Waitrose*	½ Can/135ml	92	8.1	68	0.7	2.7	6	0
Coconut, KTC*	1 Can/400ml	516	73.2	129	1.3	1.8	18.3	0
Coconut, Lighter, Sainsbury's*	¼ Can/100ml	75	6.5	75	0.9	2.9	6.5	0.5
Coconut, Organic, Canned, Coconut Merchant*	¼ Can/100g	161	17	161	1.6	2.6	17	0.5
Coconut, Organic, Tesco*	1/8 Can/49g	85	8.3	175	1.8	2.7	17	1.3
Coconut, Original, Fresh, Alpro*	1 Serving/200ml	40	1.8	20	0.1	2.7	0.9	0
Coconut, Pure, Kefir Cultures, Drink, Rhythm Health*	1 Bottle/126g	43	2.5	34	0.8	2.8	2	1.7
Coconut, Reduced Fat, Amoy*	1 Tin/400ml	440	44	110	1	2	11	1
Coconut, Reduced Fat, Average	*1 Serving/100g*	*104*	*10*	*104*	*1*	*2.4*	*10*	*0.4*
Coconut, Reduced Fat, Canned, Essential, Waitrose*	1 Can/400ml	244	24	61	0	1.8	6	0
Coconut, Rich & Creamy, Canned, Kingfisher*	¼ Can/100ml	210	20	210	2.2	5.2	20	0
Condensed, Caramel, Carnation, Nestle*	1 Serving/50g	148	3	296	5.5	55.1	6	0
Condensed, Semi Skimmed, Sweetened	*1oz/28g*	*75*	*0.1*	*267*	*10*	*60*	*0.2*	*0*
Condensed, Skimmed, Unsweetened, Average	*1oz/28g*	*30*	*1.1*	*108*	*7.5*	*10.5*	*4*	*0*
Condensed, Whole, Sweetened, Average	*1oz/28g*	*93*	*2.8*	*333*	*8.5*	*55.5*	*10.1*	*0*
Dried, Skimmed, Average	*1oz/28g*	*99*	*0.3*	*355*	*35.4*	*52.3*	*0.9*	*0*
Dried, Skimmed, Powder, Prepared, Morrisons*	100ml	35	0.1	35	3.6	5.1	0.1	0
Dried, Skimmed, Powder, Value, Tesco*	1 Serving/50g	180	0.3	361	36.1	52.9	0.6	0
Dried, Whole, Average	*1oz/28g*	*137*	*7.4*	*490*	*26.3*	*39.4*	*26.3*	*0*
Evaporated, Average	*1 Serving/85g*	*136*	*7.6*	*160*	*8.2*	*11.6*	*9*	*0*
Evaporated, Reduced Fat, Average	*1oz/28g*	*33*	*1.5*	*118*	*7.4*	*10.5*	*5.2*	*0*
Evaporated, Sainsbury's*	1 Serving/50g	80	4.5	161	8.4	11.7	9	0
Goat's, Semi Skimmed, St Helen's Farm*	1 Serving/200ml	88	3.2	44	3	4.3	1.6	0
Goat's, Skimmed, St Helen's Farm*	1 Serving/200ml	60	0.2	30	3	4.3	0.1	0
Goat's, Whole, St Helen's Farm*	1 Serving/200ml	122	7.2	61	2.8	4.3	3.6	0
Goats Semi Skimmed, Waitrose*	1 Serving/250ml	98	4	39	3	4.5	1.6	0
Goats, Pasteurised	*1 fl oz/30ml*	*18*	*1*	*60*	*3.1*	*4.4*	*3.5*	*0*
Gold Top, Original, Graham's*	1 Tbsp/15ml	12	0.8	80	3.7	4.7	5	0
Kefir, Bibi's Homemade*	1 Glass/210g	128	7.4	61	3.3	4.3	3.5	0
Life, Shot, 200, Kefir Cultures, Drink, Rhythm Health*	1 Shot/25ml	8	0.5	34	0.8	2.8	2	1.7
Life, Shot, 50, Kefir Cultures, Drink, Rhythm Health*	1 Shot/25ml	8	0.5	34	0.8	2.8	2	1.7
Oat, Original, Alpro*	1 Serving/200ml	88	3	44	0.3	6.8	1.5	1.4
Powder, Instant, Skimmed, Basics, Sainsbury's*	1 Serving/60g	209	0.4	349	35.6	50.4	0.6	0
Rice, Organic, Provamel*	1 Serving/250ml	122	3.8	49	0.1	9.5	1.5	0
Rice, Original, Alpro*	1 Glass/200ml	94	2	47	0.1	9.5	1	0
Rice, Original, Rice Dream*	1 Serving/150ml	70	1.5	47	0.1	9.4	1	0.1
Semi Skimmed, Average	*1fl oz/30ml*	*15*	*0.5*	*49*	*3.4*	*5*	*1.7*	*0*
Semi Skimmed, Long Life, Average	*1fl oz/30ml*	*15*	*0.5*	*49*	*3.4*	*5*	*1.7*	*0*
Semi Skimmed, Low Lactose, Lactofree, Arla*	1 Glass/125ml	50	1.9	40	3.6	3	1.5	0
Skimmed, Average	*1 Pint/568ml*	*194*	*0.5*	*34*	*3.3*	*5*	*0.1*	*0*
Skimmed, Lactofree, Arla*	1 Serving/200ml	66	0.8	33	3.8	3.6	0.4	0
Skimmed, Uht, Average	*1fl oz/30ml*	*10*	*0*	*34*	*3.4*	*5*	*0.1*	*0*
Soya, Banana Flavour, Provamel*	1 Serving/250ml	195	5.5	78	3.8	10.4	2.2	0.6
Soya, Choco Flavour, Provamel*	1 Serving/250ml	208	6	83	3.8	11.1	2.4	1.1
Soya, Chocolate, Alpro*	1 Serving/200ml	154	4.2	77	3.3	10.7	2.1	1
Soya, Chocolate, So Good Beverages*	1 Serving/250ml	160	2.5	64	3.6	10.8	1	0
Soya, Chocolate, UHT, Alpro*	1 Serving/200ml	122	3.6	61	3.1	7.8	1.8	0.9

M

MILK

INFO/WEIGHT	Measure	per Measure		Nutrition Values per 100g / 100ml				
		KCAL	FAT	KCAL	PROT	CARB	FAT	FIBRE
Soya, Fat Free, Original, So Good Beverages*	1 Serving/250ml	100	0.2	40	3.6	6.4	0.1	0
Soya, Flavoured, Average	*1 Glass/250ml*	*100*	*4.2*	*40*	*2.8*	*3.6*	*1.7*	*0*
Soya, Growing Up Drink, Low in Sugars, Alpro*	1 Serving/200ml	128	4.4	64	2.5	8.3	2.2	0.4
Soya, Light, Alpro*	1 Serving/200ml	54	2.4	27	2.1	1.6	1.2	0.9
Soya, Light, Fresh, Alpro*	1 Serving/200ml	44	2.4	22	2	0.1	1.2	1.2
Soya, Mild, Simply, Alpro*	1 Serving/200ml	70	3.6	35	3	1.5	1.8	0.5
Soya, No Added Sugar, Unsweetened, Average	*1 Serving/250ml*	*85*	*4.8*	*34*	*3.3*	*0.9*	*1.9*	*0.4*
Soya, Omega Original, So Good Beverages*	1 Serving/250ml	98	3.8	39	2	4.4	1.5	0
Soya, Original, Alpro*	1 Serving/200ml	88	3.8	44	3.3	3	1.9	0.6
Soya, Original, Fresh, Alpro*	1 Serving/200ml	78	3.6	39	3	2.5	1.8	0.5
Soya, Original, Fresh, Organic, Alpro*	1 Serving/200ml	76	3.4	38	3	2.4	1.7	0.5
Soya, Plain, Organic, Kirkland*	1 Glass/250ml	118	5.5	47	4	3.7	2.2	0.5
Soya, Strawberry Flavour, Provamel*	1 Serving/250ml	160	5.2	64	3.6	7.7	2.1	1.2
Soya, Strawberry, Alpro*	1 Serving/200ml	124	3.6	62	3.3	7.6	1.8	0.5
Soya, Sweetened, Actileaf, Aldi*	1 Serving/200ml	98	5.2	49	3.5	2.6	2.6	0.5
Soya, Sweetened, Average	*1 Glass/200ml*	*94*	*4.2*	*47*	*3.4*	*3.7*	*2.1*	*0.4*
Soya, Sweetened, Calcium Enriched, Average	*1 Glass/200ml*	*91*	*3.9*	*46*	*3.4*	*3.7*	*2*	*0.3*
Soya, UHT, Non Dairy, Alternative to Milk, Waitrose*	1 Serving/250ml	102	4.8	41	3.3	2.7	1.9	0.2
Soya, Unsweetened, Actileaf, Aldi*	1 Serving/200ml	68	4.2	34	3.4	0.5	2.1	0.5
Soya, Unsweetened, Organic, Waitrose*	1 Serving/60ml	19	1.1	31	3.3	0.2	1.9	0
Soya, Unsweetened, Uht, Organic, Tesco*	1 Serving/150ml	50	2.8	33	3.4	0.4	1.9	0.6
Soya, Vanilla Flavour, Organic, Provamel*	1 Serving/250ml	150	5.5	60	3.8	6.2	2.2	0.6
Soya, Vanilla, Alpro*	1 Serving/200ml	108	3.4	54	3	6.5	1.7	0.5
Soya, Vanilla, Fat Free, So Good Beverages*	1 Serving/250ml	140	0.2	56	3.6	10.4	0.1	0
Soya, Vanilla, Organic, Heinz*	1 Serving/200ml	106	3.2	53	2.6	6.9	1.6	0.2
Soya, Vanilla, So Good Beverages*	1 Serving/250ml	180	5	72	3.6	10.4	2	0
Soya, Vitasoy*	1 Serving/250ml	130	3.8	52	3	5.5	1.5	2
Soya, Wholebean, Unsweetened, Alpro*	1 Serving/200ml	66	3.6	33	3.3	0	1.8	0.6
Soya, Wholebean, Unsweetened, Fresh, Alpro*	1 Serving/200ml	66	3.6	33	3.3	0	1.8	0.6
Soya, Wholebean, Unsweetened, Organic, Alpro*	1 Serving/200ml	66	3.6	33	3.3	0	1.8	0.6
Strawberry Flavoured, Essential, Waitrose*	1 Glass/200ml	136	3.4	68	3.3	9.5	1.7	0.5
Super Milk Low Fat 1%, Avonmore*	1 Litre/1000ml	420	10	42	3.4	5	1	0
Whole, Average	*1 Serving/200ml*	*134*	*7.8*	*67*	*3.3*	*4.7*	*3.9*	*0*
Whole, Lactose Free, Lactofree, Arla*	1 Serving/200ml	114	7	57	3.4	2.8	3.5	0

MILK DRINK

INFO/WEIGHT	Measure	per Measure		Nutrition Values per 100g / 100ml				
Banana Flavour, Sterilised, Low Fat, Gulp*	1 Bottle/500ml	425	9	85	5.2	11.9	1.8	0
Chocolate Coconut, Free From, Tesco*	1 Serving/250ml	125	5.4	49	0.4	6.8	2.1	0.7
Chocolate Flavoured, Goodness for Kids, Tesco*	1 Bottlel/330ml	248	5.9	75	3.8	10.3	1.8	0.7
Chocolate Sterilised Skimmed, Happy Shopper*	1 Bottle/500ml	295	1.5	59	3.6	10.4	0.3	0
Chocolate, Break Time, Arla*	1 Bottle/500ml	290	1.5	58	3.6	10.2	0.3	0
Chocolate, Brekkie, Up & Go, Life Health Foods*	1 Carton/330ml	218	3.3	66	3.8	9.1	1	2.4
Chocolate, Spar*	1 Serving/500ml	290	1.5	58	3.6	10.2	0.3	0
Chocolatte, Cafe Met*	1 Bottle/290ml	174	4.1	60	3.7	9.1	1.4	0.3
Oat, Oat Dream*	1 Serving/200ml	56	1.4	28	0.4	4.8	0.7	0
Original, Mars*	1 Serving/330g	284	6.9	86	3.1	13.7	2.1	0
Refuel, Mars*	1 Bottle/388ml	299	5.8	77	3.1	13.5	1.5	0
Semi Skimmed, Cholesterol Lowering, Pro Activ, Flora*	1 Serving/250ml	125	4.5	50	3.6	4.8	1.8	0
Strawberry Flavoured, Goodness for Kids, Tesco*	1 Bottle/330ml	248	5.6	75	4	9.9	1.7	0.4
Strawberry, Flavoured, Asda*	1 Bottle/330ml	211	3.6	64	3.6	10	1.1	0.5

MILK SHAKE

INFO/WEIGHT	Measure	per Measure		Nutrition Values per 100g / 100ml				
Banana Flavour, Frijj*	1 Bottle/500ml	325	4.5	65	3.7	10.5	0.9	0
Banana Flavour, Shapers, Boots*	1 Bottle/250ml	201	1.9	80	5.6	12.8	0.8	1.9
Banana Flavour, Spar*	1 Bottle/500ml	250	0.5	50	3.3	9.1	0.1	0

	Measure INFO/WEIGHT	per Measure KCAL	FAT	Nutrition Values per 100g / 100ml KCAL	PROT	CARB	FAT	FIBRE
MILK SHAKE								
Banana, Diet Chef Ltd*	1 Drink/330ml	225	3	68	4.2	10.5	0.9	1.5
Banana, Shudda, Aldi*	½ Bottle/236g	163	2.1	69	3.4	12	0.9	0.5
Banana, Yazoo, Campina*	1 Bottle/200ml	120	2.4	60	3.1	9.6	1.2	0
Chocolate Flavour, BGTY, Sainsbury's*	1 Bottle/500ml	290	2.5	58	5.3	8	0.5	0.9
Chocolate Flavour, Diet Chef Ltd*	1 Drink/330ml	210	2.3	64	4.1	8.5	0.7	1.9
Chocolate Flavoured, Fresh, Thick, Frijj*	1 Bottle/500ml	350	5	70	3.5	11.7	1	0
Chocolate, Asda*	1 Serving/250ml	198	9.2	79	4.4	7	3.7	0.4
Chocolate, Extreme, Frijj*	1 Bottle/500g	425	10.5	85	3.9	12.7	2.1	0
Honeycomb Choc Swirl Flavour, The Incredible, Frijj*	1 Bottle/500ml	450	12.5	90	4	13	2.5	0.2
Mount Caramel, Frijj*	1 Bottle/500ml	360	4.5	72	3.4	12.7	0.9	0
Powder, Made Up with Semi-Skimmed Milk	*1 Serving/250ml*	*172*	*4*	*69*	*3.2*	*11.3*	*1.6*	*0*
Powder, Made Up with Whole Milk	*1 Serving/250ml*	*218*	*9.2*	*87*	*3.1*	*11.1*	*3.7*	*0*
Raspberry & Strawberry, Protein 20g, Arla*	1 Serving/225ml	171	3.6	76	9	6.5	1.6	0
Strawberry & Raspberry, Syrup, Robinson's*	1 Serving/50ml	20	0.7	39	2.9	4	1.4	0
Strawberry Flavour, Thick, Low Fat, Frijj*	1 Bottle/250ml	155	2	62	3.4	10.1	0.8	0
Strawberry, Diet Chef Ltd*	1 Drink/330g	225	3	68	4.2	10.5	0.9	1.5
Strawberry, Yazoo, Campina*	1 Bottle/475ml	300	6	60	3.1	9.5	1.2	0
Thick, Milky Way, Mars*	1 Bottle/440ml	282	4.8	64	3.4	10	1.1	0.7
Vanilla, Diet Chef Ltd*	1 Pack/330ml	225	3	68	4.2	10.5	0.9	1.5
MILKY BAR								
Buttons, Nestle*	1 Std Pack/30g	164	9.5	547	7.3	58.4	31.7	0
Chunky, Nestle*	¼ Bar/37.8g	207	12	547	7.3	58.4	31.7	0
Crunchies, Nestle*	1 Pack/30g	168	10.4	560	7	54.9	34.7	0
Eggs, Mini, Nestle*	1 Pack/100g	503	22	503	5.4	70.5	22	0.5
Funsize (17g), Mars*	1 Bar/17g	75	2.7	449	3.8	71.8	16.3	0.6
Milk & Crunchy, Nestle*	1 Bar/21g	117	7.2	557	8.5	53.5	34.3	0.1
Mini Eggs, Nestle*	5 Eggs/17g	85	3.7	501	5.4	70.1	22	0.5
Munchies, Nestle*	1 Serving/70g	392	24.3	560	7	54.9	34.7	0.1
Nestle*	1 Sm Bar/12.5g	68	4	547	7.3	58.4	31.7	0
MILKY WAY								
Fun Size, Mars*	1 Bar/17g	75	2.7	447	3.8	71.6	16.2	0
Funsize (15.5g), Mars*	1 Bar/15.5g	69	2.5	446	3.9	71.6	16.3	0.6
Mars*	1 Bar/21.5g	96	3.3	446	3.9	72.4	15.5	0.6
MINCEMEAT								
Average	*1oz/28g*	*77*	*1.2*	*274*	*0.6*	*62.1*	*4.3*	*1.3*
Sainsbury's*	1 Tbsp/20g	58	0.6	291	1.2	62.3	3.1	1.4
Traditional, Robertson*	1 Tbsp/24g	68	0.6	285	0.8	63.5	2.7	2.5
MINSTRELS								
Galaxy, Mars*	1 Serving/100g	503	22.3	503	5.2	70.3	22.3	1.1
MINT								
Dried, Average	*1 Tsp/5g*	*14*	*0.2*	*279*	*24.8*	*34.6*	*4.6*	*0*
Fresh, Average	*2 Tbsp/3.2g*	*1*	*0*	*43*	*3.8*	*5.3*	*0.7*	*0*
Spearmint, Fresh, Average	*2 Leaves/0.1g*	*0*	*0*	*44*	*3.3*	*8*	*0.7*	*7*
MINTS								
After Dinner, Dark, Elizabeth Shaw*	1 Sweet/9g	42	2.1	469	2.8	62.5	23.1	0
After Dinner, Sainsbury's*	1 Mint/7g	32	1.5	456	4.1	62.1	21.2	4.1
Butter Mintoes, M&S*	1 Sweet/9g	35	0.6	391	0	84	6.8	0
Butter Mintoes, Tesco*	1 Sweet/7g	24	0.5	349	0	71.3	7.1	0
Clear, Co-Op*	1 Sweet/6g	24	0	395	0	98	0	0
Cream, Luxury, Thorntons*	1 Sweet/13g	62	3.1	477	4.2	62.3	23.8	2.3
Creams, Bassett's*	1 Sweet/11g	40	0	365	0	91.8	0	0
Curiously Strong, M&S*	1 Sweet/1g	4	0	390	0.4	97.5	0	0
Doublemint, Sugarfree, Wrigleys*	1 Mint/3g	7	0	234	0	97.4	0	0

M

	Measure INFO/WEIGHT	per Measure KCAL	FAT	Nutrition Values per 100g / 100ml KCAL	PROT	CARB	FAT	FIBRE
MINTS								
Everton, Co-Op*	1 Sweet/6g	25	0.2	410	0.6	92	4	0
Extra Strong, Peppermint, Trebor*	1 Mint/2g	10	0	395	0.3	98.5	0	0
Extra Strong, Spearmint, Trebor*	1 Pack/44g	174	0	395	0.4	98.7	0	0
Extra, Peppermint Coolburst, Wrigleys*	1 Pack/22g	53	0.2	240	0	98	1	0
Extra, Spearmint, Sugar Free, Wrigleys*	1 Sweet/1.1g	3	0	244	0	98.5	0.8	0
Extra, Wrigleys*	1 Sweet/1.1g	3	0	240	0	64	1	0
Glacier, Fox's*	1 Sweet/5g	19	0	386	0	96.4	0	0
Humbugs, Co-Op*	1 Sweet/8g	34	0.6	425	0.6	89.9	7	0
Humbugs, Grumpy Old Gits, Spencer & Fleetwood Ltd*	1 Sweet/25g	92	0.4	366	0.2	87.5	1.5	0
Humbugs, M&S*	1 Sweet/9g	37	0.4	407	0.6	91.1	4.4	0
Humbugs, Thorntons*	1 Sweet/9g	31	0.4	340	1	87.8	4.4	0
Imperials, Co-Op*	1 Sweet/3g	12	0	395	0.3	98	0.2	0
Imperials, M&S*	1 Sweet/3g	12	0	391	0	97.8	0	0
Imperials, Sainsbury's*	1 Sweet/2.6g	10	0	374	0	92.1	0	0
Imperials, Tesco*	1 Sweet/3g	12	0	397	0.6	98.7	0	0
Mento, Sugar Free, Mentos*	1 Sweet/2g	5	0.1	260	1	87	5.5	0
Mint Assortment, M&S*	1 Sweet/7g	26	0.5	375	0.4	78.2	6.9	0
Mint Favourites, Bassett's*	1 Sweet/6g	22	0.4	367	0.9	77.4	5.9	0
Peppermints, Strong, Altoids*	1 Sweet/1g	3	0	385	0.5	96	0	0
Soft, Trebor*	1 Pack/48g	182	0	380	0	94.9	0	0
Softmints, Peppermint, Trebor*	1 Pack/48g	170	0	355	0	88.9	0	0
Softmints, Spearmint, Trebor*	1 Pack/45g	170	0	375	0	94.3	0	0
Thins, Chocolate, Waitrose*	1 Thin/5g	27	1.3	509	4.2	69.6	23.8	0.2
MIRIN								
Rice Wine, Sweetened, Average	*1 Tbsp/15ml*	*35*	*0*	*231*	*0.2*	*41.6*	*0*	*0*
MISO								
Average	*1oz/28g*	*57*	*1.7*	*203*	*13.3*	*23.5*	*6.2*	*0*
MIXED FRUIT								
Apple, Strawberry, Grape, & Blueberry, Sainsbury's*	½ Pot/120g	66	0.6	55	0.7	13.6	0.5	0
Frozen, Tesco*	1 Serving/80g	33	0.2	41	0.9	7.9	0.2	2
Grape & Strawberry, Morrisons*	1 Pot/130g	78	0.3	60	0.6	13.5	0.2	0.7
Pear, Peach & Pineapple, in Juice, Nature's Finest*	1 Pot/370g	248	0	67	0.4	15.5	0	1.4
Strawberry, Melon & Mango, Tesco*	½ Pack/113g	45	0.1	40	0.6	8.6	0.1	1.4
MIXED FRUIT & NUT								
Peanut & Rasin Mix, Alesto, Lidl*	1 Serving/25g	116	7	463	16	35	27.8	4.5
MIXED HERBS								
Average	*1 Tsp/5g*	*13*	*0.4*	*260*	*13*	*37.5*	*8.5*	*6.7*
Herbes De Provence, Dried, Schwartz*	1 Tsp/2g	7	0.1	364	12.9	65	5.8	0
MIXED NUTS								
Totally, Caffe Nero*	1 Serving/50g	317	28.1	634	16.8	12.5	56.2	5.5
Unsalted, Tesco*	1 Serving/25g	164	14.8	657	18	9.8	59.2	6.7
MIXED SPICE								
Schwartz*	1 Tsp/2g	8	0.2	390	10.4	65.8	9.5	2
MIXED VEGETABLES								
Casserole, Sliced, Diced, Washed & Ready, Chop Chop*	1 Pack/600g	294	1.8	49	1.3	9.2	0.3	2
for Bolognese, Meal Kit, As Sold, Morrisons*	¼ Pack/100g	45	0.6	45	2.1	6.3	0.6	2.8
Green, Medley, Signature, Morrisons*	½ Pack/113g	93	6.9	82	2.6	2.9	6.1	2.6
Green, Medley, Tesco*	½ Pack/80g	75	1.6	94	4.8	10.7	2	7.1
Green, with Minted Butter, Natures Pick, Aldi*	1/3 Pack/90g	76	4.9	84	3.1	4.2	5.4	3.3
Mediterranean Roasting, Tesco*	½ Pack/237g	71	0.7	30	1.1	5	0.3	1.3
Medley, Tesco*	½ Pack/113g	50	0.7	44	2.4	5.3	0.6	3.7
MOLASSES								
Average	*1 Tsp/5g*	*13*	*0*	*266*	*0*	*68.8*	*0.1*	*0*

	Measure INFO/WEIGHT	per Measure		Nutrition Values per 100g / 100ml				
		KCAL	FAT	KCAL	PROT	CARB	FAT	FIBRE
MONKEY NUTS								
without Shell, Average	*1oz/28g*	*158*	*13.4*	*565*	*25.6*	*8.2*	*48*	*6.3*
MONKFISH								
Grilled	*1oz/28g*	*27*	*0.2*	*96*	*22.7*	*0*	*0.6*	*0*
Raw	*1oz/28g*	*18*	*0.1*	*66*	*15.7*	*0*	*0.4*	*0*
MONSTER MUNCH								
Pickled Onion, Walkers*	1 Std Bag/22g	108	5.5	490	6	60	25	1.7
Roast Beef, Walkers*	1 Std Bag/22g	108	5.5	490	7	59	25	1.7
Spicy, Walkers*	1 Std Bag/25g	125	7.2	500	5	55	29	1.3
MOUSSAKA								
Beef, BGTY, Sainsbury's*	1 Pack/400g	300	10.4	75	6.1	6.8	2.6	1.2
Charlie Bigham's*	½ Pack/328g	396	24.2	121	7	7	7.4	0.9
COU, M&S*	1 Pack/340g	272	9.9	80	5.3	8.5	2.9	1.4
Lamb, Finest, Tesco*	1 Pack/335g	543	37.5	162	6.7	7.9	11.2	1.5
Lamb, Oven Cooked, NUME, Morrisons*	1 Pack/375g	368	13.5	98	8.8	5.9	3.6	3.4
Lentil, & Quinoa, Everdine*	1 Meal/450g	410	17.1	91	3.3	9.3	3.8	3.2
TTD, Sainsbury's*	1 Pack/399g	546	35.9	137	8.1	5.8	9	0.6
Vegetable, COU, M&S*	1 Pack/400g	280	10.8	70	2.7	9.1	2.7	2.4
Vegetarian, Quorn*	1 Pack/400g	364	16.4	91	3.6	9.8	4.1	1.2
MOUSSE								
Aero Chocolate, Nestle*	1 Pot/58g	101	3	174	4.8	27.3	5.1	1.1
Aero Heavenly, Nestle*	1/3 Pack/57g	115	6.7	201	4.2	19	11.7	0
Aero Twist Cappuccino & Chocolate, Nestle*	1 Pot/75g	135	8.1	180	4.2	16.8	10.8	0.2
Apricot, Lite, Onken*	1 Pot/150g	156	2.2	104	4.6	18	1.5	0.3
Banoffee, COU, M&S*	1 Pot/70g	102	1.5	145	2.9	28.8	2.1	1.5
Belgian Chocolate & Vanilla, Weight Watchers*	1 Pot/80g	106	2.2	132	4.4	22.2	2.8	0.9
Belgian Chocolate, Finest, Tesco*	1 Pot/120g	360	22.7	300	5.1	26.6	18.9	1.1
Black Cherry, Lite, Onken*	1 Pot/150g	156	2.2	104	4.6	17.9	1.5	0.2
Blackcurrant, Onken*	1 Pot/150g	210	10.2	140	5.2	14.6	6.8	0
Cadbury's Light Chocolate, St Ivel*	1 Pot/64g	79	2	123	6.2	17.3	3.2	0
Cappuccino, Essential, Waitrose*	1 Pot/100g	279	16.7	279	4.2	27.7	16.7	0.5
Caramel, Meringue, Cadbury*	1 Pot/65g	181	6.7	277	4.6	42.4	10.3	1
Chocolate	*1 Pot/60g*	*83*	*3.2*	*139*	*4*	*19.9*	*5.40*	*0*
Chocolate & Hazelnut, Onken*	1 Pot/125g	171	7.5	137	3.3	17.8	6	0
Chocolate & Mint, COU, M&S*	1 Pot/70g	84	1.8	120	6.2	18.7	2.5	1
Chocolate & Orange, COU, M&S*	1 Pot/70g	77	1.8	110	5.9	16	2.6	0.9
Chocolate & Hazelnut, Creamy, Dr Oetker*	1 Pot/115g	158	6.9	137	3.3	17.6	6	0.6
Chocolate Orange, Low Fat, Cadbury*	1 Pot/100g	110	3	110	5.6	15.1	3	0
Chocolate with Mini Chunks of, Dairy Milk, Cadbury*	1 Pot/100g	215	9.9	215	6.1	25.7	9.9	0
Chocolate with Vanilla Layer, Cadbury*	1 Pot/100g	162	6.1	162	4.8	21.9	6.1	0
Chocolate, Asda*	1 Pot/61g	134	6.1	219	3.7	26	10	1
Chocolate, Basics, Sainsbury's*	1 Pot/62.5g	94	3.8	150	5.1	18.9	6	0
Chocolate, BGTY, Sainsbury's*	1 Pot/63g	83	1.8	133	4.9	21.8	2.9	0.5
Chocolate, Cadbury*	1 Pot/55g	107	4.5	195	6.1	24.6	8.2	0
Chocolate, COU, M&S*	1 Pot/70.4g	84	1.9	120	5.2	20.3	2.7	1
Chocolate, Finest, Tesco*	1 Pot/82g	321	26.4	391	3.7	21.7	32.2	0
Chocolate, GFY, Asda*	1 Pot/60g	70	1.7	117	4.8	17.9	2.9	3.5
Chocolate, Iceland*	1 Pot/62g	113	4.3	183	4	26.3	6.9	0
Chocolate, Italian Style, Tesco*	1 Pot/90g	243	11.9	270	5	32.8	13.2	2.4
Chocolate, Light Choices, LC, Tesco*	1 Pot/62.5g	80	1.3	125	5	20.8	2.1	1.5
Chocolate, Light, Cadbury*	1 Pot/55g	60	1.9	110	4.6	14.2	3.4	0
Chocolate, Low Fat, Danette, Danone*	1 Pot/60g	73	1.1	121	5.1	20.8	1.9	1.5
Chocolate, Minty, Bubbly, Dessert, Aero, Nestle*	1 Pot/58g	108	5.9	186	4.6	18.9	10.2	0.3
Chocolate, Pere & Fils*	1 Pot/80g	282	20.3	352	8.5	20.5	25.4	0

	Measure INFO/WEIGHT	per Measure KCAL	FAT	Nutrition Values per 100g / 100ml KCAL	PROT	CARB	FAT	FIBRE
MOUSSE								
Chocolate, Sainsbury's*	1 Pot/62.5g	119	5.3	190	4.7	23.8	8.5	1
Chocolate, Shapers, Boots*	1 Pot/70g	97	1.9	138	5.3	23	2.7	1.7
Chocolate, Tesco*	1 Pot/60g	120	5	200	3.6	27.6	8.4	0.9
Chocolate, Value, Tesco*	1 Pot/63g	101	3.3	161	4.9	23.3	5.2	1.3
Chocolate, White, Bubbly, Dessert, Aero, Nestle*	1 Pot/58g	99	4.4	170	4.3	21	7.5	0.2
Layered Strawberry, Co-Op*	1 Pot/100g	120	3	120	3	19	3	0.2
Lemon Fruit Juice, Shape, Danone*	1 Pot/100g	116	2.8	116	3.5	18.6	2.8	0
Lemon with Meringue Style Sauce, Ski, Nestle*	1 Pot/60g	81	2.8	137	3.1	19.8	4.8	0
Lemon, Classic, Onken*	1 Pot/150g	210	9.4	140	5.1	15.8	6.3	0
Lemon, COU, M&S*	1 Pot/70g	91	1.8	130	3.1	23.7	2.5	0.6
Lemon, Dessert, Sainsbury's*	1 Pot/62.5g	114	5.9	182	3.6	20.7	9.4	0.6
Lemon, Low Fat, Morrisons*	1 Pot/62.5g	99	5.8	158	3.7	15.4	9.3	0.3
Lemon, Ski, Nestle*	1 Tub/60g	76	2.8	127	3.7	17.6	4.7	0
Lemon, Somerfield*	1 Pot/63g	113	5.9	181	3.5	20.7	9.4	0.6
Lemon, Tesco*	1 Pot/60g	67	1.6	111	3.4	18.2	2.7	0
Milk Chocolate, M&S*	1 Pot/90g	180	7.8	200	5.3	24.8	8.7	1.5
Mint Chocolate, Cadbury*	1 Pot/45g	90	3.6	200	6	25.6	8.1	0
Orange, Mango & Lime, Onken*	1 Pot/150g	207	9.4	138	5.1	15.3	6.3	0.1
Peach, Onken*	1 Pot/150g	204	9.4	136	5.1	15.1	6.3	0.2
Plain Chocolate, Low Fat, Nestle*	1 Pot/120g	71	0.9	59	2.4	10.4	0.8	0
Raspberry Ripple, Value, Tesco*	1 Pot/47g	70	2.9	149	2.1	21.3	6.1	0.1
Raspberry Ripple, Value, Tesco*	1 Mousse/47g	77	3.1	163	2.9	23	6.6	0.3
Raspberry, Lite, Onken*	1 Pot/150g	156	2.2	104	4.6	17.3	1.5	0.1
Rhubarb, COU, M&S*	1 Pot/70g	88	1.5	125	2.9	25.7	2.1	4.2
Rolo, Nestle*	1 Pot/50g	80	3	158	4.7	21.6	5.9	0
Strawberry & Vanilla, Weight Watchers*	1 Pot/80g	87	1.9	109	3.8	18.1	2.4	0.4
Strawberry with Strawberry Sauce, Ski, Nestle*	1 Pot/60g	79	3.1	131	3.1	18.1	5.2	0
Strawberry, Asda*	1 Pot/64g	107	5.8	167	3.5	18	9	0.2
Strawberry, Light, Muller*	1 Pot/150g	147	0.6	98	4.3	19.4	0.4	0
Strawberry, Low Fat, Waitrose*	1 Pot/95g	112	2.7	118	3.2	20	2.8	0.6
Strawberry, Sainsbury's*	1 Pot/63g	106	5.9	168	3.4	17.5	9.4	0.1
Strawberry, Shape, Danone*	1 Pot/100g	44	1.8	44	3	4	1.8	0
Strawberry, Ski, Nestle*	1 Tub/60g	77	3.1	128	3.8	16.6	5.2	0
Strawberry, Tesco*	1 Pot/63g	106	5.8	169	3.5	17.9	9.3	0.2
Summer Fruits, Light, Muller*	1 Pot/149g	143	0.6	96	4.3	18.7	0.4	0
Toffee, M&S*	1 Pot/90g	180	7.2	200	4.5	27.6	8	0.6
Vanilla, Finesse, Aero, Rowntree's*	1 Pot/57g	127	8.3	223	3.7	18.8	14.6	0
White Chocolate & Raspberry, Gu*	1 Pot/83g	225	14.6	271	1.9	28.4	17.6	4.1
White Chocolate, Finest, Tesco*	1 Pot/92g	436	34.5	474	3.9	30.2	37.5	0
MUFFIN								
All Butter, M&S*	1 Muffin/64.8g	175	4.7	270	10.3	40.8	7.3	2.1
Apple, Sultana & Cinnamon, GFY, Asda*	1 Muffin/50g	134	1.8	268	6	53	3.5	3.9
Banana & Walnut, The Handmade Flapjack Company*	1 Muffin/135g	520	30.6	385	5.3	40.5	22.7	0
Banana Pecan, Organic, Honeyrose Bakery*	1 Muffin/110g	300	12.6	273	4.1	38.3	11.5	4.3
Berry Burst, Asda*	1 Muffin/60g	139	1.4	232	6.2	46.7	2.3	1.7
Blueberry, American Style, Aldi*	1 Muffin/85g	344	17.3	405	4.3	51.2	20.3	0
Blueberry, American Style, Sainsbury's*	1 Muffin/72g	256	13.1	355	5.1	42.7	18.2	1.9
Blueberry, Asda*	1 Muffin/77g	273	13.1	353	5	45	17	1.3
Blueberry, Bakery, Tesco*	1 Muffin/82g	307	13.1	374	4.3	52.2	16	1.9
Blueberry, Big, Asda*	1 Muffin/105g	342	11.2	326	7.5	49.8	10.7	2.3
Blueberry, M&S*	1 Muffin/75g	255	12.6	340	4.9	41.9	16.8	1.3
Blueberry, McVitie's*	1 Muffin/80g	328	18.6	405	4.7	47.9	23	1.3
Blueberry, Mini, Sainsbury's*	1 Muffin/28g	82	2.3	293	6.3	48.9	8.1	1.9

MUFFIN

	Measure INFO/WEIGHT	per Measure KCAL	FAT	Nutrition Values per 100g / 100ml KCAL	PROT	CARB	FAT	FIBRE
Blueberry, Mini, Tesco*	1 Muffin/28g	104	5.4	370	5.6	43.5	19.3	1.2
Blueberry, PB, Waitrose*	1 Muffin/100g	225	2.2	225	4.6	46.5	2.2	1.8
Blueberry, Waitrose*	1 Muffin/65g	239	9.2	367	4.7	55.2	14.2	1.7
Blueberry, Wild Canadian, Fabulous Bakin' Boys*	1 Muffin/40g	140	8	349	4	39	20	1
Bran & Sultana, Weight Watchers*	1 Muffin/60g	144	1.3	240	4.5	50.7	2.1	2.3
Bran, Average	*1 Muffin/57g*	*155*	*4.4*	*272*	*7.8*	*45.6*	*7.7*	*7.7*
Cappuccino Mega, The Handmade Flapjack Company*	1 Muffin/135g	653	40	484	14	48.4	29.6	0
Caramel, Cadbury*	1 Muffin/116g	535	30.3	461	5.9	50.8	26.1	0
Caramel, Salted, TTD, Sainsbury's*	1 Muffin/113g	447	22	396	4.8	49.6	19.5	1.5
Carrot Cake, Entenmann's*	1 Muffin/105g	344	15.9	328	5.1	45.8	15.1	3
Carrot, Asda*	1 Muffin/59g	138	1.4	233	6	47	2.3	1.6
Cheese, Tesco*	1 Muffin/67g	150	1.9	224	13	36.4	2.9	3
Choc Chip, Mini, Weight Watchers*	1 Muffin/15g	47	1.3	312	6.6	52.1	8.6	3.1
Chocolate Chip, American Style, Sainsbury's*	1 Muffin/72g	284	14.4	395	5	48.8	20	2.1
Chocolate Chip, BGTY, Sainsbury's*	1 Muffin/75g	282	12.3	376	5.2	51.8	16.4	1.6
Chocolate Chip, Mini, Asda*	1 Muffin/22g	77	2.9	349	7	51	13	2.1
Chocolate Chip, Mini, BGTY, Sainsbury's*	1 Muffin/28g	91	2.4	324	6.5	55.1	8.7	1.6
Chocolate Chip, Mini, Essential, Waitrose*	1 Muffin/27g	108	5.1	399	5.9	49.8	19	2.5
Chocolate Chip, Plain, Tesco*	1 Muffin/72g	270	12.7	375	5	48.1	17.6	1.4
Chocolate Indulgence, McVitie's*	1 Muffin/75g	254	6.9	338	5.8	57.9	9.2	1.3
Chocolate, Galaxy, McVitie's*	1 Muffin/88g	319	17.1	364	5	44.5	19.5	0
Cinnamon & Sultana, Baked by Us, Morrisons*	1 Muffin/68g	166	1	244	8.3	48.2	1.4	2.9
Cranberry & White Chocolate, Sainsbury's*	1 Muffin/72g	253	13.3	352	5.7	40.7	18.5	1.5
Double Berry Burst, Entenmann's*	1 Muffin/59g	140	1.2	238	4.6	50.1	2.1	1.6
Double Chocolate Chip, American Style, Sainsbury's*	1 Muffin/72g	276	14.6	384	5.2	45	20.3	2.9
Double Chocolate Chip, Co-Op*	1 Muffin/60g	246	12.6	410	6	49	21	3
Double Chocolate Chip, Mini, Asda*	1 Muffin/19g	76	3.7	400	7.4	48.5	19.6	2.7
Double Chocolate Chip, Tesco*	1 Muffin/100g	360	17.9	360	6.1	44.9	17.9	5.4
Double Chocolate, Free From, Tesco*	1 Muffin/70g	281	12.7	402	4.7	54.8	18.2	1.7
Double Chocolate, Mini, M&S*	1 Muffin/32g	133	6.9	416	5.4	49.8	21.7	1.1
English	1 Muffin/57g	120	1	211	7	43.9	1.8	1.8
English, Butter, Tesco*	1 Muffin/67g	170	3.6	253	11.2	39.8	5.4	2
English, Egg, Cheese, & Sausage, From Restaurant	*1 Muffin/165g*	*487*	*30.9*	*295*	*13.1*	*18.8*	*18.7*	*0*
English, Gluten, Wheat & Milk Free, Free From, Livwell*	1 Muffin/50g	160	4.9	320	4.6	52.8	9.8	3.2
English, Kingsmill*	1 Muffin/75g	167	1.4	222	9.7	40.4	1.8	2.6
English, M&S*	1 Muffin/60g	135	1.1	225	11.2	43.7	1.9	2.9
English, Mild Red Cheddar Cheese, Extra Special, Asda*	1 Muffin/70g	201	4.7	288	11	45	6.7	2.7
English, Tesco*	1 Muffin/72g	171	2.3	238	11.2	41.7	3.2	2.8
English, Wholemeal, Seeded, Organic, Duchy Originals*	1 Muffin/72g	199	3.9	276	11.3	43.3	5.4	4.4
English, with Butter, From Restaurant, Average	*1 Muffin/63g*	*189*	*5.8*	*300*	*7.7*	*48.2*	*9.1*	*0*
English, with Cheese & Sausage, From Restaurant	*1 Muffin/115g*	*393*	*24.3*	*342*	*13.3*	*25.4*	*21.1*	*1.3*
Finger, Double Chocolate, Bakers Delight*	1 Muffin/25g	104	4.6	416	5.8	56.9	18.4	1.7
Fruit, Spiced, Soft, TTD, Sainsbury's*	1 Muffin/72g	205	4.3	285	8.7	47.5	6	3.2
Lemon & Blueberry, Tesco*	1 Muffin/110g	411	23	374	4	42.4	20.9	1.1
Lemon & Poppy Seed, Entenmann's*	1 Muffin/105g	417	20.3	397	5.6	52.8	19.3	2.5
Lemon & Poppy Seed, M&S*	1 Muffin/72g	281	14.3	390	6.3	46.1	19.8	1.5
Lemon & Poppy Seed, Waitrose*	1 Muffin/121g	460	23.1	380	4.3	46.8	19.1	1.8
Lemon Curd, Patisserie, TTD, Sainsbury's*	1 Muffin/108g	418	20.9	386	5.4	47.1	19.3	1.4
Lemon, Boots*	1 Muffin/110g	424	20.9	385	3.6	50	19	1.3
Lunchbox, Double Chocolate, The Fabulous Bakin' Boys*	1 Muffin/54g	218	11.8	404	5.6	46.3	21.8	1
Mini, Tesco*	1 Muffin/28g	120	6.3	428	6.4	50	22.6	1.2
Muesli, Breakfast, Love Life, Waitrose*	1 Muffin/68g	216	6.2	318	9.1	50	9.1	3.4
Orange, Apricot & Almond, Organic, Honeyrose Bakery*	1 Muffin/110g	312	11.4	284	3.5	44.2	10.4	1.9

M

MUFFIN

INFO/WEIGHT	Measure	per Measure		Nutrition Values per 100g / 100ml				
		KCAL	FAT	KCAL	PROT	CARB	FAT	FIBRE
Oven Bottom, Aldi*	1 Muffin/68g	173	1	255	10	50.4	1.5	2.2
Oven Bottom, Asda*	1 Muffin/68g	173	1	255	10	50.4	1.5	2.2
Oven Bottom, Morrisons*	1 Muffin/68g	166	0.6	245	8.9	48.8	0.9	2.9
Oven Bottom, Tesco*	1 Muffin/68g	173	1	255	10	50.4	1.5	2.2
Oven Bottom, Warburton's*	1 Muffin/63g	173	2.7	274	10.4	49.4	4.3	2.3
Plain, Co-Op*	1 Muffin/60g	135	1.1	225	11.2	41.3	1.9	2.4
Plain, Morrisons*	1 Muffin/70g	140	0.8	200	8	41.4	1.1	0
Plain, Prepared From Recipe, Average	*1 Muffin/57g*	*169*	*6.5*	*296*	*6.9*	*41.4*	*11.4*	*2.7*
Raspberry Cream, Sainsbury's*	1 Muffin/90g	314	19.8	349	3.9	33.8	22	1.3
Raspberry, PB, Waitrose*	1 Muffin/101g	220	2.1	219	4.7	45.4	2.1	3.7
Sausage, Egg & Cheese, American Style, Tesco*	1 Muffin/155g	383	20.5	247	12.2	19.9	13.2	1
Spiced Fruit, Co-Op*	1 Muffin/60g	159	1.2	265	11	52	2	3
Spiced Fruit, Toasting, Finest, Tesco*	1 Muffin/77g	215	5.2	279	9.2	43.2	6.8	3.9
Spicy Fruit, Quality Bakers*	1 Muffin/65g	146	1	225	9.4	38	1.5	3.3
Strawberry Cakelet, The Handmade Flapjack Company*	1 Muffin/135g	526	29.6	390	4.5	43.6	21.9	0
Sunblest*	1 Muffin/72g	166	1.3	230	9.6	43.9	1.8	2.2
Toasting, Warburton's*	1 Muffin/64g	138	1	216	8.9	41.4	1.6	2.9
Toasting, Warburton's*	1 Muffin/64g	138	1	216	8.9	41.4	1.6	2.9
Toffee & Pecan, Finest, Tesco*	1 Muffin/127g	551	29	434	5.4	51.8	22.8	0.9
Toffee, The Handmade Flapjack Company*	1 Muffin/135g	533	31.6	395	4.4	41.2	23.4	0
Vanilla & Choc Chip, GFY, Asda*	1 Muffin/59g	152	1.3	260	7	53	2.2	1.6
White Chocolate & Strawberry Filled, Tesco*	1 Muffin/102.5g	415	20.3	405	5.2	51.3	19.8	1.3
White Chocolate Chunk Lemon, Mini, M&S*	1 Muffin/28g	130	6.7	464	6.4	55.4	23.9	2.1
White, All Butter, Sainsbury's*	1 Muffin/67g	173	4.2	258	10.6	39.6	6.3	3.6
White, Asda*	1 Muffin/66.7g	148	1.3	222	11	40	2	2.5
White, Finest, Tesco*	1 Muffin/70g	159	0.8	227	8.4	45.7	1.2	2.1
White, M&S*	1 Muffin/60g	135	1.1	225	11.2	43.7	1.9	2.9
White, Soft, Hovis*	1 Muffin/60g	145	1.7	241	8.9	44	2.8	2.4
White, Tesco*	1 Muffin/72g	173	2.3	240	11.3	41.6	3.2	2.8
Wholemeal, Tesco*	1 Muffin/65g	130	1.3	200	12.6	32.9	2	5.7
MULBERRIES								
Raw	*1oz/28g*	*10*	*0*	*36*	*1.3*	*8.1*	*0*	*0*
MULLET								
Grey, Grilled	*1oz/28g*	*42*	*1.5*	*150*	*25.7*	*0*	*5.2*	*0*
Grey, Raw	*1oz/28g*	*16*	*0.6*	*58*	*9.9*	*0*	*2*	*0*
Red, Grilled	*1oz/28g*	*34*	*1.2*	*121*	*20.4*	*0*	*4.4*	*0*
Red, Raw, Weighed Whole, Flesh Only	*1 Portion/100g*	*25*	*0.9*	*25*	*4.3*	*0*	*0.9*	*0*
MUNCHIES								
Original, Tube, Nestle*	1 Pack/54.7g	266	12.3	487	5.4	64.6	22.5	1.4
MUSHROOMS								
Breaded, Average	*3 Mushroom/51g*	*77*	*2.9*	*152*	*4.3*	*20.8*	*5.7*	*0.6*
Breaded, Garlic, Average	*3 Mushroom/50g*	*92*	*4.9*	*183*	*5.2*	*18.7*	*9.7*	*1.7*
Buna Shimeji, Livesey Brothers*	½ Pack/75g	29	0.3	39	2.7	5.9	0.4	1.2
Button, Raw, Average	*1 Serving/50g*	*7*	*0.2*	*15*	*2.3*	*0.5*	*0.4*	*1.2*
Chestnut, Average	*1 Med/5g*	*1*	*0*	*13*	*1.8*	*0.4*	*0.5*	*0.6*
Chinese, Dried, Raw	*1oz/28g*	*80*	*0.5*	*284*	*10*	*59.9*	*1.8*	*0*
Closed Cup, Average	*1 Handful/30g*	*4*	*0.2*	*14*	*1.8*	*0.4*	*0.5*	*1.1*
Common, Boiled in Salted Water, Average	*1oz/28g*	*3*	*0.1*	*11*	*1.8*	*0.4*	*0.3*	*1.1*
Common, Fried, Average	*1oz/28g*	*44*	*4.5*	*157*	*2.4*	*0.3*	*16.2*	*1.5*
Common, Raw, Average	*1 Serving/80g*	*10*	*0.4*	*12*	*1.8*	*0.3*	*0.5*	*1.1*
Creamed, Average	*1oz/28g*	*23*	*1.5*	*82*	*1.3*	*6.8*	*5.5*	*0.5*
Crispy, M&S*	1 Serving/130g	390	33.4	300	4.2	12.5	25.7	1.8
Dried	*1oz/28g*	*45*	*1.7*	*159*	*21.8*	*4.8*	*6*	*13.3*

	Measure INFO/WEIGHT	per Measure KCAL	FAT	Nutrition Values per 100g / 100ml KCAL	PROT	CARB	FAT	FIBRE
MUSHROOMS								
Enoki, Average	*1 Serving/80g*	*34*	*0*	*42*	*3*	*7*	*0*	*3*
Flat, Large, Average	*1 Mushroom/52g*	*10*	*0.3*	*20*	*3.3*	*0.5*	*0.5*	*0.7*
Garlic, Average	*½ Pack/150g*	*159*	*14*	*106*	*2.1*	*3.7*	*9.3*	*1.7*
Oyster, Average	*1 Serving/80g*	*10*	*0.2*	*13*	*1.4*	*1.4*	*0.2*	*1.1*
Porcini, Wild, Dried, Merchant Gourmet*	1 Pack/25g	66	0.8	265	27.9	30.6	3.4	18.7
Portobello, with Spinach & Ricotta, Everdine*	1 Serving/450g	346	16.2	77	4	5.9	3.6	2.8
Shiitake & Tofu Teriyaki, Everdine*	1 Serving/450g	464	15.3	103	5.5	11.1	3.4	3
Shiitake, & Tofu, with Black Bean Sauce, Everdine*	1 Serving/450g	414	15.3	92	5	8.5	3.4	3.5
Shiitake, Cooked	*1oz/28g*	*15*	*0.1*	*55*	*1.6*	*12.3*	*0.2*	*0*
Shiitake, Dried, Raw	*1oz/28g*	*83*	*0.3*	*296*	*9.6*	*63.9*	*1*	*0*
Sliced, Average	*1oz/28g*	*3*	*0.1*	*12*	*1.8*	*0.4*	*0.3*	*1.1*
Straw, Canned, Drained	*1oz/28g*	*4*	*0.1*	*15*	*2.1*	*1.2*	*0.2*	*0*
Stuffed, Cheese, Parsley & Butter, Sainsbury's*	½ Pack/110g	246	24.2	224	4.1	2.3	22	2.6
Stuffed, Cheesy, Asda*	1 Serving/290g	322	17.4	111	4.3	10	6	0
Stuffed, Ready to Roast, Waitrose*	1 Serving/125g	94	4.6	75	3.9	6.5	3.7	1.5
Stuffed, Stilton & Leek, Portobello, Asda*	1 Mushroom/200g	292	19	146	9.2	5.5	9.5	1
Stuffed, with Leek & Wensleydale, Loved by Us, Co-Op*	1 Mushroom/100g	85	3.6	85	4.3	7.8	3.6	2.1
MUSSELS								
Boiled, Flesh Only, Average	*1 Mussel/1.9g*	*2*	*0.1*	*104*	*16.7*	*3.5*	*2.7*	*0*
Boiled, Weighed in Shell, Average	*1 Mussel/7g*	*2*	*0.1*	*28*	*4.5*	*0.9*	*0.7*	*0*
Pickled, Drained, Average	*1oz/28g*	*32*	*0.6*	*112*	*20*	*1.5*	*2.2*	*0*
Raw, Weighed in Shell, Average	*1oz/28g*	*7*	*0.2*	*23*	*3.4*	*1*	*0.7*	*0*
MUSSELS IN								
Garlic Butter Sauce, Average	*½ Pack/225g*	*179*	*11.5*	*80*	*6.4*	*2*	*5.1*	*0.2*
Oil, Smoked, Canned, Drained, John West*	1 Can/60g	117	7.3	196	19.9	1.6	12.2	0
Seasoned White Wine Sauce, Bantry Bay*	1 Serving/450g	270	9	60	6.3	4.1	2	0.1
Thai Sauce, Scottish, Waitrose*	1 Serving/250g	135	6.2	54	5.4	2.6	2.5	0.6
White Wine & Garlic Sauce , Scottish, Tesco*	1 Pouch/155g	130	6.2	84	9.8	1.9	4	0.6
White Wine Sauce, Sainsbury's*	½ Pack/250g	221	9.2	88	8	5.8	3.7	0
MUSTARD								
American, Average	*1 Tsp/5g*	*5*	*0.2*	*102*	*4.4*	*10.5*	*5*	*2.5*
Cajun, Colman's*	1 Tsp/6g	11	0.4	187	7	23	6.5	2.7
Coarse Grain, Average	*1 Tsp/5g*	*7*	*0.4*	*141*	*7.7*	*8.4*	*8.3*	*5.9*
Dijon, Average	*1 Tsp/5g*	*8*	*0.6*	*163*	*7.4*	*7.7*	*11.3*	*1.1*
English, Average	*1 Tsp/5g*	*9*	*0.4*	*173*	*6.8*	*19.2*	*7.6*	*1.2*
French, Average	*1 Tsp/5g*	*5*	*0.3*	*106*	*5.4*	*8.1*	*5.6*	*1.8*
German Style, Sainsbury's*	1 Serving/10g	9	0.6	92	5.5	2.8	6.5	0
Honey, Colman's*	1 Tsp/6g	12	0.5	208	7.4	24	8.2	0
Powder, Average	*1 Tsp/3g*	*15*	*0.9*	*452*	*28.9*	*20.7*	*28.7*	*0*
Smooth, Average	*1 Tsp/8g*	*11*	*0.7*	*139*	*7.1*	*9.7*	*8.2*	*0*
Whole Grain, Average	*1 Tsp/8g*	*11*	*0.8*	*140*	*8.2*	*4.2*	*10.2*	*4.9*
Yellow, Prepared	1 Tbsp/15ml	11	0.6	73	4	6	4	0
MUSTARD CRESS								
Raw	*1oz/28g*	*4*	*0.2*	*13*	*1.6*	*0.4*	*0.6*	*1.1*

M

	Measure INFO/WEIGHT	per Measure KCAL	FAT	Nutrition Values per 100g / 100ml KCAL	PROT	CARB	FAT	FIBRE
NACHOS								
American Chilli Beef, Asda*	1 Serving/200g	208	10	104	10	4.7	5	0.8
Cheesy with Salsa & Soured Cream, Sainsbury's*	½ Pack/170g	449	26.9	264	8.8	21.5	15.8	1.4
Chilli, Sainsbury's*	½ Pack/250g	695	32.2	278	10.9	29.5	12.9	1.3
Kit, Old El Paso*	½ Pack/260g	598	26	230	4	31	10	0
with Cheese, From Restaurant, Average	**1 Nacho/16g**	**49**	**2.7**	**306**	**8**	**32.2**	**16.8**	**0**
NASI GORENG								
Indonesian, Asda*	1 Pack/360g	778	22.7	216	7.4	32.3	6.3	1.3
Vitasia, Lidl*	1 Bowl/250g	438	11	175	7.3	25.8	4.4	1.1
NECTARINES								
Fresh, Raw, Weighed with Stone, Average	**1 Med/140g**	**50**	**0.1**	**36**	**1.2**	**8**	**0.1**	**1.1**
NESQUIK								
Chocolate Flavour, Powder, Dry Weight, Nesquik, Nestle*	1 Serving/15g	56	0.5	372	3	82.9	3.1	6.5
Strawberry Flavour, Powder, Dry Weight, Nesquik, Nestle*	1 Serving/15g	59	0	393	0	98.1	0	0
NIK NAKS								
Cream 'n' Cheesy, KP Snacks*	1 Bag/34g	196	13	575	5.2	52.7	38.1	0.2
Nice 'n' Spicy, KP Snacks*	1 Bag/30g	171	11.5	571	4.6	51.6	38.4	1.6
Rib 'n' Saucy, Golden Wonder*	1 Sm Bag/25g	143	9.4	571	4.5	53.7	37.6	0.5
Scampi 'n' Lemon, KP Snacks*	1 Bag/25g	143	9.4	573	4.9	53.1	37.5	0.1
NOODLES								
Chicken, & Mushroom, Mugfull, Batchelors*	1 Portion245g	198	1.2	81	2.5	16	0.5	0.7
BBQ, Snack, Made Up, Mug Shot, Symingtons*	1 Serving/229g	193	0.7	85	2.4	17.7	0.3	0.7
Beef, Barbecue, Instant, Asda*	1 Pack/333g	420	16	126	2.6	18	4.8	0
Beef, BBQ, Instant, Cooked, Aldi*	1 Serving/324g	515	19.4	159	3.7	21.9	6	1.1
Beef, Chilli, Finest, Tesco*	1 Pack/450g	486	8.6	108	7.7	15.2	1.9	0.9
Beef, Chilli, Ramen, M&S*	1 Pack/484g	532	17.4	110	8.1	11.9	3.6	0.8
Beef, Instant, Prepared, Heinz*	1 Pack/384g	257	0.4	67	2.1	14.4	0.1	0.6
Beef, Oriental, GFY, Asda*	1 Pack/400g	372	6.8	93	7.4	12.1	1.7	1.7
Beef, Shanghai, COU, M&S*	1 Pack/400g	380	6.4	95	6.8	13.1	1.6	1.5
Beef, Szechuan, Dry, Blue Dragon*	½ Pack/100g	350	1.2	350	10.5	72.3	1.2	0
Cellophane, Glass, Dry Weight	**1 Serving/100g**	**351**	**0.1**	**351**	**0.1**	**86.1**	**0.1**	**0.5**
Chicken, & Coconut & Lime, Fuller Longer, M&S*	1 Pack/390g	448	17.6	115	8.7	10	4.5	1.6
Chicken, & Mushroom, Pot, Prepared, NutriPot*	1 Pot/285g	300	2.8	105	7	15.7	1	2.7
Chicken, & Mushroom, Speedy, Newgate, Lidl*	1 Pot/302g	438	14.8	145	3.6	21	4.9	1.1
Chicken, & Red Thai, Easy Steam, Tesco*	1 Serving/400g	556	28.4	139	10.3	8.6	7.1	1.1
Chicken, & Sweetcorn, Snack Pot, Morrisons*	1 Pot/246.5g	249	1.5	101	4.1	19.8	0.6	1.6
Chicken, Chilli, GFY, Asda*	1 Pack/415g	461	3.3	111	6	20	0.8	1
Chicken, Chinese Style, GFY, Asda*	1 Pack/393g	295	6.7	75	6	9	1.7	0.6
Chicken, Chinese, As Consumed, Fresh Ideas, Morrisons*	1 Pot/375g	394	10.9	105	6.3	12.2	2.9	2.7
Chicken, Chinese, Asda*	1 Pot/302g	305	4.2	101	6	16	1.4	0.8
Chicken, Curry Flavour, Instant, Sainsbury's*	1 Pack/85g	167	6.2	196	4.6	27.9	7.3	0.8
Chicken, Flavour, 3 Minute, Dry, Blue Dragon*	1 Pack/85g	403	18.2	475	9.3	61.2	21.4	0
Chicken, Flavour, Dry, Princes*	1 Pack/85g	395	16	465	10	63.8	18.8	0
Chicken, Flavour, Instant, Cooked, Smart Price, Asda*	1 Serving/246g	293	11.1	111	2.8	14.9	4.2	1
Chicken, Flavour, Instant, Made Up, Tesco*	½ Pack/168g	285	10.6	170	4.1	23.7	6.3	1.5
Chicken, Flavour, Instant, Sainsbury's*	1 Pack/335g	549	21.4	164	4.4	22.3	6.4	1.3
Chicken, Flavour, Snack, Made Up, Mug Shot, Symingtons*	1 Mug/243g	175	1.2	75	2.3	14	0.5	1.2
Chicken, Instant, Basics, Sainsbury's*	½ Pack/132.3g	209	7	158	4	23.5	5.3	0.6
Chicken, Instant, Cooked, Aldi*	½ Pack/204g	318	12.6	156	3.4	21.1	6.2	1.1
Chicken, Instant, Made Up, Everyday Value, Tesco*	1 Pack/265g	437	15.6	165	3.8	19.4	5.9	3.2
Chicken, Instant, Weight Watchers*	1 Pack/385g	270	0.4	70	2.3	14.9	0.1	0.6
Chicken, Oriental Style, Instant, Cooked, Koka*	1 Serving/100g	79	3.3	79	1.7	10.7	3.3	0.4
Chicken, Sweet & Sour, Slim Fast*	1 Pot/250g	88	0.8	35	2.4	4.7	0.3	1.9
Chicken, Sweet Chilli, Cooked, My Goodness, Sainsbury's*	1 Pack/380g	321	5.5	87	5.9	11.6	1.5	2

NOODLES

	Measure INFO/WEIGHT	per Measure KCAL	per Measure FAT	Nutrition Values per 100g / 100ml KCAL	PROT	CARB	FAT	FIBRE
Chicken, Teriyaki, Pot, Tesco*	1 Pot/300g	315	4.8	105	5.8	15.9	1.6	1.8
Chicken, Teriyaki, Skinny, City Kitchen, Tesco*	1 Pack/385g	366	5	95	7.2	13	1.3	1.4
Chilli Infused, Blue Dragon*	1 Serving/150g	286	1	191	6.1	33.6	0.7	0.3
Chow Mein, Classic, As Prepared, Fusian, Maggi*	½ Pack/190g	273	11.8	144	3.3	18	6.2	1.7
Chow Mein, Instant, Made Up, Morrisons*	½ Pack/168g	210	7.9	125	3	17.1	4.7	1.2
Chow Mein, Sainsbury's*	1 Pack/125g	136	2.2	109	3.9	19.2	1.8	0.8
Chow Mein, Snack in a Pot, LC, Tesco*	1 Pot/235g	235	1.2	100	3.7	19.4	0.5	1.8
Crispy, Dry, Blue Dragon*	1 Box/125g	438	0.6	350	2.4	84	0.5	0
Curry, Instant, Dry, Asda*	1 Serving/65g	415	11	638	20	101.5	16.9	0.9
Curry, Instant, Dry, Heinz*	1 Serving/85g	261	0.3	307	9.5	66.4	0.4	2.7
Curry, Instant, from Heinz, Weight Watchers*	1 Pack/385g	266	0.4	69	2.2	14.8	0.1	0.6
Curry, Instant, Sainsbury's*	1 Pack/335g	412	15.4	123	2.6	17.8	4.6	0.1
Curry, Instant, Vitasia, Lidl*	1 Pack/108g	124	5.3	115	2.5	15.3	4.9	0
Curry, Singapore, Made Up, Naked Noodle Snack Pot*	1 Pot/329g	270	2	82	2.9	15.7	0.6	0.9
Curry, Spicy, Dry, Princes*	1 Pack/85g	395	16	465	9.6	64.1	18.8	0
Curry, Spicy, Speedy, Newgate, Lidl*	1 Pot/312g	443	13.7	142	3.6	21	4.4	2.1
Duck, Hoi Sin, Beautifully Balanced, HL, Tesco*	1 Pack/367g	341	9.2	93	4.8	12.1	2.5	1.3
Duck, Hoisin, Shredded, Tesco*	1 Pack/385g	655	18.4	170	7.1	24.4	4.8	1.4
Egg, & Bean Sprouts, Cooked, Tesco*	1 Pack/250g	238	5.2	95	4.4	14.6	2.1	1.5
Egg, Asda*	1 Pack/184g	213	12.9	116	2.3	11	7	0.6
Egg, Boiled	*1oz/28g*	*17*	*0.1*	*62*	*2.2*	*13*	*0.5*	*0.6*
Egg, Chilli & Ginger, Asian Fusion, Waitrose*	½ Pack/137g	188	3.3	137	4.4	24	2.4	0.8
Egg, Dry, Average	*1 Block/62.5g*	*218*	*1.2*	*348*	*12.1*	*70.1*	*1.9*	*2.6*
Egg, Fine Thread, Dry, M&S*	1 Serving/63g	220	0.6	350	14.3	71.6	0.9	5.1
Egg, Fine, Blue Dragon*	1 Serving/100g	356	1.7	356	13.8	70	1.7	3.4
Egg, Fine, Dry Weight, Sharwood's*	1 Block/63g	216	1.3	346	12	70	2.1	2.5
Egg, Fine, Fresh, M&S*	1 Pack/275g	330	6.1	120	4.4	20.7	2.2	1.5
Egg, Fine, Waitrose*	¼ Pack/62.5g	221	1.6	353	15	67.3	2.6	3.8
Egg, Free Range, Asda*	1 Serving/125g	205	4.9	164	5.1	27	3.9	1.8
Egg, Free Range, Fresh, Sainsbury's*	½ Pack/205g	340	7	166	5	28	3.4	1.8
Egg, Free Range, Morrisons*	1 Pack/300g	372	8.7	124	4.9	19.7	2.9	1.3
Egg, Fresh, Just Stir Fry, Sainsbury's*	½ Pack/192g	314	6.5	163	5	28.1	3.4	1.8
Egg, Fresh, Tesco*	½ Pack/205g	287	3.9	140	4.8	25.3	1.9	2
Egg, M&S*	½ Pack/110g	165	1.9	150	4.9	28.3	1.7	2.8
Egg, Medium, Asda*	1 Serving/83.3g	125	0.7	150	4.8	31	0.8	1.3
Egg, Medium, Dry Nests, Cooks' Ingredients, Waitrose*	1 Nest/54g	189	0.9	350	13.2	70.4	1.7	2.4
Egg, Medium, Dry, Blue Dragon*	1 Serving/50g	158	1.2	317	10.1	62.3	2.4	3.1
Egg, Medium, Dry, Sharwood's*	1 Serving/63g	216	1.3	346	12	70	2.1	2.5
Egg, Medium, Sainsbury's*	1 Serving/122g	168	1	138	5.7	26.9	0.8	1
Egg, Raw, Medium, Waitrose*	¼ Pack/63g	221	1.6	353	15	67.3	2.6	3.8
Egg, Thick, Dry Weight, Sharwood's*	1 Serving/63g	214	1.1	342	10.8	71	1.7	2.5
Egg, Tossed in Sesame Oil, Asda*	½ Pack/150g	174	10.5	116	2.3	11	7	0.6
Fried, Average	*1oz/28g*	*43*	*3.2*	*153*	*1.9*	*11.3*	*11.5*	*0.5*
Garlic, Chilli & Ginger, Tesco*	1 Serving/350g	508	11.2	145	4.8	24.1	3.2	2.6
Instant, Dry, Sainsbury's*	1 Pack/100g	392	14	392	9.4	57	14	0.2
Instant, Express, Dry, Blue Dragon*	1 Serving/75g	338	12.8	450	10	65	17	2
Instant, Value, Tesco*	1 Pack/265g	334	9	126	3.2	20.7	3.4	0.9
Japanese Udon, Sainsbury's*	1 Serving/150g	210	2.7	140	3.9	27.1	1.8	1.2
Medium, Soft, Ready to Wok, Asia Specialities, Aldi*	1 Serving/150g	232	0.9	155	6.6	30	0.6	1.6
Medium, Traditional, Straight to Wok, Amoy*	1 Serving/150g	243	2.2	162	4.3	34.3	1.5	1.3
Nest, Medium, Cooked, Waitrose*	1 Nest/63g	88	0.3	139	5	28.6	0.5	0.6
Oriental, Chinese, Tesco*	1 Pack/200g	184	5	92	2.8	14.7	2.5	1
Oriental, Snack Pot, Made Up, HL, Tesco*	1 Serving/238g	221	0.7	93	3.1	19.4	0.3	0.6

	Measure INFO/WEIGHT	per Measure		Nutrition Values per 100g / 100ml				
		KCAL	FAT	KCAL	PROT	CARB	FAT	FIBRE
NOODLES								
Pad Thai, Ribbon, Ready to Wok, Sharwood's*	1 Serving/150g	206	1.7	137	5	26.3	1.1	1
Plain, Boiled	*1oz/28g*	*17*	*0.1*	*62*	*2.4*	*13*	*0.4*	*0.7*
Plain, Dry	*1oz/28g*	*109*	*1.7*	*388*	*11.7*	*76.1*	*6.2*	*2.9*
Pork, Chinese, CBY, Asda*	1 Pack/400g	380	6.4	95	6.7	12.6	1.6	1.8
Prawn, Hot & Sour, King, Bowl, My Goodness, Sainsbury's*	1 Pack/360g	324	3.2	90	4.7	15.1	0.9	1.1
Prawn, Tiger, Stir Fry, Tesco*	1 Pack/400g	596	14.8	149	6	23	3.7	2.7
Rainbow Vegetable Pad Thai, Everdine*	1 Serving/450g	508	21.6	113	3.6	12.4	4.8	3
Ramen, Morrisons*	1/3 Pack/83g	289	0.7	348	11.1	72.7	0.8	2.8
Ribbon, Thai Style, Ready to Wok, Sharwood's*	1 Pack/150g	206	1.7	137	5	26.3	1.1	1
Rice, Cooked	*1 Cup/176g*	*192*	*0.4*	*109*	*0.9*	*24.9*	*0.2*	*1*
Rice, Cooked, Sharwood's*	1 Serving/200g	239	0.6	120	2	27.2	0.3	0.8
Rice, Dry, Amoy*	1oz/28g	101	0.3	361	6.5	86.6	1	0
Rice, Dry, Blue Dragon*	1 Serving/30g	113	0	376	7	84	0	0
Rice, Fresh, Sainsbury's*	½ Pack/150g	202	3.3	135	2.2	25.9	2.2	1.4
Rice, Medium, Blue Dragon*	1 Serving/63g	235	0	376	7	84	0	0
Rice, Oriental, Thai, Stir Fry, Dry Weight, Sharwood's*	1 Serving/63g	226	0.6	361	6.5	86.8	1	2.4
Rice, Stir Fry, Tesco*	½ Pack/190g	304	10.8	160	2	24.8	5.7	1
Rice, Thick, Thai, Dry, M&S*	1 Serving/100g	355	0.7	355	6.5	80.6	0.7	1.4
Rice, with Spring Onions, Fresh Tastes, Asda*	½ Pack/188g	248	4.1	132	2.2	25.9	2.2	1.4
Singapore, BGTY, Sainsbury's*	1 Pack/369g	317	10	86	7.2	8.2	2.7	2.1
Singapore, Everdine*	1 Serving/450g	414	15.8	92	2.8	10.5	3.5	3.7
Singapore, Morrisons*	1 Serving/400g	480	26.8	120	4.8	11.6	6.7	1.6
Singapore, Sainsbury's*	1 Pack/400g	432	15.6	108	6.5	11.7	3.9	2.8
Singapore, Sainsbury's*	1 Pack/400g	368	6.8	92	7.5	11.6	1.7	0.9
Singapore, Style, Asda*	1 Pack/400g	688	32	172	7	18	8	1
Singapore, Waitrose*	1 Pack/400g	476	17.6	119	7.3	12.6	4.4	2.1
Singapore, You Count, Love Life, Waitrose*	1 Pot/260g	243	5	97	5.4	13.3	2	2.2
Special, Chinese Takeaway, Iceland*	1 Pack/340g	422	10.9	124	6.5	17.2	3.2	0.6
Spicy, Sainsbury's*	1 Serving/180g	182	8.3	101	10.4	4.5	4.6	0.9
Stir Fry, Tesco*	1 Serving/150g	202	3.6	135	5.3	23	2.4	1.5
Straight to Wok, Medium, Amoy*	1 Pack/150g	240	2.2	160	5.8	31.7	1.5	0
Straight to Wok, Rice, Amoy*	1 Pack/150g	174	0.2	116	1.6	27.4	0.1	0
Straight to Wok, Singapore, Amoy*	1 Serving/150g	232	4.2	155	4.8	28.4	2.8	0
Straight to Wok, Thread, Fine, Amoy*	1 Pack/150g	237	3.9	158	5	28.7	2.6	0
Straight to Wok, Udon, Amoy*	1 Pack/150g	212	2	141	4.4	28.8	1.3	0
Super, Bacon Flavour, Dry Weight, Batchelors*	1 Pack/100g	526	23.6	526	9.4	69.2	23.6	1.6
Super, Barbecue Beef, Made Up, Batchelors*	1 Serving/100g	156	6.7	156	3.2	20.9	6.7	1.1
Super, Barbecue Beef, to Go, 98% Fat Free, Batchelors*	1 Pack/380g	308	0.6	81	2.4	17.6	0.2	0.6
Super, Chicken & Ham, Dry Weight, Batchelors*	1 Pack/100g	472	20.2	472	9.4	63.2	20.2	1.5
Super, Chicken & Herb, Low Fat, Made Up, Batchelors*	1 Pack/170g	322	1.6	189	6.1	39.2	0.9	1.2
Super, Chicken & Herb, Low Fat, Dry Weight, Batchelors*	½ Pack/43g	161	0.8	379	12.2	78.4	1.9	2.4
Super, Chicken Flavour, Made Up, Batchelors*	1 Serving/150g	264	11.8	176	3.1	23	7.9	0.4
Super, Chow Mein Flavour, Made Up, Batchelors*	½ Pack/150g	262	11.8	175	3	23	7.9	0.4
Super, Mild Curry Flavour, Made Up, Batchelors*	1 Serving/100g	157	6.7	157	3.2	20.9	6.7	1
Super, Mild Curry, Dry Weight, Batchelors*	½ Pack/50g	260	11.7	520	9.4	67.8	23.4	1.4
Super, Sweet Thai Chilli, Dry Weight, Batchelors*	1 Pack/85g	292	1	343	10.6	72.5	1.2	3
Sweet Chilli, Sainsbury's*	½ Pack/110g	172	6	156	4	24.6	5.5	1
Thai Glass, Vermicelli, Wai Wai*	1oz/28g	112	0.3	400	7.3	89.1	0.9	1.8
Thai Style, Sainsbury's*	1 Pack/340g	381	7.8	112	3.3	19.4	2.3	0.7
Thai Style, Snack, Cupshotz, Aldi*	1 Pack/55g	215	2.8	391	11.4	71.4	5.1	6.9
Thai, Spicy, Instant, Heinz*	1 Pack/385g	262	0.4	68	2.1	14.6	0.1	0.6
Thai, Spicy, Stir Fry, HL, Tesco*	½ Pack/250g	220	5.5	88	4.1	12.9	2.2	1.7
Thai, Waitrose*	1 Pack/300g	357	6.3	119	6.8	18.4	2.1	1.7

	Measure INFO/WEIGHT	per Measure KCAL	FAT	Nutrition Values per 100g / 100ml KCAL	PROT	CARB	FAT	FIBRE
NOODLES								
Udon, Japanese & Dashi Soup Stock, Yutaka*	1 Pack/230g	290	1.2	126	3	26.8	0.5	0
Udon, Style, Thick, Ready to Wok, Sharwood's*	1 Pack/150g	233	0.6	155	5.4	32.5	0.4	2.1
Udon, with Chicken, Indian Inspired, Pot, Itsu*	1 Pot/492g	295	3.4	60	2.1	10.3	0.7	1.8
Vegetable, Savoury, COU, M&S*	1 Pack/450g	270	2.7	60	2.9	11.5	0.6	1.2
Vermicelli Rice, Mama*	1 Serving/45g	166	0.4	370	7	81	1	0
Wheat, Udon, Organic, Explore Asian*	1 Serving/56g	202	1.2	361	14.3	71.4	2.1	1.8
Wholewheat, & Vegetable Stir Fry, As Prepared, Waitrose*	1 Pack/265g	257	5.2	104	4.6	14.9	2.1	3.6
Wholewheat, Cooked Weight, Sharwoods*	1 Portion/161g	215	1.5	134	5	24.8	0.9	2.7
Wholewheat, Dry, Blue Dragon*	1 Serving/65g	208	1.3	320	12.5	63	2	8
Wholewheat, Dry, Sharwoods*	1 Portion/63g	224	1.4	356	13	66.2	2.3	9.2
NOUGAT								
Average	*1 Sm Bar/28g*	*108*	*2.4*	*384*	*4.4*	*77.3*	*8.5*	*0.9*
Raspberry & Orange Hazelnut, Thorntons*	1 Sweet/9g	39	1.8	433	4.8	60	20	2.2
Soft, Bar, Bassett's*	1 Bar/25g	94	1	375	4	82	4	0
NUT ROAST								
Average	*1 Serving/200g*	*704*	*51.4*	*352*	*13.3*	*18.3*	*25.7*	*4.2*
Courgette & Spiced Tomato, Cauldron Foods*	1 Serving/100g	208	12.3	208	11.7	12.5	12.3	4.9
Lentil, Average	*1oz/28g*	*62*	*3.4*	*222*	*10.6*	*18.8*	*12.1*	*3.8*
NUTMEG								
Ground, Average	*1 Tsp/3g*	*16*	*1.1*	*525*	*5.8*	*45.3*	*36.3*	*0*
NUTS								
Assortment, Eat Well, M&S*	1 Pack/70g	441	41.2	630	16.7	8.5	58.9	5.3
Brazil, Chocolate, Dark, Bolivian, Hotel Chocolat*	½ Pack/50g	303	24	606	10	34	48	4
Cashews & Peanuts, Honey Roasted, Average	*1 Serving/50g*	*290*	*21.4*	*579*	*21.6*	*26.6*	*42.9*	*4.2*
Medley, On the Go, Sainsbury's*	1 Pack/20g	127	11.2	636	19.8	9.2	56.1	7.5
Mixed	*1 Pack/40g*	*243*	*21.6*	*607*	*22.9*	*7.9*	*54.1*	*6*
Mixed, Almonds, Brazil, Hazel & Walnuts, M&S*	1 Serving/25g	168	16	670	16	4.8	64	5.4
Mixed, Chopped, Tesco*	1 Serving/25g	149	12.6	595	23.5	10.5	50.6	6
Mixed, Delicious, Boots*	1 Pack/50g	332	29	663	16	16	58	8.1
Mixed, Natural Energy, Graze*	1 Punnet/37g	231	20.3	625	19	17	55	10
Mixed, Natural, Asda*	1 Snack/30g	197	18.8	656	18	4.3	62.7	7.4
Mixed, Natural, Luxury, Tesco*	1oz/28g	179	16.2	639	22.6	6.9	57.9	5.6
Mixed, Roasted, Salted, Waitrose*	1 Pack/200g	1252	116.8	626	13.7	11.3	58.4	4.4
Mixed, Roasted, Waitrose*	1 Serving/25g	166	16	662	15.2	6.2	64	8.2
Mixed, Unsalted, Sainsbury's*	1 Serving/50g	311	28.8	622	18.5	7.2	57.7	8.7
Mixed, Wholesome, Love Life, Waitrose*	1 Serving/30g	206	19.6	685	14.6	5	65.2	5.4
Omega Booster Seeds, Graze*	1 Punnet/34g	189	16.5	553	22.1	16.4	48.3	11.1
Peanuts & Cashews, Honey Roast, Tesco*	1 Serving/25g	145	10.7	579	21.6	26.6	42.9	4.2
Pine, Tesco*	1 Pack/100g	699	68.6	699	16.5	4	68.6	1.9
NUTS & RAISINS								
Mixed, Average	*1 Serving/30g*	*144*	*10.2*	*481*	*14.1*	*31.5*	*34.1*	*4.5*
Mixed, KP Snacks*	1 Serving/50g	273	20.2	546	21.4	24.4	40.3	5.2
Mixed, Tesco*	1 Serving/25g	115	6.9	450	18.6	32.6	26.8	12.5
Peanuts, Mixed, Average	*1 Pack/40g*	*174*	*10.4*	*435*	*15.3*	*37.5*	*26*	*4.4*
Yoghurt Coated, Waitrose*	1 Serving/50g	264	18.4	527	10.9	38.2	36.7	3
NUTS & SEEDS								
Chilli Almond Seed Shot, On the Go, Sainsbury's*	1 Pack/23g	140	11.5	609	27.3	7.1	50.2	9.6
Milk Chocolate & Salted Caramel, Graze*	1 Pack/33g	193	14.5	585	12	37	44	5.5

	Measure INFO/WEIGHT	per Measure KCAL	FAT	Nutrition Values per 100g / 100ml KCAL	PROT	CARB	FAT	FIBRE
OAT CAKES								
Cheese, Nairn's*	1 Cake/8g	39	2.3	471	13.2	43.3	27.2	6.8
Fine Milled, Nairn's*	1 Cake/7.8g	35	1.7	449	10.5	52.6	21.8	8.6
Herb & Pumpkin Seed, Nairn's*	1 Cake/10g	43	2.1	426	12.2	46.8	21.1	13
Highland, Walkers*	1 Cake/12g	54	2.5	451	10.3	56	20.6	6.7
Oatmeal, Rough, Nairn's*	1 Cake/11g	45	1.8	431	10.2	58.6	17.3	8
Oatmeal, Rough, Organic, Nairn's*	1 Cake/10.3g	43	1.7	418	10.2	57.7	16.3	7.5
Orkney, Thick, Stockan's*	1 Oatcake/27g	122	5.2	487	8.7	66.7	20.6	6.3
Orkney, Thin, Stockan's*	1 Oatcake/100g	453	23	453	11.1	50.3	23	6
Retail, Average	**1 Cake/13g**	**57**	**2.4**	**441**	**10**	**63**	**18.3**	**2**
Rough Scottish, Sainsbury's*	1 Cake/11g	51	2.1	462	12.3	59.9	19.3	6.5
Rough with Olive Oil, Paterson's*	1 Cake/12.5g	54	2.2	431	10.6	58.4	17.2	8.1
Rough, Sainsbury's*	1 Cake/11g	45	1.8	426	11.7	65.2	16.9	8.6
Rough, Scottish, Tesco*	1 Cake/10.3g	45	1.9	435	11.4	55.3	18.4	8
Scottish, Asda*	1 Oatcake/13g	58	2.3	461	11	59	18	9.8
Scottish, Rough, Waitrose*	1 Cake/12.5g	55	2.3	438	10.4	57.4	18.5	8
Scottish, Tower Gate, Lidl*	1 Oatcake/13g	60	2.5	465	10	60	19	6.8
Traditional, M&S*	1 Cake/11g	49	2	445	11	59.3	18.3	6.6
OAT DRINK								
Healthy, Enriched, Oatly*	1 Serving/250ml	112	3.8	45	1	6.5	1.5	0.8
Oat Milk, Organic, Healthy, Oatly*	1 Serving/250ml	88	1.8	35	1	6.5	0.7	0.8
OCTOPUS								
Chunks in Olive Oil, Palacio De Oriente*	1 Tin/111g	148	4	133	21.6	4.5	3.6	0
Raw	**1oz/28g**	**18**	**0.3**	**66**	**14.1**	**0**	**1**	**0**
OIL								
Active, Saffola*	1 Tbsp/15ml	14	1.5	90	0	0	10	0
Avocado, Olivado*	1 Tsp/5ml	40	4.4	802	0	0	88	0
Black Truffle, Grapeseed, Cuisine Perel*	1 Tsp/5ml	43	5	857	0	7.1	100	0
Chilli, Average	**1 Tsp/5ml**	**41**	**4.6**	**824**	**0**	**0**	**91.5**	**0**
Chinese Stir Fry, Asda*	1 Tbsp/15ml	123	13.7	823	0	0	91.4	0
Coconut, Average	**1 Tsp/5ml**	**45**	**5**	**899**	**0**	**0**	**99.9**	**0**
Cod Liver, Average	**1 Capsule/1g**	**9**	**1**	**900**	**0**	**0**	**100**	**0**
Corn, Average	**1 Tsp/5ml**	**43**	**4.8**	**864**	**0**	**0**	**96**	**0**
Cuisine, Flora*	1 Tsp/5ml	32	3.5	630	0.1	1	70.3	0
Dipping, Herb, Italian Style, Finest, Tesco*	1 Serving/5g	44	4.8	877	0.4	0.9	96.9	0.4
Dipping, with Balsamic Vinegar, Finest, Tesco*	1 Tsp/5ml	33	3.6	668	0	4.4	71.7	0
Evening Primrose, Average	**1 Serving/1g**	**9**	**1**	**900**	**0**	**0**	**100**	**0**
Fish, Average	**1 Serving/1g**	**9**	**1**	**900**	**0**	**0**	**100**	**0**
Flax Seed, Average	**1 Tbsp/15ml**	**124**	**13.9**	**829**	**0**	**0**	**92.6**	**0**
Fry Light, Bodyline*	1 Spray/0.25ml	1	0.1	522	0	0	55.2	0
Garlic, Infuse, Fry Light*	1 Spray/0.2ml	1	0.1	507	0	0.4	52.9	0
Gold, Saffola*	1 Tbsp/15ml	14	1.5	90	0	0	10	0
Grapeseed, Average	**1 Tsp/5ml**	**43**	**4.8**	**866**	**0**	**0**	**96.2**	**0**
Groundnut, Average	**1 Tsp/5ml**	**41**	**4.6**	**824**	**0**	**0**	**91.8**	**0**
Hazelnut, Average	**1 Tsp/5ml**	**45**	**5**	**899**	**0**	**0**	**99.9**	**0**
Linseed, Organic, Biona*	1 Serving/10ml	84	9.3	837	0	0	93	0
Macadamia Nut, Oz Tukka*	1 Tsp/5ml	40	4.6	805	0	0	91	0
Mustard, Average	**1 Serving/100g**	**884**	**100**	**884**	**0**	**0**	**100**	**0**
Olive, Average	**1 Tsp/5ml**	**43**	**4.7**	**855**	**0**	**0**	**94.9**	**0**
Olive, Basil Infused, Tesco*	1 Serving/20ml	180	20	900	0	0	100	0
Olive, Evo Filtered, Italian, Parioli, Cucina*	1 Serving/100ml	825	91.6	825	0	0	91.6	0
Olive, Extra Virgin, Average	**1 Tsp/5ml**	**42**	**4.7**	**848**	**0**	**0**	**94.5**	**0**
Olive, Extra Virgin, Only 1 Cal, Spray, Fry Light*	1 Spray/0.2ml	1	0.1	498	0	0	55.2	0
Olive, Garlic, Average	**1 Tbsp/15ml**	**127**	**14.1**	**848**	**0**	**0**	**94.3**	**0**

	Measure INFO/WEIGHT	per Measure KCAL	FAT	Nutrition Values per 100g / 100ml KCAL	PROT	CARB	FAT	FIBRE
OIL								
Olive, Lemon Flavoured, Sainsbury's*	1 Tbsp/15ml	123	13.7	823	0.1	0	91.4	0.1
Olive, Mild, Average	*1 Tbsp/15ml*	*129*	*14.4*	*862*	*0*	*0*	*95.7*	*0*
Olive, Spray, Average	*10 Sprays/2ml*	*10*	*1.1*	*508*	*0*	*0*	*54.6*	*0*
Olive, Spray, Fry Light*	5 Sprays/1ml	5	0.5	520	0	0	54.2	0
Palm, Average	*1 Tsp/5ml*	*45*	*5*	*899*	*0*	*0*	*99.9*	*0*
Peanut, Average	*1 Tsp/5ml*	*45*	*5*	*899*	*0*	*0*	*99.9*	*0*
Rapeseed, Average	*1 Tbsp/15ml*	*130*	*14.4*	*864*	*0*	*0*	*96*	*0*
Red Palm & Canola, Carotino*	1 Tsp/5ml	41	4.6	812	0	0	92	0
Rice Bran, Alpha One, Hansells Foods*	1 Serving/4ml	32	3.7	812	0	0	92	0
Rice Bran, Alphaone*	1 Tbsp/14g	120	13.6	880	0	0	100	0
Rice Bran, Average	*1 Tbsp/14g*	*120*	*13.6*	*884*	*0*	*0*	*100*	*0*
Safflower, Average	*1 Tsp/5ml*	*45*	*5*	*899*	*0*	*0*	*99.9*	*0*
Sesame, Average	*1 Tsp/5ml*	*45*	*5*	*892*	*0.1*	*0*	*99.9*	*0*
Soya, Average	*1 Tsp/5ml*	*45*	*5*	*899*	*0*	*0*	*99.9*	*0*
Sunflower & Extra Virgin Olive Oil 15%, Sainsbury's*	1 Tsp/5ml	41	4.6	827	0.5	0.5	91.9	0.5
Sunflower, Average	*1 Tsp/5ml*	*43*	*4.8*	*869*	*0*	*0*	*96.6*	*0*
Sunflower, Spray, Fry Light*	1 Spray/0.2ml	1	0.1	522	0	0	55.2	0
Ultimate Blend, Udo's Choice*	1 Capsule/1ml	9	1	900	1.3	0	96.8	0
Vegetable, Average	*1 Tbsp/15ml*	*129*	*14.3*	*858*	*0*	*0*	*95.3*	*0*
Virgin Coconut, Spray, Groovy Food Company*	1 Spray/0.2ml	1	0.1	475	0	0	53.3	0
Walnut, Average	*1 Tsp/5ml*	*45*	*5*	*899*	*0*	*0*	*99.9*	*0*
OKRA								
Boiled in Unsalted Water, Average	*1 Serving/80g*	*22*	*0.7*	*28*	*2.5*	*2.7*	*0.9*	*3.6*
Raw, Average	*1 Serving/80g*	*18*	*0.6*	*23*	*2.1*	*2.2*	*0.7*	*3*
Stir-Fried in Corn Oil, Average	*1 Serving/80g*	*215*	*20.9*	*269*	*4.3*	*4.4*	*26.1*	*6.3*
OLIVES								
Black & Green with Greek Feta Cheese, Tesco*	1 Pot/100g	200	20.1	200	3.4	0.3	20.1	4.6
Black, Pitted, Average	*½ Jar/82g*	*135*	*13.3*	*164*	*1*	*3.5*	*16.2*	*3.1*
Green & Harissa, Graze*	1 Punnet/44g	110	11.6	255	0.8	2	27	3
Green, Garlic Stuffed, Asda*	1 Olive/3g	6	0.6	174	1.8	3.5	17	0
Green, Lightly Flavoured with Lemon & Garlic, Attis*	1 Serving/50g	82	8.2	164	1.7	2.2	16.5	0
Green, Pimiento Stuffed, Somerfield*	1 Olive/3g	4	0.4	126	1	4	12	0
Green, Pitted, Average	*1 Olive/3g*	*4*	*0.4*	*130*	*1.1*	*0.9*	*13.3*	*2.5*
Green, Pitted, Stuffed with Anchovies, Sainsbury's*	1 Serving/50g	78	8	155	1.8	0.6	16.1	3.2
Green, Stuffed with Almonds, Pitted, Waitrose*	1 Serving/50g	90	8.4	180	3.8	3.2	16.9	2.5
Halkidiki, Stuffed with Garlic, Tesco*	¼ Pack/40g	66	6.7	164	1.3	0.3	16.8	3
Kalamata with Herbs, Graze*	1 Punnet/52g	144	15.3	277	0.6	1.7	29.4	3.1
Kalamata, Pitted, Greek, Drained, Sainsbury's*	1 Serving/15g	31	3.2	205	1.6	0.5	21.4	3.2
Manzanilla, Marinated with Chilli, Lidl*	1 Pot/140g	230	23.1	164	1.4	0.3	16.5	0
Marinated, Mixed, M&S*	1 Serving/20g	33	3	165	1.6	6.5	14.9	3
Marinated, Selection, M&S*	4 Olives/20g	44	4.4	225	1.4	3.9	22.6	2.1
Mixed, & Greek Feta, Sainsburys*	1 Serving/50g	114	10.8	227	5.8	1.3	21.6	2
Mixed, Chilli & Garlic, Asda*	1 Serving/30g	43	4.7	144	0.9	0	15.6	6.1
with Chipotle & Manchego, Unearthed*	1 Pack/184g	482	44.7	262	8.1	4	24.3	0
with Garlic And Herb, Delicious, Boots*	1 Pack/70g	113	11.9	161	1.7	0.1	17	1.9
OMELETTE								
Cheese & Mushroom, Apetito*	1 Serving/320g	486	25	152	6.2	14.4	7.8	1.9
Cheese, 2 Egg, Average	*1 Omelette/180g*	*479*	*40.7*	*266*	*15.9*	*0*	*22.6*	*0*
Cheese, Asda*	1 Omelette/119g	268	22.6	225	12	1.5	19	0
Ham & Mushroom, Farmfoods*	1 Omelette/120g	200	16.7	167	8.7	1.8	13.9	0.1
Mushroom & Cheese, Tesco*	1 Omelette/120g	248	21.5	207	9.8	1.6	17.9	0.2
Plain, 2 Egg	*1 Omelette/120g*	*229*	*19.7*	*191*	*10.9*	*0*	*16.4*	*0*
Spanish	*1oz/28g*	*34*	*2.3*	*120*	*5.7*	*6.2*	*8.3*	*1.4*

O

	Measure INFO/WEIGHT	per Measure		Nutrition Values per 100g / 100ml				
		KCAL	FAT	KCAL	PROT	CARB	FAT	FIBRE

OMELETTE
Spanish, 344, Wiltshire Farm Foods*	1 Serving/390g	515	22.6	132	5.5	13	5.8	0
Spanish, Potato, Rapido, Unearthed*	1 Pack/300g	492	32.7	164	5.2	10.5	10.9	2.2

ONION POWDER
Average	*1 Tsp/2g*	*7*	*0*	*341*	*10.4*	*79.1*	*1*	*15.2*

ONION RINGS
Battered, Oven Baked, Tesco*	1 Serving/50g	110	5	219	3.9	28.4	10	3.5
Battered, Sainsbury's*	1 Ring/12g	26	1.2	219	3.9	28.4	10	3.5
Breaded & Fried, From Restaurant	*1 Ring/12g*	*40*	*2.2*	*332*	*4.5*	*37.7*	*18.7*	*0*
Breaded, Asda*	1 Serving/10g	29	1.5	289	4.4	34	15	2.7
Breaded, Iceland*	1 Ring/11g	33	1.7	293	4.4	34.2	15.4	2.7
Oven Crisp Batter, Tesco*	1 Ring/17g	40	2.3	236	4.2	24.8	13.3	2.5

ONIONS
Baked	*1oz/28g*	*29*	*0.2*	*103*	*3.5*	*22.3*	*0.6*	*3.9*
Boiled in Unsalted Water	*1oz/28g*	*5*	*0*	*17*	*0.6*	*3.7*	*0.1*	*0.7*
Dried, Raw, Average	*1oz/28g*	*88*	*0.5*	*313*	*10.2*	*68.6*	*1.7*	*12.1*
Fried, Average	*1oz/28g*	*46*	*3.1*	*164*	*2.3*	*14.1*	*11.2*	*3.1*
Pickled, Average	*1 Onion/15g*	*3*	*0*	*19*	*0.7*	*4.1*	*0.1*	*0.6*
Raw, Average	*1 Med/180g*	*69*	*0.4*	*38*	*1.2*	*7.9*	*0.2*	*1.3*
Red, Raw, Average	*1 Med/180g*	*66*	*0.4*	*37*	*1.2*	*7.9*	*0.2*	*1.5*
Spring, Raw, Average	*1 Med/15g*	*4*	*0.1*	*24*	*1.9*	*2.9*	*0.5*	*1.4*

ORANGE CURD
Baxters*	1 Tbsp/15g	51	1.1	343	2	67	7.4	0.1
Florida, Finest, Tesco*	1 Tbsp/15g	52	1.3	348	2.9	63.8	9	0.2
Jaffa, Luxury, Waitrose*	1 Tbsp/15g	54	1.5	357	3	63.5	10.1	0.1
Sainsbury's*	2 Tsps/12g	34	0.5	282	1.1	59.2	4.4	0.4

ORANGES
Blood, Average	*1 Orange/140g*	*82*	*0*	*58*	*0.8*	*13.3*	*0*	*2.5*
Fresh, Weighed with Peel, Average	*1oz/28g*	*7*	*0*	*26*	*0.8*	*6*	*0*	*1.2*
Fresh, without Peel, Average	*1 Med/145g*	*54*	*0.1*	*37*	*1.1*	*8.5*	*0.1*	*1.7*
Peel Only, Raw, Average	*1 Tbsp/6g*	*6*	*0*	*97*	*1.5*	*25*	*0.2*	*10.6*
Ruby Red, Tesco*	1 Med/130g	51	0.1	39	1.1	8.5	0.1	1.7
Segments, in Juice, Canned, Morrisons*	1 Portion/80g	36	0.1	45	0.4	10.3	0.1	0.5

OREGANO
Dried	*1 Tsp/1g*	*3*	*0.1*	*306*	*11*	*49.5*	*10.3*	*0*
Fresh	*1 Tsp/1.3g*	*1*	*0*	*66*	*2.2*	*9.7*	*2*	*0*

OSTRICH
Steak, Fillet, Klein Karoo*	1 Fillet/125g	141	2.6	113	23.1	1	2.1	1
Steaks, in Marrakesh Marinade, South African, Deluxe*	1 Steak/150g	158	1.4	105	20	4.1	0.9	0

OVALTINE*
Chocolate, Light, Ovaltine*	1 Serving/20g	76	1.2	380	8.5	70.5	6	4.5
Chocolate, Light, Sachet, Ovaltine*	1 Sachet/25g	96	1.5	384	7.4	73	5.9	4.7
Hi Malt, Light, Instant Drink, Ovaltine*	1 Sachet/20g	72	1.2	358	9.1	67.1	5.9	2.8
Powder, Made Up with Semi-Skimmed Milk, Ovaltine*	1 Mug/227ml	179	3.9	79	3.9	13	1.7	0
Powder, Made Up with Whole Milk, Ovaltine*	1 Mug/227ml	220	8.6	97	3.8	12.9	3.8	0

OXTAIL
Raw	*1oz/28g*	*18*	*1.1*	*65*	*7.6*	*0*	*3.8*	*0*
Stewed, Bone Removed	*1oz/28g*	*68*	*3.8*	*243*	*30.5*	*0*	*13.4*	*0*

OYSTERS
Raw, Shelled, Shucked	*1 Oyster/14g*	*9*	*0.2*	*65*	*10.8*	*2.7*	*1.3*	*0*

	Measure INFO/WEIGHT	per Measure KCAL	FAT	Nutrition Values per 100g / 100ml KCAL	PROT	CARB	FAT	FIBRE
PAELLA								
Bistro, Waitrose*	1 Serving/300g	534	19.8	178	7.4	22.2	6.6	0.7
Chicken, & Chorizo, & Prawn, City Kitchen, Tesco*	1 Pack/400g	540	20	135	4.7	17	5	1.4
Chicken, & Chorizo, Asda*	1 Pack/390g	484	8.6	124	10	16	2.2	2.6
Chicken, & Chorizo, Big Dish, M&S*	1 Pack/450g	630	17.6	140	7.9	18.4	3.9	1.6
Chicken, & Prawn, Frozen, Microwaved, Slimzone, Asda*	1 Pack/459g	358	2.3	78	5.8	11	0.5	2
Chicken, & Prawn, King, Balanced for You, M&S*	1 Pack/390g	425	8.6	109	8.3	13.4	2.2	1.2
Chicken, & Prawn, Meal in a Bag, Cooked, Iceland*	½ Bag/373g	500	18.3	134	4.4	17.1	4.9	1.7
Chicken, & Prawn, with Cod, & Salmon, Sainsbury's*	1 Pack/750g	772	1.5	103	8.3	16.9	0.2	3.1
Chicken, As Prepared, My Healthy Kitchen*	1 Pack/400g	476	14.2	121	6.1	15.5	3.6	1.2
Chicken, Chorizo & King Prawn, Finest, Tesco*	1 Pack/450g	666	19.4	148	7	19.6	4.3	1.7
Chicken, Chorizo, & Prawn, Chargrilled, Gastropub, M&S*	1 Pack/375g	596	17.2	159	8.1	20.8	4.6	1.2
Chicken, King Prawns & Chorizo, Fuller Longer, M&S*	1 Pack/390g	410	11.3	105	9.8	10.1	2.9	1.6
Cooked, Quorn*	1 Pack/376g	361	8.3	96	4.1	13.6	2.2	2.9
Pepper, & Courgette, Smoky Piquillo, Tesco*	1 Pack/393g	322	4.3	82	2.1	14.8	1.1	2
Seafood, Finest, Tesco*	1 Pack/400g	756	23.6	189	6.8	27.2	5.9	1
Seafood, Sainsbury's*	1 Pack/400g	504	5.2	126	8.3	20.3	1.3	0.6
PAIN AU CHOCOLAT								
All Butter, Tesco*	1 Serving/59g	242	11.6	410	8.2	49.4	19.7	2.3
Average	*1 Pastry/60g*	*253*	*13.7*	*422*	*8*	*45.8*	*22.8*	*3.1*
Chocolate Filled, CBY, Asda*	1 Pastry/45g	198	11.3	441	7.1	44.9	25.2	2.9
M&S*	1 Pastry/60g	210	11.5	350	5.9	38	19.2	1.6
Mini, Asda*	1 Pastry/23g	96	5.5	420	8	43	24	3.3
Sainsbury's*	1 Pastry/58g	241	13.8	415	7.9	42.5	23.7	3.3
Waitrose*	1 Pastry/52.9g	230	12.6	435	8.8	45.5	23.9	3.7
PAIN AU RAISIN								
Takeaway, Average	*1 Pastry/100g*	*313*	*13.2*	*313*	*5.2*	*43*	*13.2*	*1.3*
Twist, Extra Special, Asda*	1 Pastry/110g	421	20.9	383	7	46	19	2.5
PAK CHOI								
Raw, Average	*1 Leaf/14g*	*2*	*0*	*11*	*1.3*	*1.9*	*0.2*	*0.9*
PAKORA								
Bhaji, Onion, Fried in Vegetable Oil	*1oz/28g*	*76*	*4.1*	*271*	*9.8*	*26.2*	*14.7*	*5.5*
Bhajia, Potato Carrot & Pea, Fried in Vegetable Oil	*1oz/28g*	*100*	*6.3*	*357*	*10.9*	*28.8*	*22.6*	*6.1*
Bhajia, Vegetable, Retail	*1oz/28g*	*66*	*4.1*	*235*	*6.4*	*21.4*	*14.7*	*3.6*
Chicken, Indian, Waitrose*	1 Pakora/25g	47	1.3	188	21.9	13.1	5.3	0
Chicken, Tikka, Asda*	1 Pack/350g	696	38.5	199	16	9	11	1.1
Spinach, Mini, Indian Selection, Somerfield*	1 Serving/22g	61	3.5	277	6.2	26.9	16.1	4.9
Vegetable, Indian Starter Selection, M&S*	1 Pakora/20g	43	0.6	214	1.2	4.1	3.2	0.9
Vegetable, Mini, Indian Snack Collection, Tesco*	1 Pakora/21g	36	1.9	173	6	16.8	9.1	4.9
Vegetable, Somerfield*	1 Pakora/15g	46	3.4	305	7	19	23	0
PANCAKE								
Apple & Sultana, M&S*	1 Serving/80g	160	6.3	200	2.2	30.2	7.9	1.2
Asda*	1 Pancake/23.2g	59	1.6	254	4.8	43	7	4
Big, Crafty, Genesis*	1 Pancake/70g	149	3.6	213	5.6	38.4	5.2	4.1
Blueberry, Tesco*	1 Pancake/75g	195	3.1	260	4.8	49.5	4.1	2
Chinese Style, Cherry Valley*	1 Pancake/8g	25	0.5	310	9.2	54.7	6	0
Chocolate, M&S*	1 Pancake/80g	125	4.9	156	3.1	22.1	6.1	0.2
Classic, Village Bakery, Aldi*	1 Pancake/60g	158	6	263	3.7	39	10	1
Lemon, M&S*	1 Pancake/38g	90	2.8	235	4.5	38.5	7.2	2.8
Maple & Raisin, M&S*	1 Pancake/35g	102	2.4	290	5.6	50.4	6.9	2.2
Mini, Scotch, Tesco*	1 Pancake/16g	44	0.9	277	6.7	50	5.6	1.4
Morello Cherry, Iceland*	1 Pancake/129g	204	3.7	158	3.1	29.8	2.9	2.9
Morrisons*	1 Pancake/60g	133	3	221	8.4	37.3	5	1.5
Plain, Prepared From Recipe, Average	*1 Pancake/38g*	*86*	*3.7*	*227*	*6.4*	*28.3*	*9.7*	*0*

P

	Measure INFO/WEIGHT	per Measure KCAL	FAT	Nutrition Values per 100g / 100ml KCAL	PROT	CARB	FAT	FIBRE
PANCAKE								
Raisin & Lemon, Asda*	1 Serving/30g	92	2.4	304	6	52	8	1.4
Raisin & Lemon, Sainsbury's*	1 Pancake/35.0g	95	1.5	272	6.3	51.8	4.4	2.2
Ready Made, Average	*1 Sm/30g*	*77*	*1.9*	*258*	*6.1*	*44.2*	*6.4*	*1.7*
Savoury, Made with Skimmed Milk, Average	*6"Pancake/77g*	*192*	*11.3*	*249*	*6.4*	*24.1*	*14.7*	*0.8*
Savoury, Made with Whole Milk, Average	*6"Pancake/77g*	*210*	*13.5*	*273*	*6.3*	*24*	*17.5*	*0.8*
Scotch	*1 Pancake/50g*	*146*	*5.8*	*292*	*5.8*	*43.6*	*11.7*	*1.4*
Scotch, Essential, Waitrose*	1 Pancake/31g	82	2.6	265	6.4	40.9	8.4	2.4
Scotch, Hovis*	1 Pancake/30g	88	2.5	295	5.5	48.1	8.4	2.3
Scotch, M&S*	1 Pancake/34g	95	1.4	280	6.5	54.5	4	1.6
Scotch, Sainsbury's*	1 Pancake/30g	78	1.3	260	5.9	48.7	4.4	1
Sultana & Syrup, Asda*	1 Pancake/34g	89	2.4	263	5.9	43.7	7.2	1.5
Syrup, Tesco*	1 Pancake/30g	80	2.5	265	4.7	42.1	8.2	1.5
Traditional, Tesco*	1 Pancake/62g	137	3.1	221	8.4	35.6	5	1.5
Vegetable Roll	*1 Roll/85g*	*185*	*10.6*	*218*	*6.6*	*21*	*12.5*	*0*
with Syrup, American Style, Large, Tesco*	1 Pancake/38g	102	1.3	268	5.1	54.2	3.4	0.9
PANCETTA								
Average	*½ Pack/65g*	*212*	*18.7*	*326*	*17*	*0.1*	*28.7*	*0*
PANINI								
Cheese, Tesco*	1 Panini/100g	249	9.1	249	10.5	31.3	9.1	3.1
Chicken, Arrabiata, Ginsters*	1 Panini/200g	489	16.8	245	12.8	29.4	8.4	2.4
Chicken, Chargrilled, Mozzarella, & Pesto, Udo's Choice*	1 Panini/170g	389	14.6	229	16.4	21.6	8.6	2
Ham, & Cheese, Ginsters*	1 Panini/200g	567	25.6	283	13.3	28.7	12.8	1.6
Mozzarella, & Tomato, M&S*	1 Serving/176g	484	28.5	275	11.3	21.3	16.2	2.1
Tuna, & Sweetcorn, Tesco*	1 Serving/250g	559	16.4	224	12	29.3	6.6	1.4
PANNA COTTA								
BGTY, Sainsbury's*	1 Pot/150g	150	2.8	100	2.4	18.2	1.9	1.4
Caramel, Sainsbury's*	1 Pot/120g	335	15.7	279	2.5	34.6	13.1	3.3
Raspberry, COU, M&S*	1 Pot/140g	146	3.5	104	2.6	17.5	2.5	0.6
Sainsbury's*	1 Pot/100g	304	15.7	304	3	41.5	15.7	4
Strawberry, COU, M&S*	1 Pot/145g	145	3.8	100	2.6	15.7	2.6	0.8
Vanilla, Pizza Express*	1 Serving/130g	453	40.6	348	1.6	15.5	31.2	0.1
PAPAYA								
Dried, Pieces, Nature's Harvest*	1 Serving/50g	178	0	355	0.2	85.4	0	2.6
Raw, Flesh Only, Average	*1 Serving/140g*	*37*	*0.1*	*26*	*0.4*	*6.6*	*0.1*	*1.2*
PAPPARDELLE								
Egg, Dry, Average	*1 Serving/100g*	*364*	*3.7*	*364*	*14.1*	*68.5*	*3.7*	*2.1*
Egg, Fresh, Waitrose*	¼ Pack/125g	350	3.4	280	12.9	51	2.7	1.9
with Salmon, COU, M&S*	1 Pack/358g	340	6.8	95	6.3	13	1.9	0.8
PAPRIKA								
Average	*1 Tsp/2g*	*6*	*0.3*	*289*	*14.8*	*34.9*	*13*	*0*
PARATHA								
Average	*1 Paratha/80g*	*258*	*11.4*	*322*	*8*	*43.2*	*14.3*	*4*
Lachha, Waitrose*	1 Paratha/75g	322	17.8	429	7.8	46	23.8	1.8
Roti, Plain, Crown Farms*	1 Slice/80g	250	10	312	5	46.2	12.5	1.2
PARCELS								
Beef, Chilli, Tex Mex Feast, Asda*	1 Parcel/25g	68	3.5	270	9	27	14	2.1
Beef, Steak, Sainsbury's*	½ Pack/226g	488	35.3	216	12.2	6.6	15.6	1
Butternut Squash, Moroccan, M&S*	1 Parcel/20g	54	2.6	270	4.7	33.7	13	2.9
Cheese, & Ham, Sainsbury's*	1 Pack/250g	445	19	178	7.4	19.9	7.6	1.5
Chicken, & Bacon, Finest, Tesco*	1 Pack/233g	379	21.6	163	16.1	3.7	9.3	0.5
Chicken, & Bacon, Sainsbury's*	½ Pack/170g	406	28.6	239	21.9	0.1	16.8	0
Filo, Brie & Cranberry, Finest, Tesco*	1 Parcel/22g	73	3.7	330	9.8	33.2	17	1.4
Filo, Feta & Spinach, Sainsbury's*	1 Parcel/27g	83	5.6	307	5.8	23.8	20.7	1.8

	Measure INFO/WEIGHT	per Measure KCAL	FAT	Nutrition Values per 100g / 100ml KCAL	PROT	CARB	FAT	FIBRE
PARCELS								
Filo, Mushroom, Leek & Gruyere, Finest, Tesco*	1 Serving/160g	440	33.6	275	6.9	20.5	21	1.5
Pork, & Ham Hock, Pastry, Aldi*	1 Parcel/159g	501	33.4	315	14	18	21	0.8
Salmon, Smoked, Sainsbury's*	1 Pack/115g	269	20.2	234	15.8	3.5	17.6	0.2
Salmon, Smoked, TTD, Sainsbury's*	1 Serving/58g	144	11.1	250	13.4	5.7	19.3	1
Salmon, Smoked, with Cucumber, TTD, Sainsbury's*	1 Parcel/57g	118	8.7	206	14.2	2.4	15.2	1.2
with Cheese, & Sweet Pepper Sauce, Egg, Somerfield*	½ Pack/125g	349	14.8	279	12.4	30.7	11.8	2.2
PARSLEY								
Dried	*1 Tsp/1g*	*2*	*0.1*	*181*	*15.8*	*14.5*	*7*	*26.9*
Fresh, Average	*1 Tbsp/3.8g*	*1*	*0*	*27*	*2.4*	*2.2*	*1*	*4*
PARSNIP								
Boiled, Average	*1 Serving/80g*	*53*	*1*	*66*	*1.6*	*12.9*	*1.2*	*4.7*
Honey Glazed, Roast, Baked, Aunt Bessie's*	1 Serving/80g	177	11.9	221	1.4	18.7	14.9	3.4
Honey Glazed, Roasting, Cooked, Betty Smith's*	1 Serving/80g	177	11.9	221	1.4	18.7	14.9	3.4
Honey Roasted, Tesco*	½ Pack/125g	165	6.6	130	1.3	16.7	5.2	5.2
Raw, Unprepared, Average	*1 Serving/100g*	*62*	*1*	*62*	*1.7*	*11.6*	*1*	*4.3*
PARTRIDGE								
Breast, Fillets, Raw, Skinned, Abel & Cole*	1 Serving/100g	145	4.7	145	25.8	0	4.7	0
Meat Only, Roasted	*1 Partridge/260g*	*551*	*18.7*	*212*	*36.7*	*0*	*7.2*	*0*
PASSATA								
Classic, Italian with Onion & Garlic, Sainsbury's*	1oz/28g	10	0	37	1.4	7.7	0.1	1.3
Mutti Di Pomodoro , Mutti*	1/5 Jar/140g	50	0.4	36	1.6	5.1	0.3	0
Napolina*	1 Bottle/690g	172	0.7	25	1.4	4.5	0.1	0
Smart Price, Asda*	1 Serving/100g	30	0.1	30	1.1	5.6	0.1	0.9
Tomato, Freshona, Lidl*	1 Carton/500g	170	2.5	34	1.5	4.6	0.5	1.3
PASSION FRUIT								
Raw, Fresh, Average	*1 Fruit/30g*	*11*	*0.1*	*36*	*2.6*	*5.8*	*0.4*	*3.3*
Weighed with Skin, Average	*1 Fruit/30g*	*7*	*0.1*	*22*	*1.6*	*3.5*	*0.2*	*2*
PASTA								
Basil, & Parmesan, Parcels, Fresh, Sainsbury's*	1 Serving/162g	357	13.5	220	10	26.4	8.3	3.3
Cheese, & Broccoli, Mild, Pasta n Sauce, Batchelors*	½ Pack/61g	221	2.4	363	15	67	3.9	4
Cheese, & Broccoli, Tubes, Tesco*	1 Serving/202g	319	13.9	158	5	19.1	6.9	2.3
Cheese, & Ham, Pot, Tesco*	1 Serving/208g	254	8.5	122	3.4	17.9	4.1	1.5
Cheese, Leek, & Ham, Pasta n Sauce, Batchelors*	1 Pack/120g	454	6.1	378	16.1	67	5.1	2
Cheese, Macaroni, Dry, Pasta n Sauce, Batchelors*	1 Pack/108g	402	5.1	372	17.2	65.2	4.7	2.7
Chicken & Chorizo, Average	*1 Pack/400g*	*174*	*5.7*	*174*	*10.1*	*20.3*	*5.7*	*1.5*
Chicken, & Chorizo, Quadrotti, TTD, Sainsbury's*	1 Pack/320g	616	25.3	192	9.6	19.5	7.9	2.4
Chicken, & Mushroom, Snack Pot, Asda*	1 Pot/228g	269	6.4	118	3.4	19.8	2.8	2.3
Chicken, & Mushroom, Snack Stop, Crosse & Blackwell*	1 Pot/60g	251	5.3	418	10.3	74.3	8.8	0
Chicken, Roast, As Consumed, Mug Shot, Symingtons*	1 Sachet/256g	221	2.3	86	3.2	15.9	0.9	1
Chicken, Tomato & Basil, HL, Tesco*	1 Pack/400g	264	2	66	7.9	7.5	0.5	1.1
Chicken, Tomato & Basil, Weight Watchers*	1 Pack/310g	310	4	100	6.1	15.4	1.3	1.1
Feta, & Slow Roasted Tomatoes, M&S*	1 Pack/190g	332	13.3	175	6	22.3	7	2.5
Green Pea, GF, As Prepared, Love Life, Waitrose*	1 Serving/175g	276	1.6	158	10.5	24.1	0.9	5.5
Margherite, Basil, & Pinenut, TTD, Sainsbury's*	½ Pack/150g	275	11.1	184	8.7	19.4	7.4	2.3
Meat, Cappelletti, Sainsbury's*	1 Pack/420g	816	23.9	195	10	25.8	5.7	2.3
Mushroom, Creamy, Sainsbury's*	1 Serving/63g	148	9.1	237	4.5	21.7	14.6	1.2
Mushroom, Wild, Fagottini, Sainsbury's*	½ Pack/125g	274	9.4	219	10.2	27.7	7.5	2.7
Orzo, Dry, Average	*1 Serving/100g*	*348*	*1.5*	*348*	*12.4*	*71.9*	*1.5*	*3*
Pesto, Spinach, & Pine Nuts, Tesco*	1 Pack/300g	480	22.2	160	5.2	17.1	7.4	1.5
Pumpkin, & Pine Nut, Stuffed, Fiorelli, Fresh, Waitrose*	½ Pack/125g	225	7.5	180	8	22.3	6	2.3
Pumpkin, & Sage, Quadrotti, Fresh, TTD, Sainsbury's*	½ Pack/160g	261	8	163	6.6	21.3	5	3.4
Salmon, & Broccoli, Lemon Dressed, Sainsbury's*	1 Serving/300g	486	17.7	162	6.9	20.4	5.9	2.1
Salmon, Smoked, Hot, Tesco*	1 Pack/275g	426	17	155	7.1	16.6	6.2	4.1

P

	Measure INFO/WEIGHT	per Measure KCAL	FAT	Nutrition Values per 100g / 100ml KCAL	PROT	CARB	FAT	FIBRE
PASTA								
Sausage, & Tomato, Italiano, Tesco*	1 Serving/450g	680	26.6	151	5.7	18.8	5.9	1.6
Seafood, Retail	*1 Serving/100g*	*110*	*4.8*	*110*	*8.9*	*7.6*	*4.8*	*0.4*
Spinach, & Ricotta, Tortelloni, Giovanni Rana*	½ Pack/125g	323	10.6	258	9	35	8.5	3.1
Spinach, Firenze, Lidl*	1 Serving/50g	175	1	350	12	72	2	3.5
Sweet & Sour, Mug Shot, Made Up, Symingtons*	1 Sachet/275g	239	1.9	87	2.2	19.5	0.7	1.2
Tomato 'n' Herb, Mug Shot, Symingtons*	1 Sachet/257g	265	2.1	103	2.3	21.6	0.8	1.2
Tomato, & Chilli, Pasta Vita, Dolmio*	1 Pot/300g	330	5.4	110	4.4	18.4	1.8	1.5
Tomato, & Herb, Pot, Dry, Tesco*	1 Pot/59g	207	1.4	352	11.8	70.7	2.4	2.6
Vegetable, Chargrilled, & Mozzarella, Melt, COU, M&S*	1 Pack/380g	319	8.7	84	3.8	11	2.3	1.8
Vegetable, Mediterranean, Cooked, BGTY, Sainsbury's*	1 Pack/400g	347	5.5	89	2.8	15.2	1.4	1.9
Wholewheat, Cooked, Tesco*	1 Serving/200g	284	1.8	142	5.7	27.9	0.9	4.5
PASTA BAKE								
Bacon & Leek, Average	*1 Serving/400g*	*633*	*32.3*	*158*	*6.7*	*14.8*	*8.1*	*1.3*
Bolognese, Annabel Karmel*	1 Pack/200g	180	7.6	90	6.8	7.2	3.8	1.8
Bolognese, Asda*	¼ Pack/375g	514	23.6	137	7.3	12.7	6.3	1.8
Bolognese, Penne, Sainsbury's*	1 Pack/397g	603	27.8	152	7.6	14.8	7	2
Bolognese, Weight Watchers*	1 Pack/400g	324	8	81	6.1	9.6	2	1.3
Cheese, & Bacon, Asda*	1 Serving/120g	168	14.4	140	3	5.2	12	0.3
Cheese, & Bacon, Fresh Italian, Asda*	1 Serving/250g	265	20	106	6	2.6	8	0.5
Cheese, & Tomato, Italiano, Tesco*	1 Bake/300g	354	12.6	118	3.9	16.1	4.2	1
Cheese, & Tomato, Tesco*	1 Pack/400g	388	5.6	97	3.4	17.8	1.4	1.2
Chicken, & Bacon, Asda*	¼ Pack/374.2g	610	26.2	163	9	16	7	4.1
Chicken, & Bacon, Asda*	1 Pack/400g	592	25.2	148	8.6	14.2	6.3	3
Chicken, & Bacon, Average	*1 Serving/400g*	*627*	*28.7*	*157*	*9*	*13.7*	*7.2*	*1.6*
Chicken, & Broccoli, Morrisons*	1 Pack/400g	452	16	113	6.1	13.3	4	0.6
Chicken, & Mushroom, Waitrose*	1 Pack/400g	532	30.8	133	6.7	9.1	7.7	0.8
Chicken, Bacon & Mushroom, Average	*1 Serving/400g*	*632*	*29.2*	*158*	*7.8*	*15.1*	*7.3*	*2.3*
Chicken, Weight Watchers*	1 Pack/300g	249	2.7	83	6	12.1	0.9	1.1
Creamy, Tomato, Dolmio*	1 Serving/125g	141	9	113	2.3	8.4	7.2	0
Meat Feast, Average	*1 Serving/400g*	*601*	*21.4*	*150*	*5.8*	*19.2*	*5.4*	*1.4*
Meatball, Aberdeen Angus, Waitrose*	½ Pack/350g	501	28	143	5.2	15.5	8	0.9
Sausage, Average	*1 Serving/400g*	*591*	*24*	*148*	*5.5*	*17.7*	*6*	*1.9*
Tomato, & Bacon, Creamy,Ãƒ š Italian,Ãƒ š Asda*	1 Serving/125g	131	11.2	105	2	3.9	9	0.6
Tomato, & Mozzarella, Average	*1 Serving/400g*	*500*	*12.4*	*125*	*5.3*	*17.3*	*3.1*	*1.5*
Tomato, & Mozzarella, Co-Op*	1 Pack/400g	556	224	139	5.8	15	56	2.3
Tomato, & Mozzarella, Sainsbury's*	1 Pack/400g	480	12.8	120	5	17.9	3.2	2.1
Tomato, & Pepperoni,Ãƒ š Spicy,Ãƒ š Asda*	1 Pack/440g	431	26.4	98	1.1	10	6	1.2
Tuna, & Sweetcorn, Average	*1 Pack/400g*	*423*	*22.4*	*106*	*5*	*8.6*	*5.6*	*1.9*
Tuna, Co-Op*	1 Serving/340g	306	6.8	90	7	12	2	1
Tuna, Counted, As Consumed, Eat Smart, Morrisons*	1 Pack/348g	310	5.9	89	5.2	12.4	1.7	1.5
Vegetable, M&S*	½ Pack/175g	201	8.8	115	4.1	12.6	5	2.2
Vegetable, Mediterranean, HL, Tesco*	1 Serving/450g	374	3.6	83	2.9	16	0.8	1.5
PASTA QUILLS								
Dry, Average	*1 Serving/75g*	*256*	*0.9*	*342*	*12*	*72.3*	*1.2*	*2*
GF, Salute*	1 Serving/75g	269	1.4	359	7.5	78	1.9	0
PASTA SALAD								
Basil Pesto Dressing, & Mixed Leaf, Tesco*	1 Pack/220g	528	37.6	240	4.7	16.9	17.1	0.7
Cheese, Average	*1 Serving/370g*	*782*	*56.8*	*211*	*5.5*	*12.8*	*15.4*	*1.2*
Cheese, Layered, Asda*	1 Pack/440g	647	40.9	147	4.5	11.4	9.3	0
Chicken, & Bacon Caesar, Tesco*	1 Pack/265g	442	23.6	167	10.2	10.8	8.9	1.3
Chicken, & Bacon, Tesco*	½ Pack/200g	450	29	225	6.3	16.8	14.5	3.2
Chicken, Tomato, & Basil, M&S*	1 Serving/279g	446	22	160	7	14.8	7.9	1.8
Chicken, Tomato, & Basil, Sainsbury's*	1 Pack/350g	626	27.6	179	7.4	19	7.9	1.1

	Measure INFO/WEIGHT	per Measure KCAL	FAT	Nutrition Values per 100g / 100ml KCAL	PROT	CARB	FAT	FIBRE
PASTA SALAD								
Chicken, Tomato, & Basil, Tesco*	1 Pack/300g	414	9.3	138	6.2	20.6	3.1	1.6
Chicken, Chargrilled, & Red Pepper, Tesco*	1 Pack/270g	554	24	205	9.8	20.3	8.9	3.1
Chicken, Honey & Mustard, M&S*	1 Serving/190g	304	4.8	160	8.7	26.7	2.5	1.5
Chicken, Honey & Mustard, Sainsbury's*	1 Pack/190g	344	16.9	181	7.1	18	8.9	0
Goats Cheese, & Mixed Pepper, Sainsbury's*	1 Pack/200g	366	18.8	183	6.4	18.2	9.4	1.5
Italian Style, Sainsbury's*	1/3 Pot/84g	129	5.3	153	3.5	20.5	6.3	1.4
Italian Style, Snack, Asda*	1 Pack/150g	141	6	94	3.4	11	4	4.1
Italian, Tesco*	½ Pack/225g	315	8.3	140	3.5	22.6	3.7	2.3
Mozzarella, & Sun Dried Tomato, Waitrose*	1 Serving/150g	312	18.3	208	5.8	18.8	12.2	1.3
Pesto, Creamy, Pot, Diet Chef*	1 Pot/248g	236	3.7	95	3.6	16.2	1.5	1
Pesto, Mini, 293, Oakhouse Foods Ltd*	1 Serving/225g	758	37.1	337	12.4	33.8	16.5	2.1
Pesto, Spicy Chilli, Sainsbury's*	¼ Pot/63g	170	12.3	272	3.8	20.1	19.6	1.6
Prawn Cocktail, Layered, Shapers, Boots*	1 Pot/210g	181	5.2	86	3.6	13	2.5	1.3
Prawn, Growers Selection, Asda*	1 Pack/380g	365	9.1	96	5.1	13	2.4	1.2
Tomato, & Basil, Sainsbury's*	1 Serving/62g	87	4.3	141	3.2	16.4	6.9	3.8
Tuna, & Sweetcorn, HE, Tesco*	1 Pot/200g	230	5.4	115	5.7	17	2.7	1.3
Tuna, & Sweetcorn, Sainsbury's*	1 Serving/100g	111	1.2	111	7.1	18.3	1.2	1.2
Vegetables, Chargrilled, & Tomato, Shapers, Boots*	1 Pack/175g	187	5.4	107	2.8	17	3.1	1.5
Vegetables, Chargrilled, Sainsbury's*	1 Serving/178g	192	4.8	108	2.7	15.9	2.7	4.7
PASTA SAUCE								
Amatriciana, Italiano, Tesco*	½ Pot/175g	124	6.6	71	4.1	5.3	3.8	0.9
Amatriciana, M&S*	1 Jar/340g	425	32.3	125	3.4	6.3	9.5	2.9
Arrabiata, Barilla*	1 Serving/100g	47	3	47	1.5	3.5	3	0
Arrabiata, Fresh, Co-Op*	½ Pot/150g	82	4.5	55	1	5	3	1
Arrabiata, Fresh, M Kitchen, Morrisons*	½ Pot/175g	89	4.2	51	1.4	5	2.4	1.8
Arrabiata, GFY, Asda*	1 Serving/350g	133	3.9	38	1.1	6	1.1	0
Arrabiata, M&S*	1 Jar/320g	240	17	75	1.2	6.2	5.3	0.8
Aubergine, & Mascarpone, Roasted, Stir Through, M&S*	½ Jar/95g	111	8.9	117	1	6.3	9.4	1.7
Bacon, Smoky, Loyd Grossman*	½ Jar/175g	142	8.4	81	3	6.1	4.8	0.8
Bolognese, Extra Onion & Garlic, Dolmio*	1 Serving/125g	51	0.8	41	1.4	6.6	0.6	1
Bolognese, Finest, Tesco*	1 Serving/175g	170	10.7	97	7	3.8	6.1	0.5
Bolognese, Free From, Tesco*	¼ Jar/125g	63	0.9	51	1.9	8.4	0.7	1.5
Bolognese, Garlic & Onion, Intense, Dolmio*	1 Jar/500g	210	1	42	1.7	7.4	0.2	1.8
Bolognese, Mushroom, Chunky, Dolmio*	½ Jar/375g	165	0.8	44	1.7	7.9	0.2	2
Bolognese, Organic, Seeds of Change*	1 Jar/500g	290	6	58	1.3	10.4	1.2	0.8
Bolognese, Original, Asda*	1 Serving/158g	73	2.2	46	1.4	7	1.4	0.8
Bolognese, Original, Light, Low Fat, Dolmio*	1 Serving/125g	41	0.1	33	1.2	6	0.1	1.3
Bolognese, Original, Sainsbury's*	¼ Jar/136g	90	2.9	66	1.9	9.9	2.1	1.3
Bolognese, Smooth, Hidden Vegetables, Dolmio*	1 Portion/125g	60	1	48	1.4	7.7	0.8	1.9
Bolognese, Tesco*	¼ Jar/125g	53	0.4	42	1.2	8	0.3	1.3
Bolognese, Tomato, Beef & Red Wine, Fresh, Waitrose*	1 Pot/350g	301	17.2	86	5.4	5.3	4.9	2
Bolognese, with Beef, Tesco*	½ Can/213g	179	10	84	4.9	5.5	4.7	0
Cacciatore, Fresh, Sainsbury's*	½ Pot/150g	152	8.8	101	5.4	8.1	5.9	1.5
Carbonara, Asda*	½ Pot/175g	359	29.8	205	7	6	17	0.1
Carbonara, Co-Op*	½ Pot/150g	270	25.5	180	3	4	17	0.1
Carbonara, Creamy, Dolmio Express, Dolmio*	1 Pack/150g	166	13.2	111	3.3	4.7	8.8	0.1
Carbonara, Creamy, Stir in Sauce, Dolmio*	1 Serving/75g	98	8	130	3.3	5.2	10.6	0.2
Carbonara, Italian, Fresh, Sainsbury's*	½ Pot/176g	209	16.3	119	5.4	3.4	9.3	0.9
Cheese, Four, Sainsbury's*	1 Serving/150g	296	25.5	197	6.6	4.5	17	0.8
Cheese, Fresh, PB, Waitrose*	½ Pot/175g	144	5.1	82	6.1	7.9	2.9	0.5
Cheese, Three, Co-Op*	1 Pack/300g	405	27	135	6	6	9	0.1
Garlic, & Onion, Finest, Tesco*	1 Serving/126g	43	0.5	34	0.8	6.9	0.4	1.3
Lasagne, Tomato, Red, Ragu, Knorr*	1 Jar/500g	215	0	43	1.1	9.7	0	1.1

	Measure INFO/WEIGHT	per Measure		Nutrition Values per 100g / 100ml				
		KCAL	FAT	KCAL	PROT	CARB	FAT	FIBRE
PASTA SAUCE								
Lasagne, White, Ragu, Knorr*	1 Jar/475g	755	72.2	159	0.5	5.1	15.2	0.3
Mediterranean, Fresh, Waitrose*	1 Pot/350g	214	13.6	61	1.4	5	3.9	2.4
Mushroom, & Cream, M&S*	1oz/28g	45	4	160	1.5	6.6	14.3	0.6
Mushroom, Creamy, Dolmio*	1 Pack/150g	166	15	111	1.3	3.7	10	0
Mushroom, Creamy, Express, Dolmio*	1 Serving/150g	160	14.4	107	1.4	3.8	9.6	0
Mushroom, Italian, Sainsbury's*	1 Serving/85g	56	1.8	66	2	9.8	2.1	1.7
Mushroom, Sainsbury's*	1 Serving/100g	66	2.1	66	2	9.8	2.1	1.7
Mushroom, Tesco*	1/6 Jar/120g	48	0.6	40	1.2	6.9	0.5	1.5
Napoletana, Fresh, Sainsbury's*	1oz/28g	25	1.6	91	1.9	7.9	5.8	1.1
Napoletana, Morrisons*	1 Serving/175g	82	2.6	47	2.6	6.7	1.5	0
Napoletana, Sainsbury's*	½ Pot/150g	126	8.4	84	1.9	6.6	5.6	0.9
Olive, & Tomato, Sacla*	1 Serving/95g	87	7.6	92	1.3	3.6	8	0
Pomodoro, Cirio*	1 Serving/200g	116	4.6	58	1.4	8.4	2.3	0
Puttanesca, Loyd Grossman*	½ Jar/175g	117	6	67	1.4	5.5	3.4	0.7
Puttanesca, Sainsbury's*	1 Serving/110g	132	9.7	120	2	8.1	8.8	0
Red Pepper, & Tomato, Roasted, Finest, Tesco*	1 Serving/145g	117	7.8	81	1.2	6.8	5.4	2.2
Red Pepper, Sweet, Loyd Grossman*	1 Jar/350g	304	19.6	87	1.7	7.3	5.6	1.2
Tomato, & Basil, Dolmio*	1 Serving/170g	95	3.6	56	1.4	7.9	2.1	0
Tomato, & Basil, Loyd Grossman*	½ Jar/175g	107	6	61	1.5	5.8	3.4	0.8
Tomato, & Basil, Morrisons*	½ Jar/140g	76	0.7	54	1.7	10.1	0.5	1.3
Tomato, & Basil, Sun Dried, Organic, Seeds of Change*	½ Jar/100g	155	13.1	155	1.6	7.7	13.1	0
Tomato, & Basil, Sun Ripened, Dolmio*	1 Serving/150g	117	6.9	78	1.3	7.9	4.6	0
Tomato, & Basil, Sun Ripened, Express, Dolmio*	1 Pouch/170g	88	2.7	52	1.5	7.9	1.6	0
Tomato, & Chilli, Pour Over, M&S*	1 Jar/330g	231	12.5	70	1.3	7.6	3.8	1.8
Tomato, & Chilli, Whole Cherry Tomatoes, Classic, Sacla*	½ Jar/175g	238	19.2	136	2	7.2	11	3.1
Tomato, & Garlic, CBY, Asda*	½ Jar/160g	74	0.8	46	1.6	7.9	0.5	1.7
Tomato, & Garlic, Roasted, CBY, Asda*	1 Pot/350g	122	2.1	35	1.5	5	0.6	1.7
Tomato, & Garlic, Roasted, Loyd Grossman*	½ Jar/175g	133	5.6	76	2	9	3.2	1.4
Tomato, & Mascarpone, Finest, Tesco*	1 Serving/175g	135	8.8	77	2.7	5.4	5	0.8
Tomato, & Mascarpone, Fresh, Sainsbury's*	1 Serving/150g	177	15.4	118	2.2	4.2	10.3	1.1
Tomato, & Mascarpone, Italiano, Tesco*	½ Pot/175g	168	12.2	96	2.8	5.5	7	0.7
Tomato, & Mascarpone, Sainsbury's*	½ Pot/150g	137	9.9	91	2.1	5.9	6.6	1.2
Tomato, & Mascarpone, Tesco*	1 Serving/175g	194	15.2	111	2.8	5.4	8.7	0.6
Tomato, & Mascarpone, Waitrose*	½ Pot/175g	184	14.7	105	1.9	5.5	8.4	1.1
Tomato, & Mixed Peppers, Spicy, Combino, Lidl*	¼ Jar/125g	55	0.8	44	1.5	7.3	0.6	1.6
Tomato, & Mushroom, Wild, Loyd Grossman*	½ Jar/175g	154	9.8	88	2.1	7.4	5.6	1.5
Tomato, & Onions, Original, Morrisons*	1 Serving/125g	51	1.4	41	1.4	6.3	1.1	1.2
Tomato, & Parmesan, Seeds of Change*	1 Serving/150g	100	4.4	67	2.5	7.8	2.9	1.1
Tomato, & Ricotta, Italian, Sainsbury's*	1 Pack/390g	238	11.7	61	2.5	6.1	3	1.2
Tomato, & Tuna, Loyd Grossman*	½ Jar/175g	154	7.7	88	4.4	7.5	4.4	0.8
Tomato, Bacon, & Mushroom, Asda*	½ Pot/50g	33	1.8	66	2.5	6	3.6	0
Tomato, Onion, & Garlic, Baresa, Lidl*	1 Jar/500g	240	2.5	48	2.1	7.8	0.5	1.8
Tomato, Sun Dried, Stir In, Light, Dolmio*	1 Serving/75g	62	3.5	83	1.7	9.8	4.7	0
Tomato, with Basil Pesto, Rich, Express, Dolmio*	1 Pack/170g	146	10	86	2	6.2	5.9	0
Vegetable, Chunky, Tesco*	1 Jar/500g	235	5	47	1.8	6.8	1	1.8
Vegetable, Mediterranean, Organic, Seeds of Change*	1 Jar/350g	210	10.2	60	1.2	6.6	2.9	1.4
Vegetable, Mediterranean, Tesco*	1 Serving/166g	95	2.8	57	1.4	9	1.7	1.2
Vegetable, Roasted, Sainsbury's*	½ Pot/151g	103	5.9	68	1.6	6.7	3.9	0.4
PASTA SHAPES								
Alphabetti, in Tomato Sauce, Heinz*	1 Can/200g	118	1	59	1.8	11.7	0.5	1.5
Bob The Builder in Tomato Sauce, Heinz*	1 Can/205g	111	0.6	54	1.7	11.3	0.3	1.5
Cooked, Tesco*	1 Serving/260g	356	2.1	137	5.1	26.3	0.8	1.1
Disney Princess in Tomato Sauce, Heinz*	1 Can/200g	114	0.6	57	1.8	11.9	0.3	1.5

	Measure INFO/WEIGHT	KCAL	FAT	KCAL	PROT	CARB	FAT	FIBRE
		per Measure		Nutrition Values per 100g / 100ml				

PASTA SHAPES
	Measure INFO/WEIGHT	KCAL	FAT	KCAL	PROT	CARB	FAT	FIBRE
Dried, Tesco*	1 Serving/100g	345	2	345	13.2	68.5	2	2.9
Durum Wheat, Dry, Basics, Sainsbury's*	1 Serving/75g	260	1.5	346	12	70	2	4
Spiderman with Mini Sausages in Tomato Sauce, Heinz*	1 Can/200g	178	6.2	89	3.6	11.6	3.1	0.5

PASTA SHELLS
Dry, Average	**1 Serving/75g**	**265**	**1.5**	**353**	**11.1**	**71.8**	**2**	**2**
Egg, Fresh, Average	**1 Serving/125g**	**344**	**3.6**	**275**	**11.5**	**49.8**	**2.8**	**3.4**
Wholewheat, Healthy Living, Co-Op*	1 Serving/75g	232	0.8	310	11	64	1	12

PASTA TWISTS
Dry, Average	**1oz/28g**	**99**	**0.4**	**354**	**12.2**	**71.8**	**1.5**	**2.2**
Wheat & GF, Glutafin*	1 Serving/75g	262	1.5	350	8	75	2	0.1

PASTE
Beef, Asda*	1 Serving/37g	72	5.2	194	17	0.1	14	0
Beef, Princes*	1 Serving/18g	42	3.1	231	15.2	3.4	17.4	0
Beef, Sainsbury's*	1 Jar/75g	142	9.9	189	16	1.5	13.2	1.4
Chicken, & Ham, Princes*	1 Jar/100g	233	18.6	233	13.6	2.8	18.6	0
Chicken, & Ham, Tesco*	1 Serving/19g	44	3.7	231	12.5	1.4	19.5	0
Chicken, & Mushroom, Princes*	1 Serving/50g	94	5.5	187	17.1	5	11	0
Chicken, & Stuffing, Asda*	½ Jar/35g	71	4.9	203	16	3.3	14	0
Chicken, & Stuffing, Princes*	1 Jar/100g	229	17	229	15.7	3.3	17	0
Chicken, Asda*	1 Thin Spread/7g	13	0.9	184	16	0.8	13	0
Chicken, Tesco*	1 Serving/12g	30	2.4	248	14.8	2.3	20	0.1
Chilli, Sainsbury's*	1 Tsp/6g	5	0.4	82	1	2.9	5.8	7.3
Crab, Sainsbury's*	1 Thick Spread/5g	6	0.2	115	16.5	1.7	4.7	0.5
Red Pepper, Mild, 1001 Delights, Lidl*	1 Tsp/6g	4	0	70	3	10.5	0.8	0
Salmon, & Shrimp, Tesco*	1 Jar/75g	83	2.6	111	15.1	5	3.4	0.1
Salmon, Value, Tesco*	1 Serving/10g	16	1	165	14	4.6	10.1	0.8
Sardine, & Tomato, Asda*	1 Thin Spread/9g	11	0.5	123	14	3.3	6	0
Sardine, & Tomato, Princes*	1 Jar/75g	130	8.1	173	13.9	3.4	10.8	3.2
Sardine, & Tomato, Sainsbury's*	1 Mini Pot/35g	60	3.8	170	16.9	1.2	10.8	1.3
Tuna, & Mayonnaise, Tesco*	1 Serving/15g	32	2.3	215	15.8	0.7	15.6	2.2

PASTILLES
Fruit, 30% Less Sugar, Rowntree's*	1 Sweet/3g	9	0	325	6.5	68.8	0.1	9.5
Fruit, Average	**1 Tube/33g**	**108**	**0**	**327**	**2.8**	**84.2**	**0**	**0**
Fruit, Rowntree's*	1 Tube/53g	186	0	351	4.4	83.7	0	0
Fruit, Sainsbury's*	1 Sweet/7g	23	0	332	3.4	78.7	0.1	0.1

PASTRAMI
Beef, Average	**1 Serving/40g**	**51**	**1.4**	**128**	**23.1**	**1.1**	**3.6**	**0.2**
Turkey, Average	**½ Pack/35g**	**38**	**0.5**	**107**	**21.8**	**1.7**	**1.5**	**0.5**

PASTRY
Cannoli, Shells, Hand Rolled, Large, Alessi*	1 Shell/21g	90	4.5	429	4.8	47.6	21.4	0
Case, From Supermarket, Average	**1 Case/230g**	**1081**	**58.9**	**470**	**5.8**	**55.9**	**25.6**	**1.2**
Choux, Cooked, Average	**1oz/28g**	**91**	**5.5**	**325**	**8.5**	**29.8**	**19.8**	**1.2**
Choux, Raw, Average	**1oz/28g**	**59**	**3.6**	**211**	**5.5**	**19.4**	**12.9**	**0.8**
Cinnamon Swirls, Bake it Fresh, Jus-Rol*	1 Swirl/45g	162	7.1	360	6.2	47.7	15.7	1.6
Filo, Average	**1 Sheet/45g**	**137**	**1.2**	**304**	**9**	**61.4**	**2.7**	**0.9**
Filo, Cooked, Ready Roll Sheets, Jus-Rol*	½ Sheet/7.62g	26	0.2	335	9.1	66.3	3	2.8
Filo, Frozen, Ready Roll Sheets, Jus-Rol*	1 Sheet/45g	123	1.2	273	8.1	52.1	2.7	2.1
Flaky, Cooked, Average	**1oz/28g**	**157**	**11.4**	**560**	**5.6**	**45.9**	**40.6**	**1.8**
Flaky, Raw, Average	**1oz/28g**	**119**	**8.6**	**424**	**4.2**	**34.8**	**30.7**	**1.4**
Pain Au Chocolat, Bake it Fresh, Jus-Rol*	1 Pain/46g	170	8.7	369	7.4	41	19	2.2
Puff, All Butter, Ready to Roll Blocks, Jus-Rol*	1oz/28g	110	7.3	392	5.6	33.8	26.1	1.3
Puff, All Butter, TTD, Sainsbury's*	1/6 Pack/62g	282	17.5	455	7.4	41.3	28.2	2.9
Puff, Frozen, Average	**1 Serving/47g**	**188**	**12**	**400**	**5**	**29.2**	**25.6**	**0**

P

GENERAL FOODS AND DRINKS A-Z

	Measure INFO/WEIGHT	per Measure KCAL	FAT	Nutrition Values per 100g / 100ml KCAL	PROT	CARB	FAT	FIBRE
PASTRY								
Puff, Light, Frozen, Ready Roll Sheets, Jus-Rol*	1/6 Sheet/53g	176	8.7	332	6.4	38.3	16.5	2.3
Puff, Light, Sheet, Jus-Rol*	1 Serving/50g	166	8.2	332	6.4	38.3	16.5	2.3
Shortcrust, Chilled, Ready to Roll Blocks, Jus-Rol*	1 Block/500g	2295	155	459	7	39	31	2
Shortcrust, Cooked, Average	*1oz/28g*	*146*	*9*	*521*	*6.6*	*54.2*	*32.3*	*2.2*
Shortcrust, Raw, Average	*1oz/28g*	*127*	*8.1*	*453*	*5.6*	*44*	*29.1*	*1.3*
Spring Roll Wrapper, TYJ Food Manufacturing*	1 Lge Sheet/18g	54	0	300	0	73	0	0
Wholemeal, Cooked, Average	*1oz/28g*	*140*	*9.2*	*499*	*8.9*	*44.6*	*32.9*	*6.3*
PASTY								
Cheese, & Onion, Average	*1 Pasty/150g*	*435*	*27.6*	*290*	*7.3*	*24.5*	*18.4*	*1.4*
Cheese, & Onion, Cheddar, Hand Crimped, Waitrose*	1 Pasty/200g	546	42.2	273	8.8	22.5	21.1	2.2
Cheese, & Onion, Sainsbury's*	1 Serving/150g	486	32.7	324	7.4	24.5	21.8	1.3
Cheese, & Onion, Tesco*	1 Pasty/150g	416	26.4	277	5.9	23.7	17.6	2.2
Chicken, Balti, Special Edition, Ginsters*	1 Pasty/180g	398	23.2	221	6.7	19.5	12.9	2.6
Cornish, Average	*1 Pasty/160g*	*450*	*27.7*	*281*	*7*	*24.2*	*17.3*	*1.6*
Cornish, Mini, Sainsbury's*	1 Pasty/70g	280	20.1	400	7.3	28.1	28.7	1.5
Cornish, Morrisons*	1 Pasty/200g	626	37	313	7.5	29.1	18.5	0
Cornish, Multi Pack, Ginsters*	1 Pasty/130g	358	24.3	275	6	20.6	18.7	2.6
Cornish, Original, Ginsters*	1 Pasty/227g	549	32.2	242	5.3	23.2	14.2	3.1
Cornish, Tesco*	1 Pasty/150g	466	32.7	311	6.8	21.9	21.8	1.6
Cornish, Traditional Style, Geo Adams*	1 Pasty/165g	488	30.4	296	7.1	25.4	18.4	1.3
Olive, & Cheese, Tapas, Waitrose*	1 Pack/130g	455	25.2	350	8.1	35.8	19.4	1.3
Vegetable	*1oz/28g*	*77*	*4.2*	*274*	*4.1*	*33.3*	*14.9*	*1.9*
Vegetable, Hand Crimped, Waitrose*	1 Pasty/200g	454	22.6	227	4.5	26.8	11.3	2.2
Vegetable, Tandoori, Holland & Barrett*	1 Pack/110g	232	9.4	211	4.3	29.4	8.5	1.8
Vegetarian, Cornish Style, Quorn*	1 Pasty/150g	320	15	213	6.9	22.5	10	3
Vegetarian, Country Slice, Linda McCartney*	1 Pasty/150g	373	20.2	249	5.6	26.5	13.5	2.9
PATE								
Ardennes, Asda*	1 Serving/50g	143	12	286	13.9	3.6	24	1.3
Ardennes, BGTY, Sainsbury's*	¼ Pack/50g	90	5.7	180	16.6	2.9	11.4	0
Ardennes, Reduced Fat, Waitrose*	¼ Pack/42g	94	7.1	224	15.4	2.6	16.9	0.5
Ardennes, Tesco*	1 Tbsp/15g	53	5	354	13.3	0.5	33.2	1.2
Ardennes, with Bacon, Tesco*	½ Pack/85g	241	20.6	284	11.4	5.1	24.2	1.1
Breton, Country with Apricots, Coarse, Sainsbury's*	1 Serving/21g	60	4.7	285	13.5	7	22.5	0.5
Brussels, & Garlic, Tesco*	1 Serving/40g	145	13.5	363	8.7	6	33.8	0
Brussels, 25% Less Fat, Morrisons*	¼ Pack/43g	106	8.8	249	14.2	0.7	20.6	0
Brussels, BGTY, 50% Less Fat, Sainsbury's*	1 Serving/100g	223	16	223	14.6	5.1	16	0.1
Brussels, Co-Op*	1 Serving/15g	51	4.6	340	11	4	31	2
Brussels, M&S*	1 Pot/170g	518	45.2	305	13.3	2.8	26.6	1
Brussels, Sainsbury's*	1 Pack/170g	663	64.9	390	10.6	1.1	38.2	0.1
Brussels, Smooth, Reduced Fat, Tesco*	1 Serving/40g	98	7.5	245	12	6.4	18.7	0.5
Brussels, Smooth, Reduced, Tesco*	1 Serving /40g	82	6.4	205	10.7	4.5	16	0.6
Brussels, Smooth, Spreadable, Sainsbury's*	1 Serving/30g	97	8.7	323	10.7	4.7	29	0
Butternut Squash, & Red Pepper, Roasted, Waitrose*	1 Pack/160g	259	16.8	162	2.6	12.9	10.5	2.5
Chicken, Liver, Asda*	1 Serving/65g	131	10.4	202	13	4	16	0.8
Chicken, Liver, M&S*	1oz/28g	79	6.7	281	14	1.9	24.1	0.1
Chicken, Liver, Organic, Waitrose*	½ Tub/88g	204	16.1	233	12.6	1.8	18.4	1.4
Chicken, Liver, Parfait, Specially Selected, Aldi*	1 Portion/85g	278	26.4	327	11	2.1	31	0.6
Chicken, Liver, Parfait, Waitrose*	1 Pack/100g	258	22.9	258	7.5	4.8	22.9	1.1
Chicken, Liver, with Madeira, Sainsbury's*	1 Serving/30g	84	7.3	279	13.1	1.9	24.3	0
Crab, M&S*	1oz/28g	63	4.8	225	12.1	5.9	17.3	0
Crab, Ready to Eat, Asda*	1 Pot/115g	210	13.2	183	12.7	6.9	11.5*	0.5
Crab, Terrine, Orkney, Luxury, Castle MacLellan*	1 Tub/113g	250	21.4	221	7.3	5.5	18.9	0.9
Crab, Waitrose*	1 Pot/113g	218	16.7	193	12.4	2.5	14.8	0.9

	Measure INFO/WEIGHT	per Measure KCAL	FAT	Nutrition Values per 100g / 100ml KCAL	PROT	CARB	FAT	FIBRE
PATE								
De Campagne, Sainsbury's*	1 Serving/55g	129	10	235	16.3	1.4	18.2	0
Duck, & Orange, Asda*	1 Serving/40g	94	7.2	235	16	2.2	18	0
Duck, & Orange, Smooth, Tesco*	1 Serving/50g	188	17.7	377	10.5	4	35.4	0.5
Duck, Liver, Grand Marnier & Orange Jelly, M&S*	½ Pot/75g	218	18.5	291	8.7	8.2	24.7	0.6
Farmhouse, Coarse, Organic, Sainsbury's*	1 Serving/56g	138	11	246	13.3	3.7	19.7	0.8
Farmhouse, Style, Finest, Tesco*	1 Serving/28g	83	7.3	295	11.9	3.6	25.9	1
Farmhouse, Waitrose*	½ Pack/50g	119	8.6	238	17.8	2.3	17.3	0.7
Farmhouse, with Mushrooms & Garlic, Tesco*	1 Serving/90g	256	22.8	285	13.8	0.6	25.3	1.3
Mackerel, Smoked	*1oz/28g*	*103*	*9.6*	*368*	*13.4*	*1.3*	*34.4*	*0*
Mackerel, Smoked, Sainsbury's*	½ Pot/57g	215	20.1	378	14.2	0.8	35.3	0
Mackerel, Smoked, Scottish, M&S*	½ Pot/58g	158	13.3	275	15.9	0.6	23.2	0.1
Mackerel, Tesco*	1 Serving/29g	102	9.5	353	14.3	0.5	32.6	0
Mushroom, M&S*	1 Pot/115g	224	20.1	195	4.2	4.8	17.5	1.5
Mushroom, Sainsbury's*	½ Pot/58g	89	7	153	3.3	7.8	12.1	2.1
Salmon, Smoked, Isle of Skye, TTD, Sainsbury's*	½ Pot/58g	133	9.8	231	17.5	1.8	17.1	0.2
Salmon, Smoked, Scottish, Castle MacLellan*	¼ Tub/28g	76	6.4	271	9	7	22.9	0
Salmon, Smoked, Tesco*	1 Pack/115g	282	22	245	15	3	19.1	1
Tofu, Spicy Mexican, Organic, GranoVita*	1 Serving/50g	108	10	216	6	3	20	0
Tomato, Lentil, & Basil, Cauldron Foods*	1 Pot/115g	161	7.8	140	6.8	14	6.8	3.2
Trout, Smoked, Waitrose*	½ Pot/56g	130	10.3	232	15.8	0.9	18.4	0.6
Tuna, M&S*	1oz/28g	106	9.5	380	17	0.8	33.8	0.7
Tuna, Tesco*	1 Pack/115g	332	26.7	289	19.8	0.3	23.2	0.2
Tuna, with Butter & Lemon Juice, Sainsbury's*	½ Pot/58g	209	18.3	360	19	0.1	31.6	0.3
Turkey, Pork, & Duck, Liver, Deluxe, Lidl*	1 Pack/125g	366	30.6	293	13.1	4.5	24.5	1
Vegetable	*1oz/28g*	*48*	*3.8*	*173*	*7.5*	*5.9*	*13.4*	*0*
Vegetarian, with Mushrooms, Organic, Tartex*	¼ Tube/50g	102	8	203	7.7	7	16	0
Yeast, Garlic & Herb, Tartex*	1 Serving/30g	69	5.4	230	7	10	18	0
Yeast, Wild Mushroom, GranoVita*	1oz/28g	60	4.8	213	10	5	17	0
PATTY								
Beef, Jamaican, Port Royal*	1 Patty/130g	299	13.3	230	10.2	24.4	10.2	0
Fish, Salt, Jamaican, Port Royal*	1 Patty/130g	300	13.4	231	6.8	27.8	10.3	0
Lamb, Jamaican, Port Royal*	1 Patty/130g	352	17.4	271	7.2	30.5	13.4	0
Vegetarian, Jamaican, Port Royal*	1 Patty/130g	315	13.8	242	12.5	24.1	10.6	0
PAVLOVA								
Raspberry & Lemon, Asda*	1 Serving/43g	102	1.9	235	2.8	46	4.4	0.5
Raspberry, Individual, M&S*	1 Pavlova/65g	133	1.6	205	4	41.8	2.4	0.2
Raspberry, M&S*	1 Serving/84g	193	8.1	230	2.3	33.3	9.6	0.3
Raspberry, Tesco*	1 Serving/65g	191	8.4	294	2.7	41.8	12.9	1.1
Sticky Toffee, Sainsbury's*	1/6 Pavlova/60g	249	9.8	415	3.7	63.1	16.4	0.9
Strawberry & Champagne, Mini, Co-Op*	1 Pavlova/19g	65	3.6	340	3	40	19	0.8
Strawberry, COU, M&S*	1 Pot/95g	147	2.3	155	2.4	30.5	2.4	0.8
PAW-PAW								
Raw, Fresh	*1oz/28g*	*10*	*0*	*36*	*0.5*	*8.8*	*0.1*	*2.2*
Raw, Weighed with Skin & Pips	*1oz/28g*	*6*	*0*	*20*	*0.3*	*5*	*0.1*	*1.3*
PEACH								
Dried, Average	*1 Pack/250g*	*472*	*1.6*	*189*	*2.6*	*45*	*0.6*	*6.9*
in Fruit Juice, Average	*1oz/28g*	*13*	*0*	*47*	*0.5*	*11.2*	*0*	*0.7*
in Light Syrup, Canned, As Sold	*1 Serving/100g*	*66*	*0*	*66*	*0.4*	*15.9*	*0*	*1*
in Syrup, Average	*1oz/28g*	*19*	*0*	*67*	*0.4*	*16.3*	*0.1*	*0.4*
Pieces in Strawberry Jelly, Fruitini, Del Monte*	1 Can/140g	91	0.1	65	0.3	15.3	0.1	0
Raw, Stoned, Average	*1oz/28g*	*9*	*0*	*33*	*1*	*7.6*	*0.1*	*1.5*
Raw, Weighed with Stone, Average	*1 Peach/125g*	*39*	*0.1*	*31*	*1*	*7.2*	*0.1*	*1.3*
Slices in Fruit Juice, Average	*1 Serving/100g*	*49*	*0*	*49*	*0.6*	*11.6*	*0*	*0.5*

P

	Measure INFO/WEIGHT	per Measure KCAL	FAT	Nutrition Values per 100g / 100ml KCAL	PROT	CARB	FAT	FIBRE
PEANUT BUTTER								
30% Less Fat, Tesco*	1 Tbsp/15g	86	5.7	570	18.4	37.1	37.9	3.6
Crunchy , Hi-pro*	1 Serving/15g	93	7.4	618	33.9	5.6	49.1	7.3
Crunchy, Natural, No Added Sugar or Salt, Average	*1 Tsp/5g*	*30*	*2.4*	*606*	*27.6*	*12.2*	*48.4*	*7*
Smooth, Average	*1 Serving/20g*	*125*	*10.7*	*623*	*22.6*	*13.1*	*53.7*	*5.4*
Smooth, No Added Sugar, Organic, Whole Earth*	1 Serving/20g	126	10.2	628	25.6	13.7	51.2	4.9
Whole Nut, Crunchy, Average	*1 Tsp/10g*	*61*	*5.3*	*606*	*24.9*	*7.7*	*53.1*	*6*
PEANUTS								
Chilli, Average	*½ Pack/50g*	*303*	*25.3*	*605*	*28.2*	*9.3*	*50.6*	*6.8*
Dry Roasted, Average	*1 Serving/20g*	*117*	*9.8*	*587*	*25.7*	*11.5*	*48.8*	*6.5*
Honey Roasted, Average	*1oz/28g*	*169*	*13.2*	*605*	*26.8*	*23.6*	*47*	*5.5*
Plain, Average	*10 Whole/10g*	*59*	*5*	*592*	*24.7*	*11*	*50*	*6.3*
Roast, Salted, Average	*10 Whole/12g*	*74*	*6.3*	*614*	*27.8*	*7.9*	*52.4*	*4.9*
Salted, Average	*10 Whole/6g*	*37*	*3.1*	*609*	*27*	*8.3*	*52*	*5.4*
Sweet Chilli, Nobby's*	1 Bag/40g	214	13.6	535	15	42	34	3
PEARL BARLEY								
Boiled	*1oz/28g*	*34*	*0.1*	*123*	*2.3*	*28.2*	*0.4*	*3.8*
Raw, Average	*1oz/28g*	*99*	*0.3*	*352*	*9.9*	*77.7*	*1.2*	*15.6*
PEARS								
Abate Fetel, Average	*1 Med/133g*	*48*	*0.1*	*36*	*0.4*	*8.3*	*0.1*	*2.2*
Asian, Nashi, Raw, Average	*1 Lge/209g*	*80*	*0.4*	*38*	*0.5*	*9.7*	*0.2*	*3.3*
Blush, Morrisons*	1 Sm/148g	86	0.2	58	0.4	15.5	0.1	3.1
Blush, Tesco*	1 Pear/133g	62	0.1	47	0.3	10	0.1	2.2
Comice, Raw, Weighed with Core	*1 Med/170g*	*56*	*0*	*33*	*0.3*	*8.5*	*0*	*2*
Conference, Average	*1 Lge/209g*	*88*	*0.2*	*42*	*0.3*	*10.1*	*0.1*	*2*
Dessert, Green, Sainsbury's*	1 Sm/135g	53	0.1	39	0.3	9.2	0.1	2
Dried, Average	*1 Pear Half/16g*	*33*	*0.1*	*204*	*1.9*	*48.4*	*0.5*	*9.7*
in Fruit Juice, Average	*1 Serving/225g*	*102*	*0.1*	*45*	*0.3*	*10.9*	*0*	*1.2*
in Syrup, Average	*1oz/28g*	*16*	*0*	*58*	*0.2*	*14.4*	*0.1*	*1.4*
Prickly, Raw, Fresh	*1oz/28g*	*8*	*0.1*	*30*	*0.4*	*7*	*0.2*	*0*
Raw, Weighed with Core, Average	*1 Med/166g*	*58*	*0.2*	*35*	*0.3*	*8.4*	*0.1*	*1.3*
Red, Tesco*	1 Med/180g	65	0.2	36	0.4	8.3	0.1	2.2
William, Raw, Average	*1 Med/170g*	*58*	*0.2*	*34*	*0.4*	*8.3*	*0.1*	*2.2*
PEAS								
Black, Dried, Hodmedod's*	1 Serving/80g	230	1.7	288	23.5	32.2	2.1	22.9
Dried, Boiled in Unsalted Water, Average	*1oz/28g*	*31*	*0.2*	*109*	*6.9*	*19.9*	*0.8*	*5.5*
Dried, Raw, Average	*1oz/28g*	*85*	*0.7*	*303*	*21.6*	*52*	*2.4*	*13*
Edible Podded, Raw	*1 Cup/63g*	*25*	*0.1*	*39*	*2.6*	*7.1*	*0.2*	*2.4*
Frozen, Average	*1 Serving/85g*	*62*	*0.8*	*73*	*6*	*9.7*	*1*	*4.5*
Frozen, Boiled, Average	*1 Serving/75g*	*51*	*0.7*	*68*	*6*	*9.4*	*0.9*	*5.1*
Garden, Canned with Sugar & Salt, Average	*1 Serving/90g*	*59*	*0.6*	*66*	*5.3*	*9.3*	*0.7*	*5.1*
Garden, Canned, No Sugar Or Salt, Average	*1 Can/80g*	*36*	*0.3*	*45*	*4.4*	*6*	*0.4*	*2.8*
Garden, Frozen, Average	*1 Serving/90g*	*66*	*1*	*74*	*6.3*	*9.8*	*1.1*	*3.3*
Garden, Minted, Average	*1 Serving/80g*	*59*	*0.9*	*74*	*6.3*	*9.7*	*1.1*	*5.9*
Marrowfat, Average	*1 Sm Can/160g*	*134*	*0.9*	*84*	*6.1*	*13.7*	*0.6*	*3.7*
Mushy, Average	*1 Can/200g*	*173*	*1*	*86*	*6.2*	*14.4*	*0.5*	*2.2*
Processed, Canned, Average	*1 Sm Can/220g*	*162*	*1.6*	*74*	*5.6*	*11.3*	*0.7*	*3.4*
Snow	*1 Serving/80g*	*24*	*0.2*	*29*	*3.3*	*3.9*	*0.2*	*2.1*
Sugar Snap, Average	*1 Serving/80g*	*27*	*0.2*	*33*	*3.2*	*4.8*	*0.2*	*1.4*
Wasabi, & Horseradish, Roasted, Roasters, Dilly & Wolf*	1 Portion/25g	94	3.1	378	18.8	32.9	12.3	29.7
Wasabi, Average	*1 Serving/28g*	*114*	*3.8*	*406*	*15.2*	*54*	*13.7*	*8.6*
Wasabi, Delicious, Boots*	½ Bag/25g	98	2.4	393	19	51	9.6	15
Wasabi, Ranch, Snapea Crisp, Harvest Snaps, Calbee*	1 Serving/28g	120	5	429	17.9	57.1	17.9	14.3
Wasabi, Roasted, Savoury Snack, Humdinger*	1 Portion/20g	81	2.4	404	15.8	50.3	12	15.9

	Measure INFO/WEIGHT	per Measure KCAL	FAT	Nutrition Values per 100g / 100ml KCAL	PROT	CARB	FAT	FIBRE
PEASE PUDDING								
Canned, Re-Heated, Drained	**1oz/28g**	**26**	**0.2**	**93**	**6.8**	**16.1**	**0.6**	**1.8**
PECAN NUTS								
Average	**3 Nuts/6g**	**42**	**4.2**	**692**	**10**	**5.6**	**70.1**	**4.7**
Honey, Golden, Graze*	1 Pack/26g	168	15.4	647	7.6	23.4	59.4	0
PENNE								
Arrabiata, BGTY, Sainsbury's*	1 Pack/450g	414	7.2	92	2.9	16.5	1.6	1.9
Brown Rice, GF, Pasta, Waitrose*	¼ Pack/125g	250	2.1	200	4.1	41	1.7	1.9
Chicken, & Red Wine, Italiana, Weight Watchers*	1 Pack/395g	249	2.8	63	3.7	10.1	0.7	0.6
Chicken, & Tomato, Italian, Sainsbury's*	½ Pack/350g	472	11.2	135	7.6	19	3.2	1.6
Chicken, & Vegetables, Eat Positive, Birds Eye*	1 Meal/396.3g	325	5.2	82	7.7	9.8	1.3	1.2
Chicken, & Vegetables, Tomato & Basil Sauce, Birds Eye*	1 Meal/400g	325	5.2	81	7.8	9.8	1.3	1.2
Cooked, Average	**1 Serving/185g**	**244**	**1.3**	**132**	**4.7**	**26.7**	**0.7**	**1.1**
Dry, Average	**1 Serving/100g**	**352**	**1.9**	**352**	**12.4**	**71.3**	**1.9**	**2.7**
Egg, Fresh, Average	**1 Serving/125g**	**352**	**4**	**282**	**11.1**	**52.2**	**3.2**	**2**
Free From, Tesco*	1 Serving/100g	340	2	340	8	72.5	2	2.5
Fresh, Dry, Average	**1 Serving/125g**	**222**	**2.4**	**178**	**7.3**	**32.2**	**1.9**	**1.6**
Organic, Dry, Average	**1 Serving/100g**	**352**	**1.8**	**352**	**12.4**	**71.6**	**1.8**	**1.9**
Red Pepper, Roasted, GFY, Asda*	1 Pack/400g	212	2.4	53	1.9	10	0.6	0.8
Rigate, Dry Weight, Average	**1 Serving/90g**	**318**	**1.6**	**353**	**12.3**	**72.1**	**1.8**	**1.8**
Salmon, Smoked, Bistro, Morrisons*	½ Pack/350g	612	23.8	175	9.7	18	6.8	1.4
Tomato & Basil, Sauce, Asda*	½ Pack/314g	185	11	59	0.8	6	3.5	2
Tomato & Basil, Sauce, Sainsbury's*	½ Pack/110g	118	0.7	107	3.6	21.8	0.6	1.1
Tomato & Vegetable, Roasted, Big Eat, Heinz*	1 Pot/351.3g	281	10.5	80	2.5	10.7	3	4.6
Vegetable, Roasted, Waitrose*	1 Pack/400g	424	15.6	106	2.8	15	3.9	0.8
Wholewheat, Asda*	1 Serving/100g	333	2.1	333	12.1	66.3	2.1	6.9
Wholewheat, Authentic, Italiano, Tesco*	1 Portion/75g	244	1.9	325	12.5	62.5	2.5	9
PEPERAMI*								
Firestick, Peperami*	1 Stick/25g	127	11	508	24.5	3.5	44	1.2
Hot, Peperami*	1 Stick/25g	126	11	504	24.5	2.5	44	1.2
Lunchbox Minis, 30% Less Fat, Peperami*	1 Stick/10g	40	3.1	400	26	5.5	31	3
Original, Peperami*	1 Stick/25g	126	11	504	24	2.5	44	0.1
PEPPER								
Black, Freshly Ground, Average	**1 Tsp/2g**	**5**	**0.1**	**255**	**11**	**64.8**	**3.3**	**26.5**
Cayenne, Ground	**1 Tsp/2g**	**6**	**0.3**	**318**	**12**	**31.7**	**17.3**	**0**
White	**½ Tsp/1g**	**3**	**0**	**296**	**10.4**	**68.6**	**2.1**	**26.2**
PEPPERCORNS								
Black, Schwartz*	1 Tsp/2g	11	0.4	529	13	68.7	22.5	27
Green, Average	**1 Tsp/10g**	**4**	**0.1**	**44**	**1.6**	**5.3**	**0.8**	**4.7**
PEPPERS								
Chargrilled, Spirit of Summer, M&S*	1 Pack/105g	45	1.5	43	1	5.6	1.4	2
Chilli, Crushed, Schwartz*	1 Tsp/0.5g	2	0.1	321	12	29	17	27
Chilli, Dried, Flakes, Average	**1 Tsp/3g**	**13**	**0.4**	**425**	**16**	**56**	**15**	**44**
Chilli, Green, Raw, Unprepared, Average	**1 Med/13g**	**4**	**0**	**29**	**1.5**	**6.9**	**0.1**	**1.1**
Chilli, Red, Chopped, Frozen, Sainsbury's*	1 Tsp/5g	3	0	64	2.6	10.7	0.6	2.5
Chilli, Red, Raw, Unprepared, Average	**1 Pepper/13g**	**4**	**0**	**29**	**1.5**	**6.9**	**0.1**	**1.1**
Chilli, Red, Very Lazy, The English Provender Co.*	1 Serving/15g	17	0.6	114	4.2	15.3	4	0.5
Green, Boiled in Salted Water	**1oz/28g**	**5**	**0.1**	**18**	**1**	**2.6**	**0.5**	**1.8**
Green, Raw, Unprepared, Average	**1 Med/160g**	**20**	**0.4**	**13**	**0.7**	**2.2**	**0.3**	**1.3**
Jalapeno, Raw	**1 Pepper/14g**	**4**	**0.1**	**28**	**1.2**	**5.4**	**0.6**	**2.6**
Mixed Bag, From Supermarket, Average	**1oz/28g**	**7**	**0.1**	**25**	**1**	**4.4**	**0.4**	**1.7**
Orange, Sweet, Raw, Average	**1oz/28g**	**8**	**0.1**	**30**	**1.8**	**5**	**0.3**	**1.5**
Red, Boiled in Salted Water	**1oz/28g**	**10**	**0.1**	**34**	**1.1**	**7**	**0.4**	**1.7**
Red, Ramiro, Sainsbury's*	1 Serving/100g	30	0.3	30	1.6	5.1	0.3	2.2

P

	Measure INFO/WEIGHT	per Measure KCAL	FAT	Nutrition Values per 100g / 100ml KCAL	PROT	CARB	FAT	FIBRE
PEPPERS								
Red, Raw, Unprepared, Average	*1oz/28g*	*7*	*0.1*	*27*	*0.8*	*5.3*	*0.3*	*1.3*
Red, Roasted, in Brine, Cooks & Co*	1 Serving/100g	23	0.3	23	1.6	4.5	0.3	0
Red, Sweet Pointed, Organic, Tesco*	1 Serving/100g	33	0.4	33	1	6.4	0.4	1.6
Stuffed, Cheesy Rice, Growers Selection, Asda*	1 Pack/252g	244	9.6	97	3	12	3.8	1.4
Stuffed, Cream Cheese, Sweet, Aldi*	1 Serving/60g	92	7.2	154	3.7	6.9	12	2.1
Stuffed, Mediterranean, Everdine*	1 Serving/450g	436	18.9	97	2.8	10.4	4.2	3.3
Stuffed, PB, Waitrose*	1 Pack/300g	243	7.2	81	3	11.8	2.4	1.3
Stuffed, Red, Filled, Halves, Vegetarian, M&S*	1 Pack/295g	239	9.7	81	2.4	9.7	3.3	1.6
Stuffed, with Rice Based Filling, Average	*1oz/28g*	*24*	*0.7*	*85*	*1.5*	*15.4*	*2.4*	*1.3*
Stuffed, with Vegetables, Cheese Topping, Average	*1oz/28g*	*31*	*1.9*	*111*	*3.4*	*9.8*	*6.7*	*1.5*
Yellow, Raw, Unprepared, Average	*1 Med/160g*	*35*	*0.3*	*22*	*1*	*4.4*	*0.2*	*1.4*
PERCH								
Raw, Atlantic	*1oz/28g*	*26*	*0.5*	*94*	*18.6*	*0*	*1.6*	*0*
PERNOD*								
19% Volume, Pernod*	1 Pub Shot/35ml	46	0	130	0	0	0	0
Ricard Pastis, Pernod Ricard*	1 Pub Shot/25ml	64	0	257	0	36.7	0	0
PESTO								
Aubergine, & Mushroom, Spread, Tan Rosie Foods*	1 Tbsp/20g	19	1.7	96	1.6	3	8.5	2
Aubergine, Chargrilled, Sacla*	1 Serving/30g	102	10.5	339	2.4	3.8	34.9	0
Chilli, Fiery, Sacla*	½ Jar/95g	342	29.3	360	4.8	16	30.8	3.4
Green, Alla Genovese, Finest, Tesco*	1 Serving/65g	188	25.7	290	5.7	1.5	39.6	2.8
Green, Alla Genovese, Sacla*	1 Serving/30g	116	12.1	388	5.2	0.8	40.4	5.7
Green, Asda*	1 Tsp/5g	21	2.2	429	4.7	3.5	44	1.4
Green, Average	*1 Tbsp/20g*	*103*	*9.5*	*517*	*20.4*	*2*	*47.5*	*0*
Green, Classic, Sacla*	1 Serving/40g	185	18.6	462	5.2	7.6	46.5	0
Green, Fresh, Tesco*	1oz/28g	141	13.4	505	6.5	12.2	48	0.1
Green, Less Than 60% Fat, BGTY, Sainsbury's*	¼ Jar/48g	61	5.3	128	4.2	2.6	11.2	0
Green, Organic, Sacla*	1 Serving/25g	115	12	461	5.5	1.5	48.1	0
Green, Reduced Fat, Tesco*	¼ Jar /49g	96	9.5	195	2.6	0.7	19.4	3.4
Green, Sainsbury's*	1 Tsp/5g	23	2.2	451	5.9	10.1	43	2
Green, Tesco*	¼ Jar/47.5g	192	20	405	5.6	0.6	42.2	4.4
Olive, Black, Sacla*	1oz/28g	115	11.8	409	2.9	4.3	42.2	0
Olive, Deluxe, Lidl*	1 Tsp/8g	20	2	254	2.2	4.2	24.4	0
Red, Garlic & Chilli, Jamie Oliver*	1 Jar/190g	494	48.8	260	1.1	5.6	25.7	1.1
Red, Morrisons*	1 Tbsp/15g	47	4.4	311	5.7	6.6	29	5.9
Red, Rosso, Bertolli*	1 Jar/185g	703	64.8	380	6.8	9.5	35	2
Spinach & Parmesan, Sainsbury's*	¼ Jar/46.4g	162	16	349	4.6	5.3	34.4	2.5
Sun Dried Tomato, Sacla*	1 Serving/30g	87	8.4	289	4.2	5.2	27.9	0
Wild Rocket, Sacla*	1 Serving/30g	128	13	425	5.2	3.2	43.5	4.5
PETIT POIS								
& Baby Carrots, Canned, Drained, Average	*½ Can/122g*	*58*	*0.8*	*47*	*2.9*	*7*	*0.7*	*3.2*
Canned, Drained, Average	*1 Sm Can/200g*	*125*	*1*	*63*	*4.8*	*8.9*	*0.5*	*2.6*
Fresh, Frozen, Average	*1 Serving/80g*	*51*	*0.8*	*63*	*5.4*	*7.1*	*1*	*4.8*
PHEASANT								
Breast, Fillets, Skinless, Cooked, Gressingham Foods*	1 Serving/100g	127	2.4	127	32.7	0	2.4	0
Meat Only, Roasted	*1oz/28g*	*62*	*3.4*	*220*	*27.9*	*0*	*12*	*0*
Meat Only, Roasted, Weighed with Bone	*1oz/28g*	*32*	*1.7*	*114*	*14.5*	*0*	*6.2*	*0*
Stuffed, Easy Carve, Finest, Tesco*	1 Serving/200g	540	37.4	270	23.2	2.2	18.7	0.9
PHYSALIS								
Goldenberries, Dried, Neal's Yard*	1 Serving/20g	60	1.6	302	6	42.8	8	17.4
Raw, without Husk, Average	*5 Fruits/30g*	*16*	*0.2*	*53*	*1.9*	*11.2*	*0.7*	*0.4*
PICCALILLI								
Haywards*	1 Serving/28g	18	0.1	66	1.4	13.9	0.5	0

P

	Measure INFO/WEIGHT	per Measure KCAL	per Measure FAT	Nutrition Values per 100g / 100ml KCAL	PROT	CARB	FAT	FIBRE
PICCALILLI								
Heinz*	1 Serving/10g	10	0.1	99	1	20.5	0.6	0.6
M&S*	1 Serving/20g	21	0.1	105	1.3	23	0.6	1.1
Morrisons*	1 Serving/50g	38	0.4	75	1.6	15	0.7	0.6
Sweet & Mild, Haywards*	2 Tbsp/40g	41	0.3	102	0.5	21	0.8	1
Sweet, Asda*	1 Tbsp/15g	17	0	112	0.5	27	0.2	0.6
Tesco*	1 Serving/50g	51	1.8	102	0.5	17.8	3.6	2
Three Mustard, Finest, Tesco*	1 Serving/30g	40	0.2	134	1.3	30.7	0.7	1
PICKLE								
Branston, Original, Crosse & Blackwell*	1 Serving/12g	19	0.1	157	0.5	34	0.7	1.8
Branston, Red Onion & Cranberry, Crosse & Blackwell*	1 Tbsp/14g	13	0.1	92	0.6	21.4	0.4	0.8
Branston, Red Pepper & Tomato, Crosse & Blackwell*	1 Tbsp/14g	12	0	84	1.2	17.7	0.3	1.1
Branston, Sm Chunk, Squeezy, Crosse & Blackwell*	1 Serving/15g	19	0	127	0.9	29.8	0.2	1.1
Branston, Smooth, Squeezy, Crosse & Blackwell*	1 Serving/15g	19	0	127	0.9	29.8	0.2	1.1
Branston, Sweet, Sm Chunk, Crosse & Blackwell*	1 Serving/20g	22	0	109	0.8	26.1	0.2	1.1
Brinjal, Patak's*	1 Tsp/16g	59	3.9	367	2.2	34.6	24.4	0.9
Chilli, Patak's*	1 Tsp/16g	52	5.4	325	4.3	1.3	33.7	0
Cornichons, Freshona, Lidl*	1 Serving/50g	18	0.2	35	1.2	5.5	0.3	0
Cucumber, Dill, Krakus*	1 Portion/80g	19	0	24	0	5.4	0	1.2
Garlic, Patak's*	1 Tsp/16g	42	3	261	3.6	20	18.5	1.6
Hot Chilli Jam, What A Pickle*	1 Tsp/8g	14	0	178	0.6	44	0.1	1.2
Lime, Hot, Patak's*	1 Tsp/16g	31	3	194	2.2	4	18.7	0.4
Lime, Oily	*1 Serving/39g*	*70*	*6.1*	*178*	*1.9*	*8.3*	*15.5*	*0*
Lime, Sharwood's*	1 Tbsp/20g	28	2	142	1.7	11.5	9.9	1.3
Mild Mustard, Heinz*	1 Tbsp/10g	13	0.1	129	2.2	25.7	1.3	0.9
Mixed, Drained	*1 Serving/100g*	*14*	*0.2*	*14*	*1*	*1.9*	*0.2*	*1*
Mixed, Drained, Haywards*	½ Jar/120g	22	0.4	18	1.4	2.4	0.3	0
Mixed, Patak's*	1 Serving/30g	78	7.7	259	2.3	4.7	25.7	0.8
Red Cabbage, Asda*	1 Serving/50g	16	0	32	1.6	6	0.1	0
Sandwich, Tesco*	1 Tbsp/30g	38	0	126	0.7	29.5	0.1	1.9
Sweet	*1 Tsp/10g*	*14*	*0*	*141*	*0.6*	*36*	*0.1*	*1.2*
Sweet, Batts, Lidl*	1 Serving/15g	17	0.1	114	0.8	26	0.5	1.1
Sweet, Bramwells*	1 Tbsp/15g	20	1	130	0.7	30	0.5	1.7
Sweet, Country, Morrisons*	1 Tbsp/15g	20	0	130	0.9	31.1	0.2	0
Sweet, Original, Tesco*	1 Tbsp/15g	20	0	135	0.5	31.5	0.1	2.1
Sweet, Savers, Morrisons*	1 Tbsp/15g	18	0	121	0.9	27.2	0.3	1.6
Tangy, Sandwich, Heinz*	1 Tsp/10g	13	0	134	0.7	31.4	0.2	0.9
PICNIC								
Cadbury*	1 Bar/48g	230	10.9	475	7.3	60.9	22.6	2.1
PIE								
Admiral's, Ross*	1 Pie/340g	357	15.6	105	4.8	10.9	4.6	0.7
Apple, & Blackberry, Bramley, Aunt Bessie's*	¼ Pie/137.5g	344	12.5	250	2.1	40.1	9.1	2.6
Apple, & Blackberry, Co-Op*	1 Serving/138g	338	15.2	245	3	33	11	2
Apple, & Blackberry, Fruit, Finest, Tesco*	1 Pie/95g	265	11.3	279	13.7	29.3	11.9	2.8
Apple, & Blackberry, Lattice Topped, BGTY, Sainsbury's*	¼ Pie/100g	256	7.5	256	2.8	44.4	7.5	3.1
Apple, & Blackberry, Shortcrust, M&S*	1 Serving/142g	469	17.8	330	4.3	50.2	12.5	1.1
Apple, Bramley, Aunt Bessie's*	¼ Pie/138g	386	15.1	281	2.4	42	11	1.1
Apple, Bramley, Bakery, Tesco*	1/6 Pie/87g	237	9.9	272	2.8	38.8	11.4	1.9
Apple, Bramley, Free From, Sainsbury's*	1 Pie/60g	220	7.6	367	1.1	61.8	12.6	1.2
Apple, Bramley, Individual, Mr Kipling*	1 Pie/66g	228	8.6	346	3.4	53.8	13	1.4
Apple, Bramley, Individual, Sainsbury's*	1 Pie/54g	165	5	307	3.6	52.2	9.3	1.3
Apple, Bramley, Individual, Tesco*	1 Pie/61g	210	7.9	344	3.4	53.1	13	1.5
Apple, Bramley, Large, Tesco*	1/8 Pie/87g	311	13	358	3.9	51.9	15	1.9
Apple, Commercially Prepared	*1 Slice/125g*	*296*	*13.8*	*237*	*1.9*	*34*	*11*	*1.6*

	Measure INFO/WEIGHT	per Measure KCAL	FAT	Nutrition Values per 100g / 100ml KCAL	PROT	CARB	FAT	FIBRE
PIE								
Apple, Deep Filled, Sainsbury's*	¼ Pie/137g	374	17.5	273	3.8	35.6	12.8	1.6
Apple, Pastry Top & Bottom	*1oz/28g*	*74*	*3.7*	*266*	*2.9*	*35.8*	*13.3*	*1.7*
Apple, Prepared From Recipe, Average	*1oz/28g*	*74*	*3.5*	*265*	*2.4*	*37.1*	*12.5*	*0*
Apple, Puff Pastry, M&S*	1 Pie/135g	338	17.1	250	2.4	31.3	12.7	1
Apple, Sainsbury's*	1/6 Pie/118g	314	13.6	266	3.4	37.1	11.5	0.6
Apple, with Custard	*1 Serving/217g*	*353*	*18.8*	*163*	*2.4*	*25.2*	*8.7*	*1.1*
Banoffee, Finest, Tesco*	1/6 Pie/69g	255	16.5	368	4.1	33.7	23.8	1.5
Banoffee, Mini, Waitrose*	1 Pie/26g	115	5.8	444	3.3	57	22.5	1.2
Banoffee, Tesco*	1/6 Pie/94g	365	19.7	390	3.9	45.8	21.1	1.5
Beef, & Onion, Minced, Tesco*	1 Pie/150g	454	28.5	303	5.7	27.4	19	1.7
Beef, & Onion, Pukka Pies Ltd*	1 Serving/231g	529	32.6	229	7.6	17.9	14.1	3
Beef, & Potato, Minced, Weight Watchers*	1 Pie/200g	328	12.4	164	6.7	20.2	6.2	3.6
Beef, Bourguignon, Deluxe, Lidl*	1 Pie/190g	591	37.6	311	9.6	22.7	19.8	1.8
Beef, Minced, Aberdeen Angus, Shortcrust, M&S*	1 Pie/170.6g	435	26.6	255	9.3	19.3	15.6	3
Cheese, & Onion, Hollands*	1 Pie/200g	516	24.4	258	6.3	30.9	12.2	0
Cheese, & Onion, Oven Baked, Average	*1 Serving/200g*	*654*	*40*	*327*	*8.2*	*30.4*	*20*	*1.2*
Cheese, & Potato	*1oz/28g*	*39*	*2.3*	*139*	*4.8*	*12.6*	*8.1*	*0.7*
Cheese, & Potato, Aunt Bessie's*	¼ Serving/200g	288	18.8	144	4.6	11.7	9.4	1.5
Cherry, Bakery, Tesco*	1/6 Pie/87g	240	9.7	276	2.6	40.5	11.2	1.3
Chicken, & Asparagus, McDougalls*	1 Serving/170g	394	21.9	232	7.4	21.6	12.9	1.5
Chicken, & Asparagus, Tesco*	1 Serving/170g	468	28.7	275	8.3	22.4	16.9	0.8
Chicken, & Bacon, Puff Pastry, Deep Fill, Sainsbury's*	1/3 Pie/200g	532	34	266	9.1	19.1	17	1.3
Chicken, & Broccoli, Lattice, Tesco*	½ Pie/200g	496	30.8	248	8.5	18.9	15.4	2.1
Chicken, & Chorizo, Simply Bistro, Aldi*	1 Pie/210g	647	42	308	9.9	22	20	1.3
Chicken, & Gravy, Deep Fill, Asda*	1 Serving/130g	370	22.1	285	10	23	17	0.8
Chicken, & Gravy, Just, Fray Bentos*	½ Pie/215g	267	7.3	124	5.6	17.2	3.4	0.6
Chicken, & Gravy, Roast, Deep Fill, Tesco*	1 Pie/700g	1540	68.6	220	11.2	20.2	9.8	2
Chicken, & Gravy, Shortcrust Pastry, Large, Tesco*	1 Pie/600g	1578	91.2	263	8.2	23.4	15.2	1
Chicken, & Gravy, Shortcrust Pastry, Tesco*	1 Pie/250g	618	34.5	247	6.8	23.9	13.8	1
Chicken, & Ham, & Leek, Pot, Higgidy*	1 Pie/250g	710	33.5	284	13.1	19.1	13.4	1.1
Chicken, & Ham, Deep Filled, Sainsbury's*	1 Pie/210g	594	37.2	283	8	23	17.7	1
Chicken, & Ham, Family, Farmfoods*	1oz/28g	67	3.9	241	9.9	19.4	13.8	1.2
Chicken, & Ham, Morrisons*	¼ Pie/115g	267	13.7	232	8.7	22.5	11.9	0.8
Chicken, & Ham, Tesco*	1 Serving/113g	293	17.6	259	9.4	20.2	15.6	1.2
Chicken, & Leek, & Bacon, Aldi*	1 Pie/210g	601	37.6	286	10.9	19.7	17.9	1
Chicken, & Leek, & Bacon, Deluxe, Lidl*	1/3 Pie/171g	511	30.8	299	11	22	18	2.7
Chicken, & Leek, & Ham, Morrisons*	1 Serving/113g	305	16.6	270	8.8	25.7	14.7	1.1
Chicken, & Leek, & Sweetcorn, Love Life, Waitrose*	1 Pie/421g	358	14.3	85	5.2	8.6	3.4	1.7
Chicken, & Leek, Deep Filled, Puff Pastry, Sainsbury's*	1/3 Pie/451g	1109	65.4	246	10.1	18.7	14.5	1.5
Chicken, & Leek, LC, Tesco*	1 Pie/350g	298	5.6	85	6.6	10.3	1.6	1.3
Chicken, & Leek, M&S*	1oz/28g	70	4.2	250	10.1	18.8	15.1	1.1
Chicken, & Leek, Shortcrust, TTD, Sainsbury's*	½ Pie/300g	824	48.8	275	12.2	19.8	16.3	1.1
Chicken, & Mushroom, & Potato, Filo, COU, M&S*	1 Pack/260g	273	7	105	7.5	12.1	2.7	1.5
Chicken, & Mushroom, Asda*	1 Pie/150g	384	24	256	9	19	16	1
Chicken, & Mushroom, Average	*1 Serving/200g*	*540*	*31.7*	*270*	*8*	*23.8*	*15.9*	*1*
Chicken, & Mushroom, Fray Bentos*	1 Pie/425g	684	40.4	161	6.7	11.5	9.5	0
Chicken, & Mushroom, Ginsters*	1 Pie/180g	486	31.1	270	8.3	20.2	17.3	1.3
Chicken, & Mushroom, Individual, Frozen, Tesco*	1 Pie/142g	347	17.9	245	8.9	23.5	12.6	1.2
Chicken, & Mushroom, Pukka Pies Ltd*	1 Pie/226g	475	29.2	210	7.6	15.7	12.9	3.5
Chicken, & Vegetable, PB, Waitrose*	1 Serving/375g	285	5.2	76	5.1	10.8	1.4	1.3
Chicken, & Vegetable, Value, Tesco*	1 Pie/121g	321	16.9	265	6.6	26.9	14	1.1
Chicken, & Wiltshire Ham, Finest, Tesco*	1 Pie/250g	688	37.2	275	11.6	22.7	14.9	1.1
Chicken, Aunt Bessie's*	¼ Pie/200g	474	24.2	237	10.6	21.4	12.1	2.1

PIE

	Measure INFO/WEIGHT	per Measure KCAL	per Measure FAT	Nutrition Values per 100g / 100ml KCAL	PROT	CARB	FAT	FIBRE
Chicken, Deep Filled, Puff Pastry, Sainsbury's*	1 Pie/210g	538	31.9	256	10	19.9	15.2	3.1
Chicken, Individual, Made with 100% Breast, Birds Eye*	1 Pie/153.7g	455	28.1	296	7.9	25	18.3	1
Chicken, Individual, Ready Made, Average	*1 Pie/155g*	*392*	*22.3*	*253*	*9.5*	*20.9*	*14.4*	*1.6*
Chicken, Shortcrust, M&S*	1 Pie/170g	510	29.6	300	9.7	26.2	17.4	1.7
Chicken, Shortcrust, Oven Baked, Birds Eye*	1 Pie/155g	411	23.1	267	8.5	24	15	1.2
Cod, & Haddock, Smoked, COU, M&S*	1 Pack/400g	320	9.6	80	6.1	9	2.4	1.2
Cottage, Aberdeen Angus, Bistro, M Kitchen, Morrisons*	1 Pack/700g	791	30.8	113	7	10.4	4.4	1.7
Cottage, Aberdeen Angus, Large, Chilled, Finest, Tesco*	½ Pack/400g	420	17.2	105	7.1	8.7	4.3	1.8
Cottage, Aberdeen Angus, Specially Selected, Aldi*	1 Pack/400g	547	30.3	137	7.6	8.6	7.6	1.8
Cottage, Aldi*	1 Pack/440g	484	27.3	110	4.1	9.5	6.2	0.2
Cottage, Asda*	1 Pack/400g	360	9.6	90	6.5	10.6	2.4	1
Cottage, Basics, Sainsbury's*	1 Pack/300g	228	9	76	4.4	7.9	3	1.5
Cottage, Beef, Delicious, Annabel Karmel*	1 Pack/200g	174	6	87	4.4	16.2	3	2.2
Cottage, Classic British, Sainsbury's*	1 Pack/450g	436	16.2	97	5.3	9.9	3.6	1.7
Cottage, COU, M&S*	1 Pack/400g	340	8	85	6	11	2	1.5
Cottage, Diet Chef Ltd*	1 Pack/270g	235	9.7	87	3.7	9.8	3.6	1.7
Cottage, Family, Iceland*	¼ Pack/259.1g	262	10.6	101	4.2	11.8	4.1	0.8
Cottage, Fresh, M&S*	1 Pie/400g	460	22.4	115	6.8	9.9	5.6	0.6
Cottage, Frozen, Weight Watchers*	1 Pack/320g	252	6.4	79	5.2	9.5	2	1
Cottage, Healthy Living, Co-Op*	1 Pack/400g	320	6.4	80	5	11	1.6	2
Cottage, Lentil & Vegetable, Linda McCartney*	1 Pot/398g	374	10.3	94	2.8	13.5	2.6	2.5
Cottage, Luxury, M&S*	½ Pack/310g	403	21.7	130	7.9	8.3	7	1.8
Cottage, Meal for One, M&S*	1 Pack/445g	356	16	80	5.4	6.2	3.6	1.7
Cottage, Mini, Waitrose*	1 Pack/250g	268	10.5	107	6.4	11.1	4.2	1.4
Cottage, Morrisons*	1 Pack/450g	450	18.4	100	5.2	10.7	4.1	1.2
Cottage, Ready Meals , Tesco*	1 Pack/400g	380	12	95	6.1	10.8	3	1.6
Cottage, Retail, Average	*1 Pack/400g*	*399*	*15.7*	*100*	*5.5*	*10.5*	*3.9*	*1.3*
Cottage, Vegetarian, Sainsbury's*	1 Pack/450g	328	9.9	73	3	10.2	2.2	1.8
Cottage, Waitrose*	1 Pack/400g	424	19.6	106	3.4	12.1	4.9	1.2
Cottage, with Cheddar Mash, TTD, Sainsbury's*	1 Pack/400g	601	27.6	150	9.2	11.6	6.9	2.4
Cottage,1kg, Aldi*	1 Serving/500g	460	17.5	92	5.4	9	3.5	1.5
Cumberland, Asda*	1 Pack/400g	504	22.4	126	6.3	12.7	5.6	1.5
Cumberland, M&S*	1 Pie/195g	312	20.3	160	6.9	10.1	10.4	1.1
Fish	*1 Serving/250g*	*262*	*7.5*	*105*	*8*	*12.3*	*3*	*0.7*
Fish, Asda*	1 Pack/450g	558	28.4	124	7.3	9.5	6.3	1
Fish, Charlie Bigham's*	½ Pack/328g	499	29.9	152	8.4	9.6	9.1	0
Fish, Co-Op*	1 Pack/400g	380	16	95	4	12	4	0.9
Fish, Creamy, Classics, Large, Finest, Tesco*	½ Pack/350g	402	19.6	115	6.4	8.6	5.6	0.9
Fish, Crunchy Topped, Menu, Waitrose*	1 Pack/400g	444	19.2	111	7.5	8.4	4.8	1.8
Fish, Cumberland, M&S*	1 Pack/400g	476	18.4	119	8.5	10.5	4.6	0.9
Fish, Extra Special, Asda*	1 Pack/400g	540	30.8	135	9.8	6.5	7.7	1.1
Fish, HL, Tesco*	1 Pack/400g	352	9.5	93	6.6	10.8	2.5	0.7
Fish, Luxury, Cafe Culture, M&S*	1 Pack/660g	627	26.4	95	7.1	7.8	4	1.1
Fish, Luxury, Oven Baked (700g), Extra Special, Asda*	1 Pack/653g	666	27.4	102	8	7.4	4.2	1.1
Fish, Mariner's, Frozen, Oven Baked, Youngs*	1 Pack/340g	444	20.3	140	5.1	15.1	6.4	1
Fish, Meal for One, Oven Baked, Gastro, Youngs*	1 Pie/317g	412	20.3	130	8.5	9.2	6.4	1
Fish, Potato Topped, Mini Meal, M&S*	1 Serving/220g	216	7.7	98	7	9.1	3.5	0.9
Fish, TTD, Sainsbury's*	½ Pack/390g	386	12.9	99	7.1	10.3	3.3	1.6
Fish, with Cheese, Ross*	1 Pack/300g	321	13.5	107	4.7	12	4.5	0.8
Fish, with Grated Cheddar, Asda*	¼ Pie/250g	262	12.5	105	7	8	5	1
Fisherman's, Chilled, Co-Op*	1 Pie/300g	345	18	115	4	11	6	0.7
Fisherman's, Youngs*	1 Pack/340g	377	13.6	111	5.6	12.8	4	0.8
Fruit, Pastry Top & Bottom	*1oz/28g*	*73*	*3.7*	*260*	*3*	*34*	*13.3*	*1.8*

P

INFO/WEIGHT	Measure	per Measure KCAL	FAT	Nutrition Values per 100g / 100ml KCAL	PROT	CARB	FAT	FIBRE
PIE								
Fruit, Selection, Mr Kipling*	1 Pie/66g	232	9	350	3.5	53.5	13.6	1.3
Lamb, & Mint, Shortcrust Pasty, Tesco*	¼ Pack/150g	412	26.1	275	5.9	23.6	17.4	1.6
Lemon Meringue	*1 Portion/120g*	*383*	*17.3*	*319*	*4.5*	*45.9*	*14.4*	*0.7*
Lemon Meringue, Mini, Asda*	1 Pie/26g	101	3.3	396	3.7	66	13	1.8
Lemon Meringue, Sainsbury's*	¼ Pie/110g	351	9.9	319	2.3	57.3	9	0.5
Lemon Meringue, Tesco*	1 Pie/385g	989	28.1	257	4	43.7	7.3	0.5
Lentil, & Olive, Greek, Clive's*	1 Pie/235g	505	25.1	215	5.2	21.8	10.7	0
Macaroni Cheese, Countryside*	1 Serving/144g	282	10.1	196	4.9	28.3	7	1.2
Meat, & Potato, Hollands*	1 Pie/175g	410	19.2	234	6.1	27.5	11	0
Meat, & Potato, Tesco*	1 Serving/150g	414	26.8	276	5.1	23.6	17.9	1.6
Mince, All Butter Pastry, Extra Special, Asda*	1 Pie/70g	278	11.1	400	3.6	59	16	3.2
Mince, All Butter, 1, Waitrose*	1 Pie/61g	238	8.9	391	3.3	60	14.6	3.3
Mince, All Butter, Average	*1 Pie/65g*	*251*	*8.9*	*386*	*4*	*60.2*	*13.8*	*2.4*
Mince, All Butter, Mini, 1, Waitrose*	1 Pie/28g	111	3.8	392	3.1	63.6	13.4	2.5
Mince, All Butter, Mini, Average	*1 Pie/20g*	*78*	*2.8*	*389*	*4.3*	*61.6*	*13.8*	*2.8*
Mince, All Butter, Mini, The Best, Morrisons*	1 Pie/32g	127	4.7	402	4	62	14.9	2
Mince, All Butter, Puff Pastry, Average	*1 Pie/60g*	*228*	*10.5*	*381*	*4.3*	*51.1*	*17.4*	*2.2*
Mince, All Butter, Puff Pastry, Extra Special, Asda*	1 Pie/51g	195	10.1	386	3.8	47	20	1.3
Mince, Butter Enriched, Puff Pastry, Bakery, Sainsbury's*	1 Pie/65g	246	9.7	379	4.7	55.4	14.9	2.2
Mince, Christmas, Classic, Asda*	1 Pie/57g	229	9.1	401	3.5	59	16	3.5
Mince, Christmas, Finest, Tesco*	1 Pie/64g	255	9.4	395	4.6	60.3	14.5	1.4
Mince, Christmas, Sainsbury's*	1 Pie/37g	147	6	397	4.5	58	16.3	2.6
Mince, Deep Fill, Holly Lane, Aldi*	1 Pie/65g	265	10.4	407	3.9	61	16	3.3
Mince, Deep Filled, All Butter Pastry, Finest, Tesco*	1 Pie/65g	259	10.8	401	5	56.2	16.7	2.7
Mince, Deep Filled, All Butter, The Best, Morrisons*	1 Pie/67g	263	10.3	395	3.9	59.4	15.4	1.9
Mince, Deep Filled, Morrisons*	1 Pie/66g	257	9.7	386	3.7	57.9	14.6	4.2
Mince, Deep, Morrisons*	1 Pie/65g	243	9.1	371	3.7	57.8	13.9	1.5
Mince, Dusted, Mini, Finest, Tesco*	1 Pie/20g	76	2.4	379	7.3	62.9	12.2	5
Mince, Free From, Sainsbury's*	1 Pie/58g	226	7.5	393	2.3	64	13	2.5
Mince, Iced Top, Asda*	1 Pie/55g	220	7.7	399	2.8	63	14	4.7
Mince, Iced Top, Tesco*	1 Pie/58g	223	7.1	381	3.8	62.8	12.2	2.5
Mince, Individual, Average	*1 Pie/65g*	*260*	*11*	*400*	*4.2*	*56.3*	*17*	*1.6*
Mince, Individual, Mr Kipling*	1 Pie/66.4g	253	9.2	381	3.7	59.5	13.8	1.3
Mince, Luxury, Deep Filled, M&S*	1 Pie/65g	234	9	360	4.3	55	13.8	3.8
Mince, Luxury, Extra Special, Asda*	1 Pie/64g	247	8.9	387	4.2	60	14	2.3
Mince, Luxury, Iceland*	1 Pie/67g	263	10.3	392	4.5	57.6	15.3	3.4
Mince, Mini, Aldi*	1 Pie/31g	120	4.6	387	4.2	59	15	1.7
Mince, Mini, M&S*	1 Pie/28g	105	4	380	4.3	57.8	14.6	4
Mince, Puff Pastry, Co-Op*	1 Pie/72g	245	11.9	340	5	43.1	16.5	2.6
Mince, Puff, Tesco*	1 Pie/25g	105	4.4	420	3.3	62	17.6	2
Mince, Shortcrust, Essential, Waitrose*	1 Pie/53g	226	9.5	423	4	60.1	17.7	3.4
Mince, Star Motif, Mini, Finest, Tesco*	1 Pie/17g	62	2.1	365	3.8	59.9	12.1	3.8
Mince, Tesco*	1 Pie/47g	180	7.8	383	3.9	54.7	16.5	1.5
Mississippi Mud, Tesco*	1 Serving/104g	399	26.6	384	5.3	33.1	25.6	1.8
Mushroom, Feta, & Spinach, Little, Higgidy*	1 Pie/160g	385	24.4	241	6.8	20.1	15.3	1.3
Mushroom, Wild Shroom, Pieminister*	1 Pie/270g	513	26.2	190	5.2	19.5	9.7	2.7
Pork, & Egg, M&S*	¼ Pie/108g	379	28	351	9.7	19.8	25.9	0.8
Pork, Cheddar & Pickle, Mini, Finest, Tesco*	1 Pie/50g	185	10.8	365	10	31.3	21.4	1.9
Pork, Cheese & Pickle, Mini, Tesco*	1 Pie/49g	191	12.8	389	9.2	29.3	26.1	1.2
Pork, Crusty Bake, Mini, Sainsbury's*	1 Pie/43g	165	11.2	384	11.5	26	26	1.5
Pork, Crusty Bake, Sainsbury's*	1 Pie/75g	292	20	390	10.5	27	26.7	1
Pork, Individual	*1 Pie/75g*	*272*	*19.3*	*363*	*10.8*	*23.7*	*25.7*	*0.9*
Pork, Melton Mowbray, Cured, M&S*	1 Pie/290g	1044	71	360	10.1	25.9	24.5	1

PIE

	Measure INFO/WEIGHT	per Measure KCAL	FAT	Nutrition Values per 100g / 100ml KCAL	PROT	CARB	FAT	FIBRE
Pork, Melton Mowbray, Cured, Mini, M&S*	1 Pie/50g	192	12.2	385	9.8	32.6	24.4	1
Pork, Melton Mowbray, Individual, Sainsbury's*	1 Pie/75g	296	20.8	395	10.2	26.1	27.7	2.4
Pork, Melton Mowbray, Lattice, Sainsbury's*	1 Serving/100g	342	23.6	342	10.8	21.7	23.6	1.2
Pork, Melton Mowbray, Mini, Co-Op*	1 Pie/49g	189	13.2	385	11	24	27	2
Pork, Melton Mowbray, Mini, M&S*	1 Pie/50g	185	12.1	370	11.6	26.1	24.2	1.6
Pork, Melton Mowbray, Mini, Morrisons*	1 Pie/50g	197	12.5	393	10.9	31.3	24.9	0.9
Pork, Melton Mowbray, Mini, Tesco*	1 Pie/50g	192	12.8	383	10.6	26.9	25.6	1.5
Pork, Melton Mowbray, Mini, TTD, Sainsbury's*	1 Pie/50g	182	11.8	365	11.9	25.5	23.6	1.5
Pork, Melton, Mini, Pork Farms*	1 Pie/50g	200	14.6	399	8.9	26.2	29.2	0
Pork, Mini, Retail, Average	*1 Mini/50g*	*198*	*13.7*	*396*	*10.8*	*26.4*	*27.4*	*2.4*
Pork, Mini, Tesco*	1 Pie/45g	162	10.7	359	10.2	25.9	23.8	1
Pork, Sliced	*1 Slice/100g*	*380*	*29.9*	*380*	*10.2*	*18.7*	*29.9*	*0*
Pork, Turkey, and Cranberry, Waitrose*	1 Serving/108g	331	21.3	306	12.7	18.7	19.7	1.4
Pork, with Cheese & Pickle, Waitrose*	1 Pack/150g	568	36.9	379	10.3	29.1	24.6	2.7
Rhubarb, & Ginger, Deep Filled, Tesco*	1 Pie/64g	237	8.4	367	3.4	57.7	13	2.9
Rhubarb, Sara Lee*	1 Serving/90g	224	12.4	250	2.9	28.7	13.8	1.3
Rhubarb, Shortcrust Pastry, Bakery, Tesco*	1/6 Pie/87g	244	9.8	280	2.9	39.9	11.3	3.5
Saag Aloo Gobi, Clive's Pies*	1 Pie/185g	329	22.7	178	3.2	18.8	12.3	0
Salmon, & Broccoli, Birds Eye*	1 Pie/351g	449	21.8	128	6.6	11.4	6.2	0.7
Salmon, & Broccoli, Filo Pastry, Finest, Tesco*	1 Pie/170g	386	22.6	227	7.9	18.9	13.3	2.1
Salmon, & Broccoli, LC, Tesco*	1 Pack/400g	350	7.2	88	7	10.2	1.8	1.7
Sausage, & Onion, Tesco*	1 Pack/300g	333	18.3	111	2.3	11.7	6.1	0.5
Scotch, Co-Op*	1 Pie/132g	408	24.9	309	7.3	27.3	18.9	1.5
Scotch, Farmfoods*	1 Pie/151g	430	24.6	285	7.8	26.8	16.3	1.2
Shepherd's, Average	*1oz/28g*	*31*	*1.7*	*112*	*6*	*9.3*	*5.9*	*0.7*
Shepherd's, BGTY, Sainsbury's*	1 Pack/400g	350	8.4	92	4.2	11.9	2.2	1.7
Shepherd's, British Classic, Meal For One, Aldi*	1 Pie/450g	614	35.5	142	5.4	11	8.2	1
Shepherd's, Charlie Bigham's*	½ Pack/324g	496	28.8	153	8.1	9.6	8.9	0.9
Shepherd's, Chilled, Finest, Tesco*	½ Pack/400g	460	16.4	115	6.9	8	4.1	1.9
Shepherd's, Frozen, Tesco*	1 Pack/400g	270	9.1	68	4.1	7.6	2.3	1.2
Shepherd's, Gastropub, M&S*	½ Pack/400g	416	8.2	104	3.4	4.6	2	0.8
Shepherd's, Vegetarian, Average	*1 Serving/400g*	*371*	*14.6*	*93*	*4*	*10.4*	*3.6*	*2.5*
Shepherd's, Welsh Hill Lamb, Gastropub, M&S*	½ Pack/330g	314	11.6	95	5.4	10.2	3.5	1.5
Steak, & Ale with Chips & Gravy	*1 Serving/400g*	*825*	*42.2*	*206*	*7.2*	*20.5*	*10.6*	*0.5*
Steak, & Ale, Average	*1 Pie/200g*	*507*	*28.7*	*253*	*9.8*	*21.1*	*14.4*	*1.3*
Steak, & Ale, Charlie Bigham's*	1 Pie/300g	774	48.9	258	13.4	14.1	16.3	1.1
Steak, & Ale, Pub Style, Co-Op*	1 Pie/250g	538	30	215	9	17	12	2
Steak, & Ale, Puff Pastry, Asda*	1/3 Pie/200g	520	30.2	260	10.6	20.4	15.1	1.6
Steak, & Ale, Sainsbury's*	1 Serving/190g	445	23.4	234	8.3	22.6	12.3	0.9
Steak, & Dorset Ale, Mini, Finest, Tesco*	1 Pie/30g	92	4.9	305	7.9	31.4	16.4	1.9
Steak, & Guinness, Sainsbury's*	¼ Pie/137g	399	25.5	291	8.7	22.2	18.6	1
Steak, & Kidney with Puff Pastry, 425g, Fray Bentos*	1 Pie/425g	622	16.6	131	5.6	17.4	3.5	0.6
Steak, & Kidney, Deep Fill, Sainsbury's*	½ Pie/125g	314	18.6	251	8.4	21	14.9	2
Steak, & Kidney, Family, Iceland*	1/3 Pie/225g	502	29.2	223	10.2	16.3	13	2.1
Steak, & Kidney, Individual	*1 Pie/200g*	*646*	*42.4*	*323*	*9.1*	*25.6*	*21.2*	*0.9*
Steak, & Kidney, Premium, Tesco*	1 Serving/170g	428	26.4	252	9.9	18.3	15.5	1.2
Steak, & Kidney, Princes*	½ Pack/212g	379	19.9	179	8.8	14.8	9.4	0
Steak, & Kidney, Puff Pastry, Sainsbury's*	1 Pie/150g	423	23.6	282	8.2	26.9	15.7	0.9
Steak, & Kidney, Pukka Pies Ltd*	1 Pie/238g	488	25.9	205	9.1	17.7	10.9	3.6
Steak, & Merlot, Cooked, Specially Selected, Aldi*	1 Pie/210g	599	35.7	285	11	21	17	1.3
Steak, & Mushroom, Asda*	1 Pie/130g	350	18.1	270	9	27	14	1.4
Steak, & Mushroom, Sainsbury's*	¼ Pie/130g	372	21.3	286	8.6	26	16.4	1
Steak, & Mushroom, Tesco*	1 Pie/138g	345	19.5	250	8.3	22.2	14.1	1.8

P

	Measure INFO/WEIGHT	per Measure KCAL	per Measure FAT	Nutrition Values per 100g / 100ml KCAL	PROT	CARB	FAT	FIBRE
PIE								
Steak, & Onion, Ginsters*	1 Pie/180g	481	30.8	267	8	20.3	17.1	1.3
Steak, & Onion, Minced, Aberdeen Angus, Tesco*	½ Pie/300g	897	57.6	299	9.4	22.1	19.2	0.7
Steak, & Peppered Sauce, Gastro Style, McDougalls*	1 Pie/192g	495	28.8	258	8.9	21.4	15	0.9
Steak, & Red Wine, Puff Pastry, Pub, Sainsbury's*	1 Pie/240g	497	29.5	207	7.2	16.8	12.3	2.1
Steak, Aberdeen Angus, Top Crust, Waitrose*	½ Pie/280g	476	24.1	170	10	13.4	8.6	4.1
Steak, All, Pukka Pies Ltd*	1 Pie/233g	499	29.8	214	6.9	17.6	12.8	3.1
Steak, Deep Fill, Tesco*	¼ Pie/195g	468	25.5	240	9.7	20	13.1	1.5
Steak, Individual, British Classics, Tesco*	1 Pie/150g	450	27.6	300	9.1	23.3	18.4	2.5
Steak, M&S*	1oz/28g	64	3.6	230	10	19	12.7	1.2
Steak, Mini, Asda*	1 Serving/67g	117	5.3	176	9	17	8	0.9
Steak, Mushroom & Ale, Topcrust, Waitrose*	1 Pie/250g	500	29.5	200	11.1	12.2	11.8	1.1
Steak, Puff Pastry, Deep Filled, Sainsbury's*	1 Pie/210g	536	30	255	10.3	21.2	14.3	2
Steak, Scotch, Bell's Bakery*	1 Serving/150g	378	20.2	252	13.6	18.6	13.5	0.7
Steak, Short Crust, Sainsbury's*	½ Pie/117g	314	24.1	267	10.9	22.2	20.5	1.7
Steak, Tesco*	1 Serving/205g	556	33.8	271	7.2	23.3	16.5	1.4
Turkey, & Ham, Farmfoods*	1 Pie/147g	404	21.9	275	8.6	26.5	14.9	1.4
Vegetable	*1oz/28g*	*42*	*2.1*	*151*	*3*	*18.9*	*7.6*	*1.5*
Vegetable, & Cheese, Asda*	1 Pie/141g	330	16.2	234	5.8	26.9	11.5	1
Vegetable, & Feta, Moroccan, Little, Higgidy*	1 Pie/180g	418	22.5	232	5.1	24.7	12.5	0.6
Vegetable, Farmhouse, Linda McCartney*	1 Pie/146g	380	23.2	260	5.8	23.4	15.9	1.6
Vegetable, Retail, Average	*1 Serving/200g*	*348*	*19*	*174*	*3.7*	*18.6*	*9.5*	*1.1*
Vegetarian, Chicken Style, & Mushroom, Quorn*	1 Pie/235g	515	26.6	219	6.7	21.2	11.3	2.8
Vegetarian, Cottage, Quorn*	1 Lg Pack/500g	365	10	73	2.5	10	2	2.5
Vegetarian, Deep Country, Linda McCartney*	1 Pie/166g	413	23.6	249	5.2	24.9	14.2	2.6
Vegetarian, Mince & Potato, Quorn*	1 Pie/200g	388	16	194	6.5	22.5	8	3
Vegetarian, Mushroom & Ale, Linda McCartney*	1 Pie/200g	439	23.5	219	4.1	25	11.7	1.2
Vegetarian, Shepherd's, Linda McCartney*	1 Pack/340g	286	7.5	84	3.7	12.3	2.2	2.3
Vegetarian, Steak, Meat Free, Quorn*	1 Pie/235g	439	18.8	187	5.6	22	8	2
PIE FILLING								
Apple, Sainsbury's*	1 Serving/75g	67	0.1	89	0.1	22.1	0.1	1
Cherry	*1oz/28g*	*23*	*0*	*82*	*0.4*	*21.5*	*0*	*0.4*
Fruit	*1oz/28g*	*22*	*0*	*77*	*0.4*	*20.1*	*0*	*1*
Pistachio, Mix, Avidhipro*	1 Pack/25g	91	0.6	364	74.8	9.6	2.4	2
Summer Fruits, Fruit, Tesco*	1 Can/385g	377	0	98	0.4	24.1	0	0.9
PIGEON								
Meat Only, Roasted, Average	*1 Pigeon/115g*	*215*	*9.1*	*187*	*29*	*0*	*7.9*	*0*
Meat Only, Roasted, Weighed with Bone, Average	*1oz/28g*	*12*	*0.5*	*41*	*6.4*	*0*	*1.7*	*0*
PIKELETS								
Free From, Tesco*	1 Pikelet/30g	58	1.3	194	2.8	36.2	4.3	1.4
Tesco*	1 Pikelet/35g	68	0.2	193	5.8	40.9	0.7	1.7
PILAF								
Bulgur Wheat, Sainsbury's*	1 Pack/381.3g	347	11.1	91	3.9	12.3	2.9	6.3
Vegetables, with Coconut & Lentil, City Kitchen, Tesco*	1 Pack/385g	474	20.8	123	2.6	14.9	5.4	2.3
with Tomato, Average	*1oz/28g*	*40*	*0.9*	*144*	*2.5*	*28*	*3.3*	*0.4*
PILCHARDS								
Fillets in Tomato Sauce, Average	*1 Can/120g*	*158*	*7.8*	*132*	*16.2*	*2.2*	*6.5*	*0.1*
Fillets in Virgin Olive Oil, Glenryck*	1 Serving/92g	223	14.4	242	23.3	2	15.7	0
in Brine, Average	*½ Can/77g*	*114*	*5.6*	*148*	*20.8*	*0*	*7.3*	*0*
PIMMS*								
& Lemonade, Premixed, Canned, Pimms*	1 Can/250ml	160	0	64	0	8.4	0	0
25% Volume, Pimms*	1 Serving/50ml	80	0	160	0	5	0	0
PINE NUTS								
Average	*1 Tbsp/8g*	*56*	*5.5*	*695*	*15.7*	*3.9*	*68.6*	*1.9*

	Measure INFO/WEIGHT	KCAL	FAT	KCAL	PROT	CARB	FAT	FIBRE
PINEAPPLE								
& Papaya, Dried, Garden Gang, Asda*	1 Pack/50g	142	0.8	283	2.8	64	1.7	8
Chunks, Average	*1 Serving/100g*	*66*	*0.1*	*66*	*0.5*	*15.5*	*0.1*	*0.3*
Dried, Soft, Love Life, Waitrose*	1 Serving/30g	93	0.1	309	3	73.7	0.2	3.1
Dried, Unsweetened, Sainsbury's*	1 Bag/75g	255	1.5	340	1.7	84.7	2	6
in Juice, Canned, Average	*1 Can/106g*	*57*	*0*	*53*	*0.3*	*12.9*	*0*	*0.6*
Pieces in Light Syrup, Everyday Value, Tesco*	1 Tin/340g	255	0	75	0.5	16.8	0	0.8
Raw, Flesh Only, Average	*1 Whole/472g*	*200*	*0.9*	*42*	*0.4*	*10*	*0.2*	*1*
PISTACHIO NUTS								
Black Pepper, Graze*	1 Punnet/31g	104	9.7	331	10	5	31	3
Lightly Toasted, Graze*	1 Punnet/31g	104	9.7	331	10	5	31	3
Raw, Average, without Shells	*1 Serving/20g*	*111*	*8.9*	*557*	*20.6*	*28*	*44.4*	*10.3*
Roasted & Salted, without Shells, Average	*1 Serving/25g*	*152*	*13.6*	*608*	*19.6*	*9.9*	*54.5*	*6.1*
Salted, Roasted, Weighed with Shell	*1 Serving/100g*	*331*	*30.5*	*331*	*9.8*	*4.5*	*30.5*	*3.4*
Salted, Roasted, without Shells	*1 Serving/100g*	*601*	*55.4*	*601*	*17.9*	*8.2*	*55.4*	*6.1*
PIZZA								
American Hot, 12 Inch, Supermarket, Pizza Express*	½ Pizza/264g	562	19.8	213	10.5	25.9	7.5	2.6
American Hot, Supermarket, Pizza Express*	1 Pizza/250g	704	29.1	271	11.3	30.5	11.2	1.5
Aubergine, Spinach, & Tomato, Pizzeria, Waitrose*	½ Pizza/193g	403	7.7	209	7.8	35.4	4	3.6
Bacon, & Mushroom, Pizzeria, Sainsbury's*	1 Pizza/355g	880	24.8	248	11.7	34.5	7	3.7
Bacon, & Mushroom, Thin & Crispy, Sainsbury's*	½ Pizza/150g	396	15.9	264	12.9	29.2	10.6	1.7
Capricciosa, Pizza Express*	1 Serving/300g	753	29.3	251	13.6	29	9.8	0
Cheese, & Tomato French Bread, Findus*	1 Serving/143g	322	11.6	225	9.4	29	8.1	0
Cheese, & Tomato, Average	*1 Serving/300g*	*711*	*35.4*	*237*	*9.1*	*25.2*	*11.8*	*1.4*
Cheese, & Tomato, Baguette, Tesco*	1 Baguette/125g	275	8.5	220	11	28	6.8	2.8
Cheese, & Tomato, Deep Pan, Goodfella's*	¼ Pizza/102g	259	10.8	253	11.5	29.6	10.5	3.7
Cheese, & Tomato, Everyday Value, Tesco*	1 Pizza/150g	423	9.2	282	9.6	46	6.1	2.2
Cheese, & Tomato, Frozen, Sainsbury's*	1 Serving/122g	300	10.7	246	13.7	28	8.8	3
Cheese, & Tomato, Mini, Bruschetta, Iceland*	1 Pizza/34g	63	2.3	188	8	23	7	2.1
Cheese, & Tomato, Mini, M&S*	1 Pizza/95g	233	5.5	245	10	38.7	5.8	1.6
Cheese, & Tomato, Range, Italiano, Tesco*	1 Pizza/380g	969	35	255	11.4	31.7	9.2	3.3
Cheese, & Tomato, Retail, Frozen	*1oz/28g*	*70*	*3*	*250*	*7.5*	*32.9*	*10.7*	*1.4*
Cheese, & Tomato, Sainsbury's*	1 Pizza/247g	706	24.5	286	13.7	35.4	9.9	2.4
Cheese, & Tomato, Slice, Ross*	1 Slice/77g	148	6.6	192	6.5	22.2	8.6	2
Cheese, & Tomato, Slices, CBY, Asda*	1 Slice/13.7g	62	2.5	453	8.2	63.2	18.1	2.3
Cheese, & Tomato, Stone Bake, M&S*	1 Pizza/340g	782	28.6	230	10.8	30.1	8.4	1.6
Cheese, & Tomato, Stonebaked, Organic, Co-Op*	1 Pizza/330g	676	23.1	205	9	26	7	4
Cheese, & Tomato, Stonebaked, Thin & Crispy, Tesco*	½ Pizza/161g	388	13.8	241	11.6	29.4	8.6	2.1
Cheese, & Tomato, Thin & Crispy, Asda*	1 Pizza/366g	827	36.6	226	11	23	10	2
Cheese, & Tomato, Thin & Crispy, Sainsbury's*	1 Serving/135g	344	10	255	14.9	32.2	7.4	5
Cheese, & Tomato, Thin & Crispy, Waitrose*	1 Pizza/280g	658	28.3	235	12.3	23.6	10.1	2.3
Cheese, Feast, Deep Crust, Carlos, Aldi*	1 Pizza/155g	432	14.9	279	9.7	37.3	9.6	2.1
Cheese, Feast, Deep Pan, Asda*	½ Pizza/210g	422	18.9	201	13	17	9	2.3
Cheese, Feast, Stuffed Crust, Take Away, Carlos, Aldi*	½ Pizza/238g	650	27	273	11.8	29.4	11.3	2.7
Cheese, Feast, Thin Crust, Chilled, Tesco*	½ Pizza/175g	467	22.4	267	14.7	23.4	12.8	2.5
Cheese, Four, Finest, Tesco*	½ Pizza/230g	575	21.2	250	12.1	29.8	9.2	1.3
Cheese, Four, Stuffed Crust, Takeaway, Chicago Town*	¼ Pizza/157.5g	433	17	275	10.8	33	10.8	1.9
Cheese, Four, Thin & Crispy, Iceland*	½ Pizza/148g	354	12.6	239	10.7	29.1	8.5	1.6
Cheese, Reg Crust, From Restaurant, Average	*1 Pizza/905g*	*2018*	*46.2*	*223*	*12.2*	*32.5*	*5.1*	*0*
Cheese, Simply, Goodfella's*	¼ Pizza/82g	226	11	276	16.3	22.5	13.4	1.9
Cheese, Stuffed Crust, Sainsbury's*	1 Pizza/525g	1428	52.5	272	14	31.5	10	2
Cheese, Thick Crust, From Restaurant, Average	*1 Pizza/976g*	*2655*	*107.3*	*272*	*12*	*31.3*	*11*	*1.8*
Cheese, Thin Crust, From Restaurant, Average	*1 Pizza/627g*	*1906*	*98.3*	*304*	*14.2*	*26.5*	*15.7*	*2*
Cheese, Three, & Tomato, Stonebaked, Co-Op*	1 Pizza/415g	888	33.6	214	10	25.2	8.1	1.5

P

PIZZA

INFO/WEIGHT	Measure	per Measure KCAL	FAT	Nutrition Values per 100g / 100ml KCAL	PROT	CARB	FAT	FIBRE
Cheese, Triple, Deep Dish, Chicago Town*	1 Serving/170g	418	18.2	246	9.9	27.6	10.7	0
Chicken, & Bacon, Loaded, Tesco*	1 Serving/258g	622	25.3	241	12.8	25.4	9.8	1.9
Chicken, & Bacon, Pizzeria, Italian, Sainsbury's*	½ Pizza/169.5g	508	24.1	300	13.6	29.4	14.2	2.7
Chicken, & Chorizo, 12", TTD, Sainsbury's*	½ Pizza/290g	702	20.9	242	12.2	32.1	7.2	2.6
Chicken, & Chorizo, Sourdough, Carlos, Aldi*	½ Pizza/165g	406	14.2	246	12	29	8.6	4.7
Chicken, & Pesto, Californian Style, Asda*	½ Pizza/235g	533	16.4	227	10	31	7	2
Chicken, & Sweetcorn, Stonebaked, Tesco*	1 Serving/177g	354	9.6	200	11.9	26	5.4	2
Chicken, & Vegetable, Stone Baked, GFY, Asda*	½ Pizza/161g	349	3.7	217	13	36	2.3	1.7
Chicken, BBQ, M&S*	½ Pizza/210g	430	11.8	205	11.6	27.5	5.6	1.8
Chicken, BBQ, Stonebaked, Tesco*	½ Pizza/158g	285	9.5	180	10.5	20.9	6	3.9
Chicken, BBQ, Texan, Thin & Crispy, Co-Op*	½ Pizza/190g	418	14.1	220	11	27	7.4	2.1
Chicken, BBQ, Thin & Crispy, Sainsbury's*	½ Pizza/167g	399	12.4	238	11.4	30.4	7.4	2.2
Chicken, Cajun Style, Stonebaked, Tesco*	1 Pizza/561g	1318	55	235	11.9	24.8	9.8	1.4
Chicken, Cajun, Sainsbury's*	½ Pizza/146g	285	2.6	195	12.9	31.8	1.8	2.6
Chicken, Chargrilled, Iceland*	1 Pizza/381g	804	25.5	211	12.3	25.4	6.7	2
Chicken, Chargrilled, Thin & Crispy, Asda*	1 Pizza/373g	780	18.6	209	9	32	5	1.6
Chicken, Fajita, 10 Inch, CBY, Asda*	½ Pizza/151g	319	9.8	211	10.7	26.3	6.5	2.4
Chicken, Fajita, Thin & Crispy, Iceland*	1 Pizza/361g	729	21.3	202	9.6	26.5	5.9	1.8
Chicken, Garlic, Thin & Crispy, Stonebake, Sainsbury's*	½ Pizza/160g	386	17.3	241	10.7	25.2	10.8	3.5
Chicken, Hot & Spicy, Deep Pan, Morrisons*	½ Pizza/232.5g	521	13	224	10.5	32.9	5.6	1
Chicken, Hot & Spicy, Deep Pan, Tesco*	½ Pizza/222g	423	7.3	191	10.5	30	3.3	2.1
Chicken, Provencal, Goodfella's*	½ Pizza/143g	388	18	272	13.7	25.9	12.6	2.1
Chicken, Sweet Chilli, BGTY, Sainsbury's*	½ Pizza/138g	276	2.3	200	13	33.2	1.7	2.1
Diavolo, Pizza Express*	½ Pizza/163.5g	322	11	197	9.4	24.6	6.7	2.1
Diavolo, Romano, Main, Supermarket, Pizza Express*	1 Pizza/477g	978	52.5	205	11	20.2	11	1.6
Four Seasons, Stonebaked, Truly Irresistible, Co-Op*	½ Pizza/245g	502	16.2	205	9.5	26.6	6.6	2.6
Funghi, Ristorante, Dr Oetker*	1 Pizza/365g	847	43.4	232	7.6	22.5	11.9	1.8
Garlic Bread, Stonebaked, Italiano, Tesco*	1 Serving/117g	403	18.2	346	7.8	43.6	15.6	1.5
Giardiniera, from Supermarket, Pizza Express*	½ Pizza/144g	291	10.5	202	8.6	25.5	7.3	2.1
Ham, & Cheese, Ultra Thin, Sodebo*	1 Pizza/200g	400	8.6	200	11.3	29.1	4.3	0
Ham, & Mushroom Slices, Farmfoods*	1 Slice/89g	170	2.3	191	8	34	2.6	0.9
Ham, & Mushroom, Average	*1 Serving/250g*	*533*	*16*	*213*	*10.5*	*28.4*	*6.4*	*2.1*
Ham, & Mushroom, Finest, Tesco*	½ Pizza/240g	576	26.4	240	9.5	25.9	11	2.2
Ham, & Mushroom, Smoked, Thin & Crispy, Co-Op*	1 Pizza/400g	792	18	198	9	30.3	4.5	1.7
Ham, & Mushroom, Thin & Crispy, Asda*	1 Pizza/360g	760	25.2	211	11	26	7	2.4
Ham, & Mushroom, Thin & Crispy, Tesco*	½ Pizza/185g	380	11.1	205	11.2	25.6	6	2.3
Ham, & Pineapple, Average	*1 Serving/250g*	*555*	*16.8*	*222*	*11*	*29.2*	*6.7*	*2.1*
Ham, & Pineapple, Stone Bake, M&S*	1 Pizza/345g	690	19.7	200	10.1	28.3	5.7	1.6
Ham, & Pineapple, Stonebaked, Tesco*	1 Pizza/161g	293	9.2	182	9.2	23.5	5.7	3.5
Ham, & Pineapple, Tesco*	1/6 Pizza/56g	134	4.6	240	10.4	30.9	8.3	2.1
Ham, & Pineapple, Thin & Crispy Italian, Morrisons*	1 Pizza/375g	746	22.9	199	10.2	24.9	6.1	0
Ham, & Pineapple, Thin & Crispy, Iceland*	1 Serving/110g	301	13.1	274	9.9	31.9	11.9	3
Ham, & Pineapple, Thin & Crispy, Sainsbury's*	1 Pizza/330g	719	21.1	218	10.8	29.4	6.4	2.4
Ham, & Pineapple, Thin Crust, Tesco*	½ Pizza/175g	385	10	220	12.3	29.6	5.7	2.5
Ham, Mushroom & Tomato, BGTY, Sainsbury's*	½ Pizza/150g	309	6.1	206	11.8	30.4	4.1	1.2
Ham, Pepperoni & Milano, M&S*	1 Pizza/290g	696	28.4	240	14	23.3	9.8	1.1
Hawaiian, Stonebaked, Cucina, Aldi*	½ Pizza/165g	326	5.6	198	9.5	32	3.4	1.6
Hawaiian, Thin Crust, Tesco*	½ Pizza/192g	365	9.4	190	10.3	25.6	4.9	1.8
La Reine, 8 Inch, Supermarket, Pizza Express*	1 Pizza/290g	612	17.7	211	10.2	27.7	6.1	2.3
Margherita, 12", Finest, Tesco*	½ Pizza/255g	433	9.2	170	8.1	26.4	3.6	2.7
Margherita, Average	*1 Slice/108g*	*239*	*8.6*	*239*	*11*	*30.5*	*8.6*	*1.2*
Margherita, Cheese & Tomato, San Marco*	½ Pizza/200g	454	14.4	227	10.7	29.8	7.2	1.2
Margherita, Classico, Italiano, Tesco*	½ Pizza/191g	414	11.8	217	11.2	29.1	6.2	2.5

PIZZA

INFO/WEIGHT	Measure	per Measure KCAL	FAT	Nutrition Values per 100g / 100ml KCAL	PROT	CARB	FAT	FIBRE
Margherita, Pizzeria, Italian, Sainsbury's*	½ Pizza/168.5g	426	17.4	253	12.2	27.9	10.3	2.5
Margherita, Romana, 12", Supermarket, Pizza Express*	½ Pizza/169g	438	17.2	259	11.6	28.5	10.2	3.2
Margherita, Stone Baked, Goodfella's*	1 Slice/36g	95	4.1	263	10.9	31.9	11.4	7.6
Margherita, Stonebaked, 10", Sainsbury's*	½ Pizza/139g	359	11.3	258	12.4	32.2	8.1	3.5
Margherita, The Best, Morrisons*	½ Pizza/252g	670	27.2	266	11.5	30.6	10.8	2.2
Margherita, Thin & Crispy, Iceland*	½ Pizza/170g	391	14.4	230	12.7	25.9	8.5	2.8
Margherita, Thin Crust, Tesco*	1 Serving/170g	354	13.4	208	10.1	24.1	7.9	3.6
Meat Feast, Deep & Loaded, Sainsbury's*	½ Pizza/298g	818	30	275	13.2	32.7	10.1	2.6
Meat Feast, Italian, Thin & Crispy, Waitrose*	1 Pizza/182g	477	22.9	262	10.7	26.5	12.6	1.8
Meat Feast, Large, Tesco*	1 Pizza/735g	1904	69.1	259	10.9	32.6	9.4	2
Meat Feast, Mega, Asda*	½ Pizza/428g	1044	33.8	244	9.5	33.6	7.9	3.2
Meat Feast, Thin & Crispy, Asda*	½ Pizza/183g	410	14.6	224	11	27	8	1.4
Meat Feast, Thin Crust, Tesco*	½ Pizza/178g	430	20.2	242	13.6	21.3	11.4	2.3
Meat Mayhem, Goodfella's*	1 Pizza/436.5g	1100	41.9	252	10.6	30.9	9.6	2.5
Meats, Italian, Finest, Tesco*	½ Pizza/217g	449	8.5	207	13.6	29.4	3.9	1.3
Mini, Party, Tesco*	1 Pizza/11g	26	1.1	248	11.4	28.6	10.5	1.9
Mozzarella, & Sunblush Tomato, 12", TTD, Sainsbury's*	½ Pizza/251g	638	17.8	254	12.4	35	7.1	2.6
Mozzarella, Ristorante, Dr Oetker*	1 Pizza/335g	874	44.6	261	10.4	23.9	13.3	1.7
Mushroom, Garlic, Classico, Tesco*	½ Pizza/207.5g	415	13.9	200	10	24.9	6.7	2.6
Mushroom, Garlic, Tesco*	1 Pizza/425g	829	34	195	9.3	21.6	8	5.3
Mushroom, Garlic, Thin Crust, Tesco*	½ Pizza/163g	340	14.6	209	11	21.1	9	3.6
Napoletana, Sainsbury's*	½ Pizza/186g	424	14.3	228	9.7	29.9	7.7	3.1
Napoli, Tesco*	½ Pizza/184g	431	11.6	235	11.9	32.6	6.3	1.4
Onion, Caramelised, & Feta, & Rosemary, Bistro, Waitrose*	½ Pizza/230g	607	32	264	8.6	26.1	13.9	2.4
Pepperoni, & Cheese, Asda*	½ Pizza/150g	386	13.5	257	10	34	9	2.7
Pepperoni, & Jalapeno Chill, Asda*	1 Pizza/277g	742	22.2	268	10	39	8	1.8
Pepperoni, Aldi*	1 Serving/55g	123	4.3	224	8.7	29.5	7.9	1.4
Pepperoni, Asda*	½ Pizza/150g	386	13.5	257	10	34	9	2.7
Pepperoni, Average	*1 Serving/250g*	*671*	*28.4*	*269*	*11.8*	*29.6*	*11.4*	*2.1*
Pepperoni, Baguette, Ovenbaked, Asda*	1 Baguette/123g	243	7.3	197	9.7	25	5.9	2.4
Pepperoni, Deep & Crispy, Iceland*	1 Serving/175g	490	21	280	11.9	31.1	12	1.8
Pepperoni, Double, Thin & Crispy, Loved by Us, Co-Op*	½ Pizza/173g	389	18.9	225	10.5	27.3	10.9	3.4
Pepperoni, Hot & Spicy, Stuffed Crust, Asda*	1 Pizza/245g	666	30	272	13.9	26.5	12.2	2.4
Pepperoni, Mini, Tesco*	1 Serving/22g	71	3.7	323	11.8	30.5	16.8	2.7
Pepperoni, Mushroom, & Ham, GF, Goodfellas*	½ Pizza/175g	450	17.5	257	10	30	10	0
Pepperoni, Picante, Bella Italia*	1 Pizza/425g	1016	48.9	239	12.7	20.7	11.5	1.6
Pepperoni, Reg Crust, From Restaurant, Average	*1 Pizza/959g*	*2445*	*94*	*255*	*14.3*	*28*	*9.8*	*0*
Pepperoni, Stone Baked, Carlos*	1 Pizza/330g	832	39.6	252	13	23	12	0
Pepperoni, Stonebaked Ciabatta, Goodfella's*	½ Pizza/181g	503	26.1	278	11.9	27.4	14.4	2.4
Pepperoni, Stonebaked, 12", Sainsbury's*	¼ Pizza/103g	301	13.3	292	13.2	29.2	12.9	3.1
Pepperoni, Stonebaked, Chef Select, Lidl*	¼ Pizza/85g	209	7.4	246	11.1	29.5	8.7	2.4
Pepperoni, Thin & Crispy, Sainsbury's*	½ Pizza/132g	405	18.9	307	13.9	30.7	14.3	2.6
Pepperoni, Thin & Crispy, Cucina, Aldi*	½ Pizza/170g	503	23.8	296	12	29	14	2.4
Pepperoni, Thin & Crispy, Essential, Waitrose*	½ Pizza/133g	380	18	286	12.3	28.8	13.5	1
Pollo, ad Astra, Supermarket, Pizza Express*	½ Pizza/140g	315	8.7	218	11.3	28.9	6	1.8
Pollo, Primavera, Wood Fired, Ultra Thin, M&S*	1 Pizza/185g	414	15.9	224	10.4	25.3	8.6	1.9
Pollo, Ristorante, As Sold, Dr Oetker*	½ Pizza/183g	408	16.5	223	8.8	25.7	9	1.8
Pork, 'n' Pineapple, Punchy, Freshly Prepared, Tesco*	½ Pizza/186g	510	18	274	12.4	32.9	9.7	2.7
Prosciutto, Italian Style, Co-Op*	½ Pizza/183g	421	12.8	230	13	29	7	3
Prosciutto, Ristorante, Dr Oetker*	1 Pizza/330g	752	32.3	228	10.3	24.6	9.8	0
Quattro Formaggi, Ristorante, Dr Oetker*	½ Pizza/170g	457	23.8	269	10.8	24.1	14	1.6
Salame, Ristorante, Dr Oetker*	½ Pizza/160g	455	24.5	285	10.4	26.3	15.3	0
Salami, & Ham, Pizzeria, Waitrose*	½ Pizza/205g	443	13.7	216	10.1	28.7	6.7	1.8

	Measure INFO/WEIGHT	per Measure KCAL	FAT	Nutrition Values per 100g / 100ml KCAL	PROT	CARB	FAT	FIBRE
PIZZA								
Salami, & Pepperoni, Waitrose*	½ Pizza/190g	578	30.8	304	13.4	23.9	16.2	2.1
Salami, Napoli Diavolo, Pizza, Wood Fired, M&S*	½ Pizza/244g	549	24.9	225	10.8	21.7	10.2	1.7
Salami, Ultra Thin Italian, Tesco*	1 Serving/263g	692	25.5	263	12	31.9	9.7	1
Selection, Slices, M&S*	1 Serving/52g	120	4.1	230	9.4	30.3	7.8	1.9
Spinach, & Bacon & Mushroom, GFY, Asda*	1 Serving/270g	618	12.2	229	13	34	4.5	2.6
Spinach, & Ricotta, Classic Italian, Stonebaked, Tesco*	½ Pizza/190g	460	16.3	240	10.3	29	8.5	1.2
Spinach, & Ricotta, Extra Special, Asda*	1 Pizza/400g	940	28	235	9	34	7	1.9
Spinach, & Ricotta, Italian, Chilled, Sainsbury's*	1 Pizza/361g	859	34.7	238	9.3	28.7	9.6	2.3
Spinach, & Ricotta, Thin Crust, Italian, Tesco*	½ Pizza/190g	365	16.7	192	9.6	18.7	8.8	1.9
Supreme, Deep Dish, Individual, Chicago Town*	1 Pizza/170g	456	20.4	268	9.2	30.8	12	1
Vegetable, & Peppers, Fire Roasted, Waitrose*	½ Pizza/235g	442	16.7	188	9.8	21.3	7.1	2.7
Vegetable, & Pesto, Chargrilled, Specially Selected, Aldi*	½ Pizza/305g	756	29	248	9.2	30	9.5	2.9
Vegetable, Average	**1 Serving/250g**	**475**	**13.1**	**190**	**8.2**	**27.5**	**5.2**	**2.4**
Vegetable, Balsamic Roast, & Mozzarella, Sainsbury's*	½ Pizza/200g	444	15.6	222	8.5	29.4	7.8	2.4
Vegetable, Chargrilled, Frozen, BGTY, Sainsbury's*	1 Pizza/290g	548	13.3	189	10.2	26.7	4.6	3
Vegetable, Deep Pan, Co-Op*	1 Pizza/425g	829	29.8	195	8	25	7	2
Vegetable, Frozen, HL, Tesco*	1 Pizza/400g	604	10.8	151	8.1	23.5	2.7	4.4
Vegetable, GFY, Asda*	¼ Pizza/94g	141	2.7	150	7	24	2.9	3.7
Vegetable, Mediterranean, Pizzeria, Sainsbury's*	1 Serving/211g	397	13.5	188	8	24.7	6.4	3.2
Vegetable, Mediterranean, Stonebaked, Carlos, Aldi*	½ Pizza/173g	323	8.7	187	7.5	26.6	5	2.9
Vegetable, Mediterranean, Stonebaked, Sainsbury's*	½ Pizza/260g	622	16.4	239	9.8	35.7	6.3	3.1
Vegi Supreme, Stuffed Crust, Medium	**1 Slice/87g**	**209**	**7**	**240**	**12**	**29.3**	**8**	**2.2**
PIZZA BASE								
Deep Pan, Italian, Sainsbury's*	1 Base/220g	684	11	311	7	59.5	5	1.4
Deep Pan, Napolina*	1 Base/260g	757	7.8	291	7.9	58	3	0.2
Everyday Value, Tesco*	½ Base/125g	401	2.8	320	9.6	65.2	2.2	0.7
Garlic Bread, Sainsbury's*	¼ Base/58.7g	109	4.2	186	5.1	25.4	7.1	1.8
Gluten, Wheat & Dairy Free, Free From, Livwell*	1 Base/100g	237	2.6	237	5.2	48.3	2.6	4.7
Italian, Classic, Sainsbury's*	1 Base/150g	452	7.2	301	7.6	57	4.8	1.5
Light & Crispy, Napolina*	1 Base/150g	436	4.5	291	7.9	58	3	0.2
Mini, Napolina*	1 Base/75g	218	2.2	291	7.9	58	3	0.2
Pre Rolled, As Sold, Greenvale, Aldi*	1 Pack/400g	1048	16.4	262	9.3	46	4.1	2.6
Thin & Crispy, Tesco*	1 Serving/110g	348	8.2	316	9.2	52.9	7.5	1.5
Thin & Crispy, Sainsbury's*	1 Base/150g	504	7.8	336	9.9	62.3	5.2	4.3
with Tomato Sauce, Crosta & Mollica*	½ Pizza/135g	282	4.9	209	6	40.7	3.6	0
PIZZA BASE MIX								
Morrisons*	1 Serving/77g	313	3.8	407	12.7	77.9	5	3.6
Sainsbury's*	1 Pack/145g	486	5.5	335	12.8	62.3	3.8	2.9
PLAICE								
Fillets in Breadcrumbs, Average	**1 Serving/150g**	**331**	**17.9**	**221**	**12.8**	**15.5**	**11.9**	**0.8**
Fillets, Lightly Dusted, Average	**1 Fillet/113g**	**188**	**9.2**	**166**	**12.9**	**10.4**	**8.2**	**0.6**
Fillets, Raw, Average	**1oz/28g**	**24**	**0.4**	**87**	**18.2**	**0**	**1.5**	**0**
Goujons, Baked	**1oz/28g**	**85**	**5.1**	**304**	**8.8**	**27.7**	**18.3**	**0**
Goujons, Fried in Blended Oil	**1oz/28g**	**119**	**9**	**426**	**8.5**	**27**	**32.3**	**0**
Grilled	**1oz/28g**	**27**	**0.5**	**96**	**20.1**	**0**	**1.7**	**0**
in Batter, Fried in Blended Oil	**1oz/28g**	**72**	**4.7**	**257**	**15.2**	**12**	**16.8**	**0.5**
Steamed	**1oz/28g**	**26**	**0.5**	**93**	**18.9**	**0**	**1.9**	**0**
Whole, with Spinach & Ricotta Cheese, Sainsbury's*	1 Serving/159g	334	16.7	210	11.6	17.2	10.5	0.8
PLANTAIN								
Boiled in Unsalted Water	**1oz/28g**	**31**	**0.1**	**112**	**0.8**	**28.5**	**0.2**	**1.2**
Raw, Average	**1 Med/179g**	**218**	**0.7**	**122**	**1.3**	**31.9**	**0.4**	**2.3**
Ripe, Fried in Vegetable Oil	**1oz/28g**	**75**	**2.6**	**267**	**1.5**	**47.5**	**9.2**	**2.3**

	Measure INFO/WEIGHT	KCAL	FAT	Nutrition Values per 100g / 100ml				
				KCAL	PROT	CARB	FAT	FIBRE
PLUMS								
Average, Stewed without Sugar	*1oz/28g*	*8*	*0*	*30*	*0.5*	*7.3*	*0.1*	*1.3*
Fresh, Raw, Weighed without Stone, Average	*1 Plum/66g*	*24*	*0.1*	*36*	*0.6*	*8.6*	*0.1*	*1.9*
Soft Dried, Blue Parrot Cafe, Sainsbury's*	1 Pack/50g	118	0.2	237	2.6	55.6	0.5	7.1
Weighed with Stone, Average	*1 Plum/90g*	*31*	*0.1*	*34*	*0.5*	*8.1*	*0.1*	*1.8*
Whole, Dried, Graze*	1 Pack/60g	143	0.3	239	2.6	56	0.5	0
Yellow, Waitrose*	1 Plum/50g	20	0	39	0.6	8.8	0.1	1.5
POLENTA								
Dry, Merchant Gourmet*	1 Serving/65g	232	0.9	357	7.4	78.8	1.4	1.3
Organic, Dry, Kallo*	1 Serving/150g	543	2.7	362	8.5	78	1.8	0
POLLOCK								
Alaskan, Value, Tesco*	1 Serving/200g	150	1.2	75	16.6	0	0.6	0
Breaded, Asda*	1 Serving/97g	200	9.7	206	12	17	10	1
Fillets, Breaded, Cooked, Tesco*	1 Fillet/125g	315	12.2	250	15	24.4	9.7	2
Fillets, British, Sainsbury's*	1 Pack/218g	157	1.3	72	16.6	0	0.6	0
POLO								
Fruits, Nestle*	1 Tube/37g	142	0	383	0	96	0	0
Mints, Clear Ice, Nestle*	1 Sweet/4g	16	0	390	0	97.5	0	0
Mints, Original, Nestle*	1 Sweet/2g	8	0	402	0	98.2	1	0
Spearmint, Nestle*	1 Tube/35g	141	0.4	402	0	98.2	1.1	0
POMEGRANATE								
Raw, Fresh, Flesh Only, Average	*1 Sm Fruit/86g*	*59*	*0.3*	*68*	*1*	*17.2*	*0.3*	*0.6*
Raw, Weighed with Rind & Skin, Average	*1 Sm Fruit/154g*	*59*	*0.3*	*38*	*0.5*	*9.6*	*0.2*	*0*
POMELO								
Fresh, Raw, Weighed with Skin & Seeds	*100 Grams/100g*	*11*	*0.1*	*11*	*0.2*	*2.5*	*0.1*	*0*
Raw, Flesh Only, Average	*1 Fruit/340g*	*129*	*0.1*	*38*	*0.8*	*9.6*	*0*	*1*
POP TARTS								
Bustin' Berry, Kellogg's*	1 Tart/50g	200	6	400	4	69	12	2
Chocolate Chip Cookie Dough, Kellogg's*	1 Pastry/50g	190	5	380	4	70	10	2
Chocolate Chip, Kellogg's*	1 Pastry/52g	210	6	404	5.8	69.2	11.5	1.9
Chocolate, Kellogg's*	1 Pastry/50g	198	8.5	396	5	136	17	2
Cinnamon Roll, Kellogg's*	1 Pastry/50g	210	7	420	4	68	14	2
Cookies 'n' Creme, Kellogg's*	1 Pastry/50g	190	5	380	4	70	10	2
Frosted Blueberry, Kellogg's*	1 Pastry/52g	200	5	385	3.8	73.1	9.6	1.9
Frosted Blueberry, Mini Crisps, Kellogg's*	1 Pouch/23g	100	2.5	435	4.4	78.3	10.9	0
Frosted Brown Sugar Cinnamon, Kellogg's*	1 Tart/50g	210	7	420	6	68	14	2
Frosted Cherry, Kellogg's*	1 Pastry/52g	200	5	385	3.8	73.1	9.6	2.3
Frosted Chocolate Fudge, Kellogg's*	1 Pastry/52g	200	5	385	5.8	71.2	9.6	1.9
Frosted Cinnamon with Wholegrain, Low Fat, Kellogg's*	1 Pastry/50g	180	3	360	4	74	6	6
Frosted Hot Fudge Sundae, Kellogg's*	1 Pastry/48g	190	4.5	396	4.2	70.8	9.4	2.1
Frosted Raspberry, Kellogg's*	1 Pastry/52g	200	5	385	3.8	73.1	9.6	1.9
Frosted S'mores, Kellogg's*	1 Pastry/52g	200	5	385	5.8	69.2	9.6	1.9
Frosted Strawberry, Oatmeal Delights, Kellogg's*	1 Pastry/50g	200	5	400	4	72	10	6
Pumpkin Pie, Frosted, Kellogg's*	1 Pastry/50g	200	5	400	4	70	10	2
Strawberry Sensation, Kellogg's*	1 Tart/50g	198	5.5	395	4	70	11	2
Wild! Fruit Fusion, Frosted, Kellogg's*	1 Pastry/50g	200	5	400	4	72	10	2
Wild! Grape, Kellogg's*	1 Tart/50g	200	5	400	4	72	10	2
POPCORN								
94% Fat Free, Orville Redenbacher's*	1 Bag/76g	220	0	289	13.2	65.8	0	0
Air Popped, Plain, Average	*1 Sm Bag/17g*	*66*	*0.8*	*387*	*12.9*	*77.9*	*4.5*	*14.5*
Butter Flavour, Microwave, Popz*	1 Serving/100g	480	27.5	480	7.5	51.1	27.5	9.2
Butter Toffee, Belgian Milk Chocolate Coated, M&S*	1 Pack/100g	505	25	505	6.5	60.4	25	4.1
Butter Toffee, Snack-A-Jacks, Quaker*	1 Bag/35g	149	3.2	425	3.5	86	9	4.5
Butter Toffee, Tesco*	1 Pack/175g	709	13.5	405	2.2	81.7	7.7	4.3

P

POPCORN

INFO/WEIGHT	Measure	per Measure KCAL	FAT	Nutrition Values per 100g / 100ml KCAL	PROT	CARB	FAT	FIBRE
Butter, Microwave, 94% Fat Free, Act II*	½ Bag/41g	130	2.5	317	9.8	68.3	6.1	12.2
Butter, Microwave, Act II*	1 Bag/90g	425	16.2	472	9	69	18	9
Butter, Microwave, Butterkist*	1 Bag/100g	395	18.5	395	8.3	49.5	18.5	8.5
Caramel Crunch, Sugar Free, with Sweeteners, Free'ist*	1 Portion/26g	94	1.5	362	3.1	73.8	5.8	0
Choc Full Of, Cadbury*	¼ Bag/32g	160	7.6	495	4.5	64.5	23.5	2.9
Chocolate & Pecan, M&S*	1 Pack/27g	130	5.2	480	3.3	72.9	19.3	3.6
Chocolate Flavour, Toffee, Snack-A-Jacks, Quaker*	1 Bag/35g	126	3.4	359	2.2	65	9.8	3
Irish Cream, Epic Snacks*	1 Serving/30g	122	2.1	407	2.4	82	7.1	3.7
Lightly Salted, Snack-A-Jack, Quaker*	1 Bag/13g	48	1.3	370	12.1	58	9.9	14.6
Lightly Sea Salted, Wholegrain, Sunbites, Walkers*	1 Pack/20g	84	2.6	419	8.6	59.3	12.9	15.7
Lime & Sea Salt, Captain Theodore's, Ten Acre*	1 Pack/28g	139	7	497	5.3	63.8	25	6.1
Maize, Unpopped, Love Life, Waitrose*	1 Serving/33g	200	14.1	605	6.2	48.7	42.8	12.7
Maple, Shapers, Boots*	1 Bag/20g	94	3.6	469	12	59	18	10
Microwave, Salted, Sunsnacks*	1 Pack/100g	498	22.9	498	10.7	51.3	22.9	10.8
Organic Amaranth*	1 Serving/10g	36	0.9	365	14.6	26.8	8.8	0
Paprika, Smoked, Sainsbury's*	1 Bag/11g	53	2.9	480	8.7	46.6	26.1	12.1
Peanut & Almond, Smooth, Propercorn*	1 Serving/25g	120	5.9	481	11.9	49.4	23.5	12.2
Plain, Oil Popped, Average	*1 Bag/74g*	*439*	*31.7*	*593*	*6.2*	*48.7*	*42.8*	*0*
Popping Corn, Average	*1 Serving/30g*	*112*	*1.3*	*375*	*10.9*	*73.1*	*4.3*	*12.7*
Popping Corn, Lightly Salted, Graze*	1 Punnet/28g	127	7	454	8	44	25	13
Popping Corn, Slightly Sweet, Graze*	1 Punnet/26g	116	5.4	447	7.5	53	21	9.3
Ranch Kern Pops, Creamy, Sour Cream & Onion, Graze*	1 Punnet/25g	139	7.3	554	5	56	29	12
Ready Salted, Microwave, Popz*	1 Serving/20g	101	6	504	7	51.5	30	9.2
Salt & Vinegar, Sainsbury's*	1 Bag/11g	52	2.7	474	4.8	53.6	24.6	9.7
Salt & Vinegar, Snack-A-Jacks, Quaker*	1 Sm Pack/13g	47	1.3	360	12	55	9.9	14
Salted Caramel, Bloom's*	1 Bag/28g	135	6.6	483	4.9	60.3	23.4	5.8
Salted, Blockbuster*	1 Bowl/25g	99	2.9	397	10.6	62.2	11.7	8.6
Salted, Crunch Corn, Propercorn*	1 Serving/30g	140	7.9	468	5	52.1	26.4	12.2
Salted, Diet Chef Ltd*	1 Pack/23g	107	3.8	465	10.5	68.6	16.6	14
Salted, Light, Microwave, Act II*	1 Pack/85g	336	6.5	395	10.6	71	7.6	15.8
Salted, Lightly, Sea, Propercorn*	1 Bag/20g	88	2.9	438	9.3	61.4	14.5	11.8
Salted, M&S*	1 Pack/25g	132	7.8	530	9.4	50.4	31.1	6.4
Salted, Manhatten Peanuts Limited*	1 Bag/30g	135	4.3	450	10	70	14.3	13.7
Salted, Sold At Cinema, Playtime Popcorn*	1 Sm/74g	384	24.9	519	8.3	45.9	33.6	0
Sea Salt & Vinegar, Sainsbury's*	1 Bag/11g	52	2.7	474	4.8	53.6	24.6	9.7
Sea Salt Flavour, Skinny, Topcorn, Metcalfe's Food Co*	1 Pack/23g	108	5.6	471	6.6	63.7	24.4	15.2
Sesame & Salt, Bloom's*	1 Pack/40g	200	11.5	501	4.8	48.6	28.8	14
Sour Cream & Black Pepper, Propercorn*	1 Bag/20g	88	3.7	440	10.8	50.1	18.3	15.9
Super, Perri*	1 Pack/30g	139	7	464	8.4	55.5	23.2	8.5
Sweet & Salty, Bloom's*	1 Portion/28g	138	7	492	4	58.6	25	8.5
Sweet & Salty, M&S*	1 Bag/15g	73	3.7	488	7.7	55.4	24.4	7.8
Sweet & Salty, Shapers, Boots*	1 Bag/20g	89	3.2	443	5.8	65	16	10
Sweet & Salty, Skinny Pop*	1 Pack/23g	98	3.4	424	7.2	66.7	14.8	8.9
Sweet and Salted, Microwave, Butterkist*	½ Bag/30g	119	4.2	398	9	48.1	13.9	22.1
Sweet Maple, Diet Chef Ltd*	1 Pack/23g	111	3.6	483	9.7	75.2	15.7	13
Sweet, & Salty, Propercorn*	1 Bag/30g	129	4.7	431	6.5	64.4	15.8	9.9
Sweet, Best-In*	1 Serving/34g	161	5.8	473	7.3	72.6	17	0
Sweet, Butterkist, Butterkist*	1 Pack/120g	612	29.8	510	2.8	68.5	24.8	5.6
Sweet, Cinema Style, Basics, Sainsbury's*	1 Handful/20g	90	4.4	450	5.9	57.5	21.8	11.1
Sweet, Cinema Style, Butterkist*	1 Bag/120g	612	29.8	510	2.8	68.5	24.8	5.6
Sweet, Coconut & Vanilla, Propercorn*	1 Bag/25g	122	5.5	486	6	61.6	22.1	7.7
Sweet, Deli, Passions, Aldi*	1 Bag/27g	121	4.2	448	7	74.8	15.6	10.7
Sweet, Microwave, Butterkist*	½ Pack/50g	235	10	470	9.8	60.5	20.1	4.4

	Measure INFO/WEIGHT	per Measure		Nutrition Values per 100g / 100ml				
		KCAL	FAT	KCAL	PROT	CARB	FAT	FIBRE
POPCORN								
Sweet, Microwave, Cinema, Popz*	1 Bag/85g	420	21.7	494	6	60	25.5	8.2
Sweet, Vanilla & Sugar, Microwave, Act II*	1 Pack75g	369	18.1	492	7.9	60.8	24.1	10.4
Toffee, 90% Fat Free, Butterkist*	1 Pack/35g	142	3.3	406	2.8	77.7	9.3	0
Toffee, Butterkist*	1 Bag/30g	124	3	415	2.3	79.3	10	4.4
Toffee, Chicago Joes*	1 Serving/10g	31	0.5	314	3.1	84.6	4.8	0
Toffee, Milk Chocolate Coated, Sainsbury's*	¼ Bag/25g	130	6.6	520	6.5	64.1	26.4	1.3
Toffee, Sainsbury's*	1 Serving/50g	208	6.4	415	1.8	73.8	12.7	3.3
Toffee, Snack Pack, Butterkist*	1 Bag/25g	105	2.2	420	2.1	81.3	9	3.5
Twist of Black Pepper, Graze*	1 Punnet/28g	127	7	452	8	44	25	13
Vanilla, Cinema Sweet Microwave, Act II*	½ Pack/50g	234	8	468	9	71	16	12
Wasabi Flavour, Skinny, Topcorn, Metcalfe's Food Co*	1 Bag/25g	121	6.6	484	8.4	54.1	26.2	9.7
White Cheddar Cheese, Manhatten Peanuts Limited*	1 Bag/30g	132	4.1	440	10	70	13.7	13
Wholegrain, Sweet & Salty, Sunbites, Walkers*	1 Pack/30g	127	3.1	424	6.3	67.5	10.4	12.8
Yellow, Kernel, (Unpopped), Jolly Time*	2 Tbsp/33g	110	1	333	12.1	78.8	3	21.2
POPPADOMS								
Cracked Black Pepper, Ready to Eat, Sharwood's*	1 Poppadom/9g	41	2.4	461	16.7	37.2	27.3	7.3
Fried in Vegetable Oil, Takeaway, Average	*1 Poppadom/13g*	*65*	*5*	*501*	*11.5*	*28.3*	*38.8*	*5.8*
Garlic & Coriander, Ready to Eat, Sharwood's*	1 Puppodum/9g	39	1.9	438	18.4	43	21.4	6.5
Indian, Asda*	1 Pack/45g	232	15.7	516	14.5	36.2	34.8	7.8
Mini, Sainsbury's*	½ Pack/50g	249	16.2	498	14.9	36.9	32.3	7.6
Plain, Asda*	1 Poppadom/9g	44	2.5	484	18	40	28	0
Plain, Bilash, Aldi*	1 Poppadom/10g	46	2.2	463	15.2	48.7	22.3	0
Plain, Cook to Eat, Sharwood's*	1 Puppodum/12g	32	0.1	273	21.9	45.7	1	10.1
Plain, Indian to Go, Sainsbury's*	1 Poppadom/8g	34	1.5	405	18.4	43.4	17.5	9
Plain, Mini, Cook to Eat, Sharwood's*	1 Puppodum/4g	11	0	273	21.9	45.7	0.3	10.1
Plain, Ready to Eat, Average	*2 Poppadom/16g*	*68*	*2.8*	*427*	*19.8*	*46.6*	*17.3*	*6.6*
Plain, Ready to Eat, Sharwood's*	1 Puppodum/8g	37	1.8	461	19.4	46.3	22	5.6
Plain, Tesco*	1 Serving/9.4g	41	2	439	17.8	44.4	21.1	4.6
Plain, Waitrose*	1 Serving/9g	37	1.7	408	21	39.3	18.6	9.1
Spicy, Cook to Eat, Sharwood's*	1 Puppodum/12g	30	0.1	257	20.2	43	0.5	13
Spicy, COU, M&S*	1 Pack/26g	84	0.6	325	23.5	51.9	2.4	8.1
Tesco*	1 Poppadum/8.9g	39	1.9	440	17.8	44.4	21.1	4.6
POPPETS*								
Chocolate Raisins, Poppets*	1 Pack/35g	140	4.7	401	4.9	65.4	13.3	0
Mint Cream, Poppets*	1oz/28g	119	3.6	424	2	75	13	0
Peanut, Poppets*	1 Box/100g	544	37	544	16.4	37	37	0
Strawberry Milkshake, Payne's*	1 Box/40g	180	5.3	450	2	79.1	13.2	3.3
Toffee, Milk Chocolate, Poppets*	1 Box/100g	491	23	491	5.3	68	23	0
PORK								
Belly, Fresh, Raw, Weighed with Skin, Average	*1 Serving/100g*	*518*	*53*	*518*	*9.3*	*0*	*53*	*0*
Belly, Roasted, Lean & Fat	*1oz/28g*	*82*	*6*	*293*	*25.1*	*0*	*21.4*	*0*
Chitterlings, Raw, Average	*1 Serving/100g*	*182*	*16.6*	*182*	*7.6*	*0*	*16.6*	*0*
Chop, Lean & Fat, Boneless, Raw, Average	*1oz/28g*	*67*	*3.8*	*240*	*29.2*	*0*	*13.7*	*0*
Chopped, Canned, Pek*	1 Can/240g	497	37.2	207	16.9	0.1	15.5	0
Cooked with Herbs, Italian, Finest, Tesco*	2 Slices/50g	117	8.8	234	18	1	17.5	0
Diced, Lean, Average	*1oz/28g*	*31*	*0.5*	*109*	*22*	*0*	*1.8*	*0*
Escalope, Average	*1 Escalope/75g*	*108*	*1.7*	*144*	*31*	*0*	*2.2*	*0*
Escalope, Lean, Healthy Range, Average	*1 Escalope/75g*	*80*	*1.5*	*106*	*22*	*0*	*2*	*0*
Fillet, in a BBQ Sauce, As Consumed, Appleby's, Aldi*	1/3 Pack/200g	282	5.6	141	24	5.1	2.8	0.5
Ham, Hock, Raw, Weighed with Bone, Fat & Skin	*100g*	*124*	*5*	*124*	*18.4*	*0*	*5*	*0*
Haslet, Somerfield*	1oz/28g	57	3.4	205	15	10	12	0
Joint with Crackling, Ready to Roast, Average	*1 Joint/567g*	*1283*	*80.1*	*226*	*24.2*	*0.8*	*14.1*	*0*
Joint, Ready to Roast, Average	*½ Joint/254g*	*375*	*18*	*148*	*19.2*	*2.3*	*7.1*	*0.2*

P

	Measure INFO/WEIGHT	per Measure KCAL	FAT	Nutrition Values per 100g / 100ml KCAL	PROT	CARB	FAT	FIBRE
PORK								
Leg, Joint, Healthy Range, Average	*1 Serving/200g*	*206*	*4.4*	*103*	*20*	*0.6*	*2.2*	*0*
Loin, Applewood Smoked, Asda*	1 Slice/15g	18	0.5	122	21.8	0.5	3.6	0
Loin, Chops, Boneless, Grilled, Average	*1oz/28g*	*83*	*4.1*	*298*	*27*	*0*	*14.6*	*0*
Loin, Chops, Grilled, Lean	*1oz/28g*	*52*	*1.8*	*184*	*31.6*	*0*	*6.4*	*0*
Loin, Chops, Raw, Lean & Fat, Weighed with Bone	*1 Chop/130g*	*248*	*19.9*	*191*	*13.2*	*0*	*15.3*	*0*
Loin, Joint, Roast, Lean	*1oz/28g*	*51*	*1.9*	*182*	*30.1*	*0*	*6.8*	*0*
Loin, Joint, Roasted, Lean & Fat	*1oz/28g*	*71*	*4.3*	*253*	*26.3*	*0*	*15.3*	*0*
Loin, Medallions, Extra Lean, Ashfield Farm*	1 Pack/400g	468	9.6	117	24	0.5	2.4	0.5
Loin, Roasted with Rosemary, Arista, Sainsbury's*	1 Slice/17g	24	1.2	144	20.8	0.1	6.8	0.7
Loin, Steak, Fried, Lean	*1oz/28g*	*53*	*2*	*191*	*31.5*	*0*	*7.2*	*0*
Loin, Steak, Fried, Lean & Fat	*1oz/28g*	*77*	*5.2*	*276*	*27.5*	*0*	*18.4*	*0*
Loin, Steak, Lean, Raw, Average	*1 Serving/175g*	*345*	*19.6*	*197*	*22.7*	*0*	*11.2*	*0.4*
Loin, Stuffed, Roast, M&S*	1 Slice/12g	22	0.9	180	24.4	2.4	7.9	0
Loin, Sweet Cured, Sliced, Tesco*	1 Slice/12g	17	0.5	141	23	2.1	4.4	0.5
Medallions, Average	*1 Medallion/125g*	*140*	*2.6*	*112*	*22.6*	*0*	*2*	*0*
Mince, Lean, Healthy Range, Average	*1 Pack/400g*	*504*	*20.2*	*126*	*19.8*	*0.4*	*5*	*0.3*
Mince, Raw	*1oz/28g*	*46*	*2.7*	*164*	*19.2*	*0*	*9.7*	*0*
Mince, Stewed	*1oz/28g*	*53*	*2.9*	*191*	*24.4*	*0*	*10.4*	*0*
Pulled, BBQ, Shredded, As Consumed, Morrisons*	1 Pack/200g	336	11.2	168	23.7	5.6	5.6	0
Pulled, BBQ, with Boston Beans, Everdine*	1 Serving/450g	414	9	92	5.6	10.2	2	5.2
Pulled, BBQ, with Rice, City Kitchen, Tesco*	1 Pack/450g	613	18	136	7	17.2	4	1.8
Pulled, with BBQ Beans, Musclefood*	1 Serving/394g	485	20.5	123	14.5	3	5.2	3.2
Pulled, with BBQ Sauce, Boneless, British, Tesco*	1 Serving/150g	256	11.2	171	17.3	8.5	7.5	0
Pulled, with BBQ Sauce, Jim Beam*	½ Pack/198g	459	23.2	232	27.3	4.3	11.7	0.5
Pulled, with BBQ Sauce, Shoulder, British, Sainsbury's*	1 Serving/120g	290	18.1	242	24.6	1.6	15.1	0.5
Raw, Lean, Average	*1oz/28g*	*42*	*1.2*	*151*	*28.6*	*0*	*4.1*	*0*
Roast, Lean Only, Average	*1oz/28g*	*34*	*0.9*	*121*	*22.7*	*0.3*	*3.3*	*0*
Roast, Slices, Average	*1 Slice/30g*	*40*	*1.4*	*134*	*22.7*	*0.4*	*4.5*	*0*
Shoulder, Slices, Cured	*1oz/28g*	*29*	*1*	*103*	*16.9*	*0.9*	*3.6*	*0*
Shoulder, Steak, Boneless, Frozen, Grilled, Tesco*	1 Steak/125g	156	4.9	125	0	0	3.9	0
Shoulder, Whole, Lean & Fat, Raw, Average	*100g*	*236*	*18*	*236*	*17.2*	*0*	*18*	*0*
Shoulder, Whole, Lean Only, Roasted	*1 Serving/150g*	*345*	*20.3*	*230*	*25.3*	*0*	*13.5*	*0*
Steak, Lean & Fat, Average	*1oz/28g*	*61*	*3.8*	*219*	*23.8*	*0*	*13.7*	*0.1*
Steak, Lean, Stewed	*1oz/28g*	*49*	*1.3*	*176*	*33.6*	*0*	*4.6*	*0*
Stir Fry Strips, Lean, Healthy Range, Average	*¼ Pack/113g*	*118*	*2.3*	*104*	*21.3*	*0*	*2*	*0*
Tenderloin, Lean, Boneless, Raw, Average	*1 Serving/100g*	*109*	*2.2*	*109*	*21*	*0*	*2.2*	*0*
PORK CHAR SUI								
Roast, in a Chinese Style BBQ Sauce, M&S*	1 Pack/350g	441	22	126	10.3	6.4	6.3	1.2
Slices, CBY, Asda*	¼ Pack/49g	79	3.2	161	23	2.2	6.5	1
with Chicken & Egg Fried Rice, Tesco*	1 Serving/450g	602	16.2	134	7.1	18.3	3.6	0.9
PORK DINNER								
Roast, 103, Oakhouse Foods Ltd*	1 Dinner/400g	376	14.8	94	6.7	8.3	3.7	1.4
Roast, Birds Eye*	1 Pack/340g	410	12	121	7.6	14.7	3.5	1.6
PORK IN								
Mustard & Cream, Chops	*1oz/28g*	*73*	*6*	*261*	*14.5*	*2.4*	*21.6*	*0.3*
PORK SCRATCHINGS								
Crunch, Mr Porky*	1 Pack/30g	159	9.6	531	60.4	0.5	31.9	4.6
KP Snacks*	1 Pack/20g	125	9.6	624	47.3	0.5	48.1	0.5
PORK WITH								
Honey & Mustard Sauce, Steaks, Tesco*	½ Pack/160g	258	11.8	161	16.3	8.7	7.4	1.4
Medallions with Bramley Apple, M&S*	1 Serving/380g	418	12.9	110	17.7	2.5	3.4	0.5
Peppers, Marinated, Tapas, Waitrose*	1 Serving/105g	181	6.7	172	26.3	2.2	6.4	0.3
Sage & Onion Stuffing, Joint, BGTY, Sainsbury's*	1 Serving/150g	246	5.4	164	29.5	3.3	3.6	1.3

	Measure INFO/WEIGHT	per Measure KCAL	FAT	Nutrition Values per 100g / 100ml KCAL	PROT	CARB	FAT	FIBRE
PORT								
Average	*1 Serving/50ml*	*78*	*0*	*157*	*0.1*	*12*	*0*	*0*
White, Average	*1 Glass/125ml*	*182*	*0*	*146*	*0.1*	*11*	*0*	*0*
POT NOODLE*								
Beef & Tomato, King, Made Up, Pot Noodle*	1 Pot/420g	543	19.8	129	3.3	18.5	4.7	1.1
Beef & Tomato, Made Up, Pot Noodle*	1 Pot/320g	426	14.7	133	3.4	19.4	4.6	1.3
Beef & Tomato, Mini, Made Up, Pot Noodle*	1 Pot/190g	254	9.5	134	3.5	18.7	5	1.7
Bombay Bad Boy, King, Made Up , Pot Noodle*	1 Pot/420g	542	19.7	129	3.3	18.5	4.7	1.1
Bombay Bad Boy, Made Up, Pot Noodle*	1 Pot/320g	415	15.3	130	3.3	18.4	4.8	1.1
Chicken & Mushroom, King, Made Up, Pot Noodle*	1 Pack/420g	545	19.3	130	3.3	18.8	4.6	1
Chicken & Mushroom, Made Up, Pot Noodle*	1 Pot/305g	430	18	141	3	19	5.9	1
Chicken, Roast, in a Mug, Made Up, Pot Noodle*	1 Mug/227g	141	1.8	62	2.1	11.5	0.8	0.4
Chilli Beef, Made Up, Pot Noodle*	1 Pot/305g	384	14.6	126	3	17.7	4.8	0.8
Chow Mein Chinese, Made Up, Pot Noodle*	1 Pot/320g	416	14.7	130	3.2	19	4.6	1.3
Curry, Balti, Made Up, Pot Noodle*	1 Pot/301g	268	1.5	89	3.1	17.8	0.5	0.5
Curry, Chicken, Hot, Made Up, Pot Noodle*	1 Pot/300g	384	14.1	128	2.8	18.7	4.7	1.1
Curry, Original, King, Made Up, Pot Noodle*	1 Pot/420g	507	18.1	121	2.6	17.9	4.3	1
Curry, Original, Made Up, Pot Noodle*	1 Pot/320g	431	15	135	3.1	20	4.7	1.2
Curry, Spicy, Made Up, Pot Noodle*	1 Pot/300g	393	14.4	131	2.9	19.1	4.8	1.1
Jamaican Jerk, Made Up, Pot Noodle*	1 Pot/310g	430	15.4	140	3	21	5	1.5
Piri Piri Chicken, Made Up, Pot Noodle*	1 Pot/307g	430	15.4	140	3	20	5	0
Sweet & Sour, Oriental, Posh, Made Up, Pot Noodle*	1 Pot/300g	375	13.8	125	1.7	19.2	4.6	0.5
POTATO BOMBAY								
Average	*½ Pack/150g*	*176*	*10.2*	*117*	*2*	*13.7*	*6.8*	*1.2*
Indian, Cooked, Sainsbury's*	½ Pack/150g	132	7.4	95	1.6	7.8	5.3	4.9
Indian, Waitrose*	½ Pack/150g	125	5.4	83	1.6	9.7	3.6	3
Tesco*	1 Pack/300g	240	12.6	80	1.3	9.3	4.2	2.1
POTATO CAKES								
Average	*1 Cake/70g*	*127*	*1.2*	*180*	*3.8*	*37.5*	*1.7*	*2.4*
Fried, Average	*1oz/28g*	*66*	*2.5*	*237*	*4.9*	*35*	*9*	*0.8*
POTATO MASH								
Cheddar, Cheese, Sainsbury's*	½ Pack/225g	257	13.8	117	4.1	10	6.3	2.1
Cheddar, Davidstow, Extra Special, Asda*	1 Serving/225g	292	16.9	130	5.3	10.4	7.5	2.6
Cheddar, Irish, Finest, Tesco*	½ Pack/250g	350	19.8	140	6.3	10.2	7.9	1.4
Cheese & Onion, Eat Smart, Morrisons*	1 Pack/400g	340	6.4	85	4.4	13.2	1.6	1.3
Mashed, Fresh, Tesco*	1 Pack/500g	395	8	79	2.3	13.1	1.6	1.9
Mustard with Caramelised Onions, Finest, Tesco*	1 Serving/200g	232	9.2	116	2.6	16	4.6	1.8
with Beetroot, Microwaved, Sainsbury's*	½ Pack/200g	130	3.2	65	2.1	9.4	1.6	2.1
with Cracked Pepper & Sea Salt, Luxury, Sainsbury's*	½ Pack/225g	389	28.4	173	1.6	13.2	12.6	1
POTATO SALAD								
& Egg, with Mayonnaise, Tesco*	½ Tub/150g	115	8.5	77	2.9	3.1	5.7	1.2
& Yoghurt, Meadow Fresh, Lidl*	1 Portion/50g	72	4	144	1.8	15.4	8	1.8
Asda*	¼ Pot/57g	67	4	117	0.9	12.5	7	1.1
Baby, & Free Range Egg, Fresh Tastes, Asda*	1 Pack/305g	168	6.7	55	2.6	5.5	2.2	1.3
Charlotte, Yoghurt Dressed, Waitrose*	1 Serving/100g	183	13.9	183	1.6	12.1	13.9	1.5
Creamy, Asda*	½ Tub/150g	226	16	151	1.1	11.3	10.7	2.5
Creamy, Waitrose*	1 Serving/100g	163	11.9	163	1.3	12.7	11.9	1.1
From Restaurant, Average	*1/3 Cup/95g*	*108*	*5.7*	*114*	*1.5*	*13.5*	*6*	*0*
HL, Tesco*	1 Tub/250g	288	12	115	1.7	15.4	4.8	1.2
M&S*	1oz/28g	55	4.8	195	1.2	8.5	17.3	1.3
New, & Free Range Egg, Side, Sainsbury's*	1 Pack/290g	174	12.2	60	2.5	3.1	4.2	1.4
New, Co-Op*	1 Serving/50g	98	8	195	1	10	16	2
Reduced Calorie, Pre Packed	*1oz/28g*	*27*	*1.1*	*97*	*1.3*	*14.8*	*4.1*	*0.8*
Tesco*	1 Serving/100g	165	13.5	165	1.3	9.5	13.5	1.3

P

	Measure INFO/WEIGHT	per Measure KCAL	FAT	Nutrition Values per 100g / 100ml KCAL	PROT	CARB	FAT	FIBRE
POTATO SALAD								
with Mayonnaise, Retail	**1oz/28g**	**80**	**7.4**	**287**	**1.5**	**11.4**	**26.5**	**0.8**
with Onions & Chives, Co-Op*	1 Serving/50g	80	6	160	1	12	12	1
POTATO SKINS								
American Style, Loaded, Asda*	1 Serving/78g	294	18	375	15	27	23	2.4
¼ Cut, Deep Fried, McCain*	1oz/28g	52	1.7	186	3	30.1	6	0
Cheese & Bacon, Loaded, Asda*	½ Pack/125g	275	15	220	13	15	12	3.3
Cheese & Bacon, Loaded, Tesco*	1 Skin/59g	150	9.1	255	9.2	19.5	15.5	3
Cheese & Chive, Sainsbury's*	2 Skins/150g	286	17.8	191	7.7	13.3	11.9	2.8
Cheese & Ham, Iceland*	2 Skins/108.4g	155	4.9	143	6.3	19.3	4.5	2
Cheese & Onion, Loaded, Tesco*	1 Skin/60g	114	6.5	190	5.8	17.6	10.8	1.4
with Sour Cream	**1 Serving/275g**	**541**	**34.6**	**197**	**7.2**	**13.8**	**12.6**	**2.2**
POTATO WAFFLES								
Frozen, Cooked	**1oz/28g**	**56**	**2.3**	**200**	**3.2**	**30.3**	**8.2**	**2.3**
Frozen, Grilled, Asda*	1 Waffle/57g	104	5.8	183	2	21	10.1	1.7
Mini, Sainsbury's*	1 Waffle/11g	27	1.8	242	2.8	20.1	16.7	1
Oven Baked, Mini, McCain*	1oz/28g	62	2.4	221	3.9	32	8.6	0
Uncooked, Average	**1 Waffle/62g**	**113**	**5.1**	**182**	**2.4**	**24.4**	**8.3**	**1.8**
POTATO WEDGES								
Aldi*	1 Serving/100g	150	6.8	150	2.1	20.2	6.8	0
BBQ Flavour, Asda*	1 Serving/100g	185	9	185	2.9	23	9	1.7
BGTY, Sainsbury's*	½ Pack/190g	179	3.4	94	3	16.4	1.8	3.4
Crispy, M&S*	1 Serving/200g	340	14.2	170	1.3	25.3	7.1	1.7
Frozen, Average	**1 Serving/120g**	**145**	**4.1**	**121**	**2**	**20.5**	**3.4**	**2.2**
Garlic & Herb, COU, M&S*	1 Pack/300g	300	7.8	100	2.3	16.4	2.6	3.2
Harvest Basket, Lidl*	1 Serving/100g	147	5.7	147	2.2	20.5	5.7	0
Jacket, Spicy, American Style, Frozen, Sainsbury's*	1 Serving/125g	156	5	125	1.9	20.3	4	1.1
Jumbo, Finest, Tesco*	1 Serving/126g	145	2.6	115	1.4	22.7	2.1	1.7
Nacho Cheese Flavour, Ridged, Cooked, McCain*	1 Portion/110g	188	7	171	2.6	24	6.4	3.4
Savoury, Waitrose*	1/3 Bag/250g	350	10.8	140	2.3	22.9	4.3	1.9
Smoky Paprika, Ridged, Frozen, Mccain *	1 Serving/100g	156	6.2	156	2.4	21.1	6.2	2.8
Southern Fried Style, Tesco*	1 Serving/155g	232	14.1	150	3	14.1	9.1	2
Spicy, Asda*	1 Serving/100g	145	5.7	145	1.8	21.8	5.7	2.1
POTATOES								
Alphabites, Captain Birds Eye, Birds Eye*	9 Bites/56g	75	3	134	2	19.5	5.3	1.4
Anya, Raw, TTD, Sainsbury's*	1 Serving/100g	75	0.3	75	1.5	17.8	0.3	1.1
Baby, Herby, Microwaved, Growers Selection, Asda*	1 Pack/360g	198	4.7	55	2	7.4	1.3	2.8
Baby, New with Butter, Mint & Parsley, Organic, Asda*	1 Pack/360g	414	10.4	115	1.7	20.4	2.9	2.5
Baby, New, Ocado*	¼ Bag/188g	141	0.6	75	1.7	16.1	0.3	1.3
Baby, Pearl, As Sold, Waitrose*	½ Pack/100g	79	0.3	79	1.7	16.1	0.3	2.4
Baby, with Butter & Herbs, Sainsbury's*	¼ Pack/147.5g	103	0.9	70	1.9	14.2	0.6	2
Baby, with Herbs & Butter, Morrisons*	1 Serving/100g	94	2.3	94	1.9	14.6	2.3	1.9
Baked, & Cheese, Waitrose*	½ Pack/220g	281	8.6	128	3.7	18.1	3.9	2.6
Baked, Chilli Con Carne, COU, M&S*	1 Pack/300g	270	6.3	90	6	11.1	2.1	1.2
Baked, Chilli Con Carne, Pro Cuisine*	1 Pack/340g	347	3.4	102	4.6	18.7	1	0
Baked, Flesh & Skin, Average	**1 Med/200g**	**218**	**0.2**	**109**	**2.3**	**25.2**	**0.1**	**2.4**
Baked, Flesh Only, Weighed with Skin, Average	**1oz/28g**	**20**	**0**	**72**	**1.5**	**16.6**	**0.1**	**1.2**
Baked, Frozen, Lidl*	1 Potato/200g	184	0.8	92	2.3	18	0.4	3.4
Baked, Ham & Cheddar Cheese, Asda*	1 Pack/300g	435	11.1	145	7	21	3.7	1.6
Baked, in Microwave, Flesh & Skin, Average	**1oz/28g**	**29**	**0**	**105**	**2.4**	**24.1**	**0.1**	**2.3**
Baked, in Microwave, Flesh Only, Average	**1oz/28g**	**28**	**0**	**100**	**2.1**	**23.3**	**0.1**	**1.6**
Baked, in Microwave, Skin Only, Average	**1oz/28g**	**37**	**0**	**132**	**4.4**	**29.6**	**0.1**	**5.5**
Baked, Mature Cheddar Cheese, Finest, Tesco*	1 Potato/245g	360	18.4	147	5.4	14.6	7.5	2.3
Baked, Mature Cheddar Cheese, M&S*	½ Pack/206g	225	6.6	109	3.6	16.9	3.2	1

POTATOES

	Measure INFO/WEIGHT	per Measure KCAL	FAT	Nutrition Values per 100g / 100ml KCAL	PROT	CARB	FAT	FIBRE
Baked, Skin Only, Average	*1oz/28g*	*55*	*0*	*198*	*4.3*	*46.1*	*0.1*	*7.9*
Baked, Spicy Chilli Con Carne, Spar*	1 Pack/340g	265	5.4	78	3.4	12.4	1.6	1.5
Baked, Stuffed, Mini, Tesco*	1 Serving/108g	130	6.3	120	2.3	14.6	5.8	2.3
Baked, Tuna & Sweetcorn, Average	*1 Serving/300g*	*273*	*6.8*	*91*	*5*	*12.6*	*2.2*	*0.9*
Baked, Tuna & Sweetcorn, BGTY, Sainsbury's*	1 Pack/350g	360	9.4	103	6.5	13.2	2.7	1.3
Baked, Tuna & Sweetcorn, Morrisons*	1 Serving/300g	243	2.1	81	5.1	13.5	0.7	0
Baked, with Baked Beans, Pro Cuisine*	1 Pack/340g	374	1.4	110	4.3	22.3	0.4	0
Baked, with Beef Chilli, Asda*	1 Pack/300g	381	7.8	127	5	21	2.6	2
Baked, with Cheddar Cheese, Farmfoods*	1 Potato/143g	196	5.4	137	4.7	21	3.8	1.9
Baked, with Cheese & Bacon, Finest, Tesco*	1 Potato/245g	360	19.6	147	6	12.6	8	2.5
Baked, with Cheese & Butter, Tesco*	1 Potato/224.8g	263	11.2	117	3.1	14.9	5	2.3
Baked, with Cheese, Freshly Prepared, Tesco*	½ Pack/215g	150	3	70	3.9	9.7	1.4	2.8
Baking, Raw, Average	*1 Med/250g*	*198*	*0.2*	*79*	*2.1*	*18*	*0.1*	*1.6*
Boiled with Skin	*1 Potato/125g*	*98*	*0.1*	*78*	*2.9*	*17.2*	*0.1*	*3.3*
Boiled, Average	*1 Serving/120g*	*86*	*0.1*	*72*	*1.8*	*17*	*0.1*	*1.2*
Boulangere, M&S*	½ Pack/225g	180	2	80	2.8	15.9	0.9	0.9
Charlotte, Average	*1 Serving/184g*	*139*	*0.5*	*76*	*1.6*	*17.4*	*0.2*	*3.3*
Chorizo, Roast, Tesco*	¼ Pack/125g	189	9	151	4.8	16.4	7.2	1
Crispy Bites, Weighed Frozen, McCain*	1 Serving/100g	141	4.4	141	2.5	20.4	4.4	1.5
Crispy Slices, M&S*	1/3 Pack/159g	231	8.3	145	2.9	22.2	5.2	1.9
Crunchies, Oven, Ross*	1 Serving/100g	240	11.7	240	3.6	30	11.7	2.4
Dauphinoise, Average	*1 Serving/200g*	*335*	*23.9*	*168*	*2.2*	*12.8*	*12*	*1.5*
Dauphinoise, Cook*	1 Pack /225g	320	18.7	142	5.3	11	8.3	1.8
Dauphinoise, TTD, Sainsbury's*	½ Pack/174g	240	16.2	138	2.9	10.8	9.3	2.7
Desiree, Average	*1 Serving/200g*	*152*	*0.4*	*76*	*2.2*	*16.4*	*0.2*	*0.6*
Frites, Fries, Golden, Crunchy, M&S*	½ Pack/100g	158	6.2	158	2.2	23.4	6.2	1
Fritters, Crispy, Oven Baked, Birds Eye*	1 Fritter/20g	29	1.6	145	2	16.3	8	1.2
Hasselback, Average	*1 Serving/175g*	*182*	*1.6*	*104*	*1.9*	*22*	*0.9*	*2.9*
Hassleback, Dine in Side, Eat Well, M&S*	½ Pack/175g	195	6	110	2.1	18.3	3.4	1.9
Jacket, Ready Baked, Frozen, McCain*	1 Potato/200g	190	1	95	1.7	20.9	0.5	1.4
Jersey Royal, Canned, Average	*1 Can/186g*	*116*	*0.2*	*62*	*1.4*	*14*	*0.1*	*1.2*
Jersey Royal, New, Raw, Average	*1oz/28g*	*21*	*0.1*	*75*	*1.6*	*17.2*	*0.2*	*1.5*
Jersey Royal, with Mint Butter, Extra Special, Asda*	½ Pack/172.1g	148	5.3	86	1.6	13	3.1	1.5
King Edwards, Red, Raw, Waitrose*	1 Serving/100g	84	0.2	84	2.1	17.2	0.2	2.4
Lemon & Thyme, Roast, Heated, Finest, Tesco*	½ Pack/174g	225	5.2	129	2.4	22	3	2.3
Maris Piper, Mashed, Eat Fresh, Tesco*	½ Pack/212.5g	191	4	90	1.9	14.7	1.9	1.6
Maris Piper, Raw, Average	*1 Serving/200g*	*151*	*0.4*	*75*	*2*	*16.5*	*0.2*	*1.4*
Mashed, Buttery, Sainsbury's*	1 Pack /450g	454	25.6	101	1.3	11.1	5.7	3
Mashed, CBY, Asda*	½ Pack/250g	177	5.5	71	1	10.3	2.2	2.8
Mashed, Colcannon, Waitrose*	½ Pack/225g	207	8.6	92	1.7	12.8	3.8	1.4
Mashed, From Restaurant, Average	*1/3 Cup/80g*	*66*	*1*	*83*	*2.3*	*16.1*	*1.2*	*0*
Mashed, From Supermarket, Average	*½ Pack/200g*	*197*	*8.1*	*98*	*1.8*	*13.3*	*4.1*	*1.5*
Mashed, From Supermarket, Healthy Range, Average	*1 Serving/200g*	*160*	*3.1*	*80*	*1.8*	*14.6*	*1.6*	*1.3*
Mashed, From Supermarket, Premium, Average	*1 Serving/225g*	*305*	*17.8*	*136*	*1.7*	*14.4*	*7.9*	*1.1*
Mashed, Home Prepared with Whole Milk	*1 Cup/210g*	*162*	*1.2*	*77*	*1.9*	*17.6*	*0.6*	*2*
Mashed, Mash Direct*	½ Pack/200g	190	3.8	95	1.7	17.7	1.9	1.3
Mashed, Olive Oil, HE, Tesco*	1 Serving/100g	90	2.2	90	2.1	15.5	2.2	0.9
Mashed, with Carrot & Swede, Sainsbury's*	½ Pack/226g	125	3.9	55	0.9	8.1	1.7	1.8
Mashed, with Cream & Butter, Ultimate, M&S*	½ Pack/225g	268	13.7	119	2.5	12.8	6.1	1.2
Mashed, with Milk Cream & Butter, Fresh, Ocado*	½ Pack/225g	207	7.2	92	1.7	13.3	3.2	1.6
Mashed, with Spring Onion, Weight Watchers*	1 Serving/100g	77	2.2	77	1.9	10.9	2.2	1.4
New, Average	*1 Serving/100g*	*75*	*0.3*	*75*	*1.5*	*17.8*	*0.3*	*1.1*
New, Baby, Average	*1 Serving/180g*	*135*	*0.5*	*75*	*1.7*	*17*	*0.3*	*1.6*

	Measure INFO/WEIGHT	per Measure KCAL	FAT	Nutrition Values per 100g / 100ml KCAL	PROT	CARB	FAT	FIBRE
POTATOES								
New, Baby, Canned, Average	*1 Can/120g*	*69*	*0.2*	*58*	*1.4*	*12.9*	*0.2*	*1.4*
New, Easy Steam with Herbs & Butter, Tesco*	1 Serving/125g	94	3.5	75	1.8	9.6	2.8	1.7
New, Garlic, Herb & Parsley Butter, Co-Op*	1 Serving/100g	115	5	115	1	15	5	2
New, in a Herb Marinade, Tesco*	¼ Pack/150g	152	7.4	101	1.3	13	4.9	1.5
New, with Herbs & Butter, Asda*	½ Pack/169.8g	146	2.9	86	1.7	16	1.7	1.5
Organics, Boiled, Asda*	1 Serving/200g	152	0.2	76	1.8	16	0.1	1.2
Pan Fried, Aldi*	1 Serving/250g	182	2	73	2.7	13.7	0.8	0
Raw, Peeled, Flesh Only	*1 Serving/100g*	*75*	*0.2*	*75*	*2*	*17.3*	*0.2*	*1.4*
Red, Flesh Only, Average	*1 Serving/300g*	*218*	*0.4*	*72*	*2*	*16.4*	*0.2*	*1.2*
Roast, Basted in Beef Dripping, Waitrose*	1 Serving/165g	213	8.9	129	2.2	18	5.4	1.9
Roast, Dry, No Oil, No fat	*1 Serving/100g*	*79*	*0.1*	*79*	*2.7*	*18*	*0.1*	*1.6*
Roast, Extra Crispy, Oven Baked, Aunt Bessie's*	1 Serving/100g	223	11.8	223	2.9	26.1	11.8	3.6
Roast, Frozen, As Consumed, Harvest Basket, Lidl*	1 Serving/165g	190	4	115	2.4	20	2.4	2
Roast, Frozen, Average	*1 Potato/70g*	*105*	*3.5*	*149*	*2.6*	*23.5*	*5*	*1.4*
Roast, Frozen, Healthy Range, Average	*1 Potato/70g*	*70*	*1.7*	*100*	*2.6*	*18.2*	*2.4*	*2.1*
Roast, Garlic & Rosemary, Miniature, Tesco*	¼ Pack/125g	85	0.9	68	1.8	12.5	0.7	2.3
Roast, in Lard, Average	*1oz/28g*	*42*	*1.3*	*149*	*2.9*	*25.9*	*4.5*	*1.8*
Roast, in Oil, Average	*1oz/28g*	*42*	*1.3*	*149*	*2.9*	*25.9*	*4.5*	*1.8*
Roast, New, Rosemary, Ainsley Harriott*	1 Serving/150g	133	4	89	2	16	2.7	1.3
Roast, Roasties, Mini, Midweek, as Sold, Aunt Bessie's*	1 Serving/100g	129	2.7	129	2.1	23	2.7	2
Roast, Scrumptiously Crispy & Fluffy, Frozen, McCain*	1 Serving/200g	446	28.6	223	1.8	20.7	14.3	2
Roast, with Goose Fat, TTD, Sainsbury's*	½ Pack/185g	216	4.4	117	2.7	21.1	2.4	3
Roasting, Average	*1 Serving/150g*	*202*	*5.2*	*135*	*2.5*	*23.4*	*3.5*	*1.6*
Saute, Oven Baked, McCain*	1oz/28g	56	1.1	199	4.4	36.9	3.8	0
Saute, with Onion & Bacon, Country Supper, Waitrose*	¼ Pack/100g	112	4.3	112	1.9	16.4	4.3	1.3
Scallops, Battered, Deep Fried, Average	*1 Scallop/67g*	*216*	*14.5*	*323*	*5.4*	*27.3*	*21.6*	*0*
Slices, in Rich Crispy Batter, Crispy, Chilled, Sainsbury's*	¼ Pack/100g	223	10.8	223	2.6	27.3	10.8	2.8
Smiles, Weighed Baked, McCain*	1 Serving/100g	237	10.1	237	3.4	33.4	10.1	3.1
Smiles, Weighed Frozen, McCain*	1 Serving/100g	191	8	191	2.6	27	8	2.7
Vivaldi, Baked with Skin, TTD, Sainsbury's*	1 Potato/180g	248	0.4	138	3.8	28.8	0.2	2.7
White, Raw, Flesh & Skin	*1 Lge/369g*	*284*	*0.3*	*77*	*2*	*17.5*	*0.1*	*2.2*
White, Raw, Weighed with Skin, Flesh Only, Average	*1 Med/213g*	*153*	*0.3*	*72*	*1.9*	*16.1*	*0.2*	*1.2*
POTATOES INSTANT								
Mashed, Dry, Tesco*	1 Serving/70g	225	0.1	321	7.7	72	0.2	7.1
Mashed, Made Up with Water, Average	*1 Serving/180g*	*118*	*0.3*	*66*	*1.7*	*14.5*	*0.2*	*1.3*
Mashed, Original, Dry Weight, Smash*	1 Serving/30g	101	0.3	343	8.3	71.8	1	6.7
POUSSIN								
Meat & Skin, Raw, Average	*1oz/28g*	*57*	*3.9*	*202*	*19.1*	*0*	*13.9*	*0*
Spatchcock, British, Waitrose*	½ Poussin/225g	364	20.2	162	19	1.2	9	0
POWERADE								
Berry & Tropical Fruit, Coca-Cola*	1 Bottle/500ml	120	0	24	0	5.6	0	0
Isotonic, Sports Drink, Coca-Cola*	1 Bottle/500ml	120	0	24	0	5.6	0	0
Zero, Coca-Cola*	1 Bottle/500ml	5	0	1	0	0	0	0
PRAWN COCKTAIL								
& Orkney Crab, M&S*	1 Serving/90g	180	13.8	200	14.2	1.8	15.3	0.6
BGTY, Sainsbury's*	1 Pack/200g	268	17.4	134	9.1	4.7	8.7	0.5
Delicious, Boots*	1 Pack/250g	285	6.5	114	5.5	17	2.6	1.2
HL, Tesco*	1 Pack/170g	305	23.9	180	7.1	5.7	14.1	0.6
in Marie Rose Sauce, Rich & Creamy, Waitrose*	½ Pot/100g	338	32.2	338	9.1	2.7	32.2	0.5
LC, Tesco*	1 Pot/140g	210	16	150	7.5	4.3	11.4	1.3
Reduced Fat, M&S*	1 Pack/200g	260	15	130	11.9	3.2	7.5	0.7
Tesco*	1 Tub/170g	476	39.1	280	6.6	10.2	23	1

	Measure INFO/WEIGHT	per Measure KCAL	FAT	Nutrition Values per 100g / 100ml KCAL	PROT	CARB	FAT	FIBRE
PRAWN CRACKERS								
Asda*	1 Serving/25g	134	8.8	535	2	53	35	0
Green Thai Curry, M&S*	1 Pack/50g	250	12.9	500	3.2	62.2	25.8	1.6
M&S*	1 Bag/50g	262	15.6	525	2.8	57.4	31.3	0.8
Ready to Eat, Sharwood's*	1 Bag/60g	316	18.5	527	0.5	62	30.8	1.2
Sainsbury's*	1 Cracker/3g	16	1	537	2.4	60.4	31.7	0.8
Tesco*	1/3 Pack/20g	114	7.4	570	2.5	56.5	37.1	0.9
PRAWN TOAST								
Chinese Snack Selection, Morrisons*	1 Toast/12.5g	41	2.6	328	11.3	23.1	21.2	6.6
from Chinese Selection, Ken Hom, Tesco*	1 Toast/12g	48	3.8	385	13.3	11.5	30.5	4
Mini, Oriental Selection, Party, Iceland*	1 Toast/15.1g	52	3.6	345	10.5	22	23.9	2.1
Oriental Selection, Waitrose*	1 Toast/14g	38	2.4	272	11.1	18.3	17.2	2.1
Sesame Prawn, Toasted Triangles, M&S*	1 Pack/220g	616	39.6	280	12.4	17.3	18	2
Sesame, Oriental Snack Selection, Sainsbury's*	1 Toast/12g	40	2.7	335	9.3	23	22.9	5.1
PRAWNS								
Batter Crisp, Lyons*	1 Pack/160g	350	20.3	219	8	18.2	12.7	1.1
Boiled	*1 Prawn/3g*	*3*	*0*	*99*	*22.6*	*0*	*0.9*	*0*
Cooked & Peeled, Average	*1oz/28g*	*21*	*0.2*	*77*	*17.6*	*0.2*	*0.6*	*0*
Filo Wrapped, Ovenbaked, Iceland*	1 Prawn/11g	31	1.1	270	8.5	36	9.6	2.7
Hot & Spicy, Average	*1 Serving/170g*	*461*	*26.9*	*271*	*9.4*	*22.8*	*15.8*	*2.2*
Icelandic, Raw, Average	*1oz/28g*	*30*	*0.4*	*106*	*22.7*	*0*	*1.6*	*0*
King, Breaded	*1 Prawn/13g*	*33*	*1.8*	*260*	*15.1*	*17.8*	*14*	*1.2*
King, Crevettes, Cooked & Peeled, Sainsbury's*	1 Pack/225g	205	1.1	91	21.8	0.1	0.5	0.3
King, in Filo, Finest, Tesco*	1 Prawn/20g	38	0.6	189	13	27.8	2.9	1.6
King, Raw, Average	*1 Bag/200g*	*145*	*1.9*	*72*	*15.8*	*0.2*	*1*	*0.1*
King, Tandoori, Average	*1 Prawn/59g*	*33*	*0.6*	*55*	*5.7*	*5.9*	*1.1*	*0.7*
North Atlantic, Peeled, Cooked, Average	*1oz/28g*	*22*	*0.3*	*80*	*17.5*	*0*	*1.1*	*0*
North Atlantic, Raw, Average	*1oz/28g*	*17*	*0.1*	*62*	*14.4*	*0*	*0.4*	*0*
Tempura, Jumbo, As Consumed, Iceland*	1 Prawn/12g	31	1.7	259	9.4	23.6	13.9	1
Tiger, Cooked & Peeled, Average	*1 Pack/180g*	*151*	*2*	*84*	*18.4*	*0.1*	*1.1*	*0*
Tiger, Jumbo, Average	*1 Serving/50g*	*39*	*0.2*	*78*	*18.2*	*0.3*	*0.5*	*0*
Tiger, Raw, Average	*1 Prawn/30g*	*19*	*0.2*	*64*	*14.2*	*0*	*0.7*	*0*
PRAWNS CHILLI								
& Coriander, Cooked & Peeled, Tesco*	1 Pack/160g	144	3.4	90	16.7	0.2	2.1	0.5
& Coriander, King, Sainsbury's*	1 Pack/140g	112	1.8	80	16.6	0.4	1.3	0.5
Crispy, with Sweet Chilli Dipping Sauce, M&S*	1 Pack/240g	490	20.2	204	8.2	23.6	8.4	0.6
King, Chilli & Coriander, Marinated, Just Add, M&S*	1 Pack/80g	82	2.1	102	19	0.1	2.6	0
King, in Sweet Chilli Sauce with Noodles, COU, M&S*	1 Pack/400g	260	1.6	65	4.8	10.3	0.4	1.5
King, with a Sweet Chilli Sauce, Succulent, Birds Eye*	1 Serving/140g	251	17.2	179	10.5	6.5	12.3	0.1
Skewers, Sweet Chilli, King, BBQ Favourites, Asda*	1 Skewer/48g	48	0.5	100	16.6	5.4	1.1	1
Sweet, Thai, King, Sainsbury's*	1 Serving/150g	177	6.1	118	6.4	13.9	4.1	1.9
with Spicy Chilli Dip, King, Sainsbury's*	½ Pack/150g	282	10.8	188	8.6	22.2	7.2	1
PRAWNS IN								
Creamy Garlic Sauce, Youngs*	1 Serving/158g	261	22.9	165	8.5	0.3	14.5	0
PRAWNS WITH								
Chilli, Coriander & Lime, King, Waitrose*	1 Pack/140g	143	3.2	102	19.9	0.5	2.3	0.6
Garlic & Herb Butter, King, Fresh, M&S*	1 Serving/200g	330	18	165	12.5	9.1	9	0.5
Ginger & Spring Onion, King, Budgens*	1 Pack/350g	150	4.2	43	5.9	2.1	1.2	0.7
Ginger & Spring Onion, Sainsbury's*	1 Pack/300g	198	9.3	66	4.7	4.7	3.1	0.3
Honduran, & Cocktail Sauce Dipper, M&S*	1 Pack/120g	258	21.6	215	13.6	0	18	1.1
King, with a Creamy Cocktail Sauce, M&S*	1 Pack/120g	278	23.3	232	12.6	1.3	19.4	1.1
King, with Garlic Butter, M&S*	1 Serving/100g	165	9	165	12.5	9.1	9	0.5
PRESERVE								
Ginger Shred, Robertsons*	1 Tsp/15g	40	0	267	0.1	66	0	0

	Measure INFO/WEIGHT	per Measure KCAL	FAT	Nutrition Values per 100g / 100ml KCAL	PROT	CARB	FAT	FIBRE
PRESERVE								
Ginger, Asda*	1 Serving/15g	39	0.1	261	0.5	63	0.5	1.7
Greengage, Extra Fruity, Waitrose*	1 Serving/15g	36	0.1	243	0.2	59.2	0.4	0.8
Rhubarb & Ginger, Mackays Ltd*	1 Serving/10g	27	0	269	0.3	66.7	0	0
PRETZELS								
American Style, Salted, Sainsbury's*	1 Serving/50g	202	2.2	403	10.8	79.7	4.5	1.8
Cheddar Cheese, Penn State Pretzels*	1 Sm Bag/30g	124	2.8	412	10	71.6	9.3	3.8
Jumbo, Tesco*	1 Serving/50g	194	3.4	388	9.7	71.9	6.8	5.4
Mini, M&S*	1 Pack/45g	194	6	430	10.4	66.6	13.4	4.9
Salted, Average	***1 Serving/30g***	***114***	***0.8***	***380***	***10.3***	***79.8***	***2.6***	***3***
Salted, Mini, M&S*	1 Pack/25g	96	0.5	382	10.9	78	2.1	3.9
Salted, Sainsbury's*	1 Serving/50g	200	1.8	401	9.8	82.4	3.6	3.4
Snacks, Fabulous Bakin' Boys*	1 Pack/24g	96	1.2	401	9	79.5	4.9	2.5
Soft, Cheddar & Red Onion, Knot, New York Bakery Co*	1 Pretzel/59g	168	2.5	284	11.8	46.7	4.3	5.3
Soft, Cinnamon Sugar, Auntie Anne's*	1 Pretzel/112g	380	1	339	7.1	75	0.9	1.8
Soft, Salted, Original, Auntie Anne's*	1 Pretzel/112g	310	1	277	7.1	58	0.9	1.8
Sour Cream & Onion, M&S*	1 Serving/30g	136	4.4	455	11	70.9	14.5	0.7
Sour Cream & Chive, Penn State Pretzels*	1 Serving/25g	111	3.2	443	8.9	71.8	12.9	2
Wheat, GF, Trufree*	1 Bag/60g	282	12	470	0.5	72	20	0.7
PRINGLES*								
Barbecue, Pringles*	1 Serving/50g	266	18	533	4.9	48	36	5.1
BBQ Spare Rib, Rice Infusions, Pringles*	1 Pack/23g	108	5.3	469	5.1	60	23	2.6
Burger, Take Aways, Pringles*	1 Serving/25g	129	8	516	4.2	52	32	2.5
Cheese & Onion, Pringles*	1 Serving/25g	132	8.5	528	4.1	50	34	3.4
Chip n Ketchup, Pringles*	1 Serving/25g	129	8	516	3.9	52	32	2.5
Hot & Spicy, Pringles*	1 Serving/25g	132	8.5	530	4.6	49	34	3.7
Light, Aromas, Greek Cheese & Avocado Oil, Pringles*	1 Serving/25g	122	6.2	488	4.6	57	25	3.6
Light, Original, Pringles*	1 Serving/25g	121	6.2	484	4.3	59	25	3.6
Light, Sour Cream & Onion, Pringles*	1 Serving/25g	122	6.2	487	4.7	57	25	3.6
Margarita Pizza, Classic Takeaways, Pringles*	1 Serving/25g	134	8	538	3.9	53	32	2.6
Minis, Original, Pringles*	1 Pack/23g	118	6.9	514	5.1	55	30	3.7
Minis, Salt & Vinegar, Pringles*	1 Pack/23g	115	6.4	502	4.5	55	28	3.6
Minis, Sour Cream & Onion, Pringles*	1 Pack/23g	118	6.7	511	5.2	56	29	3.5
Original, Pringles*	1 Serving/25g	130	8.5	522	3.8	51	34	2.6
Paprika, Pringles*	1 Serving/25g	132	8.5	529	4.9	49	34	6.5
Prawn Cocktail, Pringles*	1 Serving/25g	130	8	518	4.1	53	32	2.5
Salt & Vinegar, Pringles*	1 Serving/25g	128	8	512	3.9	52	32	2.4
Sour Cream & Onion, Pringles*	1 Serving/30g	153	9.6	509	3.9	52	32	2.6
Texas BBQ Sauce, Pringles*	1 Serving/25g	132	8.5	527	4.2	50	34	3.5
PROFITEROLES								
12 Chocolate, Waitrose*	3 Profiteroles/65g	284	21.4	437	6	28.7	33	0.4
Asda*	1 Serving/64g	218	17.2	343	5	20	27	0
Chocolate Covered, Tesco*	1 Serving/72g	295	21.2	410	5.7	29.3	29.5	2
Chocolate, 8 Pack, Co-Op*	¼ Pack/112g	330	17.9	295	6	31	16	2
Chocolate, Sainsbury's*	1/6 Pot/95.0g	192	8.5	202	5.4	25.1	8.9	0.8
Chocolate, Stack, Sainsbury's*	¼ Pack/76g	311	19.5	409	5.3	39.3	25.6	2
Chocolate, Tesco*	1 Serving/76g	293	21.8	386	5.1	26.9	28.7	0.5
Choux & Chocolate Sauce, Tesco*	1 Serving/77g	295	22	386	5.1	26.9	28.7	0.5
Classic French, Sainsbury's*	1 Serving/90g	284	15.5	316	6.6	33.7	17.2	0.1
Dairy Cream, Co-Op*	¼ Pack/70g	242	17.5	345	6	24	25	0.5
Filled with Cream, Stack, Fresh, M&S*	1 Serving/75g	281	21.4	375	5.3	23.6	28.5	1.9
in a Pot, Waitrose*	1 Pot/80g	207	11.3	259	6.3	25.6	14.1	2.9
Savoury with Cheese & Chive, CBY, Asda*	¼ Pack/15g	95	7.7	634	9.1	32.1	51.3	3.5
Waitrose*	4 Profiteroles/75g	269	17.9	359	4.8	31.1	23.9	0.7

	Measure INFO/WEIGHT	per Measure KCAL	FAT	Nutrition Values per 100g / 100ml KCAL	PROT	CARB	FAT	FIBRE
PRUNES								
Devils on Horseback, Christmas, Waitrose*	2 Prunes/25g	88	5	352	11.5	29.5	20.1	3.5
Dried, Average	*1 Prune/7g*	*11*	*0*	*158*	*2.5*	*36.4*	*0.4*	*5.8*
in Apple Juice, Average	*1 Serving/90g*	*76*	*0.1*	*84*	*0.8*	*19.8*	*0.1*	*1.4*
in Fruit Juice, Average	1oz/28g	24	0	86	0.9	20.9	0.2	2.9
in Syrup, Average	*1oz/28g*	*25*	*0*	*89*	*0.9*	*21.5*	*0.2*	*2.6*
Stewed with Sugar	*1oz/28g*	*29*	*0.1*	*103*	*1.3*	*25.5*	*0.2*	*3.1*
Stewed without Sugar	*1oz/28g*	*23*	*0.1*	*81*	*1.4*	*19.5*	*0.3*	*3.3*
PUDDING								
Apple, & Sultana, Steamed, BGTY, Sainsbury's*	1 Pudding/110g	294	3.2	267	2.9	57.4	2.9	0.8
Beef, & Onion, Minced, Hollands*	1 Pudding/165g	353	19	214	6.5	20.6	11.5	0
Black Forest, Brilliant, Graze*	1 Punnet/37g	97	3.3	262	4	40	9	2
Bread, Retail Average	*1 Slice/120g*	*301*	*8*	*251*	*8.4*	*41.8*	*6.7*	*0.5*
Chocolate, Fudge, Pot, Pots & Co*	1 Pot/125g	495	30	396	3.8	40	24	2.4
Chocolate, Ganache, Mini Pot, Gu*	1 Pot/45g	199	16.6	442	3.3	26.4	36.8	2.3
Chocolate, M&S*	¼ Pudding/76g	265	12	350	4.1	48	15.8	2.1
Chocolate, Melt in The Middle, Frozen, Waitrose*	1 Pudding/90g	310	14.4	344	6.7	41.4	16	3.5
Chocolate, Melting Middle, Hot, Puds, Gu*	1 Pud/100g	409	26.9	409	6	36	26.9	2.7
Chocolate, Melting Middle, M&S*	1 Pudding/154.5g	510	27.8	330	5.8	36.2	18	3.1
Chocolate, Sponge with Rich Caramel Sauce, Cadbury*	1 Pudding/110g	352	16.6	320	4	41.1	15.1	1.2
Eve's, Average	*1oz/28g*	*67*	*3.7*	*241*	*3.5*	*28.9*	*13.1*	*1.4*
Golden Syrup, Steamed, Aunty's*	1 Pudding/100g	293	4.1	293	3.3	57.3	4.1	0.8
Jam, Roly Poly, Aunt Bessie's*	1 Serving/75g	290	10.4	387	3.4	62.2	13.8	0.9
Jam, Roly Poly, Sainsbury's*	¼ Pack/81g	291	11.5	359	4.4	53.3	14.2	0.5
Queen of Puddings	*1oz/28g*	*60*	*2.2*	*213*	*4.8*	*33.1*	*7.8*	*0.2*
Souffle, Hot Chocolate, Gu*	1 Pot/65g	298	23.5	458	6	24.1	36.2	2.5
Sponge, with Golden Syrup, Individual, Mr Kipling*	1 Pudding/95g	395	16.7	366	3.1	53.1	15.5	0.6
Sponge, with Raspberry Jam, Individual, Mr Kipling*	1 Pudding/108g	392	16.8	363	3.1	52.4	15.6	0.7
Sticky Toffee, Co-Op*	¼ Pudding/100g	355	20	355	3	40	20	0.7
Sticky Toffee, Deluxe, Lidl*	½ Pudding/225g	806	36	358	2.5	50	16	2.1
Sticky Toffee, Extra Special, Asda*	¼ Pudding/100g	378	18	378	1.9	52	18	1.8
Sticky Toffee, Indulgent, Specially Selected, Aldi*	¼ Pudding/112g	387	14.6	344	2.6	54	13	1.5
Sticky Toffee, Steamed, Aunty's*	1 Pudding/110g	331	5.3	301	2.6	58.4	4.8	1.2
Sticky Toffee, Tesco*	1 Serving/110g	287	14.7	261	3.3	31.8	13.4	0.7
Strawberry, Jelly Pud, with Devon Custard, Ambrosia*	1 Pot/150g	129	1.2	86	0.7	19.4	0.8	0
Suet, Average	*1oz/28g*	*94*	*5.1*	*335*	*4.4*	*40.5*	*18.3*	*0.9*
Summer Fruits, Eat Well, M&S*	1 Pudding/135g	128	0.7	95	1.7	20.8	0.5	3
Summer, BGTY, Sainsbury's*	1 Pot/110g	223	5.1	203	3.2	40.9	4.6	2.4
Summer, Waitrose*	1 Pot/120g	125	0.5	104	2	23.1	0.4	1.4
Syrup, M&S*	1 Serving/105g	370	10.5	352	3.9	61.7	10	0.8
Torte, Cheeky Little Chocolate, Gu*	1 Pud/50g	211	14.6	422	5.7	31.6	29.1	1.8
Truffle, Chocolate with Raspberry Compote, Gu*	1 Pot/80g	250	14.6	312	2.8	28.8	18.2	1.8
PUMPKIN								
Boiled in Salted Water	*1oz/28g*	*4*	*0.1*	*13*	*0.6*	*2.1*	*0.3*	*1.1*
Potimarron, Raw, Average	*1 Serving/80g*	*21*	*0.1*	*26*	*1*	*6.5*	*0.1*	*1.9*
Puree, Baking Buddy *	1 Serving/53g	92	22	174	1.7	6.7	41.7	2.5

P

	Measure INFO/WEIGHT	per Measure KCAL	FAT	Nutrition Values per 100g / 100ml KCAL	PROT	CARB	FAT	FIBRE
QUAVERS								
Cheese, Walkers*	1 Bag/20g	107	6	534	2.7	62.5	30.1	1.1
Prawn Cocktail, Walkers*	1 Bag/16.4g	88	5.1	537	2.1	62	31	1.2
Salt & Vinegar, Walkers*	1 Bag/16.4g	86	4.9	527	1.9	62	30	1.2
QUESADILLA								
Chicken, from Restaurant, Average	**1 Serving/300g**	**867**	**46.7**	**289**	**15.6**	**22.2**	**15.6**	**1.7**
QUICHE								
Asparagus, & Mushroom, Tesco*	½ Quiche/200g	474	32.8	237	5.1	17.2	16.4	1.2
Asparagus, & Vegetable, Herby Summer, Higgidy*	1 Quiche/400g	848	50	212	5.9	18.9	12.5	2.7
Bacon, & Cheese, Sainsbury's*	¼ Quiche/100g	237	15	237	7	18.6	15	0.7
Bacon, & Leek, From Our Deli, As Consumed, Morrisons*	1 Quiche/160g	435	28	272	7.8	20	17.5	1.6
Bacon, Leek & Mushroom, M&S*	¼ Quiche/100g	245	16.4	245	6.9	17.2	16.4	1.3
Bacon, Smoked & Mature Cheddar, Higgidy*	1 Quiche/400g	1096	74	274	8.4	18.6	18.5	1.5
Broccoli, Tesco*	1 Serving/100g	249	17.2	249	6	17.6	17.2	1.4
Broccoli, Tomato and Cheese, Classic, Sainsbury's*	1 Serving/100g	223	14.5	223	5.3	17.1	14.5	1.6
Cheese, & Bacon, Crustless, Tesco*	1 Serving/85g	199	12.8	234	10	14.4	15	0.6
Cheese, & Broccoli, Morrisons*	1/3 Quiche/134g	338	22.4	253	7.1	18.4	16.8	1.7
Cheese, & Egg	**1oz/28g**	**88**	**6.2**	**314**	**12.5**	**17.3**	**22.2**	**0.6**
Cheese, & Ham, Basics, Somerfield*	¼ Quiche/81g	187	11	231	7	20.1	13.6	0.7
Cheese, & Leek, & Chive, Sainsbury's*	1/3 Quiche/125g	292	20.2	234	7.1	14.9	16.2	1.3
Cheese, & Onion, Asda*	½ Quiche/200g	578	39.6	289	9	18.6	19.8	1.5
Cheese, & Onion, Caramelised Onion, Finest, Tesco*	¼ Quiche/100g	300	18.6	300	9.4	22.4	18.6	1.7
Cheese, & Onion, Co-Op*	¼ Quiche/88g	262	19.2	300	10	17	22	1
Cheese, & Onion, Crustless, Deli, Morrisons*	1 Quiche/388g	1005	68.3	259	9.7	14.9	17.6	1
Cheese, & Onion, Crustless, Weight Watchers*	1 Quiche/160g	267	12.3	167	11.3	11.1	7.7	4.3
Cheese, & Onion, Deep Filled, Sainsbury's*	¼ Quiche/100g	254	17.2	254	7.3	17.2	17.2	2.2
Cheese, & Onion, Finest, Tesco*	1 Serving/130g	346	24.3	266	9.1	15.3	18.7	2.5
Cheese, & Onion, HL, Tesco*	¼ Quiche/100g	180	7.8	180	9.4	17.6	7.8	1.8
Cheese, & Onion, Individual, Sainsbury's*	1 Quiche/180g	542	34.9	301	9.9	21.6	19.4	1.5
Cheese, & Onion, M&S*	1 Slice/100g	250	17.2	250	8.2	16.1	17.2	1.5
Cheese, & Onion, Mature Cheddar, Crustless, Higgidy*	¼ Quiche/95g	254	16.9	267	7.4	18.7	17.8	1
Cheese, & Onion, Reduced Fat, Eat Smart, Morrisons*	1 Quiche/400g	824	36.8	206	7.7	16.9	9.2	0.7
Cheese, & Onion, Retail, Average	**¼ Quiche/100g**	**262**	**17.8**	**262**	**8.4**	**17.1**	**17.8**	**1.3**
Cheese, & Onion, Value, Tesco*	½ Quiche/200g	526	36.4	263	8.6	16.1	18.2	0.7
Cheese, & Onion, Weight Watchers*	1 Quiche/165g	325	15.3	197	7	21.2	9.3	1.6
Cheese, & Tomato, Asda*	¼ Quiche/105g	274	17.8	261	8	19	17	0.9
Cheese, & Tomato, Crustless, Iceland*	¼ Quiche/203g	483	34.7	238	7.5	12.8	17.1	1.9
Cheese, & Tomato, Retail, Average	**¼ Quiche/100g**	**268**	**17.1**	**268**	**8**	**20.2**	**17.1**	**1.1**
Lorraine, Asda*	¼ Quiche/100g	246	16.2	246	6.6	18.5	16.2	4.2
Lorraine, BGTY, Sainsbury's*	1 Serving/128g	273	14	213	10.9	17.7	10.9	0.7
Lorraine, Castle Grove, Lidl*	½ Pie/200g	578	40	289	11	16	20	0.5
Lorraine, Classics, M&S*	¼ Quiche/100g	251	16.4	251	10.3	15	16.4	0.9
Lorraine, Co-Op*	¼ Quiche/100g	275	20.6	275	8.1	14.9	20.6	2.6
Lorraine, Crustless, Asda*	1 Quiche/160g	259	12.6	162	9.3	13.5	7.9	1.1
Lorraine, Crustless, LC, Tesco*	1 Pack/160g	280	13.4	175	12.6	11.8	8.4	2.5
Lorraine, Crustless, You Count, Love Life, Waitrose*	1 Quiche/160g	295	15.4	185	8.9	15.2	9.6	0.9
Lorraine, Extra Special, Asda*	¼ Quiche/100g	270	18	270	8	19	18	2.3
Lorraine, Finest, Tesco*	1 Serving/100g	330	25.1	330	8.4	17.5	25.1	1.5
Lorraine, Quiche Selection, M&S*	1 Slice/56g	160	11.5	285	12.8	12.3	20.6	2.1
Lorraine, Retail, Average	**¼ Quiche/100g**	**280**	**19.5**	**280**	**9**	**16.8**	**19.5**	**2**
Lorraine, Smoked Bacon & Cheese, M&S*	¼ Quiche/100g	270	18.4	270	9.7	16.4	18.4	1.6
Lorraine, Tesco*	½ Quiche/87.5g	249	16.6	285	9.3	18.2	19	1.9
Lorraine, TTD, Sainsbury's*	1/3 Quiche/158g	402	28.3	254	10.9	12.3	17.9	2.5
Mushroom	**1oz/28g**	**80**	**5.5**	**284**	**10**	**18.3**	**19.5**	**0.9**

	Measure INFO/WEIGHT	per Measure		Nutrition Values per 100g / 100ml				
		KCAL	FAT	KCAL	PROT	CARB	FAT	FIBRE
QUICHE								
Mushroom, Medley, Waitrose*	¼ Quiche/100g	222	15.2	222	6.4	15	15.2	2.9
Salmon, & Broccoli, Tesco*	1 Serving/133g	311	20.1	234	7.9	16.6	15.1	0.9
Salmon, & Spinach, Sainsbury's*	1/3 Quiche/125g	318	21.9	254	8.2	15.9	17.5	1
Salmon, & Spinach, Smoked, Little, Higgidy*	1 Quiche/155g	448	31.5	289	8.6	17.5	20.3	0.9
Spinach, & Red Pepper, Goats Cheese, Waitrose*	1 Serving/100g	218	14.3	218	6.5	15.8	14.3	2.6
Spinach, & Ricotta, Tesco*	¼ Quiche/100g	237	14.9	237	5.8	19.9	14.9	1
Spinach, & Roast Red Pepper, Little, Higgidy*	1 Quiche/155g	397	27.3	256	9.1	15.2	17.6	1.2
Spinach, Feta, & Roasted Red Pepper, Higgidy*	¼ Quiche/100g	253	17.7	253	8.4	17.3	17.7	1.3
Vegetable, Mediterranean Style, Classic, Sainsbury's*	1 Quiche/400g	868	50.4	217	6.2	19.8	12.6	2.2
QUINCE								
Average	*1 Avg fruit/209g*	*37*	*0.1*	*18*	*0.2*	*4.3*	*0.1*	*1.3*
QUINOA								
Black Rice & Edamame Soya Beans, Eat Well, M&S*	1 Pack/240g	283	9.4	118	4.1	13.9	3.9	5.6
Cooked, Love Life, Waitrose*	1 Serving/180g	216	3.5	120	9.9	4.4	1.9	2.8
Dry Weight, Average	*1 Serving/70g*	*258*	*4.2*	*368*	*14.1*	*64.2*	*6.1*	*7*
Red	*1 Serving/100g*	*358*	*6*	*358*	*12.9*	*62.2*	*6*	*9.7*
Red & White, with Bulgur Wheat, Tesco*	½ Pack/125g	233	4.9	186	6.7	28.9	3.9	4.6

Q

	Measure INFO/WEIGHT	per Measure KCAL	FAT	Nutrition Values per 100g / 100ml KCAL	PROT	CARB	FAT	FIBRE
RABBIT								
Meat Only, Raw	*1oz/28g*	*38*	*1.5*	*137*	*21.9*	*0*	*5.5*	*0*
Meat Only, Raw, Weighed with Bone	*1 Serving/200g*	*164*	*6.6*	*82*	*13.1*	*0*	*3.3*	*0*
Meat Only, Stewed	*1oz/28g*	*32*	*0.9*	*114*	*21.2*	*0*	*3.2*	*0*
Meat Only, Stewed, Weighed with Bone	*1oz/28g*	*11*	*0.3*	*41*	*7.6*	*0*	*1.1*	*0*
RADISH								
Black, Raw, Average	*1 Lge/9g*	*1*	*0*	*16*	*1*	*3*	*0*	*2*
Red, Unprepared, Average	*1 Radish/8g*	*1*	*0*	*11*	*0.6*	*1.7*	*0.2*	*0.8*
White, Mooli, Raw	*1oz/28g*	*4*	*0*	*13*	*0.7*	*2.5*	*0.1*	*0*
RAISINS								
& Sultanas, Jumbo, M&S*	1 Serving/80g	212	0.4	265	2.4	62.4	0.5	2.6
& Sultanas, The Fruit Factory*	1 Box/14g	43	0.1	305	3	72.3	0.5	4
Lime Infused, Tangy, Nak'd*	1 Pack/25g	68	0	272	2.1	69.3	0	0
Seedless, Average	*1 Serving/75g*	*215*	*0.4*	*287*	*2.2*	*68.5*	*0.5*	*3.2*
White Chocolate Coated, Graze*	1 Pack/30g	135	6.6	451	4.7	59.7	21.9	0
Yoghurt Coated, Fruit Bowl*	1 Pack/25g	114	4.8	455	2	67	19	3
RAITA								
Cucumber & Mint, Patak's*	1oz/28g	18	0.5	64	3.4	8.4	1.8	0
Dip, Indian, Asda*	1 Pot/70g	120	11.5	172	2.6	3.6	16.4	0.5
Plain, Average	*1oz/28g*	*16*	*0.6*	*57*	*4.2*	*5.8*	*2.2*	*0*
RASPBERRIES								
Dried, Graze*	1 Pack/30g	85	0.8	284	3.2	62	2.6	0
Freeze Dried, Simply*	1 Serving/10g	37	0	370	10	80	0	20
Fresh, Raw, Average	*1 Serving/80g*	*20*	*0.2*	*25*	*1.3*	*4.7*	*0.3*	*6.5*
Frozen, Average	*1 Serving/100g*	*27*	*0.3*	*27*	*1.3*	*4.7*	*0.3*	*5.2*
in Juice, Canned, Morrisons*	½ Can/150g	81	0.3	54	0.4	12	0.2	1.4
in Syrup, Canned	*1oz/28g*	*25*	*0*	*88*	*0.6*	*22.5*	*0.1*	*1.5*
RATATOUILLE								
Average	*1oz/28g*	*23*	*2*	*82*	*1.3*	*3.8*	*7*	*1.8*
Chicken, Finest, Tesco*	1 Pack/550g	407	11.6	74	7.8	5.9	2.1	0
RAVIOLI								
Asparagus, & Cheese, Waitrose*	1 Serving/100g	242	7.2	242	12.6	31.7	7.2	2.4
Asparagus, Waitrose*	1 Serving/150g	303	9	202	10.5	26.4	6	2
Beef	*1 Serving/300g*	*501*	*13.7*	*167*	*6.4*	*25*	*4.6*	*1.4*
Beef, & Red Wine, Italiano, Tesco*	½ Pack/200g	424	13	212	7.3	30	6.5	2.3
Beef, & Red Wine, Rich, Morrisons*	1 Pack/300g	813	20.7	271	12	42.8	6.9	2.6
Beef, in Tomato Sauce, Heinz*	½ Can/200g	147	3.2	74	2.5	12	1.6	0.8
Beef, in Tomato Sauce, Minced, Rich, Corale, Aldi*	½ Can/200g	172	2	86	2.8	16.4	1	0.5
Beef, Tesco*	1 Serving/194g	175	5	90	4.3	12.3	2.6	1.5
Cheese, Four, in Tomato Sauce, COU, M&S*	1 Pack/345g	352	7.6	102	7.5	12.3	2.2	1.5
Chicken, & Bacon, Cucina, Aldi*	1 Pack/250g	455	14	182	6.9	24.7	5.6	2.7
Chicken, & Bacon, Sainsbury's*	½ Pack/210.7g	335	11.4	159	5.5	22.2	5.4	2
Crab, & Chilli, Scottish, Cooked, Finest, Tesco*	1/3 Pack/170g	362	12.6	213	8	27.5	7.4	2.2
Garlic, & Herb, Roast, Tesco*	½ Pack/125g	342	13.6	274	12.8	31.1	10.9	1.1
Goat's Cheese, & Pesto, Asda*	½ Pack/150g	204	5.4	136	6	20	3.6	0
in Tomato Sauce, Canned, Sainsbury's*	½ Can/200g	166	2	83	3.1	15.5	1	0.5
in Tomato Sauce, Meat Free, Heinz*	1 Can/410g	308	3.3	75	2.4	14.4	0.8	0.5
Mushroom, Italiano, Tesco*	1 Serving/125g	332	16.1	266	10.4	27	12.9	3
Mushroom, Portobello, Waitrose*	½ Pack/125g	201	5.1	161	7.5	22.3	4.1	2.6
Mushroom, Tesco*	½ Pack/125g	332	16.1	266	10.4	27	12.9	3
Mushroom, Wild, Finest, Tesco*	1 Serving/200g	472	12.2	236	10.8	34.4	6.1	1.9
Pancetta, & Mozzarella, Finest, Tesco*	1 Serving/125g	344	13.2	275	12.2	32.8	10.6	1.8
Salmon, & Dill, Smoked, Sainsbury's*	1 Serving/125g	256	8.9	205	8.7	26.5	7.1	0.7
Spinach, & Ricotta, Waitrose*	1 Serving/125g	309	9	247	10.5	35	7.2	1.9

R

	Measure INFO/WEIGHT	KCAL	FAT	Nutrition Values per 100g / 100ml				
		per Measure		KCAL	PROT	CARB	FAT	FIBRE
RAVIOLI								
Vegetable, Canned, Sainsbury's*	1 Can/400g	328	2.8	82	2.6	16.3	0.7	0.7
Vegetable, Morrisons*	1 Can/400g	276	1.6	69	2.4	13.9	0.4	0
Vegetable, Roasted, Asda*	½ Pack/150g	218	0.8	145	6	29	0.5	0
Vegetable, Tesco*	½ Can/200g	164	1.4	82	2.6	16.3	0.7	0.7
RED BULL*								
Reg, Red Bull*	1 Can/250ml	112	0	45	0	11.3	0	0
REDCURRANTS								
Raw, Average	*1oz/28g*	*6*	*0*	*20*	*1.1*	*4.3*	*0*	*3.3*
Raw, Stalks Removed	*1 Serving/100g*	*21*	*0*	*21*	*1.1*	*4.4*	*0*	*0*
REEF*								
Orange & Passionfruit, Reef*	1 Bottle/275ml	179	0	65	0	9.5	0	0
RELISH								
Barbeque, Sainsbury's*	1 Serving/50g	50	1	100	1	19.3	2.1	1.1
Branston, Sweet Onion, Crosse & Blackwell*	1 Serving/10g	15	0	153	1	36.3	0.4	0.7
Burger, Caramelised Red Onion, Branston*	1 Squeeze/15g	23	0.2	151	0.8	32	1.4	1.4
Caramelised Red Onion, Tesco*	1 Serving/10g	28	0	280	0.6	69.1	0.1	0.7
Onion, M&S*	1oz/28g	46	0.8	165	1	32.1	3	1.1
Onion, Sainsbury's*	1 Serving/15g	23	0.1	151	0.9	36	0.4	0.7
Onion, Sweet, Heinz*	1 Tbsp/37.5g	38	0.2	102	1	23.5	0.4	0.6
Sweetcorn, American Style, Maryland, Tesco*	1 Serving/15g	15	0	101	1.1	23.9	0.1	0.9
Sweetcorn, Bick's*	1 Tbsp/22g	23	0	103	1.3	24.3	0.2	0
Tomato Spicy, Bick's*	1 Serving/28g	28	0.1	99	1.3	23.2	0.2	0
Tomato, M&S*	1oz/28g	36	0.1	130	1.8	30.2	0.3	1.5
Tomato, Sweet, Heinz*	1 Serving/25g	34	0	136	0.9	32.6	0.2	0.9
REVELS								
Mars*	1 Pack/35g	169	7.4	483	5.2	67.6	21	0
RHUBARB								
In Juice, Canned, Drained, Average	*1 Serving/100g*	*46*	*0*	*46*	*0.5*	*10.8*	*0*	*0.8*
Raw, Average	*1 Stalk/51g*	*4*	*0.1*	*7*	*0.9*	*0.8*	*0.1*	*1.4*
Stewed with Sugar, Average	*1oz/28g*	*32*	*0*	*116*	*0.4*	*31.2*	*0*	*2*
RIBENA*								
Apple Juice Drink, Ribena*	1 Carton/287ml	132	0	46	0	11.1	0	0
Blackcurrant Juice Drink, Ready Made, Ribena*	1 Carton/200ml	82	0	41	0	10.6	0	0
Blackcurrant, Diluted with Water, Ribena*	1 Serving/100ml	46	0	46	0	11.4	0	0
Blackcurrant, No Added Sugar, Diluted, Ribena*	1 Serving/250ml	11	0	4	0	0.6	0	0
Blackcurrant, Original, Undiluted, Ribena*	1 Serving/50ml	108	0	216	0	53	0	0
Blackcurrant, Really Light, No Added Sugar, Ribena*	1 Carton/250ml	8	0	3	0	0.8	0	0
Light, Ribena*	1 Carton/288ml	26	0	9	0.1	2.1	0	0
Orange, Juice Drink, Ribena*	1 Serving/288ml	98	0	34	0.1	8.1	0	0
Pineapple & Passion Fruit, Juice Drink, Ribena*	½ Bottle/250ml	103	0	41	0	9.9	0	0
Plus, Apple & Peach, Immunity Support, Ribena*	1 Carton/200ml	2	0	1	0	0.2	0	0
Really Light, Undiluted, Ribena*	1 Serving/25ml	20	0	80	0	2.5	0	0
Strawberry Juice Drink, Ribena*	1 Carton/288ml	130	0	45	0	10.9	0	0
RIBS								
in a Chinese Style Coating, Tesco*	1 Serving/250g	420	21.8	168	19.5	5.3	8.7	2.5
Loin, BBQ, Sainsbury's*	1 Rib/42g	104	5.5	247	24.7	7.3	13.2	0.9
Loin, Chinese, Sainsbury's*	1 Rib/42g	103	5	246	27.2	7.2	12	0.9
Loin, Chinese, Taste Summer, Sainsbury's*	1 Serving/30g	38	2.3	128	11.7	2.8	7.8	0.1
Pork, Barbecue, Meat Only, Cooked, Average	*1 Serving/130g*	*360*	*23.4*	*275*	*21.4*	*7.2*	*17.9*	*0.3*
Pork, Chinese Style, Average	*1 Serving/300g*	*736*	*44.7*	*245*	*17.9*	*10*	*14.9*	*0.7*
Pork, Chops, Raw, Lean & Fat, Weighed with Bone	*1 Chop/130g*	*241*	*16.1*	*186*	*18.5*	*0*	*12.4*	*0*
Pork, Full Rack, Sainsbury's*	1 Serving/225g	567	38.7	252	18	6.5	17.2	0.9
Pork, Rack, Szechuan BBQ, Waitrose*	½ Pack/105g	257	16.5	244	20.4	5.1	15.7	0.6

R

	Measure INFO/WEIGHT	per Measure KCAL	FAT	Nutrition Values per 100g / 100ml KCAL	PROT	CARB	FAT	FIBRE
RIBS								
Spare, Barbecue, Chinese Style, Farmfoods*	1 Pack/400g	464	25.2	116	9.3	5.6	6.3	0.1
Spare, Cantonese, Mini, Sainsbury's*	1 Rib/38g	97	5	259	17.2	17.3	13.4	1
Spare, Chinese Style, Meal Solutions, Co-Op*	1 Serving/165g	214	14.8	130	8	4	9	0.2
Spare, Chinese Style, Summer Eating, Asda*	1 Serving/116g	334	18.6	288	32	4.1	16	0.8
Spare, Sweet, Sticky, Mini, M&S*	½ Pack/75g	215	12.9	286	22.7	9.8	17.2	0.8
RICE								
Arborio, Dry, Average	**1 Serving/80g**	**279**	**0.6**	**348**	**7.1**	**78.3**	**0.8**	**0.8**
Basmati, & Wild, Cooked, Sainsbury's*	½ Pack/125g	150	0.8	120	3.1	25.7	0.6	1.3
Basmati, & Wild, Dry Weight, Tilda*	1 Serving/70g	244	0.3	349	9.4	77	0.5	1
Basmati, Boil in the Bag, Dry, Average	**1 Serving/50g**	**176**	**0.4**	**352**	**8.4**	**77.8**	**0.8**	**0.4**
Basmati, Brown, Dry, Average	**1 Serving/50g**	**177**	**1.5**	**353**	**9.5**	**71.8**	**3**	**2.2**
Basmati, Cooked, Average	**1 Serving/140g**	**189**	**1**	**135**	**3.1**	**29**	**0.7**	**0.4**
Basmati, Dry Weight, Average	**1 Serving/60g**	**212**	**0.6**	**353**	**8.1**	**77.9**	**1**	**0.6**
Basmati, Indian, Dry, Average	**1 Serving/75g**	**260**	**0.7**	**346**	**8.4**	**76.1**	**0.9**	**0.1**
Basmati, Microwave, Cooked, Average	**1 Serving/125g**	**182**	**2.3**	**146**	**2.7**	**30**	**1.8**	**0**
Basmati, White, Dry, Average	**1 Serving/75g**	**262**	**0.4**	**349**	**8.1**	**77.1**	**0.6**	**2.2**
Basmati, Wholegrain & Wild, Pouch, Tilda*	½ Pack/125g	160	2.6	128	3	23.4	2.1	1.7
Basmati, Wholegrain, Cooked, Tilda*	1 Portion/180g	203	1.6	113	3.3	23	0.9	3.2
Basmati, with Mushroom, Dine In, Veetee*	1 Pack/280g	372	6.4	133	3.3	24.4	2.3	1.2
Beef, Super, As Prepared, Savoury Rice, Batchelors*	½ Pack/116g	181	1.3	156	5	31	1.1	1.5
Black Bean, Jerk & Coconut, Pulses & Rice, Tilda*	1 Pack/140g	178	5.5	127	4	16.5	3.9	4.9
Brown, Cooked, Average	**1 Serving/140g**	**173**	**1.5**	**123**	**2.6**	**26.6**	**1.1**	**0.9**
Brown, Dry, Average	**1 Serving/75g**	**266**	**2.3**	**355**	**7.5**	**76.2**	**3**	**1.4**
Brown, Long Grain, Dry, Average	**1 Serving/50g**	**182**	**1.4**	**364**	**7.6**	**76.8**	**2.8**	**2**
Brown, Short Grain, Dry, Average	**1 Serving/50g**	**176**	**1.4**	**351**	**6.8**	**77.6**	**2.8**	**1**
Brown, Whole Grain, Cooked, Average	**1 Serving/170g**	**223**	**1.9**	**132**	**2.6**	**27.8**	**1.1**	**1.2**
Brown, Whole Grain, Dry, Average	**1 Serving/40g**	**138**	**1.2**	**344**	**7.4**	**71.6**	**2.9**	**3**
Cauliflower, & Parsley, Lets Cook, Aldi*	1 Pack/250g	85	0	34	2.9	2.1	0	2.7
Cauliflower, Frozen, Tesco*	1 Sachet/125g	30	0.2	24	1.8	2.1	0.2	3.2
Cauliflower, Garlic & Ginger, M&S*	½ Pack/138g	36	0.3	26	1.8	3.1	0.2	2.3
Cauliflower, Mediterranean, Cauli Rice*	½ Pack100g	46	1.1	46	4	5.8	1.1	2.5
Cauliflower, Microwaved, Good & Balanced, Asda*	½ Pack/200g	68	1.8	34	2.9	2.1	0.9	2.7
Cauliflower, Original, Cauli Rice*	1 Serving/100g	34	0.9	34	3.6	3	0.9	1.8
Chicken, & Sweetcorn, Savoury, Asda*	½ Pack/60g	195	1.7	325	10	65	2.8	10
Chicken, Fried, Chinese Takeaway, Iceland*	1 Pack/340g	510	15.6	150	6.5	20.7	4.6	0.6
Chicken, Savoury, Batchelors*	1 Pack/124g	455	1.9	367	8.9	79.4	1.5	2.6
Chicken, Savoury, Tesco*	1 Serving/87g	177	1.9	204	6.4	39.4	2.2	6.7
Chickpea, Harissa & Lemon, Pulses & Rice, Tilda*	1 Pack/140g	139	4.3	99	3.8	11.6	3.1	4.9
Chinese Style, Express, Uncle Ben's*	1 Pack/250g	392	5.5	157	3.4	30.9	2.2	0.4
Coconut, Thai, Sainsbury's*	½ Pack/100g	178	9.1	178	2.6	21.3	9.1	1.9
Duck, Chicken, & Pork, Fried, Celebration, Sainsbury's*	1 Pack/450g	544	16.2	121	7.9	14.2	3.6	1.5
Egg Fried, Asda*	1 Pack/228.8g	286	5.7	125	3.6	22	2.5	2.3
Egg Fried, Average	**1 Serving/300g**	**624**	**31.8**	**208**	**4.2**	**25.7**	**10.6**	**0.4**
Egg Fried, Chinese Takeaway, Tesco*	1 Serving/200g	250	3	125	4.7	23.3	1.5	1.8
Egg Fried, Express, Uncle Ben's*	½ Pack/124.9g	216	5.2	173	4	29.9	4.2	0.3
Egg Fried, M&S*	½ Pack/150g	315	10.5	210	4.2	32.4	7	0.3
Egg Fried, Micro, Tesco*	1 Pack/250g	312	9.2	125	4.6	18.3	3.7	6.4
Egg Fried, Sainsbury's*	1 Pack/250g	432	9.5	173	4.5	30.3	3.8	0.8
Egg, Fried, 2 Minute Meals, Sainsbury's*	1 Pack/250g	342	1.5	137	3.8	29.2	0.6	0.8
Golden Savoury, Dry Weight, Batchelors*	1 Pack/120g	437	3.4	364	10.1	74.7	2.8	2.4
Long Grain, & Wild, Dry, Average	**1 Serving/75g**	**254**	**1.5**	**338**	**7.6**	**72.6**	**2**	**1.7**
Long Grain, American, Cooked, Average	**1 Serving/160g**	**229**	**2.8**	**143**	**3**	**28.8**	**1.8**	**0.2**
Long Grain, American, Dry, Average	**1 Serving/50g**	**175**	**0.5**	**350**	**7.2**	**77.8**	**1.1**	**0.6**

	Measure INFO/WEIGHT	per Measure KCAL	FAT	Nutrition Values per 100g / 100ml KCAL	PROT	CARB	FAT	FIBRE
RICE								
Long Grain, Dry, Average	**1 Serving/50g**	**169**	**0.5**	**337**	**7.4**	**75.5**	**1**	**1.7**
Long Grain, Microwavable, Cooked, Average	**1 Serving/150g**	**180**	**0.9**	**120**	**2.7**	**25.8**	**0.6**	**0.7**
Mexican, Style, Cooked, Express, Uncle Ben's*	1 Pack/250g	385	4.8	154	3.2	31.1	1.9	0.7
Moroccan Inspired, Four Seasons, Aldi*	1 Bag/200g	188	1.8	94	3	16	0.9	5.3
Mushroom, & Pepper, Savoury, Cooked, Morrisons*	1 Serving/200g	204	1.6	102	2.3	21.5	0.8	0
Mushroom, Pilau, Bombay Brasserie, Sainsbury's*	1 Pack/400g	672	17.2	168	3.7	28.6	4.3	0.7
Mushroom, Pilau, Indian, Sainsbury's*	1 Serving/100g	119	2.4	119	3	21.3	2.4	1.9
Mushroom, Pilau, Sainsbury's*	1 Pack/250g	400	13.8	160	3.4	24.1	5.5	2.4
Mushroom, Savoury, Batchelors*	½ Pack/61g	217	1.3	356	10.7	73.6	2.1	2.8
Paella, Savoury, Tesco*	1 Serving/60g	220	2.8	367	8.4	72.7	4.7	4.5
Pilau, Cooked, Average	**1 Serving/200g**	**349**	**8.8**	**174**	**3.5**	**30.3**	**4.4**	**0.8**
Pilau, Dry, Average	**1oz/28g**	**101**	**0.7**	**362**	**8.4**	**78.2**	**2.4**	**3.4**
Pilau, Microwavable, Golden Sun, Lidl*	½ Pack/125g	199	3.5	159	3.7	29.3	2.8	1.1
Pinto Bean, Green Chilli & Lime, Pulses & Rice, Tilda*	1 Pack/140g	182	5.3	130	5.3	15.3	3.8	6.5
Pudding, Dry Weight, Average	**1 Serving/100g**	**356**	**1.1**	**356**	**6.9**	**82**	**1.1**	**0.4**
Risotto, Dry, Average	**1 Serving/50g**	**174**	**0.6**	**348**	**7.8**	**76.2**	**1.3**	**2.4**
Saffron, Cooked, Average	**1 Serving/150g**	**208**	**4.7**	**139**	**2.6**	**25.3**	**3.2**	**0.5**
Special Fried, Chinese Takeaway, Iceland*	1 Pack/350g	630	17.5	180	5.5	28.2	5	1.2
Special Fried, Chinese, Tesco*	1 Serving/300g	618	33.3	206	6.5	19.9	11.1	0.8
Special Fried, M&S*	1 Pack/450g	922	35.1	205	6.2	27.2	7.8	0.5
Special Fried, Sainsbury's*	1 Serving/166g	272	7.6	164	5.1	25.5	4.6	0.7
Special Fried, Waitrose*	1 Serving/350g	532	22.4	152	6.1	17.6	6.4	3.2
Spinach, & Carrot, Pilau, Waitrose*	1 Pack/350g	466	8.4	133	3.1	24.8	2.4	1.2
Spinach, Pilau, Bombay Brasserie, Sainsbury's*	1 Pack/401g	642	17.3	160	3.5	26.9	4.3	0.8
Thai, Black, Sainsbury's*	1 Serving/180g	205	2	114	3.7	20.4	1.1	3.8
Thai, Cooked, Average	**1 Serving/100g**	**136**	**1.8**	**136**	**2.5**	**27.4**	**1.8**	**0.3**
Thai, Dry, Average	**1 Serving/50g**	**174**	**0.2**	**348**	**7.1**	**78.9**	**0.4**	**0.9**
Thai, Fragrant, Dry, Average	**1 Serving/75g**	**272**	**0.5**	**363**	**7.2**	**82**	**0.7**	**0.3**
Thai, Glutinous, Sticky, White, Dry, Raw	**1 Serving/100g**	**370**	**0.6**	**370**	**6.8**	**81.7**	**0.6**	**2.8**
Thai, Sticky, Tesco*	1 Serving/250g	358	6.2	143	2.5	27.6	2.5	0.4
Thai, Style, Cooked, World Kitchen, Ainsley Harriott*	1 Pack/400g	544	6.4	136	2.3	28	1.6	2.1
Valencia, for Paella, Asda*	1 Serving/125g	435	1	348	6	79	0.8	0
Vegetable, Golden, Freshly Frozen, Asda*	1 Sachet/200g	238	2.6	119	3.2	23.6	1.3	1.3
Vegetable, Golden, Savoury, Morrisons*	1 Serving/50g	70	0.4	141	3.4	30.1	0.8	1.1
Vegetable, Golden, Savoury, Newgate, Lidl*	½ Pack/60g	70	0.4	117	2.9	24	0.7	2.1
Vegetable, Original, Birds Eye*	1oz/28g	29	0.2	105	4	20.8	0.6	1.1
Vegetable, Savoury, Mixed, Dry Weight, Tesco*	1 Pack/120g	450	3.2	375	7.8	79.1	2.7	2.9
White, Cooked, Average	**1 Serving/140g**	**182**	**1.1**	**130**	**2.6**	**28.7**	**0.8**	**0.2**
White, Cooked, Frozen, Average	**1 Serving/150g**	**168**	**0.8**	**112**	**2.9**	**23.8**	**0.6**	**1.2**
White, Flaked, Dry Weight, Average	**1oz/28g**	**97**	**0.3**	**346**	**6.6**	**77.5**	**1.2**	**0**
White, Fried	**1oz/28g**	**37**	**0.9**	**131**	**2.2**	**25**	**3.2**	**0.6**
White, Long Grain, Dry Weight, Average	**1 Serving/50g**	**181**	**1**	**362**	**7.1**	**79.1**	**1.9**	**0.4**
White, Microwave, Cooked, Average	**½ Pack/125g**	**185**	**2.4**	**148**	**3.3**	**29.4**	**1.9**	**1.4**
Whole Grain, Dry, Average	**1 Serving/50g**	**171**	**1.2**	**342**	**8.2**	**72**	**2.3**	**4**
Wholegrain, Microwave, Eat Well, M&S*	½ Pack/125g	181	1.5	145	2.5	31	1.2	2.2
Wild, Cooked, Average	**1 Cup/164g**	**166**	**0.6**	**101**	**4**	**21.3**	**0.3**	**1.8**
With Red Kidney Beans, Average	**1oz/28g**	**49**	**1**	**175**	**5.6**	**32.4**	**3.5**	**2.5**
Yellow, Ready Cooked, Tesco*	1oz/28g	32	0.4	113	2.7	27.1	1.3	0.1
RICE CAKES								
Asda*	1 Cake/8g	31	0.2	386	8.7	81.1	3	2.8
Barbecue, Sainsbury's*	1 Pack/30g	121	2.6	403	7.9	73.5	8.6	2.7
Barbeque, Tesco*	1 Cake/9g	28	0.2	328	9.6	66.8	2.5	6.2
Caramel, Flavour, Kallo*	1 Cake/10g	38	0.5	383	6.2	78.9	4.8	3.9

R

RICE CAKES

INFO/WEIGHT	Measure	per Measure KCAL	FAT	KCAL	PROT	CARB	FAT	FIBRE
RICE CAKES								
Caramel, Jumbo, Snack-A-Jacks, Quaker*	1 Cake/13g	51	0.3	390	5.5	87	2.1	1.4
Caramel, Jumbo, Tesco*	1 Cake/10g	34	0.3	340	7	74	3	5
Caramel, Less Than 3% Fat, Sainsbury's*	1 Pack/35g	134	0.6	382	5.6	86.4	1.6	1.8
Caramel, Snack, Snack-A-Jacks, Quaker*	1 Bag/30g	122	0.9	405	6	88	3	0.8
Caramel, Tesco*	1 Serving/2g	9	0.1	379	5.5	98.2	2.9	0.9
Cheese, & Onion, Namchow*	1 Serving/38g	141	1.2	377	7.2	79.5	3.3	0
Cheese, & Onion, Snack, Snack-A-Jacks, Quaker*	1 Bag/30g	120	2.2	400	6.7	77	7.5	1.5
Cheese, Jumbo, Free From, Tesco*	1 Serving/10g	44	1.8	439	8.1	62.1	17.6	3.8
Chocolate, Chip, Jumbo, Snack-A-Jacks, Quaker*	1 Cake/15g	62	1	410	6	81	7	1.7
Chocolate, Dark, Mint, Nature's Store*	1 Rice Cake/17g	82	3.9	485	6.3	61	23.1	5.1
Chocolate, Dark, Organic, Kallo*	1 Cake/12g	57	2.9	471	6.8	57.2	24.1	7.4
Chocolate, Fabulous Bakin' Boys*	1 Biscuit/17g	83	3.7	490	6.4	66.7	22	1.6
Chocolate, Flavour, Happy Shopper*	2 Portions/33g	156	6.3	469	5.1	69.9	18.8	2.4
Chocolate, Milk, Belgian, & Caramel Pieces, Kallo*	1 Biscuit/13g	63	2.8	485	6.2	65.1	21.8	1.9
Chocolate, Milk, Minis, Kids, Kallo*	1 Pack/14g	69	3.3	496	6.6	62.6	23.8	0
Chocolate, Milk, Organic, Kallo*	1 Cake/11.2g	57	3.2	509	6.5	56.2	28.7	3.5
Chocolate, Milk, Slices, Morrisons*	1 Slice/11g	53	2.5	469	7.3	58.8	22	3.3
Multigrain, Ryvita*	3 Cakes/11g	43	0.5	384	9.1	76.2	4.7	5.3
Rye, Multigrain, High Fibre, Ryvita*	1 Cake/7g	23	0.2	352	9.4	66.3	2.5	13.3
Salt, & Vinegar, Balsamic, Sea, Kallo*	1 Cake/9g	32	0.2	361	6.5	78.1	2.5	3
Salt, & Vinegar, Jumbo, Snack-A-Jacks, Quaker*	1 Cake/10g	41	0.6	391	7.4	75.4	5.7	1.6
Salt, & Vinegar, Jumbo, Tesco*	1 Cake/8.9g	31	0.2	347	8.4	72.7	2.5	6
Salt, & Vinegar, Wholegrain, Tesco*	1 Cake/9g	28	0.2	314	8.4	61.9	2.6	6
Salted, Lightly, Thick Slice, Low Fat, Kallo*	1 Cake/7.5g	28	0.2	372	8	78.7	2.8	5.1
Salted, Sea, Harvest Morn, Aldi*	1 Cake/7g	27	0.2	379	8.7	78	2.2	5.1
Salted, Slightly, Organic, Thin Slice, Kallo*	1 Cake/4.6g	17	0.1	372	8	78.7	2.8	5.1
Salted, Slightly, Thick Slice, Organic, Kallo*	1 Cake/7.5g	28	0.2	372	8	78.7	2.8	5.1
Savoury, Jumbo, HL, Tesco*	1 Cake/8.4g	31	0.2	369	11.9	75	2.4	3.6
Sesame, No Added Salt, Thick Sliced, Organic, Kallo*	1 Cake/10g	37	0.3	373	8	78	3.2	5.4
Sesame, Teriyaki, Clearspring*	1 Cake/7.4g	28	0.2	377	6.5	82.8	2.2	0
Sesame, Toasted, Ryvita*	1 Pack/11g	43	0.5	391	8.4	78.4	4.9	3.5
Sour Cream, & Chive Flavour, Snack-A-Jacks, Quaker*	1 Bag/22g	92	1.7	418	7.7	78.2	7.7	1.4
Thin Slice, No Added Salt, Organic, Kallo*	1 Cake/5g	19	0.1	372	8	78.7	2.8	5.1
Wholegrain, No Added Salt, BGTY, Sainsbury's*	1 Cake/8g	30	0.2	372	8	78.7	2.8	5.1
RICE CRACKERS								
Barbecue, Sakata*	½ Pack/50g	204	1.3	407	7.3	85.2	2.6	1.6
Cracked Pepper, Sakata*	½ Pack/50g	200	1.5	400	7.3	84.4	3	2
Japanese Style, Mix, Asda*	1 Serving/25g	96	0.2	385	6.8	88	0.6	0.5
Japanese, Mini, Sunrise*	1 Serving/50g	180	0	360	7	83	0	7
Pretzel Mix, Tesco*	1 Serving/25g	108	3	432	18	61	12	3.8
Sainsbury's*	1 Serving/20g	87	1.9	433	11.2	74.3	9.4	1
Seaweed, Woolworths Homebrand*	12 Crackers/25g	100	0.7	398	7.3	85	2.7	0
Sour Cream & Chive, Sakata*	1 Serving/25g	107	2	430	7.8	80.6	7.9	0
Sweet Chilli, The Snack Organisation, Hansells Foods*	1 Serving/25g	106	1.7	424	7.1	83	6.8	1
Thai, M&S*	1 Serving/55g	209	1.8	380	7	80.2	3.3	1.2
Thai, Wakama*	1 Cracker/2g	8	0.1	400	6.9	86.9	2.7	0.5
Thin, Blue Dragon*	3 Crackers/5g	20	0.2	395	6.1	84.4	3.7	0
RICE PUDDING								
50% Less Fat, Asda*	½ Can/212g	180	1.7	85	3.3	16.2	0.8	0.2
Apple Strudel Flavour Sauce, Muller Rice, Muller*	1 Pot/190g	205	4.4	108	3.2	18.6	2.3	0.4
Banana & Toffee (Limited Edition), Muller Rice, Muller*	1 Pot/190g	207	4.2	109	3.1	19.3	2.2	0.4
Canned, Average	***1oz/28g***	***25***	***0.7***	***89***	***3.4***	***14***	***2.5***	***0.2***
Canned, Basics, Sainsbury's*	½ Can/212.5g	157	1.7	74	3.1	13.7	0.8	1.4

R

	Measure INFO/WEIGHT	per Measure		Nutrition Values per 100g / 100ml				
		KCAL	FAT	KCAL	PROT	CARB	FAT	FIBRE
RICE PUDDING								
Canned, BGTY, Sainsbury's*	1 Can/425g	344	2.6	81	3.3	15.5	0.6	0.4
Clotted Cream, M&S*	1 Pudding/185g	431	30.7	233	3	19.2	16.6	0.2
Creamed, Canned, Ambrosia*	1 Can/425g	382	8.1	90	3.1	15.2	1.9	0
Creamed, Pot, Ambrosia*	1 Pot/150g	156	3.8	104	3.3	17	2.5	0.1
Creamed, Value, Tesco*	1 Can/425g	348	3.4	82	3.2	15.5	0.8	0
Creamy, Tesco*	1 Pudding/190g	278	14.1	146	2.3	17.5	7.4	0.1
Low Fat, Devon, Creamed, Ambrosia*	½ Can/212.5g	193	2.8	91	3.2	16.5	1.3	0.1
Low Fat, No Added Sugar, Canned, Weight Watchers*	½ Can/212g	155	3.2	73	3.7	11.4	1.5	0
Low Fat, Tesco*	1 Can/425g	404	5.5	95	3.2	16.9	1.3	0.1
My Mini Rice, Ambrosia*	1 Pot/55g	56	1.4	101	3.3	16.3	2.5	0
Original, Muller Rice, Muller*	1 Pot/190g	196	4.9	103	3.6	16.3	2.6	0.3
Pot, Ambrosia*	1 Pot/125g	126	3.1	101	3.6	16.3	2.5	0
Raspberry, Mullerice, Muller*	1 Pot/190g	201	4.4	106	3.2	18.2	2.3	0.5
Strawberry, Muller*	1 Pot/180g	191	4	106	3	18.6	2.2	0
Toffee, Smooth, Muller Rice, Muller*	1 Pot/190g	201	4.4	106	3.3	18	2.3	0.3
Vanilla Custard, Mullerrice, Muller*	1 Pot/200g	230	5	115	3.4	19.8	2.5	0.3
RICE WINE								
Sake, Average	*1 Tbsp/15ml*	*20*	*0*	*134*	*0.5*	*5*	*0*	*0*
RIGATONI								
Dry, Average	*1 Serving/80g*	*272*	*1.2*	*340*	*11.4*	*68.4*	*1.5*	*2.7*
RISOTTO								
Balls, Sun Dried Tomato, Occasions, Sainsbury's*	1 Ball/25g	71	3.8	285	6.8	30.8	15	2.9
Beetroot, & Goats Cheese, Lovely Vegetables, M&S*	1 Pack/378.5g	530	17	140	4.4	20.7	4.5	3.6
Beetroot, Feta & Lentil, Microwaved, Asda*	1 Pack/369g	402	10.3	109	5.8	13	2.8	4.6
Butternut Squash, Fresh Ideas, M Kitchen, Morrisons*	1 Pot/350g	371	11.9	106	1.8	16.8	3.4	0.7
Butternut Squash, Italian Style, Aldi*	½ Pack/252g	323	12.6	128	2.6	17	5	1.6
Cauliflower, Roasted, & Barley, Everdine*	1 Serving/450g	432	21.2	96	2.8	8	4.7	5.2
Cheese, Onion, & Wine, Rice & Simple, Ainsley Harriott*	1 Pack/140g	253	7	181	3.1	31	5	1.6
Chicken	*1 Serving/380g*	*494*	*17.4*	*130*	*7.2*	*15.2*	*4.6*	*1.3*
Chicken, & Lemon, Weight Watchers*	1 Pack/330g	327	6.9	99	6.3	13.7	2.1	0.5
Chicken, & Mushroom, Finest, Tesco*	1 Pack/400g	496	11.2	124	7.4	17.2	2.8	0.5
Chicken, & Mushroom, Italian, Microwaved, Morrisons*	1 Pack/330g	311	4	94	6.7	13.8	1.2	0.7
Chicken, & Sun Dried Tomato, Waitrose*	1 Pack/350g	385	22	110	6	7.2	6.3	0.3
Chicken, BGTY, Sainsbury's*	1 Pack/327g	356	6.2	109	7.5	15.5	1.9	1
Chicken, Chargrilled, Ready Meal, M&S*	1 Pack/365g	493	25.2	135	6.4	11.6	6.9	0.7
Chicken, Lemon & Wild Rocket, Sainsbury's*	1 Pack/360g	683	41	190	16.2	5.6	11.4	0.1
Chicken, Ready Meal, M&S*	1 Pack/360g	450	15.8	125	6.7	14.4	4.4	0.9
Green Bean, Asparagus & Pecorino, Finest, Tesco*	1 Pack/400g	460	15.6	115	4.4	15	3.9	1.5
Haddock, Smoked, Italian, Tesco*	½ Pack/350g	400	15.1	114	4.2	14.3	4.3	0.8
Mushroom, PB, Waitrose*	1 Pack/400g	384	6.4	96	4.3	16.1	1.6	2.1
Prawn, COU, M&S*	1 Pack/350g	378	7.7	108	4.3	17.3	2.2	0.8
Prawn, Pea & Mint, King, M&S*	½ Pack/300g	405	18.6	135	3.8	15.9	6.2	0.9
Red Pepper, & Italian Cheese, Roasted, M&S*	1 Pack/400g	500	13.2	125	2.9	20.4	3.3	1
Seafood, Youngs*	1 Pack/350g	424	13	121	4.5	17.4	3.7	0.1
Vegetable, & Sunblush Tomato, Roasted, Finest, Tesco*	½ Pack/200g	306	18	153	3.7	14.5	9	1.4
Vegetable, Average	*1oz/28g*	*41*	*1.8*	*147*	*4.2*	*19.2*	*6.5*	*2.2*
Vegetable, Brown Rice, Average	*1oz/28g*	*40*	*1.8*	*143*	*4.1*	*18.6*	*6.4*	*2.4*
Vegetable, Spring, M&S*	1 Serving/330g	330	13.2	100	2	14.2	4	0.9
ROCK SALMON								
Raw, Flesh Only, Average	*1oz/28g*	*43*	*2.7*	*154*	*16.6*	*0*	*9.7*	*0*
ROCKET								
Fresh, Raw, Average	*1 Serving/80g*	*12*	*0.4*	*16*	*0.8*	*1.7*	*0.5*	*1.2*

R

	Measure INFO/WEIGHT	per Measure KCAL	FAT	Nutrition Values per 100g / 100ml KCAL	PROT	CARB	FAT	FIBRE
ROE								
Cod, Average	*1 Can/100g*	96	2.8	96	17.1	0.5	2.8	0
Cod, Hard, Coated in Batter, Fried	*1oz/28g*	53	3.3	189	12.4	8.9	11.8	0.2
Cod, Hard, Fried in Blended Oil	*1oz/28g*	57	3.3	202	20.9	3	11.9	0.1
Herring, Soft, Fried in Blended Oil	*1oz/28g*	74	4.4	265	26.3	4.7	15.8	0.2
Herring, Soft, Raw	*1oz/28g*	22	0.1	78	18.2	0.5	0.4	0
ROGAN JOSH								
Chicken & Rice, Sainsbury's*	1 Pack/500g	675	27	135	6.7	14.1	5.4	2.4
Chicken Breast, Chunks, Hot, Sainsbury's*	½ Pack/114g	143	2	126	23.6	3.9	1.8	1
Chicken with Pilau Rice, Farmfoods*	1 Pack/325g	354	6.8	109	5.3	17.1	2.1	0.4
Lamb, Indian, Takeaway, CBY, Asda*	½ Pack/200g	218	12	109	8	5.1	6	1.4
Lamb, Sainsbury's*	1 Pack/400g	660	44.4	165	11.3	4.9	11.1	1.9
Lamb, Takeaway, Tesco*	½ Pack/192g	228	14	119	6.3	5.7	7.3	2.5
Lamb, Waitrose*	½ Pack/175g	242	13.3	138	12.4	5	7.6	1.3
Prawn & Pilau Rice, BGTY, Sainsbury's*	1 Pack/401g	353	3.2	88	4.8	15.3	0.8	1.9
Prawn, COU, M&S*	1 Pack/400g	360	2.4	90	4.9	16.2	0.6	0.8
ROLL								
Cheese, & Onion, Asda*	1 Serving/67g	199	12	298	7	27	18	2
Cheese, & Onion, Co-Op*	1 Roll/66g	195	11.9	295	7	26	18	2
Cheese, & Onion, Iceland*	1 Roll/67g	222	13.6	332	7.5	29.6	20.4	1.5
Cheese, & Onion, M&S*	1 Roll/25g	80	5.1	320	9.6	24.7	20.5	1.3
Cheese, & Onion, Sainsbury's*	1 Roll/67g	205	13.6	306	8	22.9	20.3	1.9
Cheese, & Onion, Tesco*	1 Roll/67g	203	12.1	305	7.3	28	18.1	1.9
Cheese, & Pickle, Sainsbury's*	1 Roll/136g	359	13.6	264	10.6	35.1	10	0
Cheese, Tomato & Onion, Sainsbury's*	1 Pack/100g	518	28.1	518	18.4	47.9	28.1	0
Chicken, & Mayonnaise, Roast, Big, Sainsbury's*	1 Pack/185g	479	27.4	259	9.6	21.8	14.8	0
Chicken, & Salad, HE, Tesco*	1 Serving/224g	289	5.8	129	10.3	16	2.6	1.1
Chicken, & Salad, Mini, Selection Pack, British, M&S*	1 Roll/61g	134	4.1	220	11.9	28.1	6.8	2.1
Chicken, & Salad, Roast, Improved, Shapers, Boots*	1 Pack/188g	302	3.6	161	11	25	1.9	1.6
Cornish, in Pastry, Pork Farms*	1 Roll/75g	226	15.1	301	6.6	24.5	20.1	0
Egg Mayo, & Cress, Fullfillers*	1 Roll/125g	266	11.8	213	10	25.7	9.4	0
Egg Mayonnaise, & Cress, Sub, Delicious, Boots*	1 Pack/204.6g	399	14.1	195	10	23	6.9	2.4
Egg Mayonnaise, & Cress, White, Soft, Somerfield*	1 Serving/211g	475	17.3	225	9.4	28.2	8.2	2.1
Egg, & Cress, HL, Tesco*	1 Pack/175g	322	6.8	184	9.6	27.7	3.9	1.2
Ham, & Cheese, Leicester, Sub, Waitrose*	1 Pack/206ml	582	31.2	282	12.6	24	15.1	13
Ham, & Salad, BGTY, Sainsbury's*	1 Roll/178g	292	3.4	164	10.8	25.9	1.9	0
Ham, & Salad, J D Gross, Lidl*	1 Roll/154g	293	9.2	190	7.7	29.1	6	1.9
Ham, & Tomato, Taste!*	1 Serving/112g	211	4.8	188	10.4	27	4.3	0
Ham, Darwins Deli*	1 Serving/125g	298	7.5	238	11	37.4	6	0
Ploughman's, Large, Ginsters*	1 Pack/140g	473	33.5	338	10.2	20.5	23.9	1.8
Pork, Stuffing, & Apple Sauce, Roast, Boots*	1 Roll/218g	602	26.2	276	10	32	12	1.8
Salmon, Oak Smoked, M&S*	1 Roll/55g	139	6.2	252	14.6	23.1	11.3	1.2
Sausage, Lincolnshire, COU, M&S*	1 Roll/175g	280	4.7	160	10	23.2	2.7	2.6
Tuna Mayo, & Cucumber, Taste!*	1 Serving/111g	274	12.5	247	9	27.3	11.3	0
Tuna Mayonnaise, with Cucumber, Yummies*	1 Serving/132g	340	18.6	257	10.4	22.5	14	0
Tuna, & Sweetcorn, with Mayonnaise, Shell*	1 Pack/180g	536	26.3	298	13.1	28.6	14.6	0
Tuna, Cheese Melt, Boots*	1 Roll/199g	612	35.8	308	13	23	18	1.2
Turkey, Salad, Northern Bites*	1 Roll/231g	323	8.3	140	8.6	19.6	3.6	3
ROLO								
Chocolate, Nestle*	2 Pieces/20g	102	5.3	509	4.1	62.6	26.6	1.3
Little, Nestle*	1 Pack/40g	196	9.4	491	4	65.5	23.5	0.5
Nestle*	1 Sweet/5g	24	1	478	4.4	68.2	20.4	1.1
ROOT BEER								
Average	*1 Can/330ml*	135	0	41	0	10.6	0	0

	Measure INFO/WEIGHT	per Measure KCAL	FAT	Nutrition Values per 100g / 100ml KCAL	PROT	CARB	FAT	FIBRE
ROSE WATER								
The English Provender Co.*	1 Tsp/5g	0	0	2	0.1	0.6	0.1	0.1
ROSEMARY								
Dried	*1 Tsp/1g*	*3*	*0.2*	*331*	*4.9*	*46.4*	*15.2*	*0*
Fresh	*1 Tsp/0.7g*	*1*	*0*	*99*	*1.4*	*13.5*	*4.4*	*0*
ROSTI								
Maris Piper & Onion, M&S*	1 Rosti/35g	77	4.2	219	1.9	24.7	12	2.4
Potato & Root Vegetable, COU, M&S*	1 Rosti/100g	85	2.7	85	1.6	13.3	2.7	1.5
Potato Cakes, Baby, M&S*	1 Rosti/23g	40	1.5	175	3.5	25.1	6.7	1.6
Potato, McCain*	1 Rosti/95g	161	8.6	169	2.2	19.6	9.1	0
Potato, Mini, Party Bites, Sainsbury's*	1 Serving/100g	218	11.5	218	2.5	26.2	11.5	3
Vegetable, Waitrose*	1 Pack/400g	248	9.2	62	1.4	8.8	2.3	1.3
ROULADE								
Black Forest, Finest, Tesco*	1/8 Roulade/74g	206	6.5	280	3.2	46.4	8.8	1
Chocolate, Finest, Tesco*	1 Serving/80g	222	4.5	277	3.4	53.2	5.6	2.3
Chocolate, Sainsbury's*	1 Serving/72g	264	15.7	367	5.7	36.9	21.8	1.8
Passion Fruit, M&S*	1oz/28g	83	2.6	295	2.8	50	9.2	0.2
Raspberry, Finest, Tesco*	1/6 Roulade/75g	220	9.2	295	2.7	41.5	12.4	2.7
Raspberry, M&S*	1oz/28g	88	3.1	315	3.3	50.3	11	0.1
Smoked Salmon & Spinach, Finest, Tesco*	1 Serving/60g	91	6.1	152	11.5	3.6	10.2	0.6
RUM								
37.5% Volume	*1 Pub Shot/35ml*	*72*	*0*	*207*	*0*	*0*	*0*	*0*
40% Volume	*1 Pub Shot/35ml*	*78*	*0*	*222*	*0*	*0*	*0*	*0*
Captain Morgans & Cola, Premixed, Canned, Diageo*	1 Can/250ml	180	0	72	0	9.1	0	0
Malibu, 21% Volume, Pernod Ricard*	1 Pub shot/25ml	50	0	200	0	29	0	0
White	*1 Pub Shot/35ml*	*72*	*0*	*207*	*0*	*0*	*0*	*0*

R

	Measure INFO/WEIGHT	per Measure KCAL	FAT	Nutrition Values per 100g / 100ml KCAL	PROT	CARB	FAT	FIBRE
SAAG								
Chicken, Masala, M&S*	½ Pack/175g	228	12.4	130	13.3	3.1	7.1	5.2
Chicken, Masala, Waitrose*	1 Pack/400g	452	20.9	113	11.7	3.8	5.2	1.8
Chicken, Microwaved, Slimming World, Iceland*	1 Pack/500g	360	7.5	72	9.9	3.8	1.5	1.6
Paneer, Sainsbury's*	1 Pack/300g	441	32.7	147	7.1	3.9	10.9	2.5
SAFFRON								
Average	*1 Tsp/1g*	*2*	*0*	*310*	*11.4*	*61.5*	*5.9*	*0*
SAGE								
Dried, Ground	*1 Tsp/1g*	*3*	*0.1*	*315*	*10.6*	*42.7*	*12.7*	*0*
Fresh	*1oz/28g*	*33*	*1.3*	*119*	*3.9*	*15.6*	*4.6*	*0*
SAGO								
Raw	*1oz/28g*	*99*	*0.1*	*355*	*0.2*	*94*	*0.2*	*0.5*
SALAD								
American, Ranch, Asda*	1 Serving/220g	253	19.8	115	2.5	6	9	2
American, Style, Sweet & Crispy, Morrisons*	1 Serving/25g	7	0.1	28	1.2	4.2	0.3	2
Artichoke, & Pepper, Roasted, M&S*	1 Serving/220g	638	53.9	290	4.1	12.8	24.5	5.1
Avocado, & Egg, Nourish Bowl, M&S*	1 Pack/285g	333	15.4	117	6.3	6.6	5.4	8.3
Avocado, & Feta, & Rice, Good to Go, Waitrose*	1 Pack/240g	340	13.2	142	3.4	18.5	5.5	2.3
Avocado, & Feta, Gourmet To Go, M&S*	1 Pack/320g	512	32	160	5.4	12.1	10	3.1
Avocado, & Grain, M&S*	1 Serving/200g	157	5.5	78	2.6	10.7	2.8	1.6
Baby Leaf, & Beetroot, Bistro, M&S*	1 Pack/165g	41	0	25	2	3.6	0	2
Baby Leaf, & Herb, Asda*	1 Serving/50g	7	0.1	14	2.3	0.7	0.2	2.4
Baby Leaf, Aldi*	1 Serving/50g	11	0	22	3.5	1	0.1	1.5
Baby Leaf, Asda*	1 Serving/80g	10	0.2	12	2.1	0.2	0.3	1.7
Baby Leaf, Florette*	1 Serving/40g	5	0.1	12	2	0.4	0.3	1
Baby Leaf, Italian Style, M&S*	1 Serving/55g	11	0.3	20	1.3	2.3	0.5	1.3
Baby Leaf, M&S*	1 Pack/100g	20	0.2	20	3	1.7	0.2	0.5
Baby Leaf, Mild, Seasonal, Tesco*	½ Pack/41.5g	9	0.3	21	1.5	1.6	0.6	1.8
Baby Leaf, Seasonal, Morrisons*	½ Pack/50g	10	0.3	21	1.4	1.6	0.6	1.8
Baby Leaf, Sweet, Seasonal, M&S*	½ Bag/60g	9	0.2	15	2.4	0.6	0.4	1.8
Baby Leaf, with Watercress, Tesco*	1 Serving/30g	6	0.2	19	1.8	1.3	0.7	1.8
Bag, Tesco*	1 Serving/200g	38	0.8	19	0.9	3	0.4	1.4
Bean, 3, Sainsbury's*	1 Tub/270g	281	6.2	104	7.1	13.6	2.3	5.9
Bean, Adzuki & Edamame, Aromatic, Waitrose*	1/3 Pack/67g	72	1.7	108	7.5	9.5	2.5	8.6
Bean, Four, Sainsbury's*	½ Pot/112.5g	121	3.2	107	6.6	11.5	2.8	4.8
Bean, M&S*	1 Serving/80g	72	0.7	90	6.4	14.3	0.9	3.9
Bean, Mexican, Sainsbury's*	1 Pot/260g	291	8.1	112	5.2	12.9	3.1	5.8
Bean, Mixed, Asda*	½ Can/145g	126	3.6	87	5	11	2.5	6
Bean, Mixed, in Water, Drained, Essential, Waitrose*	1 Serving/80g	78	0.6	97	6.5	12.9	0.8	6.2
Bean, Three, & Mint, Finest, Tesco*	½ Pack/115g	155	6.9	135	6.8	7.7	6	11.5
Bean, Three, with Mint Vinaigrette, M&S*	1 Pack/250g	250	6	100	5.9	8.2	2.4	11.1
Beef, BBQ, Burrito, Naked, Smokehouse, Tesco*	1 Pack/260g	343	14.3	132	5.4	14.4	5.5	1.4
Beetroot	*1oz/28g*	*28*	*1.9*	*100*	*2*	*8.4*	*6.8*	*1.7*
Beetroot, & Carrot, Continental, Iceland*	1 Serving/100g	24	0.2	24	1.2	4.3	0.2	2.1
Beetroot, & Lettuce, Asda*	1 Serving/30g	5	0	16	1.4	2.7	0	2.5
Beetroot, & Mint Dip, Deli, M&S*	1 Serving/200g	177	12.4	88	2.6	3.9	6.2	3.2
Beetroot, Co-Op*	1 Pack/250g	100	0.8	40	0.9	8	0.3	2
Beetroot, Cous Cous & Quinoa, Tesco*	1 Serving/100g	70	0.6	70	2.3	12.9	0.6	2.3
Beetroot, M&S*	1 Serving/225g	124	0.7	55	1	12	0.3	3
Beetroot, Morrisons*	1 Tsp/10g	6	0.1	62	0.8	10.5	1.3	2.3
Beetroot, Roast with Quinoa & Feta, Tesco*	1 Pack/400g	452	19.6	113	4.8	12.4	4.9	2.3
Beetroot, Sainsbury's*	1 Tub/200g	148	2.4	74	1.7	14.1	1.2	1.7
Beets, Squash, & Feta, Superbowl	*1 Bowl/266g*	*343*	*14.6*	*129*	*6.7*	*11.4*	*5.5*	*2.7*
Bistro, Asda*	1 Serving/180g	29	0	16	1.4	2.7	0	2.5

SALAD	Measure INFO/WEIGHT	per Measure KCAL	FAT	Nutrition Values per 100g / 100ml KCAL	PROT	CARB	FAT	FIBRE
Bistro, Sainsbury's*	1 Pack/150g	26	0.3	17	1.9	2	0.2	2
Bistro, Washed Ready to Eat, Tesco*	1 Pack/140g	22	0.7	16	1.1	1.7	0.5	1
Broccoli, & Peanut, Finest, Tesco*	½ Pack/105g	196	9.2	187	6.9	18.4	8.8	3.3
Broccoli, Kale, & Quinoa, Tenderstem, Side, Waitrose*	1 Pack/165g	173	7.6	105	6.9	6.8	4.6	4.2
Bulgur Wheat, Lentil, & Edamame Shaker, Waitrose*	1 Pack/190g	217	10.6	114	4.7	11.1	5.6	4.4
Butternut Squash, & Fennel, Roast, TTD, Sainsbury's*	1 Pack/165g	214	7.6	130	3.4	15.2	4.6	6.9
Caesar	*1 Serving/200g*	*352*	*27.8*	*176*	*4.8*	*8.1*	*13.9*	*0.7*
Caesar, Chicken, & Bacon, Gourmet, M&S*	1 Salad/250g	550	43.5	220	9	7.3	17.4	0.7
Caesar, Chicken, & Bacon, Tesco*	1 Pack/200g	506	40.2	253	6.6	11.4	20.1	1
Caesar, Chicken, Fresh, Sainsbury's*	1 Serving/200g	278	20	139	6	6.2	10	1.2
Caesar, Chicken, Lidl*	1 Salad/250g	212	12.5	85	5	5	5	0
Caesar, Chicken, Shapers, Boots*	1 Pack/200g	205	5.8	102	8.2	10	2.9	1
Caesar, Classic, M&S*	½ Pack/112g	174	14.2	155	2.9	6.8	12.7	0.5
Caesar, Kit, Asda*	½ Pack/113g	154	9	136	5	11	8	1.4
Caesar, Kit, Tesco*	½ Pack/138g	279	25.3	202	4.7	4.5	18.3	1.3
Caesar, Kit, Waitrose*	1 Bag/250g	436	36.1	174	4.4	6.1	14.4	1.3
Caesar, Morrisons*	1 Serving/115g	194	18.1	169	3.6	5.9	15.7	0.3
Caesar, with Dressing, Croutons & Parmesan, M&S*	1 Serving/115g	190	15.5	165	4.3	6.4	13.5	1.4
Caesar, with Parmigiano Reggiano, Tesco*	1 Bag/275g	552	49	201	4.1	5.8	17.8	1.3
Caponata, Organic, Florentin*	1 Serving/100g	111	12.3	111	1.5	3.7	12.3	0
Carrot, & Beetroot, with a Balsamic Dressing, Asda*	1 Pack/160g	101	6.6	63	0.9	5.6	4.1	1
Carrot, & Orange, & Ginger, Good Intentions, Somerfield*	1 Serving/250g	275	3.5	110	2	22.4	1.4	1.4
Carrot, & Sultana, Sweet, M&S*	1 Serving/100g	55	0.7	55	0.8	11.4	0.7	2.6
Cheese, Layered, M&S*	½ Pack/230g	300	20.5	130	4.6	9.3	8.9	1.2
Cheese, Ploughman's, Asda*	1 Bowl/300g	246	10.8	82	3.6	8.9	3.6	1
Chick Pea, & Butter Bean, & Tomato, Chilli, Tesco*	1 Pack/130g	146	6	112	3.4	14.3	4.6	0.5
Chick Pea, & Cous Cous, Tesco*	1 Serving/250g	245	6.5	98	3.2	15.5	2.6	0
Chick Pea, & Spinach, M&S*	1 Serving/260g	299	10.7	115	7.3	12.5	4.1	2.7
Chicken, & Avocado, & Bacon, M&S*	1 Serving/235g	235	13.6	100	8.5	2.8	5.8	2.8
Chicken, & Bacon, Carb Control, Tesco*	1 Serving/188g	244	14.7	130	13.2	1.7	7.8	0.5
Chicken, & Bacon, Ranch, Sainsbury's*	1 Pack/210g	315	15.8	150	8.4	12.1	7.5	0.9
Chicken, & Coleslaw, Roast, Boots*	1 Serving/245g	392	34.3	160	4.5	3.9	14	1.3
Chicken, & Noodle, Satay Style, Warm, Tesco*	1 Pack/235g	256	7.8	109	6.8	12.3	3.3	1.6
Chicken, & Noodle, Sweet Chilli, Shapers, Boots*	1 Pack/197g	266	5.1	135	12	16	2.6	0.9
Chicken, & Noodle, Sweet Chilli, Shapers, Boots*	1 Serving/197g	256	4.1	130	11	17	2.1	1.1
Chicken, & Noodle, Sweet Chilli, Tesco*	1 Pot/240g	245	5.3	102	5.6	14.1	2.2	1.5
Chicken, & Noodle, Sweet, Aldi*	1 Serving/295g	362	9.4	123	6.7	16	3.2	18
Chicken, Bacon, & Spinach, From Restaurant, Average	*1 Salad/330g*	*1064*	*39.6*	*322*	*12.1*	*46.1*	*12*	*0*
Chicken, Cajun, David Lloyd Leisure*	1 Pack/300g	429	10	143	11.7	17.7	3.3	1
Chicken, Chargrilled, Snack, Tesco*	1 Pot/300g	384	14.4	128	6.1	15	4.8	2.4
Chicken, Chargrilled, Tesco*	1 Serving/300g	384	14.4	128	6.1	15	4.8	2.4
Chicken, Chargrilled, Wholefood, M&S*	1 Pot/219g	230	4.2	105	10.1	11.6	1.9	4.8
Chicken, HE, Tesco*	1 Salad/216g	296	3	137	8.4	22.6	1.4	1.2
Chicken, Honey & Mustard, Bowl, Fresh, Sainsbury's*	1 Serving/300g	408	23.7	136	5.9	10.3	7.9	1.7
Chicken, Mediterranean, HL, Tesco*	1 Pack/263g	305	4.2	116	7.7	16.4	1.6	2.4
Classic, Asda*	1 Pack/185g	43	1.5	23	1	2.4	0.8	1.1
Classic, with Creamy Chive Dressing, Bowl, Sainsbury's*	½ Pack/109g	104	9.5	95	0.9	2.6	8.7	1.1
Cous Cous, & Chicken, Chargrilled, Sainsbury's*	1 Pack/240g	446	20.9	186	7.4	19.6	8.7	0
Cous Cous, & Pepper, Chargrilled, Asda*	1 Pack/325g	426	10.7	131	4.3	21	3.3	0
Cous Cous, & Pepper, Sweety Drop, Asda*	½ Pack/140g	162	0.7	116	4.2	22	0.5	2.8
Cous Cous, & Vegetable, Roasted, Waitrose*	1 Pack/220g	396	13.4	180	5.1	26.1	6.1	1.2
Cous Cous, Moroccan, Fruity, Waitrose*	1 Pack/90g	139	3.2	154	5	25.6	3.6	4.6
Crayfish, & Mango, COU, M&S*	1 Pack/250g	285	5.3	114	4.1	18.6	2.1	1.9

S

SALAD

INFO/WEIGHT	Measure	per Measure		Nutrition Values per 100g / 100ml				
		KCAL	FAT	KCAL	PROT	CARB	FAT	FIBRE
Crisp, Mixed, Morrisons*	1 Pack/230g	39	0.7	17	1	2.8	0.3	0
Crisp, Mixed, Tesco*	1 Pack/200g	40	0.6	20	1.1	3.2	0.3	2
Crispy, Co-Op*	1 Serving/80g	13	0.2	16	0.8	3	0.3	1
Crispy, Florette*	1 Portion/100g	22	0.3	22	1.5	3.4	0.3	3
Crunchy, & Crisp, Asda*	1 Pack/250g	55	1.5	22	0.8	3.3	0.6	1.4
Crunchy, Fully Prepared, Sainsbury's*	½ Pack/150g	24	0.2	16	1.1	3	0.1	1.7
Crunchy, Mini, Co-Op*	1 Pack/80g	16	0.4	20	1	2.5	0.5	1.7
Duck, & Herb, Crispy, M&S*	½ Pack/140g	378	25.6	270	20.7	3.7	18.3	1.4
Edamame, & Black Rice, Nourish Bowl, Eat Well, M&S*	1 Pack/295g	395	16.2	134	5.6	12.8	5.5	5.3
Edamame, & Petit Pois, Finest, Tesco*	½ Pack/100g	108	4.3	108	6	9.3	4.3	3.9
Edamame, Asda*	½ Pack/110g	90	3.3	82	5.9	4.8	3	5.9
Edamame, Oriental Style, Asda*	1 Pack/220g	183	8.4	83	4.8	7.3	3.8	4
Edamame, Spinach, & Teriyaki, Protein Pot, Tesco*	1 Pack/120g	123	4.7	103	7.2	8.3	3.9	2.9
Egg, & Ham, with Salad Cream Dressing, M&S*	1 Pack/240g	145	7.2	60	4.9	3.2	3	1.2
Egg, & Potato, with Salad Cream, Bowl , Aldi*	1 Pack/305g	154	6	50	1.4	6.6	2	0
Egg, & Spinach, Baby, Waitrose*	1 Pack/215g	167	13.5	78	3.5	1.8	6.3	1
Egg, & Spinach, Protein Pot, Free Range, M&S*	1 Pot/105g	152	10.7	145	12.1	1.1	10.2	0.1
Egg, Layered, Bowl, Tesco*	1 Pack/410g	726	57.8	177	4.2	8.4	14.1	1.3
English Garden, Tesco*	1 Serving/180g	22	0.4	12	0.7	1.8	0.2	0.7
Exotic, with Mango & Chilli Dressing, Co-Op*	½ Pack/65g	25	0.4	38	0.6	7.7	0.6	0.8
Falafel, & Chargrilled Red Pepper, Tabbouleh, Tesco*	1 Pack/260g	254	9.3	98	3.3	11.7	3.6	2.6
Falafel, Bulgur Wheat & Houmous, Eat Well, M&S*	1 Pack/300g	375	15.3	125	4.1	13.2	5.1	4.8
Feta, & Sunblushed Tomato, M&S*	1 Serving/190g	361	21.1	190	5.5	17.2	11.1	2.1
Fine Cut, Asda*	1 Serving/100g	24	0.3	24	1.2	4.3	0.3	2.3
Freekah, Egg, & Bulgur, Vegeree, Good to Go, Waitrose*	1 Pack/260g	302	12.5	116	5	10.2	4.8	6.1
Frilly Leaf, Tesco*	1 Pack/120g	20	0.6	17	0.8	1.7	0.5	1.4
Garden, Side, Asda*	1 Pack/175g	32	0.5	18	0.9	2.8	0.3	1.3
Garden, Sweet & Crunchy, Tesco*	1 Pack/225g	54	0.9	24	1	4.2	0.4	1.4
Greek	*1oz/28g*	*36*	*3.5*	*130*	*2.7*	*1.9*	*12.5*	*0.8*
Greek, Classic, Tesco*	1 Pack/255g	293	23.7	115	2.6	5.2	9.3	1.2
Greek, Style, Bowl, M&S*	1 Bowl/223g	212	18.3	95	2.5	2.4	8.2	0.7
Greek, Style, Feta, Tip & Mix, M&S*	1 Pack/195g	214	18.3	110	4	2.5	9.4	1.6
Green, Average	*1oz/28g*	*4*	*0.1*	*13*	*0.8*	*1.8*	*0.3*	*0.9*
Green, Complete, Sainsbury's*	1/3 Pack/55g	92	6.7	168	4.2	10.3	12.2	1.4
Green, Mixed, Average	*1 Serving/100g*	*12*	*0.3*	*12*	*0.7*	*1.8*	*0.3*	*1*
Green, Side, M&S*	1 Serving/200g	30	0.4	15	0.9	2.5	0.2	0
Ham, & Egg, Free Range, British, M&S*	1 Pack/280g	182	6.4	65	6.1	5.3	2.3	1
Ham, & Egg, Free Range, Good & Balanced, Asda*	1 Pack/265g	148	6.3	56	5.3	2.8	2.4	0.9
Ham, & Egg, with Salad Cream, Sainsbury's*	1 Pack/240g	230	15.6	96	5.2	3.5	6.5	1.1
Ham, Hock, Waitrose*	1 Pack/350g	245	9.5	70	6.6	4.8	2.7	2
Ham, Smoked, Weight Watchers*	1 Pack/181g	233	3.6	129	11	16.6	2	3
Large, Bowl, Sainsbury's*	1/6 Pack/52g	12	0.2	23	0.9	4.3	0.3	1.1
Leaves, Oriental Mix, Waitrose*	1 Bag/100g	18	0.6	18	1.5	1.7	0.6	1.9
Mediterranean, Bowl, Sainsbury's*	1 Pack/110g	30	0.3	27	1.2	4.2	0.3	1.5
Mediterranean, Style, Asda*	½ Pack/135g	22	0	16	1	3	0	0
Mixed Leaf, Essential, Waitrose*	1 Serving/30g	5	0.2	17	1	2	0.7	1.4
Mixed Leaf, Medley, Waitrose*	1 Serving/25g	4	0.1	15	0.8	1.7	0.5	1.4
Mixed Leaf, Tesco*	1 Serving/20g	3	0.1	14	0.9	1.6	0.4	0.9
Mixed Leaf, Tomato & Olive, Tesco*	1 Serving/170g	150	13.3	88	1	3.4	7.8	2
Mixed Leaf, Tomato, Feta, Boots*	1 Pack/179g	218	17	122	3.7	5.4	9.5	1
Mixed Leaf, with Beetroot, Earthy, Waitrose*	1 Bag/140g	34	0.6	24	1.5	3.6	0.4	2.1
Mixed, Bowl, Waitrose*	¼ Pack/64g	9	0.3	14	0.8	1.6	0.5	1.4
Mixed, Green Leaf, Lasting Leaf*	1 Serving/69g	12	0.3	17	0.8	1.8	0.4	1.5

SALAD

INFO/WEIGHT	Measure	per Measure KCAL	FAT	Nutrition Values per 100g / 100ml KCAL	PROT	CARB	FAT	FIBRE
Mixed, Iceland*	1 Serving/50g	12	0.1	24	1.2	4.3	0.2	2.1
Mixed, Medley, Bowl, Waitrose*	¼ Pack/60g	9	0.3	15	0.9	1.7	0.5	1
Mixed, Sweet & Crispy, Tesco*	1 Serving/200g	48	0.6	24	1	4.2	0.3	2
Mixed, Sweet & Crunchy, Lasting Leaf*	1 Serving/62g	15	0.2	24	0.8	3.6	0.3	1.9
Mixed, with Peppers & Iceberg Lettuce, Somerfield*	1 Pack/200g	50	0	25	1	5	0	0
Moroccan, Mouthwatering, Jamie Oliver*	1 Portion/125g	211	6.5	169	5.5	21.7	5.2	6.6
Mozzarella & Tomato, no Dressing	**1 Serving/105g**	**190**	**14.5**	**182**	**8**	**5.9**	**13.8**	**3.3**
Mozzarella, & Tomato, M&S*	1 Serving/310g	400	14.8	129	5.5	15.5	4.8	0.9
New Potato, Tomato, & Egg with Salad Cream, M&S*	1 Pack/300g	165	7.2	55	2.9	5.4	2.4	1.3
New Potato, Tuna, & Egg, M&S*	1 Pack/340g	255	12.9	75	3.8	6.7	3.8	0.7
Noodle, & Peanut, Oriental, Deli, Tesco*	½ Pot/180g	200	5.6	107	3.1	16	3	1.8
Orzo, & Sunbaked Tomato, BGTY, Sainsbury's*	1 Tub/275.5g	292	6.1	106	3.1	18.5	2.2	2.5
Pasta, Mediterranean Orzo, Love Life, Waitrose*	1 Pack/220g	299	10.8	136	3.9	19	4.9	3.2
Pasta, Tuna, & Sweetcorn, Morrisons*	1 Serving/100g	227	15.1	227	5	16.1	15.1	2.2
Pea Shoot, & Baby Leaves, Steve's Leaves*	1 Pack/60g	14	0.4	24	2.7	2	0.6	2
Pea Shoot, Baby Cos & Batavia Lettuce, Bagged, M&S*	1 Bag/120g	24	0.6	20	2.6	0.8	0.5	2.3
Potato, & Cheese, Pasta & Mixed Leaf, Waitrose*	1 Serving/205g	266	17.4	130	3.2	10.1	8.5	1.1
Prawn, & Avocado, M&S*	1 Serving/240g	254	16.3	106	3	2	6.8	3.1
Prawn, Cocktail, Tesco*	1 Pack/300g	360	18	120	5.7	10.9	6	0.8
Prawn, King & Rice Noodle, M&S*	1 Pack/320g	208	2.6	65	2.9	11.6	0.8	0.9
Prawn, Layer, Eat Well, M&S*	1 Pack/220g	205	8.2	93	4.1	10.3	3.7	0.6
Prawn, Layered, Co-Op*	1 Pack/300g	375	18	125	4	14	6	2
Prawn, Layered, M&S*	1 Pack/455g	410	17.7	90	4.5	8.9	3.9	1.2
Quinoa, & Avocado, Chipotle, Finest, Tesco*	½ Pack/112.5g	151	7	135	2.4	16.1	6.3	2
Rainbow, Morrisons*	½ Bowl/72g	20	0.1	27	1.4	3.7	0.2	2.5
Rice, Lentils, & Roast Aubergine, Spirit of Summer, M&S*	1 Pack/240g	350	11.5	146	3.5	19.2	4.8	6.2
Rice, Spanish Style, with Chicken, M&S*	1 Serving/220g	319	12.8	145	5.8	17.4	5.8	0.5
Rocket, & Parmesan, Wild, Italian, Sainsbury's*	1 Serving/50g	88	7.4	177	7.5	3.4	14.8	0.5
Rocket, Tesco*	1oz/28g	4	0.1	14	0.8	1.7	0.5	0.9
Salmon, Moroccan Style, Light Lunch, John West*	1 Pack/220g	299	11.7	136	11.7	8.8	5.3	3.4
Seafood, Marinated, Waitrose*	1 Tub/160g	235	10.6	147	16.3	5.5	6.6	0
Side, Garden, with Cherry Tomatoes, Waitrose*	1 Pack/170g	25	0.7	15	0.8	2	0.4	1.3
Side, Selection, M&S*	1 Serving/255g	153	12.8	60	1.1	2.5	5	1.3
Simple, Bowl, Tesco*	1 Bowl/135g	32	0.4	24	1.3	2.9	0.3	2.1
Sprouted Pea, & Bean, Mint Dressing, Eat Well, M&S*	1 Pot/165g	182	8.7	110	7.3	8.7	5.3	7.4
Sweet & Crispy, M&S*	1 Serving/140g	49	1.4	35	1.7	4.7	1	1.6
Sweet & Crispy, Side, Sainsbury's*	¼ Bag/93g	23	0.2	25	1.3	4.4	0.2	2.2
Sweet & Crunchy, Bowl, Sainsbury's*	¼ Pack	42	0.6	49	1.6	8.2	0.7	2
Sweet & Crunchy, Mixed, Prepared, Co-Op*	1 Serving/120g	42	0.4	35	1.1	5.9	0.3	1.8
Sweet & Crunchy, Side, Eat Well, M&S*	1 Pack/145g	48	0.9	33	1.5	4.3	0.6	2.3
Sweet Leaf, Fully Prepared, Fresh, Sainsbury's*	¼ Pack/75g	12	0.1	16	0.8	3	0.1	2.1
Sweet Leaf, Organic, Tesco*	1 Serving/250g	45	1	18	0.8	2.7	0.4	1.9
Sweet Potato, & Red Pepper, Deli, M&S*	1 Serving/250g	113	5.6	45	0.8	5.6	2.2	0.9
Tabbouleh, Feta, Finest, Tesco*	1 Pack/225g	266	11.7	118	4.2	13.7	5.2	0.6
Tomato, & Cucumber, Ready To eat, Morrisons*	¼ Pack/81g	17	0.2	21	0.9	3.7	0.3	2
Tomato, & Mozzarella, Finest, Tesco*	1 Pack/175g	254	21.4	145	5.6	3.3	12.2	0.7
Tomato, & Onion	**1oz/28g**	**20**	**1.7**	**72**	**0.8**	**4**	**6.1**	**1**
Tomato, Cherry, Tesco*	1 Pack/210g	136	9.4	65	0.9	4.2	4.5	1.1
Tuna, Bowl, Fresh, Asda*	1 Serving/160g	184	11.2	115	8	5	7	0
Tuna, French Style, Light Lunch, John West*	1 Pack/220g	218	6.2	99	7.5	9.8	2.8	2.5
Tuna, HE, Tesco*	1 Serving/300g	399	21.9	133	6.2	10.5	7.3	0.9
Tuna, Italian Style, Light Lunch, John West*	1 Pack/220g	205	5.7	93	7.3	9.8	2.6	0.5
Tuna, Layer, COU, M&S*	1 Pack/340g	272	8.8	80	6.2	7.5	2.6	1.5

S

	Measure INFO/WEIGHT	per Measure KCAL	FAT	Nutrition Values per 100g / 100ml KCAL	PROT	CARB	FAT	FIBRE
SALAD								
Tuna, Mediterranean Style, Light Lunch, John West*	1 Pack/220g	211	4.2	96	8.5	10	1.9	2.4
Tuna, Mediterranean Style, Nixe, Lidl*	1 Pack/220g	254	5.5	116	10	12	2.5	2.8
Tuna, Mexican Style, Nixe, Lidl*	1 Tub/220g	293	11	133	11	9.4	5	3
Tuna, Nicoise, No Mayonnaise, Shapers, Boots*	1 Pack/276g	133	3.6	48	4	5	1.3	0.8
Tuna, Nicoise, with French Dressing, Waitrose*	1 Pack/330g	297	15.5	90	5.6	5.4	4.7	1.8
Vegetable, & Cous Cous, Roasted, Sainsbury's*	1 Pot/225g	378	24.1	168	5.3	12.6	10.7	1.9
Vegetable, Canned	**1oz/28g**	**40**	**2.7**	**143**	**1.6**	**13**	**9.8**	**1.2**
Vegetable, Mixed, without Dressing, From Restaurant	**1 ½ Cups/207g**	**33**	**0.1**	**16**	**1.2**	**3.2**	**0.1**	**2.1**
Waldorf, Average	**1 Serving/100g**	**193**	**17.7**	**193**	**1.4**	**7.5**	**17.7**	**1.3**
Waldorf, with a Creamy Lemon Dressing, M&S*	1 Pack/125g	151	8.6	121	2.6	9.6	6.9	5.1
Watercress, Spinach & Rocket, Prepared , Tesco*	½ Pack/40g	10	0.3	26	2.5	1.1	0.8	2
Watercress, Spinach & Rocket, Waitrose*	1 Bag/145g	30	1.2	21	2.2	1.2	0.8	1.5
Watermelon, & Feta Cheese, Deli, M&S*	1 Serving/150g	316	28.7	211	7.5	1.8	19.1	0.7
with a Sachet of Yoghurt & Mint Dressing, Florette*	½ Pack/113g	55	2.9	49	1	4.4	2.6	2.1
with Crunchy Coleslaw, Bowl, M&S*	1 Pack/325g	455	44.8	140	1	2.5	13.8	2
SALAD CREAM								
Average	**1 Tsp/5g**	**17**	**1.4**	**335**	**1.7**	**18.6**	**27.8**	**0.1**
Reduced Calorie, Average	**1 Tsp/5g**	**6**	**0.4**	**130**	**1**	**12.9**	**7.9**	**0.2**
SALAMI								
Ardennes Pepper, Waitrose*	1 Serving/7g	30	2.7	429	18.6	1.9	38.5	1.1
Average	**1 Slice/5g**	**18**	**1.3**	**360**	**28.4**	**1.8**	**26.2**	**0**
Danish, Average	**1 Serving/17g**	**89**	**8.8**	**524**	**13.2**	**1.3**	**51.7**	**0**
German, Average	**1 Serving/60g**	**200**	**16.4**	**333**	**20.3**	**1.6**	**27.3**	**0.1**
German, Peppered, Average	**3 Slices/25g**	**86**	**6.8**	**342**	**22.2**	**2.5**	**27.1**	**0.2**
Healthy Range, Average	**4 Slices/25g**	**55**	**3.6**	**220**	**22.4**	**0.6**	**14.3**	**0**
La Rougelle, Deluxe, Lidl*	1 Slice/5g	19	1.6	386	21	1	33	0.5
Meatster, Alpenmark, Aldi*	1 Serving/25g	124	11	497	24	1	44	0.5
Mexicana, El Tequito, Lidl*	1 Pack/80g	259	19.2	324	22	3.7	24	2.6
Milano, Average	**1 Serving/70g**	**278**	**22.6**	**397**	**25.9**	**0.9**	**32.2**	**0**
Napoli, Average	**1 Slice/5g**	**17**	**1.3**	**342**	**27.1**	**0.8**	**25.5**	**0**
SALMON								
Cooked, Prepacked, Average	**1 Fillet/93g**	**180**	**11.1**	**194**	**21.8**	**0**	**11.9**	**0**
Fillets, BBQ, Kiln Roasted, Waitrose*	1 Fillet/79g	208	12.3	263	25.3	5.3	15.6	0
Fillets, Black Pepper, Kiln Roasted, Fishmonger, Aldi*	1 Fillet/93g	226	15.8	243	22	0.5	17	0.5
Fillets, Cajun, Waitrose*	1 Serving/150g	214	9.8	143	20.6	0.4	6.5	0
Fillets, Lemon & Dill Sauce, Pink, Inspirations, Birds Eye*	1 Fillet/225g	349	20.5	155	17.9	0.3	9.1	0.1
Fillets, Poached , Sainsbury's*	1 Fillet/90g	218	15.4	242	20.9	0.9	17.1	0.5
Fillets, Raw, Average	**1 Sm Fillet/120g**	**227**	**14**	**189**	**20.9**	**0.1**	**11.7**	**0.1**
Fillets, Skin On, TTD, Sainsbury's*	1 Fillet/126g	249	14.3	197	23.5	0.2	11.3	0
Fillets, Steamed, Ready to Eat, Tesco*	1 Fillet/90g	174	9	193	24.5	1	10	0.6
Fillets, Sweet Chilli, Hot Smoked, Ready to Eat, Tesco*	1 Fillet/90g	233	14.9	259	23.3	3.4	16.6	1.4
Fillets, Sweet Chilli, Kiln Roasted, Tesco*	1 Fillet/90g	233	14.9	259	23.3	3.4	16.6	1.4
Fillets, Wild Alaskan, Keta, Sainsbury's*	1 Fillet/115g	178	6.4	155	25.9	0.2	5.6	0.3
Flakes, Honey Roast, Average	**1oz/28g**	**56**	**3**	**198**	**24**	**1.9**	**10.7**	**0.2**
Flakes, Honey Roast, Sainsbury's*	½ Pack/60g	115	5.4	192	25.4	2	9	0.6
Flakes, Hot Smoked, with Honey, Tesco*	½ Pack/50g	104	5	208	22.8	6.3	10.1	0.5
Flakes, Sweet Chilli, M&S*	½ Pack/70g	143	4.6	204	24.5	11.7	6.6	0.6
Goujons, Average	**1 Pack/150g**	**321**	**16.4**	**214**	**16.4**	**12.4**	**11**	**1.1**
Gravadlax with Mustard Sauce, Waitrose*	1 Pack/200g	382	22.2	191	21.8	1	11.1	0.4
Gravadlax, Cured with Salt, Sugar & Herbs	**1 Serving/100g**	**119**	**3.3**	**119**	**18.3**	**3.1**	**3.3**	**0.4**
Grilled	**1oz/28g**	**60**	**3.7**	**215**	**24.2**	**0**	**13.1**	**0**
Hot Smoked, Average	**1 Serving/62g**	**103**	**4.4**	**166**	**24**	**0.9**	**7.2**	**0.1**
Japanese, Pot For One, Cook*	1 Bowl/310g	394	11.5	127	6.8	15.7	3.7	0

S

	Measure INFO/WEIGHT	per Measure KCAL	FAT	Nutrition Values per 100g / 100ml KCAL	PROT	CARB	FAT	FIBRE
SALMON								
Mild Oak Smoked, Average	*1 Slice/25g*	*46*	*2.5*	*182*	*22.6*	*0.1*	*10.2*	*0*
Mousse, Tesco*	1 Mousse/57g	100	7	177	13.5	2.9	12.4	0.2
Mousse, with Lemon & Dill, Hot Smoked, Waitrose*	1 Mousse/60g	146	12.6	244	11.3	2.5	21	0
Pink in Brine, Average	*1 Sm Can/105g*	*129*	*5.5*	*122*	*18.8*	*0*	*5.3*	*0*
Pink, Canned, Average	*1 Serving/125g*	*162*	*7.2*	*130*	*19.5*	*0.1*	*5.8*	*0.1*
Poached, Average	*1 Serving/90g*	*176*	*10.5*	*195*	*22.5*	*0.2*	*11.7*	*0.3*
Portions, Lemon & Pepper, Fish of the Day, Iceland*	1 Portion/130g	281	18.3	216	22.2	0	14.1	0
Red in Brine, Average	*1oz/28g*	*42*	*2.2*	*149*	*19.7*	*0*	*7.8*	*0*
Red, Average	*½ Can/90g*	*141*	*7.4*	*156*	*20.4*	*0.1*	*8.2*	*0.1*
Sashimi, Smoked, Scottish Lochmuir, M&S*	1 Pack/130g	214	11	165	18.6	3.3	8.5	0.5
Skewers, Teriyaki, Sweet, M&S*	1 Skewer/48g	96	5.9	201	17.1	5.8	12.2	0
Smoked, Average	*1 Serving/70g*	*126*	*7*	*179*	*21.9*	*0.5*	*10*	*0.1*
Smoked, Juniper & Birch, TTD, Sainsbury's*	½ Pack/60g	132	8.4	220	23.3	0.3	14	0.1
Smoked, Trimmings, Average	*1 Serving/55g*	*101*	*5.7*	*184*	*22.8*	*0.2*	*10.3*	*0*
Steaks	*1 Serving/100g*	*180*	*11*	*180*	*20.2*	*0*	*11*	*0*
Steamed	*1oz/28g*	*55*	*3.6*	*197*	*20.1*	*0*	*13*	*0*
Teriyaki, Infusions, John West*	1 Pot/80g	180	9.6	225	19	10	12	0
SALMON EN CROUTE								
Frozen, Tesco*	1 Serving/166g	365	18.4	220	10.1	19.1	11.1	1.1
M&S*	½ Pack/185g	574	40.5	310	10.4	17.3	21.9	0.6
Retail, Average	*1oz/28g*	*81*	*5.3*	*288*	*11.8*	*18*	*19.1*	*0*
with Lemon & Dill, Easy to Cook, Waitrose*	½ Pack/185g	487	31.5	263	10.7	16.9	17	2.7
SALMON IN								
Creamy Watercress Sauce, Fillets, Scottish, Seafresh*	1 Pack 300g	528	38.7	176	13.7	1.2	12.9	0.1
Dill Sauce, Youngs*	1 Pack/435g	265	10	61	6.1	4.2	2.3	0.1
Lime & Coriander, Fillets, Good Choice, Iceland*	½ Pack/150g	189	4.4	126	19.8	5.1	2.9	0.8
Tomato & Mascarpone Sauce, Fillets, Asda*	½ Pack/181g	279	19.9	154	13	0.8	11	0.6
White Wine & Cream Sauce, Tesco*	1 Serving/170g	279	19.2	164	13.5	2	11.3	1.2
SALMON WITH								
Garlic & Herb Butter, Tesco*	1 Fillet/112g	291	23.1	260	17.6	0	20.6	0
Giant Cous Cous & Lentils, Creations, John West*	1 Pack/180g	297	15.5	165	7.6	13	8.6	2.5
Scottish Lochmuir with Soy & Ginger, Fuller Longer, M&S*	1 Pack/360g	415	18	115	8	7.8	5	3.1
Sweet Chilli, Hot Smoked, Scottish, Tesco*	1 Fillet/120g	252	12.7	210	26.1	1.7	10.6	0.6
SALSA								
Chunky, Sainsbury's*	½ Pot/84g	43	1.4	51	1.1	7.8	1.7	1.2
Mediterranean, with Roasted Aubergine, Sabra*	1 Serving/30g	58	4.9	192	2	9.2	16.3	1.7
Medium Hot, Discovery*	1 Serving/30g	17	0.1	56	1.4	11.7	0.4	0.8
Mild, Original, Old El Paso*	1 Sachet/144g	60	0.7	42	1.6	9	0.5	0
Original from Dinner Kit, Old El Paso*	1 Jar/226g	71	0.7	32	1.2	6	0.3	0
Spicy Mango & Lime, Morrisons*	½ Pot/85g	62	0.3	73	1	15.9	0.4	1.3
Spicy Red Pepper, Fresh, Waitrose*	½ Pot/85g	27	0.8	32	1.9	4.1	0.9	1.6
Tomato, Chunky, Tesco*	1 Pot/170g	68	2.2	40	1.1	5.9	1.3	1.1
Tomato, Cool, Asda*	1 Pot/215g	84	1.1	39	1.4	6.4	0.5	1.5
Tomato, Onion, Coriander & Chilli, Fresh, Waitrose*	1 Tub/170g	110	5.3	65	1.3	8	3.1	1.2
Tomato, Sun Ripened, Tesco*	1 Serving/40g	46	1.7	115	5	14.2	4.2	4.6
Tomato, with Coriander & Garlic, Sainsbury's*	1 Serving/50g	31	0.9	62	1	9.9	1.8	1.2
SALT								
Alternative, Reduced Sodium, Losalt*	10g	0	0	0	0	0	0	0
Rock, Average	*¼ Tsp/1g*	*0*	*0*	*0*	*0*	*0*	*0*	*0*
Table, Average	*1 Tsp/5g*	*0*	*0*	*0*	*0*	*0*	*0*	*0*
SAMBUCA								
Average	*1 Pub Shot/35ml*	*122*	*0*	*348*	*0*	*37.2*	*0*	*0*

S

	Measure INFO/WEIGHT	per Measure KCAL	FAT	Nutrition Values per 100g / 100ml KCAL	PROT	CARB	FAT	FIBRE
SAMOSAS								
Chicken, Tikka, Indian, Sainsbury's*	1 Samosa/55g	131	5.5	237	9.4	25	10	4.6
Indian Style Selection, Co-Op*	1 Samosa/21g	50	2.7	240	5	27	13	3
Lamb, Halal, Mumtaz*	1/3 Pack/70g	172	9.8	246	10.5	22.3	14	2.9
Meat, Takeaway, Average	*1 Samosa/110g*	*299*	*19*	*272*	*11.4*	*18.9*	*17.3*	*2.4*
Vegetable, Average	*1 Samosa/110g*	*258*	*12.8*	*235*	*4.8*	*26.9*	*11.6*	*2.5*
Vegetable, Indian Starter Selection, M&S*	1 Samosa/21g	53	2.5	254	5.3	29.3	12.1	3.3
Vegetable, Large, Individual, Sainsbury's*	1 Samosa/110g	254	16.5	231	3.3	20.7	15	2.1
Vegetable, Large, Tesco*	1 Samosa/64g	148	7.9	231	4.8	25.2	12.4	3.4
Vegetable, Lightly Spiced, Sainsbury's*	1 Samosa/50.2g	112	6.3	223	4	22.5	12.5	1.2
Vegetable, M&S*	1 Samosa/45g	115	6.9	255	5.1	24.8	15.3	2.8
Vegetable, Mini, Asda*	1 Samosa/23g	52	2	233	6	32	9	2.6
Vegetable, Mini, Indian Snack Selection, Sainsbury's*	1 Samosa/25g	70	4	280	4.7	29.8	15.8	3.2
Vegetable, Mini, Indian Snack Selection, Tesco*	1 Samosa/32g	76	4.2	238	4.7	25.5	13	3.3
Vegetable, Waitrose*	1 Samosa/58g	129	6.6	223	4.5	23.8	11.4	3.8
SANDWICH								
All Day Breakfast, Shapers, Boots*	1 Pack/207g	323	5.2	156	11	23	2.5	2.2
All Day Breakfast, Tesco Classic*	1 Pack/374g	636	29.9	170	8	14.5	8	3
Argi Bhaji, Cranks*	1 Pack/204g	401	10.6	197	5.2	31.3	5.2	2.2
Bacon, & Egg, Co-Op*	1 Pack/188g	536	32	285	13	20	17	2
Bacon, & Egg, Sainsbury's*	1 Pack/160g	384	17.8	240	13	22	11.1	1.8
Bacon, & Egg, Tesco*	1 Pack/213g	494	19.6	232	14.8	21.6	9.2	1.8
Bacon, Lettuce, & Tomato, Loved by Us, Co-Op*	1 Pack/195g	410	14.2	210	10.2	25.1	7.3	2.3
Bacon, Lettuce, & Tomato, on Malted Bread, Sainsbury's*	1 Pack/190g	417	16.6	219	11.2	22.7	8.7	2.7
Bap, Ham, & Salad, Co-Op*	1 Bap/164g	295	4.9	180	8	30	3	2
Beef, & Horseradish Mayonnaise, Roast, Rare, Waitrose*	1 Pack/197g	415	15.3	211	12.2	23.1	7.8	2
Beef, & Horseradish, & Tomato, Asda*	1 Pack/169g	255	4.4	151	10	22	2.6	2.7
Beef, & Horseradish, Deep Filled, BGTY, Sainsbury's*	1 Pack/202g	313	4.8	155	11.4	22	2.4	2.4
Beef, & Horseradish, Roast, Rare, Eat Well, M&S*	1 Serving/200g	360	9.2	180	13.1	21.9	4.6	2.7
Beef, & Horseradish, Sainsbury's*	1 Pack/187g	391	12.5	209	12.5	23.8	6.7	1.5
Beef, & Pate, M&S*	1 Pack/188g	310	7.3	165	11.2	21.6	3.9	2.4
Beef, & Salad, Gibsons*	1 Pack/185g	348	10.6	188	10.6	23.5	5.7	0
Beef, & Salad, Roast, Daily Bread*	1 Pack/202g	319	8.3	158	9	21.4	4.1	0
Beef, & Horseradish, Onion Bloomer, Booths*	1 Pack/199g	493	23.9	248	1.4	20	12	1.8
Beef, Roast, Handmade, Tesco*	1 Pack/223g	439	15.8	197	12.5	20.7	7.1	1.6
Beef, Salt, with Gherkins & Mustard Mayo, Sainsbury's*	1 Pack/242g	486	18.2	201	9.3	24.1	7.5	3.1
BLT, Asda*	1 Sandwich/172g	325	11.9	189	9.9	21.8	6.9	4.6
BLT, M&S*	1 Serving/181g	381	14.7	210	10.7	23.8	8.1	1.8
BLT, on Malted Brown Bread, Tesco*	1 Pack/185g	454	21.7	245	10.9	22.9	11.7	2.4
BLT, Waitrose*	1 Pack/184.3g	398	16.4	216	9.5	24.5	8.9	2.3
BLT, with Mayo, Malted Bread, Just Tasty, Aldi*	1 Pack/186g	437	17.9	235	14	22	9.6	2.4
Brie, & Cranberry, Morrisons*	1 Pack/178g	438	20.3	246	10.4	24.4	11.4	2.2
Brie, & Grape, Finest, Tesco*	1 Pack/209g	527	31.6	252	8.5	20.6	15.1	1.5
Brie, & Wild Cranberry, Delicious, Boots*	1 Pack/168g	413	18.5	246	9.1	27	11	3.3
Cheddar, & Celery, M&S*	1 Pack/200g	540	31.8	270	9.7	22.4	15.9	1.5
Cheddar, & Ham, M&S*	1 Pack/165g	396	18.6	240	15.1	20	11.3	1.7
Cheddar, & Salad, Mature, Upper Crust*	1 Pack/225g	466	22.1	207	9.5	20.3	9.8	0
Cheddar, & Tomato, Red, Tesco*	1 Pack/165g	474	23.8	287	9.2	29.2	14.4	1.9
Cheddar, Oldfields*	1 Pack/121g	384	17.3	317	12.8	33.2	14.3	1.5
Cheddar, Red Leicester, & Onion, Tesco*	1 Pack/182g	604	38.9	332	11	23.8	21.4	2.5
Cheese, & Coleslaw, M&S*	1 Pack/186g	498	32.4	268	10.2	17.6	17.4	3.2
Cheese, & Ham, & Pickle, Healthy Range, Average	*1 Pack/185g*	*299*	*5.1*	*162*	*13.6*	*20.6*	*2.8*	*2.5*
Cheese, & Ham, & Pickle, HL, Tesco*	1 Pack/201g	312	4.2	155	13.1	21	2.1	1.7
Cheese, & Ham, & Pickle, Tesco*	1 Serving/215g	497	24.7	231	11.7	20.3	11.5	1.8

S

SANDWICH

	Measure INFO/WEIGHT	KCAL	FAT	KCAL	PROT	CARB	FAT	FIBRE
Cheese, & Ham, Smoked, Co-Op*	1 Pack/167g	334	8.4	200	15	24	5	2
Cheese, & Marmite, No Mayonnaise, Boots*	1 Pack/156g	420	20	269	12.2	26.3	12.8	1.7
Cheese, & Onion, Eat Smart, Morrisons*	1 Pack/144g	340	10.9	236	13.1	27.8	7.6	2.1
Cheese, & Onion, Essential, Waitrose*	1 Pack/158g	432	21.5	273	11.5	25.2	13.6	2
Cheese, & Onion, Reduced Fat, NUME, Morrisons*	1 Pack/142g	348	13.6	245	11.8	26.1	9.6	3.5
Cheese, & Onion, Tesco*	1 Pack/172g	505	28.3	294	10.2	24.5	16.5	3.3
Cheese, & Pickle, Shapers, Boots*	1 Pack/165g	342	8.1	207	9.8	31	4.9	2.3
Cheese, & Pickle, Tesco*	1 Pack/140g	400	19.3	286	12.7	27.8	13.8	1.4
Cheese, & Pickle, Virgin Trains*	1 Pack/158g	444	19.6	281	11.5	31.1	12.4	0
Cheese, & Salad, & Reduced Fat Mayonnaise, Waitrose*	1 Pack/180g	301	9	167	9.8	20.8	5	3.1
Cheese, & Salad, COU, M&S*	1 Pack/188g	244	3	130	12.1	17	1.6	2.4
Cheese, & Spring Onion, Three, Shell*	1 Pack/168g	672	50.9	400	11.1	20.8	30.3	0
Cheese, & Tomato, Asda*	1 Pack/154g	388	19.7	252	11	23.2	12.8	3.7
Cheese, & Tomato, Co-Op*	1 Pack/155.3g	365	18.5	235	10.6	21.8	11.9	1.9
Cheese, & Tomato, Organic, M&S*	1 Pack/165g	559	35.3	339	11.8	24.8	21.4	1.9
Cheese, & Apple Slaw, Wholemeal, Nutritious, Boots*	1 Pack/252g	400	14.3	159	8.1	17	5.7	3
Cheese, Hamwich, Iceland*	1 Hamwich/54g	165	11.9	306	11	16	22	3
Cheese, Simply, Boots*	1 Pack/138g	375	13.9	272	13.8	30.4	10.1	2.2
Chicken, & Avocado, Roast, on Soft Malted Bread, M&S*	1 Pack/200g	412	14.2	206	11.2	23	7.1	2.7
Chicken, & Avocado, Roast, Tesco*	1 Serving/202g	395	15.2	195	10.5	20.5	7.5	1.8
Chicken, & Bacon, & Avocado, M&S*	1 Pack/242g	508	28.3	210	10.7	15.8	11.7	3.2
Chicken, & Bacon, & Lettuce, No Mayo, LC, Tesco*	1 Pack/186g	326	6.9	175	15.2	19.6	3.7	2.5
Chicken, & Bacon, Club, Fully Loaded, Handmade, Tesco*	1 Pack/257g	580	21.1	225	12.1	24.3	8.2	2.3
Chicken, & Bacon, COU, M&S*	1 Pack/178.6g	250	3.6	140	13.5	15.8	2	3.8
Chicken, & Bacon, Deep Filled, Co-Op*	1 Pack/166g	556	33.2	335	16	23	20	3
Chicken, & Bacon, HE, Tesco*	1 Pack/155g	240	2.6	155	10.4	24.6	1.7	1.7
Chicken, & Bacon, Tesco*	1 Pack/195g	486	24.2	249	14.3	20	12.4	2.7
Chicken, & Chorizo, British, Finest, Tesco*	1 Pack/186g	391	12.6	210	15.7	21.2	6.8	2.7
Chicken, & Mayo, Simply, Delicious, Boots*	1 Pack/148g	318	8.6	215	14	25	5.8	2.2
Chicken, & Salad, Aldi*	1 Pack/195.4g	338	4.5	173	11.5	23.8	2.3	2
Chicken, & Salad, Co-Op*	1 Pack/195g	448	21.4	230	10	24	11	2
Chicken, & Salad, Deep Fill, Ginsters*	1 Pack/203g	364	12.4	179	10.3	20.8	6.1	2.1
Chicken, & Salad, Healthy Living, Co-Op*	1 Pack/196g	265	3.5	135	10.4	19.1	1.8	3.9
Chicken, & Salad, M&S*	1 Pack/225.8g	350	9.3	155	10.6	18.8	4.1	3
Chicken, & Salad, Roast, Pick of the Pantry, On A Roll*	1 Pack/225g	293	6.8	130	9.7	16.2	3	1.4
Chicken, & Salad, Roast, Shapers, Boots*	1 Pack/183g	274	4.4	150	12	20	2.4	3.4
Chicken, & Salad, Roast, Waitrose*	1 Pack/217g	482	24.1	222	9.4	21.1	11.1	2
Chicken, & Salad, Sainsbury's*	1 Pack/240g	425	14.2	177	12.1	18.8	5.9	0
Chicken, & Stuffing, Co-Op*	1 Pack/208g	420	13	202	13.5	22.6	6.2	2.4
Chicken, & Stuffing, Pork Sage & Onion, Tesco*	1 Pack/136.2g	376	17	276	12.1	28.1	12.5	1.4
Chicken, & Stuffing, Roast, Boots*	1 Pack/235g	669	39.9	285	12	22	17	1.9
Chicken, & Stuffing, Roast, Tesco*	1 Sandwich/200g	450	14.4	225	15	24.8	7.2	1.9
Chicken, & Stuffing, Waitrose*	1 Pack/183g	450	18.8	246	12.8	25.6	10.3	1.5
Chicken, & Sweetcorn, British, Eat Well, M&S*	1 Pack/194.3g	340	10.5	175	11.4	19.6	5.4	3.1
Chicken, & Sweetcorn, Roast, Good to Go, Waitrose*	1 Pack/189g	321	6.2	170	12.1	21.3	3.3	3.3
Chicken, & Sweetcorn, Tesco*	1 Pack/174g	355	11	204	10.8	24.6	6.3	3
Chicken, & Avocado, Limited Edition, Co-Op*	1 Pack/192g	362	11.9	188	10	21	6.2	2.9
Chicken, & Balsamic Roasted Tomatoes, COU, M&S*	1 Pack/200g	280	4.6	140	11.6	18.1	2.3	2.6
Chicken, & Stuffing, LC, Tesco*	1 Pack/172g	275	4.8	160	14.4	18.7	2.8	6.9
Chicken, Asian, Shapers, Boots*	1 Pack/190g	273	4.6	144	12	19	2.4	2.9
Chicken, Coronation, M&S*	1 Pack/210g	420	20.4	200	11.2	20.2	9.7	3.1
Chicken, Coronation, on Onion Bread, M&S*	1 Pack/260g	520	21.3	200	10.7	20	8.2	1.9
Chicken, Flame Grilled, Rustlers*	1 Pack/150g	346	14.2	231	16.3	20.1	9.5	0

S

SANDWICH

INFO/WEIGHT	Measure	per Measure KCAL	FAT	Nutrition Values per 100g / 100ml KCAL	PROT	CARB	FAT	FIBRE
Chicken, Jerk, & Sunshine Slaw, Boots*	1 Pack/202g	349	7.7	173	10	23	3.8	2
Chicken, No Mayo, M&S*	1 Pack/142g	248	3.3	175	16.6	20.6	2.3	3.2
Chicken, Pesto, Shapers, Boots*	1 Pack/181g	311	4.2	172	12	26	2.3	1.7
Chicken, Rustlers*	1 Pack/150g	346	14.2	231	16.3	20.1	9.5	0
Chicken, Tikka, & Mango Chutney, Tesco*	1 Pack/201g	352	4.8	175	11.6	25.4	2.4	2.6
Chicken, Tikka, COU, M&S*	1 Pack/185g	268	3.3	145	12.1	20.5	1.8	3.2
Chicken, Tikka, on Pepper Chilli Bread, Shapers, Boots*	1 Pack/172g	296	4.5	172	13	25	2.6	2.5
Club, New York Style, Sainsbury's*	1 Pack/212g	608	33.5	287	13.3	22.8	15.8	2.7
Corned Beef, on White, Simply, Brambles*	1 Pack/126g	325	10.8	258	14.2	30.8	8.6	1.4
Corned Beef, Tomato & Onion, Salad Garden*	1 Pack/137g	338	14.8	247	14.2	23	10.8	0
Crayfish, & Rocket, Finest, Tesco*	1 Pack/178g	365	10.5	205	9.8	27.5	5.9	2.1
Cream Cheese, & Peppers, Taste!*	1 Pack/154g	296	10.5	192	7.3	25.5	6.8	0
Deli Meat, Feast Sub, Tesco*	1 Sub/223g	502	17.8	225	12	25.3	8	1.8
Egg Mayo, & Salad, You Count, Love Life, Waitrose*	1 Pack/196g	314	10.2	160	8.8	18.5	5.2	2.2
Egg Mayo, Free Range, Asda*	1 Sandwich/178g	311	10.1	175	9.3	21.5	5.7	2.1
Egg Mayo, Free Range, on Oatmeal Bread, M&S*	1 Pack/180g	315	12.2	175	9.4	18.2	6.8	2.8
Egg Mayonnaise, & Cress, Co-Op*	1 Pack/159g	405	24	255	8.8	20.8	15.1	1.9
Egg Mayonnaise, & Cress, Go Simple, Asda*	1 Pack/169g	370	18.6	219	10	20	11	1.7
Egg Mayonnaise, & Cress, HL, Tesco*	1 Pack/149g	271	7.7	182	9	23.5	5.2	2.6
Egg Mayonnaise, & Cress, Reduced Fat, Waitrose*	1 Pack/162g	300	12.8	185	10.4	18.1	7.9	3.4
Egg, & Avocado, & Chilli Chutney, M&S*	1 Pack/209g	368	15.1	176	7.7	18.3	7.2	3.5
Egg, & Bacon, Handmade, Tesco*	1 Pack/217g	489	20.4	225	13.4	20.8	9.4	2
Egg, & Cress, BGTY, Sainsbury's*	1 Pack/145g	268	7.5	185	9.1	25.4	5.2	2.7
Egg, & Cress, Co-Op*	1 Pack/159g	398	23.8	250	9	21	15	2
Egg, & Cress, COU, M&S*	1 Pack/192g	240	5.2	125	9.8	15.5	2.7	2.8
Egg, & Cress, Free Range, M&S*	1 Pack/192g	307	9	160	10.7	17.8	4.7	3
Egg, & Cress, Free Range, Sainsbury's*	1 Pack/204g	404	16.9	198	10.5	20.3	8.3	3.3
Egg, & Cress, No Mayo, LC, Tesco*	1 Pack/160g	280	7.2	175	9.4	23.7	4.5	3
Egg, & Ham, Deli Club, Tesco*	1 Pack/220g	433	15.4	197	11.4	20.5	7	2.7
Egg, & Salad, Co-Op*	1 Pack/190g	285	7.6	150	7	22	4	4
Egg, & Salad, on Softgrain Bread, HL, Tesco*	1 Sandwich/197g	290	4.7	147	7	23.6	2.4	1.7
Egg, & Tomato & Salad Cream, M&S*	1 Pack/216g	400	14.9	185	7.4	21.7	6.9	2.3
Egg, & Watercress, Bloomer, Freshly Prepared, M&S*	1 Pack/221.4g	465	26.1	210	10.2	15.3	11.8	3
Egg, & Tomato, with Salad Cream, Delicious, Boots*	1 Sandwich/205g	410	16	200	7.8	23.4	7.8	2.6
Feta Cheese, & Salad, Tastte*	1 Pack/178g	367	13.4	206	10.6	24	7.5	0
Goat's Cheese, & Cranberry, Shapers, Boots*	1 Pack/150g	323	6.3	216	8.4	36	4.2	2.6
Ham, & Cheese, & Mayo, Brown Bread, Mattessons*	1 Pack/172g	439	18.1	255	13.8	27	10.5	2.2
Ham, & Cheese, & Pickle, & Lettuce, No Mayo, Tesco*	1 Pack/207.1g	435	16.2	210	12.2	23	7.8	2.7
Ham, & Cheese, & Pickle, Average	*1 Pack/220g*	*524*	*25.1*	*238*	*12.2*	*21.6*	*11.4*	*2.5*
Ham, & Cheese, on a Croissant, Smoked, M&S*	1 Croissant/105g	341	22.7	325	13.4	22.2	21.6	3.9
Ham, & Cheese, Salad, Pick of the Pantry, On A Roll*	1 Pack/228g	431	22.6	189	10.9	13.5	9.9	2.6
Ham, & Coleslaw, Smoked, Brambles*	1 Pack/166g	283	4.1	171	8.2	28.8	2.5	1.8
Ham, & Edam, Smoked, Shapers, Boots*	1 Pack/183g	315	11.9	172	9.3	19	6.5	2.7
Ham, & Egg, Honey Roast, Tesco*	1 Pack/192g	355	9.8	185	12.8	20.6	5.1	2.5
Ham, & Mustard, Ginsters*	1 Pack/140g	307	9.4	219	11.8	28	6.7	2.5
Ham, & Mustard, Loved by Us, Co-Op*	1 Pack/162g	310	7.9	191	13.2	22.4	4.9	1.8
Ham, & Mustard, Salad, BGTY, Sainsbury's*	1 Pack/182.5g	261	3.8	143	8.7	22.4	2.1	2.6
Ham, & Mustard, Tesco*	1 Pack/147g	437	27.9	297	10.6	20.8	19	1.2
Ham, & Mustard, Wiltshire, The Ultimate, M&S*	1 Sandwich/246g	344	11.8	140	9.8	15	4.8	1.4
Ham, & Salad, On the Go, Sainsbury's*	1 Pack/174g	244	3	140	10.1	20	1.7	2
Ham, & Salad, Shapers, Boots*	1 Pack/195g	269	2.7	138	9.4	22	1.4	1.8
Ham, & Soft Cheese, Tesco*	1 Serving/164g	333	12.1	203	11.6	22.5	7.4	2.2
Ham, & Swiss Cheese, M&S*	1 Pack/159g	393	20	247	14.7	18.9	12.6	3.3

SANDWICH

	Measure INFO/WEIGHT	per Measure KCAL	per Measure FAT	Nutrition Values per 100g / 100ml KCAL	PROT	CARB	FAT	FIBRE
Ham, & Tomato, Brambles*	1 Pack/159g	288	7.3	181	11.1	24.1	4.6	3.3
Ham, & Turkey with Salad, Co-Op*	1 Pack/188g	263	5.6	140	9	21	3	2
Ham, & Cheese, Morrisons*	1 Serving/183g	273	4.6	149	12.5	19.2	2.5	4.1
Ham, & Mustard Mayo, Smoked, Good to Go, Waitrose*	1 Pack/160g	309	8	193	12.9	23	5	2.2
Ham, No Mayo, Just Ham, Tesco*	1 Pack/122g	250	4.9	205	11.6	30.4	4	2.1
Houmous, & Carrot, Shapers, Boots*	1 Pack/204g	323	10.2	158	7.5	21	5	5.2
Ploughman's, Cheese, Cheddar, Deep Fill, Asda*	1 Pack/229g	471	22.9	206	9	20	10	4.3
Ploughman's, Cheese, Cheddar, Vintage, Sainsbury's*	1 Pack/204g	439	20.2	215	9.3	22.3	9.9	0
Ploughman's, Cheese, Deep Fill, Ginsters*	1 Pack/213g	491	24.2	231	8.4	23.8	11.4	2.2
Ploughman's, Deep Fill, Tesco*	1 Pack/245g	551	27.4	225	10.9	20.2	11.2	1.4
Prawn Mayonnaise, Co-Op*	1 Pack/154g	285	6	185	9.7	27.3	3.9	3.2
Prawn Mayonnaise, M&S*	1 Pack/156g	328	12	210	10	24.7	7.7	2.2
Prawn Mayonnaise, Malted Bread, Tesco*	1 Pack/181g	369	14.3	204	9.4	22.9	7.9	2
Prawn Mayonnaise, Morrisons*	1 Pack/157g	234	3.9	149	9	22.7	2.5	3
Prawn Mayonnaise, on Oatmeal Bread, HL, Tesco*	1 Pack/150g	249	3.8	166	11.3	23.4	2.5	2.3
Prawn Mayonnaise, on Oatmeal Bread, Sainsbury's*	1 Pack/150g	277	10	185	9.7	20.3	6.7	2.1
Prawn Mayonnaise, On Soft Malted Brown Bread, M&S*	1 Pack/197g	347	8.9	176	11.6	21.1	4.5	2.3
Prawn Mayonnaise, Shapers, Boots*	1 Pack/160g	293	7.5	183	9.4	25.6	4.7	2.5
Prawn, & Salmon, Smoked, M&S*	1 Pack/445g	1135	63.6	255	11.7	19.3	14.3	1.4
Prawn, King, Sainsbury's*	1 Pack/204g	424	16.3	208	11.6	22.3	8	0
Prawn, Marie Rose, Waitrose*	1 Pack/164g	226	5.6	138	8.8	18	3.4	1.9
Rib, BBQ, Pork, Rustlers*	1 Pack/170g	459	22.1	270	14.3	22.9	13	2
Salami, & Cheese, Migrolino*	1 Sandwich/140g	486	26.6	347	14	29	19	2
Salmon, & Cream Cheese, Smoked, Morrisons*	1 Pack/160g	342	13.1	214	11	22	8.2	4
Salmon, & Cucumber, Brown Bread, Waitrose*	1 Pack/150g	296	10.6	197	10.5	22.7	7.1	1.4
Salmon, & Cucumber, M&S*	1 Pack/168g	329	13.9	196	11	19.5	8.3	2.6
Salmon, & Cucumber, Red, Tesco*	1 Pack/144g	284	9.2	197	11.1	23.8	6.4	1.9
Salmon, & Soft Cheese, Smoked, Waitrose*	1 Pack/180g	416	18	231	11.5	22.6	10	2.2
Salmon, & Watercress, Poached, Lochmuir, M&S*	1 Pack/192g	355	11.7	185	10.3	22.3	6.1	1.6
Salmon, & Cream Cheese, Smoked, Sainsbury*	1 Pack/168g	408	17.5	243	11.7	24.5	10.4	2.2
Salmon, & Cucumber, Good to Go, Waitrose*	1 Pack/185g	316	9.2	171	12.1	18	5	2.8
Salmon, & Cucumber, LC, Tesco*	1 Pack/178g	330	5.7	185	10.1	26.8	3.2	2.3
Sausage, Pigs Under Blankets, Delicious, Boots*	1 Pack/181g	453	16.7	250	11	29	9.2	2.5
Seafood, Medley, M&S*	1 Pack/227g	468	28.1	206	7.2	16.3	12.4	3.5
Steak	**1 Sandwich/204g**	**459**	**14.1**	**225**	**14.9**	**25.5**	**6.9**	**0**
Sub, Cold Cuts, From Restaurant	**1 Sandwich/228g**	**456**	**18.6**	**200**	**9.6**	**22.4**	**8.2**	**0**
Sub, Ham, & Tomato Salad, Shapers, Boots*	1 Pack/170g	286	3.9	168	9.2	28	2.3	1.4
Sub, Tuna, & Salad, From Restaurant, Average	**1 Sandwich/256g**	**584**	**28**	**228**	**11.6**	**21.6**	**10.9**	**0**
Tastes of Christmas, Selection, M&S*	1 Pack/205g	484	21.5	236	12.3	22	10.5	1.9
Tuna Mayo, Essential, Waitrose*	1 Pack/133g	283	7.4	213	13.3	25.9	5.6	2.9
Tuna Mayonnaise, & Cucumber, Daily Bread*	1 Pack/190g	392	16.6	206	12.1	19.8	8.7	0
Tuna Mayonnaise, & Cucumber, Finest, Tesco*	1 Pack/225g	484	19.1	215	11.6	23.1	8.5	1.7
Tuna Mayonnaise, & Cucumber, Simply, Boots*	1 Pack/200g	498	26	249	12	21	13	2.4
Tuna Mayonnaise, & Salad, Serious About Sandwiches*	1 Pack/192g	305	9	159	8.6	20.5	4.7	2.9
Tuna Mayonnaise, Menu, Boots*	1 Pack/182g	451	20	248	13	23	11	1.1
Tuna Mayonnaise, Sainsbury's*	1 Sandwich/150g	314	9.9	209	11.4	24.5	6.6	2.8
Tuna, & Cucumber, & Red Onion, Brambles*	1 Pack/161.0g	264	3.9	164	11.3	24.3	2.4	1.6
Tuna, & Cucumber, BGTY, Sainsbury's*	1 Pack/178g	268	3.2	151	11.3	22.3	1.8	3.1
Tuna, & Cucumber, COU, M&S*	1 Pack/204g	294	5.1	144	9.1	20.6	2.5	1.5
Tuna, & Cucumber, Finest, Tesco*	1 Pack/169g	380	16.7	225	10.2	23.4	9.9	2.7
Tuna, & Cucumber, Healthy Living, Co-Op*	1 Pack/192g	250	3.5	130	10.9	17.9	1.8	3
Tuna, & Cucumber, NUME, Morrisons*	1 Pack/151g	255	3.5	169	12	23.7	2.3	2.5
Tuna, & Cucumber, On Oatmeal Bread, Ginsters*	1 Pack/175g	290	7.2	166	11.7	20.7	4.1	2.4

S

	Measure INFO/WEIGHT	per Measure KCAL	FAT	Nutrition Values per 100g / 100ml KCAL	PROT	CARB	FAT	FIBRE
SANDWICH								
Tuna, & Cucumber, On the Go, Sainsbury's*	1 Pack/196g	284	5.5	145	9.6	19.4	2.8	2.1
Tuna, & Cucumber, You Count, Love Life, Waitrose*	1 Pack/195g	321	5.3	165	13	21.4	2.7	1.4
Tuna, & Sweetcorn, Loved by Us, Co-Op*	1 Pack/200g	380	9.2	190	11.7	24.1	4.6	2.4
Tuna, & Sweetcorn, Malted Bread, Asda*	1 Pack/202g	365	10.7	181	11	21	5.3	2.5
Tuna, & Sweetcorn, BGTY, Sainsbury's*	1 Pack/187g	309	5.1	165	10.8	24.7	2.7	2.8
Tuna, & Sweetcorn, Ginsters*	1 Pack/169g	348	11.4	205	9.6	26.4	6.7	2.4
Tuna, & Sweetcorn, on Malt Bread, Tesco*	1 Pack/170g	425	20.4	250	11.4	22.5	12	3.3
Tuna, Crunch, HL, Tesco*	1 Pack/180g	261	4.3	145	11	19.9	2.4	0.5
Turkey, & Bacon, COU, M&S*	1 Pack/165g	256	4	155	12	21	2.4	1.7
Turkey, & Cranberry, COU, M&S*	1 Pack/180g	279	3.1	155	12.1	22.8	1.7	2.9
Turkey, & Cranberry, Salad, Fullfillers*	1 Serving/180g	319	5.8	177	13	23.3	3.2	0
Turkey, & Pastrami, HL, Tesco*	1 Pack/185g	286	4.8	155	9.6	22.1	2.6	2.6
Turkey, & Salad, Fullfillers*	1 Serving/218g	320	7	147	10.3	18.6	3.2	0
Turkey, & Salad, Healthy Eating, Wild Bean Cafe*	1 Serving/230g	315	2.5	137	10	21.5	1.1	1.8
Turkey, & Stuffing & Cranberry, Shapers, Boots*	1oz/28g	53	0.7	190	12	28	2.5	2.6
Turkey, & Trimmings, Christmas, Tesco*	1 Pack/209g	476	16.5	228	12.5	25.5	7.9	2.3
Turkey, & Trimmings, Light Choices, HL, Tesco*	1 Pack/154g	256	4.3	166	10.1	24.1	2.8	2.2
Turkey, & Stuffing, M&S*	1 Pack/190g	352	9.3	185	12.3	23.1	4.9	1.9
Vegetable, Roasted, Open, COU, M&S*	1 Pack/150g	260	2.2	173	8.4	31.3	1.5	4.4
Veggie Threesome, Cranks*	1 Pack/227g	500	20.5	220	9	24.3	9	3
SANDWICH FILLER								
Cheese & Spring Onion, M&S*	1 Serving/56g	199	18.8	355	8.5	5	33.6	0.2
Cheese & Onion, Reduced Fat, Supermarket, Average	*1 Serving/100g*	*227*	*18.1*	*227*	*11.8*	*4.4*	*18.1*	*1.7*
Cheese & Onion, Sainsbury's*	1 Tub/200g	632	59.6	316	8.7	3.2	29.8	2.2
Cheese & Onion, Supermarket, Average	*1 Serving/100g*	*405*	*38.6*	*405*	*10.2*	*4.1*	*38.6*	*1.3*
Cheese & Onion, Tesco*	1 Pack/250g	1060	106.5	424	10	0.2	42.6	1.5
Chicken & Bacon with Sweetcorn, Sainsbury's*	1 Serving/60g	123	9.4	205	12	4	15.7	0.9
Chicken & Bacon, Asda*	1 Serving/100g	341	29	341	17	3	29	0.5
Chicken Tikka, HE, Tesco*	1 Serving/100g	110	3.6	110	7.1	12.4	3.6	1
Chicken, Coronation, Deli, Meadow Fresh, Lidl*	1 Serving/30g	78	5.7	261	9.8	19	1.2	
Chicken, Sweetcorn & Bacon, Tesco*	1 Serving/50g	167	14.8	334	12.3	4.3	29.7	1.6
Coronation Chicken, Sainsbury's*	¼ Tub/60g	183	14.8	305	12.1	8.9	24.6	1.2
Coronation Chicken, Tesco*	1 Tbsp/30g	88	7	293	11.4	9.2	23.2	0.7
Egg & Bacon, Fresh, Tesco*	1 Serving/45g	112	9	248	12.7	4.2	20.1	0.6
Egg & Bacon, Free Range, Deli, Essential, Waitrose*	½ Pot/85g	267	23.6	314	12.7	3.3	27.8	0.5
Egg Mayonnaise, BGTY, Sainsbury's*	1 Serving/63g	71	4.1	113	10.2	3.4	6.5	0.1
Egg Mayonnaise, Chunky Free Range, Tesco*	1 Serving/50g	104	8.9	209	11.3	0.9	17.8	1.6
Egg Mayonnaise, Country Fresh, Aldi*	¼ Pack/50g	106	8.9	211	9.8	2.9	17.8	0
Egg Mayonnaise, Free Range, Co-Op*	1 Pack/200g	260	17.6	130	10.1	2.4	8.8	0.5
Egg Mayonnaise, Morrisons*	1 Serving/50g	71	5.3	142	10	1.7	10.6	0
Egg Mayonnaise, Tesco*	1 Serving/50g	100	7.8	199	10.9	3.5	15.6	0.5
Prawn Marie Rose, Sainsbury's*	1 Serving/60g	121	10.6	201	8.1	2.5	17.6	0.9
Prawn Mayonnaise, Deli, Asda*	1 Serving/50g	170	16.5	339	9	1.6	33	0.4
Seafood Cocktail, Sainsbury's*	½ Tub/120g	314	27.6	262	5.7	8.1	23	1
Smoked Salmon & Soft Cheese, M&S*	1 Pack/170g	450	40.6	265	11.1	4.9	23.9	0
Tuna & Sweetcorn, Reduced Fat, Supermarket	*1 Serving/100g*	*119*	*5.4*	*119*	*11.5*	*5.8*	*5.4*	*1.2*
Tuna & Sweetcorn, Supermarket	*1 Serving/100g*	*228*	*17.8*	*228*	*11.6*	*5.7*	*17.8*	*1.4*
Tuna & Sweetcorn, Tesco*	1 Serving/54g	127	9.8	235	8.6	8.1	18.1	0.6
Tuna Mayonnaise & Cucumber, Choice, Tesco*	1 Serving/200g	463	22.8	232	12.8	23.2	11.4	1.6
Tuna Mayonnaise, BGTY, Sainsbury's*	1 Serving/100g	114	3.4	114	17.6	3.5	3.4	0.1
SANDWICH SPREAD								
Beef, Classic, Shippam's Foods*	1 Pot/75g	133	8.8	177	15.5	2.2	11.8	0
Chicken Tikka, Asda*	1 Serving/50g	77	5	154	7	9	10	0.2

S

	INFO/WEIGHT	KCAL	FAT	KCAL	PROT	CARB	FAT	FIBRE
SANDWICH SPREAD								
Chicken, Classic, Shippam's Foods*	1 Serving/35g	64	4.4	182	15.5	1.8	12.5	0
Heinz*	1 Tbsp/10ml	22	1.3	220	1	24	13	1
Light, Heinz*	1 Tbsp/10g	16	0.9	161	1.1	18.2	9.2	0.9
SARDINES								
Grilled	*1oz/28g*	*55*	*2.9*	*195*	*25.3*	*0*	*10.4*	*0*
Grilled, No Added Brine, Canned, John West*	1 Can/100g	198	11.9	198	22.8	0	11.9	0.1
in Brine, Canned, Drained	*1oz/28g*	*38*	*2.1*	*136*	*17*	*0*	*7.6*	*0*
in Oil, Canned, Drained	*1oz/28g*	*51*	*3.2*	*180*	*19.1*	*0*	*11.6*	*0*
in Spring Water, Portuguese, Sainsbury's*	1 Can/90g	165	9.3	183	22.4	0	10.3	0
in Tomato Sauce, Canned	*1oz/28g*	*45*	*2.8*	*162*	*17*	*1.4*	*9.9*	*0*
Raw, Whole with Head	*1oz/28g*	*22*	*1.2*	*78*	*9.7*	*0*	*4.3*	*0*
SATAY								
Chicken with Peanut Sauce, Waitrose*	1 Pack/250g	492	27	197	18.9	6	10.8	0.5
Chicken, 12 Mini, Taste Original*	2 Skewers/18g	44	2.8	242	17.9	7.8	15.2	1.2
Chicken, Indonesian, Mini, Sainsbury's*	1 Stick/10g	17	0.7	171	23	4	7	0.7
Chicken, Sticks, Asda*	1 Stick/20g	43	2.8	216	18	4.5	14	0
Spicy Chicken & Noodles, Microwaved, Asda*	1 Portion/380g	361	10.3	95	6.4	10	2.7	1.4
SATSUMAS								
Fresh, Raw, Flesh Only, Average	*1 Sm/56g*	*21*	*0*	*37*	*0.9*	*8.6*	*0.1*	*1.3*
Weighed with Peel, Average	*1 Sm/60g*	*16*	*0*	*26*	*0.6*	*6.1*	*0.1*	*0.6*
SAUCE								
Apple, Bramley, Sainsbury's*	1 Tsp/15g	17	0	111	0.2	27.2	0.1	1.8
Apple, Everyday Value, Tesco*	1 Tbsp/15g	15	0	105	0.1	24.8	0.1	0.5
Arrabiata, Don Pomodoro*	½ Pot/185g	231	20.4	125	0.5	6	11	0
Arrabiata, Italian, Tesco*	½ Pot/175g	72	0.5	41	1.3	8.3	0.3	1.1
Balti Curry, Tesco*	1 Serving/200g	126	9.2	63	1.7	4.3	4.6	1.7
Balti, Cooking, Sharwood's*	¼ Jar/140g	120	8.3	86	1.2	7.1	5.9	1.4
Balti, Kanpur Garden, Lidl*	1 Jar/350g	388	21.7	111	1.6	11.3	6.2	1.9
Balti, Loyd Grossman*	½ Jar/175g	180	11.7	103	1.3	8.4	6.7	1.7
Barbecue, Asda*	1 Serving/135g	128	0.3	95	1.2	22	0.2	0.6
Barbeque, Cook in, Homepride*	1 Can/500g	375	7.5	75	0.7	14.6	1.5	0.6
BBQ, Heinz*	1 Serving/20g	28	0.1	139	1.1	31.7	0.3	0.5
Bearnaise, Sainsbury's*	1 Tbsp/15g	59	6.2	393	6	5	41	0
Bechamel, M&S*	1 Jar/425g	480	34.8	113	2.1	7	8.2	1.6
Bhuna, Cooking, Sharwood's*	1/3 Jar/140g	116	7.6	83	1.2	7.6	5.4	1.6
Biryani, Med & Aromati, Oven Bake, Patak's*	½ Jar/175g	135	9.3	77	1.1	6.1	5.3	1.7
Black Bean & Red Pepper, Sharwood's*	½ Jar/213g	132	3	62	1.9	10.5	1.4	1.2
Black Bean, Asda*	1 Serving/55g	55	0.8	100	2.9	19	1.4	0
Black Bean, Canton, Stir Fry, Blue Dragon*	½ Pack/60g	53	1.2	88	2.8	14.8	2	1.5
Black Bean, Stir Fry Additions, Tesco*	1 Sachet/50g	69	1.5	138	4.1	23.6	3	0
Black Bean, Stir Fry, Fresh Tastes, Asda*	1 Pack/180ml	149	5.2	83	3.7	10.4	2.9	1.4
Black Bean, Stir Fry, Sainsbury's*	½ Pack/75ml	91	3.2	121	3.3	17.6	4.3	1.7
Black Bean, Stir Fry, Sharwood's*	1 Jar/195g	127	0.6	65	2.3	12.9	0.3	0
Black Bean, Uncle Ben's*	1 Serving/125g	89	1.6	71	2	12.8	1.3	0
Bolognese, Dolmio*	1 Serving/100g	33	0.2	33	1.5	6.3	0.2	1.3
Bolognese, Loyd Grossman*	¼ Jar/106g	80	3.1	75	2	10.2	2.9	1.4
Bramley Apple, Colman's*	1 Tbsp/15ml	16	0	107	0.2	26.5	0	1.3
Branston, Rich & Fruity, Crosse & Blackwell*	1 Serving/15g	20	0.1	134	0.5	30	0.5	1.6
Bread, Christmas, Tesco*	1 Serving/60g	64	3.2	107	3.3	11.8	5.3	0.5
Bread, Made with Semi-Skimmed Milk	*1 Serving/45g*	*42*	*1.4*	*93*	*4.3*	*12.8*	*3.1*	*0.3*
Brown, Bottled	*1 Tsp/6g*	*6*	*0*	*99*	*1.1*	*25.2*	*0*	*0.7*
Brown, Bramwells, Aldi*	1 Tbsp/15g	17	0.1	115	0.5	27	0.5	1
Brown, Chop, Hammonds of Yorkshire*	1 Tbsp/15g	10	0	66	0.3	16.1	0.1	0.3

SAUCE	Measure INFO/WEIGHT	per Measure KCAL	FAT	Nutrition Values per 100g / 100ml KCAL	PROT	CARB	FAT	FIBRE
Brown, Original, HP*	1 Tbsp/15g	18	0	122	0.9	28.3	0.1	0.4
Brown, Reduced Salt & Sugar, HP*	1 Tbsp/15g	13	0	87	0.7	20	0.1	0.3
Brown, Tesco*	1 Tsp/10g	10	0	104	0.7	25.1	0.1	0.6
Brown, Value, Value, Tesco*	1 Serving/15g	13	0	86	0.7	18.8	0.1	0.3
Burger, Hellmann's*	1 Tbsp/15g	36	3.2	240	1.1	12	21	0
Butter & Tarragon, Chicken Tonight, Knorr*	¼ Jar/125g	132	13	106	1	2.1	10.4	0.7
Cantonese Chow Mein Stir Fry, Sainsbury's*	½ Jar/100g	67	1.9	67	0.4	12.1	1.9	0.8
Caramelised Orange, The Bay Tree*	1 Serving/168g	188	0.2	112	0.8	28.1	0.1	0.5
Carbonara, TTD, Sainsbury's*	½ pot/175g	347	31	198	5.2	4.5	17.7	0.5
Cheese, Fresh, Italiano, Tesco*	½ Tub/175g	236	16.1	135	6.8	6.2	9.2	0
Cheese, Fresh, Waitrose*	1 Pot/350g	458	34.3	131	5.1	5.7	9.8	0
Cheese, Instant, Morrisons*	1 Serving/14g	38	2.8	272	7.9	14.3	20.3	0
Cheese, Made with Semi-Skimmed Milk	**1 Serving/60g**	**107**	**7.6**	**179**	**8.1**	**9.1**	**12.6**	**0.2**
Cheese, Made with Whole Milk	**1 Serving/60g**	**118**	**8.8**	**197**	**8**	**9**	**14.6**	**0.2**
Cheese, Sainsbury's*	1 Serving/125g	140	9.4	112	5	6.1	7.5	1.2
Chickpea & Spinach, Asda*	1 Jar/500g	365	14	73	3.5	8.4	2.8	2
Chilli & Garlic, Blue Dragon*	1 Serving/30ml	26	0.1	85	1.1	19.7	0.2	0
Chilli & Garlic, Lea & Perrins*	1 Tsp/6g	4	0	60	1	14.9	0	0
Chilli Con Carne, Homepride*	½ Jar/250g	145	1.2	58	1.6	11.1	0.5	1.6
Chilli Con Carne, Hot, Uncle Ben's*	1 Jar/500g	295	3	59	2.3	10.9	0.6	1.7
Chilli, Barbeque, Encona*	1 Tbsp/15ml	19	0	129	1.3	30.7	0.1	0
Chilli, Hot, Blue Dragon*	1 Tbsp/15ml	14	0	96	0.5	23	0.2	0
Chilli, Hot, Mexican, Morrisons*	¼ Jar/125g	72	0.6	58	2.2	11.2	0.5	2
Chilli, Linghams*	1 Tsp/5g	4	0	79	0	17.3	0.8	0
Chilli, Mild, Tesco*	1 Jar/550g	302	1.6	55	2.3	10	0.3	3.4
Chilli, Sweet, Thai, Dipping, Original, Blue Dragon*	1 Serving/30ml	69	0.2	229	0.6	55.1	0.7	1.6
Chilli, Tesco*	1 Tsp/5ml	4	0.2	90	1.3	14	3.2	1.1
Chilli, Tomato Based, Bottled, Average	**1 Tbsp/15g**	**16**	**0**	**104**	**2.5**	**19.8**	**0.3**	**5.9**
Chimichurri, Deluxe, Lidl*	1 Tbsp/15ml	8	0.2	54	0.9	7.8	1.6	2.2
Chinese Curry, Cooking, Sharwoods*	1/3 Jar/140g	66	2.2	47	0.9	6.7	1.6	1.2
Chinese Stir Fry, Sainsbury's*	½ Sachet/75.3g	61	1.9	81	0.4	14.1	2.5	1
Chinese Style Curry, Cooking, Asda*	1 Jar/560g	465	24.1	83	1.5	9.6	4.3	1.7
Chip Shop Curry, Knorr*	1 Sachet/150ml	146	6.9	97	1.7	12.4	4.6	0.7
Chip Shop Curry, Prepared, CBY, Asda*	1 Serving/62ml	50	3	80	0.5	8.6	4.8	0.2
Chocolate, Dessert, M&S*	1 Dtsp/11g	35	1	330	2.1	59.3	9.4	1.9
Chow Mein, Stir Fry, Blue Dragon*	1 Sachet/120g	110	3.5	92	1.1	15.4	2.9	0.4
Chow Mein, Stir Fry, Straight to Wok, Amoy*	1 Pack/120g	172	7	143	0.9	21.9	5.8	0.5
Cooking, Hunters Chicken, Tesco*	1/3 Jar/163g	155	0.3	95	1.2	20.6	0.2	0.8
Country French, Chicken Tonight, Knorr*	¼ Jar/125g	110	8.8	89	0.4	5.3	7.1	0.8
Cranberry Jelly, Morrisons*	1 Tsp/12g	23	0	189	0.2	47	0	0.1
Cranberry, Sainsbury's*	1 Tsp/15g	26	0.1	170	0.5	41.5	0.5	0.5
Cranberry, Tesco*	1 Tsp/15g	23	0	156	0.1	38.8	0	0.9
Cream, GraddsÃƒ¥s, Ikea*	1 Serving/60ml	72	6.6	120	1	4	11	0
Creamy Peppercorn & Whisky, Baxters*	1 Pack/320g	422	34.6	132	1.9	6.7	10.8	0.2
Curry, Asda*	1 Tbsp/15g	62	2.1	414	13	59	14	1.3
Curry, Basics, Sainsbury's*	¼ Jar/110g	70	2.8	64	0.7	9.7	2.5	0.9
Curry, Bettabuy, Morrisons*	1 Jar/440g	295	10.1	67	0.7	10.8	2.3	1
Curry, Chinese Style, Cooking, CBY, Asda*	1 Serving/140g	89	4.3	64	1.5	7.4	3.1	3.5
Curry, Cook in, Homepride*	½ Can/250g	140	4.8	56	1.1	8.6	1.9	0.5
Curry, Green Thai, Finest, Tesco*	1 Serving/350g	420	37.1	120	1.4	4.8	10.6	0.7
Curry, Medium, Uncle Ben's*	1 Jar/500g	330	10	66	0.9	10.9	2	0
Curry, Red Thai, Finest, Tesco*	1 Jar/350g	388	31.5	111	1.3	6.2	9	0.9
Curry, Thai Coconut, Uncle Ben's*	1 Serving/125g	128	6	102	1.4	13.2	4.8	0

S

SAUCE

	Measure INFO/WEIGHT	per Measure KCAL	per Measure FAT	Nutrition Values per 100g / 100ml KCAL	PROT	CARB	FAT	FIBRE
Dhansak, Sharwood's*	1 Jar/445g	668	34.7	150	4.7	15.2	7.8	1.4
Dill & Lemon, Delicate for Fish, Schwartz*	1 Pack/300g	387	34.2	129	1.1	5.6	11.4	0.5
Dreamy Caramel, Dessert Topping, Clarks*	1 Tbsp/15g	46	0.2	308	1.5	43.8	1.5	28.2
Enchilada, Medium, Old El Paso*	1 Can/270g	92	4.6	34	0	5	1.7	0
Fajita, Asda*	¼ Jar/125g	79	5.4	63	1	5	4.3	1
Four Cheese for Pasta, Waitrose*	1 Pot/300g	392	24.8	112	6.6	5.5	7.1	0.5
Fruity Damson, Jelly, Tracklements*	1 Tsp/10g	28	0	281	0.2	70.2	0	0
Fruity, HP*	1 Tbsp/15g	20	0	135	0.9	31.5	0	0.3
Garlic & Chive, Table & Dip, Heinz*	1 Serving/10ml	32	3	323	1	12.1	29.9	0.2
Garlic, Creamy, Sainsbury's*	1 Tbsp/15g	44	4.3	296	0.5	7.6	29	1.5
Garlic, Heinz*	1 Serving/10ml	32	3	323	1	12.1	29.9	1.2
Gastro Chicken & Chorizo , Loyd Grossman*	½ Pouch/175g	178	10.7	102	3.4	7	6.1	2.7
Green Thai Curry, M&S*	½ Jar/175g	175	13.3	100	1.1	7.4	7.6	0.8
Habanero Hot Boy, Glorious!*	1 Pot/300g	342	26.4	114	1.6	6.8	8.8	1.3
Hoisin & Plum, Stir Fry, HL, Tesco*	1 Serving/250g	148	3.2	59	2.1	9.7	1.3	1.3
Hoisin & Garlic, Blue Dragon*	1 Serving/60g	80	1.6	133	1.2	26.1	2.6	0
Hoisin & Spring Onion, Stir Fry, Sharwood's*	1 Jar/165g	196	1.5	119	1.3	26.5	0.9	0.8
Hoisin, Lee Kum Kee*	1 Serving/35g	80	0.5	230	1.2	53.3	1.3	0.8
Hoisin, Sharwood's*	1 Tbsp/15g	32	0	211	2.7	49.5	0.3	0.1
Hoisin, Stir Fry, Asda*	1 Pack/120g	103	0.7	86	0.6	18	0.6	3.1
Hoisin, Stir Fry, Fresh Tastes, Asda*	½ Sachet/90ml	122	0.8	135	1.8	29.7	0.9	0
Hollandaise, Atkins & Potts*	1 Serving/30g	144	15	480	1.2	6.2	50	0.3
Hollandaise, Finest, Tesco*	1 Serving/98g	473	44.5	485	1.4	17.2	45.6	0.3
Hollandaise, Fresh, Average	*1 Pack/150g*	*342*	*32.4*	*228*	*2.4*	*6.1*	*21.6*	*0*
Hollandaise, Sainsbury's*	1 Tbsp/15g	72	7.6	478	0.2	5.9	50.4	0.4
Honey & Mustard, Chicken Tonight, Knorr*	¼ Jar/125g	132	6.6	106	1	12.6	5.3	1.8
Horseradish, Batts, Lidl*	1 Tbsp/20g	29	1.5	143	1.9	16.2	7.3	2.4
Horseradish, Colman's*	1 Tbsp/15ml	17	0.9	112	1.9	9.8	6.2	2.6
Horseradish, Creamed, M&S*	1 Tsp/5g	16	1.5	325	2.4	12.1	29.3	2.5
Horseradish, Creamed, Waitrose*	1 Tbsp/16g	30	1.6	185	2.4	19.6	9.9	2.3
Horseradish, Creamy, Sainsbury's*	1 Tsp/5g	11	0.6	223	2.8	28.9	11.8	1.6
Horseradish, Hot, Morrisons*	1 Serving/20g	22	1.1	110	1.6	10.9	5.6	1.1
Horseradish, Hot, Tesco*	1 Tsp/5g	9	0.5	185	2.3	19.7	10.6	2.3
Horseradish, Mustard, Sainsbury's*	1 Tsp/5g	8	0.5	163	7.9	18.2	6.6	3.5
Horseradish, Sainsbury's*	1 Dtsp/10g	14	0.7	145	1.5	17.8	6.6	2.4
Hot Pepper, Encona*	1 Tsp/5ml	3	0.1	52	0.5	10.5	1.2	0
Hot, Original, Cholula Hot Sauce*	1 Tsp/5ml	1	0	19	0.9	0.4	0.9	2.8
Italian Hot Chilli, Dolmio*	½ Pack/150g	104	5.8	69	1.3	7.1	3.9	0
Jalfrezi, Average	*1 Sm Jar/350g*	*326*	*23.7*	*93*	*1.3*	*6.7*	*6.8*	*1.6*
Jalfrezi, Cooking, Sainsbury's*	1 Serving/250g	160	6	64	1	9.6	2.4	1.7
Jalfrezi, Stir Fry, Patak's*	1 Jar/250g	260	18.8	104	1.4	7.6	7.5	1.4
Korma, Coconut & Cream, Mild, in Glass Jar, Patak's*	1 Jar/450g	652	50	145	1.2	9.4	11.1	0
Korma, Cooking, Sharwood's*	1 Jar/420g	680	42.8	162	1.7	15.9	10.2	2.2
Korma, Curry, Loyd Grossman*	½ Jar/175g	224	14.5	128	1.5	11.3	8.3	0.8
Korma, Curry, Uncle Ben's*	1 Jar/500g	630	42	126	1.4	11.1	8.4	0
Korma, Mild Curry, BFY, Morrisons*	¼ Jar/118g	150	7.2	127	1.3	16.8	6.1	1.5
Korma, Tesco*	¼ Jar/125g	192	14.6	154	2.4	9.9	11.7	1.3
Lemon & Ginger, Stir Fry, Finest, Tesco*	¼ Jar/85g	144	0.2	169	0.2	41.7	0.2	0.2
Madras, Aldi*	1 Serving/113g	68	2.3	60	1.5	9	2	0
Madras, Cooking, Sharwood's*	1 Tsp/2g	2	0.1	86	1.5	6.9	5.8	1.3
Madras, Cumin & Chilli, Original, in Glass Jar, Patak's*	1 Jar/540g	648	38.3	120	2.1	11.9	7.1	1.8
Marie Rose, Fresh, The Saucy Fish Co.*	1 Pack/150g	590	59.7	393	1.6	7	39.8	0
Marie Rose, Spicy, with Brandy, Extra Special, Asda*	1 Tbsp/15g	72	6.9	482	1.4	15	46	1.4

	Measure INFO/WEIGHT	per Measure KCAL	FAT	Nutrition Values per 100g / 100ml KCAL	PROT	CARB	FAT	FIBRE
SAUCE								
Mediterranean Vegetable, Chargrilled, Italiano, Tesco*	1 Pot/350g	175	3.9	50	1.6	8.4	1.1	1.3
Mint Garden, Fresh, Tesco*	1 Tsp/5g	2	0	40	2.6	3.6	0.4	1.5
Mint, Bramwells, Aldi*	1 Serving/30g	28	0.2	93	0.5	21	0.5	0
Mint, Sainsbury's*	1 Dtsp/10g	13	0	126	2.5	28.7	0.1	4
Mint, Value, Tesco*	1 Serving/10g	4	0	41	1.1	9	0.1	1.8
Mushroom, Creamy, Chicken Tonight, Knorr*	¼ Jar/125g	99	7.1	79	0.5	6	5.7	1
Napoli Tomato, Combino, Lidl*	1 Jar/500ml	325	9.5	65	1.7	8.9	1.9	0
Oriental, Cantonese, Uncle Ben's*	¼ Jar/125g	108	0.2	86	0.8	20.3	0.2	1.2
Oyster & Spring Onion, Stir Fry, Blue Dragon*	1 Sachet/120g	134	0	112	1.5	26.3	0	0
Oyster, Blue Dragon*	1 Tsp/5ml	6	0	121	3.4	26.9	0	0
Parsley, Fresh, Microwaved, Sainsbury's*	1/3 Pot/100g	78	5.4	78	1.7	5.3	5.4	0.5
Parsley, Made Up, Bisto*	1 Serving/50ml	41	2.4	82	0.6	9.2	4.8	0
Parsley, Tesco*	½ Pack/89g	85	5.1	95	2.8	8.1	5.7	1.1
Pasta Bake, Creamy Tomato & Bacon, Homepride*	1 Serving/110g	99	6.9	90	1.9	6.5	6.3	0
Pasta Bake, Creamy Tomato & Herb, Homepride*	1 Serving/125g	128	8.8	102	1.5	8.3	7	0.9
Pasta Bake, Tomato & Cheese, Dolmio*	¼ Jar/125g	70	1.5	56	2.1	9.1	1.2	1.2
Pasta Bake, Tuna, Homepride*	½ Jar/250g	208	13	83	1.4	7.6	5.2	0.9
Pasta, Tomato & Mushroom, Cucina, Aldi*	1 Jar/500g	165	1	33	1.1	5.7	0.2	1.9
Peanut, Sainsbury's*	1 Sachet/70g	185	9.2	264	1.9	34.7	13.1	1.6
Peking Lemon, Stir Fry, Blue Dragon*	1 Serving/35g	47	0.2	134	0	31.6	0.7	0.5
Pepper, As Prepared, Colman's*	1 Portion/75ml	89	4.7	119	4.7	11	6.3	0
Pepper, Creamy, Tesco*	1 Serving/85ml	128	11.4	151	1.2	6.4	13.4	0.5
Peppercorn, M&S*	1 Pack/200g	220	16.4	110	3	5.6	8.2	0
Peri Peri, Garlic, Nando's*	1 Serving/15g	9	0.5	59	0.5	6.6	3.4	0.8
Peri Peri, Hot & Zingy, Heinz*	1 Tbsp/15g	10	0.5	70	0.5	8.3	3.1	0
Prawn Cocktail, Frank Cooper*	1 Tbsp/15g	47	4	316	0.8	18.3	26.7	0.1
Prawn Cocktail, Morrisons*	1 Portion/15ml	81	8.5	540	1.4	5.5	56.9	1.1
Raspberry, Dessert, M&S*	1 Serving/20g	24	0.1	120	0.5	28.7	0.3	2.6
Red Hot Wings, Buffalo, Franks*	1 Tbsp/15g	4	0.2	30	0.8	2	1.5	2.5
Red Wine & Shallot, Rich & Velvety, Waitrose*	½ Pot/100g	46	1.9	46	1.9	5.1	1.9	0.2
Red Wine, Cooking, BGTY, Sainsbury's*	1 Serving/125g	52	0.6	42	0.5	8.8	0.5	0.8
Redcurrant, Colman's*	1 Tsp/12g	44	0	368	0.7	90	0	0
Reggae Reggae, Jerk BBQ, Levi Roots*	1 Jar/310g	375	0.3	121	1.1	28.8	0.1	0.5
Rendang, Indonesian, Seasoned Pioneers*	1 Pouch/400g	500	46.8	125	1.3	3.5	11.7	1.8
Roast Peanut Satay, Stir Fry, Straight to Wok, Amoy*	½ Pack/60g	106	6.4	176	4	16.3	10.6	1.3
Roasted Peanut Satay, Stir Fry Sensations, Amoy*	1 Pouch/160g	354	19.8	221	4.7	21.9	12.4	1
Rogan Josh, Cooking, CBY, Asda*	1/3 Jar/167g	90	5	54	1	4.6	3	2.2
Rogan Josh, Curry, The Curry Sauce Company*	1 Serving/235g	310	23.7	132	1.9	8.4	10.1	1.5
Rogan Josh, Medium, Sharwood's*	½ Jar/210g	151	7.6	72	1.4	8.6	3.6	0.5
Rogan Josh, Spice & Simmer, Asda*	1/3 Jar/120g	101	5.6	84	1.3	8.3	4.7	1.5
Salted Caramel, Dipping, Waitrose*	1 Tsp/5g	21	1.2	425	2.4	46.4	24.5	4.4
Satay, Peanut, M&S*	1 Serving/15g	33	2.3	221	6.4	8.6	15.2	12.2
Satay, Tesco*	1 Jar/180g	265	14	147	4.7	10.9	7.8	7.1
Sausage Casserole, Cook in, Homepride*	½ Jar/250g	92	0.5	37	0.7	8	0.2	0.6
Seafood, Asda*	1 Serving/10g	45	4.2	448	1.6	16	42	0.2
Seafood, Average	*1 Tsp/5g*	*20*	*1.9*	*410*	*1.4*	*15.4*	*38*	*0.2*
Seafood, Colman's*	1 Tbsp/15g	44	3.4	296	0.9	21.5	22.9	0.4
Seafood, Sainsbury's*	1 Tbsp/15g	50	4.2	330	0.7	17.6	28.2	0.1
Seafood, Tesco*	1 Serving/10g	46	4.4	465	1.8	15.6	43.5	0.3
Smoked Bacon & Tomato, Stir in, Dolmio*	½ Tub/75g	74	4.2	98	4.6	7.2	5.6	1.3
Southern Pepper Curry, The Spice Tailor*	1 Serving/100g	167	13	167	2.4	8.4	13	3.8
Soy & Garlic, Stir Fry, Fresh Tastes, Asda*	1 Pack/180g	175	6.7	97	1.7	14.1	3.7	0.5
Soy & Plum, Stir Fry Additions, COOK!, M&S*	½ Sachet/60g	48	0.2	80	1.5	17.5	0.3	1.5

S

SAUCE

	Measure INFO/WEIGHT	per Measure KCAL	FAT	KCAL	PROT	CARB	FAT	FIBRE
Soy, Average	*1 Tsp/5ml*	*3*	*0*	*64*	*8.7*	*8.3*	*0*	*0*
Soy, Dark, Amoy*	1 Tsp/5ml	5	0	106	0.9	25.6	0	0
Soy, Dark, Average	*1 Tsp/5g*	*4*	*0*	*84*	*4*	*16.7*	*0.1*	*0.2*
Soy, Dark, M&S*	1 fl oz/30ml	19	0	63	9.1	6.6	0	0
Soy, Light, Amoy*	1 Tsp/5ml	3	0	52	2.5	10.5	0	0
Soy, Naturally Brewed, Kikkoman*	1 Tbsp/15g	11	0	74	10.3	8.1	0	0
Soy, Reduced Salt, Amoy*	1 Tsp/5ml	3	0	56	4	10	0	0
Spanish Chicken, Batts, Lidl*	½ Jar/250g	122	4.8	49	1.3	5.9	1.9	1.4
Spanish Chicken, Chicken Tonight, Knorr*	¼ Jar/125g	68	2	55	1.6	7.3	1.6	2.3
Spare Rib, Lee Kum Kee*	2 Tbsp/38g	80	1	211	2.6	39.5	2.6	2.6
Spicy Sweet & Sour, Sharwood's*	1 Serving/138g	142	0.7	103	0.7	23.8	0.5	0.4
Sticky BBQ, Spread & Bake, Heinz*	¼ Jar/78g	131	0.5	168	1	39.6	0.6	1.2
Sticky Plum, Stir Fry, Blue Dragon*	1 Serving/60g	145	0.2	242	0.1	35.6	0.3	0
Stir Fry, Hoisin with Garlic & Spring Onion, Tesco*	¼ Pack/38g	46	0.4	120	2.2	25.2	1.1	0.5
Stir Fry, Pad Thai, Tesco*	1 Pack/125g	112	2.9	90	1.3	15.8	2.3	0.8
Stroganoff, Mushroom, Creamy, M&S*	1 Serving/75g	86	6.9	115	3.3	4.8	9.2	0.6
Sweet & Sour, Chinese, Sainsbury's*	½ Jar/150g	222	0.2	148	0.2	36.6	0.1	0.1
Sweet & Sour, Cook In, Glass Jar, Homepride*	1 Jar/500g	335	0.5	67	0.3	16.2	0.1	0.5
Sweet & Sour, Cooking, Chinese, Sainsbury's*	¼ Jar/125g	155	0.1	124	0.6	30.1	0.1	0.7
Sweet & Sour, Spicy, Uncle Ben's*	1 Jar/400g	364	0.4	91	0.6	22.1	0.1	0
Sweet & Sour, Stir Fry Additions, Tesco*	1 Sachet/50g	84	0.5	167	0.8	38.7	1	0.5
Sweet & Sour, Stir Fry, Asda*	1 Serving/63g	146	3.2	232	0.8	46	5	0
Sweet & Sour, Stir Fry, M&S*	1 Pack/120g	150	0.5	125	0.7	29.8	0.4	1.3
Sweet & Sour, Stir Fry, Sharwood's*	1 Jar 160g	168	0.8	105	0.6	24.5	0.5	0.8
Sweet & Sour, Stir Fry, Tesco*	½ Jar/222g	164	0.4	74	0.6	17	0.2	0.4
Sweet & Sour, Take-Away	*1oz/28g*	*44*	*1*	*157*	*0.2*	*32.8*	*3.4*	*0*
Sweet & Sour, Cooking, HL, Tesco*	½ Jar/250g	98	1	39	0.2	8.3	0.4	0.6
Sweet & Sour, Cooking, LC, Tesco*	1 Jar/510g	357	0.5	70	0.3	16.1	0.1	0.5
Sweet & Sour, Extra Pineapple, Uncle Ben's*	1 Serving/165g	147	0.3	89	0.3	21.2	0.2	0.7
Sweet & Sour, Light, Uncle Ben's*	¼ Jar/125g	71	0.1	57	0.4	12.6	0.1	0.9
Sweet & Sour, Original, Uncle Ben's*	1 Pack/300g	264	0.6	88	0.4	21.9	0.2	0.8
Sweet & Sour, Stir Fry, Pouch, Average	*1 Pouch/120g*	*148*	*2.3*	*124*	*0.8*	*25.7*	*1.9*	*1*
Sweet & Sour, Stir Fry, Sachet, Blue Dragon*	1 Sachet/120g	145	0.1	122	0.2	29.7	0.1	0.3
Sweet Chilli & Garlic, Stir Fry & Dipping, Tesco*	½ Jar/95g	78	0	82	0.3	20.1	0	0.1
Sweet Chilli, Dipping, M&S*	1 Tbsp/15g	34	0.1	225	0.9	53.2	0.7	0.6
Sweet Chilli, Garlic, Stir Fry, Blue Dragon*	1 Pack/120g	142	0.1	118	0.2	28.8	0.1	0.3
Sweet Chilli, Heinz*	1 Serving/25g	38	0.1	150	0.3	36.5	0.4	6.4
Sweet Chilli, Stir Fry, Additions, Tesco*	1 Serving/50g	106	3.8	211	0.3	35.2	7.6	0.6
Sweet Curry, Eazy Squirt, Heinz*	1 Serving/10ml	12	0	124	0.7	29	0.3	0.5
Sweet Pepper, Stir in, Dolmio*	½ Pot/75g	77	4.6	103	1.4	9.6	6.2	1.6
Szechuan Style, Stir Fry, Fresh Ideas, Tesco*	1 Sachet/50g	114	4.8	228	1.9	33.4	9.7	0.1
Szechuan, Spicy Tomato, Stir Fry, Blue Dragon*	½ Sachet/60g	59	1.8	98	1.3	15.8	3	0.9
Szechuan, Tomato, Spicy, Stir Fry, Sharwoods*	½ Jar/97.5g	56	0.3	57	1.1	12	0.3	0.8
Tabasco, Tabasco*	1 Tsp/5ml	1	0	12	1.3	0.8	0.8	0.6
Tamari, Soya, Clearspring*	1oz/28g	55	0.1	196	14	34	0.2	0
Tamarind & Lime, Stir Fry, Sainsbury's*	1 Serving/75g	88	5.6	117	1.1	11.4	7.4	0.8
Tartare	*1oz/28g*	*84*	*6.9*	*299*	*1.3*	*17.9*	*24.6*	*0*
Tartare, Colman's*	1 Tbsp/15g	45	3.7	290	1.5	17	24	0.6
Tartare, Mild & Creamy, Heinz*	1 Tbsp/15g	47	4.2	312	0.9	13.4	28.3	0.1
Tartare, Rich, Colman's*	1 Tsp/5ml	14	1.2	284	1.2	17	23	0.6
Tartare, Sainsbury's*	1 Serving/20ml	94	9.8	469	0.4	5.8	49	1
Tartare, Tesco*	1 Tbsp/15g	47	3.9	312	0.7	18.7	25.8	1.1
Teriyaki, Asda*	1 Serving/98g	99	0.1	101	2.1	23	0.1	0

S

	Measure INFO/WEIGHT	per Measure KCAL	FAT	Nutrition Values per 100g / 100ml KCAL	PROT	CARB	FAT	FIBRE
SAUCE								
Teriyaki, Japanese Grill, Kikkoman*	1 Serving/15ml	24	0	158	4.5	30.8	0.1	0
Teriyaki, Lee Kum Kee*	1 Serving/15g	27	0	178	2.2	42.4	0	0.5
Teriyaki, Stir Fry, Blue Dragon*	1 Pack/120g	131	0.2	109	0.9	25.9	0.2	0
Teriyaki, Stir Fry, Fresh Ideas, Tesco*	1 Serving/25g	33	0.6	133	1.1	26.9	2.3	0
Thai Curry, Yellow, Loyd Grossman*	1 Serving/100g	111	7.5	111	1.7	9.1	7.5	1
Thai, Sweet Chilli, Blue Dragon*	1 Serving/15g	28	0.1	188	0.5	45.5	0.6	0
Tikka Masala, Cooking, HL, Tesco*	¼ Jar/125g	78	3.1	62	0.4	9	2.5	0.7
Tikka Masala, GFY, Asda*	½ Jar/250g	190	8	76	2.9	9	3.2	0.5
Tikka Masala, Hot & Spicy in Glass Jar, Patak's*	1 Jar/350g	332	23.8	95	1.7	6.5	6.8	1.7
Tikka Masala, LC, Tesco*	¼ Jar/125g	100	3.4	80	2	11.1	2.7	1.2
Tikka Masala, Medium, Cooking, Sharwood's*	1/3 Jar/140g	150	9.7	107	1.3	9.7	6.9	0.5
Tikka Masala, Ready Made, Average	*1 Sm Jar/350g*	*422*	*28.8*	*121*	*2*	*9.6*	*8.2*	*1.2*
Toffee, GFY, Asda*	1 Serving/5g	15	0.1	306	2.2	68	2.8	0
Toffee, Luxury, Rowse*	1 Serving/20g	67	0.7	336	1.9	73.9	3.7	0.4
Tomato & Basil, Fresh, Organic, Waitrose*	¼ Pot/175g	77	3	44	1	6.2	1.7	0.8
Tomato & Marscapone, Finest, Tesco*	1 Serving/350g	270	17.5	77	2.7	5.4	5	0.8
Tomato & Marscapone, Italiano, Tesco*	1 Serving/175g	194	15.2	111	2.8	5.4	8.7	0.6
Tomato & Basil Sauce, Fresh, Tesco*	1 Pot/500g	245	9	49	1.5	6.8	1.8	0.8
Tomato & Basil, for Meatballs, Dolmio*	¼ Jar/125g	48	0.2	38	1.5	6.9	0.2	1.3
Tomato & Basil, Italian, Fresh, Asda*	½ Tub/175g	107	5.7	60	1.5	6.1	3.2	0.6
Tomato & Basil, Italian, Sainsbury's*	½ Pot/175g	102	4.4	58	1.6	7	2.5	0.7
Tomato & Garlic for Pasta, Asda*	¼ Jar/125g	80	2.9	64	2.7	8	2.3	1.1
Tomato & Garlic, for Meatballs, Dolmio*	1 Portion/125g	46	0.1	37	1.6	6.5	0.1	0
Tomato, & Aubergine, Greek Style, Eridanous, Lidl*	½ Jar/145g	161	10.4	111	1.6	8.3	7.2	3.3
Tomato, Heinz*	1 Tbsp/17g	18	0	103	0.9	24.1	0.1	0.7
Tomato, Pizza Topping, Napolina*	1 Serving/70g	34	1.5	49	0.9	6.3	2.2	0.6
Vindaloo, Hot, Patak's*	1 Jar/540g	643	46.4	119	1.7	8.5	8.6	2.1
Vongole, Sainsbury's*	½ Pot/150g	106	4.5	71	3.1	7.8	3	1.9
Watercress, & Stilton, Creamy for Fish, Schwartz*	1 Pack/300g	141	12.3	47	0.6	2	4.1	0.7
White Wine & Mushroom, BGTY, Sainsbury's*	¼ Jar/125g	81	2.5	65	2.8	9	2	0.3
White Wine & Cream, Cook in, Classic, Homepride*	¼ Can/125g	101	5.1	81	1	8	4.1	0.4
White Wine & Parsley, Pour Over, Loyd Grossman*	½ Sachet/85g	94	7.9	111	1	5.6	9.3	0.5
White, Savoury, Made with Semi-Skimmed Milk	*1oz/28g*	*36*	*2.2*	*128*	*4.2*	*11.1*	*7.8*	*0.2*
White, Savoury, Made with Whole Milk	*1oz/28g*	*42*	*2.9*	*150*	*4.1*	*10.9*	*10.3*	*0.2*
Worcestershire Sauce, Sainsbury's*	1 Tbsp/15ml	16	0	107	0.7	23.3	0.1	0.3
Worcestershire, Average	*1 Tsp/5g*	*3*	*0*	*65*	*1.4*	*15.5*	*0.1*	*0*
Worcestershire, Lea & Perrins*	1 Tsp/5ml	5	0	96	0.8	21	0.9	0
SAUCE MIX								
Beef Bourguignon, Colman's*	1 Pack/40g	136	0.8	340	7	72	2	3
Beef Stroganoff, Colman's*	1 Pack/40g	140	3.6	350	11.6	56.1	8.9	2.7
Bread, Made Up, Colman's*	1 Serving/75ml	70	1.5	95	5	14	2	0.6
Cheddar Cheese, Colman's*	1 Pack/40g	164	6	410	19	51	15	2
Cheddar Cheese, Dry Mix, Schwartz*	1 Pack/40g	144	3	361	18.4	55.1	7.4	2.3
Cheese Flavour, Dairy Free, Free & Easy*	4 Teasp/15g	4	0.1	26	0.6	4.9	0.4	0.3
Cheese, Made Up with Skimmed Milk	*1 Serving/60g*	*47*	*1.4*	*78*	*5.4*	*9.5*	*2.3*	*0*
Chicken Chasseur, Schwartz*	1 Pack/40g	126	1.8	316	9.6	59.1	4.6	6.8
Chilli Con Carne, Asda*	1 Sachet/50g	157	0.8	314	7	68	1.6	2.5
Chilli Con Carne, Recipe Mix, Bramwells, Aldi*	1 Pack/38g	130	1.1	341	6.2	70	2.8	5.3
Chilli Con Carne, Recipe Mix, Schwartz*	1 Pack/41g	133	1.5	324	8.2	60.8	3.6	0
Chip Shop Curry, Dry Weight, Bisto*	1 Dtsp/9g	38	1.6	427	3.4	63.5	17.7	1.3
Cream, for Meatballs, Ikea*	1 Pack/40g	179	9.4	448	9.6	49.2	23.6	0
Dauphinoise Potato Bake, Schwartz*	1 Pack/40g	161	10.5	402	6.8	34.7	26.3	15.8
Four Cheese, Colman's*	1 Pack/35g	127	3.9	362	17.1	48.4	11.1	1.8

	Measure INFO/WEIGHT	per Measure KCAL	FAT	Nutrition Values per 100g / 100ml KCAL	PROT	CARB	FAT	FIBRE
SAUCE MIX								
Hollandaise, Colman's*	1 Pack/28g	104	3.1	372	6.4	61.6	11.1	1.8
Hollandaise, Made Up, Schwartz*	1 Serving/79g	58	2	73	3.9	8.7	2.5	0
Lemon Butter for Fish, Schwartz*	1 Pack/38g	136	3	357	6.1	65.3	8	5.8
Mixed Herbs for Chicken, So Juicy, Maggi*	1 Pack/34g	97	1	285	8.3	53.8	2.8	5.5
Paprika For Chicken, So Juicy, Maggi*	1 Pack/34g	91	1.4	267	8.8	45.5	4	7.1
Parsley & Chive for Fish, Schwartz*	1 Pack/38g	132	3.2	348	9	58.9	8.5	7.7
Parsley, Creamy, Made Up, Schwartz*	1 Serving/79g	59	2	75	4.2	8.7	2.5	0.3
Pepper, Creamy, Schwartz*	1 Pack/25g	86	1.7	342	17.9	52	6.9	7
Peppercorn, Made Up with Water, CBY, Asda*	1 Serving/63ml	52	3.9	84	0.7	5.4	6.2	1.7
Peppercorn, Mild, Creamy, Schwartz*	1 Pack/25g	88	2.2	352	13.8	55	8.6	5
Savoury Mince, Schwartz*	1 Pack/35g	108	0.7	310	14.6	58.3	2	1.8
Shepherd's Pie, Schwartz*	1 Pack/38g	118	0.9	311	8.2	60.3	2.3	11.1
Shepherds Pie, Bramwells*	1 Pack/50g	168	3	336	8.6	62	6	6.9
Spaghetti Bolognese, Colman's*	1 Pack/40g	120	0.4	300	8.9	64.1	0.9	5.2
Spaghetti Bolognese, Schwartz*	1 Pack/40g	114	0.6	285	9.2	59	1.6	7
Spaghetti Carbonara, Schwartz*	1 Pack/32g	135	6.4	421	10.4	49.4	20.1	7.2
Stroganoff, Beef, Schwartz*	1 Pack/35g	125	3.6	358	15.6	50.8	10.3	4.4
Stroganoff, Mushroom, Schwartz*	1 Pack/35g	113	1.9	324	10	59.2	5.3	9.6
Thickening Granules, McDougalls*	1 Tbsp/10g	46	1.9	463	0	73.7	18.7	0
Tuna Napolitana, Schwartz*	1 Pack/30g	107	3.9	357	10.3	49.6	13.1	0.5
White, Dry Weight, Bisto*	1 Dtsp/9g	45	2.5	496	3.2	57.4	28.2	0.4
White, Instant, Made Up, Sainsbury's*	1 Serving/90ml	65	2.5	72	0.8	10.9	2.8	0.1
White, Made Up with Semi-Skimmed Milk	**1oz/28g**	**20**	**0.7**	**73**	**4**	**9.6**	**2.4**	**0**
White, Made Up with Skimmed Milk	**1oz/28g**	**17**	**0.3**	**59**	**4**	**9.6**	**0.9**	**0**
White, Savoury, Colman's*	1 Pack/25g	105	3.8	420	9	63	15	2
SAUERKRAUT								
Average	**1oz/28g**	**3**	**0**	**11**	**1.1**	**1.6**	**0**	**0.9**
with Wine, Bavarian Style, Hengstenberg*	1 Portion/100g	22	0.1	22	1.5	1.9	0.1	0
SAUSAGE								
Bake, Boston Bean, Microwaved, Slimzone, Asda*	1 Pack/456g	397	8.2	87	8.2	7.2	1.8	4.8
Beef, Average	**1 Sausage/60g**	**151**	**11.1**	**252**	**14.5**	**7**	**18.5**	**0.6**
Bierwurst, Average	**1 Slice/10g**	**25**	**2.1**	**252**	**14.4**	**1**	**21.2**	**0**
Billy Bear, Kids, Tesco*	1 Slice/20g	37	2.2	185	13.7	7.5	11.2	0.4
Bockwurst, Average	**1 Sausage/45g**	**114**	**10.4**	**253**	**10.8**	**0.8**	**23**	**0**
Bratwurst, Frozen, Lidl*	1 Sausage/80g	235	21.4	294	12.8	0.5	26.8	0
Bratwurst, Nuremberg, Dulano, Lidl*	1 Sausage/22g	77	7	349	14	1	32	0.5
Chicken, & Turkey, Morrisons*	1 Sausage/56.6g	86	4.1	152	16	5.8	7.2	1.1
Chicken, Debbie & Andrews*	2 Sausages/104g	141	4.5	136	22.4	1.8	4.3	0.5
Chicken, Italia, Grilled, Heck*	1 Sausage/34g	36	0.8	106	18.7	1.5	2.3	0
Chicken, Manor Farm*	1 Sausage/65g	126	8.1	194	13.7	6.6	12.5	1.2
Chicken, Sundried Tomoato & Basil, As Consumed, Mor*	1 Sausage/34g	43	1.3	127	12.4	9.6	3.9	2.2
Chipolata, Average	**1 Sausage/28g**	**81**	**6.5**	**291**	**12.1**	**8.7**	**23.1**	**0.7**
Chipolata, Chicken, Smoky Paprika, Grilled, Heck*	1 Chipolata/34g	49	0.8	142	25	6.4	2.2	0
Chipolata, Chicken, Zesty, Grilled, Heck*	1 Chipolata/34g	50	0.6	145	25.2	8.1	1.9	0
Chipolata, Lamb, & Rosemary, Tesco*	1 Sausage/31.6g	69	4.9	218	11.3	8.3	15.5	0
Chipolata, Pork, & Honey, Finest, Tesco*	2 Sausages/64g	170	12.3	265	14	8.7	19.2	0.7
Chipolata, Premium, Average	**1 Serving/80g**	**187**	**13.8**	**234**	**14.8**	**4.7**	**17.3**	**1.2**
Chipolatas, Chicken, Mediterranean, As Served, Mor*	2 Chipolatas/60g	76	2.3	127	12.4	9.6	3.9	2.2
Chorizo, Average	**1 Serving/80g**	**250**	**19.4**	**313**	**21.1**	**2.6**	**24.2**	**0.2**
Chorizo, Lean, Average	**1 Sausage/67g**	**131**	**9.2**	**195**	**15.7**	**2.3**	**13.7**	**0.8**
Chorizo, Mini, Snack Size, Noel, Tesco*	1 Pack/80g	402	34.4	502	26	2.8	43	0
Chorizo, with Red Peppers, Rich & Smokey, Waitrose*	1 Sausage/49g	136	9.8	275	19.8	3.9	19.9	0.5
Cocktail, Average	**1 Sausage/7g**	**23**	**1.9**	**323**	**12.1**	**8.6**	**26.7**	**0.9**

S

	Measure INFO/WEIGHT	per Measure KCAL	FAT	Nutrition Values per 100g / 100ml KCAL	PROT	CARB	FAT	FIBRE
SAUSAGE								
Cumberland, Average	1 Sausage/57g	167	13	293	13.8	8.6	22.8	0.8
Cumberland, Healthy Range, Average	1 Sausage/53g	75	2.1	142	17.4	9	4	0.9
Debrecziner, Spicy Smoked, Gebirgsjager*	1 Sausage/37g	118	10.4	320	16	1	28	0
Extrawurst, German, Waitrose*	1 Slice/28.3g	80	7.1	281	13	1	25	0
Free From, Wheat & Gulten, Sainsbury's*	1 Serving/23g	61	4.8	268	15.2	4.5	21	1.8
French Saucisson, Tesco*	1 Slice/5g	19	1.4	379	26.7	4.1	28.4	0
Garlic, Average	1 Slice/11g	25	2	227	15.7	0.8	18.2	0
German, Extrawurst, Selection, Sainsbury's*	1 Slice/3g	9	0.8	279	13.1	0.5	25	0.1
German, Schinkenwurst, Selection, Sainsbury's*	1 Slice/3g	8	0.7	251	13.1	0.3	21.9	0.1
German, Selection, Lidl*	1 Slice/6g	15	1.4	250	11	0.5	22.8	0.5
Irish, Average	1 Sausage/40g	119	8.3	298	10.7	17.2	20.7	0.7
Lamb, & Mint, M&S*	1oz/28g	63	4.6	225	13.3	6.6	16.3	1.7
Lincolnshire, Average	1 Sausage/42g	122	9.1	291	14.6	9.2	21.8	0.6
Lincolnshire, Healthy Range, Average	1 Sausage/50g	89	4.3	177	15.8	9	8.6	0.8
Lorne, Average	1 Sausage/25g	78	5.8	312	10.8	16	23.1	0.6
Merguez	1 Merguez/55g	165	14.3	300	16	0.6	26	0
Paprika, Mediterranean Style, Waitrose*	1 Sausage/67g	190	16.1	283	12.1	4.6	24	1.9
Pigs in Blankets, Cooked, Morrisons*	1 Roll/22g	52	2.9	235	22.9	5.2	13.3	1.5
Pigs In Blankets, Cooked, Sainsbury's*	1 Roll/15g	42	2.8	280	3.1	11.2	18.5	1
Polish Kabanos, Sainsbury's*	1 Sausage/25g	92	7.6	366	23	0.1	30.4	0.1
Pork & Beef, Average	1 Sausage/45g	133	10.2	295	8.7	13.6	22.7	0.5
Pork & Herb, Average	1 Sausage/75g	231	19.5	308	13.2	5.4	26	0.4
Pork & Herb, Healthy Range, Average	1 Sausage/59g	75	1.4	126	16	10.8	2.4	1.1
Pork & Tomato, Grilled, Average	1 Sausage/47g	127	9.7	273	13.9	7.5	20.8	0.4
Pork & Apple, Average	1 Sausage/57g	146	10.7	256	14.5	7.5	18.8	1.9
Pork, & Caramelised Onion, Thick, Cooked, Morrisons*	1 Sausage/45g	125	8.3	279	20.1	7.1	18.6	0.9
Pork, & Leek, Thick, Signature, Morrisons*	1 Sausage/55g	127	8.6	231	20.5	1.5	15.6	1.4
Pork, & Pepper, Spicy, Summer Selection, Sainsbury's*	1 Sausage/33g	86	5.7	260	20.1	6	17.3	1.6
Pork, & Sweet Chilli, Waitrose*	1 Sausage/67g	151	10.1	226	15.5	6.9	15.1	2.7
Pork, Average	1 Sausage/45g	139	11.2	309	11.9	9.8	25	0.8
Pork, Battered, Fishnchickn*	1 Sausage/100g	307	17.5	307	11.9	9.2	17.5	0
Pork, Battered, Thick, Average	1oz/28g	126	10.2	448	17.3	21.7	36.3	2
Pork, Beetroot, & Bramley Apple, Mor*	2 Sausages/118g	205	11.7	174	10	10	9.9	2.4
Pork, Extra Lean, Average	1 Sausage/54g	84	3.7	155	17.3	6.1	6.8	0.8
Pork, Frozen, Fried	1oz/28g	88	6.9	316	13.8	10	24.8	0
Pork, Frozen, Grilled	1oz/28g	81	5.9	289	14.8	10.5	21.2	0
Pork, Garlic & Herb, Average	1 Sausage/76g	203	16.5	268	12	6	21.8	1.2
Pork, Premium, Average	1 Sausage/74g	191	13.6	258	14.9	8.3	18.4	1
Pork, Reduced Fat, Chilled, Grilled	1 Sausage/45g	104	6.2	230	16.2	10.8	13.8	1.5
Pork, Reduced Fat, Healthy Range, Average	1 Sausage/57g	86	3.4	151	15.6	9	6	0.9
Pork, Roasted Pepper, & Chilli, COU, M&S*	1 Sausage/57g	57	1.1	100	15.2	7.1	2	2.1
Pork, Skinless, Average	1oz/28g	81	6.6	291	11.7	8.2	23.6	0.6
Pork, Super Green Veg & Lentil, As Consumed, Mor*	1 Serving/117g	320	18.2	192	12.2	9.7	10.9	3
Pork, Thick, Average	1 Sausage/39g	115	8.7	296	13.3	10	22.4	1
Pork, Thick, Reduced Fat, Healthy Range, Average	1 Sausage/52g	90	3.8	172	14	12.3	7.4	0.8
Premium, Chilled, Fried	1oz/28g	77	5.8	275	15.8	6.7	20.7	0
Premium, Chilled, Grilled	1oz/28g	82	6.3	292	16.8	6.3	22.4	0
Saveloy, Unbattered, Takeaway, Average	1 Saveloy/65g	192	14.5	296	13.8	10.8	22.3	0.8
Smoked, Average	1 Sausage/174g	588	52.2	338	13	4	30	0
Toulouse, M&S*	1 Sausage/57g	123	8.9	215	12.4	5.8	15.6	1.3
Toulouse, TTD, Sainsbury's*	1 Sausage/45g	146	11.5	324	21.4	2.3	25.5	0.8
Turkey & Chicken, Average	1 Sausage/57g	126	8.2	222	14.4	8.2	14.6	1.8
Turkey, Average	1 Sausage/57g	90	4.6	157	15.7	6.3	8	0

S

	Measure INFO/WEIGHT	per Measure KCAL	per Measure FAT	Nutrition Values per 100g / 100ml KCAL	PROT	CARB	FAT	FIBRE
SAUSAGE								
Tuscan, M&S*	1 Sausage/66g	145	10.6	220	14.9	4.6	16	0.6
Vegetarian, Bangers, Quorn*	1 Sausage/50g	58	2.4	116	11.7	6.6	4.8	3
Vegetarian, Best of British, Chef's Selection, Quorn*	1 Sausage/60g	111	5.7	185	11	12	9.5	3.5
Vegetarian, Cocktail, Quorn*	1 Sausage/15g	31	1.7	206	12.4	11.6	11.3	4.3
Vegetarian, Quorn*	1 Sausage/40g	71	3.1	177	10.2	13.4	7.8	6.2
Vegetarian, Tomato & Basil, Quorn*	1 Sausage/50g	51	1.2	102	14.3	6	2.3	2.8
Venison & Pork, Waitrose*	1 Sausage/64g	93	4	146	16.5	5.3	6.3	1.1
Venison & Red Wine, TTD, Sainsbury's*	1 Sausage/39g	88	5.2	228	20.7	5.8	13.6	1.7
Wiejska, Polish, Sainsbury's*	1/8 Pack/50g	78	4.5	157	18.7	0.4	9	0.5
Wild Boar	*1 Sausage/85g*	*220*	*17*	*259*	*16.5*	*1.2*	*20*	*0*
SAUSAGE & MASH								
2 British Pork & Rich Onion Gravy, M&S*	1 Pack/400g	340	6.8	85	5.7	12.2	1.7	1.3
Bangers, Morrisons*	1 Pack/300g	306	14.7	102	3	12.3	4.9	0.8
British Classic, Tesco*	1 Pack/450g	675	42.8	150	5.1	11.1	9.5	0.9
Chef Select, Lidl*	1 Pack/450g	472	26.6	105	4.7	7.6	5.9	1.4
Classic Kitchen, Tesco*	1 Meal/447g	532	25.5	119	3.7	12.5	5.7	1.5
Everyday, Value, Tesco*	1 Pack/400g	400	16.4	100	3.6	11.5	4.1	1.2
LC, Tesco*	1 Pack/400g	360	8.8	90	4.4	11.8	2.2	1.4
Lincolnshire, & Root Vegetable Mash, Weight Watchers*	1 Pack/380g	294	8	77	5.3	8.6	2.1	1.4
Vegetarian, Tesco*	1 Pack/410g	398	15.6	97	4.6	11.1	3.8	2
with Onion Gravy, Bangers, Classic, Sainsbury's*	1 Pack/450g	588	27.4	133	5.1	12.9	6.2	2.5
with Red Wine & Onion Gravy, BGTY, Sainsbury's*	1 Pack/379.5g	315	7.2	83	5	11.4	1.9	2
SAUSAGE MEAT								
Pork, Average	*1oz/28g*	*96*	*8.2*	*344*	*9.9*	*10.2*	*29.4*	*0.6*
SAUSAGE ROLL								
BGTY, Sainsbury's*	1 Roll/65g	200	11.4	308	9.6	27.9	17.6	1.4
Buffet, HE, Tesco*	1 Roll/30g	83	3.8	278	9.6	31.2	12.8	1.5
Cocktail, Average	*1 Roll/15g*	*57*	*3.7*	*378*	*8.9*	*29.4*	*24.9*	*1.9*
Cumberland, CBY, Asda*	1 Roll/66g	201	10.9	304	8.3	28.9	16.5	3.1
Frozen, Greggs Iceland Exclusive*	1 Roll /103g	349	24.7	339	8	22	24	1.5
Jumbo, Sainsbury's*	1 Roll/145g	492	34.4	339	8.2	23.2	23.7	1.5
Kingsize, Pork Farms*	½ Roll/50g	241	15.9	483	10.5	39.9	31.8	0
Large, Freshbake*	1 Roll/52g	153	9.5	294	6.6	25.9	18.3	4.6
Mini, 40 Pack, Tesco*	1 Roll/16g	60	4	375	8.4	28.5	25.1	2.5
Mini, Oven Baked, Greggs, Iceland*	1 Roll/25g	76	6	303	7.9	21	24	0
Mini, Tesco*	1 Roll/15g	53	3.7	356	9	23.9	24.9	1.5
Mini, Waitrose*	1 Roll/35g	124	9.2	353	13	16.1	26.3	1
Party Size, Value, Tesco*	1 Roll/12g	40	2.7	335	6.6	26	22.5	1.5
Party, Sainsbury's*	1 Roll/13g	54	4	422	8.7	26.7	31.1	1.2
Pork, Morrisons*	1 Roll/70g	195	9	278	9.6	31.2	12.8	1.5
Pork, Party, Ovenbaked, Iceland*	2 Rolls/63g	190	11.4	301	11.2	22.8	18	1.6
Puff Pastry	*1 Med/60g*	*230*	*16.6*	*383*	*9.9*	*25.4*	*27.6*	*1*
Snack Size, Tesco*	1 Roll/32g	118	8.8	369	9.1	21.7	27.4	2.3
Snack, GFY, Asda*	1 Roll/34g	112	7	329	9.4	26.5	20.6	0.9
TTD, Sainsbury's*	1 Roll/115g	440	31.9	383	11.9	21.3	27.8	2
SAUSAGE ROLL VEGETARIAN								
Linda McCartney*	1 Roll/52g	145	7.1	278	13.1	26	13.7	1.6
Mini, Linda McCartney*	1 Roll/14g	41	2.2	293	11.3	23.7	15.8	5.2
Vegetarian, Chilled, Quorn*	1 Roll/130g	293	12.1	225	12.3	21.2	9.3	3.8
SAUSAGE VEGETARIAN								
Asda*	1 Sausage/43g	81	3.9	189	20	7	9	2.9
Braai Flavour, Fry's Special Vegetarian*	1 Sausage/62.5g	86	4.4	138	16.5	10	7	4
Cumberland, Cauldron Foods*	1 Sausage/46g	75	4	163	14	6.5	8.6	2

S

	Measure INFO/WEIGHT	per Measure KCAL	FAT	Nutrition Values per 100g / 100ml KCAL	PROT	CARB	FAT	FIBRE
SAUSAGE VEGETARIAN								
Cumberland, Meat Free, Quorn*	1 Sausage/50g	86	3.5	172	13.5	12	7	3.5
Cumberland, Waitrose*	1 Sausage/50g	80	3.4	160	12.6	12.3	6.7	2.4
Grilled, Linda McCartney*	1 Sausage/50g	80	2.7	160	17.9	7.5	5.4	5
Italian, Tofurky*	1 Sausage/63g	167	8	270	29	12	13	8
Leek & Potato, Soysages, Dragonfly Foods*	1 Sausage/50g	89	3.7	178	3.2	22.2	7.4	5.1
Lincolnshire, Asda*	1 Sausage/56g	96	4.5	172	17	8	8	1.4
Lincolnshire, Cauldron Foods*	1 Sausage/46g	84	4.5	182	16.1	5.5	9.8	3.6
Lincolnshire, Frozen, Tesco*	1 Sausage/50g	78	2.5	155	15.5	10.8	5	3
Morrisons*	1 Serving/90g	149	8.8	165	17.2	2	9.8	8.1
Outrageously Succulent, Grilled, Linda Mccartney's*	2 Sausage/88g	148	5.3	168	18.2	8.7	6	3
Patties, Quorn*	1 Pattie/42g	53	2	127	12.8	5.8	4.9	4.7
Spinach, Leek & Cheese, Gourmet, Wicken Fen*	1 Sausage/46g	92	4.7	201	10.3	17	10.2	1.9
SCALLOPS								
Breaded, Thai Style with Plum Sauce, Finest, Tesco*	1 Serving/210g	401	14.7	191	11.5	20.6	7	0.8
Lemon Grass & Ginger, Tesco*	½ Pack/112g	90	1.1	80	15.2	2.5	1	0.6
Queen, & Minted Pea, Oven Cooked, TTD, Sainsbury's*	½ Pack/92g	98	2.3	107	10.7	9.1	2.5	2.8
Raw, Bay or Sea with Roe, Average	*1 Scallop/15g*	*13*	*0.1*	*88*	*16.8*	*2.4*	*0.8*	*0*
Steamed, Average	*1oz/28g*	*33*	*0.4*	*118*	*23.2*	*3.4*	*1.4*	*0*
SCAMPI								
& Chips, Chunky, Finest, Tesco*	1 Pack/280g	420	15.4	150	5.9	18.3	5.5	1.4
& Chips, with Peas	*1 Serving/490g*	*822*	*43.6*	*168*	*10.1*	*11.3*	*8.9*	*1.2*
Bites, Everyday, Value, Tesco*	½ Pack/125g	262	10	210	9.4	23.4	8	1.2
Breaded, Baked, Average	*½ Pack/255g*	*565*	*27.4*	*222*	*10.7*	*20.5*	*10.7*	*1*
Breaded, Fried in Oil, Average	*1 Serving/100g*	*237*	*13.6*	*237*	*9.4*	*20.5*	*13.6*	*0*
Provencale	*1 Serving/100g*	*500*	*49*	*500*	*7*	*4*	*49*	*1*
Wholetail, Crispy, in Breadcrumbs, Ocean Trader, Lidl*	½ Pack/125g	270	10.8	216	11.9	22.2	8.6	1.1
Wholetail, Jumbo, Oven Baked, Gastro, Youngs*	1 Serving/103g	228	10.1	221	9.4	23	9.8	1.6
SCHNAPPS								
Vodkat, Intercontinental Brands Ltd*	1 Serving/25ml	31	0	124	0	0.8	0	0
SCONE								
All Butter, Sultana, TTD, Sainsbury's*	1 Scone/73g	248	8.1	340	7.7	51.3	11.1	1.9
All Butter, Tesco*	1 Scone/60g	225	8.2	375	8.2	53.5	13.7	0.9
Cheese & Black Pepper, Mini, M&S*	1 Scone/18g	67	3.3	370	10.2	41.1	18.3	1.7
Cheese, Average	*1 Scone/40g*	*145*	*7.1*	*363*	*10.1*	*43.2*	*17.8*	*1.6*
Cheese, Cornish, TTD, Sainsbury's*	1 Scone/74g	267	13.8	361	12.3	36.1	18.6	2.3
Cherry, Double Butter, Genesis Crafty*	1 Scone/63g	198	4.8	314	6.8	54.5	7.6	1.4
Cherry, Genesis Crafty*	1 Scone/81g	226	5.8	279	4.9	50.5	7.1	0
Cherry, M&S*	1 Scone/60g	202	7.3	337	6.9	49.7	12.2	1.9
Clotted Cream, Cornish, TTD, Sainsbury's*	1 Scone/70g	269	12.7	384	8.4	46.6	18.2	2.1
Devon, M&S*	1 Scone/59g	225	9.6	380	7.1	50.8	16.2	1.5
Fresh Cream with Strawberry Jam, Tesco*	1 Scone/83g	290	15.6	352	4.7	40.7	18.9	1.1
Fruit, Aldi*	1 Scone/65g	239	5.8	367	6.3	64.4	9	1.6
Fruit, Average	*1 Scone/40g*	*126*	*3.9*	*316*	*7.3*	*52.9*	*9.8*	*0*
Fruit, Smart Price, Asda*	1 Scone/41g	139	4.1	338	7	55	10	3
Fruit, Waitrose*	1 Scone/59g	190	4.8	325	6.3	56.5	8.2	2.2
Plain, All Butter, Sainsbury's*	1 Scone/58g	213	7.4	366	8.1	54.1	12.7	1.6
Plain, Average	*1 Scone/40g*	*145*	*5.8*	*362*	*7.2*	*53.8*	*14.6*	*1.9*
Plain, Genesis Crafty*	1 Scone/74g	227	7.4	307	6.8	49.1	10	0
Potato, Average	*1 Scone/40g*	*118*	*5.7*	*296*	*5.1*	*39.1*	*14.3*	*1.6*
Potato, Mother's Pride*	1 Scone/37g	77	0.8	207	4.7	42	2.2	4.3
Red Berry, Mixed, Finest, Tesco*	1 Scone/110g	344	9.5	313	7.8	50.1	8.6	1.9
Strawberry, Fresh Cream, BGTY, Sainsbury's*	1 Scone/50g	154	5.6	309	5.1	47	11.2	1.1
Sultana, Finest, Tesco*	1 Scone/70g	238	7.6	340	8.9	50.9	10.9	2.1

S

	Measure INFO/WEIGHT	KCAL	FAT	Nutrition Values per 100g / 100ml				
				KCAL	PROT	CARB	FAT	FIBRE
SCONE								
Sultana, M&S*	1 Scone/66g	231	8.2	350	6.5	53	12.5	2
Sultana, Rowan Hill Bakery, Lidl*	1 Scone/60g	220	7.2	367	7.1	57	12	1.1
Sultana, Tesco*	1 Scone/60g	189	5	315	7.1	52.5	8.4	2.6
Sultana, TTD, Sainsbury's*	1 Scone/70g	239	8.1	341	6.5	52.9	11.5	2.6
Sultana, Value, Tesco*	1 Scone/40g	134	4	335	6.5	53.8	10.1	2.7
Tattie, Scottish, Nick Nairn's*	1 Scone/21g	42	0.3	199	4	34.7	1.6	0.7
Wholemeal	*1 Scone/40g*	*130*	*5.8*	*326*	*8.7*	*43.1*	*14.4*	*5.2*
Wholemeal, Fruit	*1 Scone/40g*	*130*	*5.1*	*324*	*8.1*	*47.2*	*12.8*	*4.9*
SEA BASS								
Cooked, Dry Heat, Average	*1 Fillet/100g*	*124*	*2.6*	*124*	*23.6*	*0*	*2.6*	*0*
Fillets with Lemon & Parsley Butter, Iceland*	½ Pack/110g	197	13.2	179	17.6	0.1	12	0.1
Fillets, Caramelised Ginger & Lime Butter, Sainsbury's*	1 Fillet/115g	258	18.1	224	19.9	0.5	15.7	0.5
Fillets, with Butter, Cooked, Tesco*	1 Fillet/86g	189	13	220	19.4	1	15.1	1.7
Raw, Fillet, Average	*1 Fillet/95g*	*108*	*3.4*	*113*	*20.3*	*0*	*3.5*	*0.1*
SEA BREAM								
Fillet, Cooked, Dry Heat, Average	*1 Serving/100g*	*124*	*3*	*124*	*24*	*0*	*3*	*0*
Fillets, Raw, Average	*1oz/28g*	*27*	*0.8*	*96*	*17.5*	*0*	*2.9*	*0*
SEAFOOD								
Cocktail, Average	*1oz/28g*	*24*	*0.4*	*87*	*15.6*	*2.9*	*1.5*	*0*
Selection, Asda*	1 Pack/240g	173	1.9	72	13.4	2.9	0.8	0
Selection, Fresh, Tesco*	1 Pack/234g	187	2.3	80	17.7	0.1	1	0
Selection, Mussels, King Prawns & Squid, Frozen, Tesco*	½ Pack/200g	140	3	70	13.7	0.1	1.5	0
Selection, Sainsbury's*	½ Pack/125g	85	1.2	68	14.6	0.8	1	2.5
SEAFOOD STICKS								
Average	*1 Stick/15g*	*16*	*0*	*106*	*8*	*18.4*	*0.2*	*0.2*
with Cocktail Dip, Asda*	1 Pot/95g	126	4.8	133	6	16	5	0.1
SEASONING MIX								
All Purpose, Dunns River*	1 Tbsp/15g	37	1.5	248	8.3	26.7	9.9	9.3
Cajun, Perfect Shake, As Sold, Schwartz*	1 Tbsp/1g	2	0.1	249	9.9	27.2	7	19
Chicken Provencal, Schwartz*	1 Pack/35g	104	0.7	296	9.3	55.3	2	9.9
Garlic, For Chicken, So Juicy, Maggi*	1 Pack/30g	95	0.8	316	9.4	58.9	2.8	8.7
Garlic, Papyrus Sheets, SoTender, Maggi*	1 Sheet/5.8g	25	1.9	438	6.3	24.4	32.5	11.4
Italian Herb, Schwartz*	1 Tsp/1g	3	0	338	11	64.5	4	0
Italian Herbs, Papyrus Sheets, SoTender, Maggi*	1 Sheet/5.9g	26	2	440	7.3	22.1	34.1	7.7
Jamaican Jerk Chicken, Recipe, Schwartz*	1 Pack/27g	75	0.8	276	9.8	69.8	3	17.2
Lamb Hot Pot, Colman's*	¼ Pack/10g	32	0.2	320	12	61	1.5	4
Lemon & Herb, for Chicken, Cook in Bag, Average	*1 Bag/34g*	*121*	*1.9*	*356*	*10.8*	*63.7*	*5.5*	*4.1*
Mediterranean Chicken, Season & Shake, Colman's*	1 Pack/33g	99	0.7	300	10.3	56.8	2.1	5.9
Mediterranean, for Chicken, Cook in Bag, Average	*1 Bag/33g*	*99*	*0.7*	*302*	*10.6*	*56.6*	*2*	*7*
Mexican Chicken, As Sold, So Juicy, Maggi*	1 Pack/40g	123	1.7	308	7.4	57.2	4.2	6
One Pan Rice Meal, for Chicken, Old El Paso*	¼ Pack/89g	203	4.3	228	4.4	40.9	4.8	1.7
Paprika, for Chicken, Cook in Bag, Average	*1 Bag/34g*	*96*	*1.3*	*283*	*12.3*	*45.8*	*4*	*8.1*
Paprika, Papyrus Sheets, SoTender, Maggi*	1 Sheet/5.8g	25	2	431	9.1	12.2	35.2	14.5
Potato Wedges, Garlic & Herb, Schwartz*	1 Pack/38g	106	1.9	278	11.4	47.1	4.9	11.7
Shepherd's Pie, Colman's*	1 Pack/50g	170	1	340	13	60	2	5
Smoked Paprika Chicken, As Sold, Schwartz*	1 Pack/28g	87	1.6	309	10.3	44.4	5.7	0
Spaghetti Bolognaise, Naturally Tasty, As Sold, Knorr*	1 Pack/43g	132	1.8	306	8.5	54	4.3	12
Taco, Old El Paso*	¼ Pack/9g	30	0.4	334	5.5	69	4	0
SEAWEED								
Chuka Wakame, Daiwa*	1 Serving/100g	70	3.3	70	1.3	8.8	3.3	1.4
Crispy, Average	*1oz/28g*	*182*	*17.3*	*651*	*7.5*	*15.6*	*61.9*	*7*
Mixed, Trimmed, Sea Vegetables, Waitrose*	1 Pack/80g	15	0.2	19	2.1	1	0.3	1.8
Nori, Dried, Raw	*1oz/28g*	*38*	*0.4*	*136*	*30.7*	*0*	*1.5*	*44.4*

S

	Measure INFO/WEIGHT	per Measure KCAL	FAT	Nutrition Values per 100g / 100ml KCAL	PROT	CARB	FAT	FIBRE
SEAWEED								
Snack, Honey & Sesame, Selwyn's*	1 Pack/4g	14	0.5	350	33	10.6	12.9	29.8
Spaghetti, Dry Weight, Tesco*	½ Pack/40g	89	0.2	223	10	29	0.5	31
Wakame, Dried, Raw	**1oz/28g**	**20**	**0.7**	**71**	**12.4**	**0**	**2.4**	**47.1**
SEED MIX								
Alesto, Lidl*	1 Serving/30g	175	7.1	582	23.8	10.1	23.8	8.3
Chia & Flaxseed, Sprinkles, Tesco*	1 Serving/26g	135	9.2	518	24.2	15.9	35.3	20.2
Omega, Graze*	1 Pack/25g	153	12.4	613	28.4	13.1	49.7	0
Omega, Morrisons*	¼ Pack/25g	138	11.4	554	20.9	15	45.6	6.4
Omega, Munchy Seeds*	1 Bag/30g	184	14.9	613	28.4	13.1	49.7	2.2
Original, The Food Doctor*	1 Serving/30g	157	13.3	522	28.2	3.7	44.4	17.7
Roasted Sunflower & Pumpkin, Salad Sprinkles, Tesco*	1 Serving/20g	112	8.5	561	30	9.4	42.6	10.2
Savoury Roasted Seeds, Graze*	1 Pack/34g	203	16.2	595	21.4	17.8	47.5	5.5
SEEDS								
Chia, White, The Chia Co*	1 Serving/15g	67	5.2	447	20.4	4.5	35	37.5
Chia, Whole, Natural Selection*	1 Serving/15g	63	4	423	19.5	11.1	26.6	31
Fenugreek, Average	**1 Tsp/3.7g**	**12**	**0.2**	**323**	**23**	**58.4**	**6.4**	**24.6**
Fiery, Graze*	1 Pack/34g	173	14.8	510	21.8	17.3	43.5	7.9
Flaxseed, Sunflower & Pumpkin, Milled, Linwoods*	1 Scoop/10g	54	4.9	542	22.7	2.4	49.1	16.2
Hemp, Shelled, Linwoods*	2 Tbsps/30g	178	14.8	593	35.1	7.6	49.5	5.9
Mixed, Wholesome, Love Life, Waitrose*	1 Serving/30g	166	13.6	554	21.3	15.5	45.2	8
Mustard, Average	**1 Tsp/3.3g**	**15**	**0.9**	**469**	**34.9**	**34.9**	**28.8**	**14.7**
Nigella, Average	**1 Tsp/5g**	**20**	**1.7**	**392**	**21.3**	**1.9**	**33.3**	**8.4**
Poppy, Average	**1 Tbsp/8.8g**	**47**	**3.9**	**533**	**18**	**23.7**	**44.7**	**10**
Pumpkin, Alesto, Lidl*	1 Serving/25g	128	9	511	34.5	4.2	36.2	15.2
Pumpkin, Average	**1 Tbsp/10g**	**57**	**4.6**	**568**	**27.9**	**13**	**45.9**	**3.8**
Pumpkin, Whole, Roasted, Salted, Average	**1 Serving/50g**	**261**	**21.1**	**522**	**33**	**13.4**	**42.1**	**3.9**
Sesame, Average	**1 Tsp/2g**	**12**	**1.1**	**610**	**22.3**	**3.6**	**56.4**	**7.8**
Sesame, Tesco*	1 Tsp/4g	24	2.3	598	18.2	0.9	58	7.9
Sunflower, Average	**1 Tbsp/10g**	**59**	**4.9**	**585**	**23.4**	**15**	**48.7**	**5.7**
SEMOLINA								
Average	**1oz/28g**	**98**	**0.5**	**348**	**11**	**75.2**	**1.8**	**2.1**
Pudding, Creamed, Ambrosia*	1 Can/425g	344	7.2	81	3.3	13.1	1.7	0.2
Pudding, Creamed, Co-Op*	1 Can/425g	382	8.5	90	4	15	2	0
SHALLOTS								
Pickled in Hot & Spicy Vinegar, Tesco*	1 Onion/18g	14	0	77	1	18	0.1	1.9
Raw, Average	**1 Serving/80g**	**16**	**0.2**	**20**	**1.5**	**3.3**	**0.2**	**1.4**
SHANDY								
Bavaria*	1 Can/300ml	109	0	36	0	0	0	0
Bitter, Original, Ben Shaws*	1 Can/330ml	89	0	27	0	6	0	0
Canned, Morrisons*	1 Can/330ml	36	0	11	0	1.8	0	0
Homemade, Average	**1 Pint/568ml**	**148**	**0**	**26**	**0.2**	**2.9**	**0**	**0**
Lemonade, Schweppes*	1 Can/330ml	76	0	23	0	5.1	0	0
Lemonade, Traditional Style, Tesco*	1 Can/330ml	63	0	19	0	4.7	0	0
SHARK								
Raw	**1oz/28g**	**29**	**0.3**	**102**	**23**	**0**	**1.1**	**0**
SHARON FRUIT								
Average	**1oz/28g**	**19**	**0**	**68**	**0.7**	**17.3**	**0**	**1.5**
SHERRY								
Dry, Average	**1 Glass/120ml**	**139**	**0**	**116**	**0.2**	**1.4**	**0**	**0**
Medium	**1 Serving/50ml**	**58**	**0**	**116**	**0.1**	**5.9**	**0**	**0**
Sweet	**1 Serving/50ml**	**68**	**0**	**136**	**0.3**	**6.9**	**0**	**0**
SHORTBREAD								
All Butter, Deans*	1 Biscuit/15g	77	3.8	511	4.9	65.7	25.4	1.2

S

	Measure INFO/WEIGHT	per Measure KCAL	FAT	Nutrition Values per 100g / 100ml KCAL	PROT	CARB	FAT	FIBRE

SHORTBREAD

	Measure INFO/WEIGHT	KCAL	FAT	KCAL	PROT	CARB	FAT	FIBRE
All Butter, Fingers, Highland, Sainsbury's*	2 Biscuits/40g	208	11.5	521	4.8	59.4	28.8	2.7
All Butter, Fingers, Scottish, M&S*	1 Finger/17.6g	90	4.9	510	5.7	58.9	27.8	4.7
All Butter, Petticoat Tails, Co-Op*	1 Biscuit/13g	68	3.8	520	5	60	29	2
All Butter, Round, Luxury, M&S*	1 Biscuit/20g	105	5.8	525	6.2	60	29	2
All Butter, Selection, Waitrose*	1 Biscuit/18g	95	11	527	5.3	58.3	61.1	3
All Butter, Trufree*	1 Biscuit/11g	58	3.1	524	2	66	28	0.9
Average	*1oz/28g*	*139*	*7.3*	*498*	*5.9*	*63.9*	*26.1*	*1.9*
Belgian Chocolate Chunk, Asda*	1 Biscuit/20g	106	6.2	531	7	56	31	1.8
Butter, with Real Lemons, Mini, Deluxe, Lidl*	3 Biscuits/24g	125	7	521	5.6	57.6	29.1	3.2
Caramel, Millionaires, Fox's*	1 Serving/16g	75	3.9	483	6.1	57.9	25.3	0.1
Choc Chip, Fair Trade, Co-Op*	1 Biscuit/19g	100	6	526	5.3	57.9	31.6	2.6
Chocolate Chip, Jacob's*	1 Biscuit/17g	87	4.7	513	5.2	61.2	27.5	1.8
Chocolate Chip, Tesco*	1 Serving/20g	105	6.1	525	7.5	55	30.6	3
Chocolate, Belgian, Chunky, TTD, Sainsbury's*	1 Piece/70g	353	19	505	5.5	58.8	27.2	1.4
Chocolate, Triple, Finest, Tesco*	1 Square/63g	325	18.5	516	5.8	56.3	29.4	1.5
Clotted Cream, Finest, Tesco*	1 Biscuit/20g	109	6.4	543	5.2	58	32.2	1.7
Demerara, Rounds, TTD, Sainsbury's*	1 Biscuit/22g	113	5.9	508	5.1	62.2	26.5	1.8
Double Choc Chip, Petit Four, Scottish, Tesco*	1 Serving/50g	266	15	531	5.1	60.4	30	1.7
Fingers, Asda*	1 Finger/18g	93	5.1	519	5.8	60.3	28.3	18
Fingers, Scottish, Finest, Tesco*	1 Biscuit/21g	104	5	498	5.1	65.5	23.9	2
Mini Bites, Co-Op*	1 Biscuit/10g	53	3	530	7	59	30	2
Pecan All Butter, Sainsbury's*	1 Biscuit/18g	99	6.5	548	5.3	49.9	36.3	2.5
Petticoat Tails, All Butter, Highland, Sainsbury's*	1 Biscuit/13g	64	3.6	516	6.3	58	28.8	2.2
Raspberry & Oatmeal, Deans*	1 Biscuit/20g	103	5.7	514	4.7	63.1	28.6	1.4
Rings, Handbaked, Border*	1 Biscuit/17g	86	4.9	520	6.2	61.2	29.5	0
Spotty Scottie Dogs, with Chocolate Chips, Sainsbury's*	1 Biscuit/12g	62	3.3	515	5.1	60.5	27.5	2.5

SHRIMP

	Measure INFO/WEIGHT	KCAL	FAT	KCAL	PROT	CARB	FAT	FIBRE
Boiled, Average	*1 Serving/60g*	*70*	*1.4*	*117*	*23.8*	*0*	*2.4*	*0*
Frozen, Average	*1oz/28g*	*20*	*0.2*	*73*	*16.5*	*0*	*0.8*	*0*
in Brine, Canned, Drained, Average	*1oz/28g*	*17*	*0.2*	*61*	*13.5*	*0*	*0.8*	*0*

SKATE

	Measure INFO/WEIGHT	KCAL	FAT	KCAL	PROT	CARB	FAT	FIBRE
Grilled	*1oz/28g*	*22*	*0.1*	*79*	*18.9*	*0*	*0.5*	*0*
in Batter, Fried in Blended Oil	*1oz/28g*	*47*	*2.8*	*168*	*14.7*	*4.9*	*10.1*	*0.2*
Raw, Edible Portion	*1oz/28g*	*18*	*0.1*	*64*	*15.1*	*0*	*0.4*	*0*

SKIPS

	Measure INFO/WEIGHT	KCAL	FAT	KCAL	PROT	CARB	FAT	FIBRE
Cheesy, KP Snacks*	1 Bag/17g	89	5	524	6.2	58.5	29.5	1
Prawn Cocktail, KP Snacks*	1 Bag/15g	82	4.7	532	6	58.7	30.1	1

SKITTLES

	Measure INFO/WEIGHT	KCAL	FAT	KCAL	PROT	CARB	FAT	FIBRE
Mars*	1 Pack/55g	223	2.4	406	0	90.6	4.4	0

SLICES

	Measure INFO/WEIGHT	KCAL	FAT	KCAL	PROT	CARB	FAT	FIBRE
Bacon & Cheese, Pastry, Tesco*	1 Slice/165g	480	32	291	7.4	21.7	19.4	1
Bacon & Cheese, Savoury, Pastry, Somerfield*	1 Slice/165.0g	490	33.5	297	7.4	21.2	20.3	1.5
Beef, Minced Steak & Onion, Tesco*	1 Slice/150g	424	27.2	283	8.7	21.3	18.1	1.6
Cheese & Onion, Pastry, Tesco*	1 Slice/150g	502	37	335	8	20.1	24.7	1.4
Chicken & Mushroom, Tesco*	1 Slice/165g	457	28.9	277	9.2	20.6	17.5	0.9
Chicken & Bacon, Wall's*	1 Slice/225g	576	33.5	256	10.5	19.9	14.9	0
Chicken & Mushroom, Ginsters*	1 Slice/180g	439	26.8	244	8.3	19.1	14.9	1.8
Chicken & Mushroom, Sainsbury's*	1 Slice/164g	427	26.5	259	7.3	21.3	16.1	1
Chicken Fajita, Puff Pastry, Sainsbury's*	1 Pack/180g	452	23	251	9.1	23.6	12.8	2.5
Custard, Pastry, Tesco*	1 Slice/108g	275	11.1	255	2.8	37.2	10.3	1.3
Fresh Cream, Tesco*	1 Slice/75g	311	21	414	3.5	37.4	27.9	1
Goats Cheese & Spinach, Crisp & Creamy, Waitrose*	1 Slice/100g	351	22.7	351	7.6	28.3	22.7	1.8
Ham & Cheese, Ginsters*	1 Pack/180g	511	33.7	284	8.5	20.4	18.7	2.5

	Measure INFO/WEIGHT	per Measure KCAL	FAT	Nutrition Values per 100g / 100ml KCAL	PROT	CARB	FAT	FIBRE
SLICES								
Minced Beef & Onion, Crestwood, Aldi*	1 Slice/165g	543	40.1	329	6.3	19.7	24.3	3.1
Minced Steak & Onion, Sainsbury's*	1 Slice/165g	475	29.9	288	15.2	16	18.1	2.5
Raisin, Crispy, LC, Tesco*	1 Biscuit/15g	56	0.6	370	6	76.6	3.9	5.5
Spicy Chicken, Ginsters*	1 Slice/180g	448	27.4	249	6.7	21.4	15.2	1.9
Steak, Peppered, Ginsters*	1 Slice/180g	457	27	254	8.4	21.3	15	1.6
SLIM FAST*								
Bars, Chocolate Caramel Treat, Snack, Slim Fast*	1 Bar/26g	95	2.6	360	3.5	63	10	1.5
Bars, Chocolate Peanut, Meal, Slim Fast*	1 Bar/56g	210	7.2	380	24	50	13	5
Bars, Chocolate, Nutty, Nougat, Snack, Slim Fast*	1 Bar/25g	95	3	380	4	63	12	1.5
Bars, Heavenly Chocolate Delight, Snack, Slim Fast*	1 Bar/24g	95	3.2	390	5	58	13	7
Bars, Heavenly Chocolate, Crunch Snack, Slim Fast*	1 Bar/24g	95	3.2	390	5	58	13	7
Bars, Nutty Salted Caramel, Meal, Slim Fast*	1 Bar/60g	218	6.8	364	25.4	26.9	11.3	18.7
Bars, Summer Berry, Meal, Slim Fast*	1 Bar/60g	210	5	350	23.3	51.7	8.3	5.8
Chunky Chocolate, Shake, Ready to Drink, Slimfast*	1 Shake/325ml	204	5.2	63	4.6	6.6	1.6	1.5
Crackers, Cheddar Flavour Bites, Snack Bag, Slim Fast*	1 Pack/22g	92	2	417	9.6	72.8	9.2	2.5
Milk Shake, Blissful Banana, Powder, Dry, Slim Fast*	2 Scoops/36.5g	131	2.4	359	13.4	60.2	6.7	11
Milk Shake, Chunky Chocolate, Powder, Dry, Slim Fast*	2 Scoops/37g	132	2.7	363	13.9	59	7.5	10.9
Milk Shake, Simply Vanilla, Powder, Dry, Slim Fast*	2 Scoops/36.5g	131	2.4	360	13.4	60.9	6.5	11
Milk Shake, Summer Strawberry, Powder, Dry, Slim Fast*	2 Scoops/37g	139	2.4	380	13.5	60.1	6.6	11.1
Milk Shake,Caramel Temptation, Powder, Dry, Slim Fast*	1 Serving/37g	139	2.2	380	14	62	6	11
Noodles, Chicken Tikka Masala, Box, Slim Fast*	1 Box/250g	81	2.2	33	2.3	2.7	0.9	2.5
Noodles, Spicy Thai, Slim Fast*	1 Box/240g	70	3.1	29	0.9	2.4	1.3	2.4
Pretzels, Sour Cream & Chive, Snack Bag, Slim Fast*	1 Pack/23g	99	2.2	432	9.7	74.9	9.5	4.1
Tortillas, Barbecue Flavour, Snack Bag, Slim Fast*	1 Bag/22g	96	2.6	435	6.5	73.9	11.8	3.6
SMARTIES								
Biscuits, Nestle*	1 Biscuit/5g	26	1.4	519	7.7	57.6	28.6	0
Mini Eggs, Nestle*	5 Eggs/17g	83	3.4	489	3.4	73.5	19.8	1.2
Mini, Treat Size, Smarties, Nestle*	1 Carton/14g	68	2.8	471	5	68.1	19.6	1
Nestle*	1 Tube/40g	188	7.1	469	3.9	72.5	17.7	2.4
Tree Decoration, Nestle*	1 Chocolate/18g	95	5.4	529	5.6	58.9	30.1	0.8
SMOOTHIE								
Apples & Blackcurrants for Kids, Innocent*	1 Carton/180ml	104	0.2	58	0.3	14.1	0.1	0.1
Banana Fruit with Yoghurt, Tesco*	1 Bottle/1000ml	610	7	61	2.1	11.3	0.7	0.4
Blackberries & Blueberries, Innocent*	1 Bottle/250ml	120	0.2	48	0.5	12	0.1	2.1
Cherries & Strawberries, Innocent*	1 Bottle/250ml	122	0.2	49	0.6	12.6	0.1	0
Coconut, Pineapple & Banana, Coldpress*	1 Serving/150ml	96	1.2	64	0.7	12.7	0.8	0
Cucumber, Avocado, & Lime, M&S*	1 Bottle/250ml	148	3.5	59	0.4	10.4	1.4	1.4
Fruit, & Cereal, Forest Fruits, Morning Boost , Tropicana*	1 Serving/250ml	152	0	61	0.7	13	0	2.4
Magnificent Mango, Innocent*	1 Bottle/250ml	136	0	54	0.4	12	0	1.4
Mangoes & Passion Fruits, Pure Fruit, Innocent*	1 Bottle/250ml	142	0.5	57	0.6	12.5	0.2	1.6
Mixed Berry, CBY, Asda*	1 Glass/250ml	143	0	57	0.6	12.6	0	1.6
Orange, Banana, Mango, Morning Boost, Tropicana*	1 Serving/250ml	125	0	50	0.1	9.2	0	2.3
Oranges, Mangoes & Pineapples For Kids, Innocent*	1 Carton/180ml	94	0.2	52	0.7	11.7	0.1	0.9
Peaches & Passionfruit, for Kids, Innocent*	1 Carton/180ml	95	0	53	0.6	14.7	0	0.9
Peaches, Bananas & Passionfruit, PJ Smoothies*	1 Bottle/250g	128	0.2	51	0.4	12.1	0.1	0
Pineapple, Banana & Coconut, CBY, Asda*	1 Glass/250ml	178	2.8	71	0.7	13.6	1.1	1
Pineapples, Bananas & Coconuts, Innocent*	1 Bottle/250ml	172	2.8	69	0.7	13.6	1.1	1
Pomegranates, Blueberries & Acai, Special, Innocent*	1 Serving/250ml	170	0.5	68	0.6	15.6	0.2	0.8
Protein Superfood, Mango & Banana, PhD Nutrition*	1 Serving/130g	175	7.7	135	15.4	4.2	5.9	1.4
Raspberry & Blueberry, Plus, Tesco*	1 Serving/100ml	59	0.3	59	2.6	11.6	0.3	0.5
Strawberries & Bananas, Pure Fruit, Innocent*	1 Bottle/250ml	132	0.2	53	0.7	13.1	0.1	1.3
Strawberries, Blackberries, Raspberries, Kids, Innocent*	1 Carton/180ml	81	0.2	45	0.5	9.9	0.1	1.3
Strawberry & Banana, Tesco*	1 Bottle/250ml	112	0.5	45	0.6	10.1	0.2	0.8

S

	Measure INFO/WEIGHT	per Measure KCAL	FAT	Nutrition Values per 100g / 100ml KCAL	PROT	CARB	FAT	FIBRE
SMOOTHIE								
Strawberry & Banana, Prepacked, Average	*1 Serving/250ml*	*131*	*0.2*	*53*	*0.6*	*11.9*	*0.1*	*0.9*
Super Orange, Cold Pressed, Raw Fruit & Veg, Savse*	1 Bottle/250ml	110	0.2	44	0.9	9.8	0.1	0.7
Super Red, Cold Pressed, Raw Fruit & Veg, Savse*	1 Bottle/250ml	98	0.2	39	0.8	8.4	0.1	0.7
Superfruits, Pomegranates, Blueberries & Acai, Innocent*	1 Serving/250ml	170	0.5	68	0.5	15.6	0.2	0.8
Vanilla Bean, M&S*	1 Bottle/500ml	450	13	90	3.3	13.9	2.6	0
SMOOTHIE MIX								
Banana, Kale & Mango, As Sold, Iceland*	1 Sachet/150g	90	0.4	60	1.1	12.2	0.3	2.3
Berry, Frozen, Love Life, Waitrose*	1 Serving/80g	31	0	39	1.1	7.2	0	2.9
Mango & Pineapple, CBY, Asda*	1 Portion/80g	48	0.4	59	0.6	12	0.5	1.9
Strawberry & Banana, Frozen, Love Life, Waitrose*	1 Serving/80g	37	0.3	46	0.7	8.2	0.4	3.4
Tropical, Frozen, Love Life, Waitrose*	1 Serving/80g	45	0.2	57	0.7	11.8	0.3	1.9
Yellow Frozen, Morrisons*	1 Portion/80g	41	0.2	51	0.5	10.9	0.2	1.9
SNACKS								
Corn, Original, Mister Corn*	1 Serving/30g	145	6.3	482	7.6	63	21	5.5
Mild Green Curry, Baked Pea Sticks, Yushoi *	1 Serving/21g	87	3	415	19.1	45.7	14.2	14.3
Mix, Sweet & Salty, Reese's*	½ Pack/28g	139	7.6	496	12.4	54.7	27.1	0
Pea, Malaysian Sweet Curry Flavour, Passions, Aldi*	1 Pack/21g	89	3.2	422	19	47	15	13
Pea, Thai Red Curry Flavour, Passions, Aldi*	1 Pack/21g	88	2.9	421	19	48	14	12
Slightly Salted, Baked Pea Sticks, Yushoi *	1 Serving/21g	88	0.6	419	19.2	9.9	2.9	13.4
Smoky Salt & Pepper, Baked Pea Sticks, Yushoi *	1 Serving/21g	86	2.7	409	19.3	46.5	13	14.3
Sour Cream & Onion, Lentil Curls, Passions Deli, Aldi*	1 Pack/20g	91	3.4	454	11	63	17	3.6
Soy & Balsamic Vinegar, Baked Pea Sticks, Yushoi *	1 Serving/21g	88	2.9	417	18.6	47.9	13.7	13.5
Sweet Chilli & Lemon, Baked Pea Sticks, Yushoi *	1 Serving/21g	88	3	420	19.2	46.7	14.3	13.7
Teddy Faces, Snackrite, Aldi*	1 Bag/19g	96	5.1	505	3.4	61	27	2.7
Veggie Caesar, Graze*	1 Punnet/24g	115	4.6	478	17	52	19	9.4
SNAILS								
in Garlic Butter, Average	*6 Snails/50g*	*219*	*20.8*	*438*	*9.7*	*8*	*41.5*	*1*
Raw, Average	*1 Snail/5g*	*4*	*0.1*	*90*	*16.1*	*2*	*1.4*	*0*
SNAPPER								
Red, Fried in Blended Oil	*1oz/28g*	*35*	*0.9*	*126*	*24.5*	*0*	*3.1*	*0*
Red, Weighed with Bone, Raw	*1oz/28g*	*12*	*0.2*	*42*	*9.2*	*0*	*0.6*	*0*
SNICKERS								
& Hazelnut, Snickers*	1 Bar/49g	240	11.7	489	8.1	59.5	23.9	0
Mars*	1 Single/48g	245	13.4	510	9.5	54.3	27.9	1.3
Protein, Mars*	1 Bar/51g	199	7.1	391	35.6	36.1	13.9	0
SOLE								
Fillet, Yellowfin, Lightly Dusted, Northern Catch, Aldi*	1 Fillet/114g	171	4.6	150	20	7.6	4	2.5
Yellow, Fillet, Lightly Dusted, As Consumed, Morrisons*	1 Fillet/124g	218	8.5	176	14	13.9	6.9	1
SOPOCKA								
Sliced, Cured, Pork Loin	*1 Serving/100g*	*101*	*2.9*	*101*	*17.8*	*0.8*	*2.9*	*0*
SORBET								
Blackcurrant, Yorvale Ltd*	1 Serving/100g	120	0.2	120	0	28.8	0.2	0
Exotic Fruit, Sainsbury's*	1 Serving/75g	90	1.5	120	1.2	24.1	2	0
Jamaican Me Crazy, Ben & Jerry's*	1 Serving/100g	130	0	130	0.2	32	0	0.4
Lemon	*1 Scoop/60g*	*79*	*0*	*131*	*0.9*	*34.2*	*0*	*0*
Lemon, Sainsbury's*	¼ Pot/89g	100	0	112	0	28.1	0	0.1
Lemon, Tesco*	1 Serving/75g	80	0	106	0	26.2	0	0.4
Mandarin Orange, Yorvale Ltd*	1 Serving/100g	125	0.2	125	0.1	30.5	0.2	0
Mango, Tesco*	1 Serving/100g	107	0	107	0.1	26.5	0	0.3
Mango, Waitrose*	1 Pot/100g	90	0	90	0.1	22.1	0	0.6
Orange, Del Monte*	1 Sorbet/500g	625	0.5	125	0.2	32.1	0.1	0
Passion Fruit, Yorvale Ltd*	1 Serving/100g	109	0.2	109	0.1	26.6	0.2	0
Raspberry & Blackberry, Fat Free, M&S*	1 Sorbet/125g	140	0	112	0.4	27.5	0	0.6

S

	Measure INFO/WEIGHT	per Measure KCAL	FAT	Nutrition Values per 100g / 100ml KCAL	PROT	CARB	FAT	FIBRE
SORBET								
Raspberry, Haagen-Dazs*	½ Cup/105g	120	0	114	0	28.6	0	1.9
Raspberry, Tesco*	1 Serving/70ml	97	0	138	0.5	34	0	0
SOUFFLE								
Cheese	*1oz/28g*	*71*	*5.4*	*253*	*11.4*	*9.3*	*19.2*	*0.3*
Cheese, Alizonne*	1 Serving/33g	129	3.4	392	60.5	14.5	10.2	0.2
Cheese, Mini, Waitrose*	1 Souffle/14g	32	2.4	232	16	2.9	17.4	2.4
Chocolate, Gu*	1 Pot/70g	307	24.9	439	6.3	24.4	35.6	2.9
Lemon, Finest, Tesco*	1 Pot/80g	270	20.5	338	2.9	24.1	25.6	0.2
Plain	*1oz/28g*	*56*	*4.1*	*201*	*7.6*	*10.4*	*14.7*	*0.3*
Raspberry & Amaretto, M&S*	1oz/28g	83	4.7	298	2.8	33.1	16.7	0.1
Ricotta & Spinach, M&S*	1 Serving/120g	186	13.3	155	8	6.2	11.1	2.1
Strawberry, M&S*	1 Serving/95g	171	10.1	180	1.6	19.5	10.6	0.9
SOUP								
Asparagus, Cream Of, Canned, M&S*	½ Can/200g	108	7.2	54	0.9	4.3	3.6	0.2
Asparagus, New Covent Garden Food Co*	½ Carton/300g	132	7.2	44	1.5	4.1	2.4	0.9
Asparagus, with Croutons, Aldi*	1 Sachet/229ml	96	3.7	42	0.5	6.5	1.6	0.5
Bacon & Lentil, CBY, Asda*	½ Pot/300g	177	4.2	59	3.8	7.2	1.4	1.2
Bean, Hearty, Italian Inspired, Love Life, Waitrose*	½ Pot/300g	151	6.6	50	1.5	5.2	2.2	1.8
Bean, Italian Style, Tesco*	1 Can/300g	153	3.6	51	2.8	7.3	1.2	1.1
Beef & Mushroom, Big Soup, Heinz*	1 Can/515g	216	2.6	42	2.3	7	0.5	0.7
Beef & Tomato in a Cup, Sainsbury's*	1 Serving/210ml	61	1.1	29	0.6	5.6	0.5	0.2
Beef & Tomato, Cup a Soup, Made Up, Batchelors*	1 Serving/252g	83	1.6	33	0.6	6.3	0.6	0.4
Beef & Vegetable, Big Soup, Heinz*	1 Can/400g	212	4	53	3.5	7.5	1	0.9
Beef Broth, Big Soup, Heinz*	1 Can/400g	184	2.8	46	2.5	7	0.7	0.9
Beef Broth, Classic, Heinz*	1 Can/400g	180	2	45	1.9	7.6	0.5	0.9
Beef, & Vegetables, Chunky, Newgate, Lidl*	1 Tin/400g	232	3.2	58	3.6	8.2	0.8	1.8
Beef, Chilli, Bean, & Rice, M&S*	½ Pot/300g	159	2.4	53	2.7	7.8	0.8	1.9
Big Red Tomato, Heinz*	½ Can/210g	63	0.8	30	0.5	6.4	0.4	0
Blended Sweetcorn & Yellow Pepper, Heinz*	½ Can/200g	98	4.2	49	0.9	6.6	2.1	0.6
Brazilian Super Grain, Glorious!*	½ Pot/300g	163	4.2	54	2.6	6.6	1.4	2.3
Broccoli & Stilton, Canned, Tesco*	1 Can/400g	240	14	60	1.7	5	3.5	0.4
Broccoli & Stilton, Classics, Fresh, Tesco*	½ Pot/300g	156	10.8	52	2.4	1.8	3.6	1.5
Broccoli & Stilton, Canned, Sainsbury's*	½ Can/200g	84	4	42	1.5	4.2	2	0.6
Broccoli & Stilton, Cup Soup, Ainsley Harriott*	1 Satchet/229ml	87	1.8	38	1	7	0.8	1.3
Broccoli & Stilton, Fresh, Sainsbury's*	½ Pot/300ml	141	9.9	47	2.7	1.8	3.3	1.5
Broccoli & Stilton, New Covent Garden Food Co*	1 Carton/600ml	240	14.4	40	2.2	1.9	2.4	1.1
Broccoli & Stilton, Tesco*	1 Can/400g	192	10.4	48	1.9	4.2	2.6	1.2
Broccoli & Zucinni, Cream Of, Canned, Italiamo*	½ Can/195ml	84	5.1	43	0.9	3.8	2.6	0.5
Broccoli with Kale, & Watercress, Naked Locals*	½ Pack/250ml	130	6.8	52	1.7	3.9	2.7	2.8
Broccoli, Pea & Pesto, New Covent Garden Food Co*	½ Pack/350g	182	7.4	52	2.3	5.2	2.1	1.4
Broccoli, Salmon & Watercress, Stay Full, Baxters*	1 Can/400g	244	8.8	61	3.3	5.8	2.2	2.4
Broth, Ten Vegetable, Morrisons*	1 Pot/600g	240	7.8	40	1.7	5.8	1.3	1.1
Butter Bean & Chorizo, Meal, Sainsbury's*	1 Pot/400g	257	9.6	64	3.9	5.6	2.4	2.3
Butternut Squash & Chilli, Sainsbury's*	½ Pot/300g	112	7.2	37	0.7	3.1	2.4	0.2
Butternut Squash & Red Pepper, Canned, Sainsbury's*	½ Can/195g	99	4.3	51	1	6.6	2.2	3.6
Butternut Squash & Red Pepper, Vegetarian, Baxters*	1 Can/415g	149	2.5	36	0.9	6.6	0.6	0.5
Butternut Squash & Sage, New Covent Garden Food Co*	½ Carton/300g	153	6.9	51	0.9	6.6	2.3	0.7
Butternut Squash & Tarragon, Waitrose*	½ Pot/300g	123	6.6	41	0.8	4.5	2.2	1
Butternut Squash, Creamy, New Covent Garden Food Co*	½ Carton/300g	153	7.5	51	0.8	6.4	2.5	0.9
Butternut Squash, Fresh, Waitrose*	½ Pot/300g	153	8.7	51	0.5	5.8	2.9	0.8
Butternut Squash, Soupreme, Aldi*	½ Pot/300g	60	3.3	20	0.5	1.5	1.1	1.5
Butternut Squash, Tesco*	1 Pot/600g	164	8.5	27	0.4	2.5	1.4	1.5
Cantonese Hot & Sour Noodle, Baxters*	1 Serving/215g	133	2.8	62	1.4	11.1	1.3	0.5

S

	Measure INFO/WEIGHT	per Measure KCAL	FAT	Nutrition Values per 100g / 100ml KCAL	PROT	CARB	FAT	FIBRE
SOUP								
Carrot & Coriander, Canned, BGTY, Sainsbury's*	½ Can/200g	62	2	31	0.8	4.8	1	0.9
Carrot & Coriander, Canned, M&S*	½ Can/210g	94	5	45	0.4	5.9	2.4	0.9
Carrot & Coriander, Canned, Tesco*	1 Can/400g	220	11.6	55	0.7	5.7	2.9	0.8
Carrot & Coriander, Classic Homestyle, M&S*	1 Can/425g	170	8.5	40	0.6	5.6	2	0.7
Carrot & Coriander, Fresh, Organic, Simply Organic*	1 Pot/600g	276	18	46	0.5	4.5	3	1.3
Carrot & Coriander, Less Than 5% Fat, Asda*	1 Serving/300g	96	0.9	32	1	6	0.3	0.8
Carrot & Ginger, Fresh, Sainsbury's*	1 Pot/600g	150	5.4	25	0.4	3.9	0.9	1
Carrot & Butter Bean, Vegetarian, Baxters*	1 Can/415g	237	7.9	57	1.5	7.2	1.9	2.2
Carrot & Coriander, Average	**1 Can/400g**	**167**	**8.6**	**42**	**0.6**	**4.8**	**2.2**	**1**
Carrot & Coriander, Blended, Heinz*	½ Can/200g	104	5.4	52	0.7	6.2	2.7	0.6
Carrot & Coriander, Classic, Classic, Heinz*	1 Can/400g	164	6.4	41	0.4	5.8	1.6	0.9
Carrot & Coriander, Fresh, Healthy Living, Co-Op*	1 Pot/600g	180	6	30	0.6	4.7	1	1
Carrot & Coriander, Fresh, M&S*	½ Pot/300g	90	4.5	30	0.4	4.2	1.5	0.5
Carrot & Coriander, Fresh, New Covent Garden Food Co*	1 Serving/250g	88	4.3	35	0.5	3.9	1.7	1.2
Carrot & Coriander, Fresh, Tesco*	½ Pot /300g	99	4.8	33	0.6	2.9	1.6	2.2
Carrot & Coriander, Weight Watchers*	1 Pouch/300g	102	3.9	34	0.4	5.1	1.3	0.6
Carrot & Lentil, Weight Watchers*	1 Can/295g	87	0.3	29	1.3	5.5	0.1	0.7
Carrot, Coriander & Ginger, So Organic, Sainsbury's*	½ Can/197g	75	3.3	38	0.3	5.3	1.7	0.7
Carrot, Red Lentil & Cumin, Organic, Waitrose*	1 Pack/350g	175	8.8	50	0.2	6.7	2.5	0.5
Carrot, Thai, Skinny, Aldi*	½ Pot/300g	90	4.8	30	0.5	3.3	1.6	0.6
Cauliflower & Celeriac, Love Life, Waitrose*	1 Pot/350g	79	3.1	23	1.6	1.4	0.9	1.3
Celeriac, Velvety, Waitrose*	½ Pot/300g	151	11.5	50	0.8	2.8	3.8	0.9
Chantenay Carrot & Parsnip, Fresh, Extra Special, Asda*	½ Pot/300g	153	8.4	51	1.2	4.8	2.8	0.8
Cheese, Leek & Bacon, Somerfield*	1 Carton/300g	441	36	147	5	5	12	0
Chicken & Leek, Cup a Soup, Made Up, Batchelors*	1 Serving/259g	96	4.7	37	0.5	4.7	1.8	0.7
Chicken & Mushroom in a Cup, Sainsbury's*	1 Sachet/223ml	107	4.2	48	0.7	7.1	1.9	0.1
Chicken & Sweetcorn, Canned, HL, Tesco*	½ Can/200g	70	0.6	35	1.6	6.4	0.3	0.3
Chicken & Sweetcorn, Cup Soup, Asda*	1 Sachet/200ml	109	3.9	54	0.7	8.5	2	0.3
Chicken & Sweetcorn, Light Choice, Tesco*	½ Can 200g	84	0.8	42	1.7	7.9	0.4	0.2
Chicken & Vegetable with Pasta, Select, Campbell's*	1 Can/480ml	220	1	46	2.9	7.9	0.2	0.8
Chicken & Vegetable, Fresh, Somerfield*	½ Pot/300g	177	8.4	59	2.9	5.6	2.8	3
Chicken & Vegetable, Mighty, Asda*	1 Can/410g	176	5.3	43	2.5	6.8	1.3	0.7
Chicken & Black Eyed Pea, Gumbo, Hearty, Baxters*	1 Can/400g	184	2	46	2.6	6.7	0.5	1.5
Chicken & Multigrain, Finest, Tesco*	½ Pot/298g	125	3.6	42	3.2	3.9	1.2	1.3
Chicken & Mushroom, Grain Soup , Sainsbury's*	1 Pot/600g	332	14.5	55	3.8	4.4	2.4	0.5
Chicken & Sweetcorn, Fresh, Average	**1 Serving/300g**	**146**	**3.1**	**48**	**2.4**	**7.3**	**1**	**0.6**
Chicken & Vegetable Broth, Fresh, M Kitchen, Morrisons*	½ Pot/298g	131	4.5	44	2.8	4	1.5	1.6
Chicken & Vegetable, Big Soup, Heinz*	½ Can/200g	104	2.8	52	3.3	6.7	1.4	0.8
Chicken & Vegetable, Canned, Average	**1 Can/400g**	**192**	**8.5**	**48**	**2.5**	**4.6**	**2.1**	**0.8**
Chicken & Vegetable, Chunky, Canned, Soupreme, Aldi*	1 Can/400g	184	2.4	46	3	6.4	0.6	1.3
Chicken & Vegetable, Cully & Sully*	½ Pot200g	98	6.8	49	1.9	3	3.4	0.8
Chicken & Vegetable, Fresh, M&S*	½ Pot/300g	123	5.1	41	3.5	2.3	1.7	1.2
Chicken & Vegetable, Fresh, Tesco*	½ Pack/300g	118	3.3	39	3.6	3.2	1.1	1.1
Chicken & Vegetable, Healthy, Baxters*	1 Can/415g	170	2.1	41	1.9	6.3	0.5	1.8
Chicken Balti, Meal, Sainsbury's*	1 Pack/400g	242	7.1	61	3.9	6.3	1.8	1.8
Chicken Broth, Favourites, Baxters*	1 Can/400g	140	1.2	35	1.7	5.9	0.3	1
Chicken Miso, Noodle, Waitrose*	1 Pot/400g	268	8.8	67	5.9	5.9	2.2	0.9
Chicken Mix, Telma*	1 Serving/7g	20	0.5	286	14.3	42.9	7.1	0
Chicken Noodle in a Cup, You Count, Love Life, Waitrose*	1 Cup/205ml	43	0.2	21	0.7	4.5	0.1	0.1
Chicken Noodle, Canned, Sainsbury's*	½ Can/217g	78	0.7	36	1.7	7.4	0.3	0.7
Chicken Noodle, Classic, Heinz*	1 Can/400g	124	1.2	31	1.2	6	0.3	0.2
Chicken Noodle, Clear, Weight Watchers*	1 Can/295g	51	0.6	17	0.8	3.1	0.2	0.2
Chicken Noodle, Cup Soup, Dry, Heinz*	1 Sachet/20g	48	0.5	240	8	46	2.5	1.5

	Measure INFO/WEIGHT	per Measure KCAL	FAT	Nutrition Values per 100g / 100ml KCAL	PROT	CARB	FAT	FIBRE
SOUP								
Chicken Noodle, Cup Soup, Made Up, Heinz*	1 Serving/218ml	48	0.4	22	0.7	4.3	0.2	0.1
Chicken Noodle, Dry, Nissin*	1 Pack/85g	364	14.1	428	9.5	62	16.6	3.3
Chicken Noodle, Fresh, CBY, Asda*	½ Pot/297g	98	1.2	33	2.5	4.3	0.4	0.9
Chicken Noodle, In a Cup, BGTY, Sainsbury's*	1 Sachet/59g	14	0.3	23	1.4	4.2	0.4	0.4
Chicken Noodle, Soup in a Cup, Made Up, Sainsbury's*	1 Serving/200ml	44	0.2	22	0.7	4.7	0.1	0.2
Chicken Noodle, Thai Green, Yorkshire Provender*	½ Pot/300g	159	6	53	2.9	5.6	2	0
Chicken, & Barley, Broth, Heinz*	1 Can/400g	128	1.2	32	1.3	5.9	0.3	0.8
Chicken, & Vegetable, Chunky, Canned, Asda*	½ Can/200g	90	2	45	4.3	4.3	1	0.8
Chicken, Chardonnay Wine & Tarragon, Finest, Tesco*	½ Pot/300g	171	9.6	57	3.1	3.7	3.2	0.3
Chicken, Classic, New Covent Garden*	½ Pack/213g	151	9.6	71	2.9	4.8	4.5	0.5
Chicken, Courgette & Orzo Pasta, Meal Soup, Glorious!*	½ Pot/300g	141	4.2	47	3.5	5.1	1.4	0.8
Chicken, Cream Of, Canned, Tesco*	1 Can/400g	260	15.2	65	1.2	5.5	3.8	0
Chicken, Cream of, Reduced Salt, Heinz*	1 Can/400g	216	12	54	1.7	4.9	3	0.1
Chicken, Cream of, Soupreme, Aldi*	1 Can/400g	228	15.2	57	1.8	3.8	3.8	0.4
Chicken, Green Thai, Spiced, M&S*	½ Pot/300g	195	11.4	65	2	6.3	3.8	0.6
Chicken, Green Thai, Waitrose*	1 Pot/600g	462	30	77	4.4	3.5	5	1.6
Chicken, Hot & Sour, New Covent Garden Food Co*	½ Carton/300g	69	0.6	23	1.2	3.5	0.2	1
Chicken, Jamaican Jerk & Pumpkin, Sainsbury's*	½ Pot/300g	141	5.1	47	2.7	5.1	1.7	0.2
Chicken, Moroccan Inspired, Love Life, Waitrose*	½ Pot/300g	136	2.4	45	2.7	6.1	0.8	1.4
Chicken, Mulligatawny, Finest, Tesco*	½ Pot/300g	216	7.8	72	5.2	6.5	2.6	0.9
Chicken, Mushroom & Rice, M&S*	1 Pack/350g	206	7.7	59	2.7	6.6	2.2	0.9
Chicken, Mushroom, & Potato, Big Soup, Heinz*	½ Can/200g	132	4.6	66	3.4	8.1	2.3	0.4
Chicken, Potato & Bacon, Big Soup, Heinz*	1 Can/515g	294	11.3	57	3	6.1	2.2	0.5
Chicken, Potato & Leek, Weight Watchers*	1 Can/295g	97	2.4	33	1.1	5.1	0.8	0.3
Chicken, Spicy Thai, Nupo*	1 Serving/32g	114	2.4	356	38	39	7.6	9.3
Chicken, Thai Style, Canned, Soupreme, Aldi*	1 Can/400g	200	10.8	50	2.5	3.8	2.7	1.1
Chicken, Thai Style, Thick & Creamy, in a Mug, Tesco*	1 Sachet/28g	107	4	390	3.7	61.3	14.5	5.1
Chicken, Thai, Fresh, Finest, Tesco*	½ Tub/300g	255	16.2	85	4.1	4.2	5.4	1.1
Chicken, Tomato & Red Pepper, Italian, Big Soup, Heinz*	½ Can/200g	78	1.8	39	1.6	6.2	0.9	0.7
Chicken, Weight Watchers*	1 Can/295g	97	3	33	1.6	4.4	1	0
Chilli Bean, Mexican, Tesco*	1 Carton/600g	270	6.6	45	2.2	6.4	1.1	1.9
Chilli Tomato & Pasta, COU, M&S*	1 Serving/300g	150	5.7	50	1.3	7.2	1.9	0.9
Chorizo And Butter Bean, Chunky, Sainsbury's*	½ Can/200g	150	5.6	75	3.4	7.8	2.8	2.7
Chowder, Corn, Spicy, New Covent Garden Food Co*	½ Carton/300g	132	5.4	44	1.6	4.3	1.8	2.2
Chowder, Ham & Sweetcorn, Diet Chef Ltd*	1 Pack/300g	165	3.6	55	1.9	9.2	1.2	0.9
Chowder, Smoked Haddock & Salmon, Cully & Sully*	1 Pack/400g	232	9.2	58	2.6	6.2	2.3	0.9
Chunky Beef Chilli, Greggs*	1 Serving/300g	216	5.1	72	4.1	9.7	1.7	0
Chunky Chicken Hotpot, Big Soup, Heinz*	½ Can/258g	126	3.1	49	2.3	7.4	1.2	0.8
Chunky Chilli Beef, Asda*	1 Can/400g	212	4	53	4.2	5.7	1	2.4
Chunky Lentil & Bacon, Canned, M&S*	1 Can/400g	204	2.4	51	3.3	7.2	0.6	1.8
Chunky Minestrone, Love Life, Waitrose*	1 Can/400g	166	0.4	42	1.3	8.7	0.1	1.9
Chunky Vegetable, Diet Chef Ltd*	1 Pack/300g	114	0.9	38	1.4	7.4	0.3	1.3
Chunky Vegetable, Fresh, CBY, Asda*	½ Pot/300g	117	2.1	39	1.6	5.9	0.7	1.1
Chunky, Chicken & Vegetable Meal Soup, Tesco*	1 Can/400g	184	7.2	46	2.5	4.6	1.8	1
Cock-A-Leekie, Favourites, Baxters*	1 Can/400g	116	2.4	29	1.1	4.7	0.6	0.3
Coconut, Lime, & Chilli, Glorious!*	½ Tub/300g	168	2.4	56	3.4	6.7	0.8	4.1
Country Garden, Canned, Vegetarian, Baxters*	1 Can/400g	144	2	36	1	6.2	0.5	1
Country Vegetable, Canned, Heinz, Weight Watchers*	1 Can/295g	97	0.6	33	1.2	5.9	0.2	1
Country Vegetable, Chunky, Baxters*	1 Can/400g	188	2.4	47	1.6	7.2	0.6	2
Country Vegetable, Fresh, Soupreme, Aldi*	1 Tub/600g	204	3.6	34	1.1	5.1	0.6	1.7
Country Vegetable, Hearty, Canned, Baxters*	1 Can/400g	192	2.4	48	1.9	7.5	0.6	1.9
Country Vegetable, Knorr*	1 Pack/500ml	160	3.5	32	0.9	5.5	0.7	1.2
Country Vegetable, Weight Watchers*	1 Can/295g	97	0.3	33	1.2	6.3	0.1	1

SOUP

INFO/WEIGHT	Measure	per Measure		Nutrition Values per 100g / 100ml				
		KCAL	FAT	KCAL	PROT	CARB	FAT	FIBRE
Courgette & Parmesan, Fresh, Sainsbury's*	1 Pack/300ml	198	16.8	66	1.5	2.5	5.6	0.4
Farmhouse Vegetable, Thick, Co-Op*	1 Can/400g	140	1.6	35	1	7	0.4	0.3
Fiery Mexican Spices, Cream of, Cup Soup, Heinz*	1 Cup/250g	90	1.8	36	0.5	6.6	0.7	0.2
Fire Roasted Tomato & Red Pepper, Asda*	½ Tub/265g	114	6.9	43	0.7	4.1	2.6	1
Fish, Bouillabaise, Bistro, M&S*	1 Pack/820g	2665	18	325	10	4.3	2.2	1.3
Florida Spring Vegetable, Dry, Knorr*	1 Pack/36g	104	2	290	7.8	52.2	5.6	5.2
French Onion	*1oz/28g*	*11*	*0.6*	*40*	*0.2*	*5.7*	*2.1*	*1*
French Onion & Cider, Waitrose*	1 Can/425g	94	0.4	22	0.5	4.8	0.1	0.4
French Onion & Gruyere Cheese, Fresh, Finest, Tesco*	½ Pot/300g	210	15.3	70	1.4	4.7	5.1	0.5
French Onion, Chilled, M&S*	½ Pot/300g	150	4.5	50	2	7.2	1.5	1
French Onion, Favourites, Baxters*	½ Can/200g	66	1.2	33	0.7	5.8	0.6	0.6
Garden Pea & Mint, Vegetarian, Baxters*	½ Can/200g	100	1.6	50	2.5	7.3	0.8	1.9
Golden Vegetable with Croutons Cup Soup, Co-Op*	1 Sachet/25g	120	6.5	480	4	56	26	2
Golden Vegetable, Cup, GFY, Asda*	1 Sachet/217ml	52	1.1	24	0.5	4.4	0.5	0.2
Golden Vegetable, Slim a Soup, Batchelors*	1 Sachet/207g	58	1.7	28	0.5	4.7	0.8	0.7
Green Thai Curry, Chicken Noodle, M&S*	1 Pack/256g	333	9	130	5.3	18.9	3.5	1.1
Haddock, Smoked, Chowder, M&S*	½ Pot/300g	180	7.2	60	3.1	6.4	2.4	0.8
Ham Hock & Vegetable, Broth, Crosse & Blackwell*	1 Can/400g	158	2	40	2.7	5.7	0.5	0.8
Ham Hock, Leek & Potato, Chunky, Soup Pot, Tesco*	1 Pot/350g	174	6.3	50	2.5	5.5	1.8	1
Hearty Pea & Wiltshire Cured Ham Hock, Waitrose*	½ Carton/300g	165	4.2	55	3.1	6.6	1.4	1.8
Highlander's Broth, Favourites, Baxters*	1 Can/400g	192	5.6	48	1.7	6.3	1.4	0.9
Hot & Sour	*1 Serving/233g*	*90*	*2.8*	*39*	*2.6*	*4.3*	*1.2*	*0.5*
Indian Super Spinach & Chickpea, Glorious!*	½ Pot/300g	232	6.9	77	3.4	7.9	2.3	5.4
Indian, Cauliflower, Chickpea, & Turmeric , Glorious!*	½ Pot/300g	114	2.4	38	2	4.4	0.8	2.7
Italian Plum Tomato & Basil, PB, Waitrose*	½ Pot/300g	69	1.5	23	0.9	3.8	0.5	0.9
Italian Plum Tomato & Mascarpone, Finest, Tesco*	1 Pot/600g	360	13.8	60	1.3	7.2	2.3	0.6
Italian Style Tomato & Basil, Co-Op*	1 Pack/500g	200	10	40	1	4	2	0.6
Italian Tomato with Basil, Vegetarian, Baxters*	1 Can/415g	170	3.7	41	1.4	5.7	0.9	0.6
Keralan Chicken, Sainsburys*	½ Carton/300g	252	15.3	84	3.5	5.5	5.1	1.1
Korean Spicy Pepper, & Rice, Skinny Soup, Glorious!*	½ Tub/300g	108	2.7	36	1	5.4	0.9	1.1
Lamb & Vegetable, Big Soup, Heinz*	½ Can/200g	120	2.6	60	3	9.1	1.3	1.3
Leek & Chicken, Knorr*	1 Serving/300ml	82	5.2	27	0.6	2.4	1.7	0.1
Leek & Maris Piper Potato, Chilled, M&S*	1 Serving/300g	165	11.4	55	0.6	4.5	3.8	0.9
Leek & Potato, Cup a Soup, Batchelors*	1 Sachet/28g	121	4.9	432	5.2	63.2	17.6	1.8
Leek & Potato, Soup in a Mug, HL, Tesco*	1 Serving/16g	54	0.9	336	4.3	67.1	5.6	7.4
Leek & Potato, Canned, Asda*	1 Can/400g	160	3.6	40	0.9	6.5	0.9	1
Leek & Potato, Fresh with Cream, Tesco*	½ Tub/300g	180	7.2	60	1.5	8	2.4	0.9
Leek & Potato, Fresh, Sainsbury's*	½ Pot/300ml	141	7.2	47	1	5.3	2.4	0.4
Leek & Potato, Fresh, Waitrose*	½ Pot/300g	108	5.1	36	0.7	4.6	1.7	0.9
Leek, Cream of, Favourites, Baxters*	1 Can/400g	228	16.8	57	1.1	3.8	4.2	0.7
Lentil & Bacon, Canned, Tesco*	1 Serving/200g	96	1.4	48	3.2	7.2	0.7	0.5
Lentil & Chick Pea, Fresh, Organic, Tesco*	1 Serving/300ml	117	2.4	39	1.9	6.1	0.8	0.5
Lentil & Tomato, New Covent Garden Food Co*	½ Pack/284g	162	3.1	57	3.6	8.1	1.1	0.7
Lentil & Tomato, Spicy, Chunky, Fresh, Tesco*	½ Pot/300g	195	5.4	65	2.6	9.7	1.8	1.3
Lentil & Bacon, Canned, Sainsbury's*	½ Can/200g	102	1.4	51	4.1	6.6	0.7	1
Lentil & Bacon, Classic, Heinz*	1 Can/400g	232	5.6	58	2.7	8.4	1.4	0.7
Lentil & Bacon, Favourites, Baxters*	1 Can/400g	208	2.8	52	3.4	7.3	0.7	0.8
Lentil & Smoked Bacon, Fresh, Tesco*	1 Pack/600g	420	11.4	70	3.9	8.5	1.9	1.6
Lentil & Vegetable Soup, Healthy, Baxters*	1 Can/415g	174	1.2	42	1.9	7.4	0.3	1.2
Lentil & Vegetable, LC, Tesco*	1 Can/400g	188	0.8	47	2.5	8.8	0.2	1.1
Lentil Dhal, Canned, Asda*	½ Can/200g	117	3	59	2.4	7.7	1.5	2.3
Lentil with Red Lentils, Carrots, Potato & Onion, Asda*	1 Can/400g	192	0.8	48	1.4	10.2	0.2	1.2
Lentil, & Bacon, Smoked, New Covent Garden Food Co*	1 Carton/350g	178	3.5	51	3.7	8.9	1	4.3

S

SOUP

	Measure INFO/WEIGHT	per Measure KCAL	FAT	Nutrition Values per 100g / 100ml KCAL	PROT	CARB	FAT	FIBRE
Lentil, Asda*	½ Can/202g	89	0.4	44	2.6	8	0.2	0.7
Lentil, Bacon & Mixed Bean, Low Fat, Aldi*	1 Serving/400g	260	3.6	65	4.7	9.5	0.9	1.6
Lentil, Classic, Heinz*	1 Can/400g	180	0.8	45	2.4	8.5	0.2	0.8
Lobster Bisque, Luxury, with Brandy & Cream, Baxters*	1 Can/400g	272	17.2	68	2.6	4.8	4.3	0.2
Lobster Bisque, Waitrose*	½ Carton/300g	201	13.8	67	0.9	5.5	4.6	0.6
Mediterranean Tomato & Vegetable, Fresh, Tesco*	½ Pot/300g	105	2.1	35	1	6.2	0.7	0.7
Mediterranean Tomato, Fresh, Organic, Sainsbury's*	1 Serving/250ml	78	3.5	31	1.3	3.3	1.4	1
Mediterranean Tomato, Slim a Soup, Cup, Batchelors*	1 Serving/208g	56	1.2	27	0.5	4.8	0.6	0.4
Mediterranean Tomato, Vegetarian, Baxters*	1 Can/400g	126	0.4	32	0.9	5.6	0.1	0.8
Mexican Bean, Fresh, Morrisons*	½ Pot/300g	171	3.9	57	2.1	8.3	1.3	1.9
Mexican Black Bean, Extra Special, Asda*	½ Pot/263g	194	10.8	74	2.3	7	4.1	1.7
Mexican Chilli Beef & Bean, Soups of the World, Heinz*	1 Can/515g	360	9.3	70	4.5	9	1.8	1.6
Mexican Spiced Chicken & Bean, Eat Smart, Morrisons*	1 Can/400g	200	2	50	2.9	7.3	0.5	1.9
Mexican Super Bean & Sweet Potato, Glorious!*	½ Pot/300g	137	0.6	46	2.3	6.9	0.2	3.4
Minestrone with Croutons in a Cup, Sainsbury's*	1 Sachet/225ml	72	0.9	32	0.9	6.3	0.4	0.5
Minestrone with Croutons in a Mug, Tesco*	1 Sachet/23g	83	1.9	360	9	62.6	8.1	2.7
Minestrone with Croutons, Dry, Soupreme, Aldi*	1 Serving/27g	94	1.7	349	7.6	65.3	6.4	4.4
Minestrone with Pasta, Chunky, Co-Op*	1 Pack/400g	140	2.4	35	1	6	0.6	0.7
Minestrone, Canned, Average	*1 Can/400g*	*252*	*12*	*63*	*1.8*	*7.6*	*3*	*0.9*
Minestrone, CBY, Asda*	½ Can/200g	70	1	35	0.4	6.4	0.5	1.6
Minestrone, Chunky, Classic, Fresh, Tesco*	½ Pot/300g	126	2.1	42	1.2	7.8	0.7	1.2
Minestrone, Chunky, Fresh, Sainsbury's*	½ Pot/300g	93	0.6	31	1.4	6.1	0.2	2.3
Minestrone, Classic, Heinz*	1 Can/400g	128	0.8	32	1	6.2	0.2	0.8
Minestrone, Diet Chef Ltd*	1 Pack/300g	123	1.8	41	1.4	7.5	0.6	1.2
Minestrone, Favourites, Baxters*	1 Can/400g	156	2.4	39	1.5	5.5	0.6	1.3
Minestrone, Fresh, Asda*	½ Pot/300g	138	2.1	46	1.8	8.2	0.7	1.2
Minestrone, Fresh, Average	*1 Carton/600g*	*244*	*4.9*	*41*	*1.7*	*6.8*	*0.8*	*1.2*
Minestrone, Fresh, Co-Op*	1 Pot/600g	260	8.4	43	1	6.2	1.4	1.3
Minestrone, Fresh, Morrisons*	1 Pot/506ml	182	2	36	1.9	6.4	0.4	0.2
Minestrone, Fresh, Tesco*	½ Carton/300g	132	3	44	1.8	6.3	1	1.4
Minestrone, Fresh, Waitrose*	1 Pack/600g	240	8.4	40	1.1	5.8	1.4	0.8
Minestrone, Loved by Us, Co-Op*	½ Pot/300g	135	4.2	45	1	6.2	1.4	1.3
Minestrone, Pack, Dry, Knorr*	1 Pack/61g	204	2.4	335	12	58.8	4	6.9
Minestrone, Sainsbury's*	½ Can/200g	66	0.8	33	1.1	6.3	0.4	0.9
Minted Lamb Hot Pot, Big Soup, Heinz*	1 Can/400g	228	5.2	57	2.9	8.1	1.3	1
Miso with Tofu, Instant, Kikkoman*	1 Sachet/10g	35	1	350	30	30	10	0
Miso, Japanese, Made Up, Yutaka*	1 Serving/250ml	24	0.7	10	0.6	1.1	0.3	0
Miso, Wakama*	1 Sachet/8g	27	0.6	336	18.7	48.6	7.6	0
More Bangalore, Skinnylicious, Skinny Soup, Glorious!*	½ Pot/300g	147	4.2	49	2	6.1	1.4	2.2
Moroccan Chicken & Vegetable, Love Life, Waitrose*	½ Pot/300g	192	5.7	64	3.7	7.9	1.9	1.9
Moroccan Chicken, Finest, Tesco*	½ Pot/300g	201	5.1	67	4.2	8.1	1.7	1.2
Moroccan, Inspired, Pot, Tesco*	½ Pack/266g	146	2.4	55	1.9	8.9	0.9	1.9
Moroccan, with Vegan Pieces, Quorn*	½ Pot/283g	136	1.7	48	4.2	4.4	0.6	3.7
Mulligatawny	*1 Serving/220g*	*213*	*15*	*97*	*1.4*	*8.2*	*6.8*	*0.9*
Mulligatawny, Canned, Tesco*	1 Can/400g	188	4	47	1.3	8.1	1	0.3
Mulligatawny, Classic, Heinz*	1 Can/400g	232	7.6	58	1.9	8	1.9	0.5
Mushroom & Chestnut, Fresh, Finest, Tesco*	1 Serving/250g	130	8.2	52	1.1	4.7	3.3	0.7
Mushroom Potage, Woodland Mushrooms, Baxters*	1 Can/415g	328	20.8	79	1.6	6.9	5	0.3
Mushroom with Croutons in a Cup, Waitrose*	1 Sachet/212g	102	4.2	48	0.6	6.8	2	0.5
Mushroom with Croutons, Soup in a Mug, Tesco*	1 Serving/226ml	115	4.7	51	1	6.8	2.1	0.4
Mushroom, Canned, HL, Tesco*	1 Can/400g	132	5.6	33	0.5	4.4	1.4	0.2
Mushroom, Cream Of, Canned, Tesco*	½ Can/200g	94	5.8	47	0.7	4.8	2.9	0.2
Mushroom, Cream of, Classics, Heinz*	1 Can/400g	208	11.2	52	1.5	5.2	2.8	0.1

SOUP

INFO/WEIGHT	Measure	per Measure KCAL	FAT	Nutrition Values per 100g / 100ml KCAL	PROT	CARB	FAT	FIBRE
Mushroom, Cream Of, Condensed, Batchelors*	1 Can/295g	330	25.1	112	1.3	7.5	8.5	0.2
Mushroom, Cream of, Fresh, Finest, Tesco*	½ Pot/300g	238	19	79	1.9	3.5	6.3	0.5
Mushroom, Cully & Sully*	1 Carton/400g	192	17.6	48	0.8	1.3	4.4	1
Mushroom, Diet Chef Ltd*	1 Pack/300g	105	5.1	35	1.9	3.2	1.7	0.9
Mushroom, for One, Heinz*	1 Can/290g	148	7.8	51	1.4	5.1	2.7	0.1
Mushroom, Fresh, Average	*1 Serving/300g*	*146*	*9.3*	*49*	*1.3*	*4*	*3.1*	*0.8*
Mushroom, Fresh, M&S*	½ Pack/300g	165	11.7	55	1.8	3.5	3.9	0.9
Mushroom, Wild, New Covent Garden Food Co*	1 Carton/600g	162	8.4	27	1	1.9	1.4	1.5
Noodle, Cup, Shin, Nongshim*	1 Cup/75g	326	11.2	435	7	68	15	0
Oxtail, Average	*1 Can/400g*	*163*	*4.5*	*41*	*2*	*5.8*	*1.1*	*0.4*
Oxtail, Canned	*1 Serving/220g*	*97*	*3.7*	*44*	*2.4*	*5.1*	*1.7*	*0.1*
Oxtail, Classic, Heinz*	1 Can/400g	168	2	42	1.9	7.3	0.5	0.3
Oxtail, Favourites, Baxters*	1 Can/400g	192	4.4	48	1.8	6.8	1.1	0.5
Oxtail, For One, Heinz*	1 Can/300g	126	1.5	42	1.9	7.3	0.5	0.3
Oxtail, Soupreme, Aldi*	1 Can/400g	152	2	38	2.2	6	0.5	0.5
Parsnip & Butternut Squash, The Best, Morrisons*	1 Can/400g	244	8.4	61	2.4	8.1	2.1	1.6
Parsnip & Honey, Festive, New Covent Garden Food Co*	½ Carton/350g	217	7	62	0.9	9.2	2	1.9
Parsnip & Honey, Fresh, Sainsbury's*	½ Carton/300g	192	12.6	64	1.1	5.4	4.2	1.5
Parsnip & Orchard Apple, Duchy Originals*	1 Pack/350g	116	3.2	33	0.7	5.4	0.9	1
Parsnip, Spicy, Average	*1 Serving/400g*	*212*	*11.2*	*53*	*0.9*	*6*	*2.8*	*1.6*
Pea & Mint, Fresh, M&S*	1 Serving/164g	49	0.2	30	1.8	6.3	0.1	1.5
Pea & Ham	*1 Serving/220g*	*154*	*4.6*	*70*	*4*	*9.2*	*2.1*	*1.4*
Pea & Ham Hock, Finest, Tesco*	½ Pot/300g	197	6.6	66	3.7	6.6	2.2	2.4
Pea & Ham, Canned, Favourites, Baxters*	1 Can/400g	218	4	55	3.3	7.1	1	2
Pea & Ham, Canned, Tesco*	1 Can/400g	184	2	46	3.1	6.1	0.5	2.1
Pea & Ham, CBY, Asda*	1 Pot/600g	282	6.6	47	2.9	5.6	1.1	1.4
Pea & Ham, Classic, Heinz*	1 Can/400g	252	3.2	63	2.8	10.1	0.8	1.1
Pea & Ham, Diet Chef Ltd*	1 Pack/300g	138	3.3	46	3.2	5.8	1.1	2.6
Pea & Ham, Fresh, Sainsbury's*	½ Pack/300ml	120	1.5	40	1.9	7	0.5	0.3
Pea & Ham, Fresh, Waitrose*	1 Serving/300g	196	10	65	2.9	6.2	3.3	1.6
Pea & Mint, Best of British, Crosse & Blackwell*	1 Can/400g	192	8.4	48	1.7	4.6	2.1	1.9
Pea & Mint, Canned, M&S*	½ Can/200g	96	4.2	48	1.7	4.6	2.1	1.9
Pea & Mint, Fresh, Co-Op*	½ Tub/300g	105	1.7	35	1.7	4.8	0.6	1.8
Pea & Mint, Fresh, Finest, Tesco*	1 Serving/300g	165	7.2	55	1.3	6	2.4	1.5
Pea & Mint, Fresh, Sainsbury's*	½ Pot/300g	102	2.7	34	1.4	5	0.9	1.9
Pea & Mint, Fresh, Tesco*	½ Pot/300g	145	3.3	48	2.4	6	1.1	2.4
Pea & Mint, Slimming World, Iceland*	1 Tub/500g	210	1.5	42	2.6	6	0.3	2.4
Pea & Mint, with Leek, Fresh, Waitrose*	1 Serving/300g	123	4.5	41	1.7	4.4	1.5	1.5
Pepper & Chorizo, Canned, Sainsbury's*	1 Can/400ml	172	4	43	7	2	1	0
Pepper, Sweetcorn & Chilli, Mexican, TTD, Sainsbury's*	½ Pot/300g	190	6.6	63	2.4	7.2	2.2	3
Pepper, with Chilli, Italiamo, Lidl*	1 Can/390ml	222	9.4	57	0.6	7.6	2.4	1.3
Plum Tomato & Basil, New Covent Garden Food Co*	½ Carton/300g	132	6	44	1.3	5.2	2	1.3
Potato & Leek, Classics, Canned, Heinz*	1 Can/400g	184	7.2	46	0.8	6.7	1.8	0.6
Potato & Leek	*1oz/28g*	*15*	*0.7*	*52*	*1.5*	*6.2*	*2.6*	*0.8*
Potato & Leek, Canned, Sainsbury's*	½ Can/200g	92	3.2	46	1	6.7	1.6	0.3
Potato & Leek, Favourites, Baxters*	1 Can/400g	192	7.2	48	1	6.6	1.8	0.9
Prawn Tom Yum, Cook*	1 Portion/335g	231	3	69	3.5	10.8	0.9	0
Prawn, King, & Glass Noodles, Pho, pot	*1 Pot/642g*	*212*	*2.6*	*33*	*1.8*	*5.4*	*0.4*	*0.5*
Pumpkin, & Ginger, New Covent Garden Food Co*	1 Serving/300	128	4.8	43	0.7	5.7	1.6	1.5
Pumpkin, Creamy, Very Special, Heinz*	1 Sm Can/290g	188	5.5	65	1.3	9.9	1.9	1.1
Pumpkin, Spicy, Fresh, Sainsbury's*	½ Pot/300g	87	3	29	0.9	4.2	1	1.3
Pumpkin, Sweet Potato & Red Pepper, SO, Sainsbury's*	½ Pot/300g	111	3.9	37	0.8	5.6	1.3	0.8
Red Lentil & Ham, Waitrose*	½ Pot/300g	147	3.3	49	3.9	5.8	1.1	2

	Measure INFO/WEIGHT	per Measure KCAL	FAT	Nutrition Values per 100g / 100ml KCAL	PROT	CARB	FAT	FIBRE

SOUP

	Measure INFO/WEIGHT	per Measure KCAL	FAT	KCAL	PROT	CARB	FAT	FIBRE
Red Pepper & Wensleydale, Asda*	1 Carton /600g	306	12.6	51	2.5	5	2.1	0.8
Rich Beef Broth, with Smoky Paprika, Heinz*	½ Can/200g	82	1	41	1.8	6.9	0.5	0.7
Roasted Red Pepper & Tomato, M&S*	1 Serving/150g	105	7.4	70	1.4	5	4.9	0.6
Roasted Red Pepper & Tomato, Canned, Sainsbury's*	1 Can/400g	196	6	49	1	7.5	1.5	0.9
Roasted Red Pepper, Fresh, Waitrose*	1 Pack/600g	172	9	29	0.8	3	1.5	1
Roasted Vegetable, Fresh, Sainsbury's*	½ Pot/300ml	78	1.5	26	0.5	4.8	0.5	1.2
Royal Game, Favourites, Baxters*	1 Can/400g	152	0.8	38	1.8	6.9	0.2	0.3
Scotch Broth, Canned, Tesco*	½ Can/200g	85	2.6	42	1.3	5.9	1.3	0.8
Scotch Broth, Classic, Heinz*	1 Can/400g	156	2.4	39	1.4	6.7	0.6	0.6
Scotch Broth, Favourites, Baxters*	1 Can/400g	196	6	49	1.8	6.2	1.5	1.5
Seafood Chowder, Waitrose*	1 Can/404g	226	11.3	56	2.2	5.6	2.8	0.6
Sicilian Tomato & Balsamic, Skinny Soup, Glorious!*	1 Carton/600g	216	11.4	36	1	3.3	1.9	0.7
Smoked Bacon & Bean, Diet Chef Ltd*	1 Pack/300g	162	3.3	54	2.8	8.2	1.1	2.1
Smoked Bacon & Three Bean, Chunky, Baxters*	1 Can/400g	232	4.8	58	2.9	8.8	1.2	1.8
Smoky Chipotle Beans, with Quinoa, Meal, Sainsbury's*	1 Pot/400g	369	12.8	92	3.5	10.5	3.2	3.7
Soup, Leek & Potato, Fresh, Sainsbury's*	½ Pot/300g	114	3.6	38	0.7	6.1	1.2	1.3
Spiced Lentil, High Protein, Cup a Soup, Batchelors*	1 Pack/255g	97	1.5	38	1.9	6	0.6	0.5
Spiced Spinach & Green Lentil, Asda*	½ Pot/250g	122	5	49	2.7	5	2	0
Spicy Lentil & Vegetable, Chilled, M&S*	½ Serving/300g	150	2.4	50	2.7	8	0.8	1.1
Spicy Lentil, M&S*	1 Serving/100g	50	1.1	50	2.6	6.3	1.1	2.1
Spicy Parsnip, Aldi*	1 Serving/250g	132	8.5	53	0.6	4.9	3.4	1.4
Spicy Parsnip, Vegetarian, Baxters*	1 Can/425g	212	10.6	50	0.7	5.3	2.5	1.7
Spicy Tomato & Vegetable, Healthy Living, Co-Op*	1 Can/400g	180	3.2	45	2	8	0.8	2
Spicy Tomato & Rice with Sweetcorn, Healthy, Baxters*	1 Can/414g	211	0.8	51	1.6	9.2	0.2	1
Spinach & Watercress, New Covent Garden Food Co*	½ Carton/298g	60	1.2	20	1.3	2.8	0.4	0.8
Spinach, Creme Fraiche, & Nutmeg, Organic, Waitrose*	½ Pot/300g	243	22.8	81	0.9	2.3	7.6	1.1
Split Pea & Ham, Asda*	1 Serving/300g	129	0.6	43	3.5	6.9	0.2	0.7
Split Peas, Yellow, Simply Organic*	1 Pot/600g	354	3	59	4.3	10.4	0.5	2.6
Spooky Spiced Pumpkin, New Covent Garden Food Co*	1 Serving/350g	168	5.2	48	1.8	6	1.5	1.6
Spring Vegetable, Classic, Heinz*	1 Can/400g	148	1.6	37	0.8	7	0.4	0.8
Spring Vegetable, Sainsbury's*	½ Can/200g	72	0.8	36	0.8	7.4	0.4	0.6
Squash, Butternut, Curried, & Lentil, Seeds of Change*	1 Pack/400g	164	1.2	41	2.3	7.2	0.3	1.9
Steak & Potato, Angus, Big Soup, Heinz*	½ Can/250g	120	2	48	3.1	6.8	0.8	0.6
Steak, & Ale, Chunky, Asda*	1 Can/400g	188	4.4	47	3	5.9	1.1	0.6
Stilton, Celery & Watercress, Morrisons*	1 Serving/250g	272	23	109	3.9	3.1	9.2	0.3
Sun Dried Tomato & Basil, Heinz*	1 Serving/275ml	124	5.2	45	0.6	6.5	1.9	0.1
super Broccoli, Spinach & Pea, Super, M&S*	1 Serving/300g	102	3.9	34	2.1	2.7	1.3	1.6
Super Chicken Noodle, Dry, Knorr*	1 Pack/56g	182	2.7	325	14.3	56	4.9	1.8
Superbean, Lentil & Barley, M&S*	1 Pack /600g	270	9	45	1.8	5.1	1.5	2.1
Supergreens, Seaweed, Spirulina & Quinoa, Tideford*	1 Pot/600g	198	3	33	2.5	3.9	0.5	1.3
Sweet Potato, Coconut & Chilli, TTD, Sainsbury's*	½ Pot/300g	176	5.7	59	0.9	8.5	1.9	1.8
Sweetcorn Chowder, Microwaved, Slimming World*	1 Pot/500g	160	2.5	32	1.1	5.3	0.5	0.7
Thai Pumpkin Coconut, New Covent Garden Food Co*	1 Carton/568ml	182	7.4	32	1.3	3.5	1.3	1.1
Three Bean & Vegetable, HL, Tesco*	1 Portion/200g	90	0.6	45	2.1	7.5	0.3	1.9
Three Bean & Vegetable, LC, Tesco*	½ Can/200g	110	0.6	55	2.6	9.7	0.3	1.9
Three Mushroom, Broth, Soupologie*	1 Serving/300g	48	0.6	16	0.7	2.4	0.2	0.7
Tomato & Basil, Cup a Soup, Made Up, GFY, Asda*	1 Serving/250ml	50	0.2	20	0.4	4.4	0.1	0.2
Tomato & Basil, Fresh, Finest, Tesco*	½ Pot/300g	219	14.7	73	1	6.3	4.9	0.6
Tomato & Roasted Red Pepper, COU, M&S*	1 Serving/415g	145	0.4	35	1	7.6	0.1	0.9
Tomato & Vegetable, Cup a Soup, Batchelors*	1 Serving/218g	107	2.6	49	1.1	8.5	1.2	0.6
Tomato & Basil Flavoured, CWP*	1 Serving/40g	139	3.6	348	33.5	28.5	9	8.2
Tomato & Basil, CBY, Asda*	½ Pot/297g	89	2.4	30	1	4.3	0.8	0.7
Tomato & Basil, Creamy, Cully & Sully*	1 Pack/400g	216	18.5	54	0.8	2.5	4.6	0.5

S

SOUP

INFO/WEIGHT	Measure		Nutrition Values per 100g / 100ml				
	KCAL	FAT	KCAL	PROT	CARB	FAT	FIBRE
Tomato & Basil, Cup, Co-Op*	1 Sachet/45g	158	1.8	350	2	76	4	4
Tomato & Basil, Fresh, Low Fat, Sainsbury's*	½ Carton/300ml	75	1.8	25	1.1	4.1	0.6	0.7
Tomato & Basil, Fresh, M Kitchen, Morrisons*	½ Pot/300g	115	3.6	38	1	5.5	1.2	0.7
Tomato & Basil, Fresh, M&S*	½ Pot/300g	120	5.1	40	1	5	1.7	1.3
Tomato & Basil, Italian, 99% Fat Free, Baxters*	½ Can/208g	119	2.1	57	2.6	9.3	1	1.1
Tomato & Basil, M&S*	½ Pot/300g	105	4.2	35	0.7	4.5	1.4	1
Tomato & Basil, Rich, Waitrose*	1 Serving/130g	53	1.3	41	1.3	6.3	1	0.7
Tomato & Basil, Weight Watchers*	1 Serving/295g	114	1.8	39	0.6	7.5	0.6	0.6
Tomato & Brown Lentil, Healthy, Baxters*	1 Can/415g	199	0.8	48	2.6	9	0.2	2.7
Tomato & Butter Bean, Classic, Heinz*	½ Can/200g	92	1.4	46	1.3	8.1	0.7	0.8
Tomato & Lentil, Organic, Tideford*	1 Carton/300g	120	2.7	40	2.3	8.1	0.9	0.9
Tomato & Lentil, Truly Irresistible, Co-Op*	½ Pot/300g	165	2.1	55	3.1	8	0.7	1.2
Tomato & Three Bean, Canned, BGTY, Sainsbury's*	½ Can/200g	120	2.2	60	2.8	8.4	1.1	2.4
Tomato & Three Bean, Co-Op*	½ Can/200g	130	1.8	65	3.7	10.2	0.9	2
Tomato & Three Bean, Eat Smart, Morrisons*	1 Can/400g	228	4	57	2.8	8.2	1	2.2
Tomato & Thyme, Organic, Duchy, Waitrose*	½ Pot/300g	140	8.9	47	1.2	3.3	3	1
Tomato, Borlotti Bean & Kale, Fresh, M&S*	1 Pot/600g	318	10.2	53	2	6.3	1.7	2.1
Tomato, Canned, LC, Tesco*	½ Can/200g	90	3.8	45	0.9	5.9	1.9	0.4
Tomato, Chunky, Organic, Canned, Amy's Kitchen*	1 Can/400g	212	5.6	53	1.2	8.6	1.4	1.2
Tomato, Cream of with a Hint of Basil, Heinz*	½ Can/200g	114	6	57	0.9	6.6	3	0.4
Tomato, Cream Of, Asda*	½ Can/200g	122	6.4	61	0.7	7.3	3.2	0.7
Tomato, Cream Of, Canned, Average	**1 Can/400g**	**208**	**12**	**52**	**0.8**	**5.9**	**3**	**0.7**
Tomato, Cream of, Canned, Crosse & Blackwell*	1 Can/400g	228	10	57	0.9	7.4	2.5	0.8
Tomato, Cream of, Canned, Tesco*	½ Can/192g	115	4.8	60	0.9	7.4	2.5	0.8
Tomato, Cream of, Classic, Heinz*	½ Can/200g	118	6	59	0.9	6.7	3	0.4
Tomato, Cream Of, Classics, Soupreme, Aldi*	1 Can/400g	192	8	48	0.8	6.4	2	0.8
Tomato, Cream of, Eat Well, M&S*	½ Pot/300g	189	9.9	63	0.8	7.1	3.3	0.6
Tomato, Cream of, Favourites, Baxters*	½ Can/200g	132	5.4	66	1.1	6.9	2.7	0.4
Tomato, Cream Of, for One, Heinz*	1 Can/300g	189	10.8	63	0.8	6.9	3.6	0.4
Tomato, Cream Of, Fresh, Sainsbury's*	1 Pot/600g	318	19.2	53	0.8	5.2	3.2	1.3
Tomato, Cream Of, Sainsbury's*	1 Can/400g	244	12.8	61	0.7	7.3	3.2	0.7
Tomato, Cream Of, with Spanish Chorizo, Heinz*	1 Can/400g	244	12	61	1.4	6.9	3	0.4
Tomato, Cup a Soup, Made Up, Batchelors*	1 Sachet/255.6g	92	2.3	36	0.3	6.7	0.9	0.3
Tomato, Original, Cup a Soup, Batchelors*	1 Sachet/24g	90	2.1	387	3.9	70.5	9	3.4
Tomato, Red Lentil & Pepper, CBY, Asda*	½ Pot/300g	177	3.3	59	3	8.8	1.1	0.9
Tomato, Singapore Crushed, Skinny Soup, Glorious!*	½ Pot/300g	129	5.4	43	1	5.8	1.8	1.1
Tomato, Slow Roast, New Covent Garden Food Co*	½ Carton/350g	98	1.4	28	0.9	4.4	0.4	1.5
Tomato, Smart Price, Asda*	1 Can/400g	184	7.6	46	0.6	6.5	1.9	0.9
Tomato, Weight Watchers*	1 Can/295g	76	1.5	26	0.7	4.6	0.5	0.3
Turkey Broth, Canned, Baxters*	½ Can/208g	79	1.5	38	1.3	6.5	0.7	0.7
Tuscan Bean, Canned, HL, Tesco*	½ Can/200ml	140	3.6	70	3.5	10.3	1.8	1.3
Tuscan Bean, Chunky, Love Life, Waitrose*	½ Can/200g	101	1	50	2.6	7.6	0.5	2.3
Tuscan Bean, Organic, Fresh, Sainsbury's*	1 Pack/400g	171	3.2	43	2.6	6.3	0.8	2
Tuscan Bean, Tesco*	1 Can/400g	272	3.2	68	3.6	10.3	0.8	2.6
Tuscan Bean, with Roasted Garlic & Tomatoes, Heinz*	1 Can/400g	188	3.6	47	1.3	7.7	0.9	1.1
Tuscan Chicken & Orzo, Glorious!*	½ Pot/300g	120	1.2	40	2.8	6.2	0.4	0.7
Tuscan, Chicken, Tomato, & Grains, Glorious!*	½ Pack/300g	111	2.1	37	2	4.9	0.7	1.5
Vegetable & Three Bean, Chunky, M&S*	1 Can/400g	228	3.6	57	3	7.7	0.9	3.1
Vegetable Broth, Best of British, Crosse & Blackwell*	1 Can/400g	135	1.6	34	1.1	5.9	0.4	1.1
Vegetable Broth, Hearty, Weight Watchers*	1 Can/295g	135	0.6	46	2	8.2	0.2	1.4
Vegetable Gyoza, with Miso Broth, Everdine*	1 Serving/450g	369	5	82	2.9	13.3	1.1	3.6
Vegetable, Balance, Reduced Salt, Canned, Heinz*	1 Can/400g	168	2.8	42	1.2	7.2	0.7	1.2
Vegetable, Canned	**1oz/28g**	**13**	**0.2**	**48**	**1.4**	**9.9**	**0.6**	**1.5**

S

	Measure INFO/WEIGHT	per Measure KCAL	FAT	Nutrition Values per 100g / 100ml KCAL	PROT	CARB	FAT	FIBRE
SOUP								
Vegetable, Canned, Essential, Waitrose*	½ Can/200g	103	1	52	1.9	9.2	0.5	1.4
Vegetable, Canned, Tesco*	½ Can/200g	70	1	35	1.1	5.9	0.5	1
Vegetable, Canned, Tesco*	½ Can/200g	100	2	50	1.4	8.1	1	1.3
Vegetable, Chunky, Canned, Sainsbury's*	1 Can/400g	184	2.8	46	1.5	8.3	0.7	1.2
Vegetable, Chunky, Canned, Soupreme, Aldi*	1 Can/400g	172	4	43	1.1	6.4	1	2.3
Vegetable, Chunky, Fresh, Tesco*	1 Serving/300g	123	5.7	41	0.6	5.5	1.9	1
Vegetable, Chunky, Fresh, Waitrose*	½ Pot/300g	117	5.4	39	1.3	4.5	1.8	2.1
Vegetable, Classic, Heinz*	1 Can/400g	188	3.2	47	1.1	8.3	0.8	0.9
Vegetable, Cream of, VeloutÃƒ© De LÃƒ©gumes, Liebig*	1 Portion/200ml	84	4	42	0.7	5.3	2	1
Vegetable, Cully & Sully*	1 Pack/400g	204	14.4	51	0.6	4.2	3.6	0.9
Vegetable, Cup Soup, Dry, Heinz*	1 Sachet/15.5g	54	1.1	348	5.8	64.5	7.1	3.2
Vegetable, Cup Soup, Made Up, Heinz*	1 Cup/200g	50	1	25	0.4	4.7	0.5	0.2
Vegetable, Fresh, Average	**1 Serving/300g**	**118**	**4.1**	**40**	**1.4**	**5.4**	**1.4**	**1.3**
Vegetable, Fresh, Co-Op*	1 Pack/600g	150	6	25	0.6	4	1	1
Vegetable, in a Cup, HL, Tesco*	1 Sachet/18g	66	1.4	367	7.2	66.1	7.8	2.8
Vegetable, Instant, Cup, Average	**1 Pack/19g**	**69**	**2**	**362**	**8.7**	**57.1**	**10.5**	**5.5**
Vegetable, Moroccan, Tagine, Yorkshire Provender*	½ Pot/300g	171	5.1	57	2.3	7.2	1.7	0.7
Vegetable, Soup In A Mug, Made Up, HL, Tesco*	1 Sachet/218ml	66	1.1	30	0.7	5.5	0.5	0.4
Vietnamese Super Green, Skinny Soup, Glorious!*	½ Tub/300g	117	1.2	39	2.7	4.5	0.4	3.1
Vine Tomato, Harissa & Mint, The Best, Morrisons*	1 Pot/600g	294	11.4	49	1.5	6.4	1.9	1.1
Watercress, M&S*	½ Pot/300g	75	5.1	25	1.3	1.5	1.7	0.6
Winter Vegetable, New Covent Garden Food Co*	½ Pack/300g	117	2.1	39	2	5.1	0.7	2.3
SOUP MIX								
Butternut Squash, Sainsbury's*	¼ Pack/147g	47	1	32	0.8	5.3	0.7	0.5
Leek & Potato, As Sold, Good & Balanced, Asda*	¼ Pack/125g	69	0.4	55	1.7	10.5	0.3	1.7
Minestrone & Bean, Cooks' Ingredients, Waitrose*	½ Pack/200g	118	1	59	2.7	9	0.5	3.6
Soup & Broth Mix, Dry, Wholefoods, Tesco*	¼ Pack/125g	456	2.4	365	14.7	71.4	1.9	7.3
Vegetable, Kit, Morrisons*	1 Pack/500g	220	3.5	44	1.2	6.6	0.7	3
SOUTHERN COMFORT								
37.5% Volume	**1 Pub Shot/35ml**	**72**	**0**	**207**	**0**	**0**	**0**	**0**
SOYA								
Barbeque Chilli, Vegelicious, Tesco*	1 Portion/450g	450	15.8	100	3.1	12.9	3.5	2.7
Chunks, Dried, Cooked, Sainsbury's*	1oz/28g	27	0.1	98	14	9.8	0.3	1.1
Chunks, Protein, Natural, Nature's Harvest*	1 Serving/50g	172	0.5	345	50	35	1	4
Mince, Dry Weight, Sainsbury's*	1 Serving/50g	164	0.4	328	47.2	33.2	0.8	3.6
Mince, Granules	**1oz/28g**	**74**	**1.5**	**263**	**43.2**	**11**	**5.4**	**0**
Mince, Prepared, Sainsbury's*	1 Serving/200g	164	0.4	82	11.8	8.3	0.2	0.9
SPAGHETTI								
Black Bean, Organic, Dry, Explore Asian*	1 Serving/56g	198	2	353	44	15	3.6	21
Brown Rice, GF, Organic, Dry, Dove's Farm*	1 Serving/70g	237	1	338	7.9	70.3	1.5	4.1
Carrot, Tesco*	1 Serving/80g	34	0.2	42	0.6	7.9	0.3	2.4
Cooked, Average	**1oz/28g**	**33**	**0.2**	**119**	**4.1**	**24.8**	**0.6**	**1.1**
Dry, Average	**1oz/28g**	**98**	**0.4**	**350**	**12.1**	**72.1**	**1.5**	**2.4**
Durum Wheat, Dry, Average	**1oz/28g**	**97**	**0.1**	**348**	**12.4**	**71.8**	**0.4**	**1.4**
Edamame, Organic, Dry, Explore Asian*	1 Serving/56g	204	2	365	45	18	3.6	20
Egg, Fresh, Cooked, Tesco*	½ Pack/150g	480	3.7	320	9.7	62.7	2.5	3.4
Fresh, Cooked, Average	**1 Serving/125g**	**182**	**2.2**	**146**	**6.1**	**26.9**	**1.7**	**1.8**
Fresh, Dry, Average	**1 Serving/100g**	**278**	**3**	**278**	**10.8**	**53**	**3**	**2.2**
Hoops, Canned, Smart Price, Asda*	½ Can/205g	127	0.6	62	1.7	13	0.3	0.4
Hoops, in Tomato Sauce, Heinz*	½ Can/200g	106	0.4	53	1.7	11.1	0.2	0.5
Hoops, in Tomato Sauce, Snap Pot, Heinz*	1 Pot/190g	115	0.4	61	1.7	12.6	0.2	0.6
Hoops, Tesco*	½ Can/205g	123	0.4	60	1.6	12.9	0.2	0.5
in Rich Tomato Sauce, Canned, Corale, Aldi*	½ Can/200g	114	1	57	2.1	10	0.5	2.6

S

	Measure INFO/WEIGHT	per Measure KCAL	per Measure FAT	Nutrition Values per 100g / 100ml KCAL	PROT	CARB	FAT	FIBRE
SPAGHETTI								
in Tomato Sauce with Parsley, Weight Watchers*	1 Sm Can/200g	100	0.4	50	1.8	9.9	0.2	0.6
In Tomato Sauce, Basics, Sainsbury's*	1 Can/410g	197	1.2	48	1.4	10	0.3	0.7
in Tomato Sauce, Canned	*1oz/28g*	*18*	*0.1*	*64*	*1.9*	*14.1*	*0.4*	*0.7*
in Tomato Sauce, Heinz*	½ Can/200g	120	0.6	60	1.7	12.7	0.3	2.4
Marinara	*1 Serving/450g*	*675*	*18.9*	*150*	*8*	*19*	*4.2*	*0.9*
Rings, in Tomato Sauce, Canned, Sainsbury's*	1 Serving/213g	136	0.8	64	1.9	13.3	0.4	0.5
Whole Wheat, Cooked, Average	*1oz/28g*	*32*	*0.3*	*113*	*4.7*	*23.2*	*0.9*	*3.5*
Whole Wheat, Dry, Average	*1 Serving/100g*	*324*	*2.6*	*324*	*13.5*	*62.2*	*2.6*	*8*
Whole Wheat, Dry, Napolina*	1 Serving/75g	258	1.5	344	13	64	2	9
Wholegrain, Spelt, Cooked, Sainsbury's*	1 Serving/200g	319	2	160	6.2	30.3	1	2.6
with Sausages, in Tomato Sauce, Heinz*	1 Can/400g	352	14	88	3.4	10.8	3.5	0.5
SPAGHETTI & MEATBALLS								
556, Wiltshire Farm Foods*	1 Serving/405g	456	22.5	112	4.4	10.8	5.6	1
American, Superbowl, Asda*	1 Pack/453g	594	17.7	131	11	13	3.9	1.1
Beef & Pork, Calorie Controlled, Love Life, Waitrose*	1 Pack/356g	342	9.3	96	5.5	11.9	2.6	1.3
Chicken, in Tomato Sauce, Heinz*	1 Can/400g	332	9.2	83	4.2	11.3	2.3	0.5
GFY, Asda*	1 Pack/400g	344	6	86	7	11	1.5	1.5
Italian Cuisine, Tesco*	1 Pack/400g	500	17.6	125	5.9	14.6	4.4	1.7
Little Dish*	1 Pack/200g	227	9.6	114	6.2	10.6	4.8	1.6
Low Fat, Co-Op*	1 Pack/390g	355	9	91	5.2	11	2.3	2
Meal for One, Microwaved, Iceland*	1 Meal/453g	421	4.5	93	4.4	15.7	1	1.8
Meatballs, Italian, As Prepared, Waitrose*	1 Pack/400g	520	23.8	131	6.1	12.8	6	0.8
Pork & Beef, in Tomato Sauce, Prepared, Sainsbury's*	1 Pack/401g	566	27.3	141	7.3	11.9	6.8	1.6
Ready Mea, lHealthy Range, Average	*1 Serving/400g*	*375*	*8.3*	*94*	*5.7*	*12.9*	*2.1*	*1.7*
Tesco*	1 Serving/475g	641	30.9	135	5.1	14.1	6.5	0.9
SPAGHETTI WITH								
King Prawn, Italian, Cooked, Finest, Tesco*	1 Pack/390g	485	22.9	125	5	12.2	5.9	1.3
Pulled Beef, Ragu, Everdine*	1 Serving/450g	360	8.1	80	7.7	7.2	1.8	2.1
SPAM*								
Fritters, Hormel Foods*	1 Fritter/80g	221	14.5	276	10.2	18.1	18.1	2.2
Pork & Ham, Chopped, Spam*	1 Serving/100g	289	24.3	289	15	3.2	24.3	0
SPICE MIX								
Chilli Con Carne, Tex Mex, Recipe Mix, Schwartz*	1 Sachet/35g	97	2.3	277	12.9	66.6	6.6	24.6
for Burritos, Old El Paso*	½ Pack/22.5g	68	0.9	304	13	54	4	0
for Fajitas, Old El Paso*	1 Pack/35g	107	2.1	306	9	54	6	0
for Mexican Fajitas, Discovery*	½ Pack/15g	34	1	230	8	35	6.5	17.5
Moroccan, Rub, Schwartz*	1 Serving/3g	9	0.3	309	15	36.4	11.4	19.5
Ras El Hanout, Al'fez*	1 Tsp/2g	4	0.2	217	9.8	25.7	8.3	17.5
Ras El Hanout, Blend, Finest, Tesco*	1 Tsp/5g	16	0.5	320	9.4	37.1	9.2	23.6
Thai, Blend, Sharwood's*	1 Pack 260g	424	30.9	163	1.8	12	11.9	1
Tikka, Blend, Sharwood's*	1 Pack/260g	263	14	101	2.7	10.2	5.4	1.7
Zaatar, Waitrose*	1 Serving/10g	42	3	416	14.7	8.2	30.2	26.1
SPINACH								
Baby, Average	*1 Serving/90g*	*22*	*0.7*	*25*	*2.8*	*1.6*	*0.8*	*2.1*
Boiled or Steamed, Average	*1 Serving/80g*	*17*	*0.6*	*21*	*2.6*	*0.9*	*0.8*	*2.1*
Canned, Average	*1 Serving/80g*	*16*	*0.4*	*20*	*2.8*	*1.3*	*0.5*	*2.7*
Creamed with Marscarpone Sauce, Sainsbury's*	½ Pack/147g	110	6.3	75	4.2	5	4.3	3.4
Creamed, Frozen, Weight Watchers*	1 Portion/112g	48	1.1	43	2.5	5	1	1.5
Mornay, Waitrose*	½ Pack/125g	112	8.6	90	3.3	3.6	6.9	1.6
Raw, Average	*1 Serving/80g*	*19*	*0.6*	*24*	*2.9*	*1.4*	*0.7*	*2.2*
SPIRALI								
Dry, Average	*1 Serving/50g*	*176*	*0.8*	*352*	*12.2*	*72.6*	*1.6*	*2.8*

S

	Measure INFO/WEIGHT	per Measure KCAL	FAT	Nutrition Values per 100g / 100ml KCAL	PROT	CARB	FAT	FIBRE
SPIRITS								
37.5% Volume	**1 Pub Shot/35ml**	**72**	**0**	**207**	**0**	**0**	**0**	**0**
40% Volume	**1 Shot/35ml**	**78**	**0**	**222**	**0**	**0**	**0**	**0**
Non Alcoholic, Garden, Seedlip Ltd*	1 Serving/50ml	0	0	0	0	0	0	0
Non Alcoholic, Spice 94, Botanical, Seedlip Ltd*	1 Serving/50ml	0	0	0	0	0	0	0
SPLIT PEAS								
Dried, Average	**1oz/28g**	**89**	**0.5**	**319**	**22.1**	**57.4**	**1.7**	**3.2**
Green, Dried, Average	**1 Serving/80g**	**261**	**1.3**	**326**	**22.5**	**45**	**1.6**	**20**
Green, Dried, Boiled, Average	**1 Tbsp/35g**	**40**	**0.2**	**115**	**8.3**	**19.8**	**0.6**	**3.9**
Yellow, Morrisons*	1 Serving /120g	338	1.4	282	21.3	62.2	1.2	15.6
Yellow, Wholefoods, Tesco*	1 Serving/15g	52	0.4	345	22.1	58.2	2.4	6.3
SPONGE FINGERS								
Boudoir, Sainsbury's*	1 Finger/5g	20	0.2	396	8.1	82.8	3.6	0.4
Tesco*	1 Finger/5g	19	0.2	386	7.6	80.6	3.7	1
Trifle, Average	**1 Sponge/24g**	**77**	**0.5**	**319**	**5.2**	**69.9**	**2.2**	**0.8**
SPONGE PUDDING								
Average	**1 Portion/170g**	**578**	**27.7**	**340**	**5.8**	**45.3**	**16.3**	**1.1**
Blackberry & Apple, HE, Tesco*	1 Pot/102.5g	159	1.4	155	3.1	32.6	1.4	0.7
Blackcurrant, BGTY, Sainsbury's*	1 Serving/110g	155	1	141	2.5	30.7	0.9	3.2
Canned, Average	**1 Serving/75g**	**214**	**8.6**	**285**	**3.1**	**45.4**	**11.4**	**0.8**
Cherry & Almond Flavour, Sainsbury's*	¼ Pudding/110g	334	15.7	304	3.5	40.3	14.3	0.7
Chocolate & Sauce, Co-Op*	1 Pack/225g	608	29.2	270	5	34	13	0.6
Chocolate, Cadbury*	1 Pack/370g	1276	73.3	345	4.9	36.7	19.8	0
Chocolate, Free From, Sainsbury's*	1 Pudding/110g	388	10.2	353	5.2	62	9.3	0.3
Chocolate, Less Than 3% Fat, BGTY, Sainsbury's*	1 Pudding/105g	180	2	171	4.5	34	1.9	0.9
Chocolate, M&S*	¼ Pudding/131g	524	32.2	400	6.1	38.6	24.6	1.8
Chocolate, M&S*	1 Pudding/105g	401	24.3	382	5.7	36	23.1	3.5
Chocolate, Sainsbury's*	¼ Pudding/110g	464	28.3	422	5.4	42.3	25.7	0.8
Chocolate, Tesco*	1 Pudding/115g	196	4.7	170	4.7	28.3	4.1	2.8
Chocolate, Trufree*	1 Serving/115g	374	17.2	325	2.5	44	15	2
Chocolate, Waitrose*	1 Pudding/110g	400	22.5	363	3.6	41.4	20.4	1.7
Fruit, Co-Op*	1 Can/300g	1110	48	370	3	53	16	2
Fruited with Brandy Sauce, Sainsbury's*	1 Pudding/125g	261	8.4	209	3.6	33.6	6.7	0.8
Ginger with Plum Sauce, Waitrose*	1 Pudding/120g	424	17.9	353	3.1	51.7	14.9	0.7
Golden Syrup, Co-Op*	1 Can/300g	945	39	315	2	47	13	0.6
Honey& Fig, M&S*	¼ Pudding/73g	225	12	310	3.6	34.8	16.6	3.4
Jam & Custard, Somerfield*	¼ Pudding/62g	143	5	231	3	38	8	0
Lemon Curd, Heinz*	¼ Can/78g	236	9.1	302	2.6	46.7	11.7	0.6
Lemon, COU, M&S*	1 Pudding/100g	157	2.3	157	2	32.1	2.3	1.9
Lemon, M&S*	1 Pudding/105g	326	16	310	4.3	39.4	15.2	2.3
Lemon, Waitrose*	1 Serving/105g	212	2.5	202	3.4	41.7	2.4	1.4
Milk Chocolate, Sticky Puds, Cadbury*	1 Pudding/95g	390	17.3	360	4.2	48.9	16	0.8
Mixed Berry, BGTY, Sainsbury's*	1 Pudding/110g	189	2.6	172	2.4	33.3	2.4	3.8
Pear & Ginger, COU, M&S*	1 Pudding/100g	175	0.7	175	1.9	39.8	0.7	1.1
Raspberry Jam, Asda*	½ Pudding/147g	481	16.2	327	3.1	54	11	4.1
Salted Caramel, Specially Selected, Aldi*	1 Pudding/115g	459	20.7	399	3.6	54	18	1
Sticky Ginger, Really Good Puds, M Kitchen, Morrisons*	1 Pudding/110g	372	12	338	3.5	56.2	10.9	0.5
Sticky Toffee, Microwavable, Heinz*	1 Serving/75g	233	9	311	3.3	47.4	12	0.7
Sticky Toffee, Mini, Somerfield*	1 Pudding/110g	384	14.3	349	3	54	13	0
Sticky Toffee, Somerfield*	1 Pudding/440g	1602	61.6	364	3	56	14	0
Strawberry Jam, Heinz*	¼ Can/82g	230	6.2	281	2.6	50.4	7.6	0.6
Sultana with Toffee Sauce, HL, Tesco*	1 Serving/80g	280	2.2	350	3.2	60.2	2.8	1
Summer Fruits, BGTY, Sainsbury's*	1 Serving/110g	243	4.7	221	2.7	42.9	4.3	1
Syrup & Custard, Morrisons*	1 Serving/125g	290	8.6	232	3.4	39.1	6.9	0.8

SPONGE PUDDING	Measure INFO/WEIGHT	KCAL	FAT	KCAL	PROT	CARB	FAT	FIBRE
Syrup, BGTY, Sainsbury's*	1 Pudding/110g	338	4.5	307	2.8	64.6	4.1	0.4
Syrup, Finest, Tesco*	1 Pudding/115g	330	9	287	3.1	51.2	7.8	0.6
Syrup, GFY, Asda*	1 Sponge/105g	207	4.3	197	2	38	4.1	2.6
Syrup, Individual, Tesco*	1 Pudding/110g	390	14.5	355	3.1	55.6	13.2	0.5
Syrup, Sainsbury's*	¼ Pudding/110g	408	13	371	2.7	63.5	11.8	0.4
Syrup, Value, Tesco*	1 Serving/100g	307	10.2	307	2.1	51.7	10.2	0.6
Toffee & Pecan	*½ Pudding/100g*	*395*	*18.4*	*395*	*4.3*	*52.3*	*18.4*	*1.4*
Treacle with Custard, Farmfoods*	1 Serving/145g	539	33.1	372	3.2	38.4	22.8	0.8
Treacle, Heinz*	1 Serving/160g	445	13	278	2.5	48.9	8.1	0.6
Treacle, Super Sticky, Heinz*	1 Pudding/110g	318	12.2	289	1.9	45.3	11.1	1.6
Treacle, Waitrose*	1 Pudding/105g	385	13.8	367	2.8	59.5	13.1	0.5
Vanilla, with Blackcurrant Sauce, Waitrose*	1 Pudding/105g	263	10.9	250	3.5	34.5	10.4	2.6
Very Fruity Cherry, M&S*	1 Pot/110g	286	11.3	260	3.5	38.6	10.3	1.8
with Custard	*1 Serving/200g*	*521*	*24.9*	*261*	*4.8*	*34.1*	*12.4*	*0.9*
with Dried Fruit	*1oz/28g*	*93*	*4*	*331*	*5.4*	*48.1*	*14.3*	*1.2*
with Jam or Treacle	*1oz/28g*	*93*	*4*	*333*	*5.1*	*48.7*	*14.4*	*1*
with Lyles Golden Syrup, Heinz*	½ Pudding/95g	368	14.4	386	3.1	53.3	15.1	0.5
SPOTTED DICK								
Average	*1 Serving/105g*	*343*	*17.5*	*327*	*4.2*	*42.7*	*16.7*	*1*
Individual, Tesco*	1 Pudding/121g	417	14.5	345	3.2	55.2	12	1.2
Pudding, Individual, Sainsbury's*	1 Serving/110g	346	12.9	315	3.8	48.7	11.7	2.2
with Custard	*1 Serving/210g*	*438*	*15.6*	*209*	*3.4*	*31.5*	*7.4*	*1.3*
SPRATS								
Fried	*1oz/28g*	*116*	*9.8*	*415*	*24.9*	*0*	*35*	*0*
Raw	*1oz/28g*	*33*	*2.1*	*117*	*12.4*	*0*	*7.5*	*0*
SPREAD								
Average	*1 Thin Spread/7g*	*51*	*5.7*	*726*	*0.1*	*0.5*	*81*	*0*
Butter Me Up, Light, Tesco*	1 Thin Spread/7g	24	2.7	350	0.3	0.5	38	0
Butter Me Up, Tesco*	1 Thin Spread/7g	38	4.1	540	0.8	1.2	59	0
Butter Style, Average	*1 Thin Spread/7g*	*44*	*4.8*	*627*	*0.7*	*1.1*	*68.9*	*0*
Butterlicious, Vegetable, Sainsbury's*	1 Thin Spread/7g	44	4.8	628	0.6	1.1	69	0
Buttersoft, Light, Reduced Fat, Sainsbury's*	1 Thin Spread/7g	38	4.2	544	0.4	0.5	60	0
Buttery Gold, Somerfield*	1 Thin Spread/7g	44	4.8	627	0.5	1	69	0
Buttery Taste, Benecol*	1 Thin Spread/7g	40	4.4	575	0	0.8	63.3	0
Clover, Light, Dairy Crest Ltd*	1 Serving/7g	32	3.4	455	0.7	2.9	49	0
Dairy Free, Organic, Pure Spreads*	1 Thin Spread/7g	37	4.1	533	0.5	0	59	0
Enriched Olive, Tesco*	1 Thin Spread/7g	38	4.1	540	0.2	1.2	59	0
Gold, Made with Buttermilk, Low Low, Kerry*	1 Spread/10g	48	5.3	483	0.6	0.8	53	0
Heart, Cholesterol Reducing, Dairygold	*1 Thin Spread/7g*	*24*	*2.5*	*338*	*0.7*	*2.8*	*36*	*0*
Lactofree Spreadable, Lactofree, Arla*	1 Serving/10g	68	7.5	679	0.5	0.5	75	0
Light, Benecol*	1 Thin Spread/7g	23	2.4	333	2.5	0	35	0
Lighter Than Light, Flora*	1 Serving/10g	19	1.8	188	5	1.6	18	0
Low Fat, Average	*1 Thin Spread/7g*	*27*	*2.8*	*390*	*5.8*	*0.5*	*40.5*	*0*
Olive Light, Sainsbury's*	1 Thin Spread/7g	24	2.7	348	1.5	0	38	0
Olive Oil, 55% Reduced Fat, Benecol*	1 Thin Spread/7g	35	3.8	498	0.3	0.5	55	0
Olive Oil, Bertolli*	1 Serving/10g	53	5.9	532	0.5	0.5	59	0
Olive, Light, Low Fat, HL, Tesco*	1 Thin Spread/7g	24	2.7	348	1.5	0	38	0
Olive, Low Fat, Morrisons*	1 Thin Spread/7g	24	2.7	346	0.9	0	38	0
Olive, Reduced Fat, Asda*	1 Thin Spread/7g	38	4.1	536	0.2	1.1	59	0
Olive, Waitrose*	1 Thin Spread/7g	37	4.1	534	0.2	0.5	59	0
Orange, Thick Cut, St Dalfour*	1 Spread/11g	23	0	211	0.6	52	0.1	1.6
Original, Made with Buttermilk, Low Low, Kerry*	1 Spread/10g	39	4.2	394	0.2	3	42	0
Pro Activ with Olive Oil, Flora*	1 Thin Spread/7g	23	2.4	331	0.1	4	35	0

S

	Measure INFO/WEIGHT	per Measure KCAL	FAT	Nutrition Values per 100g / 100ml KCAL	PROT	CARB	FAT	FIBRE

SPREAD

	Measure / INFO/WEIGHT	KCAL	FAT	KCAL	PROT	CARB	FAT	FIBRE
Pro Activ, Light, Flora*	1 Thin Spread/7g	23	2.4	331	0.1	4	35	0
Pro Active, Becel*	1 Serving/7g	22	1.8	320	0	0	25	0
Prutella, Musclefood*	1 Tsp/15g	49	0.9	327	19.2	68.2	6.3	26.2
Reduced Fat, Average	*1 Thin Spread/7g*	*25*	*2.7*	*356*	*0.6*	*3*	*38*	*0*
Soft, Reduced Fat, Smart Price, Asda*	1 Thin Spread/7g	32	3.5	455	0.2	1	50	0
Soft, Value, Tesco*	1 Thin Spread/7g	30	3.4	433	0	0	48.1	0
Sunflower, Average	*1 Thin Spread/7g*	*42*	*4.6*	*595*	*0.1*	*0.4*	*65.9*	*0.4*
Sunflower, Enriched, Tesco*	1 Thin Spread/7g	37	4.1	535	0.1	0.2	59	0
Sunflower, Light, BFY, Morrisons*	1 Thin Spread/7g	24	2.7	342	0	0	38	0
Sunflower, Light, BGTY, Sainsbury's*	1 Thin Spread/7g	19	2	265	0.1	0.8	29	0
Sunflower, Light, Reduced Fat, Asda*	1 Thin Spread/7g	24	2.7	347	0.3	1	38	0.1
Sunflower, Low Fat, Aldi*	1 Thin Spread/7g	26	2.7	366	0.2	5.7	38	0
Sunflower, M&S*	1 Thin Spread/7g	44	4.9	630	0	0	70	3
Sunflower, Morrisons*	1 Thin Spread/7g	37	4.1	531	0	0.2	59	0
Sunflower, Sainsbury's*	1 Thin Spread/7g	37	4.1	532	0.1	0.2	59	0
Utterly Butterly*	1 Thin Spread/7g	32	3.4	452	0.3	2.5	49	0
Vegetable, Soft, Tesco*	1 Thin Spread/7g	46	5.1	661	0.1	1	73	0
Vitalite, St Ivel*	1 Thin Spread/7g	35	3.9	503	0	0	56	0
with Soya, Dairy Free, Pure Spreads*	1 Thin Spread/7g	34	3.8	490	0.5	1	54	0
with Sunflower, Dairy Free, Organic, Pure Spreads*	1 Thin Spread/7g	42	4.7	603	0	0	67	0

SPRING ROLLS

	Measure / INFO/WEIGHT	KCAL	FAT	KCAL	PROT	CARB	FAT	FIBRE
Chicken, Asda*	1 Roll/58g	115	5.2	199	4.6	25	9	3.4
Chicken, Oriental Snack Selection, Sainsbury's*	1 Roll/15g	38	1.5	256	11.5	30.3	9.9	1.7
Chinese Takeaway, Tesco*	1 Roll/50g	100	4.3	201	4.4	26.4	8.6	1.5
Duck, M&S*	1 Roll/30g	75	3.4	250	9.8	27.7	11.2	1.5
Duck, Mini, Asda*	1 Roll/18g	47	1.9	259	8.7	32.8	10.3	1.9
Duck, Party Bites, Sainsbury's*	1 Roll/20g	49	1.8	245	10.1	31.4	8.8	1
From Restaurant, Average	*1 Roll/140g*	*344*	*14.8*	*246*	*11.1*	*23.2*	*10.6*	*0*
M&S*	1 Pack/180g	333	15.1	185	3.5	24.2	8.4	2.3
Mini Vegetable, Co-Op*	1 Roll/18g	40	1.6	220	4.1	30.9	9.1	2.7
Mini, Asda*	1 Roll/20g	35	0.6	175	3.5	33.6	3	1.9
Mini, Sainsbury's*	1 Roll/12g	27	1.2	221	4.2	28.7	9.9	1.6
Oriental Vegetable, Tesco*	1 Roll/67.5g	152	7.6	225	4	25.9	11.3	1.6
Prawn, Crispy, M&S*	1 Roll/34.1g	75	3.4	220	10	22.2	9.9	1.3
Roast Duck, M&S*	1 Roll/31g	85	4.9	275	7.8	26.2	15.7	1.4
Thai, Sainsbury's*	1 Roll/30g	69	3.4	229	2.9	28.8	11.3	3.5
Vegetable, Asda*	1 Roll/62g	126	5.6	203	3.5	27	9	2.7
Vegetable, Cantonese, Large, Sainsbury's*	1 Roll/63.4g	130	6.3	205	3.6	25.3	9.9	1.5
Vegetable, Cantonese, Sainsbury's*	1 Roll/36g	84	4.2	233	3.6	28.1	11.7	1.4
Vegetable, Chilled, Tesco*	1 Roll/67.5g	149	7.6	221	4	25.9	11.3	1.6
Vegetable, Chinese Takeaway, Sainsbury's*	1 Roll/59g	100	3.7	170	4	24.4	6.3	2.8
Vegetable, Frozen, Tesco*	1 Roll/60g	123	6.4	205	3.5	23	10.6	1.3
Vegetable, M&S*	1 Roll/37g	80	3.6	215	4.3	27.8	9.6	2
Vegetable, Mini, Nirvana*	1 Roll/26g	54	2.7	208	3.5	25.1	10.4	1.7
Vegetable, Mini, Occasions, Sainsbury's*	1 Roll/24g	52	2.3	216	4.1	28.2	9.6	2.9
Vegetable, Mini, Party Food, M&S*	1 Roll/20g	40	1.6	200	3.7	26.2	8.1	2.7
Vegetable, Mini, Tesco*	1 Roll/18g	36	1.5	205	4.4	26.4	8.6	1.5
Vegetable, Oriental Selection, Party, Iceland*	1 Roll/14.9g	36	1.4	241	4.3	34.1	9.7	2.1
Vegetable, Oriental, Waitrose*	1 Roll/36g	90	4.3	249	5.7	27.1	12	4.8
Vegetable, Parcels, Snack Selection, Oriental, Waitrose*	1 Parcel/18g	48	2	267	4.5	34.6	11.3	4.6
Vegetable, Tempura, M&S*	1 Pack/140g	280	12	200	2.8	27.9	8.6	1.8

SPRITE*

	Measure / INFO/WEIGHT	KCAL	FAT	KCAL	PROT	CARB	FAT	FIBRE
Sprite*	1 Bottle/500ml	215	0	43	0	10.5	0	0

S

	Measure INFO/WEIGHT	per Measure		Nutrition Values per 100g / 100ml				
		KCAL	FAT	KCAL	PROT	CARB	FAT	FIBRE
SPRITE*								
Zero, Lemon & Lime, Sprite*	1 Bottle/500ml	6	0	1	0	0	0	0
Zero, Sprite*	1 Can/330ml	3	0	1	0	0	0	0
SPRITZER								
Red Grape, Non-Alcoholic, Extra Special, Asda*	1 Bottle/750ml	330	0	44	0	11	0	0
Rose & Grape, Non Alcoholic, Extra Special, Asda*	1 Bottle/750ml	90	0	12	0	3	0	0
White Wine, Echo Falls*	1 Serving/125ml	78	0	39	0	0	0	0
with White Zinfadel, Echo Falls*	1 Serving/200ml	216	0	108	0	0	0	0
SPROUTING SEEDS								
Peas, and Sow On, W S Bentley*	1 Serving/80g	92	0.6	115	10.3	26.4	0.7	9.6
Salad Radish, and Sow On, W S Bentley*	1 Serving/80g	25	1.1	31	3.5	3.7	1.4	2.5
SPROUTS								
Radish, China Rose, Aconbury Sprouts*	½ Pack/65g	52	1	80	7.5	8.9	1.6	0
SQUASH								
Apple & Blackcurrant, No Added Sugar, Tesco*	1 Serving/30ml	4	0	15	0.2	2	0	0
Apple & Blackcurrant, Special R, Diluted, Robinson's*	1 Serving/30ml	2	0	8	0.1	1.1	0.1	0
Apple & Blackcurrant, Special R, Robinson's*	1 Serving/30ml	2	0	8	0.1	1.1	0	0
Apple & Mango, High Juice, Diluted, Sainsbury's*	1 Serving/250ml	88	0	35	0	8.5	0	0.2
Apple & Strawberry High Juice, Sainsbury's*	1 Serving/250ml	82	0.2	33	0.1	8.2	0.1	0.1
Apple & Blackcurrant, Fruit, Robinson's*	1 Glass/50ml	18	0	36	0.1	8	0	0
Apple, Blackcurrant, Low Sugar, Diluted, Sainsbury's*	1 Glass/250ml	5	0.2	2	0.1	0.2	0.1	0.1
Apple, Cherry & Raspberry, High Juice, Robinson's*	1 Serving/25ml	49	0	196	0.2	47.6	0.1	0
Blackcurrant, High Juice, M&S*	1 Glass/250ml	50	0	20	0.1	5.2	0	0.1
Blackcurrant, High Juice, Tesco*	1 Serving/75ml	215	0	287	0.3	70	0	0
Blackcurrant, No Added Sugar, Tesco*	1 Serving/25ml	4	0	14	0.4	1.7	0	0
Cherries & Berries, Tesco*	1 Serving/25ml	5	0	21	0.2	3.2	0	0
Cherries & Berries, Sugar Free, Diluted, Tesco*	1 Glass/250ml	5	0	2	0	0.3	0	0
Cranberry, Light, Classic, Undiluted, Ocean Spray*	1 Serving/50ml	32	0	63	0.2	14.1	0	0
Elderflower, 0%, No Added Sugar, Undiluted, Teisseire*	1 Serving/20ml	5	0	23	0.1	0.5	0.1	0
Fruit & Barley Orange, Diluted, Robinson's*	1 Serving/50ml	6	0	12	0.2	1.7	0	0.1
Fruit & Barley, No Added Sugar, Robinson's*	1 fl oz/30ml	4	0	14	0.3	2	0	0
Fruit & Barley, Tropical, No Added Sugar, Robinson's*	1 Serving/60ml	7	0	12	0.2	1.6	0	0
Grape & Passion Fruit, High Juice, Diluted, Sainsbury's*	1 Serving/250ml	100	0.2	40	0.1	9.8	0.1	0.1
Grapefruit, High Juice, No Added Sugar, Sainsbury's*	1 Serving/25ml	2	0	6	0.1	1.1	0	0
Just A dash, Apple, Concentrate, MacB*	1 Serving/25ml	0	0	1	0.1	0	0	0
Just A dash, Peach, Concentrate, MacB*	1 Serving/25ml	0	0	1	0.1	0	0	0
Lemon & Lime, Double Strength, No Added Sugar, Asda*	1 Glass/200ml	4	0	2	0	0	0	0
Lemon Barley Water, Made Up, Robinson's*	1 Serving/250ml	48	0	19	0.1	4.4	0	0
Lemon, Double Concentrate, Value, Tesco*	1 Serving/25ml	3	0	11	0.2	0.3	0	0
Lemon, High Juice, Diluted, Sainsbury's*	1 Glass /250ml	98	0.2	39	0.1	9.1	0.1	0.1
Lemon, No Added Sugar, Double Concentrate, Tesco*	1 Serving/25ml	4	0	16	0.3	0.7	0	0
Mixed Fruit, Diluted, Kia Ora*	1 Serving/250ml	5	0	2	0	0.3	0	0
Mixed Fruit, Low Sugar, Sainsbury's*	1 Glass/250ml	5	0.2	2	0.1	0.2	0.1	0.1
Mixed Fruit, Tesco*	1 Serving/75ml	13	0	17	0	3.5	0	0
Orange & Mandarin, Fruit Spring, Robinson's*	1 Serving/440ml	26	0	6	0.1	0.8	0	0
Orange & Mango, Low Sugar, Sainsbury's*	1 Serving/250ml	5	0.2	2	0.1	0.2	0.1	0.1
Orange & Mango, Special R, Diluted, Robinson's*	1 Serving/250ml	20	0	8	0.2	0.9	0	0
Orange & Pineapple, Original, Undiluted, Robinson's*	1 Serving/250ml	138	0	55	1	13	0	0
Orange & Mango, No Added Sugar, Robinson's*	1 Serving/25ml	2	0	8	0.2	0.9	0	0
Orange & Pineapple, No Sugar Added, Robinson's*	1 Serving/25ml	2	0	8	0.2	0.7	0	0.2
Orange, Hi Juice, Tesco*	1 Serving/75ml	140	0.1	187	0.3	45	0.1	0
Orange, High Juice, Undiluted, Robinson's*	1 Serving/200ml	364	0.2	182	0.3	44	0.1	0
Orange, No Added Sugar, High Juice, Sainsbury's*	1 Serving/100ml	6	0.1	6	0.1	1.1	0.1	0.1
Orange, Special R, Diluted, Robinson's*	1fl oz/30ml	2	0	8	0.2	0.7	0.1	0

S

	Measure INFO/WEIGHT	per Measure KCAL	FAT	Nutrition Values per 100g / 100ml KCAL	PROT	CARB	FAT	FIBRE
SQUASH								
Peach & Apricot, Fruit & Barley, Diluted, CBY, Asda*	1 Serving/250ml	5	0	2	0	0.2	0	0.1
Pear Drop Flavour, Diluted, Tesco*	1 Serving/50ml	3	0	6	0.1	0.5	0	0
Pink Grapefruit, High Juice, Low Sugar, Tesco*	1 Serving/75ml	12	0.1	16	0.2	3.7	0.1	0
Pink Grapefruit, High Juice, Undiluted, Robinson's*	1 Glass/250ml	455	0.2	182	0.2	43.3	0.1	0
Red Apple, No Added Sugar, Diluted, Ribena*	1 Serving/250ml	12	0	5	0	0.9	0	0
Spaghetti, Baked	*1oz/28g*	*6*	*0.1*	*23*	*0.7*	*4.3*	*0.3*	*2.1*
Spaghetti, Including Pips & Rind, Raw	*1oz/28g*	*5*	*0.1*	*20*	*0.4*	*3.4*	*0.4*	*1.7*
Summer Fruit, No Added Sugar, Sainsbury's*	1 Serving/250ml	5	0.2	2	0.1	0.2	0.1	0.1
Summer Fruits & Barley, no Added Sugar, Tesco*	1 Serving/50ml	6	0	11	0.2	1.7	0	0
Summer Fruits, High Juice, Undiluted, Robinson's*	1fl oz/30ml	61	0	203	0.1	49	0.1	0
Summer Fruits, High Juice, Waitrose*	1 Serving/250ml	102	0	41	0	10	0	0
Summer Fruits, No Added Sugar, Double Strength, Asda*	1 Serving/50ml	1	0	2	0	0.2	0	0
Summer Fruits, No Added Sugar, Made Up, Morrisons*	1 Glass/200ml	3	0	2	0	0.2	0	0
Summer Fruits, No Added Sugar, Sun Quench, Aldi*	1 Serving/25ml	5	0.1	21	0.5	2.9	0.5	0.5
Summer Fruits, Robinson's*	1 Measure/25ml	14	0	56	0.1	13	0	0
Summer, All Varieties	*1 Sm/118g*	*19*	*0.2*	*16*	*1.2*	*3.4*	*0.2*	*1.1*
Summerfruits, High Juice, Tesco*	1 Serving/50ml	12	0	23	0.2	4.5	0	0
Tropical, Double Strength, No Added Sugar, CBY, Asda*	1 Serving/100ml	2	0	2	0	0.2	0	0
Tropical, No Added Sugar, Diluted, Tesco*	1 Glass/200ml	18	0	9	0.2	0.9	0	0
Winter, Acorn, Baked, Average	*1oz/28g*	*16*	*0*	*56*	*1.1*	*12.6*	*0.1*	*3.2*
Winter, Acorn, Raw, Average	*1oz/28g*	*9*	*0*	*30*	*0.6*	*6.8*	*0.1*	*1.7*
Winter, All Varieties, Flesh Only, Raw, Average	*1oz/28g*	*10*	*0*	*34*	*1*	*8.6*	*0.1*	*1.5*
SQUID								
Calamari, Battered with Tartar Sauce Dip, Tesco*	1 Pack/210g	573	41	273	8.9	15.4	19.5	0.6
Calamari, Breaded, Whitby Seafoods*	½ Pack/100g	259	13.8	259	9.6	23.1	13.8	2.3
Calamari, Oven Baked, Gastro, Youngs*	½ Pack/97g	247	13.3	254	7.7	24.3	13.7	1.3
in Batter, Fried in Blended Oil, Average	*1oz/28g*	*55*	*2.8*	*195*	*11.5*	*15.7*	*10*	*0.5*
Pieces in Squid Ink, Palacio De Oriente*	1 Can/120g	274	21.6	228	13	3.6	18	0
Raw, Average	*1oz/28g*	*23*	*0.5*	*81*	*15.4*	*1.2*	*1.7*	*0*
Salt & Pepper Chargrilled, Cooked, Tesco*	1 Pack/80g	78	2.3	98	17.9	0	2.9	0.1
with Sweet Chilli Sauce, Pan Fried, CBY, Asda*	1 Serving/125g	229	9.3	183	9.6	19	7.4	0.9
STAR FRUIT								
Average, Tesco*	1oz/28g	9	0.1	31	0.5	7.1	0.3	1.3
STARBAR								
Cadbury*	1 Bar/53g	260	14.8	491	10.7	49	27.9	0
STARBURST								
Fruit Chews, Tropical, Mars*	1 Tube/45g	168	3.3	373	0	76.9	7.3	0
Mars*	1 Pack/45g	185	3.4	411	0.3	85.3	7.6	0
STEAK & KIDNEY PUDDING								
M&S*	1 Pudding/121g	260	13.4	215	9.2	19.4	11.1	3.2
Sainsbury's*	1 Pudding/435g	1135	62.6	261	10.5	22.3	14.4	0.8
Somerfield*	1 Pudding/190g	488	25.6	257	10.2	23.6	13.5	1
Tesco*	1 Serving/190g	437	22.6	230	10	20.7	11.9	1.2
Waitrose*	1 Pudding/223g	497	26.1	223	8.9	20.4	11.7	1.2
STEW								
Beef & Dumplings, British Classics, Tesco*	1 Pack/450g	563	29.7	125	7.9	8.6	6.6	0.5
Beef & Dumplings	*1 Serving/652g*	*766*	*32.7*	*117*	*7.4*	*10.7*	*5*	*0.8*
Beef with Dumplings, Classic British, Sainsbury's*	1 Pack/450g	531	23.4	118	7.7	10.2	5.2	0.5
Beef with Dumplings, COU, M&S*	1 Pack/454g	431	11.8	95	8.9	9.1	2.6	0.8
Beef with Dumplings, Sainsbury's*	1 Pack/450g	603	27.4	134	9.5	6.1	6.1	0.7
Beef, & Dumplings, Aldi*	1 Pack/450g	567	27.9	126	8	8.6	6.2	2
Beef, & Dumplings, Frozen, Tesco*	1 Serving/400g	380	12.8	95	5.7	10.5	3.2	1.5
Beef, Asda*	½ Can/196g	178	4.9	91	10	7	2.5	1.5

	Measure INFO/WEIGHT	per Measure KCAL	FAT	Nutrition Values per 100g / 100ml KCAL	PROT	CARB	FAT	FIBRE
STEW								
Beef, Meal for One, M&S*	1 Pack/440g	350	8.4	80	7	8.7	1.9	2
Beef, Value, Tesco*	1 Serving/200g	170	9.8	85	4	6.2	4.9	1
Chicken & Dumplings, Birds Eye*	1 Pack/320g	282	8.6	88	7	8.9	2.7	0.5
Chicken & Dumplings, Tesco*	1 Serving/450g	567	29.7	126	7.6	9.1	6.6	0.7
Chicken, Morrisons*	1 Pack/400g	492	7.6	123	17.6	8.9	1.9	0.5
Chickpea, Roast Sweet Potato, & Feta, Stewed!*	½ Pot/250g	188	7.2	75	3.3	8.8	2.9	2.7
Irish, Tesco*	1 Can/400g	308	11.2	77	7	5.9	2.8	0.8
Lentil & Vegetable, Organic, Simply Organic*	1 Pack/400g	284	6	71	3.5	11	1.5	1.3
Moroccan, Vegetable, Slimfree, Aldi*	1 Pack/500g	155	2.5	31	1.2	4.7	0.5	1.9
Tuscan Bean, Tasty Veg Pot, Innocent*	1 Pot/400g	320	7.6	80	3.1	12.5	1.9	3.6
STIR FRY								
Bean Sprout & Vegetable with Red Peppers, Asda*	1 Pack/350g	126	3.9	36	1.8	4.7	1.1	2.3
Beef, BGTY, Sainsbury's*	½ Pack/125g	156	5.1	125	22	0.1	4.1	0
Cabbage, Carrot, Broccoli & Onion, Vegetable, Tesco*	1 Serving/100g	31	0.4	31	1.9	4.9	0.4	2.6
Chicken Chow Mein, Fresh, HL, Tesco*	1 Pack/400g	312	4.8	78	5.7	11.4	1.2	1.3
Chicken, Chinese, Meal Kit, Aldi*	½ Pack/210g	277	8.6	132	16	7.6	4.1	1.2
Chinese Chicken, As Consumed, Iceland*	½ Pack/371g	353	2.6	95	6.5	15.2	0.7	1
Chinese Mushroom, Sainsbury's*	1 Serving/175g	66	4.2	38	1.7	2.4	2.4	1.7
Chinese Prawn, Iceland*	1 Pack/340g	235	4.4	69	3.1	11.1	1.3	2.1
Chinese Style Rice with Vegetables, Tesco*	1 Serving/550g	495	13.8	90	2.2	14.8	2.5	0.3
Chinese Vegetables, Oriental Express*	½ Pack/200g	44	0.4	22	1.4	3.7	0.2	2.2
Edamame Bean & Mixed Vegetables, Morrisons*	¼ Pack/80g	31	1.4	39	2.4	1.9	1.8	2.9
Family Pack, Vegetables & Beansprouts, Fresh, Tesco*	1 Pack/600g	108	0.6	18	2	2.2	0.1	2.1
Green Vegetable, M&S*	1 Pack/220g	165	13	75	3.1	2.5	5.9	2.2
Hot & Spicy, Mixed Vegetables, Cooked, Sainsbury's*	½ Pack/149g	85	4.6	57	1.2	4.9	3.1	2.2
Mixed Pepper, Sainsbury's*	1 Pack/300g	188	12.9	70	1.5	4.6	4.8	1.2
Mixed Pepper, Tesco*	1/3 Pack/100g	23	0.1	23	1.9	3.7	0.1	1.9
Mixed Vegetable & Beansprout, Tesco*	1 Bag/320g	170	6.1	53	2.5	5.1	1.9	2.5
Mushroom, Just Stir Fry, Sainsbury's*	1 Pack/350g	172	9.4	49	2.8	3.3	2.7	2.8
Noodles & Bean Sprouts, Tesco*	½ Pack/125g	131	2.6	105	4.2	16.1	2.1	0.7
Oriental Mix, Quick & Easy, Frozen, Cooked, CBY, Asda*	1 Pack/500g	130	1	26	1.1	3.5	0.2	3
Oriental Style Pak Choi, M&S*	1 Pack/220g	165	12.5	75	2.2	3.5	5.7	2.4
Oriental Style, Vegetables, Sainsbury's*	1 Pack/300g	195	14.4	65	1.5	4.1	4.8	2.1
Rice, Quinoa & Vegetable, Waitrose*	½ Pack/134g	199	7.8	148	5.4	15.6	5.8	6
Vegetable & Mushroom, Asda*	½ Pack/160g	59	2.4	37	2.4	3.4	1.5	3.4
Vegetable Mix, As Consumed, Tesco*	½ Pack/128g	72	3	56	1.9	5.5	2.3	3
Vegetable, Chop Suey, Chinese, Sharwood's*	1 Pack/310g	223	3.4	72	1.5	13.9	1.1	0.6
Vegetable, Oriental Mix, Tesco*	½ Pack/126g	88	4.4	70	2.6	5.7	3.5	2.7
Vegetable, Oriental, Just Stir Fry, Sainsbury's*	½ Pack/135g	94	7.2	70	2.2	3.4	5.3	1.3
Vegetable, Rainbow, Fresh Tastes, Asda*	½ Pack/225g	119	5	53	1.8	4.6	2.2	3.8
Vegetable, Ready Prepared, M&S*	½ Pack/150g	38	0.4	25	2.2	3.5	0.3	2.2
Vegetable, Sweet & Crunchy, Waitrose*	1 Pack/300g	69	0.3	23	1.8	3.6	0.1	1.4
Vegetable, Thai Style, Tesco*	½ Pack/135g	42	0.7	31	2.3	4.2	0.5	2.1
Vegetables, Frozen, Farm Foods*	1 Pack/650g	208	3.2	32	1.9	4.9	0.5	2.2
Vegetables, Mixed with Slices of Pepper, Cooked, Tesco*	½ Pack/125g	58	1.6	47	2.4	5.6	1.3	2.4
STOCK								
Beef, Cooks' Ingredients, Waitrose*	1 Jar/500g	110	2.5	22	3.2	0.9	0.5	0.5
Beef, Fresh, Sainsbury's*	¼ Pot/113g	27	0.6	24	5.1	0.5	0.5	0.5
Beef, Fresh, Tesco*	1 Serving/300ml	54	0.9	18	2.1	1.6	0.3	0.5
Beef, Made Up, Stock Pot, Knorr*	1 Serving/100ml	10	0.4	10	0.2	1	0.4	0
Beef, Pots, Unprepared, Sainsbury's*	1 Pot/28g	31	1.7	112	4.1	8.5	6.2	2.9
Beef, Rich, Stock Pot, Knorr*	1 Pot/28g	42	1.1	150	3	27	4	0.8
Beef, Simply Stock, Knorr*	1 Serving/100ml	6	0	6	1.4	0.1	0	0

S

	Measure INFO/WEIGHT	per Measure KCAL	FAT	Nutrition Values per 100g / 100ml KCAL	PROT	CARB	FAT	FIBRE
STOCK								
Beef, Slow Cooked, Finest, Tesco*	¼ Pouch/113ml	18	0.2	16	2	1.6	0.2	0
Beef, Slowly Prepared, Sainsbury's*	1 Serving/100g	7	0.3	7	0.7	0.3	0.3	0.5
Chicken, As Sold, Stock Pot, Knorr*	1 Pot/28g	45	1.1	160	4	26	4	0.8
Chicken, Asda*	½ Pot/150g	26	1.4	17	1.8	0.7	0.9	0.2
Chicken, Concentrated, M&S*	1 Tsp/5g	16	0.9	315	25.6	12.2	18.1	0.8
Chicken, Cooks' Ingredients, Waitrose*	1 Pack/500ml	75	0.5	15	3.2	0.3	0.1	0.2
Chicken, Fresh, Sainsbury's*	½ Pot/142ml	23	0.1	16	3.7	0.1	0.1	0.3
Chicken, Fresh, Tesco*	1 Serving/300ml	27	0.3	9	1.6	0.5	0.1	0.5
Chicken, Granules, Knorr*	1 Tsp/4.5g	10	0.2	232	13.1	36.5	3.7	0.4
Chicken, Home Prepared, Average	*1fl oz/30ml*	*7*	*0.3*	*24*	*3.8*	*0.7*	*0.9*	*0.3*
Chicken, Made Up, Stock Pot, Knorr*	1 Serving/125ml	15	0.3	12	0.2	1.6	0.2	0
Chicken, Prepared, Tesco*	1 Serving/300ml	54	0.3	18	2.4	1.8	0.1	0.5
Chicken, Slow Roasted, Fresh, Extra Special, Asda*	1 Serving/100g	21	0.5	21	4.2	0.5	0.5	0.5
Chicken, Slowly Prepared, Sainsbury's*	1 Pot/300g	27	0.3	9	0.6	1.3	0.1	0.5
Fish, Fresh, Finest, Tesco*	1 Serving/100g	10	0	10	0.6	1.8	0	0.5
Fish, Home Prepared, Average	*1 Serving/250ml*	*42*	*2*	*17*	*2.3*	*0*	*0.8*	*0*
Rich Beef, with Onion & Rosemary, As Prepared, Oxo*	1 Serving/100ml	7	0.5	7	0.5	0.9	0.5	0.5
Roast Chicken, Diluted Concentrate, Finest, Tesco*	½ Pot/150g	39	0	26	4.9	1	0	1
Vegetable, 3 Peppercorn, Flavour Pot , Knorr*	1 Pot/9g	14	0.6	160	0.9	22	7	4.5
Vegetable, As Sold, Stock Pot, Knorr*	1 Serving/100ml	9	0.5	180	6	19	9	1.5
Vegetable, Campbell's*	1 Serving/250ml	38	1.8	15	0.3	2	0.7	0
Vegetable, Cooks Ingredients, Waitrose*	1 Pouch/500ml	15	0.5	3	0.2	0.4	0.1	0.5
Vegetable, Granules, Knorr*	2 Tsp/9g	18	0.1	199	8.5	39.9	0.6	0.9
Vegetable, Made Up, Stock Pot, Knorr*	1 Serving/100ml	10	0.5	10	0.4	1	0.5	0.1
STOCK CUBES								
Beef Flavour, Made Up, Oxo*	1 Cube/188.9ml	17	0.4	9	0.6	1.3	0.2	0.1
Beef, Dry Weight, Bovril*	1 Cube/5.9g	12	0.2	197	10.8	29.3	4.1	0
Beef, Dry Weight, Oxo*	1 Cube/5.8g	15	0.3	265	17.3	38.4	4.7	1.5
Beef, Knorr*	1 Cube/10g	31	2.3	310	5	19	23	0
Beef, Organic, Kallo*	1 Cube/12g	25	1	208	16.7	16.7	8.3	0
Beef, Smart Price, Asda*	1 Cube/11g	31	2.5	279	10	8	23	0
Beef, Tesco*	1 Cube/7g	17	0.2	260	9.7	48.9	2.8	1.3
Beef, Value, Tesco*	1 Cube/10g	14	0.4	135	11.1	12.9	3.9	6.6
Chicken	*1 Cube/6g*	*14*	*0.9*	*237*	*15.4*	*9.9*	*15.4*	*0*
Chicken, Dry, Average	*1 Cube/10g*	*29*	*1.8*	*293*	*7.3*	*25.5*	*18*	*0.4*
Chicken, Dry, Oxo*	1 Cube/7g	17	0.2	249	10.9	44	3.3	0.9
Chicken, Just Bouillon, Kallo*	1 Cube/12g	30	1.3	247	11.8	26.1	10.6	1
Chicken, Knorr*	1 Cube/10g	31	2	310	4	29	20	0
Chicken, Made Up, Average	*1 Pint/568ml*	*43*	*1*	*8*	*0.4*	*1.1*	*0.2*	*0.1*
Chicken, Made Up, Sainsbury's*	1 Cube/200ml	16	0.2	8	0.3	1.4	0.1	0.1
Chicken, Prepared, Oxo*	1 Cube/100ml	9	0.1	9	0.4	1.5	0.1	0.1
Chicken, Tesco*	1 Cube/11g	32	2.5	290	10.5	11.1	22.6	0.7
Chicken, Value, Tesco*	1 Cube/10g	15	0.6	150	9.4	14.3	5.9	0.8
Fish, Knorr*	1 Cube/10g	32	2.4	321	8	18	24	1
Fish, Sainsbury's*	1 Cube/11g	31	2.2	282	19.1	7.3	20	0.9
Ham, Knorr*	1 Cube/10g	31	1.9	313	11.8	24.4	18.7	0
Ham, Quixo*	1 Cube/450ml	18	2.2	4	0.5	0.5	0.5	0.5
Lamb, Made Up, Knorr*	1 Serving/100ml	5	0.6	5	0.3	0.3	0.6	0.1
Vegetable Bouillon, Vegetarian, Amoy*	1 Cube/10g	30	2	300	0	20	20	0
Vegetable Bouillon, Yeast Free, Made Up, Marigold*	1 Serving/250ml	19	1.6	8	0	0.5	0.6	0
Vegetable, Average	*1 Cube/7g*	*18*	*1.2*	*253*	*13.5*	*11.6*	*17.3*	*0*
Vegetable, Dry, Oxo*	1 Cube/6g	17	0.3	251	10.4	41.4	4.9	1.4
Vegetable, Knorr*	1 Cube/10g	33	2.4	330	10	25	24	1

S

	Measure INFO/WEIGHT	per Measure KCAL	FAT	Nutrition Values per 100g / 100ml KCAL	PROT	CARB	FAT	FIBRE
STOCK CUBES								
Vegetable, Low Salt, Organic, Made Up, Kallo*	1 Serving/500ml	50	3.5	10	0.3	0.7	0.7	0.2
Vegetable, Made Up, Organic, Kallo*	2 Cubes/100ml	7	0.4	7	0.1	0.5	0.4	0.1
Vegetable, Made up, Oxo*	1 Cube/100ml	9	0.2	9	0.4	1.4	0.2	0.1
Vegetable, Organic, Yeast Free, Dry, Kallo*	1 Cube/11g	37	3.1	334	11.4	8.2	27.8	2.3
Vegetable, Smart Price, Asda*	1 Cube/11g	27	2.1	243	6	12	19	0
Vegetable, Value, Tesco*	1 Cube/9.7g	14	0.3	145	10.6	17.4	3.3	3.6
STOLLEN								
Bites, Betty's*	1 Bite/11g	46	2.5	420	7.3	41	23	0
Bites, Marzipan, Holly Lane, Aldi*	1 Bite/27g	111	4.8	412	5.9	55	18	1.9
Bites, with Jamaican Rum, Aldi*	1 Bite/23g	92	4.4	400	6.2	51	19	2.4
STOVIES								
Chef Select, Lidl*	1 Pack/412g	346	3.7	84	4.6	13	0.9	2.9
STRAWBERRIES								
Dried, Urban Fresh Fruit*	1 Pack/35g	111	0.1	318	1.6	77	0.4	5.9
Fresh, Raw, Average	*1 Berry/12g*	*3*	*0*	*28*	*0.8*	*6*	*0.1*	*1.4*
Frozen, Average	*1 Serving/100g*	*30*	*0.2*	*30*	*0.8*	*6.3*	*0.2*	*1*
in Fruit Juice, Canned, Average	*1/3 Can/127g*	*58*	*0*	*46*	*0.4*	*11*	*0*	*1*
in Syrup, Canned, Average	*1 Serving/100g*	*63*	*0*	*63*	*0.4*	*15.2*	*0*	*0.6*
Lightly Yoghurt Coated, Bites, Yu!*	1 Bag/18g	70	1.8	389	3	61.3	9.9	10.2
STROGANOFF								
Beef & Rice, TTD, Sainsbury's*	1 Pack/410g	595	20.9	145	9.6	15.2	5.1	1.7
Beef with Long Grain & Wild Rice, Somerfield*	1 Pack/400g	485	16.4	121	7.3	13.8	4.1	1.6
Beef with Rice 'n' Peppers, Tesco*	1 Pack/450g	562	19.8	125	7.5	13.1	4.4	0.4
Beef, 115, Oakhouse Foods Ltd*	1 Meal/400g	428	19.6	107	5	10.8	4.9	0.6
Beef, 604, Wiltshire Farm Foods*	1 Serving/360g	466	22	129	6	11	6.1	0
Beef, Asda*	1 Serving/120g	276	20.4	230	16	3.3	17	0.6
Beef, BGTY, Sainsbury's*	1 Pack/400g	416	10.4	104	5.6	14.6	2.6	0.6
Beef, Eat Smart, Morrisons*	1 Pack/400g	344	9.2	86	5	11.2	2.3	0.9
Beef, Finest, Tesco*	½ Pack/200g	330	13.4	165	9.4	16.2	6.7	0.7
Beef, HL, Tesco*	1 Pack/400g	400	8.8	100	7	13	2.2	1.3
Beef, M&S*	1 Pack/400g	380	9.6	95	7.3	10.3	2.4	1.4
Beef, Weight Watchers*	1 Pack/330g	297	7.6	90	4.3	13	2.3	0.1
Beef, with White & Wild Rice, Heated, Finest, Tesco*	1 Pack/426g	591	21.3	139	10.3	12	5	2.2
Beef, with White & Wild Rice, Low Fat, Waitrose*	1 Pack/401g	429	6.4	107	7.9	15.3	1.6	1
Chicken with Rice, BGTY, Sainsbury's*	1 Pack/415g	448	5.4	108	7	17.1	1.3	1.1
Mushroom with Rice, BGTY, Sainsbury's*	1 Serving/450g	418	6.8	93	3.3	16.6	1.5	1
Mushroom with Rice, Vegetarian, LC, Tesco*	1 Pack/450g	420	7.5	95	2.6	16.4	1.7	1.1
Mushroom, Diet Chef Ltd*	1 Pouch/250g	202	14.8	81	2.6	4.5	5.9	1.7
Mushroom, Eat Smart, Morrisons*	1 Pack/400g	312	4.4	78	2.6	14.3	1.1	1
Pork with Rice, HE, Tesco*	1 Pack/450g	482	8.1	107	7	15.8	1.8	0.5
Pork, Classic Kitchen, Tesco*	½ Pack/222g	284	13.5	128	12.9	4.6	6.1	1.2
STRUDEL								
Apple & Mincemeat, Tesco*	1 Serving/100g	322	16.7	322	3.3	39.6	16.7	2
Apple with Sultanas, Tesco*	1/6 Strudel/100g	245	12	245	2.9	30.9	12	0.7
Apple, Co-Op*	1 Slice/100g	225	12	225	3	28	12	3
Apple, Frozen, Sainsbury's*	1 Serving/100g	283	15.4	283	3.2	32.8	15.4	1.9
Apple, Ovenbaked, CBY, Asda*	1 Slice/100g	249	12	249	2.7	31.6	12	1.7
Apple, Plum & Custard, Heavenly Desserts, Aldi*	1/6 Strudel/94g	265	13.2	282	4	35	14	2
Apple, Sainsbury's*	1/6 Strudel/90g	255	13.9	283	3.2	32.8	15.4	1.9
Apple, Tesco*	1 Serving/150g	432	21.6	288	3.3	36.4	14.4	2.8
Tesco*	1 Serving/150g	370	19.4	247	2.9	29.8	12.9	4.7
Woodland Fruit, Sainsbury's*	1/6 Strudel/95g	276	14.8	290	3.7	34	15.5	2
Woodland Fruit, Tesco*	1 Serving/100g	257	13.1	257	3.2	31.5	13.1	1.8

S

	Measure INFO/WEIGHT	per Measure KCAL	FAT	Nutrition Values per 100g / 100ml KCAL	PROT	CARB	FAT	FIBRE
STUFFING								
Apple & Apricot, Tray, As Sold, Mr Crumb *	1 Serving/45g	84	3	186	2.8	27.5	6.6	2.3
Leek, Pancetta & Thyme, Parcels, Cooked, Finest, Tesco*	1 Parcel/39g	103	7.8	263	12.9	7.2	20	1.4
Olde English Chestnut, Sainsbury's*	1 Serving/110g	216	12.8	196	9.4	13.5	11.6	2.1
Parsley & Thyme, Co-Op*	1 Serving/28g	95	0.8	340	10	67	3	6
Pork, Chestnut & Onion, Cooked, Finest, Tesco*	1/8 Pack/41g	108	6.9	263	12.9	13.6	16.8	2.4
Pork, with Chestnuts & Leek, Waitrose*	1 Serving/100g	192	8.8	192	12.5	14.9	8.8	1.3
Sage & Onion with Lemon, Paxo*	1 Serving/50g	61	0.6	122	3.4	24.2	1.2	1.9
Sage & Onion, for Chicken, Paxo*	1 Serving/50g	60	0.6	120	3.4	22.8	1.3	1.7
Sausagemeat & Thyme, Made Up, Celebrations, Paxo*	1 Serving/50g	80	1.8	160	6.3	25.8	3.5	4
Sausagemeat, Pork, Gourmet, British, Cooked, Waitrose*	1 Serving/59g	134	6.4	229	20	12.7	10.9	0.5
Sausagemeat, Sainsbury's*	1 Serving/100g	175	4.2	175	7	27	4.2	2.3
STUFFING BALLS								
British Pork, Sage & Onion, Cooked, Finest, Tesco*	2 Balls/49g	110	5	224	13.9	17.4	10.2	2.2
Pork, Sausagemeat, Aunt Bessie's*	1 Ball/25.9g	55	2.1	212	7.2	27.3	8.2	3
Sage & Onion, Aunt Bessie's*	1 Ball/26g	63	2.3	243	6.4	34.4	8.9	3.1
Sage & Onion, Meat-Free, Aunt Bessie's*	1 Ball/28g	54	1.9	193	5.4	28	6.7	1.7
Sage & Onion, Tesco*	1 Serving/20g	64	4.4	322	10	21.1	22	1.9
Tesco*	1 Ball/20.6g	65	4.1	315	9.6	23.5	20	1.4
STUFFING MIX								
Apple & Herb, Special Recipe, Sainsbury's*	1 Serving/41g	68	0.9	165	3.8	32.4	2.2	2.2
Apricot & Walnut, Made Up, Celebrations, Paxo*	1 Serving/50g	80	1.8	161	4.3	28	3.5	2.8
Chestnut & Cranberry, Celebration, Paxo*	1 Serving/25g	35	0.5	141	4	26.7	2	2.4
Chestnut, Morrisons*	1 Serving/20g	33	0.7	165	4.6	29.1	3.4	3.7
Dry, Average	*1 Serving/25g*	*84*	*1*	*338*	*9.6*	*70.1*	*3.8*	*5.3*
Herb & Onion, GF, Allergycare*	1 Serving/12g	43	0.3	360	7.9	76.8	2.4	0
Parsley, Thyme & Lemon, Sainsbury's*	1 Pack/170g	240	2.2	141	4.2	28.2	1.3	1.3
Sage & Onion, Asda*	1 Serving/27g	29	0.2	107	3.4	22	0.6	1.3
Sage & Onion, Co-Op*	1 Serving/28g	94	0.6	335	10	68	2	6
Sage & Onion, Prepared, Tesco*	1 Serving/100g	50	0.4	50	1.5	10.1	0.4	0.9
Sage & Onion, Smart Price, Asda*	1/4 Pack/75g	262	2.8	349	11	68	3.7	4.7
Sage & Onion, Dry Weight, Tesco*	1 Std Pack/170g	578	4.1	340	10.3	69.3	2.4	6.3
Sage & Onion, Free From, Tesco*	1 Pack/170g	197	18.5	116	0.8	3.6	10.9	0.3
Sage & Onion, Value, Tesco*	1 Ball/38g	133	1.1	350	10.2	70.7	2.9	5.1
Sage & Onion, with Apple, Made Up, Paxo*	1 Serving/50g	69	0.8	138	3.8	26	1.6	2.2
Sausage Meat, Morrisons*	1 Serving/20g	35	0.5	174	6.8	30.8	2.6	2.9
SUET								
Beef, Tesco*	1 Serving/100g	854	91.9	854	0.6	6.2	91.9	0.1
Vegetable, Average	*1oz/28g*	*234*	*24.6*	*836*	*1.2*	*10.1*	*87.9*	*0*
SUGAR								
Brown, Soft, Average	*1 Tsp/4g*	*15*	*0*	*382*	*0*	*96.5*	*0*	*0*
Brown, Soft, Light, Average	*1 Tsp/5g*	*20*	*0*	*393*	*0.2*	*97.8*	*0.1*	*0*
Caster, Average	*1 Tsp/5g*	*20*	*0*	*399*	*0*	*99.8*	*0*	*0*
Cubes, Rogers*	2 Cubes/6g	22	0	375	0	100	0	0
Dark Brown, Muscovado, Average	*1 Tsp/7g*	*27*	*0*	*380*	*0.2*	*94.8*	*0*	*0*
Dark Brown, Soft, Average	*1 Tsp/5g*	*18*	*0*	*369*	*0.1*	*92*	*0*	*0*
Demerara, Average	*1 Tsp/5g*	*18*	*0*	*368*	*0.2*	*99.2*	*0*	*0*
Fructose, Fruit Sugar, Tate & Lyle*	1 Tsp/4g	16	0	400	0	100	0	0
Golden, Unrefined, Average	*1 Tsp/4g*	*16*	*0*	*399*	*0*	*99.8*	*0*	*0*
Granulated, Organic, Average	*1 Tsp/4g*	*16*	*0*	*398*	*0.2*	*99.7*	*0*	*0*
Icing, Average	*1 Tsp/4g*	*16*	*0*	*394*	*0*	*102.2*	*0*	*0*
Light Or Diet, Average	*1 Tsp/4g*	*16*	*0*	*394*	*0*	*98.5*	*0*	*0*
Maple, Average	*1 Tsp/5g*	*18*	*0*	*354*	*0.1*	*90.9*	*0.2*	*0*
Muscovado, Light, Average	*1 Tsp/5g*	*19*	*0*	*384*	*0*	*96*	*0*	*0*

	Measure INFO/WEIGHT	per Measure KCAL	FAT	Nutrition Values per 100g / 100ml KCAL	PROT	CARB	FAT	FIBRE
SUGAR								
White Plus Stevia Blend, Light at Heart, Tate & Lyle*	1 Serving/2g	8	0	398	0	99.6	0	0
White, Granulated, Average	*1 Tsp/5g*	*20*	*0*	*398*	*0*	*100*	*0*	*0*
SULTANAS								
Average	*1oz/28g*	*82*	*0.1*	*291*	*2.8*	*69.2*	*0.4*	*2*
SUNDAE								
Blackcurrant, M&S*	1 Sundae/53g	212	10.2	400	3	54.2	19.2	1.9
Caramel, From Restaurant, Average	*1 Sundae/155g*	*304*	*9.3*	*196*	*4.7*	*31.8*	*6*	*0*
Chocolate & Vanilla, HL, Tesco*	1 Sundae/120g	193	3.1	161	2.8	31.5	2.6	0.6
Chocolate & Vanilla, Tesco*	1 Sundae/70g	140	6	199	2.8	27.5	8.6	0.5
Chocolate & Cookie, Weight Watchers*	1 Pot/82g	128	2.8	156	2.5	30.3	3.4	2.2
Chocolate Brownie, Finest, Tesco*	1 Serving/215g	778	56.5	362	2.7	28.7	26.3	2.3
Chocolate Mint, COU, M&S*	1 Pot/90g	108	2.3	120	5.4	17.8	2.6	0.5
Chocolate Nut	*1 Serving/70g*	*195*	*10.7*	*278*	*3*	*34.2*	*15.3*	*0.1*
Chocolate, Sainsbury's*	1 Pot/140g	393	29.8	281	2.5	19.3	21.3	0.6
Hot Fudge, Two Scoop, Baskin Robbins*	1 Serving/203g	530	29	261	3.9	30.5	14.3	0
Ice Cream	*1 Serving/170g*	*482*	*15.4*	*284*	*5.9*	*45.3*	*9.1*	*0.3*
Raspberry, PB, Waitrose*	1 Pot/175ml	150	1	86	1.7	18.9	0.6	0
Strawberry & Vanilla, Tesco*	1 Serving/68g	120	3.9	177	2	29.5	5.7	0.1
Strawberry & Vanilla, Weight Watchers*	1 Pot/105g	148	2.2	141	1.2	29.1	2.1	0.3
Strawberry, M&S*	1 Sundae/45g	173	8	385	3.4	53.3	17.8	1
Strawberry, Tesco*	1 Sundae/48g	194	8.7	408	3.3	57.6	18.3	1.3
Toffee & Vanilla, Tesco*	1 Serving/70g	133	4.5	189	2.1	30.7	6.4	0.1
Toffee, Asda*	1 Serving/120g	322	19.2	268	2.1	29	16	0
Toffee, Good Puds, M Kitchen, Morrisons*	1 Pot/138g	268	13.4	194	3.6	22.9	9.7	0.4
Toffee, Sainsbury's*	1 Sundae/140g	378	27.2	270	3.1	20.2	19.4	0.9
Vanilla Caramel, Aldi*	1 Sundae/72g	159	7.4	221	2.6	29.2	10.3	0.7
SUNNY DELIGHT*								
Florida Style, Sunny Delight*	1 Serving/200ml	70	0.2	35	0.4	7.4	0.1	0.2
Original, Sunny Delight*	1 Glass/200ml	88	0.4	44	0.1	10	0.2	0
SUPPLEMENT								
Acai Shake, Fruitein, Nature's Plus*	1 Scoop/34g	110	0	324	29.4	44.1	0	2.9
Argi+ L Arginine & Vitamin Complex, Forever Aloe*	1 Scoop/10g	40	0	400	50	30	0	0
Baobab, Aduna*	1 Serving/10g	25	0.1	253	1.9	38.8	0.9	46.9
Barley Grass, Powder, Creative Nature*	1 Tsp/10g	25	0.2	250	29	5.4	2.5	39
BCAA Power Punch, Ultimate Sports Nutrition*	2 Tsp/13g	40	0	304	0	3	0	0
Beyond Greens, Udo's Choice*	1 Dsp/5g	21	0.8	423	25	46.2	16.3	20
Cacao Powder, Organic, Naturya*	1 Serving/25g	92	3	370	27	26	12	26
Chocolate Shake, Micellar Casien, Reflex Nutrition Ltd*	1 Serving/45g	159	0.7	354	80	4	1.5	0
Chocolate, Forever Lite, Ultra, Powder, Forever Living*	1 Scoop/25g	90	1	360	68	16	4	4
Fibre, Powder, Benefibre*	1 Tsp/3.2g	6	0	200	0.5	15	0	85
Fibre, Sachets, Celebrity Slim *	1 Sachet/8g	15	0	188	1.7	3.4	0.1	87
Fruits & Fibres, Ortis*	1 Cube/10g	27	0.2	266	3.9	53	1.7	16
Green Apple, Vitamin Drink, Low Calorie, Vit Hit*	1 Serving/100ml	8	0.1	8	0.1	1.4	0.1	0.1
Green Berry, Superfood, Amazing Grass*	2 Tsp/8g	30	1	375	25	50	12.5	25
Green, Powder, Superblend, Funktional Foods*	1 Tbsp/15g	45	0.4	301	38	16	2.7	30
GU Energy Gel, Chocolate Outrage, TCL Sports*	1 Pack/32g	100	2	312	0	62.5	6.2	0
GU Energy Gel, Vanilla Bean, TCL Sports*	1 Pack/32g	100	0	312	0	78.1	0	0
Hemp, Protein Powder, Raw, Sevenhills Wholefoods*	1 Serving/20g	75	2.1	374	49.6	10.4	10.5	19.5
High Protein Powder, Sanatogen*	2 Tsp/7g	25	0.1	360	81	5.8	1.2	0
IMO Powder, VitaFibre*	1 Tbsp/15g	30	0	202	0	96	0	91
Inulin Powder, NOW Foods*	1 Level Tsp/3g	5	0	179	0	96.4	0	89.3
Inulin, Powder, Prebiotic, Organic, Golden Greens*	1 Tsp/5g	10	0	200	0	94.7	0	91
Malt Extract, Holland & Barrett*	1 Tbsp/24g	72	0	300	5.3	70	0	0

S

	Measure INFO/WEIGHT	per Measure KCAL	FAT	Nutrition Values per 100g / 100ml KCAL	PROT	CARB	FAT	FIBRE
SUPPLEMENT								
Moringa Powder, Raw Organic, MRM*	2 Tsps/4g	15	0	375	25	50	0	50
Myofusion Protein Shake, Gaspari*	1 Scoop/35g	158	3	450	71.4	14.3	8.6	2.9
Powder, Daily Fibre Boost, Arbonne*	1 Scoop/30g	56	0	188	0	93.8	0	75
Pro Peptide, Cnp*	1 Scoop/32.5g	115	1.5	354	69.2	9.2	4.6	0
Pro Recover, Cnp*	2 Scoops/80g	297	1	371	29.5	60.6	1.3	0
Protein Shake, Coconut, Purition*	1 Serving/40g	240	16	480	41	7.8	32	17.2
Protein Shake, Macadamia & Vanilla, Purition*	1 Serving/40g	198	14	495	39.1	8.6	35	15.6
Protein Shake, Pistachio, Purition*	1 Serving/40g	192	12.8	481	40.5	9.9	32	15.7
Protein Shake, Powder, Chocolate, Thrive , Phyto Pro*	3 Tbsps/30g	112	1.9	374	60	2	6.3	8.3
Protein Shake, Protein Haus*	1 Bottle/330ml	275	8	83	7.2	5.7	2.4	0
Protein Shake, Vegan Hemp, Chocolate, Purition*	1 Serving/40g	194	12.1	484	35.4	11.3	30.3	27.3
Protein Shake, Vegan Hemp, Original, Purition*	1 Serving/40g	200	12.9	501	36.8	10.8	32.3	26.4
Protein Shake, Vegan Hemp, Vanilla, Purition*	1 Serving/40g	199	12.8	497	36.2	11	31.9	26.6
Protein, Hot Chocolate, Easy Body*	1 Serving/20g	74	0.2	370	70.7	19.2	1.2	0
Protein, Total Gainer, Myprotein*	1 Serving/100g	411	9.8	411	34.7	46	9.8	3.3
Protein, Vanila, Precision, EAS*	1 Scoop/25.5g	91	0.5	357	78.4	4.7	2	0
Psyllium Husk, Average	*1 Tsp/5g*	*19*	*0*	*377*	*0.4*	*89*	*0.4*	*58*
Shake, Diet, Chocolate Delight Flavour, Maxitone*	1 Serving/50g	209	6.4	418	33.2	40	12.8	4.4
Shake, Strawberry, Max Elle True Diet, Myprotein*	1 Scoop/28g	106	2.1	378	63.6	14.7	7.4	3.3
Soya Protein Isolate Powder, Holland & Barrett*	1 Scoop/28g	109	1.3	391	86.6	1	4.5	0
Sport Gel, Smart Berry Flavour, Science in Sport*	1 Sachet/60ml	86	0	144	0	36	0	0
Super Green Detox, Super Eleven*	1 Scoop/30g	11	0.4	37	1.5	4.6	1.2	1.8
Tablet, Berocca*	1 Tablet/4.5g	5	0	109	0	5.7	0.1	0
Total Superfood, Powder, Nutriseed*	1 Serving/10g	40	1.7	405	22.2	29.2	17.1	18.3
Wheat Grass Powder, Organic, Daylesford*	1 Pack/100g	284	3.5	284	24	20.3	3.5	37.8
Whey Powder, Molkosan Vitality, Vogel*	1 Serving /28g	56	0	200	1	20	0.1	61
Whey Protein Isolate, Musashi*	2 Scoop/30g	111	0.2	371	88.7	1.2	0.6	0
Whey Protein, Body Fortress*	1 Scoop/25g	98	2.2	392	70.5	7.9	8.9	2.1
Whey Protein, Body Supreme*	1 Serving/28g	109	3.3	389	68.2	13.9	11.8	2.5
Whey Protein, Define*	1 Serving/40g	165	3.8	412	71.5	10.3	9.4	0.5
Whey protein, Holland & Barrett*	1 Serving/24g	94	1.9	392	73.3	7.1	7.9	0
Whey Protein, Super, Precision*	1 Scoop/24g	94	2	390	71.5	7.3	8.3	0
Whey, Chocolate, White, Diet, PhD Nutrition*	1 Serving/50g	195	2.5	390	70	12.5	5	3.7
Whey, Instant, Strawberry Flavour, Reflex Nutrition Ltd*	1 Serving/25g	98	1.4	394	80	6	5.5	0.2
SUSHI								
California Roll Selection, Classics, M&S*	1 Pack/225g	326	6.1	145	7	23.2	2.7	1.1
California Rolls 8 Pack	*1 Pack/206g*	*354*	*9.3*	*172*	*5.1*	*27.5*	*4.5*	*1.4*
California Set, Waitrose*	1 Pack/120g	223	9.1	186	3.8	25.2	7.6	1.7
Californian Roll & Nigiri, Selection, M&S*	1 Pack/215g	355	5.8	165	7.1	28	2.7	1.1
Chicken & Duck, Asian Inspired, Selection, Tesco*	1 Pack/205g	333	6.3	163	4.4	28.9	3.1	0.7
Fish & Veg Selection, Tesco*	1 Pack/150g	248	3.4	165	6.7	29.2	2.3	0.4
Fish Roll, Nigiri & Maki Selection, M&S*	1 Pack/210g	315	4.8	150	6.5	25.8	2.3	1
Fish Selection, Large, Tesco*	1 Pack/218g	365	6.8	167	5.3	29	3.1	0.9
Fish, Selection, Asda*	1 Pack/153g	242	2.6	158	5.3	30	1.7	0.6
Fish, Selection, Medium, Sainsbury's*	1 Pack/157g	256	3.9	163	5.6	28.6	2.5	1.9
Fish, Snack, Tesco*	1 Pack/104g	159	2.6	153	4.5	28	2.5	1.5
Komachi Set with Salmon, Whiting & Handroll, Waitrose*	1 Pack/257g	447	13.9	174	5.3	25.8	5.4	1.2
Medium Pack, Tesco*	1 Pack/139g	211	3.2	152	6.3	26.6	2.3	2.3
Naniwa, Box, Lidl*	1 Pack/190g	262	3.8	138	4.6	25	2	0.6
Nigiri Set, Taiko, Salmon & Tuna, Waitrose*	1 Pack/113g	174	2.3	154	6.3	26	2	0.6
Roll Selection, Sainsbury's*	1 Pack/217.4g	363	8	167	5	28.4	3.7	0.5
Salmon & Roll Set, Sainsbury's*	1 Serving/101g	167	2.6	165	4.9	30.4	2.6	0.8
Salmon & Prawn, Nigiri, M&S*	1 Pack/125g	186	1.4	149	7	27.2	1.1	1

S

	Measure INFO/WEIGHT	per Measure KCAL	FAT	Nutrition Values per 100g / 100ml KCAL	PROT	CARB	FAT	FIBRE
SUSHI								
Salmon & Tuna, Tesco*	1 Pack/151g	248	5.6	164	6.9	25.6	3.7	0.5
Salmon Wrap, Taiko Foods*	1 Pack/200g	284	4.6	142	5.1	24.8	2.3	0
Salmon, Smoked, Snack Pack, Tesco*	1 Pack/69g	114	1.9	165	5	29.1	2.7	0.9
Snack Selection, Eat Well, M&S*	1 Pack/96g	134	0.7	140	5.3	28.7	0.7	0.8
Taiko, California, Waitrose*	1 Pack/140g	246	10.1	176	4.1	22	7.2	4.1
Taiko, Fuji Set, Waitrose*	1 Pack /332g	515	10	155	5	28	3	1
Tuna, to Snack Selection, Food to Go, M&S*	1 Serving/150g	225	3.9	150	5.2	26.4	2.6	2.3
Vegetable Selection Pack, M&S*	1 Pack/154g	215	2.8	140	2.8	28.1	1.8	1.3
Vegetable, Mixed, Pick & Mix, Snack Pack, Tesco*	1 Pack/85g	132	2	155	3.7	28.6	2.4	1.4
Vegetable, Morrisons*	1 Pack/75g	126	2.9	168	3.4	29.2	3.9	1.4
Vegetable, Selection, Aldi*	1 Pack/149g	238	5.1	160	3.1	29	3.4	1.1
Vegetarian with Pickled Vegetables, Waitrose*	1 Pack/135g	244	4.9	181	5	27.8	3.6	1.7
Vegetarian, Snack Selection, Tesco*	1 Pack/85g	106	2.8	125	3.7	20.1	3.3	0.6
Yo!, Bento Box, Sainsbury's*	1 Pack/208g	530	6.2	255	8.4	48.7	3	0.9
SWEDE								
Boiled, Average	*1oz/28g*	*3*	*0*	*11*	*0.3*	*2.3*	*0.1*	*0.7*
Raw, Flesh Only, Peeled	*1 Serving/100g*	*24*	*0.3*	*24*	*0.7*	*5*	*0.3*	*1.6*
Raw, Unprepared, Average	*1oz/28g*	*5*	*0.1*	*18*	*0.7*	*3.8*	*0.3*	*1.6*
SWEET & SOUR								
Chicken Balls, Chinese Takeaway, Iceland*	1 Pack/255g	311	3.3	122	9.9	17.5	1.3	6
Chicken with Egg Fried Rice, Chilled, HL, Tesco*	1 Pack/400g	389	4.2	103	6.9	15.5	1.1	1.9
Chicken with Long Grain Rice, Weight Watchers*	1 Pack/330g	300	1.6	91	5.4	15.5	0.5	1.4
Chicken with Noodles, Steamed, HE, Tesco*	1 Pack/370g	289	0.7	78	8.3	10.8	0.2	0.6
Chicken with Rice, Chilled, BGTY, Sainsbury's*	1 Pack/400g	344	3.6	86	6	13.5	0.9	1
Chicken without Batter, Cantonese, Chilled, Sainsbury's*	1 Pack/350g	410	4.9	117	8.5	17.6	1.4	1
Chicken, & Noodles, Chinese Takeaway, Tesco*	1 Pack/350g	350	0.7	100	5.7	18.8	0.2	0.2
Chicken, Breaded, Fried, From Restaurant, Average	*6 Pieces/130g*	*346*	*18*	*266*	*13*	*22.3*	*13.8*	*0*
Chicken, Chinese Takeaway, Sainsbury's*	1 Pack/264g	515	16.9	195	13.1	21.3	6.4	1
Chicken, Crispy, Fillets, Tesco*	1 Pack/350g	508	19.6	145	7.2	15.3	5.6	0.9
Chicken, in Batter, Cantonese, Chilled, Sainsbury's*	1 Pack/350g	560	21	160	8.9	22.4	6	0.9
Chicken, M&S*	1 Pack/300g	465	10.8	155	6.6	24.4	3.6	0.8
Chicken, Take It Away, M&S*	1 Pack/200g	200	1.6	100	9.4	13.2	0.8	1.2
Pork	*1oz/28g*	*48*	*2.5*	*172*	*12.7*	*11.3*	*8.8*	*0.6*
Pork with Rice, 229, Oakhouse Foods Ltd*	1 Meal/400g	484	12	121	5.1	18.4	3	0.7
Pork, Battered, Sainsbury's*	½ Pack/175g	306	8.8	175	7.3	25.1	5	0.6
with Long Grain Rice, Rice Time, Uncle Ben's*	1 Pot/300g	393	2.4	131	1.9	28.4	0.8	0.7
SWEET POTATO								
Baked, Flesh Only, Average	*1 Med/130g*	*150*	*0.5*	*115*	*1.6*	*27.9*	*0.4*	*3.3*
Boiled in Salted Water, Average	*1 Med/200g*	*168*	*0.6*	*84*	*1.1*	*20.5*	*0.3*	*2.3*
Mash, Frozen, As Consumed, Aunt Bessie's*	1 Serving/80g	70	1.1	88	0.8	17	1.4	2.3
Mash, Tesco*	½ Pack/190g	206	6.5	108	1.9	16.2	3.4	2.7
Raw, Peeled, Average	*1 Sm/130g*	*112*	*0.1*	*86*	*1.6*	*20.1*	*0*	*3*
Raw, Unprepared, Average	*1 Potato/200g*	*146*	*0.5*	*73*	*1*	*17.9*	*0.3*	*2*
Roasted, So Organic, Sainsbury's*	1 Serving/176g	216	0.9	123	2.9	24.7	0.5	4.2
Steamed, Average	*1 Med/200g*	*168*	*0.6*	*84*	*1.1*	*20.4*	*0.3*	*2.3*
Wedges, Eat Well, M&S*	½ Pack/150g	123	2.2	82	1.4	14.5	1.5	2.6
Wedges, Spicy & Zesty Chilli & Lime, Waitrose*	½ Pack/195g	205	7	105	1.3	15.2	3.6	3.5
SWEETBREAD								
Lamb, Fried	*1oz/28g*	*61*	*3.2*	*217*	*28.7*	*0*	*11.4*	*0*
SWEETCORN								
Baby, Frozen, Average	*1oz/28g*	*7*	*0.1*	*24*	*2.5*	*2.7*	*0.4*	*1.7*
Boiled, Average	*1oz/28g*	*31*	*0.6*	*111*	*4.2*	*19.6*	*2.3*	*2.2*
Canned with Sugar & Salt, Average	*1 Lge Can/340g*	*369*	*4*	*108*	*3.2*	*21.5*	*1.2*	*1.9*

S

	Measure INFO/WEIGHT	per Measure KCAL	FAT	Nutrition Values per 100g / 100ml KCAL	PROT	CARB	FAT	FIBRE
SWEETCORN								
Frozen, Average	*1 Serving/80g*	*84*	*1.7*	*105*	*3.8*	*17.9*	*2.1*	*1.8*
No Sugar & Salt, Canned, Average	*½ Can/125g*	*99*	*1.3*	*79*	*2.7*	*15*	*1.1*	*1.6*
with Peppers, Canned, Average	*1 Serving/50g*	*40*	*0.2*	*79*	*2.6*	*16.4*	*0.3*	*0.6*
SWEETENER								
Aspartamo, Artificial Sugar, Zen*	1 Tbsp/2g	8	0	383	1.8	94	0	0
Calorie Free, Truvia*	1 Sachet/1.5g	0	0	0	0	99	0	0
Canderel*	1 Tbsp/2g	8	0	379	24.7	7	0	5.3
Canderel, Spoonful, Canderel*	1 Tsp/0.5g	2	0	384	2.9	93	0	0
Granulated, Low Calorie, Splenda*	1 Tsp/0.5g	2	0	391	0	97.7	0	0
Granulated, Silver Spoon*	1 Tsp/0.5g	2	0	387	1	96.8	0	0
Granulated, Tesco*	1 Tsp/1g	4	0	383	1.8	94	0	0
Low Calorie, Somerfield*	1 Tsp/1g	2	0	380	3	92	0	0
Lucuma Powder, Navitas*	1 Tbsp/15g	60	0	400	6.7	86.7	0	0
Natural Syrup, Fruit, Dark, Sweet Freedom*	1 Tsp/5g	13	0	292	0	79	0	0
Silver Spoon*	1 Tablet/0.1g	0	0	325	10	71	0	0
Simply Sweet*	1 Tbsp/2g	8	0	375	1.4	92.3	0	0
Slendasweet, Sainsbury's*	1 Tsp/1g	4	0	395	1.8	97	0	0.1
Slendersweet, Sainsbury's*	1 Tsp/1g	4	0	395	1.8	97	0	0.1
Spoonfull, Low Calorie, SupaSweet*	1 Tsp/1g	4	0	392	3	95	0	0
Sweet' N Low*	1 Sachet/1g	3	0	368	0	92	0	0
Tablet, Average	*1 Tablet/0.1g*	*0*	*0*	*355*	*8.7*	*73*	*0*	*0.8*
Tablets, Low Calorie, Canderel*	1 Tablet/0.1g	0	0	342	13	72.4	0	0
Tablets, Splenda*	1 Tablet/0.1g	0	0	345	10	76.2	0	1.6
Tablets, Tesco*	1 Tablet/1g	0	0	20	2	2	0.5	0
The Pantry, Aldi*	1 Tsp1g	4	0	376	0.5	94	0.5	0.5
Xylosweet, Xylitol*	1 Serving/4g	10	0	240	0	100	0	0
SWEETS								
Almonds, Sugared, Dragee*	1 Sweet/3.5g	17	0.6	472	10	68.3	17.9	2.5
Alphabet Candies, Asda*	1 Pack/80g	306	0	382	0.5	95	0	0
Banana Split Eclairs, Walker's Nonsuch Ltd*	1 Serving/40g	200	8.9	501	2.7	72.4	22.2	0
Banana, Baby Foam, M&S*	1/3 Pack/34g	131	0	385	4.1	92.7	0	0
Big Purple One, Quality Street, Nestle*	1 Sweet/39g	191	9.9	490	4.7	60.5	25.5	0.7
Black Jacks & Fruit Salad, Bassett's*	1 Serving/190g	760	11.8	400	0.7	84.9	6.2	0
Blackcurrant & Liquorice, M&S*	1 Sweet/8g	32	0.3	400	0.6	89	4.3	0
Body Parts, Rowntree's*	1 Pack/42g	146	0	348	4.3	82.9	0	0
Bon Bons, Strawberry, Classic Favourites, Asda*	1 Sweet/5g	20	0.3	402	0	88	5.6	0
Butter Candies, Original, Werther's*	1 Sweet/5g	21	0.4	424	0.1	85.7	8.9	0.1
Butterscotch Candies, Weight Watchers*	1 Box/42g	95	0	226	0	81.9	0	14.5
Candy Cane, Average	*1 Cane/13g*	*50*	*0*	*386*	*0*	*96*	*0*	*0.2*
Candy Cane, Peppermint, Sainsbury's*	1 Cane/12g	48	0	386	0	96.5	0	0
Candy Corn, Brachs*	19 Pieces/39g	140	0	359	0	92.3	0	0
Candy Floss, Asda*	1 Tub/75g	292	0	390	0	100	0	0
Candy Foam Shapes, Fun Fruits, Value, Tesco*	1 Serving/25g	94	0	374	3.1	90.3	0.1	0.5
Cherry Lips, Chewits*	1 Serving/100g	319	0.2	319	5.6	72.1	0.2	0
Chew	*1oz/28g*	*107*	*1.6*	*381*	*1*	*87*	*5.6*	*1*
Chewits, Blackcurrant, Leaf*	1 Chew/3g	12	0.1	385	0.2	87.5	3	0
Chewits, Cola, Leaf*	1 Chew/3g	12	0.1	385	0.2	87.5	3	0
Chewits, Fruit Salad, Leaf*	1 Chew/3g	12	0.1	385	0.2	87.5	3	0
Chewits, Strawberry, Leaf*	1 Chew/3g	12	0.1	385	0.2	87.5	3	0
Chewitts, Blackcurrant	*1 Pack/33.1g*	*125*	*0.9*	*378*	*0.3*	*86.9*	*2.7*	*0*
Chews, Calcium, Ellactiva*	1 Sweet/7g	24	1.1	350	1.4	51.4	15.7	0
Chews, Just Fruit, Fruit-tella*	1 Serving/43g	170	2.8	400	0.9	79.5	6.5	0
Chews, Spearmint, Victoria, Aldi*	1 Sweet/9.9g	40	0.8	405	0.3	83.8	7.6	0

SWEETS

INFO/WEIGHT	Measure	per Measure		Nutrition Values per 100g / 100ml				
		KCAL	FAT	KCAL	PROT	CARB	FAT	FIBRE
Chews, Strawberry Mix, Starburst*	1 Sweet/3.8g	15	0.3	401	0	83.9	7.3	0
Choco & Mint, Mentos*	1 Pack/38g	156	3.2	410	2.8	79	8.5	0
Choco Toffee, Sula*	1 Sweet/7.8g	21	1.2	267	3.3	31.7	15.8	0
Chocolate Caramels, Milk, Tesco*	1 Sweet/3g	15	0.5	444	2.7	72.1	16.1	0.1
Chocolate Eclairs, Cadbury*	1 Sweet/8g	36	1.4	455	4.5	68.9	17.9	0
Chocolate Eclairs, Co-Op*	1 Sweet/8g	38	1.6	480	3	71	20	0.6
Chocolate Limes, Pascall*	1 Sweet/8g	27	0.2	333	0.3	77.2	2.5	0
Cocoa & Orange, Super Bites, Truffles, Good 4u*	1 Bag/40g	153	6.1	383	10.8	46.9	15.2	7.7
Cola Bottles, Asda*	1 Serving/100g	329	0.2	329	9	73	0.2	0
Cola Bottles, Barratt*	1 Sweet/10g	34	0.1	337	1.3	82	0.4	0.1
Cola Bottles, Fizzy Wizzy, Woolworths*	1 Bag/100g	336	0	336	3.5	77.2	0	0
Cola Bottles, Fizzy, M&S*	1 Pack/200g	650	0	325	6.4	75	0	0
Cough, Herbs, Swiss, Orginal, Ricola*	1 Pack/37g	148	0	400	0	98	0	0
Cream Caramel, Sula*	1 Sweet/3g	10	0	297	0.4	86.1	0	0
Creme Caramel, Sugar Free, Be Light, Aldi*	1 Sweet/2.7g	7	0.2	275	0.2	90.2	6.3	0.1
Crunchies, Fruit, Fruit-tella*	1 Box/23g	90	1.2	390	0.7	86	5	0
Dolly Mix, Bassett's*	1 Bag/45g	171	1.4	380	3	85.1	3.1	0.4
Dolly Mixtures, M&S*	1 Pack/115g	431	1.6	375	1.8	89.2	1.4	0
Dolly Mixtures, Sainsbury's*	1 Serving/10g	40	0.2	401	1.4	94.4	1.9	0.1
Dolly Mixtures, Smart Price, Asda*	1 Sweet/3g	11	0	380	0.5	91	1.6	0
Dolly Mixtures, Tesco*	1 Pack/100g	376	1.5	376	1.6	88.9	1.5	0
Double Lolly, Swizzels Matlow*	1 Lolly/10g	41	0.3	407	0	92.4	3.4	0
Drops, Lemon & Orange, M&S*	1 Pack42g	97	0	230	0	61	0	0
Drumstick, Matlow's*	1 Pack/40g	164	2.2	409	0.4	88.3	5.5	0
Drumstick, Squashies, Swizzels*	1 Bag/160g	568	0.2	355	3.4	83.5	0.1	0
Edinburgh Rock, Gardiners of Scotland*	1 Piece/2.2g	8	0	380	0.1	94.4	0.3	0.8
Fizzy Mix, Tesco*	½ Bag/50g	166	0	332	5.2	75.2	0	0
Fizzy Pop, M&S*	1 Sweet/4g	14	0	352	0.1	88.7	0.5	0.5
Flumps, Bassett's*	1 Serving/5g	16	0	325	4	77	0	0
Flumps, Fluffy Mallow Twists, Fat Free, Bassett's*	1 Twist/13g	30	0	230	4.1	77.1	0	0
Flying Saucers, Tesco*	½ Pack/9g	34	0.1	380	1.3	90.8	1	1.2
Foamy Mushrooms, Chewy, Asda*	1 Sweet/2.6g	9	0	347	4.2	82	0.2	0
Fruit Gums & Jellies	**1 Tube/33g**	**107**	**0**	**324**	**6.5**	**79.5**	**0**	**0**
Fruit, Mentos*	1 Sweet/3g	10	0	333	0	100	0	0
Fruities, Lemon & Lime, Weight Watchers*	1 Sweet/2g	3	0	134	0	54	0	33
Fruity Chews, Starburst*	1 Sweet/8.3g	34	0.6	404	0	83.4	7.4	0
Fruity Frogs, Rowntree's*	1 Serving/40g	128	0.1	321	4.7	74.5	0.2	0
Gobstoppers, Everlasting, Wonka*	9 Pieces/15g	60	0	400	0	93.3	0	0
Gummy Bears	**10 Bears/25g**	**80**	**0**	**320**	**8**	**76**	**0**	**0**
Gummy Mix, Tesco*	1 Pack/100g	327	0.1	327	5.9	75.7	0.1	0
Gummy Worms	**10 Worms/74g**	**286**	**0**	**386**	**0**	**98.9**	**0**	**98.9**
Gummy Zingy Fruits, Bassett's*	1 Sm Bag/40g	135	0	337	5.1	79.2	0	0
Ice Cream Sundae, Asda*	1 Sweet/2.3g	9	0	387	4.9	70	0.5	0.5
Jellies, Fruit, Ringtons*	4 Jellies/44g	150	0.2	341	0.1	84	0.4	0.7
Jellies, Very Berry, Rowntrees*	1 Sweet/3.7g	12	0	326	5	74.8	0.2	0.1
Jelly Babies, Morrisons*	1 Serving/227g	781	0	344	5.3	80.7	0	0
Jelly Beans, Lucozade*	1 Pack/30g	111	0	370	0	92	0	0
Jelly Beans, Tesco*	¼ Bag/63g	243	0.2	385	0.1	94.5	0.3	0.3
Jelly Bears, Co-Op*	1 Sweet/3g	10	0	325	6	76	0.1	0
Jelly Bunnies, Bassetts, Maynards*	4 Sweets/26g	87	0	330	3.5	78	0.1	0
Jelly Tots, Rowntree's*	1 Pack/42g	145	0	346	0.1	86.5	0	0
Kisses, Hershey*	1 Sweet/5g	28	1.6	561	7	59	32	0
Laces, Apple Flavour, Tesco*	5 Laces/15g	52	0.5	347	3.6	74.8	3.2	2.1

S

SWEETS

INFO/WEIGHT	Measure	per Measure KCAL	FAT	Nutrition Values per 100g / 100ml KCAL	PROT	CARB	FAT	FIBRE
Laces, Strawberry, Fizzy, Somerfield*	1 Pack/100g	380	2	380	3	86	2	0
Laces, Strawberry, Sainsbury's*	1 Serving/25g	94	1.2	377	3.3	76.3	4.6	0.1
Laces, Strawberry, Tesco*	1 Serving/75g	260	2.4	347	3.6	74.8	3.2	2.1
Lances, Fizzy, Strawberry, Somerfield*	1 Sweet/4g	13	0.1	362	2.8	79.8	2.7	1.5
Lances, Strawberry & Cream Flavour, Tesco*	1 Bag/75g	276	0.9	368	3.2	86.1	1.2	2.1
Lances, Strawberry Flavour, Fizzy, Tesco*	½ Pack/50g	177	1.3	354	2.8	79.8	2.6	1.8
Lemon Mint Flavour, Herb Drops, Sugar Free, Ricola*	1 Sweet/3g	7	0	235	0	96	0	0
Liquorice, Boiled, Sugar Free, Sula*	1 Sweet/3g	7	0	227	0.2	93	0	0.2
Lovehearts, Giant, Swizzels*	1 Pack/42g	165	0	393	0	100	0	0
Lovehearts, Swizzels*	1oz/28g	100	0	359	0.7	88.2	0	0
Maoam Sour, Haribo*	1 Pack/22g	85	1.4	386	1.2	80	6.5	0.1
Maynards Sours, Bassett's*	1 Pack/52g	169	0	325	6.1	75	0	0
Midget Gems, Maynards*	1 Sweet/1g	3	0	340	8.7	76.2	0	0
Midget Gems, Value, Tesco*	1 Serving/40g	130	0.1	324	4.5	76.1	0.2	0
Milk Chocolate Eclairs, Sainsbury's*	1 Sweet/8g	33	1.1	442	2.1	75.7	14.5	0.5
Milk Chocolate Eclairs, Value, Tesco*	1 Bag/200g	918	32.6	459	2.6	75.2	16.3	1
Milk Duds, Hershey*	13 Pieces/33g	170	6	510	3	84	18	0
Mini Macs, CBY, Asda*	2 Sweets/96g	420	12.6	437	1.9	77.7	13.1	0.1
Mini Marti, Mushrooms, Asda*	1 Sweet/3g	10	0	340	3.8	81.1	0.1	0
Original, Chocolate Soft Caramel, Speciality, Werther's*	1 Piece/6g	30	1.5	480	5.1	61.5	23.5	1
Paradise Fruits, Dominion, Aldi*	1 Sweet/6g	23	0	382	0	95.5	0	0
Parma Violets, Swizzlers*	1 Sm Tube/10g	41	0	406	0.9	99.1	0	0
Percy Pig & Pals, Soft, M&S*	1 Sweet/8g	30	0	344	5.8	80	0.1	0
Pic 'n' Mix, Woolworths*	1 Serving/180g	750	6	417	0	96.7	3.3	0
Randoms, Rowntree's*	1 Pack/50g	164	0.2	328	4.9	75.7	0.3	0.6
Refreshers, Candyland, Barratt*	1 Tube/34g	129	0.5	380	0	89.1	1.4	0
Rhubarb & Custard, Sainsbury's*	1 Sweet/8g	28	0	351	0.1	87.7	0	0
Rhubarb & Custards, Tesco*	1 Sweet/9g	36	0	396	0.3	97.6	0.5	0.1
Rotella, Haribo*	1 Sweet/12.5g	43	0	343	1.5	84	0.2	0
Santa Babies, Berry Mix, Bassetts*	1 Bag/165g	544	0	330	3.5	78.5	0	0
Scary Mix, Tesco*	1 Bag/100g	327	0.5	327	9.5	71.1	0.5	0.3
Scary Sours, Rowntree's*	1 Serving/100g	321	0	321	3.5	74.7	0	0
Sherbert Dib Dab with Strawberry Lolly, Barratt*	1 Pack/23g	90	0	385	0.1	95.6	0.1	0
Sherbert Lemons, M&S*	1 Serving/20g	76	0	380	0	93.9	0	0
Sherbert Lemons, Weight Watchers*	1 Box/35g	84	0.2	239	0	94.7	0.5	0
Sherbet Lemons, Bassett's*	1 Sweet/6.7g	25	0	375	0	93.9	0	0
Shrimps & Bananas, Sainsbury's*	½ Pack/50g	188	0	376	2.5	91.3	0.1	0.5
Snakes, Bassett's*	1 Sweet/9.4g	30	0	320	3.5	76.8	0.1	0
Soft Fruits, Trebor*	1 Roll/45g	165	0	367	0	90.9	0	0
Sour Apple Sticks, Fizzy Wizzy, Woolworths*	1 Sweet/5g	18	0.1	358	2.8	79.8	2.7	0
Strawberry & Cream, Sugar Free, Sula*	1 Sweet/3.2g	9	0.2	267	0.2	90.5	5.4	0
Strawberry Laces, CBY, Asda*	1 Pack/50g	184	1.2	367	3.3	82	2.5	1.6
Sugar Free, Sula*	1 Sweet/3g	7	0	231	0	96.1	0	0
Sweetshop Favourites, Bassett's*	1 Sweet/5g	17	0	340	0	84.3	0	0
Tic Tac, Cool Cherry, Ferrero*	1 Pack/18g	69	0.1	382	0.2	92.2	0.7	0
Tootsie Roll, Sm Midgees, Tootsie*	1 Sweet/7g	23	0.5	350	2.5	70	7.5	0
Tooty Frooties, Rowntree's*	1 Bag/28g	111	1	397	0.1	91.5	3.5	0
Wiggly Worms, Sainsbury's*	1 Serving/10g	32	0	317	5.6	72.7	0.4	0.2
Wine Gummies, Matlow, Swizzels*	1 Pack/16g	52	0	324	0	58.7	0	0
Yo Yo's, All Flavours, 100% Fruit, We Are Bear*	1 Roll/10g	28	0	275	1.9	63.4	0.2	12
Yo Yo's, Strawberry 100% Fruit, We Are Bear*	1 Roll/10g	28	0	275	1.9	63.4	0.2	12
York Fruits, Terry's*	1 Sweet/9g	29	0	320	0	78.5	0	0.5

S

	Measure INFO/WEIGHT	per Measure KCAL	FAT	Nutrition Values per 100g / 100ml KCAL	PROT	CARB	FAT	FIBRE
SWORDFISH								
Grilled, Average	*1oz/28g*	*39*	*1.5*	*139*	*22.9*	*0*	*5.2*	*0*
Raw, Average	*1oz/28g*	*42*	*2*	*149*	*21.1*	*0*	*7.2*	*0*
SYRUP								
Amaretto, Sugar Free, Monin*	1 Serving/30ml	0	0	0	0	13.3	0	0
Artificial Maple Flavour, Sugar Free, Cary's*	1 Serving/60ml	30	0	50	0	20	0	0.5
Balsamic, Merchant Gourmet*	1 Tsp/5g	12	0	232	0.4	60	0.1	0
Butterscotch, Monin*	1 Serving/30ml	100	0	333	0	80	0	0
Caramel, for Coffee, Lyle's*	2 Tsps/10ml	33	0	329	0	83	0	0
Caramel, Sugar Free, Monin*	1 Serving/30ml	0	0	0	0	13.3	0	0
Chocolate Mint, Monin*	1 Serving/30ml	100	0	333	0	80	0	0
Cinnamon, Monin*	1 Serving/30ml	100	0	333	0	80	0	0
Corn, Dark, Average	*1 Tbsp/20g*	*56*	*0*	*282*	*0*	*76.6*	*0*	*0*
Gingerbread, Monin*	1 Serving/30ml	90	0	300	0	76.7	0	0
Golden, Average	*1 Tbsp/20g*	*61*	*0*	*304*	*0.4*	*78.2*	*0*	*0*
Hazelnut, Monin*	1 Serving/30ml	90	0	300	0	73.3	0	0
Maple, Average	*1 Tbsp/20g*	*52*	*0*	*262*	*0*	*67.2*	*0.2*	*0*
Maple, Flavour, Zero Calorie, Bulk Powders*	1 Tsp/5g	0	0	4	0	0	0	1.2
Organic Rice Malt, Clearspring*	2 Tbsp/42g	133	0.2	316	1.5	76.8	0.4	0
Peppermint, Monin*	1 Serving/30ml	96	0	320	0	80	0	0
Praline, Monin*	1 Serving/30ml	94	0	313	0	76.7	0	0
Strawberry, Aardbeien Siroop, Plein Sud, Lidl*	1 Serving/20ml	56	0	280	0	71	0	0
Sugar	*1 Tbsp/20g*	*64*	*0*	*319*	*0*	*83.9*	*0*	*0*
Toffee Nut, Monin*	1 Serving/30ml	90	0	300	0	70	0	0
Vanilla, Fabbri*	1 Serving/20ml	70	0	349	0	86	0	0
Vanilla, Monin*	1 Shot/35ml	119	0	340	0	84.4	0	0
Vanilla, Sugar Free, Monin*	1 Serving/30ml	0	0	0	0	13.3	0	0

S

	Measure INFO/WEIGHT	per Measure KCAL	FAT	Nutrition Values per 100g / 100ml KCAL	PROT	CARB	FAT	FIBRE
TABOULEH								
Average	*1oz/28g*	*33*	*1.3*	*119*	*2.6*	*17.2*	*4.6*	*0*
Harissa & King Prawn, Everdine*	1 Serving/450g	320	7.2	71	4.3	7.9	1.6	3.7
TACO KIT								
Garlic & Paprika, Crunchy, As Sold, Old El Paso *	1 Taco/26g	77	3.6	296	3.8	37.3	13.8	2.7
TACO SHELLS								
Corn, Crunchy, Old El Paso*	1 Taco/10g	51	2.6	506	7	61	26	0
Old El Paso*	1 Taco/12g	57	2.7	478	7.4	60.8	22.8	0
Taco, Crunchy, Taco Bell *	1 Serving/78g	133	7.8	170	8	13	10	1
Traditional, Discovery*	1 Taco/11g	55	3.2	489	5.7	53.4	28.1	6
TAGINE								
Beef, Slow Cooked, Cook*	1 Portion/325g	462	15.6	142	13.5	11.2	4.8	1.3
Chicken & Chickpeas, Men's Health *	1 Pack/422g	394	5.5	93	9	10.2	1.3	2.5
Chickpea & Vegetable, Everdine*	1 Serving/450g	351	9	78	1.9	10.9	2	3.9
Chickpeas, Creationz, Heinz*	½ Can/196g	176	5.1	90	4	11	2.6	3.4
Lamb, Moroccan Style with Couscous, COU, M&S*	1 Pack/400g	340	5.6	85	8.9	8.3	1.4	1.6
Moroccan, Allplants*	½ Pack/370g	370	16.3	100	3.3	9.3	4.4	5
TAGLIATELLE								
Dry, Average	*1 Serving/100g*	*356*	*1.8*	*356*	*12.6*	*72.4*	*1.8*	*1*
Egg & Spinach, M&S*	1 Serving/100g	365	2.7	365	15.5	69.6	2.7	3
Egg, Dry, Average	*1 Serving/75g*	*272*	*2.5*	*362*	*14.2*	*68.8*	*3.3*	*2.3*
Egg, Fresh, Dry, Average	*1 Serving/125g*	*345*	*3.5*	*276*	*10.6*	*53*	*2.8*	*2.1*
Fresh, Dry, Average	*1 Serving/75g*	*211*	*2*	*281*	*11.4*	*53.3*	*2.6*	*2.6*
Garlic & Herb, Fresh, Sainsbury's*	1 Serving/125g	184	2.2	147	6.5	26.2	1.8	1.9
Ham & Mushroom, Asda*	1 Pack/340g	469	12.9	138	6	20	3.8	0.2
Ham & Mushroom, BGTY, Sainsbury's*	1 Pack/400g	368	4.8	92	4.2	15.5	1.2	1.1
Ham & Mushroom, Eat Smart, Morrisons*	1 Pack/400g	340	10	85	3.2	12.3	2.5	0.9
Ham & Mushroom, Italian, Waitrose*	1 Pack/400g	585	24	151	7.1	16.3	6.2	1
Ham & Mushroom, LC, Tesco*	1 Pack/400g	400	8.8	100	6	13.8	2.2	1.8
Lamb Ragu, Slow Cooked, Finest, Tesco*	1 Pack/400g	560	19.2	140	8.5	14.9	4.8	1.1
Smoked Salmon, Ready Meals, M&S*	1 Pack/360g	612	40.3	170	6.2	10.6	11.2	0.9
Vegetables, Retail	*1oz/28g*	*21*	*0.8*	*74*	*1.6*	*11*	*3*	*0.7*
Verdi, Fresh, Average	*1 Serving/125g*	*171*	*1.8*	*137*	*5.5*	*25.5*	*1.5*	*1.8*
Wholewheat, Fresh, Uncooked, Essential, Waitrose*	1 Portion/125g	278	4.1	222	10.9	33.6	3.3	7.6
TAHINI PASTE								
Average	*1 Tsp/6g*	*36*	*3.5*	*607*	*18.5*	*0.9*	*58.9*	*8*
TANGERINES								
Fresh, Raw	*1oz/28g*	*10*	*0*	*35*	*0.9*	*8*	*0.1*	*1.3*
Fresh, Raw, Weighed with Peel, Average	*1 Med/70g*	*13*	*0.1*	*18*	*0.5*	*4.2*	*0.1*	*0.7*
TANGO*								
Cherry, Britvic*	1 Bottle/500ml	55	0	11	0	2.4	0	0
Orange, Britvic*	1 Can/330ml	63	0	19	0.1	4.4	0	0
Orange, Sugar Free, Britvic*	1 Can/330ml	13	0	4	0	0	0	0
TAPAS								
Basque Beef, (Estofado Vasco), Tapas at, Tesco*	½ Pack/80g	80	3.1	100	9.5	6.4	3.9	1.5
Champinones Al Ajillo, Tapas at, Tesco*	½ Pack/85g	123	11.6	145	2.3	2.5	13.6	1.5
Chorizo & Cheese Croquettes, Tapas at, Tesco*	½ Pack/117g	263	11.1	225	5.4	28.6	9.5	2.6
Pollo Con Salsa, Tapas at, Tesco*	½ Pack/75g	94	6.5	125	9.4	2.1	8.7	0.7
TAPENADE								
Black Olive, Specially Selected, Aldi*	1 Tbsp/20g	46	4.6	231	1.4	2.7	23	4.4
Sundried Tomato & Jalapeno Pepper, Finest, Tesco*	1 Jar/90g	392	36.9	436	3.4	13.1	41	5
TAPIOCA								
Creamed, Ambrosia*	½ Can/213g	159	3.4	75	2.6	12.6	1.6	0.2
Raw	*1oz/28g*	*101*	*0*	*359*	*0.4*	*95*	*0.1*	*0.4*

T

	Measure INFO/WEIGHT	per Measure KCAL	FAT	Nutrition Values per 100g / 100ml KCAL	PROT	CARB	FAT	FIBRE
TARAMASALATA								
Average	*1 Tbsp/30g*	*143*	*14.4*	*478*	*4.2*	*7.9*	*47.9*	*1.1*
Reduced Fat, Waitrose*	1 Pack/170g	522	48.3	307	4	8.9	28.4	1.5
TARRAGON								
Dried, Ground	*1 Tsp/2g*	*5*	*0.1*	*295*	*22.8*	*42.8*	*7.2*	*0*
Fresh, Average	*1 Tbsp/3.8g*	*2*	*0*	*49*	*3.4*	*6.3*	*1.1*	*0*
TART								
Apple & Custard, Asda*	1 Tart/84g	227	11	270	3.1	35	13.1	0.1
Aubergine & Feta, Roast Marinated, Sainsbury's*	1 Serving/105g	227	15.2	216	4.8	16.6	14.5	1.7
Bakewell, Average	*1 Tart/50g*	*228*	*14.8*	*456*	*6.3*	*43.5*	*29.7*	*1.9*
Bakewell, Cherry, Morrisons*	1 Tart/46g	198	9.8	430	4.6	54.9	21.4	1.3
Bakewell, Large, Tesco*	1 Serving/57g	247	11.2	433	4.3	59.5	19.7	1.7
Bakewell, Lemon, Average	*1 Tart/46g*	*206*	*9.7*	*447*	*3.7*	*60.9*	*21.1*	*0.9*
Bakewell, Lyons*	1/6 Tart/52g	205	8.9	397	3.8	56.7	17.2	0.9
Bakewell, Toffee, Morrisons*	1 Tart/47g	201	7.4	422	3	67.2	15.5	0.9
Blackcurrant Sundae, Asda*	1 Tart/55g	227	10.4	413	3.5	57	19	2.3
Brie, Pear & Hazelnut Crowns, Luxury	*1 Serving/110g*	*242*	*14*	*220*	*8*	*18*	*12.7*	*1.2*
Cherry Tomato & Mascarpone, Asda*	1 Tart/160g	290	18	181	4.4	15.6	11.2	1.1
Chocolate, Co-Op*	1 Tart/22g	102	6.8	465	4	42	31	0.7
Custard, Individual, Average	*1 Tart/94g*	*260*	*13.6*	*277*	*6.3*	*32.4*	*14.5*	*1.2*
Date Pecan & Almond, Sticky, Sainsbury's*	1/8 Tart/75g	298	10.3	397	5	63.5	13.7	1.7
Egg Custard, Asda*	1 Tart/80g	215	10.4	269	9	29	13	1.2
Egg Custard, Free Range, Sainsbury's*	1 Tart/85g	232	10	273	6.3	35	11.8	0.9
Egg Custard, Twin Pack, Tesco*	1 Tart/90g	238	11.2	265	6	32	12.4	0.9
Feta Cheese & Spinach, Puff Pastry, Tesco*	1 Tart/108g	306	19.2	283	7.1	23.5	17.8	0.9
Frangipane, Apple, The Best, Morrisons*	1/6 Tart/75g	264	12.7	352	5.1	43.9	16.9	1.7
Gruyere Pancetta & Balsamic Onion, Finest, Tesco*	¼ Tart/106.3g	320	21.9	301	7.7	21.3	20.6	3.3
Jam, Assorted, Tesco*	1 Tart/35g	123	5	351	3.4	51.9	14.4	1.2
Jam, Average	*1 Slice/90g*	*342*	*13.4*	*380*	*3.3*	*62*	*14.9*	*1.6*
Jam, Real Fruit, Mr Kipling*	1 Tart/35g	136	5.2	388	3.8	67.9	14.9	1.7
Jam, Real Fruit, Sainsbury's*	1 Tart/37g	142	5.2	383	3.4	60.9	14	1.4
Lemon & Raspberry, Finest, Tesco*	1 Tart/120g	360	16.8	300	5.2	38.4	14	2.9
Lemon Curd, Asda*	1 Tart/30g	121	4.5	402	2.8	64	15	2.2
Lemon, M&S*	1/6 Tart/50g	208	14.6	415	5	32.7	29.3	0.9
Lemon, Sainsbury's*	1/8 Tart/56g	258	15.8	459	4.4	47	28.1	0.6
Mince, Gluten & Wheat Free, Florentines, Lovemore*	1 Tart/45g	183	8.3	407	4.5	55.7	18.4	2.5
Mixed Fruit, Fresh, Waitrose*	1 Tart/129g	351	17.4	272	4.2	32.8	13.5	1.5
Pineapple, Individual, Waitrose*	1 Tart/54g	216	6.1	400	2.2	77.2	11.3	0.5
Plum, Seriously Fruity, Waitrose*	1/6 Tart/95g	183	5.9	192	2.9	30.2	6.2	1.9
Pulled Beef, Open, Gastropub, M&S*	½ Pack/152g	351	21.9	231	9.8	14.8	14.4	1.4
Raspberry & Blueberry, Tesco*	1 Serving/85g	168	7.5	198	2.7	27	8.8	2.8
Roasted Vegetable, Finest, Tesco*	¼ Tart/113g	213	10.4	188	2.9	22.5	9.2	2.1
Salted Caramel & Chocolate, Waitrose*	1/12 Tart/79g	349	18.5	443	5.1	52.2	23.5	1.2
Seriously Fruit & Almond, Waitrose*	1 Slice/64g	195	10	303	4.9	34.3	15.6	2.7
Spinach & Ricotta, Individual, TTD, Sainsbury's*	1 Quiche/170g	466	33.7	274	7.5	16.5	19.8	1.4
Strawberry & Fresh Cream, Finest, Tesco*	1 Tart/129g	350	19.1	271	3.3	31.1	14.8	1.2
Strawberry Custard, Asda*	1 Tart/100g	335	15	335	3.1	47	15	0
Strawberry, Fresh, M&S*	1 Tart/119.6g	305	18.4	255	3.1	26.4	15.4	2.4
Toffee Pecan, Waitrose*	¼ Tart/133g	564	19.1	423	4.3	69.3	14.3	1.6
Treacle with Custard	*1 Serving/251g*	*586*	*23.5*	*233*	*3.1*	*36.1*	*9.4*	*0.8*
Treacle, Average	*1 Portion/125g*	*460*	*17.6*	*368*	*3.7*	*60.4*	*14.1*	*1.1*
Treacle, Tesco*	1 Slice/63g	228	7.6	362	3.9	58.5	12.1	1.7
Treacle, Waitrose*	¼ Tart/106g	302	11	285	2.8	45	10.4	0.6
Triple Choc, Brompton House*	1 Slice/25g	124	7	498	4	55	28	7

T

	Measure INFO/WEIGHT	per Measure		Nutrition Values per 100g / 100ml				
		KCAL	FAT	KCAL	PROT	CARB	FAT	FIBRE
TART								
Vegetable & Feta, Deli, M&S*	½ Tart/115g	315	18.4	274	5	20	16	6
Zesty Lemon, Tesco*	1/6 Tart/64g	260	15.5	405	5.3	41	24.2	0.7
TARTE								
Au Chocolat, Seriously Chocolatey, Waitrose*	1/6 Tarte/70g	348	22.8	497	6	43.8	32.6	2.6
Au Citron, Frozen, TTD, Sainsbury's*	1/6 Tarte/80g	232	13.4	290	4.7	40.7	16.8	7.7
Au Citron, Waitrose*	1 Tarte/100g	325	18.1	325	4.9	35.7	18.1	1
Bacon, Leek & Roquefort, Bistro, Waitrose*	¼ Tarte/100g	277	18.2	277	8.4	19.8	18.2	0.6
TARTLETS								
Brie & Cranberry, Filo, Waitrose*	1 Tartlet/16g	44	2.2	275	8.9	26.9	13.9	3.5
Butternut Squash & Goats Cheese, Linda McCartney*	1 Tartlet/150g	405	25	270	6.3	24.2	16.7	1.2
Goats Cheese & Caramelised Onion, Aldi*	1 Tartlet/150g	402	26	268	7.3	20.7	17.3	1.2
Lemon, Petit, Bonne Maman*	1 Tartlet/14g	61	2.4	439	5	66	17	0
Raspberry, Mini, M&S*	1 Tartlet/27g	90	5.4	330	4.3	34.4	19.6	0.5
Red Onion & Goats Cheese, Sainsbury's*	1 Tartlet/113g	335	21.8	297	7	23.7	19.3	1.5
Tomato & Goats Cheese, Waitrose*	1 Tartlet/130g	295	19	227	6.6	17.4	14.6	2
TEA								
A Moment of Calm, herbal Infusion, Brewed, Twinings*	1 Mug/200ml	4	0	2	0	0.3	0	0
Apple & Cinnamon, Made Up, Heath And Heather*	1 Serving/250ml	8	0	3	0.1	0.7	0	0
Assam, Blended, TTD, Sainsbury's*	1 Serving/2g	0	0	0	0	0	0	0
Blackberry & Nettle, Twinings*	1 Cup/250ml	5	0	2	0	0.3	0	0
Blackcurrant, Fruit Creations, Typhoo*	1 Sm Cup/100ml	5	0	5	0.2	0.8	0	0.2
Camomile, Pure, Classic Herbal, Twinings*	1 Serving/200ml	4	0	2	0	0.3	0	0
Chai Latte, Skinny Blend, Drink Me Chai*	1 Serving/15g	62	1.2	415	7.5	77.7	8	1.3
Chai, Twinings*	1 Cup/200ml	2	0	1	0.1	0	0	0
Chamomile & Spiced Apple, Warming, Twinings*	1 Cup/100ml	2	0	2	0	0.3	0	0
Cranberry & Elderflower, Boost, Tetley*	1 Serving/225ml	5	0	2	0.1	0.6	0	0
Damask, Rose, Chinese, Choi Time*	1 Mug/500ml	0	0.3	0	0	0	0.1	0
Darjeeling Infusion, with Raspberry Juice, M&S*	1 Bottle/500ml	170	0	34	0	8.5	0	0
Decaf, Tetley*	1 Cup/100ml	1	0	1	0	0.3	0	0
Earl Grey, Green, Twinings*	1 Cup/200ml	2	0	1	0	0.2	0	0
Earl Grey, Infusion with Water, Average	*1 Mug/250ml*	*2*	*0*	*1*	*0*	*0.2*	*0*	*0*
Fruit Or Herbal, Made with Water, Twinings*	1 Mug/200ml	8	0	4	0	1	0	0
Fruit, Green, Infusion, Eat Well, M&S*	½ Pack/150g	80	1.2	53	1.4	9.8	0.8	0.6
Fruit, Twinings*	1 Mug/227ml	4	0	2	0	0.4	0	0
Fruits of the Forest, Westminster Tea*	1 Bag/250ml	5	0	2	0	0.6	0	0
Ginger, Herbal, Brit & Tang*	1 Tea Bag/1.8g	5	0	278	0	55.6	0	0
Green Tea, Apple & Cucumber, Super, Beauty, Tetley*	1 Teabag/200ml	2	0	1	0	0.3	0	0
Green with Citrus, Twinings*	1 Serving/200ml	2	0	1	1	0.2	0	0
Green with Jasmine, Twinings*	1 Serving/100ml	1	0	1	0	0.2	0	0
Green with Jasmine, Wellbeing Selection, Flavia*	1 Cup/200ml	0	0	0	0	0	0	0
Green with Lemon, Jackson's*	1 Serving/200ml	2	0	1	0	0.2	0	0
Green with Mango, Brewed with Water, Twinings*	1 Cup/200ml	2	0	1	0	0.2	0	0
Green with Mint, Whittards of Chelsea*	1 Cup/100ml	1	0	1	0.2	0.1	0	0
Green with Pomegranate, Twinings*	1 Serving/200ml	2	0	1	0	0.2	0	0
Green, Powder, Matcha*	1 Serving/10g	30	0	300	0	50	0	30
Green, with Yerba Mate & Honey, Herbal Mist*	1 Serving/240ml	80	0	33	0	8.3	0	0
Herbal, Wellbeing Blends, Infusions, Twinings*	1 Serving/200ml	4	0	2	0	0.3	0	0
Ice with Lemon, Lipton*	1 Bottle/325ml	91	0	28	0	6.9	0	0
Ice with Mango, Lipton*	1 Bottle/500ml	165	0	33	0	8.1	0	0
Ice with Peach, Lipton*	1 Bottle/500ml	140	0	28	0	6.8	0	0
Iced, Green, Orange, Lipton*	1 Bottle/500ml	100	0	20	0	5	0	0
Iced, No Sugar Peach Flavour, Nestle*	1 Glass/100ml	1	0	1	0	0.1	0	0
Iced, Peach, Twinings*	1 Serving/200ml	60	0.2	30	0.1	7.3	0.1	0

	Measure INFO/WEIGHT	per Measure KCAL	FAT	Nutrition Values per 100g / 100ml KCAL	PROT	CARB	FAT	FIBRE
TEA								
Iced, Raspberry, Bottle, Lipton*	1 Serving/250ml	48	1.3	19	0.5	4.6	0.5	0
Lemon & Earl Grey Flavour, Sainsbury's*	1 Serving/250ml	7	1.2	3	0.5	0.7	0.5	0.5
Lemon & Ginger, Lipton*	1 Cup/200ml	8	0	4	0.5	0.5	0	0
Lemon, Iced, Diet, Nestea*	1 Glass/250ml	3	0	1	0	0	0	0
Lemon, Instant, Original, Lift*	1 Serving/15g	53	0	352	0	87	0	0
Lemon, Instant, Tesco*	1 Serving/7g	23	0	326	1	80.5	0	0
Lemon, with Yerba Mate, Herbal Mist*	1 Serving/240ml	80	0	33	0	8.8	0	0
Light & Delicate, Green with Lemon, Twinings*	1 Cup/100ml	1	0.1	1	0.1	0.2	0.1	0.1
Made with Water	*1 Mug/227ml*	*0*	*0*	*0*	*0.1*	*0*	*0*	*0*
Made with Water with Semi-Skimmed Milk, Average	*1 Cup/200ml*	*14*	*0.4*	*7*	*0.5*	*0.7*	*0.2*	*0*
Made with Water with Skimmed Milk, Average	*1 Mug/270ml*	*16*	*0.5*	*6*	*0.5*	*0.7*	*0.2*	*0*
Made with Water with Whole Milk, Average	*1 Cup/200ml*	*16*	*0.8*	*8*	*0.4*	*0.5*	*0.4*	*0*
Mango, with Yerba Mate, Herbal Mist*	1 Serving/240ml	70	0	29	0	7.5	0	0
Morning Detox, Twinings*	1 Serving/200ml	5	0	2	0	0.3	0	0
Nettle & Peppermint, Twinings*	1 Cup/200ml	2	0	1	0	0.2	0	0
Nettle & Sweet Fennel, Twinings*	1 Cup/200ml	4	0	2	0	0.3	0	0
Orange & Mango, Herbal, Organic, Honest, Coca-Cola*	1 Bottle/500ml	96	0	19	0	4.7	0	0
Peach, with Yerba Mate, Herbal Mist*	1 Serving/240ml	80	0	33	0	9.2	0	0
Peppermint, Made with Water, Average	*1 Serving/200ml*	*3*	*0*	*2*	*0*	*0.2*	*0*	*0*
Raspberry & Cranberry, T of Life, Tetley*	1 Serving/100ml	36	0	36	0	9	0	0
Raspberry, with Yerba Mate, Herbal Mist*	1 Serving/240ml	80	0	33	0	9.2	0	0
Red Berries, Brewed, PG Tips*	1 Cup/200ml	5	0	2	0	0.6	0	0
Red Bush, Made with Water, Tetley*	1 Mug/250ml	2	0	1	0	0.1	0	0
Sleep, Herbal Infusion, Brewed, Twinings*	1 Mug/200ml	4	0	2	0	0.3	0	0
TEACAKES								
Average	*1 Teacake/60g*	*178*	*4.5*	*296*	*8*	*52.5*	*7.5*	*0*
Caramel, Highlights, Mallows, Cadbury*	1 Teacake/15g	61	1.9	408	6.2	69.1	12.4	3.6
Currant, Sainsbury's*	1 Teacake/72g	204	2.9	284	8.2	53.7	4	2.5
Fruited, Co-Op*	1 Teacake/62g	160	2	258	9.7	46.8	3.2	3.2
Fruity, Warburton's*	1 Teacake/62.5g	160	2.2	256	8.7	48	3.5	2.7
Large, Sainsbury's*	1 Teacake/100g	291	6.8	291	8.3	49.1	6.8	3.4
Large, TTD, Sainsbury's*	1 Teacake/90g	264	3.5	293	7.5	57	3.9	2.6
Marshmallow, Milk Chocolate, Tunnock's*	1 Teacake/24g	106	4.6	440	4.9	61.9	19.2	2.4
Mini Bites, M&S*	1 Bite/6g	29	1.2	484	3.2	72.6	20.3	2.1
Morrisons*	1 Teacake/64g	172	1.9	268	9.9	50.7	2.9	2.8
Richly Fruited, Waitrose*	1 Teacake/72g	205	2.7	285	7.8	55	3.7	2.2
Sainsbury's*	1 Teacake/70g	171	2.5	244	8	45	3.6	2.6
Tesco*	1 Teacake/61g	163	2.1	267	7.8	51.1	3.5	2.4
Toasted, Average	*1 Teacake/60g*	*197*	*5*	*329*	*8.9*	*58.3*	*8.3*	*0*
with Orange Filling, M&S*	1 Teacake/20g	80	2.8	410	4.5	66.6	14.2	0.9
TEMPEH								
Average	*1oz/28g*	*46*	*1.8*	*166*	*20.7*	*6.4*	*6.4*	*4.3*
TEQUILA								
Average	*1 Pub Shot/35ml*	*78*	*0*	*224*	*0*	*0*	*0*	*0*
TERRINE								
Ham Hock, M&S*	1 Slice/70g	98	4.1	140	22.5	0.1	5.8	0.5
Lobster & Prawn, Slices, M&S*	1 Serving/55g	107	7.4	195	18.2	0.7	13.4	0.7
Salmon & King Prawn, Waitrose*	1 Serving/75g	98	4	130	19.3	1.3	5.3	0
Salmon & Crayfish, Slice, Finest, Tesco*	1 Serving/110g	148	5.7	135	21.9	0.1	5.2	0.1
Salmon & Lemon, Luxury, Tesco*	1 Serving/50g	98	7.8	196	10.6	3.2	15.7	0.8
Salmon, Poached, Tesco*	1 Pack/113g	349	30.6	309	15.5	0.8	27.1	0
Salmon, Three, M&S*	1 Serving/80g	168	12.2	210	17.6	0.8	15.3	0.9

T

	Measure INFO/WEIGHT	per Measure KCAL	FAT	Nutrition Values per 100g / 100ml KCAL	PROT	CARB	FAT	FIBRE
THYME								
Dried, Average	*1 Tsp/1g*	*3*	*0.1*	*276*	*9.1*	*45.3*	*7.4*	*0*
Fresh, Average	*1 Tsp/1g*	*1*	*0*	*95*	*3*	*15.1*	*2.5*	*0*
TIA MARIA								
Original	*1 Pub Shot/35ml*	*105*	*0*	*300*	*0*	*0*	*0*	*0*
TIC TAC								
Extra Strong Mint, Ferrero*	2 Tic tacs/1g	4	0	381	0	95.2	0	0
Fresh Mint, Ferrero*	2 Tic Tacs/1g	4	0	390	0	97.5	0	0
Lime & Orange, Ferrero*	2 Tic Tacs/1g	4	0	386	0	95.5	0	0
Orange, Ferrero*	2 Tic Tacs/1g	4	0	385	0	95.5	0	0
Spearmint, Ferrero*	1 Box/16g	62	0	390	0	97.5	0	0
TIKKA MASALA								
Chicken, & Pilau Basmati Rice, Frozen, Patak's*	1 Pack/400g	580	20	145	9.9	15.1	5	0.2
Chicken, & Pilau Rice, BGTY, Sainsbury's*	1 Pack/400g	380	4.8	95	8.1	13	1.2	1.1
Chicken, & Pilau Rice, Waitrose*	1 Pack/500g	797	34.5	159	8.2	16.1	6.9	0.8
Chicken, & Rice, Ready Meal, Healthy Range, Average	*1 Serving/400g*	*390*	*6.4*	*98*	*6.6*	*14.3*	*1.6*	*1.1*
Chicken, & Vegetable, HL, Tesco*	1 Pack/450g	360	12.2	80	6.8	6.9	2.7	1.8
Chicken, & Pilau Rice, Meal for One, M&S*	1 Pack/400g	592	20.4	148	8.9	15.3	5.1	2.7
Chicken, & Pilau Rice, Takeaway, Asda*	1 Pack/560.5g	852	27.5	152	7	20	4.9	1.5
Chicken, & Rice, Be Light, Aldi*	1 Pack/400g	516	10	129	9.8	16	2.5	1.5
Chicken, Asda*	1 Pack/340g	388	20.4	114	9	6	6	1.5
Chicken, Breast, GFY, Asda*	1 Pack/380g	486	14.4	128	19	4.5	3.8	0.2
Chicken, Chef Select, Lidl*	1 Pack/450g	707	31	157	8.7	13.1	6.9	4
Chicken, Frozen, Microwaved, Slimzone, Asda*	1 Pack/443g	350	5.8	79	13	3.3	1.3	1.2
Chicken, Hot, Sainsbury's*	1 Pack/400g	604	37.2	151	13.2	3.6	9.3	1.5
Chicken, Indian Takeaway, Iceland*	1 Pack/400g	484	28.4	121	8.9	6	7.1	1.9
Chicken, Indian Takeaway, Tesco*	1 Serving/125g	100	3.2	80	8.9	4.9	2.6	2.1
Chicken, Indian, Medium, Sainsbury's*	1 Pack/400g	848	61.2	212	13.2	5.3	15.3	0.1
Chicken, M&S*	½ Pack/200g	288	15.6	144	13.5	4.7	7.8	0.7
Chicken, Weight Watchers*	1 Pack/331g	344	4.6	104	7	15.8	1.4	0.2
Chicken, with Pilau Rice, Frozen, Waitrose*	1 Pack/400g	676	32.4	169	9.3	14.6	8.1	2.1
Chicken, with White Rice, Good Choice, Iceland*	1 Serving/400g	356	4	89	5.4	14.7	1	0.6
Spicy, with Long Grain Rice, Rice Time, Uncle Ben's*	1 Tub/300g	328	4.8	109	2	21.1	1.6	0.8
Vegetable, Waitrose*	1 Serving/196g	149	4.3	76	3.6	10.5	2.2	3.8
Vegetarian, Chef's Selection, Quorn*	½ Pack/170g	274	17	161	6	10	10	3.5
TILAPIA								
Raw, Average	*100g*	*95*	*1*	*95*	*20*	*0*	*1*	*0*
TIME OUT								
Break Pack, Cadbury*	1 Serving/20g	108	6.3	530	6.2	58.3	30.7	0
Chocolate Fingers, Cadbury*	2 Fingers/35g	186	10.6	530	7.1	57.3	30.3	1.1
Orange, Snack Size, Cadbury*	1 Finger/11g	61	3.6	555	5	59.4	32.9	0
TIRAMISU								
Asda*	1 Pot/100g	252	11	252	4.3	34	11	0.5
Classic, Sainsbury's*	1 Serving/84g	209	8.5	250	4.2	31.7	10.2	1.1
Dine in Dessert, M&S*	½ Dessert/145g	515	36.7	355	2.6	28.8	25.3	0.7
Family Size, Tesco*	1 Serving/125g	356	18.1	285	4.3	34.5	14.5	4.3
Morrisons*	1 Pot/90g	248	9.9	276	4	38	11	0
Single Size, Tesco*	1 Pot/100g	290	12.9	290	3.8	35.1	12.9	4.5
Waitrose*	1 Pot/90g	221	11.2	246	6.4	27.2	12.4	0
TOAD IN THE HOLE								
Average	*1 Serving/231g*	*640*	*40.2*	*277*	*11.9*	*19.5*	*17.4*	*1.1*
Frozen, Cooked, CBY, Asda*	1 Slice/72g	168	7.5	232	9.2	24.2	10.4	2.6
Large, Great Value, Asda*	¼ Pack/81g	238	13.8	293	10	25	17	2.3

T

	Measure INFO/WEIGHT	per Measure KCAL	FAT	Nutrition Values per 100g / 100ml KCAL	PROT	CARB	FAT	FIBRE
TOAD IN THE HOLE								
Mini, Aunt Bessie's*	1 Serving/62g	118	6.8	191	11	12	11	3.6
Mini, Christmas, Ovenbaked, Asda*	1 Toad/20g	57	2.8	283	13	25	14	2.5
Tesco*	1 Serving/188g	461	28.4	245	8.5	18.7	15.1	2.6
with Three Sausages, Asda*	1 Pack/150g	435	27	290	10	22	18	1
TOASTIE								
All Day Breakfast, M&S*	1 Serving/174g	375	13.8	215	11.2	25	7.9	1.7
Cheese & Pickle, M&S*	1 Toastie/136g	320	9.1	235	10.4	33.5	6.7	2.6
Cheese & Ham, Tayto*	1 Serving/50g	260	14.8	519	6.8	58	29.7	0
Cheese & Onion, Ginsters*	1 Toastie/122g	330	12.3	269	10.9	33.1	10	1.5
Chicken, Bacon, & Three Cheese, Greggs*	1 Toastie/223g	617	29	277	19	20	13	0
Ham & Cheddar, British, M&S*	1 Pack/128g	269	8.6	210	15.5	22.3	6.7	1.3
Ham & Cheese, Tesco*	1 Serving/138g	388	18.2	281	11.5	29.1	13.2	1
Ham & Cheese, White Bread	*1 Toastie/150g*	*409*	*14.9*	*273*	*14.5*	*31.3*	*9.9*	*0.9*
Ham, & Three Cheese, Greggs*	1 Toastie/175g	451	19.2	258	16	25	11	0
TOFFEE APPLE								
Average	*1 Apple/141g*	*188*	*3*	*133*	*1.2*	*29.2*	*2.1*	*2.3*
TOFFEE CRISP								
Biscuit, Nestle*	1 Original/44g	228	12.1	519	3.7	62.8	27.6	1.4
Bitesize, Nestle*	1 Serving/20g	101	5.4	518	3.8	63	27.6	1.3
TOFFEES								
Assorted, Bassett's*	1 Toffee/8g	35	1.1	434	3.8	73.1	14	0
Assorted, Sainsbury's*	1 Sweet/8g	37	1.3	457	2.2	76.5	15.8	0.2
Brazil Nut, Diabetic, Thorntons*	1 Serving/20g	93	7	467	3.2	49	35.1	0.5
Butter, Smart Price, Asda*	1 Toffee/8g	37	1.3	440	1.3	75	15	0
Chewy, Werther's*	1 Toffee/5g	22	0.8	436	3.5	71.3	15.2	0.1
Dairy, Smart Price, Asda*	1 Sweet/9g	37	1.3	407	1.3	68.4	14.2	0
Dairy, Waitrose*	1 Toffee/8g	37	1.1	458	2	80.2	14.3	0.5
Devon Butter, Thorntons*	1 Sweet/9g	40	1.5	444	1.7	72.2	16.7	0
English Butter, Co-Op*	1 Toffee/8g	38	1.6	470	2	71	20	0
Everyday Value, Tesco*	3 Toffees/22.5g	101	3.3	450	2.1	77.3	14.8	0.3
Liquorice, Thorntons*	1 Bag/100g	506	29.4	506	1.9	58.8	29.4	0
Milk Chocolate Covered, Thorntons*	1 Bag/215g	1120	66	521	4.1	57.2	30.7	0.9
Milk Chocolate Smothered, Thorntons*	1 Pack/125g	655	38.5	524	4.3	57.5	30.8	1.1
Mixed, Average	*1oz/28g*	*119*	*5.2*	*426*	*2.2*	*66.7*	*18.6*	*0*
Original, Thorntons*	1 Bag/100g	514	30.1	514	1.8	59.3	30.1	0
Squares, No Added Sugar, Russell Stover*	1 Piece/15g	57	3.9	380	6	49.3	26	1.3
TOFU								
Average	*1 Pack/250g*	*297*	*16.5*	*119*	*13.4*	*1.4*	*6.6*	*0.1*
Beech Smoked, Organic, Cauldron Foods*	½ Pack/110g	124	7.8	113	10.9	1	7.1	0.5
Firm Silken Style, Blue Dragon*	1 Pack/216g	134	5.8	62	6.9	2.4	2.7	0
Fried, Average	*1oz/28g*	*75*	*4*	*268*	*28.6*	*9.3*	*14.1*	*0*
Original, Organic, Cauldron Foods*	¼ Pack/99g	84	4.2	85	10	1.9	4.2	0.9
Pieces, Marinated, Organic, Cauldron Foods*	1 Pack/160g	363	27.2	227	17.5	1	17	2.7
Smoked, Organic, Evernat*	1oz/28g	36	1.8	127	16.3	0.8	6.6	0
TOMATILLOS								
Raw	*1 Med/34g*	*11*	*0.3*	*32*	*1*	*5.8*	*1*	*1.9*
TOMATO PASTE								
Average	*1 Tbsp/20g*	*19*	*0*	*96*	*5*	*19.2*	*0.2*	*1.5*
Sun Dried, Average	*1 Hpd Tsp/10g*	*38*	*3.5*	*385*	*3.2*	*13.8*	*35.2*	*0*
TOMATO PUREE								
Average	*1 Tsp/5g*	*4*	*0*	*76*	*4.5*	*14.1*	*0.2*	*2.3*
Double Concentrate, Average	*1 Tbsp/15g*	*13*	*0*	*85*	*4.9*	*14.9*	*0.2*	*3.6*

T

	Measure INFO/WEIGHT	per Measure KCAL	FAT	Nutrition Values per 100g / 100ml KCAL	PROT	CARB	FAT	FIBRE
TOMATO PUREE								
Sun Dried, & Olive Oil & Herbs, GIA*	1 Serving/20g	41	4.3	204	2.6	0.5	21.6	0
TOMATOES								
Cherry, Average	*1 Tomato/15g*	*3*	*0*	*18*	*0.7*	*3*	*0.3*	*0.5*
Cherry, Canned, TTD, Sainsbury's*	½ Can/204g	47	0.4	23	1.4	4	0.2	0.9
Cherry, on the Vine, Average	*1 Serving/80g*	*15*	*0.3*	*18*	*0.7*	*3.1*	*0.3*	*1.2*
Chopped with Basil, Canned, Freshona, Lidl*	½ Can/200g	64	0.4	32	1.1	5.3	0.2	1.3
Chopped, Canned, Average	*1 Can/400g*	*77*	*0.6*	*19*	*1.1*	*3.3*	*0.2*	*0.9*
Chopped, Canned, Branded Average	*1 Serving/130g*	*27*	*0.2*	*21*	*1.1*	*3.8*	*0.1*	*0.8*
Chopped, Italian, Average	*½ Can/200g*	*47*	*0.2*	*23*	*1.3*	*4.4*	*0.1*	*0.9*
Chopped, with Garlic, Average	*½ Can/200g*	*43*	*0.3*	*21*	*1.2*	*3.8*	*0.1*	*0.8*
Chopped, with Herbs, Average	*½ Can/200g*	*42*	*0.3*	*21*	*1.1*	*3.8*	*0.1*	*0.8*
Chopped, with Olive Oil & Roasted Garlic, Sainsbury's*	1 Pack/390g	187	8.2	48	1.3	5.9	2.1	1
Fresh, Raw, Average	*1 Med/123g*	*22*	*0.2*	*18*	*0.9*	*3.9*	*0.2*	*1.2*
Fried in Blended Oil	*1 Med/85g*	*77*	*6.5*	*91*	*0.7*	*5*	*7.7*	*1.3*
Grilled, Average	*1 Med/85g*	*17*	*0.3*	*20*	*0.8*	*3.5*	*0.3*	*1.5*
Plum, Baby, Average	*1 Serving/50g*	*9*	*0.2*	*18*	*1.5*	*2.3*	*0.3*	*1*
Plum, in Tomato Juice, Average	*1 Can/400g*	*71*	*0.4*	*18*	*1*	*3.3*	*0.1*	*0.7*
Plum, in Tomato Juice, Premium, Average	*1 Can/400g*	*93*	*1.2*	*23*	*1.3*	*3.8*	*0.3*	*0.7*
Pome Dei Moro, Waitrose*	1 Serving/80g	16	0.2	20	0.7	3.1	0.3	1.2
Pomodorino, TTD, Sainsbury's*	1 Tomato/8g	1	0	17	0.7	3.1	0.4	1.3
Ripened on the Vine, Average	*1 Med/123g*	*22*	*0.4*	*18*	*0.7*	*3.1*	*0.3*	*0.7*
San Marzano, on the Vine, Mini, Finest, Tesco*	1 Serving/80g	16	0.2	20	0.7	3.1	0.3	1
Santini, M&S*	1 Serving/80g	16	0.2	20	0.7	3.1	0.3	1
Stuffed with Rice Based Filling, Average	*1oz/28g*	*59*	*3.8*	*212*	*2.1*	*22.2*	*13.4*	*1.1*
Sugardrop, Finest, Tesco*	1 Tomato/14g	3	0	20	0.7	3.1	0.3	1
Sun Dried in Oil	*100g*	*301*	*24.8*	*301*	*5.8*	*13.5*	*24.8*	*7*
Sun Dried, Average	*3 Pieces/20g*	*43*	*3.2*	*214*	*4.7*	*13*	*15.9*	*3.3*
Sun Dried, Moist, Waitrose*	1 Serving/25g	44	0.5	175	11.8	27.4	2	7.2
Sweet, Baby, Mixed, Finest, Tesco*	½ Pack/125g	25	0.4	20	0.7	3.1	0.3	1
TONGUE								
Lunch, Average	*1oz/28g*	*51*	*3*	*181*	*20.1*	*1.8*	*10.6*	*0*
Ox from Deli Counter, Sainsbury's*	1 Serving/100g	195	13.3	195	18.3	0.5	13.3	0.1
Slices, Average	*1oz/28g*	*56*	*3.9*	*201*	*18.7*	*0*	*14*	*0*
TONIC WATER								
Average	*1 Glass/250ml*	*82*	*0*	*33*	*0*	*8.8*	*0*	*0*
Diet, Asda*	1 Glass/200ml	2	0	1	0	0	0	0
Indian with Lime, Low Calorie, Tesco*	1 Glass/250ml	5	0	2	0	0	0	0
Indian, Britvic*	1 Mini Can/150ml	39	0.2	26	0.1	6.2	0.1	0.1
Indian, Diet, Schweppes*	1 Glass/100ml	1	0	1	0	0	0	0
Indian, Fever-Tree*	1 Bottle/200ml	72	0	36	0	8.9	0	0
Indian, Schweppes*	1 Serving/500ml	110	0	22	0	5.1	0	0
Indian, Slimline, Schweppes*	1 Serving/188ml	3	0	2	0.4	0	0	0
Indian, Sugar Free, Essential, Waitrose*	1 Serving/50ml	1	0	2	0	0	0	0
Low Calorie, Tesco*	1 Serving/200ml	4	0	2	0	0.5	0	0
Quinine, Schweppes*	1 Glass/125ml	46	0	37	0	9	0	0
TONIC WINE								
Original, Sanatogen*	1 Bottle/700ml	889	0	127	0	124.4	0	0
TOPIC								
Mars*	1 Bar/47g	234	12.3	498	6.2	59.6	26.2	1.7
TORTE								
Chocolate & Pecan Brownie, Gu*	1/6 Torte/67g	292	17.7	436	5.3	45.1	26.4	3.1
Chocolate Brownie, Belgian, TTD, Sainsbury's*	1 Slice/90g	360	24.6	400	5.6	32.5	27.3	0.8
Chocolate Fondant, Gu*	1/8 Torte/62g	264	18.9	423	5.7	32	30.2	1.8

T

	Measure INFO/WEIGHT	per Measure KCAL	FAT	Nutrition Values per 100g / 100ml KCAL	PROT	CARB	FAT	FIBRE
TORTE								
Chocolate Orange & Almond, Gu*	1 Serving/65g	273	19.8	420	5	28.2	30.5	2.7
Chocolate Truffle, Waitrose*	1 Serving/116g	359	20.1	309	4.6	30.1	17.3	1.4
Chocolate, Tesco*	1 Serving/50g	126	6	251	3.6	32.3	11.9	1
Lemon & Mango, Waitrose*	1 Serving/80g	142	2.4	177	3.9	33.6	3	0.6
TORTELLINI								
Beef & Red Wine, Italian, Asda*	½ Pack/150g	242	4.2	161	9	25	2.8	0
Beef & Red Wine, Italiano, Tesco*	1 Serving/150g	324	4.8	216	11.7	35.3	3.2	3.3
Cheese & Ham, Italiano, Tesco*	½ Pack/150g	396	12.3	264	12.8	34.8	8.2	3
Cheese, Tomato & Basil, Cooked, Tesco*	1 Serving/270g	551	15.1	204	6.7	30.5	5.6	2.5
Ham & Cheese, Fresh, Asda*	½ Pack/150g	255	9	170	6	23	6	1.7
Meat, Italian, Tesco*	1 Serving/125g	332	9.5	266	10.6	38.9	7.6	2.3
Mushroom, Asda*	1 Serving/125g	218	5.2	174	6	28	4.2	2.3
Pesto & Goats Cheese, Fresh, Sainsbury's*	½ Pack/150g	310	12.2	207	8.9	24.6	8.1	2.6
Ricotta & Spinach, Giovanni Rana*	½ Pack/125g	319	10	255	9	35.5	8	10
Sausage & Ham, Italiano, Tesco*	1 Pack/300g	816	27.9	272	13.1	34	9.3	3.7
Spicy Pepperoni, Asda*	½ Pack/150g	252	6	168	7	26	4	0
Spinach & Ricotta, Italian, Asda*	½ Pack/150g	189	3.6	126	5	21	2.4	0.6
Tomato & Mozzarella, Fresh, Sainsbury's*	½ Pack/150g	291	12	194	7.5	23	8	3.4
TORTELLONI								
Arrabiata, Sainsbury's*	½ Pack/210g	407	11.8	194	7.1	28.8	5.6	2.6
Cheese & Smoked Ham, As Consumed, Tesco*	½ Pack/270g	535	17.3	198	8.4	25.8	6.4	1.8
Chicken & Bacon, As Consumed, Italiano, Tesco*	½ Pack/280g	567	14	202	6.8	30.7	5	3.7
Mozzarella, Tomato & Basil, Italian, Somerfield*	½ Pack/125g	314	5.1	251	10.5	43.1	4.1	1.9
Mushroom, Fresh, Sainsbury's*	1 Pack/400g	656	10.8	164	5.9	27.9	2.7	2.3
Pasta, Fresh, Cream Cheese, Garlic & Herb, Morrisons*	1 Serving/150g	400	9	267	10.3	46.1	6	3.2
Sausage & Ham, As Consumed, Italiano, Tesco*	½ Pack/270g	515	18.9	191	8.5	22.5	7	1.8
Spinach & Ricotta Cheese, Co-Op*	½ Pack/126g	315	6.3	250	10	41	5	4
Spinach & Ricotta, Chilled, Italiano, Tesco*	½ Pack/150g	412	12.8	275	10.4	38.1	8.5	3.3
Spinach & Ricotta, Fresh, Waitrose*	½ Pack/150g	239	5.3	159	6.3	24.4	3.5	2.5
Spinach & Ricotta, Sainsbury's*	½ Pack/150g	326	10.8	217	7.8	30.2	7.2	2.4
Tomato & Mozzarella, Sainsbury's*	1 Serving/175g	340	14	194	7.5	23	8	3.4
Wild Mushroom, Italian, Sainsbury's*	½ Pack/150g	309	12.3	206	7.7	25.4	8.2	2.3
TORTIGLIONI								
Dry, Average	*1 Serving/75g*	*266*	*1.4*	*355*	*12.5*	*72.2*	*1.9*	*2.1*
TORTILLA CHIPS								
Aldi*	¼ Pack/50g	234	9.5	469	6.3	66	19	4.2
Chilli, with Chopped Jalapeno, Tyrrells*	1 Serving/30g	154	8.3	512	5.9	57.3	27.5	0
Cool Flavour, BGTY, Sainsbury's*	1 Pack/22g	94	2.7	425	7.1	71.4	12.3	4.5
Cool Flavour, Sainsbury's*	1 Serving/50g	232	9.4	463	5.7	68.1	18.7	3.7
Cool, Tesco*	1 Serving/40g	190	9.9	474	6.3	56.7	24.7	7.8
Easy Cheesy!, Sainsbury's*	1 Serving/50g	249	13	498	7.1	58.7	26.1	4.5
Lightly Salted, M&S*	1 Serving/20g	98	4.8	490	7.2	61.5	24.1	4.5
Lightly Salted, Smart Price, Asda*	¼ Bag/50g	251	13	502	7	60	26	5
Lightly Salted, Tesco*	1 Serving/50g	248	13.8	495	4.8	56.8	27.6	7.5
Lightly Salted, Waitrose*	1 Serving/40g	187	8.6	468	7.1	61.2	21.6	6.5
Lighty Salted, Basics, Sainsbury's*	½ Pack/50g	242	11.9	483	6.5	60.7	23.8	5.3
Nacho Cheese Flavour, Morrisons*	1 Serving/25g	126	6.6	504	7.2	59.4	26.4	3.6
Plain	*1 Serving/100g*	*486*	*21.1*	*486*	*6.8*	*62*	*21.1*	*4.2*
Salsa, M&S*	½ Bag/75g	364	18.8	485	5.7	59.1	25.1	6.1
with Guacamole	*1 Serving/100g*	*515*	*30.8*	*515*	*6*	*53*	*30.8*	*6.3*
TORTILLAS								
Corn, Soft, Mexican, Discovery*	1 Tortilla/40g	119	2.8	297	7.4	51	7.1	2.3
Corn, Soft, Old El Paso*	1 Tortilla/37.5g	129	2.6	343	10	60	7	0

T

	Measure INFO/WEIGHT	per Measure KCAL	FAT	Nutrition Values per 100g / 100ml KCAL	PROT	CARB	FAT	FIBRE
TORTILLAS								
Flour, From Dinner Kit, Old El Paso*	1 Tortilla/42g	144	4.9	344	8.7	51.1	11.7	0
Flour, Soft, Discovery*	1 Tortilla/40g	119	2.8	298	8	49.6	7.1	2.4
Flour, Wheat, Waitrose*	1 Tortilla/62g	203	6.1	327	8.5	51.5	9.8	0
Plain, Wheat, Waitrose*	1 Tortilla/43g	134	3.5	311	8.1	51.5	8.1	3
TREACLE								
Black, Average	**1 Tbsp/20g**	**51**	**0**	**257**	**1.2**	**67.2**	**0**	**0**
TRIFLE								
Average	**1 Portion/170g**	**272**	**10.7**	**160**	**3.6**	**22.3**	**6.3**	**0.5**
Black Forest, Asda*	1 Serving/100g	237	9	237	3.1	36	9	0
Chocolate , Tesco*	1 Pot /120g	218	10.6	182	3.7	21.8	8.8	0.4
Chocolate, M Kitchen, Morrisons*	¼ Trifle/138g	266	12.5	193	3.1	24.2	9.1	1.1
Chocolate, Tesco*	1 Serving/125g	312	19	250	4.3	24	15.2	0.7
Fruit Cocktail, Individual, M&S*	1 Pot/135g	205	9.2	150	2.7	19.3	6.7	0.7
Fruit Cocktail, Individual, Tesco*	1 Pot/113g	175	8.8	155	1.7	19.6	7.8	0.6
Fruit Cocktail, Sainsbury's*	1 Trifle/150g	241	9	161	1.8	24.8	6	0.4
Lemon Drizzle, Tesco*	¼ Trifle/141g	400	23.8	284	3	29.7	16.9	0.5
Peach & Zabaglione, COU, M&S*	1 Glass/130g	150	3	115	2.8	20.6	2.3	0.8
Raspberry & Sherry, Waitrose*	1 Pot/120g	223	14.3	186	2.5	16.9	11.9	0.7
Raspberry, Co-Op*	1 Trifle/125g	206	10	165	2	22	8	0.3
Raspberry, Tesco*	1 Pot/150g	210	9.8	140	1.7	18.5	6.5	1
Strawberry, Aldi*	1/3 Trifle/153g	193	8	126	1.9	18	5.2	0.7
Strawberry, Co-Op*	1 Serving/120g	175	9.1	146	1.7	16.7	7.6	1.4
Strawberry, Essential, Waitrose*	¼ Pot/155g	274	15.7	177	2.3	19.1	10.1	0.8
Strawberry, Everyday Value, Tesco*	¼ Trifle/118g	157	6.4	133	1.4	18.5	5.4	2.4
Strawberry, Individual, Waitrose*	1 Pot/150g	206	8.6	137	1.8	19.7	5.7	1
Strawberry, Low Fat, COU, M&S*	1 Pot/140g	148	3.5	106	2.9	17.6	2.5	0.8
Strawberry, Tesco*	1 Trifle/605g	998	55.7	165	1.5	19.1	9.2	0.8
Summer Fruit, Sainsbury's*	¼ Trifle/125g	196	9.4	157	1.8	20.1	7.5	0.9
TRIPE								
& Onions, Stewed	**1oz/28g**	**26**	**0.8**	**93**	**8.3**	**9.5**	**2.7**	**0.7**
TROMPRETTI								
Fresh, Waitrose*	1 Serving/125g	339	3	271	11.7	50.6	2.4	2
TROUT								
Brown, Steamed, Average	**1 Serving/120g**	**162**	**5.4**	**135**	**23.5**	**0**	**4.5**	**0**
Fillets, Scottish, Hot Smoked, TTD, Sainsbury's*	½ Pack/63g	85	3.4	136	20.8	1	5.4	0.5
Fillets, with Juniper Berries, Ocean Sea, Lidl*	1 Serving/63g	87	3.5	138	22	0	5.5	0
Grilled, Weighed with Bones & Skin	**1 Serving/100g**	**98**	**3.9**	**98**	**15.7**	**0**	**3.9**	**0**
Rainbow, Grilled, Average	**1 Serving/120g**	**162**	**6.5**	**135**	**21.5**	**0**	**5.4**	**0**
Rainbow, Raw, Average	**1oz/28g**	**33**	**1.3**	**118**	**19.1**	**0**	**4.7**	**0**
Rainbow, Smoked, Average	**1 Pack/135g**	**190**	**7.6**	**140**	**21.7**	**0.8**	**5.6**	**0**
Raw, Average	**1 Serving/120g**	**159**	**6.5**	**132**	**20.6**	**0**	**5.4**	**0**
Smoked, Average	**2 Fillets/135g**	**187**	**7.1**	**138**	**22.7**	**0.3**	**5.2**	**0.1**
TUMS								
Extra 750, Sugar Free, Tums*	2 Tablets/2g	5	0	250	0	50	0	0
Extra 750, Tums*	2 Tablets/2g	10	0	500	0	100	0	0
Reg, Tums*	1 Tablet/2g	2	0	125	0	25	0	0
Smoothies, Extra Strength 750, Tums*	2 Tablets/2g	10	0	500	0	100	0	0
TUNA								
Bluefin, Cooked, Dry Heat, Average	**1 Serving/100g**	**184**	**6.3**	**184**	**29.9**	**0**	**6.3**	**0**
Chunks in Brine, Drained, Value, Morrisons*	1 Can/120g	122	0.6	102	23.1	1	0.5	0
Chunks with a Little Sunflower Oil, No Drain, John West*	1 Can/120g	185	7.1	154	25.2	0	5.9	0
Chunks, in Brine, Average, Drained	**1 Can /130g**	**141**	**0.7**	**108**	**25.9**	**0**	**0.5**	**0**
Chunks, in Brine, Drained, Average	**1 Can /130g**	**141**	**0.7**	**108**	**25.9**	**0**	**0.5**	**0**

	Measure INFO/WEIGHT	KCAL	FAT	KCAL	PROT	CARB	FAT	FIBRE
TUNA								
Chunks, in Spring Water, Average, Drained	**1 Sm Can/56g**	**60**	**0.4**	**108**	**25.4**	**0**	**0.6**	**0.1**
Chunks, in Sunflower Oil, Average, Drained	**1 Can/138g**	**260**	**12.6**	**188**	**26.5**	**0**	**9.2**	**0**
Chunks, Skipjack, in Brine, Average	**1 Can/138g**	**141**	**0.8**	**102**	**24.3**	**0**	**0.6**	**0**
Chunks, with a Little Brine, No Drain, 120g, John West*	1 Can/120g	130	1.1	108	25	0	0.9	0
Chunks, with a Little Brine, No Drain, 60g, John West*	1 Can/60g	55	0.5	91	21	0	0.8	0
Coronation Style, Canned, Average	**1 Can/80g**	**122**	**7.6**	**152**	**10.2**	**6.5**	**9.5**	**0.6**
Coronation, BGTY, Sainsbury's*	1 Can/80g	90	2.1	112	16.5	5.7	2.6	1
Flakes, in Brine, Average	**1oz/28g**	**29**	**0.2**	**104**	**24.8**	**0**	**0.6**	**0**
in a Light Mayonnaise, Slimming World, Princes*	1 Can/80g	96	3.3	120	17.3	3.6	4.1	0
in a Tomato & Herb Dressing, Weight Watchers*	1 Can/80g	79	2.9	99	11.6	5.1	3.6	0.5
in Coronation Style Dressing, Weight Watchers*	1 Can/80g	75	2	94	9.3	8.7	2.5	0.4
in Water, Average	**1 Serving/120g**	**126**	**1**	**105**	**24**	**0.1**	**0.8**	**0**
Lime & Black Pepper, John West*	1 Serving/85g	133	7.8	156	15.6	2.8	9.2	0
Mexican Style, Spreadables, John West*	1 Can/80g	149	9.8	186	13.1	5.6	12.3	1.3
Steak in Sunflower Oil, Canned, Drained, Nixe, Lidl*	1 Can/140g	252	11.2	180	27	0	8	0
Steaks, Chargrilled, Italian, Sainsbury's*	1 Serving/125g	199	8	159	25.1	0.2	6.4	0.5
Steaks, in Brine, Average	**1 Sm Can/99g**	**106**	**0.5**	**107**	**25.6**	**0**	**0.6**	**0**
Steaks, in Olive Oil, Average	**1 Serving/111g**	**211**	**10.7**	**190**	**25.8**	**0**	**9.6**	**0**
Steaks, in Sunflower Oil, Average	**1 Can/150g**	**269**	**12.6**	**179**	**26**	**0**	**8.4**	**0**
Steaks, in Water, Average	**1 Serving/200g**	**215**	**0.8**	**107**	**25.6**	**0**	**0.4**	**0**
Steaks, Raw, Average	**1 Serving/140g**	**179**	**2.7**	**128**	**27.6**	**0.1**	**1.9**	**0.2**
Steaks, Skipjack, in Brine, Average	**½ Can/75g**	**73**	**0.4**	**98**	**23.2**	**0**	**0.6**	**0**
Steaks, with a Little Brine, No Drain, John West*	1 Can/60g	68	0.5	113	26	0	0.8	0
Steaks, with a Little Olive Oil, No Drain, John West*	1 Can/130g	209	7	161	28.2	0	5.4	0
Steaks, with a Little Sunflower Oil, No Drain, John West*	1 Can/120g	212	8.2	177	26.4	0	6.8	0
Tangy Jalapeno, Infusions, John West*	1 Can/80g	142	6.1	177	24.1	3	7.6	0
with a Little Spring Water, No Drain, Canned, John West*	1 Can/120g	137	1.1	114	26.4	0.1	0.9	0
with a Twist, French Dressing, John West*	1 Pack/85g	135	8.2	159	15.2	2.8	9.7	0.1
with Lemon & Black Pepper, Tesco*	1 Can/85g	144	6.5	170	21.2	4	7.6	0.5
Yellowfin, Cooked, Dry Heat, Average	**1 Serving/100g**	**139**	**1.2**	**139**	**30**	**0**	**1.2**	**0**
TUNA MAYONNAISE								
& Sweetcorn, Canned, BGTY, Sainsbury's*	1 Can/80g	78	1.8	97	15.2	4	2.3	0.7
Light, Slimming World*	1 Serving/80g	96	3.3	120	17.3	3.6	4.1	0
with Sweetcorn, John West*	½ Can/92g	231	19	251	12	4.5	20.6	0.2
TUNA WITH								
Wild Rice & Lentils, Indian Style, Creations, John West*	1 Sachet/180g	250	8.5	139	9.5	14	4.7	1.2
TURBOT								
Grilled	**1oz/28g**	**34**	**1**	**122**	**22.7**	**0**	**3.5**	**0**
Raw	**1oz/28g**	**27**	**0.8**	**95**	**17.7**	**0**	**2.7**	**0**
TURKEY								
Breast Golden Norfolk, Bernard Matthews*	1 Slice/20g	22	0.2	109	23.8	0.9	1.1	0.8
Breast Slices, Bernard Matthews*	1 Slice/20g	21	0.5	103	19.2	0.9	2.5	0.5
Breast, Butter Basted, Average	**1 Serving/75g**	**110**	**3.6**	**146**	**23.7**	**1.9**	**4.9**	**0.4**
Breast, Chunks, Bernard Matthews*	1 Serving/55g	64	0.5	116	26.1	0.9	0.9	1.6
Breast, Diced, Healthy Range, Average	**1oz/28g**	**30**	**0.4**	**108**	**23.8**	**0**	**1.3**	**0**
Breast, Honey Roast, Sliced, Average	**1 Serving/50g**	**57**	**0.7**	**114**	**24**	**1.6**	**1.4**	**0.2**
Breast, Joint, Raw, Average	**1 Serving/125g**	**134**	**2.6**	**108**	**21.3**	**0.7**	**2.1**	**0.6**
Breast, Pieces, Raw, Everyday, Value, Tesco*	1 Pack/525g	574	4.7	110	24.4	0	0.9	0
Breast, Raw, Average	**1oz/28g**	**33**	**0.6**	**117**	**24.1**	**0.5**	**2**	**0.1**
Breast, Roast, British, Sliced, Finest, Tesco*	1 Slice/30g	41	0.5	136	29.8	0.5	1.6	0.5
Breast, Roast, Slices, Specially Selected, Aldi*	1 Slice/46g	51	0.5	111	26	0.5	1	0.5
Breast, Roasted, Average	**1oz/28g**	**37**	**0.9**	**131**	**24.6**	**0.7**	**3.3**	**0.1**
Breast, Roll, Cooked, Average	**1 Slice/10g**	**9**	**0.1**	**92**	**17.6**	**3.5**	**0.8**	**0**

T

	Measure INFO/WEIGHT	per Measure KCAL	FAT	Nutrition Values per 100g / 100ml KCAL	PROT	CARB	FAT	FIBRE
TURKEY								
Breast, Slices, Cooked, Average	*1 Slice/20g*	*23*	*0.3*	*114*	*24*	*1.2*	*1.4*	*0.3*
Breast, Smoked, Sliced, Average	*1 Slice/20g*	*23*	*0.4*	*113*	*23.4*	*0.7*	*2*	*0*
Breast, Steaks, in Crumbs, Average	*1 Steak/76g*	*217*	*14.1*	*286*	*13.7*	*16.4*	*18.5*	*0.2*
Breast, Steaks, Raw, Average	*1oz/28g*	*30*	*0.3*	*107*	*24.3*	*0*	*1.1*	*0*
Breast, Strips, for Stir Fry, Average	*1 Serving/175g*	*205*	*2.7*	*117*	*25.6*	*0.1*	*1.6*	*0*
Breast, Stuffed, Just Roast, Sainsbury's*	1 Serving/100g	155	6.6	155	21.1	2.9	6.6	0.6
Butter Roasted, Carvery, Morrisons*	1 Slice/22g	25	0.3	113	24	1.2	1.3	0
Dark Meat, Raw, Average	*1oz/28g*	*29*	*0.7*	*104*	*20.4*	*0*	*2.5*	*0*
Drummers, Golden, Bernard Matthews*	1 Drummer/57g	147	10.3	258	13.1	11	18	1.1
Escalope, Average	*1 Escalope/138g*	*341*	*19.3*	*247*	*13.5*	*16.7*	*14*	*0.6*
Escalope, Golden Breaded, Baked, Bernard Matthews*	1 Escalope/123g	322	18.6	262	13.7	16.6	15.1	2.4
Escalope, Lemon & Pepper, Average	*1 Escalope/143g*	*371*	*22.6*	*260*	*12.6*	*16.7*	*15.8*	*0.4*
Goujons, Cooked, Bernard Matthews*	4 Goujons/128g	355	23.3	277	11.8	16.6	18.2	1.1
Leg, Dark Meat, Raw , Average, Weighed with Bone	*1 Serving/100g*	*73*	*1.8*	*73*	*14.3*	*0*	*1.8*	*0*
Light Meat, Raw, Average	*1oz/28g*	*29*	*0.2*	*105*	*24.4*	*0*	*0.8*	*0*
Light Meat, Roasted	*1 Cup/140g*	*163*	*3.3*	*116*	*22.1*	*0*	*2.4*	*0*
Mince, 7%, Sainsbury's*	1 Serving/150g	210	10.5	140	18.9	0.5	7	0
Mince, Average	*1oz/28g*	*45*	*2*	*161*	*23.9*	*0*	*7.2*	*0*
Mince, Lean, Healthy Range, Average	*1oz/28g*	*33*	*1.1*	*118*	*20.3*	*0*	*4.1*	*0*
Mince, Thigh, Essential, Waitrose*	1 Serving/100g	118	3.5	118	20.9	0.5	3.5	0.5
Pudding, Christmas	*1 Serving/175g*	*312*	*10.9*	*178*	*26.4*	*3.7*	*6.2*	*1*
Rashers, Average	*1 Rasher/26g*	*26*	*0.4*	*101*	*19.1*	*2.3*	*1.6*	*0*
Rashers, Smoked, Average	*1 Serving/75g*	*76*	*1.4*	*101*	*19.8*	*1.5*	*1.8*	*0*
Roast Dinner, 105, Oakhouse Foods Ltd*	1 Dinner/430g	624	16.3	145	7	9.4	3.8	1.4
Roast, Breast, Wafer Thin, M&S*	½ Pack/50g	52	0.6	105	23.2	0.1	1.2	0.1
Roast, Meat & Skin, Average	*1oz/28g*	*48*	*1.8*	*171*	*28*	*0*	*6.5*	*0*
Roast, Meat Only, Average	*1 Serving/100g*	*157*	*3.2*	*157*	*29.9*	*0*	*3.2*	*0*
Roast, Wafer Thin, Tesco*	1 Slice/8g	8	0.2	105	20	1.5	2	0
Smoked, Applewood, 1, Waitrose*	½ Pack/40g	48	0.4	121	27.3	0.5	1.1	0.1
Strips, Stir-Fried, Average	*1oz/28g*	*46*	*1.3*	*164*	*31*	*0*	*4.5*	*0*
Thigh, Diced, Average	*1oz/28g*	*33*	*1.2*	*117*	*19.6*	*0*	*4.3*	*0*
Vegetarian, Slices, Deli, with Stuffing, Quorn*	½ Pack/50g	60	1.2	120	16	8.9	2.3	4
Vegetarian, Slices, with Sage, Meat Free, Quorn*	¼ Pack/25g	32	0.6	128	16	8.9	2.3	4
Wafer Thin, Cooked, Average	*1 Slice/10g*	*12*	*0.4*	*122*	*19*	*3.2*	*3.7*	*0*
Wafer Thin, Honey Roast, Average	*1 Slice/10g*	*11*	*0.2*	*109*	*19.2*	*4.2*	*1.7*	*0.2*
Wafer Thin, Smoked, Average	*1 Slice/10g*	*12*	*0.4*	*119*	*18.1*	*3.6*	*3.7*	*0*
TURKEY DINNER								
Roast, Asda*	1 Pack/400g	344	6.4	86	7	11	1.6	2
Roast, Meal for One, M&S*	1 Pack/370g	462	16.3	125	9.1	12.4	4.4	2.7
Roast, Sainsbury's*	1 Pack/450g	354	9	79	6.8	8.4	2	1.9
Traditional, Birds Eye*	1 Pack/340g	292	7.8	86	6.1	10.3	2.3	1.7
TURKEY HAM								
Average	*1 Serving/75g*	*81*	*2.9*	*108*	*15.6*	*2.8*	*3.9*	*0*
TURKISH DELIGHT								
Dark Chocolate Covered, Thorntons*	1 Chocolate/10g	39	1.1	390	2.7	69	11	2
Fry's*	1 Bar/51g	195	3.4	385	1.4	74.6	6.7	1.3
Milk Chocolate, M&S*	1 Pack/55g	220	4.7	400	1.6	79	8.5	0
with Mixed Nuts, Hazer Baba*	1 Piece/12g	47	0.2	389	1.6	88.5	1.7	0
with Rose, Hazer Baba*	1 Square/18g	70	0.3	389	1.6	88.6	1.7	0
Woolworths*	1 Bar/50g	232	9.8	463	5.3	70.6	19.7	0
TURMERIC								
Powder	*1 Tsp/3g*	*11*	*0.3*	*354*	*7.8*	*58.2*	*9.9*	*0*

T

	Measure INFO/WEIGHT	per Measure KCAL	FAT	Nutrition Values per 100g / 100ml KCAL	PROT	CARB	FAT	FIBRE
TURNIP								
Boiled, Average	*1oz/28g*	*3*	*0.1*	*12*	*0.6*	*2*	*0.2*	*1.9*
Greens, Leaves, Cooked	*1 Serving/80g*	*16*	*0.2*	*20*	*1.1*	*4.4*	*0.2*	*3.5*
Mashed, Mash Direct*	1 Pack/400g	148	2.3	37	0.8	6	0.6	2.5
Raw, Unprepared, Average	*1oz/28g*	*5*	*0.1*	*17*	*0.7*	*3.5*	*0.2*	*1.8*
Turnip, As Sold, Sainsbury's*	1 Serving/80g	23	0.4	29	0.9	4.7	0.5	1.8
TURNOVER								
Apple, Bramley & Cream, Sainsbury's*	1 Turnover/78g	243	13.6	312	3.9	34.3	17.4	1.3
Apple, Co-Op*	1 Turnover/77g	308	20.8	400	4	35	27	1
Apple, Fresh Cream, Sainsbury's*	1 Turnover/84g	292	20.9	347	4.1	26.9	24.8	2.5
Apple, Puff Pastry, Bakery, Tesco*	1 Turnover/83g	263	13	317	4.3	38.6	15.7	1.8
Raspberry, Fresh Cream, Asda*	1 Turnover/100g	411	23	411	6	45	23	2.1
Raspberry, Tesco*	1 Turnover/84g	290	20.2	345	4	27.2	24.1	2.1
TWIGLETS								
Original, Jacob's*	1 Bag/30g	115	3.5	383	12.7	57	11.6	11.8
TWIRL								
Cadbury*	1 Finger/22g	118	6.8	535	7.6	56	30.9	0.8
Treat Size, Cadbury*	1 Bar/21g	115	6.6	535	7.6	56	30.9	0.8
TWIX								
'Xtra, Mars*	1 Pack/85g	416	20.1	490	4.7	65.5	23.7	1.5
Fun Size, Mars*	1 Bar/20g	99	4.8	495	4.5	64.6	24	1.5
Standard, Mars*	1 Pack/58g	284	13.7	490	4.7	65.5	23.7	1.5
Top, Mars*	1 Bar/28g	143	7.8	511	5.2	60.2	27.7	0
Twixels, Mars*	1 Finger/6g	31	1.6	513	5	64	26.1	0
TZATZIKI								
Asda*	1 Serving/50g	54	4.2	108	3.8	4.6	8.5	1.2
Average	*1 Tbsp/15g*	*11*	*0.8*	*76*	*3.4*	*3.4*	*5.5*	*0.2*
Fresh, Sainsbury's*	1/5 Pot/46g	59	4.8	129	4.4	4.4	10.4	0.2
Tesco*	¼ Pack/50g	72	6	145	4	5.1	12	0.2
Waitrose*	1 Serving/50g	54	2.6	108	6.7	8.4	5.3	0.8

T

	Measure INFO/WEIGHT	per Measure KCAL	FAT	Nutrition Values per 100g / 100ml KCAL	PROT	CARB	FAT	FIBRE
VANILLA								
Bean, Average	**1 Pod/2g**	**6**	**0**	**288**	**0**	**13**	**0**	**0**
VANILLA EXTRACT								
Average	**1 Tbsp/13g**	**37**	**0**	**288**	**0.1**	**12.6**	**0.1**	**0**
VEAL								
Chop, Loin, Raw, Weighed with Bone, Average	**1 Chop/195g**	**317**	**17.8**	**163**	**18.9**	**0**	**9.1**	**0**
Diced, Lean, British, Waitrose*	1 Pack/275g	300	7.4	109	21.1	0	2.7	0
Escalope, Breaded, M&S*	1 Escalope/130g	292	13.9	225	13.6	18.7	10.7	0.4
Escalope, Fried, Average	**1oz/28g**	**55**	**1.9**	**196**	**14.3**	**0**	**6.8**	**0**
Mince, Raw, Average	**1oz/28g**	**40**	**2**	**144**	**20.3**	**0**	**7**	**0**
Shoulder, Lean & Fat, Roasted, Average	**1oz/28g**	**41**	**1.8**	**145**	**20.1**	**0**	**6.5**	**0**
Shoulder, Lean Only, Roasted, Average	**1oz/28g**	**35**	**1.3**	**125**	**19.9**	**0**	**4.4**	**0**
Sirloin, Lean & Fat, Roasted, Average	**1oz/28g**	**43**	**2.2**	**152**	**18.9**	**0**	**7.8**	**0**
Sirloin, Lean Only, Roasted, Average	**1oz/28g**	**33**	**1.2**	**118**	**18.4**	**0**	**4.4**	**0**
VEGEMITE								
Australian, Kraft*	1 Tsp/5g	9	0	173	23.5	19.7	0	0
VEGETABLE CHIPS								
As Sold, Aunt Bessie's*	1 Serving/125g	189	11	151	2.1	13	8.8	5.3
Cassava, Average	**1oz/28g**	**99**	**0.1**	**353**	**1.8**	**91.4**	**0.4**	**4**
Oven Cooked, Aunt Bessie's*	1 Serving/125g	205	11.9	164	2.2	14	9.5	5.8
Parsnip, Golden, Kettle Chips*	½ Pack/50g	258	18.8	515	4.6	39.5	37.6	8.4
Sweet Potato, Kettle Chips*	½ Pack/50g	242	16.4	483	2.4	44.4	32.8	9.3
VEGETABLE FINGERS								
Crispy Crunchy, Dalepak*	1 Finger/28g	62	3.1	223	4.2	26.7	11	15
Crispy, Birds Eye*	2 Fingers/60g	107	4.8	179	3.2	23.5	8	2.3
Sweetcorn, Tesco*	1 Finger/28g	66	3.5	236	7.7	23	12.6	3
VEGETABLE MEDLEY								
Carrots, Sweetcorn, Peas, Broccoli, Four, Tesco*	¼Pack/84g	51	0.9	61	3.6	7.2	1.1	3.9
Frozen, M&S*	1 Pack/500g	175	4	35	3.4	3.9	0.8	3.1
Green, Peas, Broccoli, Beans & Leek, Mint Butter, Co-Op*	½ Pack/130g	99	5.8	76	2.9	4.2	4.5	3.7
Green, Sainsbury's*	1 Pack/220g	178	14.3	81	3	2.5	6.5	2.9
Roasted, Waitrose*	½ Pack/200g	282	15.6	141	1.2	16.4	7.8	3.7
VEGETABLES								
& Bean, Stew Mix, Cooks' Ingredients, Waitrose*	½ Pack /200g	166	3.8	83	4.2	10.2	1.9	4.3
Broccoli, Leek & Cabbage, Prepared Fresh, Waitrose*	1 Serving/80g	29	0.6	36	3.2	2.7	0.8	2.8
Carrots & Peas, Chilled, Fresh Tastes, Asda*	1 Serving/200g	76	0.8	38	2.4	4.8	0.4	2.9
Casserole, Cooks' Ingredients, Waitrose*	¼ Pack/125g	38	0.4	30	1	5.9	0.3	4
Chilli Mix, Tesco*	1 Serving/50g	50	1	99	3.3	13.8	2.1	5.7
Chunky Mediterranean, Cooked, Sainsbury's*	¼ Pack/150g	83	2.6	55	1.1	7.9	1.7	2
Collard Greens, Raw, Average*	1 Serving/80g	26	0.5	32	3	5	0.6	4
Colourful, Ribbon, Stir Fry, Waitrose*	½ Pack/116g	57	2.4	49	1.3	5	2.1	2.3
Farmhouse, Mixed, Frozen, Boiled in Salted Water, Tesco*	1 Portion /75g	32	0.5	42	3.2	5.8	0.7	3.3
Grilled Mix, Frozen, Essential, Waitrose*	1 Serving/80g	34	0.2	42	1.8	8.1	0.3	2.4
Grilled, Frozen, Sainsbury's*	1 Serving/80g	42	2.9	52	1.2	3.8	3.6	1.5
Indian Spiced, HL, Tesco*	1 Pack/347g	267	5.5	77	3	11.5	1.6	2.7
Layered, with Butter, Waitrose*	1 Pack/280g	207	16.2	74	1.7	3.6	5.8	2.4
Mediterranean Roasted, Sainsbury's*	1 Serving/150g	118	5.4	79	2.2	9.5	3.6	3.4
Mediterranean, Ready to Roast, Waitrose*	1 Serving/200g	128	8	64	1.3	5.6	4	1.6
Medley, Tender, Green, Sainsbury's*	1 Pack/160g	62	0.8	39	2.9	4.3	0.5	3.6
Mix, Steamer, Love Life, Waitrose*	1 Bag/160g	83	1.8	52	2.8	7.7	1.1	2.8
Mixed, Baby, Steam, Fresh, Tesco*	1 Pack/160g	72	1.3	45	2.7	6.7	0.8	3.8
Mixed, Bag, M&S*	1 Serving/200g	70	0.4	35	2.9	5.6	0.2	0
Mixed, Broccoli & Cauliflower Florets, Baby Carrots, Asda*	1 Serving/113g	28	0.7	25	2.2	2.6	0.6	2.4
Mixed, Broccoli, Peas & Green Beans, Co-Op*	1 Serving/80g	36	0.3	45	4.8	3.8	0.4	3.6

V

VEGETABLES

	Measure INFO/WEIGHT	per Measure KCAL	FAT	Nutrition Values per 100g / 100ml KCAL	PROT	CARB	FAT	FIBRE
Mixed, Broccoli, Sweetcorn & Peas, Rice, Birds Eye*	1 Bag/160g	181	5.3	113	3.5	17.3	3.3	2.1
Mixed, Carrot, Cauliflower & Broccoli, Prepared, Co-Op*	1 Pack/250g	100	1.5	40	2.4	5	0.6	2.7
Mixed, Carrot, Cauliflower, & Broccoli, Fresh, Tesco*	1 Serving/80g	26	0.2	32	2.6	3.9	0.2	2.8
Mixed, Carrots, Broccoli & Sweetcorn, Sainsbury's*	1 Pack/120g	67	1.4	56	2.6	8.7	1.2	2
Mixed, Carrots, Broccoli & Sweetcorn, Steam Veg, Tesco*	1 Sachet/160g	80	1.8	50	2.5	7.5	1.1	3
Mixed, Carrots, Cauliflower & Broccoli, Waitrose*	1 Serving/100g	35	0.6	35	2.4	4.9	0.6	2.9
Mixed, Carrots, Peas, Green Beans & Sweetcorn, Tesco*	1 Serving/80g	45	0.6	56	3.1	7.3	0.7	3.9
Mixed, Casserole with Baby Potatoes, Fresh, M&S*	½ Pack/350g	140	1	40	1.2	7.8	0.3	2.1
Mixed, Casserole, Tesco*	1 Pack/440g	176	1.3	40	1.2	8	0.3	2.3
Mixed, Chunky, Frozen, Sainsbury's*	1 Serving/85g	31	0.6	37	2.9	4.7	0.7	3.1
Mixed, Farmhouse, Frozen, Four Seasons, Aldi*	1oz/28g	10	0.2	34	2.8	4.3	0.7	0
Mixed, Fresh, Asda*	1oz/28g	7	0.2	26	1.9	3	0.7	1
Mixed, Freshly Frozen, Asda*	1 Serving/80g	42	0.6	52	3.2	8	0.8	3
Mixed, Freshly Frozen, Iceland*	1 Serving/100g	54	0.8	54	3.3	8.3	0.8	3.7
Mixed, Frozen, Cooked, Sainsbury's*	1 Serving/80g	45	0.6	56	2.9	7.5	0.7	4
Mixed, Layered, Classics, M&S*	½ Pack/160g	112	6.2	70	1.2	7.3	3.9	1.2
Mixed, Peas & Carrots, Buttery & Tender, Tesco*	½ Pack/150g	138	6.1	92	3.7	7.9	4.1	4.5
Mixed, Roast, Four Seasons*	1 Serving/187g	79	0.4	42	1.2	8.8	0.2	0
Mixed, Special, Freshly Frozen, Morrisons*	1 Serving/100g	48	0.8	48	3.2	7.2	0.8	0
Mixed, Special, Sainsbury's*	1 Serving/120g	68	1.2	57	3.2	8.9	1	2.9
Peas & Leeks, with a Lemon & Herb Butter, Cook*	1 Portion/145g	202	17.1	139	3.1	5.3	11.8	3.2
Roasted Root, Extra Special, Asda*	½ Pack/205g	160	3.1	78	1.1	15	1.5	6
Roasted Root, Ready to Roast, Mash Direct*	1 Pack/350g	200	7.4	57	0.8	5.8	2.1	5.9
Roasted, Italian, M&S*	1 Serving/95g	218	20	230	1.8	7.1	21	1.7
Roasted, Mediterranean, Tesco*	½ Pack/172.7g	95	3.1	55	1.3	7.6	1.8	2
Root, for Mashing, Eat Fresh, Tesco*	1 Pack/720g	238	2.9	33	0.7	5.4	0.4	2.7
Root, Mashed, Microwaved, Growers Selection, Asda*	½ Pack/200g	116	4.4	58	0.7	7.2	2.2	2.7
Root, Rainbow, Collection, M&S*	Half Pack/176g	67	2.5	38	0.7	3.9	1.4	3.6
Selection, Lightly Buttered & Seasoned, M&S*	½ Pack/150g	122	7.5	81	1.5	6.2	5	2.6
Selection, Roasted, COU, M&S*	1 Pack/250g	88	2	35	1.2	6.1	0.8	0.6
Stir Fry, Frozen, Sainsbury's*	1 Serving/80g	19	0.2	24	1.3	3.9	0.3	2
Stir Fry, Hot, & Spicy, Natures Pick, Aldi*	1 Serving/100g	37	0.5	37	1.6	5.3	0.5	2.3
Stir Fry, Tesco*	1 Serving/150g	38	0.2	25	0.9	5	0.1	1.4
Winter Soup Mix, Sainsbury's*	1 Portion/149g	61	0.3	41	1.1	7.9	0.2	1.7

VEGETABLES MIXED

	Measure INFO/WEIGHT	per Measure KCAL	FAT	Nutrition Values per 100g / 100ml KCAL	PROT	CARB	FAT	FIBRE
Mediterranean, Ovenbaked, Growers Selection, Asda*	1 Pack/400g	260	9.6	65	1.9	7.1	2.4	3.6
Red Pepper, Butternut, Courgette, & Red Onion, M&S*	½ Pack/142.5g	48	0.3	34	1.2	5.9	0.2	1.9
Roasting, Selection, Sweet & Colourful, Waitrose*	½ Pack/300g	147	3	49	1	7.5	1	2.8

VEGETARIAN

	Measure INFO/WEIGHT	per Measure KCAL	FAT	Nutrition Values per 100g / 100ml KCAL	PROT	CARB	FAT	FIBRE
Chicken Style Pieces, Sainsbury's*	1 Pack/375g	754	26.2	201	25.5	9	7	0.6
Chicken Style Pieces, Vivera*	1 Pack/175g	208	0.9	119	19.4	6.4	0.5	0
Chicken Style, Southern Fried, Pieces, VegiDeli*	1 Pack/150g	489	32.7	326	16.4	17.3	21.8	4.2
Chicken Style, Strips, Meat Free, Fry's*	1 Serving/95g	226	12.3	238	20.4	10	13	5.6
Duck, Shredded Hoisin, Cooked, Linda McCartney*	½ Pack/167g	317	12.9	190	22.1	5.9	7.7	3.9
Fingers, Fish Style, Breaded, The Redwood Co*	1 Finger/36g	94	5.2	262	16.5	16	14.5	0
Mixed Vegie Bites, Australian Eatwell*	½ Pack/112g	171	1.5	153	6	22	1.3	6.5
Nut & Date Roast with Gravy, Asda*	1 Serving /196g	300	12.7	153	4.7	16.1	6.5	5.5
Roast, Chicken Style, Vegeroast, Realeat*	4 Slices/113.5g	211	10.2	186	23	3.2	9	1.5
Schnitzel, Breaded, Tivall*	1 Schnitzel/100g	172	8	172	16	9	8	5
Slices, Sage & Onion, Vegi Deli, The Redwood Co*	1 Slice/10g	23	1.4	233	21.4	5	14.1	0.5
Slices, Vegetable, Tesco*	1 Slice/165g	452	30.5	274	5.6	21.4	18.5	3.3
Smokey BBQ Pulled Veggie, Vivera*	½ Pack/88g	98	0.4	111	14.6	10	0.4	4.4

V

	Measure INFO/WEIGHT	per Measure KCAL	FAT	Nutrition Values per 100g / 100ml KCAL	PROT	CARB	FAT	FIBRE
VEGETARIAN MINCE								
Chicken Style Pieces, Realeat*	¼ Pack/87.5g	119	1.4	136	29	1.5	1.6	4.4
Easy Cook, Linda McCartney*	1oz/28g	35	0.1	126	21.4	9.3	0.4	1.7
Frozen, Meatfree, Improved Recipe, Sainsbury's*	1 Pack/454g	799	31.8	176	18.3	10.7	7	6.7
Meat Free, Boiled, CBY, Asda*	1 Serving/75g	83	2.5	111	13.7	6.7	3.3	4.4
Vegemince, Realeat*	1 Serving/125g	218	12.5	174	18	3	10	3
VENISON								
Grill Steak, Average	*1 Steak/150g*	*178*	*3.8*	*119*	*19*	*5*	*2.5*	*1*
in Red Wine & Port, Average	*1oz/28g*	*21*	*0.7*	*76*	*9.8*	*3.5*	*2.6*	*0.4*
Minced, Cooked, Average	*1 Serving/100g*	*187*	*8.2*	*187*	*26.4*	*0*	*8.2*	*0*
Minced, Raw, Average	*1 Serving/100g*	*157*	*7.1*	*157*	*21.8*	*0*	*7.1*	*0*
Raw, Haunch, Meat Only, Average	*1 Serving/100g*	*103*	*1.6*	*103*	*22.2*	*0*	*1.6*	*0*
Roasted, Average	*1oz/28g*	*46*	*0.7*	*165*	*35.6*	*0*	*2.5*	*0*
Steak, Raw, Average	*1oz/28g*	*30*	*0.5*	*108*	*22.8*	*0*	*1.9*	*0*
VERMICELLI								
Dry	*1oz/28g*	*99*	*0.1*	*355*	*8.7*	*78.3*	*0.4*	*0*
Egg, Cooked, Average	*1 Serving/185g*	*239*	*2.6*	*129*	*5*	*24*	*1.4*	*1*
VERMOUTH								
Dry	*1 Shot/50ml*	*54*	*0*	*109*	*0.1*	*3*	*0*	*0*
Sweet	*1 Shot/50ml*	*76*	*0*	*151*	*0*	*15.9*	*0*	*0*
VIMTO*								
Cordial, No Added Sugar, Diluted, Vimto*	1 Glass/250ml	6	0.2	2	0.1	0.4	0.1	0
Cordial, No Added Sugar, Undiluted, Vimto*	1 Serving/50ml	2	0	4	0	0.7	0	0
Cordial, Original, Diluted, Vimto*	1 Serving/200ml	60	0	30	0	7.4	0	0
Cordial, Original, Undiluted, Vimto*	1 Serving/50ml	49	0	98	0	23.6	0	0
Grape, Blackcurrant & Raspberry Drink, Fizzy, Vimto*	1 Can/330ml	147	0	44	0	11	0	0
Mango, Strawberry & Pineapple, Remix, Diluted, Vimto*	1 Serving/200ml	4	0	2	0	0.2	0	0
Raspberry, Orange & Passionfruit, Remix, Vimto*	1 Serving/200ml	4	0	2	0	0.2	0	0
VINAIGRETTE								
Balsamic Vinegar & Pistachio, Finest, Tesco*	1 Tbsp/15ml	56	5.9	370	0.2	2.8	39.2	0
Balsamic, Hellmann's*	1 Tbsp/15ml	12	0.4	82	0.1	9.6	2.7	0.6
Cider Vinegar, Maille*	1 Tsp/5ml	20	2	400	0.5	7	40	0
Fat Free, Hellmann's*	1 Serving/15ml	8	0	50	0.1	11	0	0.3
French Style, Finest, Tesco*	1 Tbsp/15ml	93	9.8	620	0.6	6.3	65.3	0.2
French, Real, Briannas*	2 Tbsp/30ml	150	17	500	0	0	56.7	0
Luxury French, Hellmann's*	1 Tsp/5ml	15	1.3	305	0.8	16	26.1	0.4
Olive Oil & Lemon, Amoy*	½ Sachet/15ml	38	3.6	250	0.3	3	24	0
PB, Waitrose*	1 Tsp/5ml	4	0	89	0.4	20.9	0.4	0.5
Raspberry, Fat Free, Love Life, Waitrose*	1 Serving/15ml	9	0.1	62	0.8	13.2	0.5	0.5
VINDALOO								
Chicken, Average	*1 Serving/410g*	*787*	*51.2*	*192*	*18.5*	*2.6*	*12.5*	*0.3*
Chicken, Sainsbury's*	1 Pack/400g	460	16.8	115	14.6	4.8	4.2	0.6
Chicken, Scorching Hot, Microwaved, CBY, Asda*	1 Pack/450g	414	14.4	92	7.4	7.5	3.2	1.8
Chicken, Waitrose*	1 Pack/340g	398	18.4	117	10.6	6.4	5.4	1.6
VINE LEAVES								
Stuffed with Rice	*1oz/28g*	*73*	*5*	*262*	*2.8*	*23.8*	*18*	*0*
Stuffed with Rice & Mixed Herbs, Sainsbury's*	1 Leaf/37g	44	1.8	120	2.6	16.3	4.9	1.2
Stuffed with Rice, Palirria*	½ Pack/140g	186	9	133	2.2	16.6	6.4	0
Stuffed, Mediterranean Deli, M&S*	1 Leaf/37g	39	1.5	105	2.6	14.2	4.1	1.2
Stuffed, Sainsbury's*	1 Parcel/37.5g	46	2.1	124	2.9	15.3	5.7	3.1
VINEGAR								
Aged, Balsamic, Finest, Tesco*	1 Tbsp/15ml	34	0	230	0.5	51.4	0	0
Balsamic, Average	*1 Tsp/5ml*	*6*	*0*	*115*	*0.9*	*26*	*0*	*0*
Balsamic, of Modena, So Organic, Sainsbury's*	1 Tsp/5g	6	0	111	1.4	26.3	0.1	0.1

V

	Measure INFO/WEIGHT	per Measure KCAL	per Measure FAT	Nutrition Values per 100g / 100ml KCAL	PROT	CARB	FAT	FIBRE
VINEGAR								
Cider	*1 Tbsp/15ml*	*2*	*0*	*14*	*0*	*5.9*	*0*	*0*
Malt, Average	*1 Tbsp/15g*	*1*	*0*	*4*	*0.4*	*0.6*	*0*	*0*
Red Wine, Average	*1 Tbsp/15ml*	*3*	*0*	*19*	*0*	*0.3*	*0*	*0*
Rice Wine, Shaoxing, Waitrose*	1 Tbsp/15ml	18	0	121	1.6	4.1	0	0
VODKA								
& Diet Coke, Average	*1 Serving/150ml*	*68*	*0*	*45*	*0*	*0*	*0*	*0*
& Tonic, Ready Mixed, M&S*	1 Can/250ml	202	0	81	0	6.3	0	0
37.5% Volume	*1 Pub Shot/35ml*	*72*	*0*	*207*	*0*	*0*	*0*	*0*
40% Volume	*1 Pub Shot/35ml*	*78*	*0*	*222*	*0*	*0*	*0*	*0*
Bullett & Cola, Premixed, Canned, Diageo*	1 Can/250ml	218	0	87	0	10.6	0	0
Cookies & Cream, Sidekick, Halewood International Ltd*	1 Serving/30ml	48	0.5	160	0.3	7.7	1.6	0
Smirnoff & Cola, Premixed, canned, Diageo*	1 Can/250ml	178	0	71	0	8.9	0	0
Smirnoff & Cranberry, Premixed, Canned, Diageo*	1 Can/250ml	175	0	70	0	8.5	0	0
Smirnoff & Diet Cola, Premixed, Canned, Diageo*	1 Can/250ml	100	0	40	0	0	0	0
Smirnoff & Schweppes Tonic, Premixed, Canned, Diageo*	1 Can/250ml	158	0	63	0	6.4	0	0
VOL AU VENTS								
Chicken & Mushroom, M&S*	1oz/28g	98	6.8	350	7.7	25.2	24.3	2.1
Deluxe, Lidl*	1 Pastry/7g	40	2.8	567	7.8	41.5	40.7	1.5
Garlic Mushroom, Mini, Asda*	1 Serving/17g	59	4.6	347	5	21	27	0
Mushroom & Roast Garlic, M&S*	1 Serving/19g	65	4.6	345	6.2	25.2	24.3	1.9
Mushroom, Sainsbury's*	1 Serving/14g	49	3.1	350	6.9	30.8	22.1	1.4
Seafood, Party, Youngs*	1 Serving/17g	60	4.2	354	8.3	26	24.8	1

V

	Measure INFO/WEIGHT	per Measure KCAL	FAT	Nutrition Values per 100g / 100ml KCAL	PROT	CARB	FAT	FIBRE
WAFERS								
Cafe Curls, Rolled, Askeys*	1 Wafer/5g	21	0.4	422	5.8	80.3	8.6	0
Caramel Log, Tunnock's*	1 Wafer/32g	150	6.7	468	4.2	65.7	21	3.4
Caramel, Dark Chocolate, Tunnock's*	1 Wafer/26g	128	6.6	492	5.2	60.7	25.4	0
Caramel, Tunnock's*	1 Wafer/26g	116	4.5	448	3.6	69.2	17.4	2.5
Chewy Caramel, Tesco*	1 Bar/28g	132	5.6	472	5	66.7	20	2.6
Cream, Tunnock's*	1 Wafer/20g	103	5.6	513	6.6	63.2	28	0
Filled, Average	*1oz/28g*	*150*	*8.4*	*535*	*4.7*	*66*	*29.9*	*0*
for Ice Cream, Askeys*	1 Wafer/1.5g	6	0	388	11.4	79	2.9	0
Hazelnut, Elledi*	1 Wafer/8g	38	1.9	493	6.3	62.4	24.3	0
Timeout, Cadbury*	1 Bar/21g	111	6	524	6.7	60	28.3	2.1
WAFFLES								
Belgian Sugar, Aldi*	1 Waffle/55g	249	12.6	452	5.7	54	23	2
Belgian, TTD, Sainsbury's*	1 Waffle/25g	122	7.3	490	6	50.6	29.3	1.2
Caramel, Asda*	1 Waffle/8g	37	1.8	459	3.3	62	22	1.1
Classic, Frozen, Hello Morning, Birds Eye*	1 Waffle/30g	97	4.3	319	7	40	14	2.6
Milk Chocolate, Tregroes*	1 Waffle/49g	220	20.5	450	4.5	57	42	0.5
Sweet, American Style, Sainsbury's*	1 Waffle/35.0g	160	8.9	457	7.2	50.6	25.3	1.1
Toasting, McVitie's*	1 Waffle/24.9g	118	6.3	474	6	52.6	25.5	0.6
Toffee, Tregroes, Aldi*	1 Waffle/34.6g	160	6.2	463	3.5	71.7	18	2.2
WAGON WHEEL								
Chocolate, Original, Epic Inside, Burton's*	1 Biscuit/39g	172	5.7	441	5.1	68.7	14.5	2.1
Jammie, Burton's*	1 Biscuit/40g	168	5.6	420	5.1	67.7	14.1	1.9
WAHOO								
Fresh, Raw	*1 Serving/113g*	*110*	*1*	*97*	*23*	*0*	*0.9*	*0*
WALNUT WHIP								
Nestle*	1 Whip/35g	173	8.8	494	5.3	61.3	25.2	0.7
The, Classics, M&S*	1 Whip/26g	127	7.1	490	7.2	54.9	27.4	1.1
Vanilla, Nestle*	1 Whip/34g	165	8.4	486	5.7	60.5	24.6	0
WALNUTS								
Average	*1 Nut/7g*	*48*	*4.8*	*688*	*14.7*	*3.3*	*68.5*	*3.5*
Cocoa Cream, Dusted, Julian Graves*	1 Bag/200g	1124	70.6	562	8.2	52.9	35.3	2
Halves, Average	*1 Half/3g*	*23*	*2.3*	*669*	*17.4*	*6.3*	*65*	*4.7*
Pickled, in Malt Vinegar, Drained, Opies*	1 Walnut/25g	23	0	92	0.8	23	0	3.4
Wholesome, Organic, Kernels, Love Life, Waitrose*	1 Serving/30g	207	20.6	689	14.7	3.3	68.5	6.8
WASABI								
Paste, Ready Mixed, Japanese, Yutaka*	1 Tsp/5g	14	0.4	286	2.7	53	7	0
WATER								
Apple & Raspberry Flavour, Sparkling, Spar*	1 Glass/250ml	2	0	1	0	0	0	0
Apple & Strawberry Flavoured, Morrisons*	1 Serving/200ml	3	0	2	0.2	0.1	0	0
Blackberry & Strawberry, Sparkling, Strathmore*	1 Glass/250ml	45	0	18	0	4.3	0	0
Cactus, Truenopal*	1 Serving/330ml	30	0	9	0	2.2	0	0
Cranberry & Raspberry Flavoured, Morrisons*	1 Serving/200ml	3	0	2	0.2	0.1	0	0
Elderflower & Pear, Detox, V Water*	1 Bottle/500ml	40	0	8	0	1.9	0	0
Elderflower Presse, Bottle Green*	1 Serving/250ml	88	0	35	0	8.9	0	0
Elderflower, Presse, Sparkling, M&S*	1 Bottle/330ml	99	0.3	30	0.1	7.4	0.1	0.5
Grapefruit, Slightly Sparkling, Tesco*	1 Serving/200ml	4	0	2	0	0.2	0	0
Juicy Spring, Blackcurrant & Apple, Drench*	1 Serving/250ml	98	0	39	0	9.2	0	0
Lemon & Lime, Sugar Free, Touch of Fruit, Volvic*	1 Bottle/150ml	2	0	1	0	0	0	0
Lemon & Lime Flavour Sparkling Spring, Co-Op*	1 Serving/200ml	2	0	1	0	0	0	0
Lemon & Lime Flavoured, Strathmore*	1 Bottle/500g	85	0	17	0	4	0	0
Lemon & Lime, Sparkling, M&S*	1 Bottle/500ml	15	0	3	0	0.4	0	0
Lemon & Lime, Still, M&S*	1 Bottle/500ml	5	0	1	0	0.2	0	0
Lemon, Vittel*	1 Bottle/500ml	6	0	1	0	0	0	0

W

	Measure INFO/WEIGHT	per Measure KCAL	per Measure FAT	Nutrition Values per 100g / 100ml KCAL	PROT	CARB	FAT	FIBRE
WATER								
Lemons & Limes, Spring Water, This Juicy Water*	1 Bottle/420ml	160	0.4	38	0.2	9.5	0.1	0
Mango Lime, Carbonated, Henniez, Nestle*	1 Bottle/50ml	7	0	14	0	3.2	0	0
Mineral Or Tap	*1 Glass/200ml*	*0*	*0*	*0*	*0*	*0*	*0*	*0*
Mineral, Apple & Elderflower, Hedgerow*	1 Serving/250ml	85	0	34	0	8.2	0	0
Orange & Passion Fruit, Vital V, V Water*	1 Bottle/500ml	45	0	9	0	2.1	0	0
Peach & Raspberry, Still, M&S*	1 Bottle/500ml	10	0	2	0	0	0	0
Peach & Orange Flavoured, Morrisons*	1 Serving/200ml	3	0	2	0.2	0.1	0	0
Peach, Slightly Sparkling, Tesco*	1 Serving/200ml	4	0	2	0	0.2	0	0
Raspberry & Apple, Still, Shapers, Boots*	1 Serving/250ml	10	0	4	0	0.8	0	0
Sparkling, Fruit, Aqua Libra*	1 Glass/200ml	54	0	27	0	5.1	0	0
Sparkling, San Pellegrino*	1 Glass/200ml	0	0	0	0	0	0	0
Sparkling, Smart Price, Asda*	1 Glass/300ml	0	0	0	0	0	0	0
Sparkling, Strawberry & Kiwi, Sugar Free, Perfectly Clear*	1 Glass/250ml	2	0	1	0	0	0	0
Spring, Apple & Cherry Flavoured, Sparkling, Sainsbury's*	1 Glass/250ml	5	0.2	2	0.1	0.2	0.1	0.1
Spring, Apple & Mango, Sparkling, Asda*	1 Glass/200ml	2	0	1	0	0.2	0	0
Spring, Apple & Raspberry, Sparkling, Tesco*	1 Glass/330ml	7	0	2	0	0.5	0	0
Spring, Cranberry & Raspberry, Drench*	1 Bottle/440ml	146	0.4	33	0.1	7.7	0.1	0
Spring, Lemon & Lime Flavoured, Sparkling, Sainsbury's*	1 Glass/250ml	4	0.2	2	0.1	0.1	0.1	0.1
Spring, Lemon & Lime, Slightly Sparkling, Tesco*	1 Serving/200ml	4	0.2	2	0.1	0.2	0.1	0.1
Spring, Orange & Passionfruit, Drench*	1 Serving/250ml	95	0.5	38	0.1	9	0.2	0
Spring, Strawberry & Aloe Vera, Botanical, M&S*	1 Bottle/500ml	5	0	1	0	0.2	0	0
Spring, Strawberry & Kiwi, Still, Shapers, Boots*	1 Glass/250ml	2	0	1	0	0.1	0	0.9
Spring, Strawberry, Sparkling, Tesco*	1 Bottle/1000g	20	0	2	0	0.2	0	0
Spring, White Grape & Blackberry, Tesco*	1 Glass/200ml	4	0	2	0	0.5	0	0
Spring, with a Hint of Orange, Slightly Sparkling, Tesco*	1 Serving/250ml	5	0	2	0	0.2	0	0
Still Raspberry & Apple Spring, WaterVit, Shapers, Boots*	1 Bottle/500ml	5	0	1	0	0	0	0
Still, Cranberry & Apple, Sugar Free, Blue Keld*	1 Serving/200ml	2	0	1	0	0.1	0	0
Still, Raspberry & Mango, Shapers, Boots*	1 Bottle/500g	5	0	1	0	0	0	0
Strawberry & Guava, Still, M&S*	1 Glass/250ml	5	0	2	0	0.1	0	0
Strawberry & Kiwi, Flavoured, Loved by Us, Co-Op*	1 Serving/250ml	2	0	1	0	0	0	0
Strawberry, Original, Touch of Fruit, Volvic*	1 Bottle/500ml	99	0	20	0	4.8	0	0
Strawberry, Sugar Free, Touch of Fruit, Volvic*	1 Bottle/500ml	7	0	1	0	0.1	0	0
Tonic, Indian, Low Calorie, Vive, Aldi*	1 Serving/250ml	3	0	1	0	0	0	0
Vitamin, XXX, Triple Berry, Glaceau, Coca-Cola*	1 Bottle/500ml	65	0	13	0	3	0	0
WaterVit, Refresh & Revive, Shapers, Boots*	1 Bottle/500ml	10	0	2	0	0.2	0	0
WATER CHESTNUTS								
Raw, Average	*1oz/28g*	*8*	*0*	*29*	*0.8*	*6.6*	*0*	*0.1*
Whole, in Water, Drained, Sainsbury's*	1 Can/140g	25	0.1	18	0.8	3.4	0.1	0.4
with Bamboo Shoots, Sainsbury's*	1 Serving/50g	29	0.1	58	2	12	0.2	1.1
WATERCRESS								
Raw, Trimmed, Average	*1 Sprig/2.5g*	*1*	*0*	*22*	*3*	*0.4*	*1*	*1.5*
WATERMELON								
Flesh Only, Average	*1 Serving/250g*	*75*	*0.8*	*30*	*0.4*	*7*	*0.3*	*0.4*
Raw	*1 Wedge/286g*	*48*	*0.6*	*17*	*0.3*	*3.7*	*0.2*	*0.3*
Raw, Weighed with Skin, Average	*1 Wedge/286g*	*49*	*0.5*	*17*	*0.2*	*4*	*0.2*	*0.2*
Spiced Pickle, Pickled Pink Foods*	1 Piece/28g	30	0	107	0	25	0	0
WHEAT								
Whole Grain, Split, Average	*1 Serving/60g*	*205*	*1*	*342*	*11.3*	*75.9*	*1.7*	*12.2*
WHEAT BRAN								
Average	*1 Tbsp/7g*	*14*	*0.4*	*206*	*14.1*	*26.8*	*5.5*	*36.4*
Coarse, Holland & Barrett*	1 Tbsp/4g	8	0.2	206	14.1	26.8	5.5	36.4
Natural, Jordans*	1 Tbsp/7g	13	0.4	188	16.3	17.4	5.9	44.5

	Measure INFO/WEIGHT	per Measure KCAL	FAT	Nutrition Values per 100g / 100ml KCAL	PROT	CARB	FAT	FIBRE
WHEAT GERM								
Average	*1oz/28g*	*100*	*2.6*	*357*	*26.7*	*44.7*	*9.2*	*15.6*
Natural, Jordans*	2 Tbsp/16g	54	1.5	340	28	36	9.3	13.1
WHELKS								
Boiled, Weighed without Shell	*1oz/28g*	*25*	*0.3*	*89*	*19.5*	*0*	*1.2*	*0*
WHISKEY								
Irish, Jameson*	1 Shot/25ml	58	0	233	0	0	0	0
Jack Daniel's*	1 Pub Shot/35ml	78	0	222	0	0	0	0
WHISKY								
37.5% Volume	*1 Pub Shot/35ml*	*72*	*0*	*207*	*0*	*0*	*0*	*0*
40% Volume	*1 Pub Shot/35ml*	*78*	*0*	*222*	*0*	*0*	*0*	*0*
Bells & Ginger Ale, Premixed, Canned, Diageo*	1 Can/250ml	170	0	68	0	7.6	0	0
Scots, 37.5% Volume	*1 Pub Shot/35ml*	*72*	*0*	*207*	*0*	*0*	*0*	*0*
Scots, 40% Volume	*1 Pub Shot/35ml*	*78*	*0*	*224*	*0*	*0*	*0*	*0*
Teacher's*	1 Pub Shot/35ml	78	0	222	0	0	0	0
WHITE PUDDING								
Average	*1oz/28g*	*126*	*8.9*	*450*	*7*	*36.3*	*31.8*	*0*
WHITEBAIT								
in Flour, Fried	*1oz/28g*	*147*	*13.3*	*525*	*19.5*	*5.3*	*47.5*	*0.2*
Raw, Average	*1 Serving/100g*	*172*	*11*	*172*	*18.3*	*0*	*11*	*0*
WHITING								
in Crumbs, Fried in Blended Oil	*1 Serving/180g*	*344*	*18.5*	*191*	*18.1*	*7*	*10.3*	*0.2*
Raw	*1oz/28g*	*23*	*0.2*	*81*	*18.7*	*0*	*0.7*	*0*
Steamed	*1 Serving/85g*	*78*	*0.8*	*92*	*20.9*	*0*	*0.9*	*0*
WIENER SCHNITZEL								
Average	*1oz/28g*	*62*	*2.8*	*223*	*20.9*	*13.1*	*10*	*0.4*
WINE								
Cherry, Lambrini*	1 Glass/125ml	80	0	64	0	0	0	0
Diet, Lambrini*	1 Glass/125ml	43	0	35	0	0	0	0
Elderberry & Lemon, Ame*	1 Glass/125ml	46	0	37	0	6.4	0	0
Fruit, Average	*1 Glass/125ml*	*115*	*0*	*92*	*0*	*5.5*	*0*	*0*
Grape & Apricot, Ame*	1 Glass/125ml	49	1.2	39	1.3	6.7	1	0
Light, made with Italian Pinot Grigio, First Cape*	1 Serving/125ml	51	0	41	0	0	0	0
Madeira, Henriques & Henriques*	1 Glass/100ml	130	0	130	0	0	0	0
Mulled, Homemade, Average	*1 Glass/125ml*	*245*	*0*	*196*	*0.1*	*25.2*	*0*	*0*
Mulled, Sainsbury's*	1 Glass/125ml	112	0	90	0	8.6	0	0
Mulled, Vinglogg, Average*	1 Glass/125ml	162	0	130	0	14	0	0
Original, Lambrini*	1 Glass/125ml	88	0	70	0	0	0	0
Red, Alcohol Free, Winemakers' Selection, Sainsbury's*	1 Glass/125ml	32	0	26	0.5	6	0	0.5
*Red, Amarone, Average**	*1 Glass/125ml*	*120*	*0*	*96*	*0.1*	*3*	*0*	*0*
Red, Average	*1 Glass/125ml*	*104*	*0*	*83*	*0*	*2*	*0*	*0*
Red, Burgundy, 12.9% Abv, Average	*1 Glass/125ml*	*110*	*0*	*88*	*0.1*	*3.7*	*0*	*0*
Red, Cabernet Sauvignon, 13.1% Abv, Average	*1 Glass/125ml*	*105*	*0*	*84*	*0.1*	*2.6*	*0*	*0*
Red, Cabernet Sauvignon, Non Alcoholic, Eisberg*	1 Glass/125ml	26	0	21	0	4.5	0	0
Red, Cabernet Sauvigon, Non Alcoholic, Ariel*	1 Serving/240ml	50	0	21	0	4.8	0	0
Red, California, Blossom Hill*	1 Glass/175ml	132	0	75	0	0.9	0	0
Red, Claret, 12.8% Abv, Average	*1 Glass/125ml*	*105*	*0*	*84*	*0.1*	*3*	*0*	*0*
Red, Cooking, Asda*	1 Serving/100ml	94	0	94	0	23	0	0
Red, Gamay, 12.3% Abv, Average	*1 Glass/125ml*	*99*	*0*	*79*	*0.1*	*2.4*	*0*	*0*
Red, Merlot, 13.3% Abv, Average	*1 Glass/125ml*	*105*	*0*	*84*	*0.1*	*2.5*	*0*	*0*
Red, Non Alcoholic, Ame*	1 Glass/125ml	42	0	34	0	5.7	0	0
Red, Petit Sirah, 13.5% Abv, Average	*1 Glass/125ml*	*108*	*0*	*86*	*0.1*	*2.7*	*0*	*0*
Red, Pinot Noir, 13% Abv, Average	*1 Glass/125ml*	*104*	*0*	*83*	*0.1*	*2.3*	*0*	*0*
Red, Sangiovese, 13.6% Abv, Average	*1 Glass/125ml*	*109*	*0*	*87*	*0.1*	*2.6*	*0*	*0*

	Measure INFO/WEIGHT	per Measure KCAL	FAT	Nutrition Values per 100g / 100ml KCAL	PROT	CARB	FAT	FIBRE
WINE								
Red, Syrah, 13.1% Abv, Average	*1 Glass/125ml*	*105*	*0*	*84*	*0.1*	*2.6*	*0*	*0*
Red, Zinfandel, 13.9% Abv, Average	*1 Glass/125ml*	*111*	*0*	*89*	*0.1*	*2.9*	*0*	*0*
Rose, Alcohol Free, Eisberg*	1 Glass/200ml	52	0	26	0	5.9	0	0
Rose, GarnachaLow Alcohol	*1 Glass/125ml*	*58*	*0*	*46*	*0*	*10.9*	*0*	*0*
Rose, Medium, Average	*1 Glass/125ml*	*98*	*0*	*79*	*0*	*2.1*	*0*	*0*
Rose, Refreshing, Weight Watchers*	1 Glass/125ml	80	0	64	0	1.6	0	0
Rose, Sparkling, Average	*1 Glass/125ml*	*102*	*0*	*82*	*0*	*2.5*	*0*	*0*
Rose, The Pink Chill, Co-Op*	1 Glass/125ml	85	0	68	0	0	0	0
Rose, White Grenache, Blossom Hill*	1 Glass/125ml	105	0	84	0	3.2	0	0
Rose, White Zinfandel, Ernest & Julio Gallo*	1 Glass/125ml	101	0	81	0.2	2.7	0	0
Saki, Sawanotsuru*	1 Serving/60ml	57	0	95	0.4	3.5	0	0
Sangria, Average	*1 Glass/125ml*	*95*	*0*	*76*	*0.1*	*9.9*	*0*	*0.1*
Sauvignon Blanc, Low Alcohol, Featherweight*	1 Serving/200ml	88	0	44	0	0	0	0
Strong Ale Barley	*1 Can/440ml*	*290*	*0*	*66*	*0.7*	*6.1*	*0*	*0*
Vie, Rose, Low Alcohol, Blossom Hill*	1 Glass/175ml	93	0	53	0	3.9	0	0
White, Average	*1 Glass/125ml*	*95*	*0*	*76*	*0*	*2.4*	*0*	*0*
White, Californian, Chardonnay, LC, Tesco*	1 Bottle/181ml	96	0	53	0	1.8	0	0
White, Chardonnay, Southern Australia, Kissing Tree*	1 Bottle/185ml	85	0	46	0	0	0	0
White, Chenin Blanc, 12% Abv, Average	*1 Glass/125ml*	*101*	*0*	*81*	*0.1*	*3.3*	*0*	*0*
White, Dry, Average	*1 Glass/125ml*	*88*	*0*	*70*	*0.1*	*0.6*	*0*	*0*
White, Fume Blanc, 13.1% Abv, Average	*1 Glass/125ml*	*104*	*0*	*83*	*0.1*	*2.3*	*0*	*0*
White, Gewurztraminer, 12.6% Abv, Average	*1 Glass/125ml*	*102*	*0*	*82*	*0.1*	*2.6*	*0*	*0*
White, Late Harvest, 10.6% Abv, Average	*1 Glass/125ml*	*141*	*0*	*113*	*0.1*	*13.4*	*0*	*0*
White, Medium, Average	*1 Glass/125ml*	*92*	*0*	*74*	*0.1*	*3*	*0*	*0*
White, Muller-Thurgau, 11.3% Abv, Average	*1 Glass/125ml*	*96*	*0*	*77*	*0.1*	*3.5*	*0*	*0*
White, Muscat, 11% Abv, Average	*1 Glass/125ml*	*104*	*0*	*83*	*0.1*	*5.2*	*0*	*0*
White, Non Alcoholic, Trocken , Carl Jung*	1 Glass/175ml	5	0	3	0	0	0	0
White, Pinot Blanc, 13.3% Abv, Average	*1 Glass/125ml*	*102*	*0*	*82*	*0.1*	*0*	*0*	*0*
White, Pinot Grigio, 13.4% Abv, Average	*1 Glass/125ml*	*105*	*0*	*84*	*0.1*	*2.1*	*0*	*0*
White, Riesling, 11.9% Abv, Average	*1 Glass/125ml*	*101*	*0*	*81*	*0.1*	*3.7*	*0*	*0*
White, Sauvignon Blanc, 13.1% Abv, Average	*1 Glass/125ml*	*102*	*0*	*82*	*0.1*	*2*	*0*	*0*
White, Semillon, 12.5% Abv, Average	*1 Glass/125ml*	*104*	*0*	*83*	*0.1*	*3.1*	*0*	*0*
White, Sparkling, Alcohol Free, Eisberg*	1 Glass/125ml	31	0	25	0	6.3	0	0
White, Sparkling, Average	*1 Glass/125ml*	*92*	*0*	*74*	*0.3*	*5.1*	*0*	*0*
White, Summer, Light, 5.5%, Miranda Wines*	1 Glass/125ml	45	1.2	36	1	1.5	1	0
White, Sweet, Average	*1 Glass/120ml*	*113*	*0*	*94*	*0.2*	*5.9*	*0*	*0*
WINE GUMS								
Average	*1 Sweet/6g*	*19*	*0*	*315*	*5*	*73.4*	*0.2*	*0.1*
Haribo*	1 Pack/175g	609	0.4	348	0.1	86.4	0.2	0.4
Mini, Rowntree's*	1 Sm Bag/36g	125	0	348	6.7	80.5	0	0
Sour, Bassett's*	¼ Bag/50g	160	0	319	3.7	78	0	0
WISPA								
Bite, with Biscuit in Caramel, Cadbury*	1 Bar/47g	240	13.4	510	6.4	56.9	28.6	0
Cadbury*	1 Bar/40g	220	13.6	550	7.3	52.5	34	1
Gold, Cadbury*	1 Bar/52g	265	15.1	510	5.3	56	29	0.7
WONTON								
Prawn, Crispy from Selection, Modern Asian, M&S*	1 Wonton/25g	65	3.3	250	9.5	23.4	12.7	2
Prawn, Dim Sum Selection, Sainsbury's*	1 Wonton/10g	26	1.2	259	11.3	26.8	11.8	1.3
Prawn, Oriental Selection, Waitrose*	1 Wonton/18g	45	2	252	9.1	29.2	11	1.1
Prawn, Oriental Snack Selection, Sainsbury's*	1 Wonton/20g	53	2.7	265	10.6	25.6	13.4	2
WOTSITS								
Baked, Really Cheesy, Walkers*	1 Bag/22.5g	123	7.4	546	5.5	56	33	1.1
Really Cheesy, Big Eat, Walkers*	1 Bag/36g	197	11.9	547	5.5	56	33	1.1

WRAP

INFO/WEIGHT	Measure	per Measure		Nutrition Values per 100g / 100ml				
		KCAL	FAT	KCAL	PROT	CARB	FAT	FIBRE
BBQ Chicken, No Mayo, Tesco*	1 Pack/154g	367	8.6	239	12.5	33.7	5.6	1.7
Butternut Squash, COU, M&S*	1 Pack/181.5g	245	4.7	135	4.3	22.2	2.6	2.9
Cajun Chicken, Sandwich King*	1 Pack/138g	386	19.9	279	12.3	25	14.4	0
Cheese, & Bean, Tesco*	1 Pack/105g	235	9.4	224	7	28.6	9	1
Chicken & Bacon, Caesar, Just Tasty, Aldi*	1 Pack/196g	459	18	234	12.8	24	9.2	1.5
Chicken Caesar, Ginsters*	1 Pack/180g	440	21.1	244	11.1	23.5	11.7	1.8
Chicken Fajita, Morrisons*	1 Pack/214g	430	16.5	201	9.5	22.5	7.7	1.9
Chicken Korma, Rainbow, Co-Op*	1 Wrap/198g	348	8.5	176	8.6	24	4.3	2.4
Chicken Tikka, Average	*1 Wrap/200g*	*403*	*15.1*	*202*	*9.5*	*23.6*	*7.6*	*4.4*
Chicken, & Bacon, Caesar Salad, Asda*	1 Pack/160g	565	35.2	353	18	20.8	22	0.9
Chicken, & Bacon, Caesar, COU, M&S*	1 Pack/170g	260	4.2	153	10.6	22	2.5	2.1
Chicken, & Bacon, Simple Solutions, Tesco*	1 Pack/300g	474	23.4	158	20.7	1.2	7.8	0.5
Chicken, BBQ, Shapers, Boots*	1 Wrap/156g	278	4.5	178	11	26	2.9	1.8
Chicken, Caesar, Tesco*	1 Pack /215g	516	24.3	240	11.6	23	11.3	1.2
Chicken, Cajun, Tesco*	1 Pack/175g	357	13.8	204	9.4	22.6	7.9	2.3
Chicken, Coronation , Waitrose*	1 Pack/164g	283	8.3	173	10.1	21.3	5.1	2.2
Chicken, Fajita, M&S*	1 Pack/213g	394	15.1	185	8.8	20.1	7.1	2.5
Chicken, Fajita, Omelette, Tesco*	1 Pack/161g	289	16.6	179	16.7	4	10.3	1.5
Chicken, Fajita, PB, Waitrose*	1 Serving/218g	368	5.7	169	10.5	26	2.6	1.9
Chicken, Fillets, with Cheese, & Bacon, Asda*	1 Pack/164g	366	21.3	223	25	1.4	13	0
Chicken, Lemon, & Herb, Delicious, Boots*	1 Pack/173g	351	13.1	203	7.9	24	7.6	3
Chicken, M&S*	1 Pack/247g	530	24.9	215	8.2	23.4	10.1	1.6
Chicken, Mexican Style, Co-Op*	1 Pack/163g	367	14.7	225	11	26	9	3
Chicken, Moroccan, BGTY, Sainsbury's*	1 Pack/207g	315	3.1	152	9.4	25.3	1.5	0
Chicken, Salad, Free From Gluten, CBY, Asda*	1 Pack/187g	352	11	188	9.6	23	5.9	2.3
Chicken, Salad, Roast, Sainsbury's*	1 Pack/214g	443	19.9	207	10	20.9	9.3	2.5
Chicken, Southern Fried, CBY, Asda*	1 Pack/210g	452	17	215	7.1	27	8.1	2.7
Chicken, Sweet Chilli , Sainsbury's*	1 Pack/209g	434	11.5	208	8.5	30.1	5.5	1.8
Chicken, Sweet Chilli, Shapers, Boots*	1 Pack/194.6g	302	3.7	155	10	24	1.9	3
Duck, Hoisin, Delicious, Boots*	1 Pack/160g	295	4.3	184	11	28	2.7	2
Duck, Hoisin, M&S*	1 Pack/225g	405	8.3	180	8.4	27.7	3.7	1.5
Feta, Salad, Greek , Shapers, Boots*	1 Pack/158g	241	5.7	153	6.4	24	3.6	1.2
Ham, Cheese, & Pickle Tortilla, Weight Watchers*	1 Pack/170g	296	4.8	174	10.9	26.4	2.8	1.2
Hoisin Duck, No Mayo, Tesco*	1 Pack/168g	382	13.1	227	10.3	27.7	7.8	2.6
King Prawn, Sweet Chilli , M&S*	1 Pack/155g	225	3.1	145	8	24.2	2	2.1
Minted Lamb, Darwins Deli*	1 Pack/250g	287	6.3	115	3.2	19.9	2.5	0
Pulled Pork, Mexican Spiced, Good to Go, Waitrose*	1 Pack/189g	339	14.2	179	7.2	19.8	7.5	1.8
Roast Turkey, Ranch & Bacon, Arby's*	1 Wrap/279g	620	31	222	13.3	14	11.1	1.4
Salmon, Smoked, & Prawn, Finest, Tesco*	1 Serving/59g	84	5.3	143	14.3	1	9.1	0
Sausage, & Bacon, Cooked, Sainsbury's*	1 Wrap/12g	38	2.6	315	17.7	12.1	21.7	0
Soft Cheese, & Spinach, to Go*	1 Serving/250g	278	6.7	111	4.5	17.4	2.7	0
Tuna, Sweetcorn, & Red Pepper, BGTY, Sainsbury's*	1 Pack/178g	306	8.2	172	11.5	21.2	4.6	2.1
Turkey, Bacon, & Cranberry, COU, M&S*	1 Pack/144g	230	2.2	160	9.6	27.1	1.5	2.3

	Measure INFO/WEIGHT	per Measure KCAL	FAT	Nutrition Values per 100g / 100ml KCAL	PROT	CARB	FAT	FIBRE
YAM								
Baked	**1oz/28g**	**43**	**0.1**	**153**	**2.1**	**37.5**	**0.4**	**1.7**
Boiled, Average	**1oz/28g**	**37**	**0.1**	**133**	**1.7**	**33**	**0.3**	**1.4**
Raw	**1oz/28g**	**26**	**0.1**	**92**	**1.2**	**22.8**	**0.2**	**1.1**
YEAST								
Extract	**1 Tsp/9g**	**16**	**0**	**180**	**40.7**	**3.5**	**0.4**	**0**
Extract, Reduced Salt, Sainsbury's*	1 Tsp/4g	10	0	246	41.2	17.6	0.5	4.3
Quick, Doves Farm*	1 Serving/8g	24	0.5	301	43.5	19	5.7	27
YOGHURT								
0.1% Fat, Lidl*	1 Pot/150g	118	0.2	79	4	15.6	0.1	0
Activia, Danone*	1 Pot/132.4g	125	4.2	94	3.5	12.8	3.2	2
After Dinner Mint, Limited Edition, Mullerlight, Muller*	1 Pot/165g	91	0.8	55	4.3	7.6	0.5	0
Apple & Pear, Low Fat, Sainsbury's*	1 Pot/125g	115	1.9	92	4.3	15.2	1.5	0.2
Apple & Prune, Fat Free, Yeo Valley*	1 Pot/125g	98	0.1	78	5.1	14.1	0.1	0.2
Apple & Berry Pie, Dessert Recipe, Weight Watchers*	1 Pot/120g	58	0.1	49	4.1	6.8	0.1	0.3
Apple & Peach, Bircher Muesli, Moma Foods*	1 Pot/170g	224	4.1	132	4.3	24.3	2.4	1.7
Apple, & Quince, Spiced, Yeo Valley*	¼ Pot/113g	115	4.3	102	4.6	12.3	3.8	0
Apple, Spiced, 6% Fat, TTD, Sainsbury's*	1 Pot/15g	16	0.6	107	2.7	15.6	3.8	0.5
Apricot & Mango, Thick & Creamy, Sainsbury's*	1 Pot/150g	178	5.4	119	4.3	17.3	3.6	0.2
Apricot & Passion Fruit, Fat Free, Yeo Valley*	1 Pot/125g	94	0.1	75	5.3	13.2	0.1	0.1
Apricot, Bio Activia, Danone*	1 Pot/125g	121	4	97	3.7	13.3	3.2	1.7
Apricot, Fat Free, Weight Watchers*	1 Pot/110g	45	0.1	41	4	5	0.1	0.2
Apricot, Fruity, Mullerlight, Muller*	1 Pot/175g	88	0.2	50	4.2	7.5	0.1	0.1
Apricot, Low Fat, Brooklea, Aldi*	1 Pot/125g	99	1	79	2.8	15.1	0.8	0
Apricot, Low Fat, Sainsbury's*	1 Pot/124g	108	1.6	87	4.2	14.3	1.3	0.5
Apricot, Low Fat, Tesco*	1 Pot/125g	112	2.2	90	4.3	14.1	1.8	0
Apricot, Summer Fruits, Benecol*	1 Pot/120g	109	2	91	3.7	15	1.7	0.2
Banana & Custard, Smooth, Mullerlight, Muller*	1 Pot/175g	94	0.2	54	4.1	8.6	0.1	0.6
Banana & Custard, Yeo Valley*	1 Serving/100g	109	4.3	109	4.6	13	4.3	0
Banana Choco Flakes, Crunch Corner, Muller*	1 Pot/135g	193	6.9	143	4.3	19.3	5.1	0.3
Banana, Low Fat, Average	**1 Serving/100g**	**98**	**1.4**	**98**	**4.6**	**16.7**	**1.4**	**0.1**
Banoffee, Snackpot, Activia, Danone*	1 Pot/155g	116	0.2	75	5	13.3	0.1	0.3
Berry & Apple, Low Fat, Breakfast Pot, Tesco*	1 Pot/215g	233	2.6	108	0	14.5	1.2	2.4
Bio, Low Fat, Spelga*	1 Pot/125g	125	2.1	100	3.9	17	1.7	0
Black Cherries & Cream, The Best, Morrisons*	1 Pot/150g	218	9.4	146	3.2	19	6.3	0
Black Cherry, 0%, Greek Style, Yeo Valley*	1 Serving/150g	108	0	72	6.6	10.7	0	0
Black Cherry, Average	**1 Serving/100g**	**96**	**2.2**	**96**	**3.4**	**16.5**	**2.2**	**0.1**
Black Cherry, Extremely Fruity, Bio, M&S*	1 Pot/150g	165	2.2	110	4.9	18.4	1.5	0.2
Black Cherry, Fat Free, Benecol*	1 Pot/120g	78	0.6	65	3	11	0.5	2.1
Black Cherry, Garden Fruits, Fat Free, Benecol*	1 Pot/125g	79	0.6	63	3	11	0.5	2.1
Black Cherry, Greek Style, Corner, Muller*	1 Pot/150g	172	4.5	115	5	16.2	3	0.1
Black Cherry, Low Fat, Average	**1 Serving/100g**	**69**	**0.6**	**69**	**3.8**	**12.2**	**0.6**	**0.3**
Black Cherry, Swiss, Finest, Tesco*	1 Pot/150g	195	8.8	130	3.5	15.7	5.9	0.5
Black Cherry, Thick & Creamy, Waitrose*	1 Pot/125g	139	3.1	111	3.7	18.3	2.5	0.4
Blackberry & Raspberry, Fruit Corner, Muller*	1 Pot/150g	158	5.8	105	3.8	13.1	3.9	0.9
Blackberry, Soya, Alpro*	1 Pot/125g	94	2.4	75	3.6	9.7	1.9	1.1
Blackcurrant, & Elderflower, Soya, Alpro*	1 Pot/125g	92	2.4	74	3.6	9.5	1.9	1.1
Blackcurrant, Garden Fruits, Low Fat, Tesco*	1 Pot/125g	120	2.4	95	3.8	15.1	1.9	0.3
Blackcurrant, Longley Farm*	1 Pot/150g	168	5.6	112	4.9	14.7	3.7	0
Blackcurrant, Probiotic, Organic, Yeo Valley*	1 Pot/150g	152	5.8	101	4.1	12.4	3.9	0.2
Blackcurrant, Soya, Go On, Alpro*	1 Pot/150g	122	4.2	81	5.1	7.5	2.8	2
Blueberries & Cream, Made Up, Easiyo*	1 Serving/100g	105	4.1	105	3.9	13.7	4.1	0
Blueberry, Bursting, Intensely Creamy, Activia, Danone*	1 Pot/110g	112	3.3	102	5	13.4	3	0.5
Blueberry, Fat Free, Probiotic, Organic, Yeo Valley*	1 Serving/100g	73	0.1	73	5.1	12.9	0.1	0.4

Y

YOGHURT

	Measure INFO/WEIGHT	per Measure KCAL	FAT	KCAL	PROT	CARB	FAT	FIBRE
Blueberry, Fruit Corner, Muller*	1 Pot/150g	156	5.7	104	3.8	12.9	3.8	0.4
Blueberry, Longley Farm*	1 Pot/150g	168	8	112	4.1	12.8	5.3	0
Blueberry, Soya, Alpro*	1 Pot/125g	91	2.5	73	3.6	9.4	2	1.2
Blueberry, Soya, Free From, Tesco*	1 Pot/100g	76	2.1	76	3.7	10.5	2.1	0.3
Blueberry, with Crunchy Granola, Organic, Yeo Valley*	1 Yoghurt/135g	217	7.7	161	5.6	21.1	5.7	0
Bramble & Apple, Virtually Fat Free, Longley Farm*	1 Pot/150g	118	0.2	79	5.5	13.9	0.1	0
Bramley Apple & Gooseberry, M&S*	1 Pot/150g	186	10.6	124	2.8	12.3	7.1	0.5
Breakfast Crunch, Strawberry, Corner, Muller*	1 Pot/135g	163	3.5	121	5.5	0	2.6	0
British Rhubarb, Yeo Valley*	1 Serving/100g	102	3.8	102	4.6	12.3	3.8	0
Caramel, Indulgent Layered, Specially Selected, Aldi*	1 Pot/150g	276	16.5	184	2.3	19	11	1.4
Cereals, Fibre, Bio Activia, Danone*	1 Pot/120g	119	4.1	99	3.7	13.5	3.4	3
Champagne Rhubarb, Finest, Tesco*	1 Pot/150g	212	11.6	141	3.4	14.1	7.7	0.7
Cherry, Bio, Low Fat, Benecol*	1 Pot/150g	122	0.9	81	3.8	15.2	0.6	0
Cherry, Charmer, Greek Style, Light & Free, Danone*	1 Pot/115g	59	0.1	51	4.7	7.7	0.1	0.1
Cherry, Fat Free, Activia, Danone*	1 Pot/125g	76	0.1	61	4.8	9.8	0.1	0.9
Cherry, Fat Free, Milbona, Aldi*	1 Pot/175g	50	0.1	29	2.3	4.5	0.1	0.1
Cherry, Fruit, Biopot, Onken*	1 Serving/100g	107	2.7	107	3.7	16.7	2.7	0.2
Cherry, Fruity, Mullerlight, Muller*	1 Pot/175g	86	0.2	49	4.3	7	0.1	0.2
Cherry, Greek Style, Fruitopolis, Mullerlight, Muller*	1 Pot/130g	90	0.1	68	4.8	11.4	0.1	0
Cherry, Light, Fat Free, Muller*	1 Pot/175g	88	0.2	50	3.9	7.9	0.1	0.2
Cherry, Low Fat, CBY, Asda*	1 Pot/125g	90	1.6	72	3.6	11.4	1.3	0.3
Cherry, Low Fat, Milbona, Lidl*	1 Pot/125g	110	1.1	88	3.6	16	0.9	0
Cherry, Luscious, Intensely Creamy, Activia, Danone*	1 Pot/110g	109	3.3	99	5	12.8	3	0.2
Cherry, Soya, Alpro*	1 Pot/125g	91	2.5	73	3.6	9.4	2	1.2
Cherry, Whip n Mix, Oykos, Danone*	1 Pot/92g	144	5.4	156	3.2	22.4	5.9	0.2
Coconut & Lemon, Dairy Free, Koko*	1 Pot/125g	141	6.9	113	0.7	15.1	5.5	0.3
Coconut & Vanilla, Greek Style, Fat Free, Brooklea, Aldi*	1 Pot/125g	65	0.6	52	4.9	7.6	0.5	0.5
Coconut, Greek Style, Brooklea, Aldi*	1 Serving/150g	212	12.9	141	3.7	12	8.6	0.5
Coconut, Greek Style, Milbona, Lidl*	1 Pot/150g	236	14.7	157	3.9	13	9.8	0.5
Coconut, Low Fat, Tesco*	1 Portion/150g	150	4	100	5	13.8	2.7	0.1
Cranberry, Bio Activia, Danone*	1 Pot/125g	115	4	92	3.6	12.3	3.2	1.7
Drink, Actimel, Peach & Mango, Danone*	1 Bottle/100g	28	0.1	28	2.7	3.1	0.1	0.4
Fat Free, Greek Style, Counted, Eat Smart, Morrisons*	¼ Pot/125g	95	0.6	76	7	10.9	0.5	0
Fat Free, Vanilla, Onken*	½ Pot/225g	166	0.2	74	4.4	12.6	0.1	0.3
Fig, Bio, Activia, Danone*	1 Pot/125g	124	4.2	99	3.6	13.4	3.4	0.2
Forest Fruits, Greek Style, Layered, Shapers, Boots*	1 Pot/150g	86	2.1	57	3.2	7.9	1.4	2.2
Forest Fruits, Soya, Dairy Free, Alpro*	1 Serving/100g	79	2.2	79	3.8	10.1	2.2	1.2
French Set, Low Fat, Iceland*	1 Pot/125g	100	1.5	80	3.6	13.6	1.2	0
Fruit Whole Milk	**1 Pot/150g**	**158**	**4.2**	**105**	**5.1**	**15.7**	**2.8**	**0**
Fruit, Low Fat, Average	**1 Pot/125g**	**112**	**0.9**	**90**	**4.1**	**17.9**	**0.7**	**0**
Fruits with Cherries, Bio, 0% Fat, Danone*	1 Pot/125g	65	0.1	52	3.6	9.1	0.1	0
Fruity Favourites, Organic, Yeo Valley*	1 Pot/125g	126	4.9	101	4.1	12.4	3.9	0.2
Fudge, Devonshire Style, Finest, Tesco*	1 Pot/150g	206	9.2	137	4	16.4	6.1	0.4
Fudge, Devonshire Style,, Specially Selected, Aldi*	1 Pot/150g	234	12	156	3.2	18	8	0.5
Ginger, Greek Style, Bio, Live, Rachel's Organic*	1 Serving/100g	137	7.4	137	3.2	14.4	7.4	0
Goat's Milk, Honey, Blossom, Live, St Helen's Farm*	1 Pot/125g	166	8	133	4.9	14	6.4	0
Goat's Milk, Natural, Fat Free, St Helen's Farm*	1 Serving/150g	63	0.2	42	6	4.3	0.1	0
Goat's Milk, Natural, St Helen's Farm*	1 Serving/150g	158	11	105	5.5	4.3	7.3	0
Goats Whole Milk	**1 Carton/150g**	**94**	**5.7**	**63**	**3.5**	**3.9**	**3.8**	**0**
Gooseberry & Elderflower, Fragrant, Creamy, Waitrose*	1 Pot/150g	188	9.9	125	2.6	13.8	6.6	0.5
Gooseberry, Bio Live, Rachel's Organic*	1 Pot/450g	450	15.3	100	4	13.3	3.4	0.2
Gooseberry, Garden Fruits, Low Fat, Tesco*	1 Pot/125g	115	2.4	90	3.3	14.9	1.9	0.3
Gooseberry, Low Fat, Average	**1 Serving/100g**	**90**	**1.4**	**90**	**4.5**	**14.5**	**1.4**	**0.2**

YOGHURT

INFO/WEIGHT	Measure KCAL	FAT	KCAL	PROT	CARB	FAT	FIBRE
Gooseberry, Virtually Fat Free, Longley Farm*	1 Pot/150g	122	0.2	81	4.2	15.7	0.1	0
Greek Style, Brooklea, Aldi*	1 Serving/100g	109	8.5	109	2.9	5.3	8.5	0.5
Greek Style, Low Fat, M&S*	1 Serving/100g	75	2.7	75	6.1	6.9	2.7	0.5
Greek Style, Luxury, Loseley*	1 Pot/175g	226	17.8	129	4.8	4.5	10.2	0
Greek Style, Natural, Milbona, Lidl*	1 Serving/150g	183	15	122	4.6	3.2	10	0
Greek Style, Strained, 0%, Glenisk Organic Dairy Co*	1 Pot/150g	84	0	56	10	4	0	0
Greek Style, Vanilla, 0% Fat, COU, M&S*	1 Pot/140g	81	0.3	58	6.8	7.2	0.2	0.5
Greek, 0% Fat, Strained, Authentic, Total, Fage*	¼ Pot/125g	71	0	57	10.3	4	0	0
Greek, 0%, Mevgal*	1 Serving/100g	52	0	52	8	5	0	0
Greek, 2% Fat, Strained, Authentic, Total, Fage*	1 Pot/170g	124	3.4	73	9.9	3.8	2	0
Greek, Authentic, Natural, Strained, Waitrose*	1 Serving/125g	164	12.8	131	5.9	3.7	10.2	0.3
Hazelnut, Longley Farm*	1 Pot/150g	201	8.5	134	5.5	16	5.7	0
Hazelnut, Sainsbury's*	1 Serving/150g	183	3.4	122	5	20.3	2.3	0.2
Honey & Muesli, Breakfast Break, Tesco*	1 Pot/170g	207	4.6	122	3.9	20.5	2.7	0.6
Honey & Ginger, West Country, Luxury, M&S*	1 Pot/150g	219	11.6	146	3.6	15.6	7.7	0
Honey Breakfast Pot, Activia, Danone*	1 Pot/160g	192	4.2	120	4.9	18.8	2.6	0.7
Honey, Greek Style, 0% Fat, Tesco*	1/3 Pot/150g	122	0.3	81	6.8	13.1	0.2	0
Honey, Greek Style, Milbona, Lidl*	1 Yoghurt/100g	145	8.3	145	3.8	13.5	8.3	0.5
Honey, Greek Style, Strained, 0% Fat, Liberte, Yoplait*	1 Pot/100g	92	0.1	92	7.7	14.1	0.1	0.1
Icelandic Style, Strained, Honey, Fat Free, Skyr, Arla*	1 Serving/150g	110	0.2	73	9.4	7.8	0.1	0
Icelandic Style, Strained, Natural, Fat Free, Skyr, Arla*	1 Serving/150g	98	0.3	65	11	4	0.2	0
Icelandic Style, Strained, Natural, Fat Free, Skyr, Arla*	1 Serving/150g	98	0.3	65	11	4	0.2	0
Icelandic Style, Strained, Strawberry, Fat Free, Skyr, Arla*	1 Pot/150g	112	0.3	75	9.4	8	0.2	0.2
Juicy Raspberry, Intensely Creamy, Activia, Danone*	1 Pot/110g	109	3.3	99	4.8	12.7	3	0.6
Kiwi, Bio, Activia, Danone*	1 Pot/125g	122	4.2	98	3.6	12.9	3.4	0.3
Kiwi, Cereal, Fibre, Bio Activia, Danone*	1 Pot/120g	124	4	103	3.8	14.5	3.3	3
Lemon Cheesecake, Average	*1 Serving/100g*	*55*	*0.2*	*55*	*4.3*	*8.8*	*0.2*	*0.2*
Lemon Curd, Deluxe, Lidl*	1 Pot/150g	250	12.3	167	3	20	8.2	0.5
Lemon Curd, Handmade, Specially Selected, Aldi*	1 Pot/140g	188	8.7	134	3.3	16	6.2	0.5
Lemon Curd, West Country, Extra Special, Asda*	1 Pot/150g	252	13	168	3.2	19	8.7	0
Lemon Curd, West Country, TTD, Sainsbury's*	1 Pot/150g	243	10	162	3.7	21.6	6.7	0.5
Lemon Curd, Whole Milk, Yeo Valley*	1 Pot/120g	153	5.3	128	4.8	17.2	4.4	0.2
Lemon, Greek Style, Brooklea, Aldi*	1/3 Pot/150g	195	12.5	130	3.5	10	8.3	0.5
Lemon, Greek Style, Whipped, Bliss Corner, Muller*	1 Pot/110g	177	6.5	161	4	22.2	5.9	0
Lemon, Lavish, Greek Style, Light & Free, Danone*	1 Pot/115g	56	0.1	49	4.9	7.1	0.1	0.1
Lemon, Longley Farm*	1 Pot/150g	159	5.6	106	5	13.4	3.7	0
Lemon, Sicilain, The Best, Morrisons*	1 Pot/150g	235	12.1	157	3.4	17.5	8.1	0
Lemon, Summer, Biopot, Onken*	1 Pot/150g	154	3.9	103	3.9	15.9	2.6	0.1
Low Calorie	*1 Pot/120g*	*49*	*0.2*	*41*	*4.3*	*6*	*0.2*	*0*
Luscious Lemon, Greek Style, Mullerlight, Muller*	1 Pot/125g	75	0.2	60	6.3	7.5	0.2	0
Madagascan Vanilla, West Country, TTD, Sainsbury's*	1 Pot/150g	197	11.8	132	3.1	11.9	7.9	0.5
Mandarin, Fat Free, Mullerlight, Muller*	1 Pot/175g	95	0.2	54	4.2	8.5	0.1	0
Mandarin, Llaeth Y Llan, Village Dairy*	1 Pot/125g	130	3.5	104	5.6	14.3	2.8	0.1
Mandarin, Longley Farm*	1 Pot/150g	141	5.7	94	4.9	13.3	3.8	0
Mango & Apple, Fat Free, Onken*	1 Serving/150g	132	0.2	88	4.4	16	0.1	0.2
Mango & Passion Fruit, Low Fat, Sainsbury's*	1 Pot/125g	105	1.6	84	4.2	13.5	1.3	0.5
Mango Flavour, Bio Live, Yeo Valley*	1 Pot/120g	84	1.7	70	4.5	10	1.4	0
Mango, Bio, Activia, Danone*	1 Pot/125g	124	4.2	99	3.5	13.5	3.4	0.2
Mango, Soya, Go On, Alpro*	1 Pot/150g	129	4.2	86	5	9.1	2.8	1.3
Mellow Vanilla, Protein, Snack Pot, Arla*	1 Pot/220g	249	9.9	113	9.5	8.2	4.5	2
Mixed Berries, Jogood, Imlek*	1 Pot/200g	172	4.4	86	2.9	13.4	2.2	0
Morello Cherry, Specially Selected, Aldi*	1 Pot/150g	171	7.5	114	2.5	15	5	0.5
Muesli Nut, Low Fat	*1 Pot/120g*	*134*	*2.6*	*112*	*5*	*19.2*	*2.2*	*0*

Y

YOGHURT

INFO/WEIGHT	Measure	per Measure KCAL	per Measure FAT	Nutrition Values per 100g / 100ml KCAL	PROT	CARB	FAT	FIBRE
Natural with Cow's Milk, Greek Style, Tesco*	1 Pot/150g	214	16.4	143	4.5	6.6	10.9	0
Natural with Honey, Greek Style, Sainsbury's*	1 Sm Pot/150g	243	14.1	162	4	15.4	9.4	0
Natural, 0.1% Fat, Stirred, Biopot, Onken*	1 Serving/100g	48	0.1	48	5.4	6.4	0.1	0
Natural, Almond Milk, Dairy Free, Nush Foods*	1 Pot/125g	165	10	132	4	3	8	0
Natural, Bio Activia, Individual Pots, Danone*	1 Pot/125g	86	4.2	69	4.2	5.5	3.4	0
Natural, Bio Live, Low Fat, Organic, Waitrose*	¼ Pot/125g	81	1.2	65	5.8	8.3	1	0
Natural, Bio Set, Low Fat, Sainsbury's*	1 Pot/150g	78	2.2	52	3.9	5.7	1.5	0
Natural, Bio, BFY, Morrisons*	1 Serving/100g	65	0.2	65	6.5	9.4	0.2	0
Natural, Bio, HL, Tesco*	1 Serving/100g	55	0.1	55	5.4	7.6	0.1	0
Natural, Bio, Lancashire Farm*	3 Dstsps/40g	32	1.4	80	5.2	7	3.5	0.5
Natural, Bio, Lge Pot, Activia, Danone*	¼ Pot/112g	64	0.1	57	5.4	7.4	0.1	0
Natural, Bio, Virtually Fat Free, HL, Tesco*	1 Serving/100g	47	0.2	47	5.5	5.8	0.2	0.1
Natural, Danone*	1 Pot/125g	71	3.6	57	3.2	3.8	2.9	0
Natural, Fat Free, Biopot, Dr Oetker*	¼ Pot/125g	60	0.1	48	5.4	6.4	0.1	0
Natural, Fat Free, Eat Smart, Morrisons*	1 Pot/150g	88	0.3	59	7	7.2	0.2	0
Natural, Fat Free, Lancashire Farm Dairies*	1 Serving/100g	48	0.1	48	5	7.3	0.1	0.9
Natural, Fat Free, Onken*	1 Serving/100g	46	0.1	46	5.4	4.3	0.1	0
Natural, Fat Free, Rachel's Organic*	1 Pot/500g	180	0.5	36	3.9	4.8	0.1	0
Natural, Greek Style, Average	***1 Serving/100g***	***138***	***10.6***	***138***	***4.7***	***6.1***	***10.6***	***0***
Natural, Greek Style, Bio Live, Rachel's Organic*	1 Pot/450g	518	40.5	115	3.6	4.9	9	0
Natural, Greek Style, Bio Live, Tims Dairy*	1 Serving/50g	65	5	130	5.7	4.9	10	0
Natural, Greek Style, Fat Free, CBY, Asda*	1 Tub/200g	114	0.4	57	7.9	5.8	0.2	0.1
Natural, Greek Style, Fat Free, Essential, Waitrose*	1 Serving/125g	68	0.5	54	7.8	4.8	0.4	0
Natural, Greek Style, Fat Free, Tesco*	1 Pot/100g	55	0.2	55	7.5	4.8	0.2	0.4
Natural, Greek Style, HL, Tesco*	1 Serving/100g	80	2.7	80	5.7	8.2	2.7	0
Natural, Greek Style, Low Fat, Average	***1 Serving/100g***	***77***	***2.7***	***77***	***6.1***	***7.3***	***2.7***	***0.2***
Natural, Greek Style, Low Fat, Tesco*	1 Serving/100g	77	3	77	5.5	7	3	0
Natural, Greek Style, Milbona, Lidl*	1 Pot/125g	135	10.6	108	3.2	4.3	8.5	0.5
Natural, Greek Style, Organic, Tesco*	1 Pot/500g	665	50	133	4.5	6.2	10	0
Natural, Greek Style, Probiotic, Unsweetened, M&S*	1 Serving/150g	195	15.2	130	5.5	4.6	10.1	0.1
Natural, Greek Style, Strained, 0% Fat, Liberte, Yoplait*	¼ Pot/125g	70	0.1	56	9.6	3.2	0.1	0.1
Natural, Live, No Added Sugar, Glenilen Farm*	1 Portion/100g	73	3.6	73	4.3	3.7	3.6	0
Natural, Longley Farm*	1 Pot/150g	118	5.2	79	4.8	7	3.5	0
Natural, Low Fat, Average	***1 Med Pot/125g***	***75***	***1.6***	***60***	***5.4***	***7***	***1.3***	***0***
Natural, Low Fat, Everyday Value, Tesco*	1 Pot/125g	78	1.9	62	5	7.2	1.5	0
Natural, Low Fat, Live, Waitrose*	1 Pot/175g	114	1.8	65	5.8	8.2	1	0
Natural, Low Fat, Organic, Average	***1 Serving/100g***	***87***	***1.2***	***87***	***5.7***	***7.7***	***1.2***	***0***
Natural, Probiotic, Fat Free, Organic, Yeo Valley*	1 Pot/150g	87	0.2	58	5.9	8.4	0.1	0
Natural, Probiotic, Organic, Yeo Valley*	1 Pot/120g	98	5	82	4.6	6.5	4.2	0
Natural, Whole Milk, Set, Biopot, Onken*	1 Serving/125g	85	4.4	68	4.5	4.1	3.5	0
Natural, Wholemilk, Live Bio, Organic, Waitrose*	1 Serving/100g	88	4.4	88	5.1	7.1	4.4	0
Nectarine, Fat Free, Weight Watchers*	1 Pot/110g	45	0.1	41	4.1	4.8	0.1	0.3
Orange Blossom Honey, Finest, Tesco*	1 Pot/150g	237	10.6	158	3.5	20.1	7.1	0
Orange with Chocolate Flakes, Fat Free, Brooklea, Aldi*	1 Pot/165g	84	0.8	51	3.5	8.3	0.5	0.5
Orange, Low Fat, Tesco*	1 Pot/125g	114	2.2	91	4.3	14.5	1.8	0
Orange, Sprinkled with Dark Chocolate, Brooklea, Aldi*	1 Pot/165g	73	0.8	44	3.5	6.9	0.5	0.5
Orange, Sprinkled with Dark Chocolate, Light, Muller*	1 Pot/165g	91	0.8	55	4.3	7.4	0.5	0.1
Original, Dairy Free, Koko*	1 Serving/100g	79	4.9	79	0.6	8	4.9	0.2
Passion Fruit, Greek Style, Luxury, Oykos, Danone*	1 Pot/110g	163	9.1	148	2.9	15.4	8.3	0.1
Passion Fruit, Soya, Go On, Alpro*	1 Pot/150g	126	4.4	84	5.2	8.5	2.9	1.4
Peach & Apricot, HL, Tesco*	1 Pot/92g	42	0.1	46	4	7.4	0.1	1
Peach & Mango, Thick & Creamy, Waitrose*	1 Pot/125g	136	3.1	109	3.7	17.8	2.5	0.3
Peach & Passion Fruit, Layers, Mullerlight, Muller*	1 Pot/175g	94	0.2	54	3.1	9.7	0.1	0.2

YOGHURT

INFO/WEIGHT	Measure	per Measure		Nutrition Values per 100g / 100ml				
		KCAL	FAT	KCAL	PROT	CARB	FAT	FIBRE
Peach & Vanilla, Thick & Creamy, Co-Op*	1 Pot/150g	180	6.9	120	3.6	16	4.6	0.1
Peach & Apricot, Fruit Corner, Muller*	1 Pot/150g	160	5.7	107	3.9	13.5	3.8	0.5
Peach & Pineapple, Fat Free, Mullerlight, Muller*	1 Pot/175g	89	0.2	51	4.3	7.7	0.1	0.2
Peach Melba, Low Fat, Average	*1 Serving/100g*	*75*	*0.7*	*75*	*2.6*	*14.5*	*0.7*	*0*
Peach, & Pear, Soya, No Bits, Alpro*	1 Pot/125g	99	2.5	79	3.7	10.7	2	1
Peach, Bio, Activia, Fat Free, Danone*	1 Sm Pot/125g	71	0.1	57	4.7	9.3	0.1	1
Peach, Dairy Free, Organic, Yofu, Soya, Provamel*	1 Serving/125g	100	2.8	80	3.9	10.3	2.2	0.8
Peach, Garden Fruits, Fat Free, Benecol*	1 Pot/125g	79	0.6	63	3	11	0.5	2.2
Peach, Greek Style, Luxury, Oykos, Danone*	1 Pot/110g	154	8.9	140	3.1	13.4	8.1	0.3
Peach, Low Fat, Average	*1 Serving/100g*	*86*	*1.1*	*86*	*4.5*	*14.6*	*1.1*	*0.2*
Peach, Summer Fruits, Weight Watchers*	1 Pot/120g	58	0.1	48	4.1	6.8	0.1	0.2
Peaches & Cream, Intensely Creamy, Activia, Danone*	1 Pot/120g	118	3.6	98	4.8	13	3	0.3
Pineapple & Peach, Fruity, Mullerlight, Muller*	1 Pot/175g	89	0.2	51	4.2	7.7	0.1	0.2
Pineapple, Average	*1 Serving/100g*	*73*	*1.1*	*73*	*4.4*	*11.3*	*1.1*	*0.5*
Pineapple, Low Fat, Average	*1 Serving/100g*	*89*	*1.2*	*89*	*4.6*	*14.7*	*1.2*	*0*
Pineapple, Virtually Fat Free, Tesco*	1 Pot/125g	55	0.2	44	4.1	6.5	0.2	0.9
Plain, Go On, Alpro*	1 Portion/100g	71	3.6	71	6.2	2.5	3.6	1.5
Plain, Low Fat, Average	*1 Serving/100g*	*63*	*1.6*	*63*	*5.2*	*7*	*1.6*	*0*
Plain, Soya, Average	*1oz/28g*	*20*	*1.2*	*72*	*5*	*3.9*	*4.2*	*0*
Plain, Soya, Simply, Alpro*	1 Tbsp/20g	10	0.5	50	4	2.1	2.3	1
Plain, Whole Milk, Average	*1oz/28g*	*22*	*0.8*	*79*	*5.7*	*7.8*	*3*	*0*
Plain, with Almond, Soya, Alpro*	1 Tbsp/20g	11	0.6	54	3.9	2.3	2.8	1.1
Plain, with Coconut, Soya, Alpro*	1 Tbsp/20g	11	0.6	55	3.9	2.3	3	0.8
Plum, & Custard, Greek Style, 0% Fat, COU, M&S*	1 Pot/141g	83	0.3	59	6.4	8	0.2	0.5
Plum, BGTY, Sainsbury's*	1 Pot/125g	69	0.1	55	4.8	8.8	0.1	0.1
Pomegranate, Soya, Alpro*	1 Pot/125g	92	2.4	74	3.6	9.5	1.9	1.1
Protein Greens, Mango, Kale, & Lime, 20g, Arla*	1 Pot /200g	155	1.2	77	10.1	8	0.6	0
Prune, Bio, Activia, Danone*	1 Pot/125g	122	4.1	98	3.6	13.1	3.3	0.8
Prune, Live, M&S*	1 Pack/159g	254	6.5	160	5.4	24.4	4.1	1.7
Prune, Vitality, Low Fat, with Omega 3, Muller*	1 Pot/150g	144	2.8	96	4.7	15	1.9	1.1
Raspberries & Cream, The Best, Morrisons*	1 Pot/150g	205	9.7	137	3.2	16.2	6.5	0.3
Raspberry & Cranberry, Very Low Fat, Ann Forshaw's*	1 Pot/125g	91	0.1	73	4.6	14.2	0.1	0.2
Raspberry & Cranberry, Fat Free, Milbona, Lidl*	1 Yoghurt/174g	87	0.2	50	4.2	7.8	0.1	0.5
Raspberry & Cranberry, Fat Free, Mullerlight, Muller*	1 Pot/175g	91	0.2	52	4.3	7.8	0.1	0.5
Raspberry & Cranberry, Granola, Duo, Brooklea, Aldi*	1 Pot/135g	178	6.1	132	3.8	18.5	4.5	0.8
Raspberry or Strawberry, Smooth (No Bits), Ski, Nestle*	1 Pot/120g	118	3.2	98	3.9	13.6	2.7	0
Raspberry, & Cranberry, Soya, Alpro*	1 Pot/125g	94	2.4	75	3.6	9.7	1.9	1.1
Raspberry, Bio Live, Low Fat, Rachel's Organic*	1 Pot/125g	114	2	91	4.1	15.1	1.6	0.1
Raspberry, Bio, Activia, Danone*	1 Pot/125g	112	3.5	90	3.5	12.8	2.8	2
Raspberry, Bio, Activia, Fat Free, Danone*	1 Pot/125g	68	0.1	54	4.7	7.2	0.1	2.6
Raspberry, Bio, Low Fat, Benecol*	1 Pot/125g	99	0.8	79	3.8	14.5	0.6	0
Raspberry, Bio, Low Fat, Sainsbury's*	1 Pot/150g	146	1.7	97	4.7	17	1.1	0.7
Raspberry, Extremely Fruity, M&S*	1 Pot/200g	190	3	95	5	15.6	1.5	0.5
Raspberry, Fat Free, Average	*1 Serving/100g*	*64*	*0.1*	*64*	*4.9*	*11*	*0.1*	*1.7*
Raspberry, Fat Free, Probiotic, Organic, Yeo Valley*	1 Pot/125g	98	0.1	78	5.2	14	0.1	0.4
Raspberry, Lactose Free, Lactofree, Arla*	1 Pot/125g	130	3.4	104	3.3	16.5	2.7	0.7
Raspberry, Low Fat, Average	*1 Serving/100g*	*83*	*1.1*	*83*	*4.1*	*14.1*	*1.1*	*0.8*
Raspberry, Low Fat, Stapleton*	1 Serving/150g	105	0.8	70	3.3	13.6	0.5	2
Raspberry, Organic, Yeo Valley*	1 Pot/150g	152	5.8	101	4.2	12.3	3.9	0.4
Raspberry, Probiotic, Live, Yeo Valley*	1 Pot/125g	106	1.2	85	5.1	14	1	0.4
Raspberry, Probiotic, Low Fat, Organic, M&S*	1 Pot/170g	128	2.4	75	4.4	11.5	1.4	0.4
Raspberry, Razzle, Greek Style, Light & Free, Danone*	1 Pot/115g	61	0.1	53	4.7	7.8	0.1	1.1
Raspberry, Scottish, The Best, Morrisons*	1 Pot/150g	208	10.4	139	3.6	15.6	6.9	1.3

Y

YOGHURT

INFO/WEIGHT	Measure	per Measure KCAL	per Measure FAT	Nutrition per 100g KCAL	PROT	CARB	FAT	FIBRE
Raspberry, Summer Fruits, Benecol*	1 Pot/120g	109	2	91	3.7	15	1.7	0.4
Raspberry, Summer, Biopot, Onken*	1/5 Pot/90g	91	2.4	101	3.8	15	2.7	0.6
Red Berry, Vitality, Low Fat, with Omega 3, Muller*	1 Pot/150g	138	2.8	92	4.3	13.8	1.9	0.7
Red Cherry, Fruit Corner, Muller*	1 Pot/150g	158	5.8	105	3.8	13	3.9	0.5
Red Cherry, Summer Fruits, Benecol*	1 Pot/120g	103	2	86	3.7	14	1.7	0.1
Rhubarb & Beetroot, Icelandic Style, Skyr, Arla*	1 Tub/149g	103	0.3	69	9.4	7.1	0.2	0.6
Rhubarb & Fiery Ginger, Greek Style , Brooklea, Aldi*	1/3 Pot/150g	207	11	138	3	15	7.3	0.5
Rhubarb & Vanilla, Gourmet, The Collective Dairy*	1 Bowl/100g	124	5	124	4.9	14.7	5	0
Rhubarb Crumble, Inspired, Mullerlight, Muller*	1 Pot/172g	86	0.2	50	4.1	7.5	0.1	0
Rhubarb, Bio Live, Low Fat, Luscious, Rachel's Organic*	1 Pot/125g	104	2	83	4	13.1	1.6	0.1
Rhubarb, Eat Smart, Morrisons*	1 Pot/190g	79	0.2	42	4.1	6.1	0.1	1.4
Rhubarb, Fruity, Mullerlight, Muller*	1 Pot/175g	91	0.2	52	4.2	7.9	0.1	0
Rhubarb, Longley Farm*	1 Pot/150g	165	5.6	110	4.9	14.3	3.7	0
Rhubarb, Low Fat, Average	*1 Serving/100g*	*83*	*1.2*	*83*	*4.6*	*13.3*	*1.2*	*0.2*
Rhubarb, Low Fat, Garden Fruits, Tesco*	1 Pot/125g	119	2.4	95	3	15.5	1.9	0.3
Rhubarb, Natural, Live, Glenilen Farm*	1 Pot/160g	133	4.6	83	3.5	12.6	2.9	0
Rhubarb, Spiced, Thick & Creamy, COU, M&S*	1 Pot/170g	68	0.2	40	4.3	5.8	0.1	0.5
Salted Caramel, Greek Style, Luxury, Oykos, Danone*	1 Pot/110g	172	9.2	157	2.7	17.6	8.4	0
Senga Strawberry, Deluxe, Lidl*	1 Pot/150g	196	9.8	131	2.7	15	6.5	0.6
Sicilian Lemon, Italian Dream, Corner, Muller*	1 Pot/150g	170	5.7	113	3.9	15.1	3.8	0
Skinny Latte, Fat Free, Mullerlight, Muller*	1 Pot/165g	84	0.2	51	4.1	7.7	0.1	0
Smooth Toffee, Fat Free, Mullerlight, Muller*	1 Pot/175g	89	0.2	51	4.1	7.9	0.1	0
Strawberries & Cream, 0.06% Fat, TTD, Sainsbury's*	1 Pot/150g	183	8.2	122	3.5	14.7	5.5	0.4
Strawberries & Cream, Finest, Tesco*	1 Pot/150g	206	10.4	137	3.4	15.4	6.9	0.5
Strawberries & cream, The Best, Morrisons*	1 Pot/150g	196	9.4	131	3	15.5	6.3	0
Strawberry & Raspberry, High In Protein , Go On, Alpro*	1 Pot/150g	128	4.2	85	5.1	8.8	2.8	1.2
Strawberry Crumble, Crunch Corner, Muller*	1 Pot/150g	234	8.4	156	3.6	22.9	5.6	0.5
Strawberry Rice, Low Fat, Muller*	1 Pot/180g	193	4.1	107	3.2	18.4	2.3	0.4
Strawberry Shortcake, Crunch Corner, Muller*	1 Pot/135g	212	8	157	4.1	21.2	5.9	0.1
Strawberry, & Banana, Soya, No Bits, Alpro*	1 Pot/125g	99	2.5	79	3.7	10.7	2	1
Strawberry, Active, Fat Free, Optifit, Aldi*	1 Tub/125g	54	0.5	43	3	7.1	0.4	0.4
Strawberry, Bio, Activia, Danone*	1 Pot/125g	124	4.1	99	3.6	13.6	3.3	0.2
Strawberry, Bio, Low Fat, Dale Farm*	1 Pot/125g	125	2.1	100	3.9	17	1.7	0.2
Strawberry, Eat Smart, Morrisons*	1 Pot/200g	116	0.6	58	5.7	8.5	0.3	0.3
Strawberry, Everyday Low Fat, Co-Op*	1 Pot/125g	88	0.9	70	3	13	0.7	0
Strawberry, Fat Free, Average	*1 Serving/100g*	*66*	*0.1*	*66*	*4.9*	*11.1*	*0.1*	*0.6*
Strawberry, Fat Free, Probiotic, Organic, Yeo Valley*	1 Pot/125g	108	1.2	86	5.1	14.1	1	0.1
Strawberry, Greek Style, 0% Fat, Liberte, Yoplait*	1 Pot/100g	79	0.2	79	8	11	0.2	0.4
Strawberry, Greek Style, Fat Free, Brooklea, Aldi*	1 Pot/125g	72	0.3	57	4.9	8.8	0.2	0.2
Strawberry, Greek Style, Fruitopolis, Mullerlight, Muller*	1 Pot/130g	84	0.1	65	4.8	10.8	0.1	0
Strawberry, Greek Style, Luxury, Oykos, Danone*	1 Pot/110g	159	8.9	145	3.2	14.6	8.1	0.3
Strawberry, Greek Style, Milbona, Lidl*	1 Pot/125g	160	7.8	128	2.4	15.5	6.2	0.5
Strawberry, Happy Shopper*	1 Pot/150g	130	0.4	87	3	18.5	0.3	0
Strawberry, Lactose Free, Lactofree, Arla*	1 Pot/125g	126	3.2	101	3.5	15.9	2.6	0.4
Strawberry, Light, Brooklea, Aldi*	1 Pot/200g	154	0.2	77	6.1	12.9	0.1	0.4
Strawberry, Low Fat, Average	*1 Serving/100g*	*81*	*1*	*81*	*4.5*	*13.6*	*1*	*0.2*
Strawberry, Low Fat, Probiotic, Organic, M&S*	1 Pot/170g	136	2.4	80	4.8	11.6	1.4	0.4
Strawberry, Milbona, Lidl*	1 Pot/175g	175	5.2	100	3	15	3	0
Strawberry, Organic, Yeo Valley*	1 Pot/150g	159	5.7	106	4.7	13.2	3.8	0.1
Strawberry, Probiotic, Organic, Yeo Valley*	1 Pot/125g	125	5	100	4.4	11.7	4	0.1
Strawberry, Protein 20g, Arla*	1 Pot/200g	140	0.4	70	10	6.5	0.2	0
Strawberry, Smooth Set French, Low Fat, Sainsbury's*	1 Pot/125g	112	4	90	3.7	11.8	3.2	0
Strawberry, Summer Fruits, Benecol*	1 Pot/120g	102	2	85	3.7	13	1.7	0.2

Y

YOGHURT

INFO/WEIGHT	Measure			Nutrition Values per 100g / 100ml				
		KCAL	FAT	KCAL	PROT	CARB	FAT	FIBRE
Strawberry, Thick & Creamy, Co-Op*	1 Pot/150g	182	6.9	121	3.6	16.4	4.6	0.1
Strawberry, Totally, Low Fat, CBY, Asda*	1 Pot/125g	104	1.2	83	4.1	14.2	1	0.4
Strawberry, Virtually Fat Free, Average	*1 Serving/100g*	*65*	*0.2*	*65*	*4.7*	*11.3*	*0.2*	*0.2*
Strawberry, Yoplait*	1 Pot/125g	61	0.2	49	4.2	7.6	0.2	0.9
Tempting Toffee, Greek Style, Muller Light *	1 Pot/120g	84	0.1	70	6.3	10.1	0.1	0
Timperley Rhubarb, TTD, Sainsbury's*	1 Pot/150g	170	9.9	113	3.2	10.1	6.6	0.5
Toffee & Vanilla, Fat Free, Multipack, Weight Watchers*	1 Vanilla/120g	53	0.1	45	4.2	6	0.1	0.6
Toffee with Chocolate Hoops, Crunch Corner, Muller*	1 Pot/135g	209	7.8	155	4.2	20.8	5.8	0.2
Toffee, Light, HL, Tesco*	1 Pot/200g	80	0.2	40	3.9	5.9	0.1	1
Toffee, Low Fat, Average	*1 Pot/125g*	*136*	*3.1*	*109*	*4.3*	*19.5*	*2.4*	*0.1*
Toffee, Low Fat, Deliciously Silky, Waitrose*	1 Pot/151g	143	3	95	4.6	14.5	2	0.5
Total 0% Greek with Blueberries, Total, Fage*	1 Serving/150g	123	0	82	8.3	12.3	0	0
Tropical Fruit, Bio, Granola, Corner, Muller*	1 Pot/135g	161	3.2	119	5.4	18.2	2.4	0.6
Tropical, Granola, Duo, Brooklea, Aldi*	1 Pot/135g	177	6.2	131	3.6	18.5	4.6	0.8
Turkish Cream, Yayla*	1 Serving/100g	83	6	83	3.6	3.7	6	0
Vanilla Choco Balls, Crunch Corner, Muller*	1 Pot/135g	201	7.4	149	4.1	20.2	5.5	0.2
Vanilla Flavour, Weight Watchers*	1 Pot/120g	47	0.1	39	4.2	5.2	0.1	0.2
Vanilla, & Chocolate Sprinkles, Fat Free, Milbona, Lidl*	1 Pot/175g	93	0.9	53	3.9	7.6	0.5	0.1
Vanilla, Average	*1 Serving/120g*	*100*	*5.4*	*83*	*4.5*	*12.4*	*4.5*	*0.8*
Vanilla, Cashew Milk, Dairy Free, Nush Foods*	1 Pot/125g	88	5.2	70	2	3	4.2	0
Vanilla, Creamy, with Mini Smarties, Nestle*	1 Pot/120g	182	6.5	152	3.6	21.5	5.4	0
Vanilla, Fat Free, Skyr*	1 Pot/170g	95	0.3	56	9.8	3.7	0.2	0.5
Vanilla, Low Fat, Probiotic, Organic, M&S*	1 Serving/100g	85	1.8	85	6.2	10.9	1.8	0
Vanilla, Madagascan, Deluxe, Lidl*	1 Pot/150g	212	10.2	141	2.7	17	6.8	0.5
Vanilla, Onken*	1 Serving/100g	100	2.7	100	3.1	15.9	2.7	0
Vanilla, Organic, Probiotic, Fat Free, Yeo Valley*	1 Pot/500g	400	0.5	80	5.4	14.2	0.1	0
Vanilla, Proviact, Milbona, Lidl*	1 Pot/150g	154	4.2	103	4	14.6	2.8	0
Vanilla, Smooth, Light, Fat Free, Mullerlight, Muller*	1 Pot/175g	88	0.2	50	4.3	7.2	0.1	0
Vanilla, Soya, Alpro*	1oz/28g	21	0.6	75	3.7	9.5	2.2	1
Vanilla, Soya, Pots, Eat Well, M&S*	1 Pot/86g	74	1.9	86	4	12.6	2.2	0.1
Vanilla, Sprinkled with Dark Chocolate, Brooklea, Aldi*	1 Pot/165g	82	0.8	50	3.5	8.2	0.5	0.5
Vanilla, Thick & Creamy, Channel Island, M&S*	1 Pot/150g	188	6.6	125	4.5	17.5	4.4	1
Vanilla, Virtually Fat Free, Yeo Valley*	1 Pot/150g	122	0.2	81	5.1	15	0.1	0
Velvety Vanilla, Intensely Creamy, Activia, Danone*	1 Pot/120g	116	3.6	97	4.8	12.7	3	0.1
Wild Berry, Oatie Breakfast, Moma Foods*	1 Pot/235g	317	4.2	135	4.3	25.6	1.8	2.7
Wild Blackberry, Seriously Fruity, Waitrose*	1 Pot/125g	120	1.3	96	4.4	17.2	1	0.4
with Blueberry, Icelandic Style, Skyr, Brooklea, Aldi*	1 Pot/150g	122	0.8	81	7.7	12	0.5	0.5
with Golden Honey, Greek Style, Activia, Danone*	1 Pack/126g	122	3.5	97	5	13	2.8	0.1
with Honey, Greek Style, Morrisons*	1/3 Pot/150g	236	14.3	157	4.1	13.5	9.5	0.7

YOGHURT DRINK

INFO/WEIGHT	Measure			Nutrition Values per 100g / 100ml				
Actimel, Blueberry, Danone*	1 Bottle/100g	74	1.5	74	2.6	11.8	1.5	0.5
Average	*1fl oz/30ml*	*19*	*0*	*62*	*3.1*	*13.1*	*0*	*0*
Blueberry & Blackcurrant, Skyr, Arla*	1 Bottle/350ml	214	0.7	61	5.8	8.1	0.2	0
Cholesterol Lowering, Asda*	1 Bottle/100g	76	1.4	76	2.9	13	1.4	1
Fruit, Mixed, Actimel, Danone*	1 Bottle/100ml	88	1.5	88	2.7	16	1.5	0
Light, Benecol*	1 Bottle/67.5g	40	1.4	60	2.8	7.3	2.1	0.1
Light, Yakult*	1 Bottle/65ml	27	0	42	1.4	10.2	0	1.8
Multi Fruit, Actimel, Danone*	1 Bottle/100g	85	1.5	85	2.7	14.4	1.5	0.1
Orange, Pro Activ, Cholesterol, Flora*	1 Bottle/100g	45	1.5	45	3.2	5.6	1.5	1.1
Original, 0.1% Fat, Actimel, Danone*	1 Bottle/100g	28	0.1	28	2.8	3.3	0.1	1.9
Peach & Apricot, Benecol*	1 Bottle/67.5g	38	1.5	56	2.8	6.2	2.2	0
Strawberry, Actimel, Danone*	1 Bottle/100g	74	1.5	74	2.9	11.5	1.5	0
Strawberry, Benecol*	1 Bottle/67.5g	38	1.4	56	3.2	6.2	2	0

	Measure INFO/WEIGHT	per Measure KCAL	FAT	Nutrition Values per 100g / 100ml KCAL	PROT	CARB	FAT	FIBRE
YOGHURT DRINK								
Yakult*	1 Pot/65ml	43	0.1	66	1.3	14.7	0.1	0
YORKIE								
Honeycomb, Nestle*	1 Bar/65g	331	16.8	509	5.7	63.6	25.8	0
King Size, Nestle*	1 Bar/83g	445	26.1	537	6.1	57.3	31.5	0
Original, Nestle*	1 Bar/55g	302	17.4	546	6.2	57.9	31.5	1.9
Peanut, Rowntree*	1 Bar/43g	248	16.5	576	10.8	45.4	38.3	3.1
Raisin & Biscuit, Nestle*	1 Bar/66.5g	338	16.9	508	5.3	61.9	25.4	1.7
YORKSHIRE PUDDING								
& Beef Dripping, M&S*	4 Puddings/100g	410	30.4	410	9.4	25.2	30.4	3.2
3", Baked, Aunt Bessie's*	1 Pudding/36g	91	2.8	252	9	36.4	7.9	1.7
4 Minute, Aunt Bessie's*	1 Pudding/18g	52	2	291	10.5	36.6	11.3	2.2
7", Baked, Aunt Bessie's*	1 Pudding/110g	290	9.9	264	8.5	37.4	9	2
Average	***1 Pudding/30g***	***62***	***3***	***208***	***6.6***	***24.7***	***9.9***	***0.9***
Baked, Frozen, 4 Pack, Morrisons*	1 Pudding/34g	82	2.3	241	8.4	36.7	6.7	1.6
Batters, in Foils, Ready to Bake, Frozen, Aunt Bessie's*	1 Pudding/17g	47	1.8	276	9.1	32.6	10.8	1.4
Beef Dripping, Cooked, Specially Selected, Aldi*	1 Pudding/44g	129	5.7	293	9.4	32	13	3
Beef, Mini, Waitrose*	1 Pudding/14g	33	1.3	234	13.5	23.2	9.4	1.3
Frozen, Ovenbaked, Iceland*	1 Pudding/20g	53	1.8	262	7.4	36.8	8.8	3.1
Fully Prepared, M&S*	1 Pudding/22g	63	2.9	285	9.4	31.6	13.2	1.2
Giant, As Consumed, Morrisons*	1 Pudding/104g	264	7.9	254	9.1	36.3	7.6	2.1
Giant, Aunt Bessie's*	1 Pudding/115g	291	7.2	253	9.1	39	6.3	2.3
Home Bake, Rise in 20 Minutes, Baked, Aunt Bessie's*	1 Pudding/25g	43	1.7	174	6	20	7	3.1
Large, The Real Yorkshire Pudding Co*	1 Pudding/34g	103	4.1	304	11.5	37.3	12.1	2.5
Mini, Co-Op*	1 Serving/16g	50	2	312	6.2	43.8	12.5	2.5
Mini, Farmfoods*	1 Pudding/3g	8	0.2	281	9.6	43.2	7.7	1.9
Ready Baked, Smart Price, Asda*	1 Pudding/12g	36	1.1	297	10	44	9	2.8
Ready to Bake, Baked, Aunt Bessie's*	1 Pudding/17g	42	1.4	246	8.5	35.1	8	1.7
Ready to Bake, Sainsbury's*	1 Pudding/18g	48	1.6	263	9.9	35.9	8.9	1.3
Sainsbury's*	1 Pudding/14g	43	2	309	7.9	37.5	14.1	2.9
The Best, Morrisons*	1 Pudding/22g	60	1.8	271	8.3	43	8	1.6
Traditional, Giant, Asda*	1 Pudding/110g	310	11	282	10	38	10	2.3
YULE								
Christmas Roulade	***1 Serving/77g***	***265***	***14.2***	***344***	***4.9***	***38.9***	***18.4***	***1.8***
YULE LOG								
Belgian Chocolate, Finest, Tesco*	1 Slice/93g	294	14.6	316	4.7	38.2	15.7	1.8
Chocolate, Iceland*	1 Serving/75g	243	14.4	324	7.1	29.7	19.2	2.3
Chocolate, Sainsbury's*	1 Slice/35g	153	7.7	432	5	51.6	21.8	4.6
Christmas Range, Tesco*	1 Serving/30g	131	6.4	442	4.9	56.8	21.7	2.8
Mini, M&S*	1 Cake/36g	165	8.4	460	5.7	56.9	23.3	1.1
Penguin, Mini, McVitie's*	1 Roll/24g	107	5.3	453	5.2	58.6	22.3	1.6

ALL BAR ONE

BEEF

	KCAL
Steak, & Frites	1089

BREAD

Rustic, with Olive Oil	711
Rustic, with Olive Oil	711

BREAKFAST

Sausage, Egg, Beans, & Toast, Sm Appetites	469
Vegetarian	838

BREAKFAST - FULL ENGLISH

& Toasted Sourdough	1005
with Spinach & Potato Hash, & Toasted Sourdough	1419

BREAKFAST - PROTEIN POWER UP

Salmon, Egg, Avocado, & Grapefruit, with Salad	372

BREAKFAST CEREAL

Bircher, Blueberry	528

BROWNIES

Chocolate, with Bourbon Vanilla Ice Cream	727
Chocolate, with Vanilla Ice Cream, Sm Appetites	459

BRUSCHETTA

Avocado, & Tomato, Crushed	545

BURGERS

Beef, Classic	967
Beef, Sliders, Sm Appetites	303
Beef, The Californian	1267
Beef, The French	1166
Beef, The Hipster	1243
Beef, The Skinny	549
Beef, The Smoky	1399
Beef, The Spanish	1205
Beef, The Wagyu	1403
Chicken, Grilled, Classic	850
Chicken, Grilled, Sm Appetites	187
Chicken, Grilled, The Californian	1150
Chicken, Grilled, The French	1049
Chicken, Grilled, The Hipster	1126
Chicken, Grilled, The Skinny	432
Chicken, Grilled, The Smoky	1282
Chicken, Grilled, The Spanish	1089

BURGERS VEGETARIAN

Tomato, Beetroot, & Mozzarella	905
Tomato, Beetroot, & Mozzarella, The Californian	1205
Tomato, Beetroot, & Mozzarella, The French	1104
Tomato, Beetroot, & Mozzarella, The Hipster	1181
Tomato, Beetroot, & Mozzarella, The Skinny	487
Tomato, Beetroot, & Mozzarella, The Smoky	1337
Tomato, Beetroot, & Mozzarella, The Spanish	1144

BURRITO

Chicken	776
Chicken, with Fries	1179
Chicken, with House Salad	967

CAKE

Chocolate, Mascarpone, & Orange, Mousse	250
Raspberry, & Pistachio, Traybake	150

ALL BAR ONE

CHEESECAKE

	KCAL
Lemon, Sicilian, with Blueberry Compote, Baked	558

CHICKEN

Skewers, Teriyaki, Ginger	335
Wings, Buttermilk	657

CHICKEN KATSU

Main	702

CHICKEN PIRI PIRI

Half	450
Half, with Fries	853
Half, with House Salad	641

CROISSANT

with Butter, & Jam	662

DOUGHNUTS

Churros	867

DUMPLINGS

Duck, Crispy	400

EGGS

Benedict	733
Benedict, with Avocado	1009
Florentine	728
Florentine, with Avocado	1004
Poached, with Mushrooms, on Toasted Sourdough	461
Royale	807
Royale, with Avocado	1083

EGGS - SCRAMBLED ON TOAST

with Smoked Salmon, on Toasted Sourdough	722

FISH & CHIPS

Main	918

FISH - BATTERED COD

with Mushy Peas, & Tartare Sauce, Sm Appetites	301

FISH CAKES

Haddock, Smoked, & Mustard	291
Haddock, Smoked, & Mustard, with Fries	694
Haddock, Smoked, & Mustard, with House Salad	482

FLATBREAD

Garlic, Stonebaked	1053
Houmous, & Kale	615

FRIES

Potato	403
Potato	403
Potato, Sm Appetites	177
Sweet Potato	505
Sweet Potato	505
Trio	1180

FRUIT

Strawberries, & Bananas, Fresh, Sm Appetites	128

HASH

Potato, Pan Fried, with Spinach & Onion	414
Potato, Spinach, & Onion, Pan Fried	414

HOUMOUS

Duo	715

ALL BAR ONE

ICE CREAM
Trio	318
Vanilla, 2 Scoops, Sm Appetites	243

KEBAB
Chorizo, & Halloumi, Skewers	515

LAMB
Kibbeh	553

MEZZE
Little, Sm Appetites	738

MUFFIN
Blueberry Cheesecake	463
Carrot Cake	459
Chocolate, Triple	505
Lemon, & White Chocolate	462

NACHOS
Original	912
with BBQ Pulled Pork	1425

NOODLES
Pad Thai	523
Pad Thai, Little, Sm Appetites	391
Pad Thai, with Chicken Breast	808
Pad Thai, with Pan Fried King Prawns	707
Pad Thai, with Sliced Beef Fillet	775

ONION RINGS
Tempura	861
Tempura	861

PAIN AU CHOCOLAT
Pastry	425

PANCAKES - BUTTERMILK
with Maple Syrup, Banana, & Berries	491
with Maple Syrup, & Smoked Bacon	568

PASTRY
Spinach & Feta, Bourek	303

PIE
Pecan, Bourbon, with Cinnamon Ice Cream	5470

PLATTER
Brunch Board, for Two, Breakfast, ½ Board	1137
Deli Board, Sharing, Whole Board	1826
Grazing Board, Sharing, Whole Board	2074
Mezze Board, Sharing, Whole Board	1645

POTATOES
Patatas Bravas	283

PRAWNS
King, Pan Fried, Add On	104
King, Pan Fried	410

QUESADILLA
Chicken	423

RIBS
BBQ, Smoked	1494

RICE
Miso, Bowl	474
Miso, Bowl, with Chicken Breast	670
Miso, Bowl, with Pan Fried King Prawns	585

ALL BAR ONE

RICE
Miso, Bowl, with Sliced Beef Fillet	726
Steamed, Sm Appetites	179

ROLL
Bacon, Sour Cream, Chilli Tomato Jam, & Coriander	716

SALAD
Chicken, & Avocado, Chargrilled	618
Duck, Crispy	568
Feta, Carrot, & Quinoa	626
House	191
Side	191
Small Appetites	96
Superfood	440
Superfood, with Chicken Breast	634
Superfood, with Garlic & Lemon Marinated Halloumi	634
Superfood, with Pan Fried King Prawns	654

SANDWICH
Chicken, Grilled, Focaccia	610
Steak, Fillet	606

SORBET
Raspberry, 2 Scoops, Sm Appetites	158
Raspberry	236

SOUP
Tomato, Vegetable, & Quinoa	122

SQUID
Calamari, Salt & Pepper	404

TOAST
Sourdough, with Avocado, & Feta	446

TORTE
Chocolate, Salted Caramel, with Hazelnut Ice Cream	535

TORTILLA
Huevos Rancheros	585

WRAP
Fish Finger	553

ASK ITALIAN

ARANCINI
Pumpkin, Risotto, with Tomato Dip	285

AUBERGINE
Melanzane Al Forno, Main	578
Melanzane Al Forno, Starter	301

BOLOGNESE
Spaghetti, Vegan	849

BREADS / NIBBLES
Fonduta, with Dough Sticks	771
Garlic Bread	588
Garlic Bread Speciale - with Balsamic Onions	838
Garlic Bread Speciale - with Purple Pesto	801
Garlic Bread with Mozzarella	784
Italian Olives	204
Rosemary, & Sea Salt	499

BREADSTICKS
& Tomato, Dip, Tiny Tums, Kids Menu	159

	KCAL		KCAL

ASK ITALIAN

CAKE
Pistachio, & Olive Oil, Vanilla Gelato	452

CALZONE
Con Carne Piccante	970
Pollo	899

CANNELLONI
Sausage, Ragu, Baked, with Creme Fraiche	658

CARBONARA
Linguine	1060
Tagliatelle	882

CHEESECAKE
Honeycomb. with Vanilla Gelato	719

CHICKEN
Pollo, Milanese	480
Pollo, Milanese, with Chips	1051

DESSERTS
Fruity Ice Lolly - Apple, & Raspberry, Kids Menu	43
Panna Cotta	190
Tiramisu	419
Chocolate, Eton Mess, Melting	472
Chocolate Etna	767
Frutti, Kids Menu	14
Fruity Ice Lolly - Orange & Apple, Kids Menu	45
Chocolate Pizza, Kids Menu	244

DESSERTS - GELATO
Chocolate, 2 Scoops	225
Hazelnut	283
Pistachio, 2 Scoops	273
Salted Caramel	252
Strawberry	266
Vanilla	242
Gelato Gondola, Chocolate, & Nut	628
Gelato Gondola, Salted Caramel	536

DESSERTS - MAKE YOUR OWN SUNDAE
Ice Cream, Chocolate, Kids Menu	109
Sauce, Chocolate, Kids Menu	302
Ice Cream, Strawberry, Kids Menu	102
Ice Cream, Vanilla, Kids Menu	117
Sauce, Choconut, Kids Menu	57
Sauce, Strawberry, Kids Menu	22

DESSERTS - SORBET
Mango	179
Rasperry	166

FETTUCCINE
Bolognese	692

GIRASOLE
Spinach, & Ricotta	743

GNOCCHI
Chocolate, Baked	473

LASAGNE
Beef, & Pork, Ragu	717

LINGUINE
Seafood, Con Frutti Di Mare	703

ASK ITALIAN

NUTS
Chilli, Nuts	291

PASTA
with Tomato Sauce, & Cheese, Dip, & Dunk	459
in Tomato Sauce, Tiny Tums, Kids Menu	201
with Butter, Tiny Tums, Kids Menu	245

PASTA CARTWHEELS
in Bolognese Sauce, Kids Menu	424
in Cheese Sauce, Kids Menu	504
in Perfect Pesto Sauce, Kids Menu	509
in Tomato Sauce, Kids Menu	396

PENNE
Arrabiata	759
Arrabiata, with Chicken	869
Chicken, Al Pollo Della Casa	842
in Bolognese Sauce, Kids Menu	452
in Cheese Sauce, Kids Menu	352
in Perfect Pesto Sauce, Kids Menu	537
in Tomato Sauce, Kids Menu	424

PIZZA
	PER PIZZA
Beef, & Gorgonzolla, Prima	948
Black Olives, & Chicken, Kids Menu	480
Black Olives, & Extra Cheese, Kids Menu	594
Black Olives, & Ham, Kids Menu	470
Black Olives, & Mushrooms, Kids Menu	450
Black Olives, & Pepperoni, Kids Menu	529
Black Olives, & Roasted Red Peppers, Kids Menu	444
Black Olives, Kids Menu	136
Caprina, Prima	973
Chicken, & Extra Cheese, Kids Menu	625
Chicken, & Ham, Kids Menu	501
Chicken, & Mushrooms, Kids Menu	481
Chicken, & Pepperoni, Kids Menu	560
Chicken, & Roasted Red Pepper, Kids Menu	475
Chicken, Kids Menu	467
Ham, & Extra Cheese, Kids Menu	615
Ham, & Roasted Red Peppers, Kids Menu	465
Ham, & Smoked Scarmorza Cheese, Prima	1082
Ham, Kids Menu	457
Margherita, Classic	802
Margherita, Extra Cheese, Red Peppers, Kids Menu	589
Margherita, Extra Cheese, Kids Menu	581
Margherita, No Topping, Kids Menu	423
Margherita, Speciale, Alto Base	1137
Mushrooms, & Extra Cheese, Kids Menu	595
Mushrooms, & Ham, Kids Menu	471
Mushrooms, & Roasted Red Pepper, Kids Menu	445
Mushrooms, Kids Menu	437
Pepperoni, & Extra Cheese, Kids Menu	674
Pepperoni, & Ham, Kids Menu	550
Pepperoni, & Mushrooms, Kids Menu	530
Pepperoni, & Roasted Red Pepper, Kids Menu	524
Pepperoni, Alto Base	1338

ASK ITALIAN

PIZZA

	PER PIZZA
Pepperoni, Kids Menu	516
Pollo Picante Con Pancetta, Prima	878
Roasted Red Peppers, Kids Menu	431
Salami, Misti, Prima	1011
Salsiccia, Sausage, Spicy, Prima	1116
Stromboli, Classic	881
Verdure, Classic	793

PORK

Belly, Porchetta	1143

RIGATONI

Meatballs, Ragu, Mozzarella, Al Manzo Piccante	718

RISOTTO

Con Pollo E Funghi	818

SALAD

Caesar, Chicken	815
Cheese, Burrata, Tomatoes, Rocket, Caprese	303
Insalata Di Pollo E Pancetta	743
Mozzarella, & Mixed Grain	501
Salmon, Roast, & Mixed Grain	624

SEA BASS

Al Forno	584

SEAFOOD

Calamari, Breaded	476

SIDES

Baked Broccoli with Chilli Cheese Crumb	147
Chips Garlic & Cheese	892
Mixed Salad	18
Plum Tomatoes, Kids Menu	4
Broccoli, Kids Menu	13
Side Salad, Kids Menu	44
Courgette Sticks, Battered	281
with Mayo, Side	863

SORBET

Lemon	144

SPAGHETTI

Al Pomodoro, with Mozzarella	672
in Bolognese Sauce, Kids Menu	483
in Cheese Sauce, Kids Menu	563
in Perfect Pesto Sauce, Kids Menu	568
in Tomato Sauce, Kids Menu	455

STARTERS & SHARES

Mushrooms Al Forno	540
Chicken Lecca-Lecca	675
Bruschetta, Marinated Tomatoes, Basil, & Ricotta	321
Baked Dough Ball - Fontal Cheese and Chilli	711
Antipasti - Fritto	1105
Butterfly King Prawns	416
Plain	550
Meatballs Picante	718
Antipasti - Classico, The Mixed One	1310
Tuscan Bean Soup	433

ASK ITALIAN

TAGLIATELLE

Beef, Brisket, Rago	630
Lobster, & Prawn, Aragosta E Gamberoni	652
Pesto, Genovese, Purple	926

TART

Chocolate, & Blood Orange	451
Pear, with Raspberries, & Cream	415

TORTELLINI

Cheese, & Vegetable, with Tomato Sauce, & Cheese	281

VEGETABLES

Vegetable Sticks with Bread Soldiers, Kids Menu	175

BEEFEATER RESTAURANT

BEANS

Baked, in Tomato Sauce, Side, Kids Menu	51
BBQ, Spiced, Side	157

BEEF

Duo	1437
Slow Cooked, Kids, Sunday Lunch Menu	644
Slow Cooked, Sunday Lunch Menu	897

BEEF - STEAK

Fillet, 8oz, with Chips	813
Fillet, 8oz, with Chips & Salad	831
Fillet, 8oz, with Side Salad	461
Fillet, 8oz, with Veg Medley	505
Flat Iron, 6oz, with Chips	747
Flat Iron, 6oz, with Chips & Salad	765
Flat Iron, 6oz, with Side Salad	395
Flat Iron, 6oz, with Veg Medley	439
Porterhouse, 18oz, with Chips	1503
Porterhouse, 18oz, with Chips & Salad	1521
Porterhouse, 18oz, with Side Salad	1151
Porterhouse, 18oz, with Veg Medley	1197
Rib-eye, 10oz, with Chips	975
Rib-eye, 10oz, with Chips & Salad	993
Rib-eye, 10oz, with Side Salad	624
Rib-eye, 10oz, with Veg Medley	668
Ribs, & Prawn, Combo	1720
Rump, 10oz, Daytime Saver Menu	898
Rump, 10oz, Daytime Saver Menu	898
Rump, 10oz, with Chips	947
Rump, 10oz, with Chips & Salad	966
Rump, 10oz, with Veg Medley	651
Rump, 10oz, with Side Salad	595
Sirloin, 8oz, Daytime Saver Menu	758
Sirloin, 8oz, with Chips	789
Sirloin, 8oz, with Chips & Salad	808
Sirloin, 8oz, with Salad	437
Sirloin, 8oz, with Veg Medley	482
Tomahawk, 35oz, Sharing, Summer BBQ Specials	3215
with Chips, Kids Menu	461

BREAD

Brown, Buttered, Extra	257
Flatbread, Garlic, & Dips	912

BEEFEATER RESTAURANT

BREAD

Flatbread, Garlic, Strips	1013
Garlic	218
Garlic, Kids Menu	112
White, Buttered, Extra	254

BROWNIES

Chocolate	557
Chocolate, Daytime Saver Menu	570

BURGERS

Beef, Bacon & Cheese, Double	1373
Beef, Bacon & Cheese, Triple	1697
Beef, Kids Menu	587
Steak, Daytime Saver Menu	939
Steak, Double, Daytime Saver Menu	1152
Steak, with Cheese & Bacon, Daytime Saver Menu	1080
Steak, with Cheese & Bacon	1081
Chicken, Tabasco, Crispy	1059
Steak, Smoky BBQ, Summer BBQ Specials	1463

BURGERS VEGETARIAN

Main	910

CAKE

Trio of Sponges, with Custard	695

CAULIFLOWER CHEESE

Sunday Lunch Menu	281

CHEESECAKE

Vanilla, Baked	675

CHICKEN

BBQ, with Half Rack Of Ribs	1025
BBQ, with Whole Rack Of Ribs	1432
Breast, Kids, Sunday Lunch Menu	471
Breast, Plain	693
Breast, Smoky Paprika, Grilled	724
Breast, Smoky Paprika, Grilled, Daytime Saver Menu	632
Escalope, Breast, Breaded	1309
Goujons, Buttermilk, Summer BBQ Specials	742
Half, Roasted, Sunday Lunch Menu	1121
Melt, BBQ Sauce, Grilled	858
Poppin, with Chips, & Beans, Kids Menu	400
Wings, with BBQ, Spicy, 3, Side	160
Wings, with BBQ, Crispy, 5	260
Wings, with BBQ, Crispy, 8	401
Wings, with Piri Piri, Crispy, 5	252
Wings, with Piri Piri, Crispy, 8	394
Wings, with Piri Piri, Spicy, 3, Side	153

CHIPS

Side, Kids Menu	187
Triple Cooked, Side	418
Triple Cooked, Spicy, Side	420

COD

Bites, Breaded, Kids Menu	517

CORN

Cob, Mini, Side	61
Cob, Mini, Side, Kids Menu	29

BEEFEATER RESTAURANT

CRUMBLE

Apple, Toffee, Salted	596

DESSERT

Caramel Apple Betty, with Custard	454
Caramel Apple Betty, with Ice Cream	446
Caramel Apple Betty, with Pouring Cream	488
Caramel Apple Betty, with Whipped Cream	413
Chocolate Challenge, Mini, Kids Menu	342
Mississippi Mud Pie	991

DOUGHNUTS

Mini, Kids Menu	249

FISH & CHIPS

Beer Battered, Daytime Saver Menu	1197

FRIES

Skinny, Side	328
Skinny, Spicy, Side	329

FROZEN YOGHURT

Strawberry	235
Strawberry, Kids Menu	197

FRUIT SALAD

Mixed, Kids Menu	49

GAMMON

Blackened, with Egg, Daytime Saver Menu	751
Blackened, with Pineapple, Daytime Saver Menu	729
Steak, Blackened, in Spicy Rub	1034
Steak, Chargrilled, with Egg & Pineapple	1026
Steak, with Egg, Daytime Saver Menu	746
Steak, with Pineapple, Daytime Saver Menu	723

HADDOCK

Beer Battered, with Chips & Mushy Peas	1031
Beer Battered, with Chips & Peas	993

ICE CREAM

Vanilla, with Caramel Sauce, Kids Menu	254
Vanilla, with Chocolate Sauce, Kids Menu	253
Vanilla, with Raspberry Sauce, Kids Menu	253
with Chocolate Sauce	279
with Chocolate Sauce, Sunday Lunch Menu	275

KEBAB

Pork & Beef, Kofta, Grilled	444

LAMB

Rump, Minted, Grilled	720
Rump, Sunday Lunch Menu	901

LASAGNE

Beef, & Pork, with Chips, Daytime Saver Menu	860
Beef, & Pork, with Salad, Daytime Saver Menu	530

LINGUINE

Roast Vegetable, in Tomato Sauce	563
Roast Vegetable, In Tomato Sauce, with Chicken	718
Roast Vegetable, in Tomato Sauce, with Salmon	1010

MEATBALLS

Arrabiata, in Tomato Sauce, with Ciabatta	336
Arrabiata, Linguine	821

BEEFEATER RESTAURANT

MIXED GRILL
Rump Steak, Chicken Breast, Gammon, Sausage	1741
Flat Iron Steak, Chicken Breast, Gammon, Sausage	1498
Sirloin Steak, Chicken Breast, Gammon, Sausage	1583

MUSHROOMS
Crispy, Flat Cap, in Breadcrumbs	489

NACHOS
with Cheesy Yoghurt Dip, Kids Menu	235

ONION RINGS
Beer Battered, Crispy, Side	221

PASTA
Penne, in Tomato Sauce, Kids Menu	347

PATE
Duck, with Ciabatta	430

PEAS
Side, Kids Menu	47

PIE
Banoffee	701
Beef, & Cheddar, with Mash & Gravy	1397

PLATTER
The Beefeater, Sharing	1400
The Beefeater, with Ribs, Sharing	1807

POTATO MASH
Side, Kids Menu	131

POTATOES
Crushed, Garlic, Side	344
Dauphinoise, Sunday Lunch Menu	320
Dippers, With Cheese, & Bacon, Loaded	587
Dippers, with Cheese, Loaded	482
Dippers, with Cheese, Sharing	1262
Dippers, with Cheese & Spring Onion, Loaded	517
Jacket, Side	438

PRAWN COCKTAIL
Classic, with Ciabatta	423

PRAWNS
Garlic, with Ciabatta	371
King, Garlic, 3, Side	151

PROFITEROLES
Main Menu	490
Daytime Saver Menu	504

RIBS
BBQ, Sticky, Summer BBQ Specials	451
Pork, Sticky Bourbon BBQ, Grill	1320

RISOTTO
Chicken, & Mushroom, Creamy	833
Chicken, & Mushroom, Daytime Saver Menu	831
Mushroom, Creamy	678
Mushroom, Daytime Saver Menu	676

SALAD
BLT, with Egg, Daytime Saver Menu	328
Caesar, Chicken, Goujons, Summer BBQ Specials	986
Caesar, Salmon, Blackened, Summer BBQ Specials	1076
Caesar, Summer BBQ Specials	421

BEEFEATER RESTAURANT

SALAD
Chicken, Jerk, Mango, Summer BBQ Specials	323
Chunky Slaw, Side	149
Greek, Crunchy, Side	173
Halloumi, Jerk, Mango, Summer BBQ Specials	421
Mixed, Large, Side	68
Mixed Bean	604
Salmon, Jerk, Mango, Summer BBQ Specials	621
Side, Kids Menu	6
Steak, with Pear	778

SALMON
Grilled	1014

SANDWICH
Steak, Open, with Fries, Daytime Saver Menu	1066

SAUCE
Bearnaise, Steak Sauces	135
Beef, Rich, Steak Sauces	42
Cheddar, Pulled Ham, & Mushroom, Steak Sauces	98
Peppercorn, Triple, Steak Sauces	41
Prawn & Lobster, Steak Sauces	67

SAUSAGE & MASH
Bangers, Kids Menu	391
Main	835
Vegetarian, Bangers, Kids Menu	361

SEA BASS
Oven Baked, with Crunchy Greek Salad	451

SORBET
Lemon Curd	242

SOUP
Tomato	368

SPAGHETTI BOLOGNAISE
Kids Menu	345

SPINACH
Creamy, Side	123

SUNDAE
Cookie Dough	694
Funny Face, Kids Menu	265
Rocky Road	791

TRIFLE
Strawberry, Pimms, Summer BBQ Specials	699

VEGETABLE MEDLEY
Side	112

VEGETABLES
Sticks, Side, Kids Menu	28
Sticks, with Yoghurt Dip	51

WAFFLES
Apple, Salted, Toffee, Summer BBQ Specials	881

WELLINGTON
Vegetable, Sunday Lunch Menu	1179

WRAP
Chicken Breast, Cheese, Vegetables, Kids Menu	540
Quorn Sausage, Cheese, Vegetables, Kids Menu	540
Salmon, Cheese, Vegetables, Kids Menu	605

BEEFEATER RESTAURANT
YOGHURT

Strawberry, Kids Menu	127

BILL'S
BEEF

Steak, Flat Iron	694
Steak, Minute, with Chips, & Egg, & Garlic Butter	950
Steak, Minute, with Chips, & Garlic Butter	785
Steak, no Chips, Kids	359
Steak, Ribeye, 14oz	830
Steak, Sirloin, 10oz	617
Steak, with Chips, Kids	534

BREAD

Basket, with Butters, ½ Basket	730
Basket, without Butters, Whole Basket	956
Flatbread, Smoky, Italian, ½ Bread	333
Garlic, & Herb, Flatbread, ½ Bread	237
Tortilla, Corn, Spiced, with Guacamole	516
Tortilla, Corn, Spiced, without Guacamole	441

BREAKFAST

with Toast	807
Kids	598

BREAKFAST - BAKED EGGS

with Spicy Beans, & Chorizo	444
with Spicy Beans, & Chorizo, & Flatbread	564

BREAKFAST - FULL ENGLISH

with Toast	1110

BROCCOLI

Long Stem	121

BROWNIES

Chocolate, Warm, no Ice Cream	617
Chocolate, Warm, no Ice Cream, Kids	218
Chocolate, Warm, with Ice Cream	724
Chocolate, Warm, with Ice Cream, Kids	325

BUNS

Bacon	584
Sausage, Cumberland, Breakfast	565

BURGERS

Chicken, Buttermilk, no Chipotle Mayo	772
Chicken, Buttermilk, with Chipotle Mayo	986
Chicken, Fillet, Kids	365
Halloumi	888
Hamburger	696
Hamburger, no Mayo, Kids	372
Hamburger, with Mayo, Kids	522
Lamb, no Tzatziki	804
Lamb, with Tzatziki	833
Naked, with Salad, & Tzatziki, no Bun	525

CAKE

Victoria Sponge	598

CAULIFLOWER CHEESE

for Two, ½ Portion	119

CHEESE

Halloumi, Sticks, Crispy, with Lemon Garlic Mayo	962

BILL'S
CHEESE

Halloumi, Sticks, Crispy, with Lemon Garlic Mayo	962
Halloumi, Sticks, Crispy, no Lemon Garlic Mayo	675

CHEESECAKE

Banana, & Honeycomb	827

CHICKEN

Milanese, with Salad	738
Paillard	596
Mojo Marinated, with Dressed Salad	619

CHICKEN - SKEWERS

Dakkochi	462
Mojo Marinated, with Dressed Salad, & Flatbread	771
Mojo Marinated, with Salad, & Flatbread	674
Mojo Marinated, with Salad	522

CHOCOLATES

Truffles, Salted Caramel, 3 Truffles	168

CRAB CAKES

Baked, with Tartare Sauce	567
Baked, without Tartare Sauce	417
with Egg, & Asparagus	655

CREME BRULEE

Coconut, & Orange Rice	344

CRUMBLE

Plum, & Apple, no Ice Cream	606
Plum, & Apple, with Ice Cream	713

CURRY

Chicken, Thai Green, with Rice	790
Chicken, Thai Green, without Rice	563

DESSERT

Chocolate Bombe, Meltin	862

DHAL - AUBERGINE

Lentil, & Chickpea, Roasted	543
Lentil, & Chickpea, Roasted, with Flatbread	695

DOUGHNUTS - CINNAMON

Mini, Warm, no Sauce	483
Mini, Warm, Salted Caramel & Chocolate Sauce	649

DUMPLINGS

Pork, Sesame, Golden Fried, with Dipping Sauce	451

EGGS

Benedict, with Hollandaise	863
Benedict, without Hollandaise	549
on Toast, Kids	333
Royale, with Hollandaise	909
Royale, without Hollandaise	595
Scrambled, on Toast	555
Scrambled, on Toast, with Bacon	745
Scrambled, on Toast, with Salmon	698

FISH FINGERS

Cod, Kids	271

FRIES

Potato	349
Potato, Kids	175
Sweet Potato	510

BILL'S

FRUIT
Strawberries, & Banana, no Sauce, Kids	93
Strawberries, & Banana, Chocolate Sauce, Kids	198

GNOCCHI
Diablo	928

KALE
Sauteed	104

MACARONI
Kids	502

MACARONI CHEESE
with Mushroom, & Leek	1167

MAYONNAISE
Chipotle	216

MERINGUE
Eton Mess, Lemon	690

MEZZE
Sharing, for 4, ¼ Mezze	302
Veggie, Sharing, for 4, ¼ Mezze	275

MUSHROOMS
Garlic, Sauteed, Chestnut	180

OLIVES
Green, Giant, Gordal	161

OMELETTE
Summer	488

PANCAKES - BUTTERMILK
Kids	326
with Bacon, & Syrup, 3 Stack	844
with Bacon, & Syrup, 5 Stack	932
with Banana, Berries, with Syrup, 3 Stack	548
with Banana, Berries, with Syrup, 5 Stack	820

PATE
Chicken Liver, Oak Smoked, Parfait, with Toast	809
Chicken Liver, Oak Smoked, Parfait, without Toast	528

PIE
Fish	942

RIBS
BBQ, Kids	305
Main	791

SALAD
Caesar, Chicken, without Dressing	627
Halloumi, Grilled, & Pesto Toast, with Dressing	706
Halloumi, Grilled, with Dressing	548
Halloumi, Grilled, no Dressing	356
Halloumi, Grilled, & Pesto Toast, no Dressing	514
Mixed, no Dressing	24
Mixed, with Dressing	121
Salmon, Seared	728
Summer	695
Summer, with Flatbread	815

SANDWICH
Bacon, Kids	512
Fish Finger	725
Sausage, Kids	482

BILL'S

SAUCE
Bearnaise, for Steak	267
Chimichuri, for Steak	173
Garlic Butter, for Steak	193
Peppercorn, for Steak	46

SAUSAGE
Cumberland, Mini, Glazed	696

SAUSAGES
Cumberland, Kids	619

SCONE
with Jam, & Clotted Cream, Warm	709
with Jam, Warm	562

SEA BASS
Pan Fried, with Rosti	147
Pan Fried, without Rosti	465

SOUP
Tomato, Roasted, with Cream	209
Tomato, Roasted, with Cream & Pesto Toast	367
Tomato, Roasted, with Pesto Toast	250
Tomato, Roasted, without Cream & Pesto Toast	92

SQUID
Calamari, Crispy, with lemon Garlic Mayonnaise	756
Calamari, Crispy, without lemon Garlic Mayonnaise	469

SUNDAE
Granola, Breakfast	412
Ice Cream, Vanilla, Kids	292

TART
Ricotta, Red Pepper, & Cheddar, no Dressing	664
Ricotta, Red Pepper, & Cheddar, with Dressing	761

TEACAKES
Toasted, no Butter	267
Toasted, with Butter	527

TOAST
& Butter, Bloomer	356
with Avocado, & Bacon	687
with Avocado, & Poached Eggs	676
with Avocado, & Salmon	640
with Avocado	497
with Beans, Kids	220

TOASTIE
Ham, & Cheese, Kids	478

TORTILLA CHIPS
Corn, Crispy, Kids	247

YOGHURT
Strawberries, Banana, & Honey, Kids	108

BREWERS FAYRE

BEANS
Baked, in Tomato Sauce, Side, Kids Menu	51

BEEF
Steak, Rib-eye, BBQ	1372
Steak, Rib-eye, with Hollandaise Sauce	1443
Steak, Rib-eye, with Peppercorn Sauce	1361
Steak, Rib-eye, with Tennessee Whisky Sauce	1425

BREWERS FAYRE

BEEF
Steak, Rump, Grilled	920
Steak, Sirloin, Grilled	933
Steak & Eggs	1041

BHAJI
Sweet Potato	58

BREAD
Garlic, Kids Menu	110
Garlic, Side, Kids Menu	106
Garlic, with Cheese, Side	316
Naan, Garlic	48
Naan, Plain	38

BROWNIES
Chocolate, with Ice Cream	562

BUBBLE & SQUEAK
Side	348

BURGERS
Chicken, Breaded, The South Western	980
Beef, Bash Street, Kids Menu	697
Beef, Black & Blue, with Chips	1379
Beef, Black & Blue, with Sweet Potato Fries	1312
Beef, Cheese, & Mushroom	1157
Beef, Extra	303
Brie, & Bacon	1443
Chicken, Extra	211
Cluck 'N' Ale, with Chips	1563
Cluck 'N' Ale, with Sweet Potato Fries	1497
Halloumi, Heaven, with Chips	1136
Halloumi Heaven, with Sweet Potato Fries	1069
Smash 'N' Stack, with Chips	1010
Smash 'N' Stack, with Sweet Potato Fries	943
The New Yorker	1161

BURGERS VEGETARIAN
Hot 'N' Spicy, Nacho Burger	1233

BURRITO
Bowl, with Salad	550
Chicken, Bowl	705

CAULIFLOWER CHEESE
Side	281

CHEESE
Brie, Breaded, Bites	326
Halloumi, & Red Pepper, Grilled	235
Mozzarella, Sticks, Extra	330
Mozzarella, Sticks, Side	330

CHEESECAKE
Raspberry, & Prosecco	502

CHICKEN
BBQ, with Full Rack of Ribs, Combo	1743
BBQ, with Half Rack of Ribs, Combo	1375
Bites, Breaded, Kids Menu	525
Breast, Garlic, Breaded	1326
Breast, Smoky Paprika, Grilled	430
Breast, Smothered, BBQ Sauce,	953

BREWERS FAYRE

CHICKEN
Goujons, Southern Fried	477
Half, Roasted, with Chips, BBQ	954
Half, Roasted, with Chips	974
Skewers, Jerk	292

CHICKEN & RIBS COMBO
Full Rack Ribs, with Chips, Coleslaw, & Salad	1637
Half Rack Ribs, with Chips, Coleslaw, & Salad	1322

CHICKEN KATSU
Curry	1037

CHICKEN TIKKA
with Rice	863

CHILLI
Beef, Mexican, with Rice	716

CHIPS
Side	416
Smothered, Creamy Cheese Sauce, Side	551
Smothered, Curry Sauce, Side	467
Smothered, Gravy, Side	436

COD
Bites, Breaded, Kids Menu	642

COLESLAW
Side	139
Side, Kids Menu	40

CORN
Cob, Mini, Side, Kids Menu	29

CRUMBLE
Apple, Toffee, Salted	670

DESSERT
Caramel Apple Betty	454
Chocolate, Mini, Mash Up, Kids Menu	344
Dirty Mud Pie	995
Fondue, Chocolate Fudge, Caramel Sauce, Sharing	1707

DIP
Dessicated Coconut	158

DOUGHNUTS
Cinnamon	547

EMPANADAS
Cheese	401

FISH
Battered	149

FISH & CHIPS
with Mushy Peas	1286
with Peas	1248

FISH CAKES
Single	126

FRIES
Sweet Potato, Side	350
Sweet Potato, Side	350

FROZEN YOGHURT
Strawberry	274

FRUIT SALAD
Kids Menu	49

BREWERS FAYRE

GAMMON
Steak, With Egg, Grilled	917
Steak, with Egg & Pineapple, Grilled	895
Steak, with Pineapple, Grilled	873

GRILLS
Ultimate, Summer	1781
Ultimate, Summer, with Prawns	1983

HADDOCK
Battered, with Chips & Mushy Peas, Atlantic, Giant	1113
Battered, with Chips & Peas, Atlantic, Giant	1075

HOT DOG
The Big Bad Dog, Kids Menu	612

ICE CREAM
Vanilla, with Caramel Sauce, Kids Menu	259
Vanilla, with Chocolate Sauce, Kids Menu	256
Vanilla, with Raspberry Sauce, Kids Menu	256
with Caramel Sauce	271
with Raspberry Sauce	267

LAMB
Shank, Slow Cooked, in Gravy	623

LASAGNE
Beef, & Pork, with Side Salad	634
Sweet Potato & Feta, with Side Salad	742

MIXED GRILL - FLAT ITRON STEAK
Gammon, Chicken Breast, & Sausage	1413

MIXED GRILL - RUMP STEAK
Gammon, Chicken Breast, & Sausage, Ultimate	1657

MUSHROOMS
Garlic, & Herb, Breaded	389

NACHOS
with Cheesy Yoghurt Dip, Kids Menu	230

ONION RINGS
Battered, Side	442

PASTA
in Tomato Sauce, Kids Menu	344

PATE
Chicken Liver, with Toast	388

PEAS
Side, Kids Menu	47

PIE
Chicken, & Chorizo, Creamy Sauce	536
Fish	823
Lemon Meringue, with Cream	606

PIZZA
Chocolate, Kids Menu	375

POPPADOMS
Single	32

POTATOES
Dippers, Crispy	488
Dippers, Loaded, Sharing	1052
Dippers, with Spicy Cheese Sauce, Loaded, Sharing	987

PRAWN COCKTAIL
Starter	343

BREWERS FAYRE

PRAWNS
King, Tempura, with Sweet Chilli	475

PROFITEROLES
with Salted Caramel Sauce	422

PUDDING
Beef, & Doom Bar Ale	1300
Bread & Butter, Summer Berry	587
Jaffa, Sharing	1034
Sticky Toffee	671

RIBS
Full Rack, BBQ	1261
Pork, Full Rack, in Whisky Glaze	1160

SALAD
Chicken, & Bacon, Grilled	434
Chicken, Coronation	549
Halloumi, Grilled	396
Mixed, Side	51
Prawn, Sweet Chilli, Battered	718
Salmon	384

SALMON
Baked, with Hollandaise Sauce	754

SAMOSAS
Vegetable	191

SANDWICH
Chicken, Strip, Spicy, Brown Bread	688
Chicken, Strip, Spicy, White Bread	682
Fish, Goujons, Brown Bread	682
Fish, Goujons, White Bread	676
Ham, & Cheese, Brown Bread	630
Ham, & Cheese, White Bread	624
Prawn, Brown Bread	589
Prawn, White Bread	583

SAUCE
Hollandaise	128
Peppercorn	46
Tennessee Whisky Glaze, Jack Daniels	84

SAUSAGE
Egg, & Chips	996
Pork, Battered	159

SAUSAGES & MASH
Bangers, Kids Menu	391
Vegetarian, Bangers, Kids Menu	364

SCAMPI
Wholetail, Breaded, with Mushy Peas	966
Wholetail, Breaded, with Peas	928

SOUP
Tomato	234

SPAGHETTI BOLOGNAISE
Beano-ese, Kids Menu	320

SUNDAE
Choc-a-block, Cadbury	709
Funny Face, Kids Menu	268

BREWERS FAYRE

	KCAL
SUNDAE	
Salted Caramel, Brownie, & Popcorn	714
TRIFLE	
Strawberry Pimms	634
VEGETABLES	
Green, Medley, Side	112
Sticks, & Cucumber Yoghurt Dip, Kids Menu	49
Sticks, Side, Kids Menu	28
WAFFLES	
Belgian, with Chocolate Honeycomb Ice Cream	604
Belgian, with Salted Caramel Ice Cream	604
WRAP	
Chicken, Build Your Own, Kids Menu	491
Salmon, Build Your Own, Kids Menu	495
Sausage, Quorn, Build Your Own, Kids Menu	491
YORKSHIRE PUDDING	
with Sausage & Mash, Giant	1335

BURGER KING

	KCAL
BITES	
Cheese, Chilli, 4 Bites	238
BREAKFAST - CROISSAN'WICH	
Bacon, Egg, & Cheese	404
Sausage, Bacon, Egg, Cheese, Double	540
Sausage, Egg, & Cheese	600
BROWNIES	
Chocolate, Hottie, with Real Ice Cream	449
BURGERS	
Angus, Angry	760
Angus, Classic	579
Bacon, Double Cheese, XL	890
Big King, Long	620
Big King, XL	1010
Cheeseburger	303
Cheeseburger, Double	431
Cheeseburger, Kids	301
Cheeseburger. Bacon, Double	380
Chicken	392
Chicken, Royale, Bacon, & Cheese	680
Chicken, Tendercrisp, Angry	660
Chicken, Tendercrisp	639
Chicken Royale	567
Chilli Cheese, Long	480
Hamburger	263
Hamburger, Kids	260
King Fish	440
Steakhouse	760
Steakhouse	760
Texas BBQ, Long	540
Veggie, Kids	330
Whopper, Angry	710
Whopper	500
Whopper, Double	840
Whopper, JR	330

BURGER KING

	KCAL
BURGERS VEGETARIAN	
Veggie Bean	547
CHEESE	
Mozzarella, Sticks, 5	340
Mozzarella, Sticks,3	210
CHICKEN	
Nuggets, 4	190
Nuggets, 6	290
Nuggets, 9	440
Strips, Crispy	410
COFFEE	
Cappuccino, Frappe, Iced	360
Cappuccino, Large	360
Cappuccino, Reg	280
Latte	140
DOUGHNUTS	
Chocolate	330
Glazed	210
FRIES	
Apple	28
Large	395
Reg	277
Small	222
Super	469
HASH BROWNS	
Single	276
ICE CREAM	
Cone	120
Oreo, Fusions	264
MILK SHAKE	
Chocolate	430
Oreo	570
Strawberry	430
MUFFIN	
Bacon, King	320
Blueberry Filled	430
Chocolate Filled	482
Sausage, King	428
ONION RINGS	
Large, 12	535
Reg, 5	232
Super, 16	713
PANCAKE	
& Maple Syrup, Mini	268
& Maple Syrup, Mini, 9	360
SALAD	
Chicken, Crispy	210
Garden, Side	15
SANDWICH	
Bacon, Butty	210
SMOOTHIE	
Strawberry, Banana, Iced Fruit, Large	279
Strawberry, Banana, Iced Fruit, Reg	208

BURGER KING

SMOOTHIE
Tropical Mango, Iced Fruit, Large	295
Tropical Mango, Iced Fruit, Reg	221

SUNDAE
Caramel	90
Chocolate	237
Strawberry	223

WAFFLES - WARM BELGIAN
with Real Dairy Ice Cream, & Chocolate Sauce	400
with Whipped Cream, & Chocolate Sauce	364

WRAP
Chicken, BLT	384

CAFFE NERO

BARS
Granola, Organic	278
Oat, with Fruit Seeds & Honey	259
Rocky Road	268

BISCUITS
Amaretti	40
Biscotti, Almond, Organic	147
Biscotti, Chocolate, Organic	136
Double Chocolate	126
Rocco Reindeer, Christmas Special	338
Stem Ginger	264

BOLOGNESE
Pasta, Beef, Oven Bake	521

BREAD
Ciabatta, Roll	180

BREAKFAST CEREAL
Porridge, with Semi Skimmed Milk, no Topping	234
Porridge, with Skimmed Milk, no Topping	210
Porridge, with Soya Milk, no Topping	232

BROWNIES
Chocolate, Belgian	324
Chocolate, Double, GF	319

CAKE
Banana & Walnut Loaf, Wheat Free	236
Blackcurrant & Earl Grey	502
Bruno Bear, Milk & White Chocolate	250
Cappuccino	486
Carrot, & Raisin, Organic, Wrapped	290
Carrot	531
Carrot & Raisin, Wheat Free	292
Chocolate Crunch	308
Chocolate Fudge	500
Chocolate Fudge, Festive	547
Lemon Drizzle, Organic	247
Lemon Drizzle, Slice, Organic, Wrapped	248
Panettone, Classic, Mini	374
Panettone, Mini Chocolate	404
Raspberry & Vanilla Sponge	385
Red Velvet	414
Red Velvet	408

CAFFE NERO

CHEESECAKE
Lemon, Sicilian	341
White & Dark Chocolate	420

CHOCOLATE
Bar, Dark, 50% Cocoa	213
Bar, Milk	223
Bar, Milk, with Hazelnuts	229
Coins	109
Dark, Venezuelan Gold, Willies Cacao, Bar	139
Milk, of the Gods, Willies Cacao, Bar	146
White, El Blanco, Willies Cacao, Bar	159

COFFEE - CAPPUCCINO
Semi Skimmed, Grande	92
Skimmed Milk, Grande	68
Soya Milk, Grande	90
Semi Skimmed, Reg	37
Skimmed Milk, Reg	27
Soya Milk, Reg	36

COFFEE - LATTE
Amaretto, No Cream, Skimmed Milk, Reg	143
Amaretto, Whipped Cream, Skimmed Milk, Reg	315
Caramel, Semi Skimmed Milk	274
Semi Skimmed Milk, Grande	138
Skimmed Milk, Grande	102
Soya Milk, Grande	135
Iced, Semi Skimmed	155
Iced, with Sugar Free Vanilla Syrup	84
Iced, with Vanilla Syrup	205
Praline, No Cream, Skimmed Milk, Reg	154
Praline, with Whipped Cream, Skimmed Milk, Reg	325
Semi Skimmed, Shot of Syrup, Reg	191
Semi Skimmed Milk, Reg	69
Semi Skimmed Milk, Shot Sugar Free Syrup, Reg	74
Skimmed Milk, Reg	51
Soya Milk, Reg	68
Spiced Orange, Reg	155
Spiced Orange, with Cream, Reg	326
Winter Berry, Grande	557
Winter Berry, Reg	488

COFFEE - MOCHA
Semi Skim Milk, no Cream, Reg	150
Skimmed Milk, no Cream, Reg	132
Soya Milk, no Cream, Reg	148
Semi Skimmed Milk, with Whipped Cream, Reg	302
White Chocolate, Semi Skimmed Milk	414

COFFEE BEANS
Chocolate Coated	133

COOKIES
Chocolate, Triple	336
Chocolate Chip, Wrapped	266
Chocolate Chunk, Milk	344
Oat & Raisin	332
Oat & Raisin, Wrapped	241

CAFFE NERO

CRISPS

Cheddar & Spring Onion, Mature	202
Sea Salt	205
Sea Salt & Balsamic Vinegar	199

CROISSANT

Almond	350
Apricot	260
Butter	204
Cheddar & Tomato	305
Cheese Twist	316
Chocolate Twist	320
Ham & Cheddar Cheese	354
Pain au Raisin	320

CUPCAKES

Chocolate	311
Lemon	340
Raspberry	295

DANISH PASTRY

Maple Pecan	312

DESSERT

Triple Chocolate Cup, Luxury	315

DRIED FRUIT & NUTS

Pack	236

FLATBREAD

Mozzarella, & Chargrilled Vegetable	274
Mozzarella, Tomato, & Pesto	306

FRUIT SALAD

Fresh	78

GINGERBREAD

Man, Ginger Giovanni, Iced	189
Man, Gino, Christmas Special	289

HOT CHOCOLATE

Amaretto, No Cream, Reg	284
No Cream, Semi Skimmed Milk, Reg	288
Amaretto, with Whipped Cream, Reg	456
with Whipped Cream, Semi Skimmed Milk, Reg	460
Luxury, No Cream, Reg	199
Luxury, with Cream, Reg	352
Milano, with Whipped Cream	424
Mint, Reg, Whipped Cream, Semi Skimmed Milk	437
No Cream, Semi Skimmed Milk, Reg	235
No Cream, Skimmed Milk, Reg	217
No Cream, Soya Milk, Reg	229
Whipped Cream, Semi Skimmed Milk, Reg	352
with Whipped Cream, Reg	388
No Cream, Semi Skimmed Milk, Reg	290
with Whipped Cream, Semi Skimmed Milk, Reg	462
Spiced Orange, Reg	285
with Cream, Reg	457

JUICE

Apple, Organic, Carton	94
Mango & Passionfruit, Booster	220
Orange, 100% Squeezed, Fresh	95

CAFFE NERO

JUICE

Orange, Lemon & Lime, Booster	207
Raspberry & Orange, Booster	236
Strawberry & Raspberry, Booster	206

LEMONADE

Crushed Raspberry, Iced	96
Iced, Italian	328

MARSHMALLOWS

for Hot Chocolate	20

MILK SHAKE

Banana	315
Banana, Skimmed Milk	284
Banana, with Cream & Sprinkles	402
Chocolate	386
Coffee & Caramel, Creme	367
Double Chocolate, Cream, & Sprinkles	411
Double Chocolate, Skimmed Milk	290
Latte, Caramel	274
Latte, Caramel, Cream, & Sprinkles	369
Latte, Cream, & Sprinkles	334
Latte, Semi Skimmed Milk	225
Mocha Latte, Skimmed Milk	290
Raspberry & White Chocolate, Creme	452
Strawberry	285
Strawberry, with Cream, & Chocolate Sprinkles	403

MILK SHAKE - FRAPPE

Latte, Skimmed Milk	198
Latte, Soya Milk	101
Mint	399
Mint, Semi Skimmed Milk	310
Mint, Skimmed Milk	281
Mocha Latte, Cream, & Sprinkles	386
Mocha Latte, Semi Skimmed Milk	317
Vanilla	266
Vanilla, Skimmed Milk	285
Vanilla, with Cream, & Chocolate Sprinkles	402
Creme, Banana & Caramel	460
Creme, Coconut & Chocolate	516
Creme, Strawberry & Vanilla	469

MINTS

Peppermints, Sugar Free	35

MUFFIN

Apple, & Pecan, Spiced	522
Bacon, & Tomato Sauce, English	277
Blueberry	415
Blueberry, Reduced Fat	351
Chocolate, Triple	503
Chocolate Orange, Filled	486
Cranberry & Orange, Reduced Fat	322
Egg Mayo, with Cheese & Mustard, English	314
Gingerbread Filled	516
Ham, & Egg Mayo, with Cheese, English	314
Lemon Poppyseed	461

CAFFE NERO

MUFFIN

	KCAL
Raisin, Multiseed	475
Raspberry & White Chocolate	422

PAIN AU CHOCOLAT

Pastry	270

PANINI

All Day Breakfast	480
Bacon, & Tomato Sauce, Breakfast	263
Brie, Bacon, & Caramelised Onion	624
Brie & Cranberry, Christmas Special	489
Chicken, Bacon, & Arrabiata Sauce	422
Chicken, Pesto Genovese	424
Chicken, Piri Piri, Seasonal Special	353
Chicken Milanese	428
Chorizo, & Mozzarella, Spicy	461
Four Cheese, & Cranberry Chutney	544
Goats Cheese & Grilled Red Pepper	426
Ham, & Egg Mayo, Breakfast	326
Ham, & Mozzarella	447
Ham, Mozzarella, & Emmental, Tostati	225
Il Genovese	424
Meatball, & Mozzarella, Napoletana	511
Mozzarella, & Tomato, with Pesto	438
Mozzarella, Cheddar, & Tomato, Tostati	220
Mozzarella, Red Pepper, & Roast Tomato	432
Mushroom, Mozzarella & Cheddar	348
Mushroom, with Gorgonzola Cheese	377
Pepperoni, Mozzarella, & Tomato	472
Salami, & Grilled Peppers	451
Three Cheese, & Roasted Tomato, Tostati	170
Tuna, & Mozzarella, Melt	431
Turkey, Stuffing & Cranberry	409

PASTA

Chicken Pesto, Oven Bake	524
Vegetable Arrabiata	434

PIE

Lemon Meringue	299
Mince	361

POPCORN

Sea Salt, Propercorn	88
Sea Salt & Sweet Brown Sugar, Propercorn	129

RISOTTO

Mushroom & Spinach, Creamy	503

SALAD

Chicken with Caesar Dressing	156
Falafel & Tabbouleh	390
Mozzarella & Cherry Tomato, Red Pesto Dressing	276

SANDWICH

Bacon, on Bloomer Bread	365
BLT	442
Cheddar & Pickle, Mature, Malted Wheatgrain Bread	434
Chicken, Salad, & pesto, Roll, GF	359
Chicken, Salad, Malted Wheatgrain Bread	309

CAFFE NERO

SANDWICH

	KCAL
Chicken, with Rosemary Mayonnaise	309
Egg, Bacon & Sausage, on Bloomer Bread	410
Egg Mayonnaise, Free Range	323
Brie & Cranberry, & Turkey & Cranberry, Festive	412
Ham, & Cheddar, Malted Wheatgrain Bread	454
Tuna Mayo, & Cucumber, Less Than 300 Calories	258
Tuna Salad	268

SAUCE

Berry Compote, Topping, for Porridge	47
Maple, Topping, for Porridge	94

SCONE

Fruit, Sultana	287

SHORTBREAD

Bars, Crunchy, All Butter	264

SLICES

Caramel Shortcake	330
Coconut & Raspberry, Gluten & Dairy Free	286
Tiramisu	378

SOUP

Carrot & Coriander	150
Chicken, Cream Of	75
Potato & Leek, Low Fat	129
Spanish Chorizo & Lentil	233
Tomato, Sundried, & Basil	192

SYRUP

Vanilla	122
Vanilla, Sugar Free	5

TART

Apple & Blackcurrant	279
Custard, Portuguese	184
Lemon	331

TEA

Chai Latte, Semi Skimmed Milk	281
Chai Latte, Skimmed Milk	239

TEACAKES

Rich Fruit, Toasted, with Butter	302

WAFFLES

Caramel	356

WRAP

Chicken, Fajita	418
Chicken Caesar	434
Houmous, & Falafel	455
Spicy Bean Fajita	382

YOGHURT

Berry & Granola	223
Blackcurrant, Greek Style, Bio	224
Blueberry, Greek Style, Brunch Pot	198
Blueberry Bircher Muesli, Greek Style, Half Fat	236
Honey, Greek Style, Bio	264
Raspberry, Greek Style	236

	KCAL		KCAL

COSTA

APPLES

	KCAL
Fresh	43

BANANA

Fresh	51

BARS

Granola, Square, Traybake	335

BISCUITS

Biscotti, Almond	77
Fruit, & Oat	224
Ginger, Stem	248
Gingerbread	162
Jammy, Ultimate	310

BREAD

Focaccia, Halloumi, & Roasted Pepper	411

BREAKFAST

Bacon, Roll	389
Bloomer	493
Croissant, Ham, & Emmenthal	358
Oats, Instant, Porridge Pot	294
Porridge	219

BROWNIES

Chocolate	373
Chocolate, GF	418
Mocha, Mini	160

BUTTER

Salted, Extra	48

CAKE

Brioche, Maple, & Pecan, Swirl	267
Caramel, Crisp, Traybake	410
Carrot, Layered	593
Chocolate, Tiffin	457
Fruity, Caramel, Crispie, Bites	536
Lemon, Drizzle, Loaf	322
Peach, Melba, Loaf	332
Raspberry, & Almond, Traybake	465
Raspberry, Brioche, Fingers	141
Sponge, Victoria	537
Sticky Toffee, Brownie, Cakesplosion	501

CHAI

Powder	50

CHOCOLATE

Belgian, Lattice	32
Dark, Blossoms	52
Dusting	8
Flake	44
Gianduja, Milk	47
Magic Dust, Powder	8

CHOCOLATES

Dark, Belgian, Stirrer	55

COFFEE - AMERICANO

No Milk, Massimo	10
No Milk, Medio	8
No Milk, Primo	6

COSTA

COFFEE - AMERICANO

	KCAL
Skimmed Milk, Massimo	27
Skimmed Milk, Medio	16
Skimmed Milk, Primo	12
Soya Milk, Massimo	27
Soya Milk, Medio	21
Soya Milk, Primo	15
Whole Milk, Massimo	38
Whole Milk, Medio	29
Whole Milk, Primo	18

COFFEE - BABYCCINO

Chocolate, with Flake, Skimmed Milk	143
Chocolate, with Flake, Soya Milk	121
Chocolate, with Flake, Whole Milk	143
Chocolate, with Marshmallow, Skimmed Milk	93
Chocolate, with Marshmallow, Soya Milk	102
Chocolate, with Marshmallow, Whole Milk	124
with Marshmallow, Skimmed Milk	64
with Marshmallow, Soya Milk	73
with Marshmallow, Whole Milk	95

COFFEE - CAPPUCCINO

Whole Milk, Massimo, Iced	150
Whole Milk, Medio, Iced	119
Whole Milk, Primo, Iced	85
Popcorn, Full Fat Milk, Medio, Iced	127
Popcorn, Full Fat Milk, Primo, Iced, Costa	92
Popcorn, Skimmed Milk, Massimo, Iced	119
Popcorn, Skimmed Milk, Medio, Iced	95
Popcorn, Skimmed Milk, Primo, Iced	69
Popcorn, Soya Milk, Massimo, Iced	133
Popcorn, Soya Milk, Medio, Iced	106
Popcorn, Soya Milk, Primo, Iced	77
Skimmed Milk, Massimo	111
Skimmed Milk, Massimo, Takeaway	120
Skimmed Milk, Medio	90
Skimmed Milk, Medio, Takeaway	90
Skimmed Milk, Primo	60
Skimmed Milk, Primo, Takeaway	70
Soya Milk, Massimo, Takeaway	150
Soya Milk, Massimo	139
Soya Milk, Massimo, Iced	128
Soya Milk, Medio	112
Soya Milk, Medio, Iced	100
Soya Milk, Medio, Takeaway	112
Soya Milk, Primo	74
Soya Milk, Primo, Iced	71
Soya Milk, Primo, Takeaway	87
Whole Milk, Massimo	209
Whole Milk, Massimo, Takeaway	223
Whole Milk, Medio	168
Whole Milk, Medio, Takeaway	168
Whole Milk, Primo	109
Whole Milk, Primo, Takeaway	129

COSTA

COFFEE - CORTADO

	KCAL
Whole Milk, Solo, Iced	75
Skimmed Milk, Solo	42
Skimmed Milk, Solo, Iced	46
Skimmed Milk, Solo, Takeaway	53
Soya Milk, Solo	55
Soya Milk, Solo, Iced	56
Soya Milk, Solo, Takeaway	69
Whole Milk, Solo	85
Whole Milk, Solo, Takeaway	108

COFFEE - CORTADO, CARAMEL

	KCAL
Skimmed Milk	73
Skimmed Milk, Takeaway	84
Soya Milk	84
Soya Milk, Takeaway	98
Whole Milk	111
Whole Milk, Takeaway	132

COFFEE - ESPRESSO

	KCAL
Decaff, Doppio	6
Decaff, Solo	3
Doppio, Iced	40
Ristretto, Doppio, Iced	38
Ristretto, Solo, Iced	19
Shot	4
Solo, Iced	20
Old Paradise Street, Doppio	6
Old Paradise Street, Solo	3

COFFEE - ESPRESSO, MACCHIATO

	KCAL
Whole Milk, Doppio, Iced	41
Whole Milk, Solo, Iced	21
Skimmed Milk, Doppio, Iced	40
Skimmed Milk, Solo, Iced	20
Soya Milk, Doppio, Iced	41
Soya Milk, Solo, Iced	21

COFFEE - FLAT WHITE

	KCAL
Skimmed Milk, Primo	75
Skimmed Milk, Primo, Takeaway	89
Soya Milk, Primo	98
Soya Milk, Primo, Takeaway	116
Whole Milk, Primo	152
Whole Milk, Primo, Takeaway	178

COFFEE - LATTE

	KCAL
Skimmed Milk, Massimo	132
Skimmed Milk, Massimo, Takeaway	139
Skimmed Milk, Medio	102
Skimmed Milk, Medio, Takeaway	102
Skimmed Milk, Primo	66
Skimmed Milk, Primo, Takeaway	75
Soya Milk, Massimo	175
Soya Milk, Massimo, Takeaway	184
Soya Milk, Medio	135
Soya Milk, Medio, Takeaway	135
Soya Milk, Primo	86

COSTA

COFFEE - LATTE

	KCAL
Soya Milk, Primo, Takeaway	97
Whole Milk, Massimo	269
Whole Milk, Massimo, Takeaway	283
Whole Milk, Medio	207
Whole Milk, Medio, Takeaway	207
Whole Milk, Primo	133
Whole Milk, Primo, Takeaway	149
Whole Milk, Massimo, Iced	263
Whole Milk, Medio, Iced	205
Whole Milk, Primo, Iced	152
Skimmed Milk, Massimo, Iced	179
Skimmed Milk, Medio, Iced	129
Skimmed Milk, Primo, Iced	94
Soya Milk, Massimo, Iced	200
Soya Milk, Medio, Iced	156
Soya Milk, Primo, Iced	115

COFFEE - LATTE, CARAMEL

	KCAL
Skimmed Milk, Massimo, Speciality	190
Skimmed Milk, Massimo, Speciality, Takeaway	355
Skimmed Milk, Medio, Speciality	147
Skimmed Milk, Medio, Speciality, Takeaway	147
Skimmed Milk, Primo, Speciality	96
Skimmed Milk, Primo, Speciality, Takeaway	106
Skimmed Milk, Primo, Speciality, Takeaway	125
Soya Milk, Massimo, Speciality	228
Soya Milk, Massimo, Speciality, Takeaway	240
Soya Milk, Medio, Speciality	176
Soya Milk, Medio, Speciality, Takeaway	176
Soya Milk, Primo, Speciality	114
Soya Milk, Medio, Takeaway	136
Whole Milk, Massimo, Speciality	319
Whole Milk, Massimo, Speciality	267
Whole Milk, Massimo, Speciality, Takeaway	335
Whole Milk, Medio, Speciality	246
Whole Milk, Medio, Speciality, Takeaway	246
Whole Milk, Primo, Speciality	160
Whole Milk, Primo, Speciality, Takeaway	175

COFFEE - LATTE, CARAMEL, ICED

	KCAL
Whole Milk, Massimo, Speciality	257
Whole Milk, Medio, Speciality	203
Whole Milk, Primo, Speciality	150
Skimmed Milk, Massimo, Speciality	161
Skimmed Milk, Primo, Speciality	84
Soya Milk, Massimo, Speciality	195
Soya Milk, Medio, Speciality	151
Soya Milk, Primo, Speciality	112

COFFEE - LATTE, CARAMEL, ICED, SUGAR FREE

	KCAL
Whole Milk, Massimo, Speciality	199
Whole Milk, Medio, Speciality	157
Whole Milk, Primo, Speciality	120
Skimmed Milk, Massimo, Speciality	103
Skimmed Milk, Medio, Speciality	81

COSTA

COFFEE - LATTE, CARAMEL, ICED, SUGAR FREE

Skimmed Milk, Primo, Speciality	62
Soya Milk, Massimo, Speciality	137
Soya Milk, Medio, Speciality	108
Soya Milk, Primo, Speciality	83

COFFEE - LATTE, CARAMEL, SUGAR FREE

Skimmed Milk, Massimo	138
Skimmed Milk, Massimo, Takeaway	168
Skimmed Milk, Medio	106
Skimmed Milk, Medio, Takeaway	106
Skimmed Milk, Primo	68
Skimmed Milk, Primo, Takeaway	78
Soya Milk, Massimo	176
Soya Milk, Massimo, Takeaway	185
Soya Milk, Medio	136
Soya Milk, Primo	87
Soya Milk, Primo, Takeaway	97
Whole Milk, Massimo	267
Whole Milk, Massimo, Takeaway	280
Whole Milk, Medio	206
Whole Milk, Medio, Takeaway	206
Whole Milk, Primo	132
Whole Milk, Primo, Takeaway	147

COFFEE - LATTE, CINNAMON, ICED

Whole Milk, Massimo, Speciality	261
Whole Milk, Medio, Speciality	204
Whole Milk, Primo, Speciality	151
Skimmed Milk, Massimo, Speciality	164
Skimmed Milk, Medio, Speciality	127
Skimmed Milk, Primo, Speciality	93
Soya Milk, Massimo, Speciality	199
Soya Milk, Medio, Speciality	154
Soya Milk, Primo, Speciality	114

COFFEE - LATTE, GINGERBREAD

Skimmed Milk, Massimo, Speciality	195
Skimmed Milk, Massimo, Speciality, Takeaway	205
Skimmed Milk, Medio, Speciality	150
Skimmed Milk, Medio, Speciality, Takeaway	150
Skimmed Milk, Primo, Speciality	96
Skimmed Milk, Primo, Speciality, Takeaway	106
Soya Milk, Massimo, Speciality	233
Soya Milk, Massimo, Speciality, Takeaway	245
Soya Milk, Medio, Speciality	180
Soya Milk, Medio, Speciality, Takeaway	180
Soya Milk, Primo, Speciality	116
Soya Milk, Primo, Speciality, Takeaway	128
Whole Milk, Massimo, Speciality	324
Whole Milk, Massimo, Speciality, Takeaway	340
Whole Milk, Medio, Speciality	250
Whole Milk, Medio, Speciality, Takeaway	250
Whole Milk, Primo, Speciality	160
Whole Milk, Primo, Speciality, Takeaway	178

COSTA

COFFEE - LATTE, GINGERBREAD, ICED

Whole Milk, Massimo, Speciality	264
Whole Milk, Medio, Speciality	206
Whole Milk, Primo, Speciality	152
Skimmed Milk, Massimo, Speciality	167
Skimmed Milk, Medio, Speciality	129
Skimmed Milk, Primo, Speciality	95
Soya Milk, Massimo, Speciality	201
Soya Milk, Medio, Speciality	156
Soya Milk, Primo, Speciality	115

COFFEE - LATTE, GINGERBREAD, ICED, SUGAR FREE

Sugar Free, Full Fat Milk, Massimo, Speciality	198
Sugar Free, Full Fat Milk, Medio, Speciality	156
Sugar Free, Full Fat Milk, Primo, Speciality	120
Sugar Free, Skimmed Milk, Massimo, Speciality	102
Sugar Free, Skimmed Milk, Medio, Speciality	80
Sugar Free, Skimmed Milk, Primo, Speciality	62
Sugar Free, Soya Milk, Massimo, Speciality	136
Sugar Free, Soya Milk, Medio, Speciality	107
Sugar Free, Soya Milk, Primo, Speciality	82

COFFEE - LATTE, ROASTED HAZELNUT

Skimmed Milk, Massimo, Speciality	190
Skimmed Milk, Massimo, Speciality, Takeaway	200
Skimmed Milk, Medio, Speciality	147
Skimmed Milk, Medio, Speciality, Takeaway	147
Skimmed Milk, Primo, Speciality	78
Soya Milk, Massimo, Speciality	228
Soya Milk, Massimo, Speciality, Takeaway	240
Soya Milk, Medio, Speciality	176
Soya Milk, Medio, Speciality, Takeaway	176
Soya Milk, Primo, Speciality	114
Soya Milk, Primo, Speciality, Takeaway	125
Whole Milk, Massimo, Speciality	319
Whole Milk, Massimo, Speciality, Takeaway	335
Whole Milk, Medio, Speciality	246
Whole Milk, Medio, Speciality, Takeaway	246
Whole Milk, Primo, Speciality	160
Whole Milk, Primo, Speciality, Takeaway	175

COFFEE - LATTE, ROASTED HAZELNUT, ICED

Full Fat Milk, Massimo, Speciality	259
Full Fat Milk, Medio, Speciality	202
Full Fat Milk, Primo, Speciality	150
Skimmed Milk, Massimo, Speciality	162
Skimmed Milk, Medio, Speciality	125
Skimmed Milk, Primo, Speciality	92
Soya Milk, Massimo, Speciality	202
Soya Milk, Medio, Speciality	152
Soya Milk, Primo, Speciality	112

COFFEE - LATTE, VANILLA

Skimmed Milk, Massimo, Speciality	195
Skimmed Milk, Massimo, Speciality, Takeaway	205
Skimmed Milk, Medio, Speciality	150
Skimmed Milk, Medio, Speciality, Takeaway	150

COSTA

COFFEE - LATTE, VANILLA

Skimmed Milk, Primo, Speciality	98
Skimmed Milk, Primo, Speciality, Takeaway	106
Soya Milk, Massimo, Speciality	233
Soya Milk, Massimo, Speciality, Takeaway	245
Soya Milk, Medio, Speciality	180
Soya Milk, Medio, Speciality, Takeaway	180
Soya Milk, Primo, Speciality	116
Soya Milk, Primo, Speciality, Takeaway	128
Whole Milk, Massimo, Speciality	324
Whole Milk, Massimo, Speciality, Takeaway	340
Whole Milk, Medio, Speciality	250
Whole Milk, Medio, Speciality, Takeaway	250
Whole Milk, Primo, Speciality	162
Whole Milk, Primo, Speciality, Takeaway	178

COFFEE - LATTE, VANILLA, ICED

Whole Milk, Massimo, Speciality	260
Whole Milk, Medio, Speciality	203
Whole Milk, Primo, Speciality	151
Skimmed, Massimo, Speciality	164
Skimmed, Medio, Speciality	127
Skimmed, Primo, Speciality	93
Soya, Massimo, Speciality	198
Soya, Medio, Speciality	154
Soya, Primo, Speciality	113

COFFEE - MACCHIATO

Skimmed Milk, Solo	9
Soya Milk, Solo	10
Whole Milk, Solo	13

COFFEE - MOCHA

Italia, Espresso, Doppio	6
Italia, Espresso, Solo	3
Skimmed Milk, Massimo	362
Skimmed Milk, Massimo, Takeaway	367
Skimmed Milk, Medio	237
Skimmed Milk, Medio, Takeaway	237
Skimmed Milk, Primo	159
Skimmed Milk, Primo, Takeaway	168
Soya Milk, Massimo	390
Soya Milk, Massimo, Takeaway	396
Soya Milk, Medio	261
Soya Milk, Medio, Takeaway	261
Soya Milk, Primo	175
Soya Milk, Primo, Takeaway	186
Whole Milk, Massimo	456
Whole Milk, Massimo, Takeaway	469
Whole Milk, Medio	317
Whole Milk, Medio, Takeaway	317
Whole Milk, Primo	209
Whole Milk, Primo, Takeaway	228

COFFEE - MOCHA CORTADO

Skimmed Milk	53
Skimmed Milk, Takeaway	71

COSTA

COFFEE - MOCHA CORTADO

Skimmed Milk, Takeaway	84
Soya Milk	85
Soya Milk, New Recipe	61
Soya Milk, Takeaway	85
Soya Milk, Takeaway	100
Whole Milk	114
Whole Milk	82
Whole MilkTakeaway	118
Whole Milk, Takeaway	138

COFFEE - MOCHA CORTADO, ICED

Whole Milk, Solo	102
Skimmed Milk, Solo	77
Soya Milk, Solo	86

COFFEE - MOCHA LATTE

Skimmed Milk, Massimo	390
Skimmed Milk, Massimo, Takeaway	396
Skimmed Milk, Medio	261
Skimmed Milk, Medio, Takeaway	261
Skimmed Milk, Primo	177
Skimmed Milk, Primo	162
Skimmed Milk, Primo, Takeaway	189
Soya Milk, Massimo	342
Soya Milk, Massimo, Takeaway	441
Soya Milk, Medio	289
Soya Milk, Medio, Takeaway	289
Soya Milk, Primo	197
Soya Milk, Primo, Takeaway	215
Whole Milk, Massimo	523
Whole Milk, Massimo, Takeaway	536
Whole Milk, Medio	362
Whole Milk, Medio, Takeaway	362
Whole Milk, Primo	243
Whole Milk, Primo, Takeaway	271

COFFEE - MOCHA LATTE, ICED

Whole Milk, Massimo	399
Whole Milk, Medio	307
Whole Milk, Primo	220
Skimmed Milk, Massimo	302
Skimmed Milk, Medio	231
Soya Milk, Massimo	336
Soya Milk, Medio	258
Soya Milk, Primo	183

COFFEE - MOCHA, ICED

Whole Milk, Massimo	347
Whole Milk, Medio	269
Whole Milk, Primo	190
Skimmed Milk, Massimo	279
Skimmed Milk, Medio	213
Skimmed Milk, Primo	148
Soya Milk, Massimo	303
Soya Milk, Medio	233
Soya Milk, Primo	163

COSTA

COFFEE BEANS
Chocolate Coated	221

COOKIES
Chocolate, Belgian, All Butter	428
Chocolate Chip	377
Chocolate Chip, Triple	368

CREAM
Clotted, Extra	234
Whipping	80

CROISSANT
Almond	351
Plain	314

CRUMBLE
Fruity, Gluten, & Dairy Free	282

CRUMPETS
No Butter, Breakfast	210

CUPCAKES
Banoffee	431

DOUGHNUTS
Choc O Crunch, Milk	275
Choc O Crunch, White	262

DRIED FRUIT
Mango	120

FLAPJACK
Fruity	380
Nutty	425

FROSTINO
Latte, Caramel, Skimmed, Milk, Primo	155
Latte, Caramel, Skimmed Milk, Medio	210

FRUIT & NUT
Mix	204

FRUIT SALAD
Breakfast	80

HONEY
Extra	64

HOT CHOCOLATE
Lindt	163
Powder, Costa*	49
Skimmed Milk, Massimo	353
Skimmed Milk, Massimo, Takeaway	355
Skimmed Milk, Medio	232
Skimmed Milk, Medio, Takeaway	232
Skimmed Milk, Primo	150
Skimmed Milk, Primo, Takeaway	162
Skimmed Milk, Primo, Takeaway	162
Soya Milk, Massimo	387
Soya Milk, Massimo, Takeaway	395
Soya Milk, Medio	258
Soya Milk, Medio, Takeaway	258
Soya Milk, Primo	168
Soya Milk, Primo, Takeaway	183
Whole Milk, Massimo	476
Whole Milk, Massimo	476

COSTA

HOT CHOCOLATE
Whole Milk, Massimo, Takeaway	488
Whole Milk, Medio	328
Whole Milk, Medio, Takeaway	328
Whole Milk, Primo	210
Whole Milk, Primo, Takeaway	233

HOT CHOCOLATE - WITH CREAM & MARSHMALLOWS
Skimmed Milk, Primo, Takeaway	283
Medio, Takeaway	477
Skimmed Milk, Massimo	576
Skimmed Milk, Massimo, Takeaway	542
Skimmed Milk, Medio	380
Skimmed Milk, Medio, Takeaway	392
Skimmed Milk, Primo	276
Soya Milk, Massimo	609
Soya Milk, Massimo, Takeaway	574
Soya Milk, Medio	408
Soya Milk, Medio, Takeaway	416
Soya Milk, Primo	294
Soya Milk, Primo, Takeaway	303
Whole Milk, Massimo	690
Whole Milk, Massimo, Takeaway	656
Whole Milk, Medio	472
Whole Milk, Primo	334
Whole Milk, Primo, Takeaway	480

JAM
Strawberry, Extra	75

JUICE DRINK
Blackberry, & Raspberry, Fruit Cooler, Massimo	310
Blackberry, & Raspberry, Fruit Cooler, Medio	250
Blackberry, & Raspberry, Fruit Cooler, Primo	189
Cherry, & Orange, Cooler, Massimo	292
Cherry, & Orange, Cooler, Medio	230
Cherry, & Orange, Cooler, Primo	172
Mango & Passionfruit, Fruit Cooler, Massimo	295
Mango & Passionfruit, Fruit Cooler, Medio	234
Mango & Passionfruit, Fruit Cooler, Primo	177
Tropical, Cooler, Massimo	257
Tropical, Cooler, Medio	205
Tropical, Cooler, Primo	156

KETCHUP
Sachet, Extra	7

LEMON
Slices	32

LEMONADE
Original, Massimo	145
Original, Medio	115
Original, Primo	87
Raspberry, Massimo	145
Raspberry, Medio	115
Raspberry, Primo	87

MACARONI CHEESE
Box	598

COSTA		COSTA	
MARMALADE		**SANDWICH**	
Extra	75	BLT	405
MARMITE*		Chicken, Salad, Roast	396
Extra	20	Chicken, Salad, Roast, GF	355
MILK		Chicken, Salad, Roast, GF	355
Full Fat, Whole	25	Egg, Free Range	342
Skimmed	13	Egg, Free Range	342
Soya	18	Salmon, Smoked, & Soft Cheese	372
MILK DRINK		Selection	436
Chocolate, Full Fat Milk, Massimo, Iced	351	**SAUCE**	
Chocolate, Full Fat Milk, Medio, Iced	271	Belgian Chocolate	54
Chocolate, Full Fat Milk, Primo, Iced	194	Brown, Sachet, Extra	12
Chocolate, Skimmed Milk, Massimo, Iced	275	Cherry	82
Chocolate, Skimmed Milk, Medio, Iced	210	White Chocolate	214
Chocolate, Skimmed Milk, Primo, Iced	147	**SAUSAGE**	
Chocolate, Soya Milk, Massimo, Iced	302	Bap, Breakfast	488
Chocolate, Soya Milk, Medio, Iced	232	**SCONE**	
Chocolate, Soya Milk, Primo, Iced	163	Fruit	258
MIXED NUTS		**SHORTBREAD**	
Chilli, & Lime, Mix	204	Bites, Mini	52
MUFFIN		Caramel, Traybake	404
Banana & Pecan Breakfast Loaf	442	**SMOOTHIE**	
Blueberry	448	Coffee, Oats, & Banana, Superday	258
Caramel, Salted	483	Passion Fruit, Mango, & Peach, Superday	206
Chocolate, Triple	422	Spinach, Mango, Pineapple, & Banana, Superday	154
Gingerbread	496	Strawberry, & Banana, Superday	136
Lemon	454	**SPREAD**	
Mini, Chocolate, & Raspberry & White Chocolate	75	Sunflower, Extra	43
NUTELLA		**SUGAR**	
Extra	81	Brown	10
PANETTONE		White, Granulated	10
Classic	374	**SWEETENER**	
PANINI		Sweet 'n' Low	4
Bacon, British, & Brie	499	**SYRUP**	
Goats Cheese, & Sweet Chilli, Chutney	420	Amaretto, No Added Sugar	1
Ham, British, & Cheese	427	Caramel	16
Mozzarella, Tomato, & Basil	519	Caramel, Sugar Free	2
Salami, & Tomato	449	Cinnamon	32
Tuna, Melt	483	Gingerbread	33
PASTA		Gingerbread, No Added Sugar	1
Meatball	466	Gomme	17
PASTRY		Honeycomb	15
Chocolate, Twist	396	Maple, Sachet	62
Pain Aux Chocolat	266	Marshmallow	1
Pain Aux Raisins	292	Popcorn	32
PEANUT BUTTER		Roasted Hazelnut	16
Extra	92	Vanilla	17
SALAD		**TART**	
Chicken, Roast	223	Apple, & Blackberry, Crumble	266
Cous Cous, Moroccan Styles	392	Bakewell, Cherry	392
Pasta, Feta, Tomato	472	Bakewell, Mini	137
Tuna, Nicoise	219	Lemon	351

COSTA

TEA

	KCAL
Chai Latte, Skimmed Milk, Massimo	352
Chai Latte, Skimmed Milk, Medio	221
Chai Latte, Skimmed Milk, Primo	141
Chai Latte, Soya Milk, Massimo	402
Chai Latte, Soya Milk, Medio	254
Chai Latte, Whole Milk, Massimo	522
Chai Latte, Whole Milk, Medio	334
Chai Latte, Whole Milk, Primo	209
Citrus, & Ginger, Twist	6
English Breakfast, Decaff	3
Everyday	3
Green, Simply Sencha	3
Iced, Lemon, Massimo	181
Iced, lemon, Medio	136
Iced, Lemon, Primo	91
Iced, Peach, Massimo	175
Iced, Peach, Medoi	131
Iced, Peach, Primo	88
Chai Latte, Whole Milk, Massimo, Iced	426
Chai Latte, Whole Milk, Medio, Iced	327
Chai Latte, Whole Milk, Primo, Iced	231
Chai Latte, Skimmed, Massimo, Iced	350
Chai Latte, Skimmed, Medio, Iced	266
Chai Latte, Skimmed, Primo, Iced	184
Chai Latte, Soya Milk, Massimo, Iced	376
Chai Latte, Soya Milk, Medio, Iced	288
Chai Latte, Soya Milk, Primo, Iced	201
The Earl	3
Thoroughly Minted	3

TEACAKES

Fruit, No Butter, Breakfast	311

TOAST

Brown, Seeded	350
Fruit	288
White, No Butter	251

TOASTIE

Cheddar, & Tomato, Slow Roasted	443
Chicken, & Bacon	418
Emmenthal, & Mushroom	443
Ham, British, & Cheese	307
Ham, Wiltshire, & Mature Cheddar	409
Sausage, Cumberland, with Red Onion	493

VANILLA

Powder	26

WRAP

Chicken, Fajita, Roast	428
Meatball	582

YOGHURT

with Raspberry, & Strawberry, Compote, Breakfast	109

DOMINO'S PIZZA

BREAD

Garlic, Italiano, ¼ Bread	228

DOMINO'S PIZZA

BREAD

	KCAL
Garlic, Pizza, 1 Slice	156

BROWNIES

Chocolate	147

CAKE

Chocolate Melt	374

CHICKEN

Chick n Mix Box, ½ Box	324
Kickers, Combo Box, ¼ Box	177
Kickers, 1 Kicker	53
Strippers, Combo Box, ¼ Box	160
Strippers, 1 Stripper	43
Wings, Combo Box, ¼ Box	220
Wings, 1 Wing	78
Wings, Red Hot, Franks, 1 Wing	65
Wings, Spicy BBQ, 1 Wing	72

COLESLAW

Half Pot	155

COOKIES

Warm, 1 Cookie	182

DIP

BBQ, Big	188
BBQ	47
Garlic & Herb	169
Honey & Mystard	109
Red Hot, Franks, Big	24
Red Hot, Franks	6
Salsa, Tangy	41

DIP & DIPPERS

Cinni, ½ Box	400

DOUGH BALLS

Twisted, Pepperoni, ½ Box	305
Twisted, with Cheese and Herb Sauce, ½ Box	326

MEATBALLS

Meltin', ½ Box	191

NACHOS

no Jalapenos, ½ Box	243
with Jalapenos, ½ Box	244

OIL

Chilli Infused	127

PIZZA

Chocolate, Lotta, ½ Pizza	204

PIZZA - AMERICAN HOT

	PER SLICE
BBQ Stuffed Crust, Delight Mozzarella, Large	236
BBQ Stuffed Crust, Delight Mozzarella, Medium	222
BBQ Stuffed Crust, Large	251
BBQ Stuffed Crust, Medium	245
Classic Crust, Delight Mozzarella, Large	189
Classic Crust, Delight Mozzarella, Medium	175
Classic Crust, Delight Mozzarella, Personal	130
Classic Crust, Delight Mozzarella, Small	157
Classic Crust, Large	196
Classic Crust, Medium	181

DOMINO'S PIZZA

PIZZA - AMERICAN HOT

	PER SLICE
Classic Crust, Personal	134
Classic Crust, Small	160
Double Decadence, Delight Mozzarella, Large	261
Double Decadence, Delight Mozzarella, Medium	239
Double Decadence, Large	265
Double Decadence, Medium	243
GF Crust, Delight Mozzarella, Small	138
GF Crust, Small	134
Italian Style Crust, Delight Mozzarella, Large	173
Italian Style Crust, Delight Mozzarella, Medium	155
Italian Style Crust, Delight Mozzarella, Small	137
Italian Style Crust, Large	153
Italian Style Crust, Medium	58
Italian Style Crust, Small	122
Stuffed Crust, Delight Mozzarella, Large	230
Stuffed Crust, Delight Mozzarella, Medium	216
Stuffed Crust, Large	255
Stuffed Crust, Medium	240
Thin & Crispy, Delight Mozzarella, Large	160
Thin & Crispy, Delight Mozzarella, Medium	149
Thin & Crispy, Large	168
Thin & Crispy, Medium	157

PIZZA - AMERICANO

	PER SLICE
BBQ Stuffed Crust, Delight Mozzarella, Large	269
BBQ Stuffed Crust, Delight Mozzarella, Medium	246
BBQ Stuffed Crust, Large	269
BBQ Stuffed Crust, Medium	253
Classic Crust, Delight Mozzarella, Large	213
Classic Crust, Delight Mozzarella, Medium	197
Classic Crust, Delight Mozzarella, Personal	147
Classic Crust, Delight Mozzarella, Small	182
Classic Crust, Large	221
Classic Crust, Medium	204
Classic Crust, Small	183
Double Decadence, Delight Mozzarella, Large	287
Double Decadence, Delight Mozzarella, Medium	263
Double Decadence, Large	288
Double Decadence, Medium	264
GF Crust, Delight Mozzarella, Small	159
GF Crust, Small	166
Italian Style Crust, Delight Mozzarella, Large	192
Italian Style Crust, Delight Mozzarella, Medium	172
Italian Style Crust, Delight Mozzarella, Small	153
Italian Style Crust, Large	197
Italian Style Crust, Medium	176
Italian Style Crust, Small	156
Stuffed Crust, Delight Mozzarella, Large	256
Stuffed Crust, Delight Mozzarella, Medium	240
Stuffed Crust, Large	263
Stuffed Crust, Medium	247
Thin & Crispy, Delight Mozzarella, Large	183
Thin & Crispy, Delight Mozzarella, Medium	171

DOMINO'S PIZZA

PIZZA - AMERICANO

	PER SLICE
Thin & Crispy, Large	191
Thin & Crispy, Medium	179
Classic Crust, Personal	152

PIZZA - BACON DOUBLE CHEESE

	PER SLICE
BBQ Stuffed Crust, Delight Mozzarella, Large	249
BBQ Stuffed Crust, Delight Mozzarella, Medium	230
BBQ Stuffed Crust, Large	267
BBQ Stuffed Crust, Medium	256
Classic Crust, Delight Mozzarella, Large	202
Classic Crust, Delight Mozzarella, Medium	183
Classic Crust, Delight Mozzarella, Personal	140
Classic Crust, Delight Mozzarella, Small	160
Classic Crust, Large	212
Classic Crust, Medium	192
Classic Crust, Personal	146
Classic Crust, Small	165
Double Decadence, Delight Mozzarella, Large	274
Double Decadence, Delight Mozzarella, Medium	247
Double Decadence, Large	281
Double Decadence, Medium	254
GF Crust, Delight Mozzarella, Small	141
GF Crust, Small	140
Italian Style Crust, Delight Mozzarella, Large	185
Italian Style Crust, Delight Mozzarella, Medium	163
Italian Style Crust, Delight Mozzarella, Small	140
Italian Style Crust, Large	169
Italian Style Crust, Medium	149
Italian Style Crust, Small	128
Stuffed Crust, Delight Mozzarella, Large	242
Stuffed Crust, Delight Mozzarella, Medium	224
Stuffed Crust, Large	271
Stuffed Crust, Medium	251
Thin & Crispy, Delight Mozzarella, Large	173
Thin & Crispy, Delight Mozzarella, Medium	158
Thin & Crispy, Large	184
Thin & Crispy, Medium	168

PIZZA - CHEESE & TOMATO

	PER SLICE
BBQ Stuffed Crust, Delight Mozzarella, Large	197
BBQ Stuffed Crust, Delight Mozzarella, Medium	183
BBQ Stuffed Crust, Large	214
BBQ Stuffed Crust, Medium	208
Classic Crust, Delight Mozzarella, Large	150
Classic Crust, Delight Mozzarella, Medium	136
Classic Crust, Delight Mozzarella, Personal	112
Classic Crust, Delight Mozzarella, Small	133
Classic Crust, Large	159
Classic Crust, Medium	145
Classic Crust, Personal	118
Classic Crust, Personal	118
Classic Crust, Small	139
Double Decadence, Delight Mozzarella, Large	220
Double Decadence, Delight Mozzarella, Medium	199

DOMINO'S PIZZA

PIZZA - CHEESE & TOMATO

	PER SLICE
Double Decadence, Large	227
Double Decadence, Medium	205
GF Crust, Delight Mozzarella, Small	115
GF Crust, Small	113
Italian Style Crust, Delight Mozzarella, Large	132
Italian Style Crust, Delight Mozzarella, Medium	115
Italian Style Crust, Delight Mozzarella, Small	105
Italian Style Crust, Large	119
Italian Style Crust, Medium	103
Italian Style Crust, Small	88
Stuffed Crust, Delight Mozzarella, Large	191
Stuffed Crust, Delight Mozzarella, Medium	178
Stuffed Crust, Large	217
Stuffed Crust, Medium	202
Thin & Crispy, Delight Mozzarella, Large	116
Thin & Crispy, Delight Mozzarella, Medium	106
Thin & Crispy, Large	126
Thin & Crispy, Medium	115

PIZZA - CHICKEN & RASHER BACON

	PER SLICE
BBQ Stuffed Crust, Delight Mozzarella, Large	228
BBQ Stuffed Crust, Delight Mozzarella, Medium	211
BBQ Stuffed Crust, Large	243
BBQ Stuffed Crust, Medium	235
Classic Crust, Delight Mozzarella, Large	181
Classic Crust, Delight Mozzarella, Medium	165
Classic Crust, Delight Mozzarella, Personal	127
Classic Crust, Delight Mozzarella, Small	145
Classic Crust, Large	188
Classic Crust, Medium	171
Classic Crust, Personal	174
Classic Crust, Small	147
Double Decadence, Delight Mozzarella, Large	253
Double Decadence, Delight Mozzarella, Medium	144
Double Decadence, Large	257
Double Decadence, Medium	233
GF Crust, Delight Mozzarella, Small	126
GF Crust, Small	121
Italian Style Crust, Delight Mozzarella, Large	164
Italian Style Crust, Delight Mozzarella, Medium	144
Italian Style Crust, Delight Mozzarella, Small	124
Italian Style Crust, Large	145
Italian Style Crust, Medium	128
Italian Style Crust, Small	110
Stuffed Crust, Delight Mozzarella, Large	222
Stuffed Crust, Delight Mozzarella, Medium	206
Stuffed Crust, Large	247
Stuffed Crust, Medium	230
Thin & Crispy, Delight Mozzarella, Large	152
Thin & Crispy, Delight Mozzarella, Medium	139
Thin & Crispy, Large	160
Thin & Crispy, Medium	147

DOMINO'S PIZZA

PIZZA - CHICKEN FEAST

	PER SLICE
BBQ Stuffed Crust, Delight Mozzarella, Large	223
BBQ Stuffed Crust, Delight Mozzarella, Medium	208
BBQ Stuffed Crust, Large	238
BBQ Stuffed Crust, Medium	232
Classic Crust, Delight Mozzarella, Large	177
Classic Crust, Delight Mozzarella, Medium	161
Classic Crust, Delight Mozzarella, Personal	121
Classic Crust, Delight Mozzarella, Small	141
Classic Crust, Large	184
Classic Crust, Medium	167
Classic Crust, Personal	125
Classic Crust, Small	143
Double Decadence, Delight Mozzarella, Large	249
Double Decadence, Delight Mozzarella, Medium	225
Double Decadence, Large	253
Double Decadence, Medium	229
GF Crust, Delight Mozzarella, Small	122
GF Crust, Small	117
Italian Style Crust, Delight Mozzarella, Lge	160
Italian Style Crust, Delight Mozzarella, Medium	141
Italian Style Crust, Delight Mozzarella, Small	120
Italian Style Crust, Lge	141
Italian Style Crust, Medium	124
Italian Style Crust, Small	106
Stuffed Crust, Delight Mozzarella, Large	217
Stuffed Crust, Delight Mozzarella, Medium	202
Stuffed Crust, Large	243
Stuffed Crust, Medium	226
Thin & Crispy, Delight Mozzarella, Large	147
Thin & Crispy, Delight Mozzarella, Medium	136
Thin & Crispy, Large	156
Thin & Crispy, Medium	143

PIZZA - CHIPOTLE PULLED PORK

	PER SLICE
BBQ Stuffed Crust, Delight Mozzarella, Large	218
BBQ Stuffed Crust, Delight Mozzarella, Medium	204
BBQ Stuffed Crust, Large	233
BBQ Stuffed Crust, Medium	227
Classic Crust, Delight Mozzarella, Large	172
Classic Crust, Delight Mozzarella, Medium	157
Classic Crust, Delight Mozzarella, Personal	117
Classic Crust, Delight Mozzarella, Small	139
Classic Crust, Large	178
Classic Crust, Medium	163
Classic Crust, Personal	121
Classic Crust, Small	141
Delight Mozzarella, Large	244
Double Decadence, Delight Mozzarella, Medium	221
Double Decadence, Large	248
Double Decadence, Medium	225
GF Crust, Delight Mozzarella, Small	120
GF Crust, Small	116
Italian Style Crust, Delight Mozzarella, Large	155

DOMINO'S PIZZA

PIZZA - CHIPOTLE PULLED PORK	PER SLICE
Italian Style Crust, Delight Mozzarella, Medium	137
Italian Style Crust, Delight Mozzarella, Small	118
Italian Style Crust, Large	136
Italian Style Crust, Medium	120
Italian Style Crust, Small	104
Stuffed Crust, Delight Mozzarella, Large	212
Stuffed Crust, Delight Mozzarella, Medium	198
Stuffed Crust, Large	238
Stuffed Crust, Medium	222
Thin & Crispy, Delight Mozzarella, Large	142
Thin & Crispy, Delight Mozzarella, Medium	131
Thin & Crispy, Large	151
Thin & Crispy, Medium	139

PIZZA - DELUXE	PER SLICE
BBQ Stuffed Crust, Delight Mozzarella, Large	234
BBQ Stuffed Crust, Delight Mozzarella, Medium	220
BBQ Stuffed Crust, Large	249
BBQ Stuffed Crust, Medium	244
Classic Crust, Delight Mozzarella, Large	188
Classic Crust, Delight Mozzarella, Medium	174
Classic Crust, Delight Mozzarella, Personal	129
Classic Crust, Delight Mozzarella, Small	156
Classic Crust, Large	195
Classic Crust, Medium	180
Classic Crust, Personal	132
Classic Crust, Small	158
Double Decadence, Delight Mozzarella, Large	260
Double Decadence, Delight Mozzarella, Medium	238
Double Decadence, Large	264
Double Decadence, Medium	241
GF Crust, Delight Mozzarella, Small	137
GF Crust, Small	133
Italian Style Crust, Delight Mozzarella, Large	171
Italian Style Crust, Delight Mozzarella, Medium	153
Italian Style Crust, Delight Mozzarella, Small	135
Italian Style Crust, Large	152
Italian Style Crust, Medium	137
Italian Style Crust, Small	121
Stuffed Crust, Delight Mozzarella, Large	228
Stuffed Crust, Delight Mozzarella, Medium	215
Stuffed Crust, Large	254
Stuffed Crust, Medium	239
Thin & Crispy, Delight Mozzarella, Large	158
Thin & Crispy, Delight Mozzarella, Medium	148
Thin & Crispy, Large	167
Thin & Crispy, Medium	156

PIZZA - EXTRAVAGANZA	PER SLICE
BBQ Stuffed Crust, Delight Mozzarella, Large	253
BBQ Stuffed Crust, Delight Mozzarella, Medium	237
BBQ Stuffed Crust, Large	271
BBQ Stuffed Crust, Medium	263
Classic Crust, Delight Mozzarella, Large	207

DOMINO'S PIZZA

PIZZA - EXTRAVAGANZA	PER SLICE
Classic Crust, Delight Mozzarella, Medium	190
Classic Crust, Delight Mozzarella, Personal	148
Classic Crust, Delight Mozzarella, Small	168
Classic Crust, Large	217
Classic Crust, Medium	199
Classic Crust, Personal	153
Classic Crust, Small	174
Double Decadence, Delight Mozzarella, Large	279
Double Decadence, Delight Mozzarella, Medium	254
Double Decadence, Large	286
Double Decadence, Medium	261
GF Crust, Delight Mozzarella, Small	150
GF Crust, Small	148
Italian Style Crust, Delight Mozzarella, Large	190
Italian Style Crust, Delight Mozzarella, Medium	170
Italian Style Crust, Delight Mozzarella, Small	148
Italian Style Crust, Large	174
Italian Style Crust, Medium	156
Italian Style Crust, Small	136
Stuffed Crust, Delight Mozzarella, Large	247
Stuffed Crust, Delight Mozzarella, Medium	231
Stuffed Crust, Large	276
Stuffed Crust, Medium	258
Thin & Crispy, Delight Mozzarella, Large	177
Thin & Crispy, Delight Mozzarella, Medium	164
Thin & Crispy, Large	189
Thin & Crispy, Medium	175

PIZZA - FARMHOUSE	PER SLICE
BBQ Stuffed Crust, Delight Mozzarella, Large	216
BBQ Stuffed Crust, Delight Mozzarella, Medium	197
BBQ Stuffed Crust, Large	226
BBQ Stuffed Crust, Medium	220
Classic Crust, Delight Mozzarella, Large	164
Classic Crust, Delight Mozzarella, Medium	150
Classic Crust, Delight Mozzarella, Personal	113
Classic Crust, Delight Mozzarella, Small	132
Classic Crust, Large	171
Classic Crust, Medium	156
Classic Crust, Personal	117
Classic Crust, Small	135
Double Decadence, Delight Mozzarella, Large	236
Double Decadence, Delight Mozzarella, Medium	214
Double Decadence, Large	240
Double Decadence, Medium	218
GF Crust, Delight Mozzarella, Small	113
GF Crust, Small	109
Italian Style Crust, Delight Mozzarella, Large	148
Italian Style Crust, Delight Mozzarella, Medium	130
Italian Style Crust, Delight Mozzarella, Small	112
Italian Style Crust, Large	128
Italian Style Crust, Medium	113
Italian Style Crust, Small	97

DOMINO'S PIZZA

PIZZA - FARMHOUSE	PER SLICE
Stuffed Crust, Delight Mozzarella, Large	205
Stuffed Crust, Delight Mozzarella, Medium	191
Stuffed Crust, Large	230
Stuffed Crust, Medium	215
Thin & Crispy, Delight Mozzarella, Large	135
Thin & Crispy, Delight Mozzarella, Medium	124
Thin & Crispy, Large	143
Thin & Crispy, Medium	132

PIZZA - FOUR VEGI	PER SLICE
BBQ Stuffed Crust, Delight Mozzarella, Large	205
BBQ Stuffed Crust, Delight Mozzarella, Medium	192
BBQ Stuffed Crust, Large	220
BBQ Stuffed Crust, Medium	216
Classic Crust, Delight Mozzarella, Large	159
Classic Crust, Delight Mozzarella, Medium	145
Classic Crust, Delight Mozzarella, Personal	110
Classic Crust, Delight Mozzarella, Small	126
Classic Crust, Large	166
Classic Crust, Medium	152
Classic Crust, Personal	115
Classic Crust, Small	129
Double Decadence, Delight Mozzarella, Large	231
Double Decadence, Delight Mozzarella, Medium	210
Double Decadence, Large	235
Double Decadence, Medium	213
GF Crust, Delight Mozzarella, Small	107
GF Crust, Small	103
Italian Style Crust, Delight Mozzarella, Large	142
Italian Style Crust, Delight Mozzarella, Medium	125
Italian Style Crust, Delight Mozzarella, Small	106
Italian Style Crust, Large	123
Italian Style Crust, Medium	108
Italian Style Crust, Small	91
Stuffed Crust, Delight Mozzarella, Large	199
Stuffed Crust, Delight Mozzarella, Medium	186
Stuffed Crust, Large	225
Stuffed Crust, Medium	210
Thin & Crispy, Delight Mozzarella, Large	129
Thin & Crispy, Delight Mozzarella, Medium	120
Thin & Crispy, Large	138
Thin & Crispy, Medium	127

PIZZA - FULL HOUSE	PER SLICE
BBQ Stuffed Crust, Delight Mozzarella, Large	235
BBQ Stuffed Crust, Delight Mozzarella, Medium	220
BBQ Stuffed Crust, Large	250
BBQ Stuffed Crust, Medium	244
Classic Crust, Delight Mozzarella, Large	188
Classic Crust, Delight Mozzarella, Medium	174
Classic Crust, Delight Mozzarella, Personal	137
Classic Crust, Delight Mozzarella, Small	155
Classic Crust, Large	195
Classic Crust, Medium	180

DOMINO'S PIZZA

PIZZA - FULL HOUSE	PER SLICE
Classic Crust, Personal	142
Classic Crust, Small	158
Double Decadence, Delight Mozzarella, Large	260
Double Decadence, Delight Mozzarella, Medium	238
Double Decadence, Large	264
Double Decadence, Medium	241
GF Crust, Delight Mozzarella, Small	136
GF Crust, Small	132
Italian Style Crust, Delight Mozzarella, Large	172
Italian Style Crust, Delight Mozzarella, Medium	153
Italian Style Crust, Delight Mozzarella, Small	135
Italian Style Crust, Large	153
Italian Style Crust, Medium	136
Italian Style Crust, Small	120
Stuffed Crust, Delight Mozzarella, Large	229
Stuffed Crust, Delight Mozzarella, Medium	215
Stuffed Crust, Large	255
Stuffed Crust, Medium	238
Thin & Crispy, Delight Mozzarella, Large	159
Thin & Crispy, Delight Mozzarella, Medium	148
Thin & Crispy, Large	167
Thin & Crispy, Medium	156

PIZZA - HAM & PINEAPPLE	PER SLICE
BBQ Stuffed Crust, Delight Mozzarella, Large	212
BBQ Stuffed Crust, Delight Mozzarella, Medium	198
BBQ Stuffed Crust, Large	227
BBQ Stuffed Crust, Medium	221
Classic Crust, Delight Mozzarella, Large	165
Classic Crust, Delight Mozzarella, Medium	151
Classic Crust, Delight Mozzarella, Personal	114
Classic Crust, Delight Mozzarella, Small	133
Classic Crust, Large	172
Classic Crust, Medium	157
Classic Crust, Personal	118
Classic Crust, Small	136
Double Decadence, Delight Mozzarella, Large	237
Double Decadence, Delight Mozzarella, Medium	215
Double Decadence, Large	241
Double Decadence, Medium	219
GF Crust, Delight Mozzarella, Small	114
GF Crust, Small	110
Italian Style Crust, Delight Mozzarella, Large	149
Italian Style Crust, Delight Mozzarella, Medium	131
Italian Style Crust, Delight Mozzarella, Small	136
Italian Style Crust, Large	129
Italian Style Crust, Medium	114
Italian Style Crust, Small	98
Stuffed Crust, Delight Mozzarella, Large	206
Stuffed Crust, Delight Mozzarella, Medium	192
Stuffed Crust, Large	231
Stuffed Crust, Large	231
Stuffed Crust, Medium	216

DOMINO'S PIZZA

PIZZA - HAM & PINEAPPLE	PER SLICE
Thin & Crispy, Delight Mozzarella, Large	136
Thin & Crispy, Delight Mozzarella, Medium	125
Thin & Crispy, Large	144
Thin & Crispy, Medium	133

PIZZA - HAMROCK	PER SLICE
BBQ Stuffed Crust, Delight Mozzarella, Large	228
BBQ Stuffed Crust, Delight Mozzarella, Medium	212
BBQ Stuffed Crust, Large	243
BBQ Stuffed Crust, Medium	236
Classic Crust, Delight Mozzarella, Large	181
Classic Crust, Delight Mozzarella, Medium	162
Classic Crust, Delight Mozzarella, Personal	122
Classic Crust, Delight Mozzarella, Small	144
Classic Crust, Large	188
Classic Crust, Medium	172
Classic Crust, Personal	126
Classic Crust, Small	144
Classic Crust, Small	146
Double Decadence, Delight Mozzarella, Large	253
Double Decadence, Delight Mozzarella, Medium	229
Double Decadence, Large	257
Double Decadence, Medium	233
GF Crust, Delight Mozzarella, Small	125
GF Crust, Small	121
Italian Style Crust, Delight Mozzarella, Large	165
Italian Style Crust, Delight Mozzarella, Medium	165
Italian Style Crust, Delight Mozzarella, Medium	145
Italian Style Crust, Delight Mozzarella, Small	123
Italian Style Crust, Large	146
Italian Style Crust, Medium	128
Italian Style Crust, Small	109
Stuffed Crust, Delight Mozzarella, Large	222
Stuffed Crust, Delight Mozzarella, Medium	206
Stuffed Crust, Large	248
Stuffed Crust, Medium	230
Thin & Crispy, Delight Mozzarella, Large	152
Thin & Crispy, Delight Mozzarella, Medium	140
Thin & Crispy, Large	160
Thin & Crispy, Medium	143

PIZZA - HAWAIIAN	PER SLICE
BBQ Stuffed Crust, Delight Mozzarella, Large	212
BBQ Stuffed Crust, Delight Mozzarella, Medium	198
BBQ Stuffed Crust, Large	227
BBQ Stuffed Crust, Medium	222
Classic Crust, Delight Mozzarella, Large	166
Classic Crust, Delight Mozzarella, Medium	152
Classic Crust, Delight Mozzarella, Personal	114
Classic Crust, Delight Mozzarella, Small	133
Classic Crust, Large	173
Classic Crust, Medium	158
Classic Crust, Personal	119
Classic Crust, Small	136

DOMINO'S PIZZA

PIZZA - HAWAIIAN	PER SLICE
Double Decadence, Delight Mozzarella, Large	238
Double Decadence, Delight Mozzarella, Medium	216
Double Decadence, Large	242
Double Decadence, Medium	219
GF Crust, Delight Mozzarella, Small	115
GF Crust, Small	110
Italian Style Crust, Delight Mozzarella, Large	149
Italian Style Crust, Delight Mozzarella, Medium	131
Italian Style Crust, Delight Mozzarella, Small	113
Italian Style Crust, Large	130
Italian Style Crust, Medium	115
Italian Style Crust, Small	99
Stuffed Crust, Delight Mozzarella, Large	206
Stuffed Crust, Delight Mozzarella, Medium	193
Stuffed Crust, Large	232
Stuffed Crust, Medium	217
Thin & Crispy, Delight Mozzarella, Large	136
Thin & Crispy, Delight Mozzarella, Medium	126
Thin & Crispy, Large	145
Thin & Crispy, Medium	134

PIZZA - HOT & SPICY	PER SLICE
BBQ Stuffed Crust, Delight Mozzarella, Large	207
BBQ Stuffed Crust, Delight Mozzarella, Medium	193
BBQ Stuffed Crust, Large	222
BBQ Stuffed Crust, Medium	217
Classic Crust, Delight Mozzarella, Large	161
Classic Crust, Delight Mozzarella, Medium	146
Classic Crust, Delight Mozzarella, Personal	111
Classic Crust, Delight Mozzarella, Small	128
Classic Crust, Large	504
Classic Crust, Medium	152
Classic Crust, Personal	115
Classic Crust, Small	130
Double Decadence, Delight Mozzarella, Large	233
Double Decadence, Delight Mozzarella, Medium	210
Double Decadence, Large	237
Double Decadence, Medium	214
GF Crust, Delight Mozzarella, Small	109
GF Crust, Small	105
Italian Style Crust, Delight Mozzarella, Large	144
Italian Style Crust, Delight Mozzarella, Medium	126
Italian Style Crust, Delight Mozzarella, Small	107
Italian Style Crust, Large	125
Italian Style Crust, Medium	109
Italian Style Crust, Small	93
Stuffed Crust, Delight Mozzarella, Large	201
Stuffed Crust, Delight Mozzarella, Medium	187
Stuffed Crust, Large	227
Stuffed Crust, Medium	211
Thin & Crispy, Delight Mozzarella, Large	131
Thin & Crispy, Delight Mozzarella, Medium	120
Thin & Crispy, Large	140

DOMINO'S PIZZA

PIZZA - HOT & SPICY	PER SLICE
Thin & Crispy, Medium	128

PIZZA - HOUSE SPECIAL ROAST CHICKEN	PER SLICE
BBQ Stuffed Crust, Delight Mozzarella, Large	268
BBQ Stuffed Crust, Delight Mozzarella, Medium	250
BBQ Stuffed Crust, Large	286
BBQ Stuffed Crust, Medium	277
Classic Crust, Delight Mozzarella, Large	221
Classic Crust, Delight Mozzarella, Medium	203
Classic Crust, Delight Mozzarella, Personal	160
Classic Crust, Delight Mozzarella, Small	180
Classic Crust, Large	231
Classic Crust, Medium	213
Classic Crust, Personal	166
Classic Crust, Small	186
Double Decadence, Delight Mozzarella, Large	293
Double Decadence, Delight Mozzarella, Medium	268
Double Decadence, Large	300
Double Decadence, Medium	274
GF Crust, Delight Mozzarella, Small	162
GF Crust, Small	160
Italian Style Crust, Delight Mozzarella, Large	205
Italian Style Crust, Delight Mozzarella, Medium	183
Italian Style Crust, Delight Mozzarella, Small	160
Italian Style Crust, Large	189
Italian Style Crust, Medium	169
Italian Style Crust, Small	148
Stuffed Crust, Delight Mozzarella, Large	262
Stuffed Crust, Delight Mozzarella, Medium	244
Stuffed Crust, Large	291
Stuffed Crust, Medium	271
Thin & Crispy, Delight Mozzarella, Large	192
Thin & Crispy, Delight Mozzarella, Medium	178
Thin & Crispy, Large	203
Thin & Crispy, Medium	188

PIZZA - HOUSE SPECIAL TANDOORI	PER SLICE
BBQ Stuffed Crust, Delight Mozzarella, Medium	251
BBQ Stuffed Crust, Large	287
BBQ Stuffed Crust, Medium	278
Classic Crust, Delight Mozzarella, Large	222
Classic Crust, Delight Mozzarella, Medium	204
Classic Crust, Delight Mozzarella, Personal	158
Classic Crust, Delight Mozzarella, Small	174
Classic Crust, Large	233
Classic Crust, Medium	214
Classic Crust, Personal	163
Classic Crust, Small	177
Double Decadence, Delight Mozzarella, Large	294
Double Decadence, Delight Mozzarella, Medium	269
Double Decadence, Large	302
Double Decadence, Medium	275
GF Crust, Delight Mozzarella, Small	155
GF Crust, Small	152

DOMINO'S PIZZA

PIZZA - HOUSE SPECIAL TANDOORI	PER SLICE
Italian Style Crust, Delight Mozzarella, Large	206
Italian Style Crust, Delight Mozzarella, Medium	184
Italian Style Crust, Delight Mozzarella, Small	153
Italian Style Crust, Large	222
Italian Style Crust, Medium	170
Italian Style Crust, Small	140
Stuffed Crust, Delight Mozzarella, Large	263
Stuffed Crust, Delight Mozzarella, Medium	246
Stuffed Crust, Large	292
Stuffed Crust, Medium	272
Thin & Crispy, Delight Mozzarella, Large	193
Thin & Crispy, Delight Mozzarella, Medium	179
Thin & Crispy, Large	205
Thin & Crispy, Medium	189

PIZZA - MEAT LOVERS	PER SLICE
BBQ Stuffed Crust, Delight Mozzarella, Large	249
BBQ Stuffed Crust, Delight Mozzarella, Medium	233
BBQ Stuffed Crust, Large	264
BBQ Stuffed Crust, Medium	256
Classic Crust, Delight Mozzarella, Large	202
Classic Crust, Delight Mozzarella, Medium	186
Classic Crust, Delight Mozzarella, Personal	136
Classic Crust, Delight Mozzarella, Small	167
Classic Crust, Large	209
Classic Crust, Medium	192
Classic Crust, Personal	141
Classic Crust, Small	170
Double Decadence, Delight Mozzarella, Large	274
Double Decadence, Delight Mozzarella, Medium	250
Double Decadence, Large	278
Double Decadence, Medium	254
GF Crust, Delight Mozzarella, Small	148
GF Crust, Small	144
Italian Style Crust, Delight Mozzarella, Large	185
Italian Style Crust, Delight Mozzarella, Medium	166
Italian Style Crust, Delight Mozzarella, Small	147
Italian Style Crust, Large	166
Italian Style Crust, Medium	149
Italian Style Crust, Small	132
Stuffed Crust, Delight Mozzarella, Large	243
Stuffed Crust, Delight Mozzarella, Medium	227
Stuffed Crust, Large	268
Stuffed Crust, Medium	251
Thin & Crispy, Delight Mozzarella, Large	173
Thin & Crispy, Delight Mozzarella, Medium	160
Thin & Crispy, Large	181
Thin & Crispy, Medium	168

PIZZA - MEATEOR	PER SLICE
BBQ Stuffed Crust, Delight Mozzarella, Large	280
BBQ Stuffed Crust, Delight Mozzarella, Medium	255
BBQ Stuffed Crust, Large	280
BBQ Stuffed Crust, Medium	262

DOMINO'S PIZZA

PIZZA - MEATEOR	PER SLICE
Classic Crust, Delight Mozzarella, Large	224
Classic Crust, Delight Mozzarella, Medium	207
Classic Crust, Delight Mozzarella, Personal	170
Classic Crust, Delight Mozzarella, Small	191
Classic Crust, Large	232
Classic Crust, Medium	214
Classic Crust, Personal	175
Classic Crust, Small	192
Double Decadence, Delight Mozzarella, Large	298
Double Decadence, Delight Mozzarella, Medium	273
Double Decadence, Large	298
Double Decadence, Medium	273
GF Crust, Delight Mozzarella, Small	169
GF Crust, Small	175
Italian Style Crust, Delight Mozzarella, Large	203
Italian Style Crust, Delight Mozzarella, Medium	182
Italian Style Crust, Delight Mozzarella, Small	162
Italian Style Crust, Large	207
Italian Style Crust, Medium	186
Italian Style Crust, Small	166
Stuffed Crust, Delight Mozzarella, Large	266
Stuffed Crust, Delight Mozzarella, Medium	250
Stuffed Crust, Large	274
Stuffed Crust, Medium	257
Thin & Crispy, Delight Mozzarella, Large	194
Thin & Crispy, Delight Mozzarella, Medium	181
Thin & Crispy, Large	202
Thin & Crispy, Medium	188

PIZZA - MEATILICIOUS	PER SLICE
BBQ Stuffed Crust, Delight Mozzarella, Large	242
BBQ Stuffed Crust, Delight Mozzarella, Medium	226
BBQ Stuffed Crust, Large	257
BBQ Stuffed Crust, Medium	250
Classic Crust, Delight Mozzarella, Large	195
Classic Crust, Delight Mozzarella, Medium	180
Classic Crust, Delight Mozzarella, Personal	144
Classic Crust, Large	202
Classic Crust, Medium	186
Classic Crust, Personal	198
Classic Crust, Small	164
Double Decadence, Delight Mozzarella, Large	267
Double Decadence, Delight Mozzarella, Medium	244
Double Decadence, Large	271
Double Decadence, Medium	247
GF Crust, Delight Mozzarella, Small	142
GF Crust, Small	138
Italian Style Crust, Delight Mozzarella, Large	179
Italian Style Crust, Delight Mozzarella, Medium	159
Italian Style Crust, Delight Mozzarella, Medium	141
Italian Style Crust, Large	160
Italian Style Crust, Medium	143
Italian Style Crust, Small	126

DOMINO'S PIZZA

PIZZA - MEATILICIOUS	PER SLICE
Stuffed Crust, Delight Mozzarella, Large	236
Stuffed Crust, Delight Mozzarella, Medium	221
Stuffed Crust, Large	262
Stuffed Crust, Medium	245
Thin & Crispy, Delight Mozzarella, Large	166
Thin & Crispy, Delight Mozzarella, Medium	154
Thin & Crispy, Large	174
Thin & Crispy, Medium	162

PIZZA - MEATZZA	PER SLICE
BBQ Stuffed Crust, Delight Mozzarella, Large	245
BBQ Stuffed Crust, Delight Mozzarella, Medium	231
BBQ Stuffed Crust, Large	260
BBQ Stuffed Crust, Medium	254
Classic Crust, Delight Mozzarella, Large	198
Classic Crust, Delight Mozzarella, Medium	184
Classic Crust, Delight Mozzarella, Personal	134
Classic Crust, Delight Mozzarella, Small	166
Classic Crust, Large	205
Classic Crust, Medium	190
Classic Crust, Personal	138
Classic Crust, Small	168
Double Decadence, Delight Mozzarella, Large	270
Double Decadence, Delight Mozzarella, Medium	248
Double Decadence, Large	274
Double Decadence, Medium	252
GF Crust, Delight Mozzarella, Small	147
GF Crust, Delight Mozzarella, Small	147
GF Crust, Small	143
Italian Style Crust, Delight Mozzarella, Large	182
Italian Style Crust, Delight Mozzarella, Medium	163
Italian Style Crust, Delight Mozzarella, Small	145
Italian Style Crust, Large	162
Italian Style Crust, Medium	249
Italian Style Crust, Small	131
Stuffed Crust, Delight Mozzarella, Large	239
Stuffed Crust, Delight Mozzarella, Medium	225
Stuffed Crust, Large	265
Stuffed Crust, Medium	249
Thin & Crispy, Delight Mozzarella, Large	169
Thin & Crispy, Delight Mozzarella, Medium	158
Thin & Crispy, Large	177

PIZZA - MEXICAN HOT	PER SLICE
BBQ Stuffed Crust, Delight Mozzarella, Large	242
BBQ Stuffed Crust, Delight Mozzarella, Medium	227
BBQ Stuffed Crust, Large	260
BBQ Stuffed Crust, Medium	253
Classic Crust, Delight Mozzarella, Large	196
Classic Crust, Delight Mozzarella, Medium	180
Classic Crust, Delight Mozzarella, Personal	128
Classic Crust, Delight Mozzarella, Small	159
Classic Crust, Large	206
Classic Crust, Medium	189

DOMINO'S PIZZA

PIZZA - MEXICAN HOT

	PER SLICE
Classic Crust, Personal	134
Classic Crust, Personal	134
Classic Crust, Small	164
Double Decadence, Delight Mozzarella, Large	268
Double Decadence, Delight Mozzarella, Medium	244
Double Decadence, Large	275
Double Decadence, Medium	251
GF Crust, Delight Mozzarella, Small	140
GF Crust, Small	138
Italian Style Crust, Delight Mozzarella, Large	179
Italian Style Crust, Delight Mozzarella, Medium	160
Italian Style Crust, Delight Mozzarella, Small	139
Italian Style Crust, Large	163
Italian Style Crust, Medium	146
Italian Style Crust, Small	127
Stuffed Crust, Delight Mozzarella, Large	236
Stuffed Crust, Delight Mozzarella, Medium	221
Stuffed Crust, Large	265
Stuffed Crust, Medium	248
Thin & Crispy, Delight Mozzarella, Large	166
Thin & Crispy, Delight Mozzarella, Medium	154
Thin & Crispy, Large	178
Thin & Crispy, Medium	165

PIZZA - MIGHTY MEATY

	PER SLICE
BBQ Stuffed Crust, Delight Mozzarella, Large	247
BBQ Stuffed Crust, Delight Mozzarella, Medium	232
BBQ Stuffed Crust, Large	262
BBQ Stuffed Crust, Medium	256
Classic Crust, Delight Mozzarella, Large	200
Classic Crust, Delight Mozzarella, Medium	186
Classic Crust, Delight Mozzarella, Personal	135
Classic Crust, Delight Mozzarella, Small	167
Classic Crust, Large	207
Classic Crust, Medium	192
Classic Crust, Personal	139
Classic Crust, Small	170
Double Decadence, Delight Mozzarella, Large	272
Double Decadence, Delight Mozzarella, Medium	250
Double Decadence, Large	276
Double Decadence, Medium	253
GF Crust, Delight Mozzarella, Small	148
GF Crust, Small	144
Italian Style Crust, Delight Mozzarella, Large	184
Italian Style Crust, Delight Mozzarella, Medium	165
Italian Style Crust, Delight Mozzarella, Small	147
Italian Style Crust, Large	164
Italian Style Crust, Medium	148
Italian Style Crust, Small	133
Stuffed Crust, Delight Mozzarella, Large	241
Stuffed Crust, Delight Mozzarella, Medium	227
Stuffed Crust, Large	266
Stuffed Crust, Medium	250

DOMINO'S PIZZA

PIZZA - MIGHTY MEATY

	PER SLICE
Thin & Crispy, Delight Mozzarella, Large	171
Thin & Crispy, Delight Mozzarella, Medium	160
Thin & Crispy, Large	179
Thin & Crispy, Medium	168

PIZZA - MIXED GRILL

	PER SLICE
BBQ Stuffed Crust, Delight Mozzarella, Large	244
BBQ Stuffed Crust, Delight Mozzarella, Medium	229
BBQ Stuffed Crust, Large	259
BBQ Stuffed Crust, Medium	252
Classic Crust, Delight Mozzarella, Large	197
Classic Crust, Delight Mozzarella, Medium	182
Classic Crust, Delight Mozzarella, Personal	138
Classic Crust, Delight Mozzarella, Small	163
Classic Crust, Large	204
Classic Crust, Medium	188
Classic Crust, Personal	143
Classic Crust, Small	166
Double Decadence, Delight Mozzarella, Large	269
Double Decadence, Delight Mozzarella, Medium	246
Double Decadence, Large	273
Double Decadence, Medium	250
GF Crust, Delight Mozzarella, Small	144
GF Crust, Small	140
Italian Style Crust, Delight Mozzarella, Large	181
Italian Style Crust, Delight Mozzarella, Medium	162
Italian Style Crust, Delight Mozzarella, Small	143
Italian Style Crust, Large	161
Italian Style Crust, Medium	145
Italian Style Crust, Small	129
Stuffed Crust, Delight Mozzarella, Large	238
Stuffed Crust, Delight Mozzarella, Medium	223
Stuffed Crust, Large	264
Stuffed Crust, Medium	247
Thin & Crispy, Delight Mozzarella, Large	168
Thin & Crispy, Delight Mozzarella, Medium	156
Thin & Crispy, Large	176
Thin & Crispy, Medium	164

PIZZA - NEW YORKER

	PER SLICE
BBQ Stuffed Crust, Delight Mozzarella, Large	242
BBQ Stuffed Crust, Delight Mozzarella, Medium	227
BBQ Stuffed Crust, Large	257
BBQ Stuffed Crust, Medium	251
Classic Crust, Delight Mozzarella, Large	196
Classic Crust, Delight Mozzarella, Medium	180
Classic Crust, Delight Mozzarella, Personal	132
Classic Crust, Delight Mozzarella, Small	162
Classic Crust, Large	203
Classic Crust, Medium	187
Classic Crust, Medium	164
Classic Crust, Personal	136
Double Decadence, Delight Mozzarella, Large	268
Double Decadence, Delight Mozzarella, Medium	245

DOMINO'S PIZZA

PIZZA - NEW YORKER	PER SLICE
Double Decadence, Large	272
Double Decadence, Medium	248
GF Crust, Delight Mozzarella, Small	143
GF Crust, Small	139
Italian Style Crust, Delight Mozzarella, Large	179
Italian Style Crust, Delight Mozzarella, Medium	160
Italian Style Crust, Delight Mozzarella, Small	141
Italian Style Crust, Large	160
Italian Style Crust, Medium	143
Italian Style Crust, Small	127
Stuffed Crust, Delight Mozzarella, Large	236
Stuffed Crust, Delight Mozzarella, Medium	221
Stuffed Crust, Large	262
Stuffed Crust, Medium	245
Thin & Crispy, Delight Mozzarella, Large	166
Thin & Crispy, Delight Mozzarella, Medium	155
Thin & Crispy, Large	175
Thin & Crispy, Medium	163

PIZZA - PEPPERONI PASSION	PER SLICE
BBQ Stuffed Crust, Delight Mozzarella, Large	263
BBQ Stuffed Crust, Delight Mozzarella, Medium	248
BBQ Stuffed Crust, Large	281
BBQ Stuffed Crust, Medium	274
Classic Crust, Delight Mozzarella, Large	216
Classic Crust, Delight Mozzarella, Medium	201
Classic Crust, Delight Mozzarella, Personal	150
Classic Crust, Delight Mozzarella, Small	180
Classic Crust, Large	226
Classic Crust, Medium	210
Classic Crust, Personal	156
Classic Crust, Small	185
Double Decadence, Delight Mozzarella, Large	288
Double Decadence, Delight Mozzarella, Medium	265
Double Decadence, Large	295
Double Decadence, Large	295
Double Decadence, Medium	272
GF Crust, Delight Mozzarella, Small	161
GF Crust, Small	160
Italian Style Crust, Delight Mozzarella, Large	200
Italian Style Crust, Delight Mozzarella, Medium	181
Italian Style Crust, Delight Mozzarella, Small	160
Italian Style Crust, Large	184
Italian Style Crust, Medium	167
Italian Style Crust, Medium	178
Stuffed Crust, Delight Mozzarella, Large	257
Stuffed Crust, Delight Mozzarella, Medium	242
Stuffed Crust, Large	286
Stuffed Crust, Medium	269
Thin & Crispy, Delight Mozzarella, Large	187
Thin & Crispy, Delight Mozzarella, Medium	175
Thin & Crispy, Large	198
Thin & Crispy, Medium	186

DOMINO'S PIZZA

PIZZA - RANCH BBQ	PER SLICE
BBQ Stuffed Crust, Delight Mozzarella, Large	273
BBQ Stuffed Crust, Delight Mozzarella, Medium	248
BBQ Stuffed Crust, Large	273
BBQ Stuffed Crust, Medium	255
Classic Crust, Delight Mozzarella, Large	217
Classic Crust, Delight Mozzarella, Medium	199
Classic Crust, Delight Mozzarella, Personal	148
Classic Crust, Delight Mozzarella, Small	183
Classic Crust, Large	225
Classic Crust, Medium	207
Classic Crust, Personal	153
Classic Crust, Small	184
Double Decadence, Delight Mozzarella, Large	291
Double Decadence, Delight Mozzarella, Medium	265
Double Decadence, Large	292
Double Decadence, Medium	266
GF Crust, Delight Mozzarella, Small	160
GF Crust, Small	167
Italian Style Crust, Delight Mozzarella, Large	196
Italian Style Crust, Delight Mozzarella, Medium	174
Italian Style Crust, Delight Mozzarella, Small	154
Italian Style Crust, Large	201
Italian Style Crust, Medium	178
Italian Style Crust, Small	157
Stuffed Crust, Delight Mozzarella, Large	260
Stuffed Crust, Delight Mozzarella, Medium	242
Stuffed Crust, Large	267
Stuffed Crust, Medium	249
Thin & Crispy, Delight Mozzarella, Large	187
Thin & Crispy, Delight Mozzarella, Medium	173
Thin & Crispy, Large	196
Thin & Crispy, Medium	181

PIZZA - SCRUMMY	PER SLICE
BBQ Stuffed Crust, Delight Mozzarella, Large	273
BBQ Stuffed Crust, Delight Mozzarella, Medium	256
BBQ Stuffed Crust, Large	288
BBQ Stuffed Crust, Medium	280
Classic Crust, Delight Mozzarella, Large	227
Classic Crust, Delight Mozzarella, Medium	209
Classic Crust, Delight Mozzarella, Personal	166
Classic Crust, Delight Mozzarella, Small	189
Classic Crust, Large	234
Classic Crust, Medium	216
Classic Crust, Personal	169
Classic Crust, Small	192
Double Decadence, Delight Mozzarella, Large	299
Double Decadence, Delight Mozzarella, Medium	274
Double Decadence, Large	303
Double Decadence, Medium	277
GF Crust, Delight Mozzarella, Small	170
GF Crust, Small	166
Italian Style Crust, Delight Mozzarella, Large	210

DOMINO'S PIZZA

PIZZA - SCRUMMY	PER SLICE
Italian Style Crust, Delight Mozzarella, Medium	189
Italian Style Crust, Delight Mozzarella, Small	169
Italian Style Crust, Large	191
Italian Style Crust, Medium	172
Italian Style Crust, Small	154
Stuffed Crust, Delight Mozzarella, Large	267
Stuffed Crust, Delight Mozzarella, Medium	250
Stuffed Crust, Large	293
Stuffed Crust, Medium	274
Thin & Crispy, Delight Mozzarella, Large	197
Thin & Crispy, Delight Mozzarella, Medium	184
Thin & Crispy, Large	206
Thin & Crispy, Medium	191

PIZZA - SIZZLER	PER SLICE
BBQ Stuffed Crust, Delight Mozzarella, Large	246
BBQ Stuffed Crust, Delight Mozzarella, Medium	231
BBQ Stuffed Crust, Large	263
BBQ Stuffed Crust, Medium	247
Classic Crust, Delight Mozzarella, Large	206
Classic Crust, Delight Mozzarella, Medium	190
Classic Crust, Delight Mozzarella, Personal	141
Classic Crust, Delight Mozzarella, Small	169
Classic Crust, Large	212
Classic Crust, Medium	195
Classic Crust, Personal	145
Classic Crust, Small	174
Double Decadence, Delight Mozzarella, Large	280
Double Decadence, Delight Mozzarella, Medium	256
Double Decadence, Large	275
Double Decadence, Medium	252
GF Crust, Delight Mozzarella, Small	150
GF Crust, Small	158
Italian Style Crust, Delight Mozzarella, Large	184
Italian Style Crust, Delight Mozzarella, Medium	165
Italian Style Crust, Delight Mozzarella, Small	145
Italian Style Crust, Large	187
Italian Style Crust, Medium	167
Italian Style Crust, Small	146
Stuffed Crust, Delight Mozzarella, Large	240
Stuffed Crust, Delight Mozzarella, Medium	226
Stuffed Crust, Large	258
Stuffed Crust, Medium	242
Thin & Crispy, Delight Mozzarella, Large	174
Thin & Crispy, Delight Mozzarella, Medium	162
Thin & Crispy, Large	182
Thin & Crispy, Medium	170

PIZZA - SPANISH SIZZLER	PER SLICE
BBQ Stuffed Crust, Delight Mozzarella, Large	238
BBQ Stuffed Crust, Delight Mozzarella, Medium	220
BBQ Stuffed Crust, Large	253
BBQ Stuffed Crust, Medium	244
Classic Crust, Delight Mozzarella, Large	191

DOMINO'S PIZZA

PIZZA - SPANISH SIZZLER	PER SLICE
Classic Crust, Delight Mozzarella, Medium	174
Classic Crust, Delight Mozzarella, Personal	129
Classic Crust, Delight Mozzarella, Small	153
Classic Crust, Large	198
Classic Crust, Medium	180
Classic Crust, Personal	133
Classic Crust, Small	156
Double Decadence, Delight Mozzarella, Large	263
Double Decadence, Delight Mozzarella, Medium	238
Double Decadence, Large	267
Double Decadence, Medium	241
GF Crust, Delight Mozzarella, Small	134
GF Crust, Small	130
Italian Style Crust, Delight Mozzarella, Large	175
Italian Style Crust, Delight Mozzarella, Medium	153
Italian Style Crust, Delight Mozzarella, Small	133
Italian Style Crust, Large	155
Italian Style Crust, Medium	137
Italian Style Crust, Small	119
Stuffed Crust, Delight Mozzarella, Large	232
Stuffed Crust, Delight Mozzarella, Medium	215
Stuffed Crust, Large	257
Stuffed Crust, Medium	239
Thin & Crispy, Delight Mozzarella, Large	162
Thin & Crispy, Delight Mozzarella, Medium	148
Thin & Crispy, Large	170
Thin & Crispy, Medium	156

PIZZA - TANDOORI HOT	PER SLICE
BBQ Stuffed Crust, Delight Mozzarella, Large	215
BBQ Stuffed Crust, Delight Mozzarella, Medium	200
BBQ Stuffed Crust, Large	230
BBQ Stuffed Crust, Medium	224
Classic Crust, Delight Mozzarella, Large	168
Classic Crust, Delight Mozzarella, Medium	153
Classic Crust, Delight Mozzarella, Personal	115
Classic Crust, Delight Mozzarella, Small	134
Classic Crust, Large	175
Classic Crust, Medium	160
Classic Crust, Personal	119
Classic Crust, Small	137
Double Decadence, Delight Mozzarella, Large	240
Double Decadence, Delight Mozzarella, Medium	218
Double Decadence, Large	244
Double Decadence, Medium	221
GF Crust, Delight Mozzarella, Small	115
GF Crust, Small	111
Italian Style Crust, Delight Mozzarella, Large	152
Italian Style Crust, Delight Mozzarella, Medium	133
Italian Style Crust, Delight Mozzarella, Small	114
Italian Style Crust, Large	133
Italian Style Crust, Medium	116
Italian Style Crust, Small	99

DOMINO'S PIZZA

PIZZA - TANDOORI HOT

	PER SLICE
Stuffed Crust, Delight Mozzarella, Large	209
Stuffed Crust, Delight Mozzarella, Medium	194
Stuffed Crust, Large	235
Stuffed Crust, Medium	218
Thin & Crispy, Delight Mozzarella, Large	139
Thin & Crispy, Delight Mozzarella, Medium	128
Thin & Crispy, Large	147
Thin & Crispy, Medium	136

PIZZA - TEXAS BBQ

	PER SLICE
BBQ Stuffed Crust, Large	247
BBQ Stuffed Crust, Medium	230
Classic Crust, Large	199
Classic Crust, Medium	181
Classic Crust, Personal	139
Classic Crust, Small	158
Double Decadence, Large	266
Double Decadence, Medium	240
GF Crust, Small	141
Italian Style Crust, Large	175
Italian Style Crust, Medium	153
Italian Style Crust, Small	132
Stuffed Crust, Large	241
Stuffed Crust, Medium	224
Thin & Crispy, Large	169
Thin & Crispy, Medium	155

PIZZA - TUNA DELIGHT

	PER SLICE
BBQ Stuffed Crust, Delight Mozzarella, Large	217
BBQ Stuffed Crust, Delight Mozzarella, Medium	201
BBQ Stuffed Crust, Large	232
BBQ Stuffed Crust, Medium	225
Classic Crust, Delight Mozzarella, Large	170
Classic Crust, Delight Mozzarella, Medium	154
Classic Crust, Delight Mozzarella, Personal	116
Classic Crust, Delight Mozzarella, Small	135
Classic Crust, Large	177
Classic Crust, Medium	161
Classic Crust, Personal	120
Classic Crust, Small	137
Double Decadence, Delight Mozzarella, Large	242
Double Decadence, Delight Mozzarella, Medium	218
Double Decadence, Large	246
Double Decadence, Medium	222
GF Crust, Delight Mozzarella, Small	116
GF Crust, Small	112
Italian Style Crust, Delight Mozzarella, Large	154
Italian Style Crust, Delight Mozzarella, Large	134
Italian Style Crust, Delight Mozzarella, Medium	134
Italian Style Crust, Delight Mozzarella, Small	114
Italian Style Crust, Large	134
Italian Style Crust, Medium	117
Italian Style Crust, Small	100
Stuffed Crust, Delight Mozzarella, Large	211

DOMINO'S PIZZA

PIZZA - TUNA DELIGHT

	PER SLICE
Stuffed Crust, Delight Mozzarella, Medium	195
Stuffed Crust, Large	236
Stuffed Crust, Medium	219
Thin & Crispy, Delight Mozzarella, Large	141
Thin & Crispy, Delight Mozzarella, Medium	129
Thin & Crispy, Large	149
Thin & Crispy, Medium	136

PIZZA - VEG-A-ROMA

	PER SLICE
BBQ Stuffed Crust, Delight Mozzarella, Large	212
BBQ Stuffed Crust, Delight Mozzarella, Medium	197
BBQ Stuffed Crust, Large	229
BBQ Stuffed Crust, Medium	213
Classic Crust, Delight Mozzarella, Large	171
Classic Crust, Delight Mozzarella, Medium	156
Classic Crust, Delight Mozzarella, Personal	125
Classic Crust, Delight Mozzarella, Small	137
Classic Crust, Large	177
Classic Crust, Medium	161
Classic Crust, Personal	126
Classic Crust, Small	142
Double Decadence, Delight Mozzarella, Large	245
Double Decadence, Delight Mozzarella, Medium	222
Double Decadence, Large	241
Double Decadence, Medium	218
GF Crust, Delight Mozzarella, Small	117
GF Crust, Small	125
Italian Style Crust, Delight Mozzarella, Large	150
Italian Style Crust, Delight Mozzarella, Medium	131
Italian Style Crust, Large	152
Italian Style Crust, Medium	133
Italian Style Crust, Small	113
Stuffed Crust, Delight Mozzarella, Large	206
Stuffed Crust, Delight Mozzarella, Medium	191
Stuffed Crust, Large	223
Stuffed Crust, Medium	208
Thin & Crispy, Delight Mozzarella, Large	139
Thin & Crispy, Large	147
Thin & Crispy Crust, Medium	136

PIZZA - VEGI SUPREME

	PER SLICE
BBQ Stuffed Crust, Delight Mozzarella, Large	205
BBQ Stuffed Crust, Delight Mozzarella, Medium	191
BBQ Stuffed Crust, Large	220
BBQ Stuffed Crust, Large	215
Classic Crust, Delight Mozzarella, Large	159
Classic Crust, Delight Mozzarella, Medium	144
Classic Crust, Delight Mozzarella, Personal	109
Classic Crust, Delight Mozzarella, Small	126
Classic Crust, Large	166
Classic Crust, Medium	151
Classic Crust, Personal	113
Classic Crust, Small	128
Double Decadence, Delight Mozzarella, Large	231

DOMINO'S PIZZA

PIZZA - VEGI SUPREME	PER SLICE
Double Decadence, Delight Mozzarella, Medium	208
Double Decadence, Large	235
Double Decadence, Medium	212
Double Decadence, Medium	212
GF Crust, Delight Mozzarella, Small	107
GF Crust, Small	103
Italian Style Crust, Delight Mozzarella, Large	142
Italian Style Crust, Delight Mozzarella, Medium	124
Italian Style Crust, Delight Mozzarella, Small	105
Italian Style Crust, Large	123
Italian Style Crust, Medium	107
Italian Style Crust, Small	91
Stuffed Crust, Delight Mozzarella, Large	199
Stuffed Crust, Delight Mozzarella, Medium	185
Stuffed Crust, Large	225
Stuffed Crust, Medium	209
Thin & Crispy, Delight Mozzarella, Large	129
Thin & Crispy, Delight Mozzarella, Medium	119
Thin & Crispy, Large	138
Thin & Crispy, Medium	126

PIZZA - VEGI VOLCANO	PER SLICE
BBQ Stuffed Crust, Delight Mozzarella, Large	220
BBQ Stuffed Crust, Large	238
BBQ Stuffed Crust, Large	231
Classic Crust, Delight Mozzarella, Large	173
Classic Crust, Delight Mozzarella, Medium	157
Classic Crust, Delight Mozzarella, Personal	117
Classic Crust, Delight Mozzarella, Small	136
Classic Crust, Large	183
Classic Crust, Medium	167
Classic Crust, Personal	123
Classic Crust, Small	142
Double Decadence, Delight Mozzarella, Large	245
Double Decadence, Delight Mozzarella, Medium	222
Double Decadence, Large	252
Double Decadence, Medium	228
GF Crust, Delight Mozzarella, Small	118
GF Crust, Small	116
Italian Style Crust, Delight Mozzarella, Large	157
Italian Style Crust, Delight Mozzarella, Medium	137
Italian Style Crust, Delight Mozzarella, Small	116
Italian Style Crust, Large	140
Italian Style Crust, Medium	123
Italian Style Crust, Small	93
Stuffed Crust, Delight Mozzarella, Large	214
Stuffed Crust, Delight Mozzarella, Medium	198
Stuffed Crust, Large	243
Stuffed Crust, Medium	225
Thin & Crispy, Delight Mozzarella, Large	144
Thin & Crispy, Delight Mozzarella, Medium	132
Thin & Crispy, Large	155
Thin & Crispy, Medium	142

DOMINO'S PIZZA

POTATO WEDGES	
Half Box	168

RIBS	
BBQ, 1 Rib	140

SALAD	
Caesar, ½ Box	95

WRAP	
Chicken, & Bacon, Wrapzz	192
Meatball Feast, Wrapzz	302
Meatball Mayhem, 6, Wrapzz	208
Meatball Mayhem, 8, Wrapzz	246
Pepperoni Passion, 12, Wrapzz	242
Pepperoni Passion, 8, Wrapzz	195
Tandoori Hot, Wrapzz	121
Texas BBQ, Wrapzz	180
Veggie Supreme, Wrapzz	91

EAT

BAGEL	
Smoked Salmon & Cream Cheese	444

BAGUETTE	
Brie, Tomato, & Basil	455
Chicken, Bacon & Avocado	552
Chicken, Pulled, BBQ, The Brooklyn	421
Ham, & Emmental	566
Ham, & Emmental, Half	282
Ham, & Emmental, Rustic	622
Ham, Brie, & Chilli Jam	588
Ham, Brie, & Cranberry	634
Ham Hock, & Egg, The Bronx, Breakfast	439
Prosciutto, Italian	435
Red Pepper Tapenade, Avocado, & Feta, Rustic	526
Reuben, Veggie, The Staten	418
Salmon, & Egg, The Manhattan, Breakfast	484
Tuna, & Cucumber	583
Turkey, Stuffing, & Crispy Onion	635

BARS	
Dried Fruit, Nuts, & Seeds, GF	237

BEANS	
Fava, Chickpea, & Pumpkin Seeds	156

BISCUITS	
Milk Chocolate, Tiffin, Tin	346

BREAD	
Banana	349

BREAKFAST	
Mango, & Coconut, Chia, Pot	309
Poached Egg, & Avocado, with Feta, Pot	313
Poached Egg, & Avocado, with Ham Hock, Pot	307
Poached Egg, BBQ Beans, & Smoked Ham, Hot Pot	334

BREAKFAST CEREAL	
Muesli, Apple, & Berry, Bircher	312
Porridge, Plain, Sm	137
Porridge, Quinoa, & Coconut	441
Porridge, with Banana, & Honey, Big	284

EAT	KCAL
BREAKFAST CEREAL	
Porridge, with Banana, & Honey, Small	210
Porridge, with Banana, Big	234
Porridge, with Banana, Small	162
BROWNIES	
Chocolate, GF	310
BUTTER	
Almond, Porridge Topping	95
CAKE	
Jaffa	253
CROISSANT	
All Butter	347
Almond	365
Chocolate	380
Egg, & Bacon	444
Ham, & Emmental Cheese	513
CURRY	
Chicken, Red Thai, with Noodles	292
DESSERT	
Avocado, & Chocolate, Pot	213
Bakewell, Slice	408
Carrot, Cake	265
Carrot, Caramel, & Pecan, Cake	443
Cheesecake, Sicilian Lemon	284
Coffee, & Walnut, Cake	371
Cookie, Oat, & Fruit	329
Cookie, Triple Chocolate	394
Lemon Drizzle Cake	555
Mincemeat, Merry, Crumble, Slice	350
Red Velvet, Cake	263
Tiffin, Milk Chocolate & Brazil Nut	374
EGGS	
Free Range, & Chilli Greens	116
FLAPJACK	
with Sultanas, Apricots, & Orange, GF	263
FLATBREAD	
Butternut, Chickpea, & Harissa	506
Chilli, Beef, & Cheese	509
Chipotle, Cheddar, & Black Bean	499
FRUIT	
Grape, Bag	80
Mango, & Lime, Pot	86
FRUIT COMPOTE	
Apple, & Cinnamo, Porridge Topping	55
FRUIT SALAD	
Clementine, Blackberry, & Redcurrant	70
Rainbow	95
FUDGE	
Scottish, Handmade	194
HOT POT	
Mac 'N' Cheese, Kids	232
Mac 'N' Cheese, Large	790
Mac 'N' Cheese, Reg	544

EAT	KCAL
HOT POT	
Pigs in Blankets, Mash, & Gravy	498
Pigs in Blankets	237
Turkey, Festive, Full Works	504
HOUMOUS	
Turmeric, & Dip Sticks	237
MISO	
Wakame, Mushroom, & Noodles	147
NOODLES	
Chicken, Ramen	262
NUT & SEED MIX	
Chocolate Almonds, Raisins, Sunflower Seeds	380
NUTS	
Natural, Mix	222
PAIN AU RAISIN	
Pastry	383
PEANUTS	
Honey Coated, with Chilli	204
PIE	
Cauliflower, & Kale, Cheese, Pie Only	678
Cauliflower, & Kale, Cheese, with Mash, & Gravy	926
Chicken, & Mushroom, Pie Only	685
Chicken, & Mushroom, with Mash, & Gravy	931
Mince, Famous	310
Steak, & Ale, Pie Only	553
Steak, & Ale, with Mash, & Gravy	799
PIZZA	
Chicken, Grill	533
POPCORN	
Salted, Rock Salt	105
Sweet, & Salty	136
ROLL	
Bacon, British Back, Rustic	321
Bacon, Poached Egg, British Back, Rustic	336
SALAD	
Beetroot, Squash, & Feta	359
Chicken, Caeser Mayonnaise, Four Leaf Salad	347
Chicken, Noodle, Spicy, Less Than 5% Fat	429
Crayfish, Spicy, Noodles, Less Than 5% Fat	380
Houmous, & Falafel, Mezze, with Dressing	473
Houmous, & Falafel, Mezze, without Dressing	371
Jerk Chicken, with Dressing	313
Jerk Chicken, without Dressing	266
Miso, & Beef, Tahini, with Dressing	463
Miso, & Beef, Tahini, without Dressing	335
Quinoa, Black Rice, & Nuts, Super Nutty, Fit Box	342
Salmon, Smoked, & Egg, Fit Box	260
Tuna, Nicoise, with Dressing	345
Tuna, Nicoise, & without Dressing	188
SANDWICH	
Butternut Squash, Stuffing, & Slaw	445
Cheese, Marmite, Morning Melt	458
Cheese, Tomato, Soft Grain	391

EAT
SANDWICH

Chicken, & Bacon	457
Chicken, Roast, Salad	616
Chicken, Smoked, & Basil, on Stonebaked Ciabatta	458
Chicken & Chorizo	371
Egg Mayo, & Watercress, Chunky, Malted Bread	403
Emmenthal, Simple, Kids	435
Full Works, Festive, White Bloomer	599
Ham, & Egg, Free Range	567
Ham, & Mature Cheddar	474
Ham, Simple, Kids, on Malted Granary Bread	326
Pastrami, New York	525
Salmon, Smoked, Soft Cheese, Malted Granary	367
Tuna, Mayonnaise, & Cucumber	365
Turkey, & Cranberry, Less Than 5% Fat	359

SHORTBREAD

Millionaires	441

SOUP

Bacon, & Potato, Fully Loaded, Sm	250
Beef, Rendang, Malaysian, without Garnish, Sm	261
Beef Ragu, Reg	283
Beef Ragu, Small	217
Beef Ragu, Very Big	425
Broth, Shot	33
Butternut Squash, Thai, Sm	168
Cauliflower Cheese, Sm	219
Chicken, & Garden Vegetable, Sm	123
Chicken, & Kale Dahl, Big	251
Chicken, & Kale Dahl, Small	192
Chicken & Kale Dahl, Very Big	405
Chicken, Chipotle, & Black Bean	247
Chicken, Jerk, without Garnish, Sm	282
Chicken, Laksa, without Salad Garnish, Sm	256
Chicken, Mushroom, & Barley, with Garnish, Sm	216
Chicken, Pot Pie, no Pastry, Sm	216
Chicken, Pot Pie, with Pastry, Big	413
Chicken, Pot Pie, with Pastry, Small	343
Chicken, Pot Pie, with Pastry, Very Big	576
Chicken, Thai Green Curry, no Garnish, Sm	243
Chicken Noodle, Coconut, Sm	313
Duck, Hoi Sin, Gyoza, Pho, Pot	392
French Onion with Garnish	267
Leek, & Potato, Sm	210
Lentil, Spiced, Spinach, & Sweet Potato	279
Meatball, Italian, without Garnish, Sm	228
Mushroom, Wild, & Chestnut, Sm	240
Red Pepper, & Goats Cheese, Fire Roasted, Sm	141
Sweet Potato, & Chilli, Sm	261
Sweetcorn, Creamy, Sm	315
Tomato, & Basil, Spicy, Sm	78
Tomato, Slow Roasted, Creamy, Sm	240
Vegetable Gyoza, Wok Pot, Broth	300

KCAL

EAT
SPONGE

Chocolate, Cookie Buttercream, & Chocolate Button	451

SWEETS

Midget Gems	174

TOAST

Avocado, Sourdough	338
Avocado, with Feta, Sourdough	392
Avocado, with Ham Hock, Sourdough	376
Ham, Cheese, Dijon Mustard, Stonebaked Ciabatta	551
Mozzarella, Pesto, & Tomato, Stonebaked Ciabatta	539
Sourdough, with Butter	218

TOASTIE

British Beef & English Mustard Grill	506
Tuna, & Cheddar Melt, on Ciabatta Bread	650

TORTILLA CHIPS

Guacamole, Creamy, & Chipotle Bean Salsa	233

WRAP

Beetroot, & Feta	401
Chicken, Mexican	427
Chicken, Salad	491
Duck, Hoisin	421
Houmous, & Falafel	492
Houmous, & Falafel, Half	246
Simple Houmous, & Salad	377

YOGHURT

Honey, Grapenuts, & Banana	349
with Berry Compote	136
with Granola, & Berry Compote	303

YULE LOG

Festive	173

FIVE GUYS
BURGERS

Bacon, Bunless	628
Bacon	888
Bacon, Little, Bunless	383
Bacon, Little	643
Cheeseburger, Bacon, Bunless	708
Cheeseburger, Bacon	968
Cheeseburger, Bacon, Little, Bunless	423
Cheeseburger, Bacon, Little	683
Cheeseburger, Bunless	570
Cheeseburger	830
Cheeseburger, Little, Bunless	285
Cheeseburger, Little	545
Hamburger, Bunless	490
Hamburger, Bunless, Little	245
Hamburger	750
Hamburger, Little	505

FRIES

Large	1314
Little	526
Reg	953

	KCAL		KCAL

FIVE GUYS
HOT DOG
Bacon, & Cheese, Bunless	388
Bacon, & Cheese	648
Bacon, Bunless	348
Bacon	608
Cheese, Bunless	250
Cheese	510
Original, Bunless	210
Original	470
SANDWICH
BLT	642
Cheese, Grilled	470
Veggie, Cheese	372
Veggie	292
TOPPING
BBQ Sauce	45
Green Peppers	4
Jalapenos	2
Lettuce	4
Mayonnaise	93
Mushrooms	6
Onions	9
Relish	18
Tomatoes	9

GOURMET BURGER KITCHEN
BACON
Crispy, Extras	54
BURGERS
Beef, Avocado, & Bacon	875
Beef, Blue Cheese, with Blue Cheese Mayo	935
Beef, Blue Cheese, with Blue Cheese Mayo, Small	645
Beef, Blue Cheese, with Cheese Slice	817
Beef, Blue Cheese, with Cheese Slice, Small	582
Beef, Bourbon Street	885
Beef, Cheese, & Bacon, with American Cheese	942
Beef, Cheese, & Bacon, with Cheddar	982
Beef, Cheese, & Bacon, with Red Leicester	980
Beef, Cheese, & Bacon, with Smoked Applewood	982
Beef, Classic	692
Beef, Classic, Small	533
Beef, Classic, with American Cheese	815
Beef, Classic, with American Cheese, Small	595
Beef, Classic, with Cheddar	855
Beef, Classic, with Cheddar, Small	614
Beef, Classic, with Red Leicester	853
Beef, Classic, with Red Leicester, Small	613
Beef, Classic, with Smoked Applewood	855
Beef, Classic, with Smoked Applewood, Small	696
Beef, Habanero	839
Beef, Junior	538
Beef, Kiwiburger	996
Beef, Major Tom	922
Beef, Taxidriver	875

GOURMET BURGER KITCHEN
BURGERS
Beef, the Don	867
Beef, The Mighty	1328
Beef, The Stack	1010
Buffalo	811
Chicken, & Bacon, Pesterella	860
Chicken, & Bacon, Pesterella, Panko	1041
Chicken, Cajun Blue	583
Chicken, Cajun Blue, Panko	757
Chicken, Cam & Cranberry	622
Chicken, Cam & Cranberry, Panko	803
Chicken, Classic	445
Chicken, Classic, Panko	627
Chicken, Classic, Panko, Small	579
Chicken, Classic, Small	360
Chicken, Grilled, Junior	348
Chicken, Panko, Junior	499
Chicken, Satay	552
Chicken, Satay, Panko	795
Lamb, Herman the Lamb	845
Lamb, Psychobilly	676
BURGERS VEGETARIAN
Californian	802
Classic	513
Classic, Small	406
Classic, with American Cheese	635
Classic, with American Cheese, Small	468
Classic, with Cheddar	676
Classic, with Cheddar, Small	488
Classic, with Red Leicester	674
Classic, with Red Leicester, Small	487
Classic, with Smoked Applewood	676
Classic, with Smoked Applewood, Small	489
Dippy Hippy	598
Falafel	550
Johnny Be Goat	485
Junior	467
CHEESE
American, Extras	123
Cheddar, Extras	163
Halloumi, Bites	418
Red Leicester, Extras	161
Smoked Applewood, Extras	163
CHICKEN
Bites, Chilli Fried	289
Skewers, with Smoked Chilli Mayo	466
COLESLAW
Blue Cheese Slaw	412
Homeslaw	49
FRIES
Chunky	635
Skinny	454
Sweet Potato	405

GOURMET BURGER KITCHEN

FRIES
Sweet Potato, with Baconnaise	632
Truffle Cheese	756

MILK SHAKE
Banana	627
Banana, Junior	313
Chocolate	752
Chocolate, Junior	376
Honeycomb	722
Honeycomb, Junior	361
Lime	640
Lime, Junior	320
Oreo	850
Oreo, Junior	425
Peanut Butter	912
Peanut Butter, Junior	456
Salted Caramel	681
Salted Caramel, Junior	340
Strawberry	631
Strawberry, Junior	315
The Nutter	1034
The Nutter, Junior	517
Vanilla	624
Vanilla, Junior	312

MUSHROOMS
Bourbon Glazed, Extras	30

ONION RINGS
Extras	171
House	514

PEPPERS
Jalapeno, Extras	22

PICKLE
Dill, Extras	13

PINEAPPLE
Extras	48

SALAD
Chicken, Chilli Chick	507
Simple	81
Siperfood	669

SAUCE
Chilli Salsa	37
Mayo, Baconnaise	227
Mayo, Basil	245
Mayo, Blue Cheese	225
Mayo, Garlic	241
Mayo, Smoked Chilli	202
Mayo, Sriracha	219

SWEETCORN
with Butter, 1 Piece	73

GREGGS

BAGUETTE
Bacon, & Egg, Omelette, Free Range, Hot	544
Bacon, & Sausage, Hot	617

GREGGS

BAGUETTE
Bacon, Hot	540
Cheese, & Ham	541
Cheese, & Ham, Hot	542
Cheese, & Salad	492
Chicken, Club	491
Chicken, Southern Fried, Hot	585
Chicken, Tandoori	494
Chicken Mayonnaise	488
Egg, Omelette, Free Range, Hot	454
Meatball, Spicy, Aberdeen Angus, Hot	558
Prawn Mayonnaise	473
Sausage, & Egg, Omelette, Free Range, Hot	593
Sausage, Hot	604
Tuna, Crunch	462

BAKE
Chicken	426
Sausage, Bean, & Cheese, Melt	453
Steak	405

BARS
Granola	296

BISCUITS
Bunny	269
Gingerbread, Man	180
Jammy Heart	285
Shortbread, Caramel	297

BREAD
Brown, Bloomer	98
Oatmeal, Loaf	190
Rolls, Corn Topped	190
Rolls, Oval Bite	230
Rolls, Sub, Seeded	270
Rolls, Sub, White	230
Stottie	347
White, Bloomer, Loaf	138

BREAKFAST CEREAL
Porridge, Creamy Oats, Simply	253
Porridge, Golden Syrup	248
Porridge, Red Berry	250

BROWNIES
Chocolate, Mini	90

BUNS
Belgian	403
Cinnamon	425
Easter Ring	246
Hot Cross	176
Iced, Christmas Ring	210
Iced, Finger	111
Ring, Novelty	243

CAKE
Christmas Slice	360
Crispy Cornfake	280
Easter, Crispy nest	326

GREGGS

CAKE

Raspberry, & Almond, Bake	63
Rocky Road, Belgian Chocolate	362
Vanilla Slice	359
Victoria Sponge, Mini	497

COFFEE

Americano, Large	11
Americano, Reg	9
Black, Decaf, Large	7
Black, Decaf, Reg	6
Cappuccino, No Chocolate Topping, Large	111
Cappuccino, No Chocolate Topping, Reg	90
Espresso, Double	11
Espresso, Shot	8
Latte, Large	133
Latte, Reg	111
Mocha, Large	300
Mocha, Reg	233
White, Decaf, Large	24
White, Decaf, Reg	19
White, Large	45
White, Reg	34

COLA

Coca-Cola	139
Coke Zero, Coca-Cola	3
Diet, Coca-Cola	3

COOKIES

Chocolate, Chunk, Triple	374
Chocolate, Milk	380
Chocolate, White	382
Fruit & Oat	341

CROISSANT

All Butter	298
Almond	343

CUPCAKES

Chocolate	280
Easter	393
Foundation	320
Ice Cream	270
Sweet Lemon	380

DOUGHNUTS

Caramel	303
Chocolate, & Vanilla, Triple	341
Chocolate, Milk, Ring	223
Cream, Finger	334
Cream, Toffee, Finger	379
Glazed, Ring	191
Iced, Ring	226
Jam	242
Mini	64
Pink, Jammie	334
Sugar Strand	246
Yum Yum	291

GREGGS

DOUGHNUTS

Yum Yum, Mini	120

DRIED FRUIT

Sweet Mango	88

DRIED FRUIT MIX

Berries & Cherries	81

ECLAIR

with Cream Filling	347

FANTA

Fanta	150

FLAPJACK

Fruity, Mini	110

FRUIT

Medley	72
Summer Berry Pot	91
Tropical, Fingers	70

GRAPES

Mixed	92

HOT CHOCOLATE

Large	281
Reg	219

IRN BRU

Diet	2
Original	215

JUICE

Apple, Fairtrade	220
Orange, Fairtrade	220

JUICE DRINK

Citrus Punch, Oasis	90
Summer Fruits, Oasis	90

LEMONADE

Raspberry, Sparkling	10

LUCOZADE

Energy Orange	350
Sport	140

MIXED NUTS

Naked	156

MUFFIN

Chocolate, Triple	507
Jam & Toast, Breakfast	381
Lemon, Sicilian	500
Sticky Toffee	530

PAIN AU CHOCOLAT

Pastry	297
with Belgian Chocolate	393

PASTA

Cheese & Tomato, with Mixed Herbs, Pot	381
Fajita Chicken, in Tomato Sauce, Spicy, Pot	345

PASTA SALAD

Cheese, & Tomato	399
Cheese, Tomato, & Basil	328
Chicken, Mexican	375
Tuna, Crunch	283

GREGGS

PASTRY
	KCAL
Greggsnut, Caramel & Pecan	457

PASTY
Beef, & Vegetable	509
Cheese, & Onion	434
Steak, & Cheese, Roll	340

PIE
Mince, Sweet	290
Mince, Sweet, Iced	230

PIZZA
Margherita, Thin & Crispy, Slice	365
Pepperoni, Thin & Crispy, Slice	444

PUDDING
Bread	118

RIBENA*
Original	215

ROLL - CORN TOPPED
Bacon, & Egg, Omelette, Free Range, Hot	363
Bacon, & Sausage, Hot	437
Bacon, Hot	359
Sausage, & Egg, Omelette, Free Range	394
Sausage, Hot	407

ROLL - OVAL BITES
Chicken, & Salad, Honey Mustard Mayo, Seeded	389
Chicken, Mexican, & Salad, Fajita Mayo, Seeded	393
Egg, Omelette, Free Range, Hot	380

SALAD
Chicken, & Bacon, Layered	327
Chicken, Chargrill	200
Chicken, Chargrill	200
Chicken, Chargrill, Roasted Vegetables, & Grains	235
Chicken, Coconut, Lime & Chilli	220
Chicken, Teriyaki, & Noodle	256
Falafel, & Houmous	316
Ham, & Egg, Honey Roast	238

SANDWICH
Cheese, & Onion	366
Egg Mayonnaise, Free Range	348
Ham, & Egg, with Salad, Honey Roast	347
Tuna Mayonnaise, & Cucumber	350

SAUSAGE ROLL
Freshly Baked	349
Mini	81

SCONE
Derby	268

SEED MIX
Super	135

SLICES
Toffee Apple, Lattice	277

SMOOTHIE
Mango & Orange	145
Raspberry & Banana	135

GREGGS

SOUP
	KCAL
Tomato, Cream of	213
Tomato	240

SPRITE*
Original	220

SUBS
Chicken Mayonnaise	342
Ham, & Salad	332
Tuna Mayonnaise	336

TART
Egg Custard	257
Strawberry	180
Strawberry, with Fresh Cream	300

TEA
White, Large	12
White, Reg	9

TEACAKES
Bakery	206

TURNOVER
Apple, Fresh Cream	540

WATER
Cranberry or Raspberry	5

WRAP
Bacon, & Cheese	320
Chicken, & Bacon, Caesar	450
Chicken, Chargrilled	410
Chicken, Chilli, Coconut, & Lime	340
Chicken, Katsu	394
Moroccan Tagine Chicken	354

YOGHURT
Mango, & Passionfruit	162
Strawberry, & Granola, Natural	226
Strawberry, & Granola, with Almonds & Seeds	194

HARVESTER RESTAURANT

BEANS
Baked, Side, Kids Menu	52
Green, Fried, Cajun, Tapas	421

BEEF
Rib, Short, Bourbon, Glazed	1112
Steak, & Eggs	972
Steak, Fillet, 8oz	935
Steak, Rump, 12oz	1216
Steak, Rump, 4oz, Kids Menu	189
Steak, Rump, 8oz	1026
Steak, Sirloin, 10oz	1170

BREAD
Garlic, Cheesy, Tapas	695
Garlic, Tapas	331

BREAKFAST
Harvester, Recommends,	1077
Vegetarian, Harvester, Recommends	607

BROWNIES
Chocolate, Rocky Horror	729

HARVESTER RESTAURANT

BUNS

Fish Finger	1050
Steak, Rib-eye, Brioche	1151

BURGERS

Beef, Cheese, & Bacon	1254
Beef, Chicken, Breast, with Half Rack Ribs	1714
Beef, Classic	1055
Beef, Extra	329
Beef, Pulled Pork, BBQ	1395
Beef, with Cheese, Kids Menu	556
Beef, with Guacamole, Kids Menu	441
Beef, with Pineapple, Kids Menu	400
Beef, with Salsa, Kids Menu	403
Chicken, Breast, Grilled, Classic	934
Chicken, Breast, Peri Peri	1447
Chicken, Extra	207
Chicken, with Cheese, Kids Menu	500
Chicken, with Guacamole, Kids Menu	385
Chicken, with Pineapple, Kids Menu	344
Chicken, with Salsa, Kids Menu	347

BURGERS VEGETARIAN

Beetroot, & Halloumi	1122
Beetroot, Classic	809
Beetroot, Extra	82

CAKE

Chocolate, Fudge	1221

CHEESE

Halloumi, Battered, & Chips	1015
Halloumi, Skewers, Tapas	380

CHEESECAKE

Vanilla, & Lemon, Baked	684

CHICKEN

Breast, BBQ, Grilled, Kids Menu	306
Breast, Buttermilk, Fried, Tapas	511
Breast, Cajun, & Chorizo, Grilled	873
Breast, Grilled, Bacon, & Buttermilk, Fried, Combo	1440
Breast, Grilled, Kids Menu	185
Breast, with King Prawns, Spicy	1105
Fried, & Waffles	1401
Fried, Buttermilk, Kids Menu	340
Grilled, with Jacket Potato	540
Half, Rotisserie	1194
Half, Rotisserie, with Half Rack Ribs, Combo	1532
Penne, Arrabiata, Spicy	931
Quarter, Rotisserie, Kids Menu	252
Quarter, Rotisserie, Triple, Combo	1343
Quarter, Rotisserie, with Ribs, Combo	1354
Strips, Kids Menu, Sm Bites	92
Whole, Rotisserie	2390
Wings, Sticky, Tapas	210
Wings, with BBQ, Sticky, Tapas	266
Wings, with Peri Peri, Sticky, Tapas	367

HARVESTER RESTAURANT

CHICKEN CARIBBEAN

with Golden Rice & Beans, & Grilled Pepper	635

COD

Fillet, Battered, Kids Menu	431

CORN

Buttered, Side	214
Cobette, Side, Kids Menu	95
Cobettes	96

CUSTARD

& Banana, with Chocolate Sauce, Kids Menu	441
Extra	90

DESSERT

Chocolate Cookie Pizza, Build Your Own, Kids Menu	721
Eton Mess, Strawberry	693
Key Lime Pie	674
Knickerbocker Glory	595
Mango, & Passionfruit, Blizzard	651
Millionaires Shortbread	964
Mississippi Mud Pie, Baileys	953
Mississippi Mud Pie, no Baileys	872
Salted Caramel, & Chocolate, Bar	485

EGGS

Benedict	716
Poached, Breakfast Muffin, Avocado, California	455
Royale	700

FALAFEL

& Houmous, Tapas	329

FISH & CHIPS

with Mushy Peas	1505
with Peas	1446

FISH FINGERS

Kids Menu	220
Kids Menu, Sm Bites	166

FRIES

Sage, & Onion, Side	400
Side	399
Side, Kids Menu	216
Sweet Potato, Side	503

FRUIT SALAD

with Greek Yoghurt, & Granola	172
with Strawberry Yoghurt, Kids Menu	108

GAMMON

Steak, 7oz	773
Steak, 7oz, Egg, & Pineapple	917
Steak, 7oz, with Egg	890
Steak, 7oz, with Pineapple	800

ICE CREAM

Extra	119

ICE LOLLY

Strawberry, & Banana, Kids Menu	33

JAMBALAYA

Sweet Potato	735

HARVESTER RESTAURANT

JELLY

	KCAL
Orange, Fruitypot, Kids Menu	100

MACARONI CHEESE

Bites, Tapas	388
Side	367
with Veg, Kids Menu	220

MEATBALLS

Pork, Tapas	235

MIXED GRILL

Steak, Rib-eye, 5oz, Chicken, Gammon, Sausage	1464
Steak, Rump, 4oz, Chicken, Gammon, Sausage	1360

MUSHROOMS

Portabello, Battered	218
Portobello, Tapas	567

NACHOS

Cheese, Guacamole, Salsa, Tapas	595
Cheese, Guacamole, Salsa & Sour Cream	438

OMELETTE

Cheese, & Tomato, Kids Menu	218
Kids Menu	145
Kids Menu, Sm Bites	139
with Cheese, Kids Menu, Sm Bites	212

PASTA

Greek Style	368
In Tomato Sauce, Kids Menu, Sm Bites	240

PEAS

Side, Kids Menu	26

PENNE

Arrabiata	559

PEPPER

Jalapeno, Cream Cheese, Poppers, Tapas	455
Red, Stuffed	1037

PIE

Cherry, Sweet	568

PORK

Belly, Maple, Glazed, Smoked	1637

POTATO MASH

Side	187
Side, Kids Menu	83

POTATO SKINS

Cheese, & Bacon, Tapas	389
Cheese, Tapas	278

POTATOES

Jacket, Side	273
Jacket, Side, Kids Menu	245
Jacket, with Sour Cream, Side	355

PRAWNS

King, Garlic, Tapas	248
King, in Garlic Butter	165
Spicy, Crackerjack	150
Spicy, Crackerjack, Tapas	413

PUDDING

Sticky Toffee	492

HARVESTER RESTAURANT

RIBS

	KCAL
Half Rack, BBQ Sauce	747
Half Rack, Kids Menu	348
Half Rack, with BBQ Sauce	321
Pork, Full Rack, Slow Cooked, in BBQ Sauce	1427
Smoked, St Louis, with BBQ Sauce	1704

RICE

Cheese, & Tomato, Side, Kids Menu	192
Spicy, Side	231

RICE PUDDING

Coconut, & Raspberrry	405

SALMON

Grilled, Kids Menu	192
Grilled, with Jacket Potato	895

SAUCE - STEAK

Bacon, Smoked, Red Wine & Mushroom	49
Bearnaise	210
Peppercorn	76
Whisky, & Mushroom	86

SAUSAGE

Chorizo, Grilled, Tapas	287
Whirl, Mini	191
Whirl, Mini, Kids Menu	375
Whirl, Mini, Kids Menu, Sm Bites	185

SAUSAGE & MASH

Main	985

SAUSAGE VEGETARIAN

BBQ, Chargrilled, Kids Menu	280
with Gravy, Kids Menu, Sm Bites	161

SCAMPI

Extra	250
Wholetail, Crispy	1021

SEA BASS

& Chorizo, Stack, Spicy	956

SUNDAE

Best, Kids Menu	270
Build Your Own, Kids Menu	474
Chocolate, Brownie, Rocky Horror, Kids Menu	482
Vanilla, with Belgian Chocolate Sauce	348
Vanilla, with Butterscotch Sauce	351
Vanilla, with Raspberry Sauce	347
Vanilla, with Strawberry Sauce	347

SWEET POTATO

Fries, Side, Kids Menu	268

SWEETS

Munchies, Sundae, Extra	146
Oreo, Crumb, Sundae, Extra	134
Skittles, Sundae, Extra	120

TAGINE

Aubergine, & Red Lentil	1010
Aubergine, & Red Lentil, Kids Menu	303

VEGETABLES

Side, Kids Menu	59

	KCAL		KCAL
HARVESTER RESTAURANT		**HUNGRY HORSE**	
VEGETABLES		**BURGERS**	
Steamed, Side	59	CBA	1309
Sticks, Side, Kids Menu	44	Chicken, Double, Hot Mama	2381
WAFFLES		Dirty Dip	1853
Belgian, with Bacon, Egg, & Maple Syrup	1110	**BURGERS VEGETARIAN**	
Blueberry	886	Falafel, Double	1490
WRAP		Falafel	1238
Chicken, Breast, Cajun, Grilled	527	**BURRITO**	
Chicken, Breast, Grilled	528	Chicken, BBQ,	807
Chicken, Build Your Own, Kids Menu	609	Vegetable, Open	604
Chicken, Fried	775	**CAKE**	
Falafel, Build Your Own, Kids Menu	613	Chocolate, Fudge	973
Falafel	514	**CHEESE**	
YOGHURT		Camembert, with Bread	634
Strawberry, Kids Menu	99	**CHEESECAKE**	
HUNGRY HORSE		Lemon Meringue, with Ice Cream	415
BEEF		Millionaires	665
Rump, 5oz	883	**CHICKEN**	
BEEF - ROAST		BBQ, Jerk, Big Plate Specials	1655
Sunday	993	BBQ, Jerk	749
Sunday, Big Plate Special	1501	Breast, Roast, Sunday, Kids Menu	477
Sunday, Kids	493	Breast, Skewer, Extra	208
with Gravy, All Week	808	Crispy, Jumbo, Big Plate Specials	1661
BEEF - STEAK		Fillet, Roast, Sunday	809
Rump, 24oz, Megasaurus, Big Plate Specials	1794	Fillet, Roast, Sunday, Big Plate Special	1317
Rump, 12oz, Big Plate Specials	1360	New Yorker, Big Plate Special	1758
Rump, 8oz	988	New Yorker	1193
Rump, 8oz, Smothered, Sizzler, Big Plate Specials	1399	Roast, with Gravy, All Week	668
Sirloin, 9oz, Big Plate Specials	1340	Southern Fried, Skewer, Extra	422
BREAD		Wings, 10	640
Brown, Buttered, Side	303	**CHICKEN TIKKA**	
Garlic, Cheesy, Ciabatta	602	Masala, Big Plate Specials	2329
Garlic, Ciabatta	438	Masala, with Rice	821
White, Buttered, Side	330	**CHIPS**	
BREAKFAST		& Cheese, Side	582
All Day, Big Plate Specials	1094	Side	418
BROWNIES		**COD & CHIPS**	
Choc Ice	500	Jumbo, Big Plate Specials	1610
BUNS		**COLESLAW**	
Lamb Kofta, Steamed	969	Side	75
Oriental, Steamed	459	**CORN**	
BURGERS		Cob, Side	174
Beef, & Chicken, Quadzilla, Big Plate Specials	3211	Creamed, Cheesy, Side	373
Beef, Bacon, & Cheese, Double	2027	**CRUMBLE**	
Beef, Bacon, & Cheese	1536	Apple	411
Beef, Cheese, Double	1982	**CURRY - CHICKEN**	
Beef, Cheese	1491	with Rice, Big Plate Specials	2213
Beef, Classic, Double	1900	with Rice	705
Beef, Classic	1409	**CURRY - CHICKPEA**	
Beef, Double Daddy	2923	& Sweet Potato, with Rice, Big Plate Specials	2237
Beef, Pit	1852	& Sweet Potato, with Rice	730
Beef, The Elvis	1948	**EGGS**	
Black & Blue	1585	Fried, Steak Topper	202

HUNGRY HORSE

FAJITA
Chicken, Piri Piri, Big Plate Special	1407

FRIES
Side	546
Sweet Potato, Side	410

GAMMON
Gigantic, Big Plate Specials	1316
Grilled	734

KORMA
Chicken, with Rice, Big Plate Specials	2316
Chicken, with Rice	808

LAMB
Rump, Big Plate Specials	1075
Shank, Minted, with Mash	529

LASAGNE
Beef, Oven Baked	780

MACARONI CHEESE
Main	569
Side	281

MEZZE
Board, for Two	1443

MIXED GRILL
Full Monty, Big Plate Special	1754
Mini	1154

MUSHROOMS
& Stilton, Topper	171
Garlic, Creamy	374

NACHOS
Cheese, Salsa, Guacamole, Sharing	1049
Chilli, Topper	198

ONION RINGS
Side	342
Stacker, 20	1584

PASTA
Pesto, & Vegetable, Creamy	471
Pesto, & Vegetable, Creamy, with Chicken	675

PEPPERS
Jalapeno, Battered, Crispy, Side	116

PIE
Beef, & Ale	1530
Beef, Gravy, Rich, Big Plate Specials	1873
Beef, Gravy, Rich, with Chips, Big Plate Specials	2447
Beef, Gravy, Rich, with Mash, Big Plate Specials	2122
Cheese, Onion, & Potato, Big Plate Specials	1349
Ham, Hock, & Mushy Pea	1073

PUDDING
Sticky Toffee	968

RIBS
BBQ, Half Rack, Side	342

RICE
Mexican, Side	192

RISOTTO
Goats Cheese	453

HUNGRY HORSE

RISOTTO
Topper	204

SALAD
Side, Dressed	22

SAUCE
BBQ, Beer Can, Steak Sauce	206
BBQ, Jerk, Steak Sauce	226
Beef, Gravy, Steak Sauces	149
Lemon, & Garlic, Steak Sauce	160
Peppercorn, & Stilton, Steak Sauce	149
Peppercorn, Steak Sauce	64

SAUSAGE & MASH
Pork	772
Quorn	1376

SCAMPI
Chicken Wings & Goujons, Mushrooms, & Nachos	2366
Jumbo, Big Plate Specials	1519
Wholetail, Steak Topper	172

SOUP
Tomato, & Thyme	342

SPONGE
Syrup	665

SQUID
Calamari, Breaded	371

SUBS
Chicken, Club	874

SUNDAE
Sweetshop, Mania	637
Sweetshop, Mania, Ultimate	1495
Vanilla, Chocolate, Candy, Mania	794
Vanilla, Chocolate, Candy, Mania, Ultimate	1724

TORTE
Chocolate, & Coconut Milk	433

VEGETARIAN
Fish, & Chips	1596
Roast, Sunday,	1707
Roast, Sunday	1211
Roast, Sunday, Kids Menu	987

YORKSHIRE PUDDING
Roast Beef, Burrito	1387

ITSU

BEANS
Edamame	124
Edamame, Yoghurt Coated, ½ Pack	110

BREAD
Wrap, Khobez, for Salad & Sandwich Box	178

CHICKEN &
Coconut, Noodle Pot	299

CHICKEN TERIYAKI
On a Bed, Low Carb	423
Potsu, Hot	446

DRESSING
Caesar	57

ITSU

DRESSING

	KCAL
for Salad Boxes	41
Green Herb	37
Peanut, Bang Bang	53
Teriyaki	39

DRIED FRUIT & NUTS

Superseeds, Frogo	359

DUMPLINGS

Vegetable, with Rice	382

EGGS

Benedict, with Brown & Red Rice	363
Florentine, with Brown & Red Rice	289

FRUIT

Fresh, Pot	102

FRUIT COCKTAIL

Melon, Pineapple, Mango, Apple & Red Grapes	80

FRUIT SALAD

Hawaii 5 0	113

MIXED FRUIT

Yoghurt Fruit & Goji Berries	211

NOODLES

Pot, Chicken	409
Vegetable Festival, Crystal Noodle Cup	160

POPCORN

Sea Salt Flavour	115
Wasabi	121

POTSU

Ricebowl, Superbowl, Large	525
Superbowl, 7 Vegetables with Rice	525

PUDDING

Lemon Zinger	234
White Chocolate Dream, Pot	293

RICE CAKES

Chocolate, Dark	85
Chocolate, Milk	249
Yoghurt	240

RICE CRACKERS

Peanut, Snack	239

SALAD

Box, Smoked Chicken	425
Chicken, Avocado & Hard Boiled Egg, Low Carb	345
Chicken, Avocado & Poached Egg	399
Chicken, Smoked, Low Carb, Box	269
Chicken & Avocado	340
Duck Hoisin & Quinoa	488
Egg, Avo & Quinoa, with Spicy Sauce, Go Go Pot	192
Egg & Muki 'Go .Go'	149
Greens & Beans, with Zero Noodles	176
Ham Hock	404
Hip & Healthy, Box	230
Lobster, Freshwater & Poached Egg, Go Go Pot	79
Low Carb Salmon & Tuna Tartar, Box	173
Miso Salmon, with Zero Noodles, & Green Beans	198

ITSU

SALAD

	KCAL
Roast Beef Vietnam, Double Bed	618
Salmon & Tuna Tartare, Low Carb	160
Salmon Supreme, Omega 3	367
Satay Chicken, Zero Noodles	191
Special Salmon	402
Special Salmon & Poached Egg	314
Tokyo Caesar, on a Bed	352
Tuna, Low Carb	169
Tuna, No Lettuce	169
Tuna Rice Oise	333

SALMON

& Avocado, Spicy, Maki Box	458
& Egg, Special, Go Go Pot	219
Poached, Cooked Rare	370
Sashimi, Muki Beans, Wakame & Wasabi	198

SANDWICH

Crab, California, Maki Boxes & Sushi Sandwiches	327
Duck & Pomegranate, without Khobez Bread	163
Salmon Supreme, Sushi	202
Tangy Tuna, Salad, No Mayo	256
Tuna Sushi, Sushi	179
Veggie Club, Sushi	175

SAUCE

Hot Su Potsu	6

SEAWEED

Crispy Thins, Snack	24
Crispy Thins, Wasabi Flavour	22
Thins, Sweet Soy & Sea Salt Flavour	22

SMOOTHIE

Raw Veg Cleanse	162

SOUP

Chicken Noodle, Classic	219
Miso	96
Miso, Noodle, Detox	223
Miso, Original, from Supermarket	44
Teriyaki Chicken with Rice, Potsu	627
Thai Duck Hot, Potsu	397

SUSHI

Best of Its	413
Crab, California Rolls	194
Health & Happiness, Box	447
It Box	284
Maki, Spicy Tuna	151
Maki Roll, Duck Hoisin	197
Omega 3 Salmon Supreme	459
Salad, Box	488
Salmon, Super, Light	403
Salmon & Avo, Maki Rolls	242
Salmon & Salmon	518
Salmon & Tuna, Junior Pack	165
Salmon Sushi	203
Slim Salmon	288

ITSU

SUSHI

Super Salmon 3 Ways	586
Tuna, Lots of Ginger	141
Tuna & Salmon, Sashimi Box	240
Tuna & Salmon Junior	174
Tuna & Salmon Sushi	245

WATER

Vitsu Water, Lemon Ninja	60

YOGHURT

Strawberry & Blueberry, Coulis, Greek Style, Pot	141
Chocolate with GF Brownie, Greek Style, Geisha	255
with, Superseeds & Blueberries, Pot	375
with, Superseeds & Strawberries, Pot	374

J D WETHERSPOON

AVOCADO

Burger Topping	62

BACON

Maple Cured, Burger Topping	77

BAGEL - BREAKFAST CLUB

Avocado, Smashed	349
Avocado, Smashed, with Bacon	510
Avocado, Smashed, with Poached Egg	406
Salmon, & Cream Cheese, with Rocket, Smoked	409
with Cream Cheese	298

BAGEL - DELI DEALS

Avocado, Smashed	349
Pastrami, New York Style	389
Salmon, Cream Cheese, & Rocket, Smoked	409

BALTI

Chicken, Pilau Rice, Naan Bread, & Poppadoms	961

BEANS

Baked, on Toast, Breakfast Club	554

BEEF - STEAK

& Eggs, with Chips, Rump, Brunch	1110
& Eggs, with Chips, Sirloin, Brunch	1172
Rump, 14oz, Chips, Peas, Tomato, & Mushrooms	834
Rump, 8oz, Chips, Peas, Tomato, & Mushroom	1135
Rump, Skinny, with Quinoa Salad, & Dressing	627
Sirloin, 8oz, Chips, Peas, Tomato, & Mushrooms	1196
Sirloin, Skinny, with Quinoa Salad, & Dressing	688

BHAJI

Onion, 1, Curry Club	185
Onion, 2, Curry Club	371

BREAD

& Butter	457
Garlic, Ciabatta, Plain, Side	402
Garlic, Ciabatta, Single Slice	201
Garlic, Ciabatta, with Cheese, Side	558
Garlic, Ciabatta, with Cheese, Single Slice	279
Naan, Garlic & Coriander, Curry Club	303

BREAKFAST

All Day, Brunch, Pub Classics	1375
All Day, Brunch, Vegetarian	1171

J D WETHERSPOON

BREAKFAST

American, Breakfast Club	1509
Brunch, All Day	1375
Brunch, All Day, Vegetarian	1171
GF, Breakfast Club	496
Large, with Two Toast	1629
Traditional, with One Toast	971
Vegetarian, Children's	547
Vegetarian, Large, with Two Toast	1433
Vegetarian, with One Toast	993

BREAKFAST CEREAL

Porridge, with Banana, & Honey, Moma!	490
Porridge, with Blueberries, & Brown Sugar, Moma!	310

BROWNIES - CHOCOLATE

Double, Warm, with Vanilla Ice Cream, Children's	674
Warm, with Ice Cream, & Belgian Chocolate Sauce	974

BRUSCHETTA

with Rocket, & Balsamic Glaze, Sm Plates	304

BUNS

Chicken, Pulled, Brioche, with Rocket, & Red Onion	556

BURGERS - BEEF

& Pastrami, New York Deli, Chips, & Onion Rings	1753
6oz, Classic	680
6oz, Highland	1198
Asian, with Chips, & Onion Rings	1807
BBQ, with Chips, & Onion Rings	2103
Brie, Bacon, & Cranberry, Chips, & Onion Rings	2053
Brunch, with Cheese, Bacon, & Fried Egg	998
Empire State, with Chips & Onion Rings	2222
Original Gourmet, with Bacon, Blue Cheese Sauce	929
Rarebit, with Chips, & Onion Rings	2062
Tennessee	919
Texan, Chilli Con Carne, Cheese, Chips, Onion Rings	1887
Ultimate, with Chips, & Onion Rings	2121
Cornish Cheese, & Bacon, with Chips, & Onion Rings	1876

BURGERS - CHICKEN

Asian, with Chips, & Onion Rings	1564
BBQ, with Chips, & Onion Rings	1860
Breaded, Buttermilk, Fried	584
Breast, Children's	942
Breast, Grilled	437
Brunch, with Cheese, Bacon, & Fried Egg	755
Buttermilk, Asian, with Chips, & Onion Rings	1710
Buttermilk, BBQ, with Chips, & Onion Rings	2006
Buttermilk, Brunch, with Cheese, Bacon, & Fried Egg	901
Buttermilk, Original Gourmet, Monterey Cheese	812
Original Gourmet, with Monterey Cheese	666
Skinny, with Salad	450
Tennessee	676

BURGERS - VEGETARIAN

Vegetable, Children's	1059
Texan, Five Bean Chilli, Cheese, Chips, Onion Rings	1660
Vegetable, with Chips	1129

J D WETHERSPOON

BURRITO

Chicken, Pulled	1099
Chicken, Pulled, Naked, Lower Carb	504
Chilli Con Carne	1345
Chilli Con Carne, Naked, Lower Carb	750
Five Bean Chilli	1084
Five Bean Chilli, Naked, Lower Carb	489
Plain	893
Plain, Naked, Lower Carb	298
Pork, BBQ, Pulled	1182
Pork, BBQ, Pulled, Naked, Lower Carb	587

CAKE

Carrot	387
Chocolate Fudge, with Ice Cream, Warm	977

CHEESE

American, Burger Topping	82
Brie, Breaded, with Cranberry Sauce, & Rocket	503
Cheddar, Burger Topping	78
Halloumi, Grilled, Burger Topping	416
Halloumi, Grilled, with Sweet Chilli Sauce, & Rocket	475

CHEESECAKE

Vanilla, Madagascan, with Berry Compote	635
Vanilla, Madagascan, with Caramel Sauce	544

CHICKEN & RIBS COMBO

Half Rack BBQ Ribs, Chips, Onion Rings, Coleslaw	1941

CHICKEN - BALMORAL

with Macsween Haggis	1198

CHICKEN - BBQ MELT

Cheese, Bacon, & BBQ Sauce, Grilled	615

CHICKEN - BITES

Breast, Battered, Chicken Club	379
Breast, Battered, with Sticky Soy Sauce	378
Tandoori, Yoghurt & Mint Sauce	325

CHICKEN - BREAST, GRILLED

Chicken Club	332

CHICKEN - NUGGETS

with Chips, & Beans, Children's	730
with Chips, & Peas, Children's	694
with Mashed Potato, & Peas, Children's	484

CHICKEN - ROAST, HALF

Peri Peri, with Chips, & Coleslaw	1658

CHICKEN - SKEWERS

Peppers, Peri Peri Sauce, & Side Salad	501

CHICKEN - STRIPS

Southern Fried, Sm Plates	572
Southern Fried, Honey Glaze, Chips, Coleslaw	1080

CHICKEN - TRIPLE FEAST

with Coleslaw, & Chips	1799

CHICKEN - WINGS

Spicy, 10, Chicken Club	1197
with Sriracha Hot Sauce, & Blue Cheese Dip	1341

CHILLI

Con Carne, with Rice, & Tortilla Chips, British Beef	699

J D WETHERSPOON

CHILLI

Five Bean, Children's	297
Five Bean, with Rice, & Tortilla Chips, Pub Classics	491

CHIPS

Bowl, Side	955
Topped, with Cheese, Bacon, Sour Cream, Loaded	1422
Topped, with Curry Sauce, Chip Shop Style	1057
with Curry Sauce, Bowl, Side	1057
with Garlic Mayo, Side	1066

COLESLAW

Side	127

CRUMBLE

Apple, Bramley, with Custard, British	536
Apple, Bramley, with Ice Cream, British	713

CURRY - CHICKEN, FLAMING DRAGON

Chicken, Flaming Dragon, Curry Club	378
with Pilau Rice, Naan Bread, & Poppadoms	900

CURRY - SWEET POTATO, CHICKPEA, & SPINACH

Curry Club	355
Pub Classics	355
with Pilau Rice, Naan Bread, & Poppadoms	877

DESSERT

Eton Mess	604

EGGS

Benedict, Breakfast Club	585
Fried	82
Royale, Breakfast Club	597
Scrambled, on Toast, Breakfast Club	790

FALAFEL

& Houmous, with Tomato, Onion, & Coriander	509

FISH & CHIPS - COD, BATTERED

with Garden Peas, Pub Classics	1205
with Garden Peas, Sm Meal, Pub Classics	831
with Mushy Peas, Pub Classics	1268
with Mushy Peas, Sm Meal, Pub Classics	890
with Mushy Peas, Children's	814

FISH & CHIPS - HADDOCK, BATTERED

with Garden Peas, Pub Classics	1246
with Mushy Peas, Pub Classics	1308

FRUIT

Fresh, Breakfast Club	200
Fresh, Greek Style Yoghurt, Honey, Breakfast Club	385

FRUIT SALAD

Fresh, with Ice Cream	501

GAMMON WITH

Egg, & Chips, 5oz, Afternoon Deals	962
Eggs, 10oz, Chips, Peas, Tomato, & Mushrooms	1312

GRAVY

Extra	29

HAGGIS

& Whisky Sauce, Side	691
Bites, Sm Plates	474
Neeps, & Tatties	1084

J D WETHERSPOON

HAM

& Fried Egg, with Chips, Wiltshire Cured, Children's	624
with Egg, & Chips, Wiltshire Cured, Pub Classics	890

HOT DOG

Bombay, with Chips, & Onion Rings	1643
Children's	766
Chilli, with Chips, & Onion Rings	1789
Pork, in a Brioche Bun, Classic, with Chips	1128
Scottie, with Macsween Haggis, & Whisky Sauce	1019
State, with Chips, & Onion Rings	1645

ICE CREAM

& Bluberries, Children's	165
Vanilla, with Chocolate or Toffee Sauce, Children's	462

ICE LOLLY

Strawberry, & Yoghurt, Claudi & Fin, Children's	50

JALFREZI - CHICKEN

Curry Club	413
with Pilau Rice, Naan, & Poppadoms, Curry Club	935

KORMA - CHICKEN

Curry Club	556
with Pilau Rice, Naan, & Poppadoms, Curry Club	1078

LAMB SHANK

Roasted Veg, Mash, Rosemary & Redcurrant Gravy	1217

LASAGNE

Beef, with Side Salad, & Dressing	890
Vegetable, Mediterranean, Side Salad, & Dressing	775

MACARONI CHEESE

with Chips	1320
with Garlic Bread	850

MADRAS - BEEF

Curry Club	653
with Pilau Rice, Naan, & Poppadoms, Curry Club	1175

MAKHANI

Chicken, & Paneer, Curry Club	1088

MAYONNAISE

Garlic	112

MIXED GRILL

Gammon, Pork , Rump Steak, Lamb, & Sausage	1496
Gammon, Pork , Rump Steak, Lamb, & Sausage, Lge	2092

NACHOS

BBQ Pulled Pork, Large, Sharer	1630
Chilli Con Carne, Large, Sharer	1516
Five Bean Chilli, Large, Sharer	1437
Plain, Large, Sharer	1341
Plain, Small, Sm Plates	671

NOODLES

Shanghai	363
Shanghai, with Chicken	569

ONION RINGS

Beer Battered, Side, 12	675
Beer Battered, Side, 6	338

ONIONS

Crispy, Burger Topping	61

J D WETHERSPOON

PANCAKES - AMERICAN STYLE

with Bacon, & Maple Flavour Syrup, Breakfast Club	672
with Ice Cream, & Berry Compote	844
with Ice Cream, & Maple Flavour Syrup	793

PANINI

Cheese, & Tomato, Deli Deals	546
Chicken, Bacon, & Cheese, BBQ, Deli Deals	617
Ham, & Cheese, Wiltshire Cured, Deli Deals	530
Tuna, & Cheese, Melt, Deli Deals	701

PASTA

Cheesy, Children's	333
Superfood	522

PIE - BEEF & DOOM BAR ALE

with Chips, Mushy Peas, & Gravy, Pub Classics	1593
with Mash, Mushy Peas, & Gravy, Pub Classics	1263

PLATTER

Sharer, Wetherspoon, 1 Platter	2643

POPPADOMS

with Chutney and Dips, Curry Club	377

POTATO BOMBAY

Curry Club	272

POTATOES

Jacket, with Beans, & Salad	461
Jacket, with Beans, Children's	409
Jacket, with Cheese, & Salad	651
Jacket, with Cheese, Children's	459
Jacket, with Chicken Tikka Masala, & Salad	661
Jacket, with Chilli Con Carne, & Salad	584
Jacket, with Coleslaw, & Salad	613
Jacket, with Five Bean Chilli, & Salad	455
Jacket, with Tuna, Children's	728
Jacket, with Tuna Mayo, & Salad	782

PRAWNS

King, Spicy Coated, with Sweet Chilli Sauce	456

PUDDING

Steak & Kidney, Chips, Peas, & Gravy, Pub Classics	1344
Sticky Toffee, with Custard, Cartmel	678

RIBS

Pork, BBQ, with Chips, Onion Rings, & Coleslaw	2232

RICE

with Naan, & Poppadoms, for Curries	522
with Naan, & Poppadoms, Side, Curry Club	522

ROGAN JOSH

Lamb, Curry Club	488
Lamb, Pilau Rice, Naan, & Poppadoms, Curry Club	1010

ROLL

Bacon, Breakfast Club	354
Breakfast, with Black Pudding, Breakfast Club	444
Breakfast, with Fried Egg, Breakfast Club	277
Breakfast, with Haggis, Breakfast Club	353
Sausage, Breakfast Club	546
Sausage, Quorn, Vegetarian, Breakfast Club	400

J D WETHERSPOON

SALAD

Caesar, Chicken	487
Chicken, & Quinoa, Chicken Club	665
Chicken, Avocado, Bacon, Balsamic Vinaigrette	438
Chicken, Tandoori, Yoghurt & Mint Dressing	382
Quinoa, Side	233
Quinoa, with Dressing	459
Side, with Dressing	95
Steak, & Quinoa, Rump, Skinny, Steak Club	627
Steak, & Quinoa, Sirloin, Skinny, Steak Club	688

SAMOSAS

Vegetable, 1, Curry Club	220
Vegetable, 2, Curry Club	440

SANDWICH

Cookie Dough, Salted Caramel Filling, & Ice Cream	1154

SAUCE

BBQ, Burger Topping	108
Blue Cheese, & Spring Onion, Cashel Blue	212
Blue Cheese, & Spring Onion, Shropshire	95
Cheese, & Leek, Caerphilly, Burger Topping	144
Cheese, Bacon, & BBQ	247
Garlic & Parsley Butter	90
Honey Glaze, with Jack Daniels Tennessee Honey	78
Peppercorn, Creamy	120
Peri Peri, Burger Topping	21
Rarebit	126
Whisky, & Peppercorn, Irish, Jameson	67
Whisky	83

SAUSAGE & MASH

with Beans, Children's	287
with Peas, Children's	685

SCAMPI

& Chips, with Peas, Children's	663
Breaded, with Chips, & Peas, Whitby, Pub Classics	906
for Steak and Grills, Surf & Turf	242

SOUP

Broccoli, & Shropshire Blue Cheese, Bloomer Bread	580
Butternut Squash, Bloomer Bread	544
Lentil, & Bacon, Bloomer Bread	553
Tomato, & Basil, Italian, Bloomer Bread	434

SPAGHETTI BOLOGNAISE

Children's	228

SUNDAE

Cornish	932
Ice Cream, Chocolate, Chocolate Brownie Chunks	981
Knickerbocker Glory	796
Millionaire	1352

SWEET POTATO

Baked, Side	212
Baked, with Beans, & Salad	409
Baked, with Cheese, & Salad	598
Baked, with Chicken Tikka Masala, & Salad	608
Baked, with Chilli Con Carne, & Salad	582

J D WETHERSPOON

SWEET POTATO

Baked, with Coleslaw, & Salad	559
Baked, with Five Bean Chilli, & Salad	498
Baked, with Tuna Mayo, & Salad	726

TIKKA MASALA - CHICKEN

Curry Club	601
Pub Classics	601
Pilau Rice, Naan Bread, & Poppadoms, Curry Club	1123

TOAST

& Preserves, Breakfast Club	529

TOASTIE

Cheese, & Tomato, Deli Deals	415
Ham, & Cheese, Wiltshire Cured, Deli Deals	474

VINDALOO - CHICKEN

Curry Club	469
Pilau Rice, Naan Bread, & Poppadoms, Curry Club	991

WRAP

Breakfast	776
Breakfast, Vegetarian	730
Chicken, & Avocado, with Mayonnaise	1265
Chicken, Southern Fried, with Smoky Chipotle Mayo	569
Chicken, Tandoori, with Yoghurt & Mint Sauce	1178
Falafel, & Houmous, with Mango Chutney	509
Halloumi, Grilled, & Sweet Chilli	1342

KFC

BEANS

Baked, BBQ, Large	245
Baked, BBQ, Reg	105

BURGERS - CHICKEN

Big Daddy, Box Meal	1430
Fillet, Bacon, Deluxe	515
Fillet, Box Meal	1080
Fillet	440
Fillet, Kids Meal	375
Fillet, Meal	750
Fillet, Mini	280
Fillet, Tower	620
Fillet, Tower, Meal	920
Fillet, with Skin On Fries, Meal	710
The Daddy	641
Zinger, Bacon, Cheese, with Skin On Fries, Box Meal	1110
Zinger, Box Meal	1010
Zinger	450
Zinger, Meal	760
Zinger, Tower	620
Zinger, Tower, Meal	925
Zinger, Tower, with Skin On Fries	580
Zinger, with Skin On Fries, Meal	720

BURRITO

Chicken, Original Recipe	700
Chicken, Original Recipe, Meal	1025
Chicken, Original Recipe, with Skin On Fries, Meal	985
Chicken, Zinger	705

KFC

BURRITO

	KCAL
Chicken, Zinger, Meal	1015
Chicken, Zinger, with Skin On Fries, Meal	720

CHICKEN

	KCAL
& Fries, Dipping, Feast, 12 Piece	985
Fillet, Bacon, 1 Piece, Box Meal	1210
Fillet, Bacon, 2 Hot Wings, Box Meal	1130

CHICKEN - BONELESS

	KCAL
with Dips, 3 Piece	515
with Dips, 4 Piece	650
with Dips, Meal, 3 Piece	515
with Dips, Meal, 4 Piece	650
Banquet	975

CHICKEN - DOUBLE DOWN

	KCAL
Cheese, BBQ Sauce, & Bacon	580
Cheese, BBQ Sauce, & Bacon, Meal	885
Cheese, BBQ Sauce	560
Cheese, BBQ Sauce, Meal	865
Fillet, Cheese, 1 Piece, Box Meal	1190
Fillet, Cheese, 2 Hot Wings, Box Meal	1110

CHICKEN - FILLET

	KCAL
Bacon, Cheese, with Skin On Fries, Box Meal	1105
with Skin On Fries, Streetwise Snack Box	1355
Mini, Snack Box	740
Mini, Streetwise Lunch Box	925
Mini, with Skin On Fries, Streetwise Lunch Box	545

CHICKEN - MIGHTY BUCKET

	KCAL
For One, Meal	1275
For One, with Skin On Fries, Meal	1235

CHICKEN - ORIGINAL RECIPE

	KCAL
Original Recipe, Single Piece	245
& Fries, Bargain Bucket, 10 Piece	915
& Fries, Bargain Bucket, 14 Piece	1155
& Fries, Bargain Bucket, 6 Piece	670
Family Feast, 10 Piece	1020
Family Feast, 6 Piece	780
Hot Wings, & Fries, Mini Variety Pack	720
Hot Wings, & Mini Fillets, Wicked Variety, 10 Piece	1200
Hot Wings, & Mini Fillets, Wicked Variety, 6 Piece	990
Kids Meal	345
Meal, 2 Piece	795
Meal, 3 Piece	1035
Ricebox	500
Ricebox, Meal	800
Ricebox, with Skin on Fries, Meal	1070
Snack Box	860
with Skin On Fries, Meal, 2 Piece	755
with Skin On Fries, Meal, 3 Piece	1000
with Skin On Fries, Streetwise Snack Box	790

CHICKEN - POPCORN

	KCAL
& Fries, Dipping, Feast, 8 Piece	855
Kids Meal	255
Large	465

KFC

CHICKEN - POPCORN

	KCAL
Meal	595
Meal, Large	775
Small	135
Snack Box	755
with Skin On Fries, Box Meal, Large	735
with Skin On Fries, Box Meal, Reg	555
with Skin On Fries, Streetwise Snack Box	685

CHICKEN - WINGS

	KCAL
Hot, with Skin On Fries, Streetwise Snack Box	715
Hot, 2	165
Hot, 3	225
Hot, Meal, 6 Piece	810
Hot, Snack Box	785

CHICKEN - ZINGER

	KCAL
Ricebox	485
Ricebox, Meal	790
Ricebox, with Skin On Fries, Meal	750

COFFEE

	KCAL
Americano, Black	5
Americano, White	50
Cafe Mocha	295
Cappuccino	95
Espresso	5
Latte, Caramel	175
Latte	85
Latte, Vanilla	125

COLESLAW

	KCAL
Large	290
Reg	145

COOKIES

	KCAL
Chocolate Chip	375

CORN

	KCAL
Cob, Large	170
Cobette	85

FRIES

	KCAL
Large	450
Reg	310
Skin On, Kids	270
Skin On, Large	445
Skin On, Reg	270

GRAVY

	KCAL
Large	275
Reg	120

HOT CHOCOLATE

	KCAL
Plain	355

ICE CREAM

	KCAL
Caramel, Fudge, Kream Ball	360
Chocolate, Kream Ball	375

MILK SHAKE

	KCAL
Maltesers, Krushems	315
Oreo, Krushems	380
Skittles, Krushem	325

KFC

MILK SHAKE

Milky Bar, Krushems	435

SALAD POT

Plain	185
Plain, Meal	525
with Chicken, Original Recipe, & Skin On Fries, Meal	645
with Chicken, Original Recipe	405
with Chicken, Popcorn	320
with Chicken, Popcorn, Meal	660
with Chicken, Zinger	380
with Chicken, Zinger, Meal	720

SUNDAE

Strawberry	190
Toffee	195

VEGETARIAN

Ricebox	307
Ricebox, Meal	675

WRAP - CHICKEN

BBQ, & Popcorn Chicken, Streetwise All Stars	775
BBQ	270
Flamin', & Popcorn Chicken, Streetwise All Stars	775
Flamin'	305
Original Recipe, Toasted, Twister	480
Twister, Toasted, Meal	790
Twister, Toasted, with Skin On Fries, Box Meal	750
Zinger, Twister	520
Zinger, Twister, Meal	755

KRISPY KREME

DOUGHNUTS

Apple Pie	296
Blueberry, Powdered, Filled	307
Butterscotch Fudge	372
Chocolate, Glazed, Ring	237
Chocolate	340
Chocolate Dreamcake	351
Chocolate Iced, Creme Filled	372
Chocolate Iced, Custard Filled	289
Chocolate Iced, Ring, Glazed	278
Chocolate Iced, with Creme Filling	350
Chocolate Iced, with Sprinkles	262
Chocolate Praline Fudge Cake	346
Cinnamon Apple, Filled	269
Cookie Crunch	261
Cookies & Kreme	379
Cruller, Glazed	353
Glazed, Original	200
Glazed, with a Creme Filling	309
Lemon Filled, Glazed	218
Maple Iced, Crunch	250
Millionaires Shortbread	349
Orange Sundae Gloss	338
Raspberry, Glazed	324
Salted Caramel, Cheesecake	367

KRISPY KREME

DOUGHNUTS

Strawberries & Kreme	326
Strawberry Filled, Powdered	248
Strawberry Gloss	244
Vanilla	315
White Chocolate & Almond	421

MCDONALD'S

BAGEL

with Bacon, Egg & Cheese	480
with Sausage, Egg & Cheese	562

BREAD

Bagel, Plain, Toasted	216

BREAKFAST CEREAL

Porridge, Oat So Simple, Apple & Cherry	228
Porridge, Oat So Simple, Plain	194

BURGERS

Beef, & Cheese, Feast	833
Beef, Signature Collection, The BBQ	782
Beef, Signature Collection, The Classic	698
Beef, Signature Collection, The Spicy	635
Big Mac	508
Cheeseburger, Double	445
Cheeseburger	301
Chicken, BLC	399
Chicken, Christmas Warmer	560
Chicken Legend, with Bacon, & BBQ Sauce	535
Chicken Legend, with Bacon, & Hot & Spicy Mayo	569
Chicken Legend, with Bacon, Cool Mayo	580
Chicken Legend, with BBQ Sauce	484
Chicken Legend, with Cool Mayo	529
Chicken Legend, with Hot & Spicy Mayo	519
Filet-O-Fish	329
Hamburger	250
Mayo Chicken	319
McChicken Sandwich	388
Quarter Pounder, with Cheese	518

BURGERS VEGETARIAN

Vegetable, Deluxe	400
Vegetable Deluxe, Spicy	412

CARROTS

Sticks	34

CHEESE

Melt, Dippers	257

CHICKEN

McNuggets, 6 Pieces	259
McNuggets, 9 Pieces	388
Nuggets, Sharebox, 20	863
Selects, 3 Pieces	359
Selects, 5 Pieces	599

COFFEE

Black, Large	8
Black, Medium	6
Cappuccino, Large	124

MCDONALD'S

COFFEE

Cappuccino, Medium	94
Espresso, Double Shot	1
Espresso, Single Shot	1
Latte, Large	192
Latte, Medium	142
Latte, Spiced Cookie, Large	219
Latte, Spiced Cookie, Medium	174
Latte, Toffee, Large	227
Latte, Toffee	183
White, Large	40
White, Medium	30

COLA

Coca-Cola, Diet	2
Coca-Cola	170
Coke, Zero	1

COOKIES

Triple Chocolate	368

DOUGHNUTS

Chocolate Donut	254
Sugared Donut	189

FANTA

Orange	48

FLATBREAD

Cheesy, Bacon	298

FRIES

French, Large	444
French, Medium	337
French, Small	237

FRUIT

Bag, Apple & Grape	46
Bag, Happy Meal	46

FRUIT SHOOT

Robinsons	10

HAPPY MEAL

Cheeseburger with Carrot Sticks	335
Cheeseburger with Fruit Bag	347
Cheeseburger with Sm Fries	538
Chicken McNuggets with Carrot Sticks	207
Chicken McNuggets with Fruit Bag	219
Chicken McNuggets with Sm Fries	410
Crispy Chicken Wrap, with Carrot Sticks	277
Crispy Chicken Wrap, with Fruit Bag	289
Crispy Chicken Wrap, with Sm Fries	289
Fish Fingers with Carrot Sticks	228
Fish Fingers with Fruit Bag	240
Fish Fingers with Sm Fries	431
Hamburger with Carrot Sticks	284
Hamburger with Fruit bag	296
Hamburger with Sm Fries	487

HASH BROWNS

BLANK	136

MCDONALD'S

HOT CHOCOLATE

Large	231
BLANK	173

ICE CREAM CONE

BLANK	145
with Flake	190

IRN BRU

BLANK	170

JUICE

Tropicana	108

JUICE DRINK

Oasis	42

LEMONADE

Sprite, Zero	5

MCFLURRY

Chocolate Orange	408
Crunchie	323
Dairy Milk	332

MCMUFFIN

Bacon & Egg, Double	401
Bacon & Egg	348
Egg, & Cheese	295
Sausage & Egg, Double	565
Sausage & Egg	430

MILK SHAKE

Banana, Large	495
Banana, Medium	386
Banana, Small	203
Chocolate, Large	488
Chocolate, Medium	380
Chocolate, Small	200
Strawberry, Large	488
Strawberry, Medium	379
Strawberry, Small	200
Vanilla, Large	483
Vanilla, Medium	377
Vanilla, Small	198

MUFFIN

Blueberry	401
Chocolate	515

PANCAKE

& Sausage, with Syrup	670
& Syrup	535

PIE

Apple, Hot	250

ROLL

Bacon, with Brown Sauce	323
Bacon, with Tomato Ketchup	319

SALAD

Chicken, No Bacon, Grilled	133
Chicken, with Bacon, Grilled	184
Crispy Chicken, No Bacon	265
Crispy Chicken, with Bacon	316

MCDONALD'S	KCAL
SALAD	
Side, Shaker	18
SMOOTHIE	
Berry Burst, Large	208
Berry Burst, Medium	159
Mango & Pineapple, Iced, Large	236
Mango & Pineapple, Iced, Medium	187
SUNDAE	
Strawberry	168292
Toffee	344
TEA	
with Milk, Large	12
with Milk	6
WRAP	
Breakfast, Bacon, & Egg Snack, Brown Sauce	281
Breakfast, Bacon, & Egg Snack, Ketchup	279
Breakfast, Egg, & Cheese, Snack, Brown Sauce	256
Breakfast, Egg, & Cheese, Snack, Ketchup	253
Breakfast, Sausage, & Egg Snack, Brown Sauce	323
Breakfast, Sausage, & Egg Snack, Ketchup	321
Breakfast, with Brown Sauce	609
Breakfast, with Tomato Ketchup	605
Chicken, Spicy, Snack	322
Chicken & Bacon One, Crispy, BBQ	500
Chicken & Bacon One, Grilled, BBQ	366
Chicken One, Crispy, Garlic Mayo	479
Chicken One, Crispy, Hot Peri Peri	488
Chicken One, Crispy, Sweet Chilli	474
Chicken One, Grilled, Garlic Mayo	345
Chicken One, Grilled, Hot Peri Peri, Big Flavour	353
Chicken One, Grilled, Sweet Chilli	340
NANDO'S	
AVOCADO	
Burger Add-On	80
Salad Extra	161
BREAD	
Garlic, Roll, Kids Menu	218
Garlic, Large, Side	672
Garlic, Side	336
BROWNIES	
Salted Caramel	389
BURGERS	
Beanie, Peri Peri, Extra Hot	614
Beanie, Peri Peri, Hot	573
Beanie, Peri Peri, Lemon & Herb	542
Beanie, Peri Peri, Mango & Lime	555
Beanie, Peri Peri, Medium	552
Beanie, Plain	532
Chicken, Breast, Peri-Peri, Extra Hot	449
Chicken, Breast, Peri-Peri, Hot	408
Chicken, Breast, Peri-Peri, Lemon & Herb	377
Chicken, Breast, Peri-Peri, Mango & Lime	390
Chicken, Breast, Peri-Peri, Medium	387

NANDO'S	KCAL
BURGERS	
Chicken, Breast, Plain, Kids Menu	289
Chicken, Breast, Plain	367
Chicken, Butterfly Burger, Peri Peri, Extra Hot	629
Chicken, Butterfly Burger, Peri Peri, Hot	588
Chicken, Butterfly Burger, Peri Peri, Lemon & Herb	557
Chicken, Butterfly Burger, Peri Peri, Mango & Lime	570
Chicken, Butterfly Burger, Peri Peri, Medium	567
Chicken, Butterfly Burger, Plain	547
Chicken, Double, Peri Peri, Extra Hot	579
Chicken, Double, Peri Peri, Hot	538
Chicken, Double, Peri Peri, Lemon & Herb	507
Chicken, Double, Peri Peri, Mango & Lime	520
Chicken, Double, Peri Peri, Medium	517
Chicken, Double, Plain	497
Chicken, Sunset Burger, Peri Peri, Extra Hot	683
Chicken, Sunset Burger, Peri Peri, Hot	642
Chicken, Sunset Burger, Peri Peri, Lemon & Herb	611
Chicken, Sunset Burger, Peri Peri, Mango & Lime	624
Chicken, Sunset Burger, Peri Peri, Medium	621
Chicken, Sunset Burger, Plain	601
Mushroom, & Halloumi, Peri Peri, Extra Hot	729
Mushroom, & Halloumi, Peri Peri, Hot	688
Mushroom, & Halloumi, Peri Peri, Lemon & Herb	657
Mushroom, & Halloumi, Peri Peri, Mango & Lime	670
Mushroom, & Halloumi, Peri Peri, Medium	667
Mushroom, & Halloumi, Plain	647
Supergreen, Peri Peri, Extra Hot	484
Supergreen, Peri Peri, Hot	443
Supergreen, Peri Peri, Lemon & Herb	412
Supergreen, Peri Peri, Mango & Lime	425
Supergreen, Peri Peri, Medium	422
Supergreen, Plain	402
Sweet Potato, & Butternut, Kids Menu	333
Sweet Potato, & Butternut, Pattie Only, Kids Menu	219
Sweet Potato, & Butternut, Peri Peri, Extra Hot	511
Sweet Potato, & Butternut, Peri Peri, Hot	470
Sweet Potato, & Butternut, Peri Peri, Lemon & Herb	439
Sweet Potato, & Butternut, Peri Peri, Mango & Lime	452
Sweet Potato, & Butternut, Peri Peri, Medium	449
Sweet Potato, & Butternut, Plain	429
CAKE	
Carrot, Four High	711
Choc-A-Lot	535
CHEESE	
Cheddar, Burger Add-on	78
Halloumi, Grilled, Burger Add-On	177
CHEESECAKE	
Gooey Caramel	434
Raspberrry	508
CHICKEN	
Butterfly, Crispy, Peri Peri, Extra Hot	392
Butterfly, Crispy, Peri Peri, Hot	351

NANDO'S

CHICKEN

	KCAL
Butterfly, Crispy, Peri Peri, Lemon & Herb	320
Butterfly, Crispy, Peri Peri, Mango & Lime	333
Butterfly, Crispy, Peri Peri, Medium	330
Butterfly, Crispy, Plain	310
Half, Peri-Peri, Extra Hot	639
Half, Peri-Peri, Hot	598
Half, Peri-Peri, Lemon & Herb	567
Half, Peri-Peri, Mango & Lime	580
Half, Peri-Peri, Med	577
Half, Plain	557
Quarter, Breast, & Wing, Peri-Peri, Extra Hot	360
Quarter, Breast, & Wing, Peri-Peri, Hot	319
Quarter, Breast, & Wing, Peri-Peri, Lemon & Herb	288
Quarter, Breast, & Wing, Peri-Peri, Mango & Lime	301
Quarter, Breast, & Wing, Peri-Peri, Medium	298
Quarter, Breast, & Wing, Plain	278
Quarter, Leg, & Thigh, Peri-Peri, Extra Hot	361
Quarter, Leg, & Thigh, Peri-Peri, Hot	320
Quarter, Leg, & Thigh, Peri-Peri, Lemon & Herb	289
Quarter, Leg, & Thigh, Peri-Peri, Mango & Lime	302
Quarter, Leg, & Thigh, Peri-Peri, Medium	299
Quarter, Leg, & Thigh, Plain	279
Strips, Plain, Kids Menu	130
Thighs, Deboned, Peri-Peri, Extra Hot	653
Thighs, Deboned, Peri-Peri, Hot	612
Thighs, Deboned, Peri-Peri, Lemon & Herb	581
Thighs, Deboned, Peri-Peri, Mango & Lime	594
Thighs, Deboned, Peri-Peri, Medium	591
Thighs, Deboned, Plain	571
Thighs 2, Salad Extra, Peri Peri, Extra Hot	368
Thighs 2, Salad Extra, Peri Peri, Hot	327
Thighs 2, Salad Extra, Peri Peri, Lemon & Herb	296
Thighs 2, Salad Extra, Peri Peri, Mango & Lime	309
Thighs 2, Salad Extra, Peri Peri, Medium	306
Thighs 2, Salad Extra, Plain	286
Whole, Peri-Peri, Extra Hot	1196
Whole, Peri-Peri, Hot	1155
Whole, Peri-Peri, Lemon & Herb	1124
Whole, Peri-Peri, Mango & Lime	1137
Whole, Peri-Peri, Medium	1134
Whole, Plain	1114
Wings, Peri-Peri, Extra Hot, 10	1017
Wings, Peri-Peri, Extra Hot, 3	362
Wings, Peri-Peri, Extra Hot, 5	549
Wings, Peri-Peri, Hot, 10	976
Wings, Peri-Peri, Hot, 3	321
Wings, Peri-Peri, Hot, 5	508
Wings, Peri-Peri, Lemon & Herb, 10	945
Wings, Peri-Peri, Lemon & Herb, 3	290
Wings, Peri-Peri, Lemon & Herb, 5	477
Wings, Peri-Peri, Mango & Lime, 10	958
Wings, Peri-Peri, Mango & Lime, 3	303

NANDO'S

CHICKEN

	KCAL
Wings, Peri-Peri, Mango & Lime, 5	490
Wings, Peri-Peri, Medium, 10	955
Wings, Peri-Peri, Medium, 3	300
Wings, Peri-Peri, Medium, 5	487
Wings, Plain, 10	935
Wings, Plain, 3	280
Wings, Plain, 5	467

CHIPS

Kids Menu	336
Large, Side	1256
Peri Salted, Large, Side	1260
Peri Salted, Reg, Side	467
Reg, Side	465

COFFEE

Americano	0
Cappuccino	73
Espresso	0
Latte	63

COLESLAW

Large, Side	535
Side	268

CORDIAL

Green, Kids Menu	29

CORN

Cob, Kids Menu	72
Cob, Flame-Grilled, 2, Side	288
Cob, Flame-Grilled, Side	144

DIP

Red Pepper, & Chilli, with Pitta	462

DRINK

Mango Quencher	129
Rubro	92

FROZEN YOGHURT

Chocolate	91
Mango	71
Strawberry	70
Vanilla	71

HOT CHOCOLATE

Original	291

HOUMOUS

Peri Drizzle, & Pitta	800

ICE CREAM

Chocolate	145
Coconut	161
Mango	95
Vanilla, Kids Menu	158
Vanilla	161

ICE LOLLY

Chilly Billy	29

JUICE

Orange	118

NANDO'S

LEMONADE
Cloudy	137

MASH
Creamy, Side	294
Large, Side	588
Sweet Potato, Kids Menu	124
Sweet Potato, Side	248

MILK
Organic, Kids Menu	113

MUSHROOMS
Portabello, Roasted, Burger Add-On	105

NUTS
Peri-Peri	793

OLIVES
Mixed, Spicy	138

PEAS
Macho, Large, Side	283
Macho, Side	141

PINEAPPLE
Slice, Grilled, Burger Add-On	37

POTATO WEDGES
Sweet Potato, Kids Menu	87
Sweet Potato, Side	330
Sweet Potato, with Peri Peri Salt, Side	333

RELISH
Chilli, Jam, Burger Add-On	59

RICE
Portuguese, Large, Side	453
Portuguese, Side	227

ROLL - CHICKEN, LIVER
Portuguese, Peri Peri, Extra Hot	551
Portuguese, Peri Peri, Hot	510
Portuguese, Peri Peri, Lemon & Herb	479
Portuguese, Peri Peri, Mango & Lime	492
Portuguese, Peri Peri, Medium	489
Portuguese, Plain	469

ROLL - STEAK, FILLET
Prego, Peri Peri, Extra Hot	446
Prego, Peri Peri, Hot	405
Prego, Peri Peri, Lemon & Herb	374
Prego, Peri Peri, Mango & Lime	387
Prego, Peri Peri, Medium	384
Prego, Plain	364

SALAD - CAESAR
no Chicken	334

SALAD - CAESAR, CHICKEN
& Extra Grilled Chicken, Peri-Peri, Extra Hot	546
& Extra Grilled Chicken, Peri-Peri, Hot	505
& Extra Grilled Chicken, Peri-Peri, Lemon & Herb	474
& Extra Grilled Chicken, Peri-Peri, Mango & Lime	487
& Extra Grilled Chicken, Peri-Peri, Med	484
Chicken	464

NANDO'S

SALAD - MEDITERRANEAN
Plain	288
with Grilled Chicken, Peri-Peri, Extra Hot	499
with Grilled Chicken, Peri-Peri, Hot	458
with Grilled Chicken, Peri-Peri, Lemon & Herb	641427
with Grilled Chicken, Peri-Peri, Mango & Lime	440
with Grilled Chicken, Peri-Peri, Medium	437
with Grilled Chicken	417

SALAD - MIXED LEAF
with Chicken Breast, Peri Peri, Extra Hot	236
with Chicken Breast, Peri Peri, Hot	195
with Chicken Breast, Peri Peri, Lemon & Herb	164
with Chicken Breast, Peri Peri, Mango & Lime	177
with Chicken Breast, Peri Peri, Medium	174
with Chicken Breast, Plain	154

SALAD - QUINOA & AVOCADO
Plain	460
with Grilled Chicken, Peri-Peri, Extra Hot	672
with Grilled Chicken, Peri-Peri, Hot	631
with Grilled Chicken, Peri-Peri, Lemon & Herb	600
with Grilled Chicken, Peri-Peri, Mango & Lime	613
with Grilled Chicken, Peri-Peri, Med	610
with Grilled Chicken	590

SALAD - SUPERGRAIN
Kids Menu	114
Plain	377
Side, Large	359
Side, Reg	188
with Chicken Breast, Peri Peri, Extra Hot	589
with Chicken Breast, Peri Peri, Hot	548
with Chicken Breast, Peri Peri, Lemon & Herb	517
with Chicken Breast, Peri Peri, Mango & Lime	530
with Chicken Breast, Peri Peri, Medium	527
with Chicken Breast, Plain	507

SANDWICH - BEANIE
Peri Peri, Extra Hot, Pitta	628
Peri Peri, Hot, Pitta	587
Peri Peri, Lemon & Herb, Pitta	556
Peri Peri, Mango & Lime, Pitta	569
Peri Peri, Medium, Pitta	566
Plain, Pitta	546

SANDWICH - CHICKEN
Breast, Peri-Peri, Extra Hot, Pitta	463
Breast, Peri-Peri, Hot, Pitta	422
Breast, Peri-Peri, Lemon & Herb, Pitta	391
Breast, Peri-Peri, Mango & Lime, Pitta	404
Breast, Peri-Peri, Medium, Pitta	401
Breast, Plain, Pitta	381
Double, Pitta, Peri Peri, Extra Hot	592
Double, Pitta, Peri Peri, Hot	551
Double, Pitta, Peri Peri, Lemon & Herb	520
Double, Pitta, Peri Peri, Mango & Lime	533
Double, Pitta, Peri Peri, Medium	530

NANDO'S

SANDWICH - CHICKEN

Thigh, Fino Pitta, Peri Peri, Extra Hot	875
Thigh, Fino Pitta, Peri Peri, Hot	834
Thigh, Fino Pitta, Peri Peri, Lemon & Herb	803
Thigh, Fino Pitta, Peri Peri, Mango & Lime	816
Thigh, Fino Pitta, Peri Peri, Medium	813
Thigh, Fino Pitta, Plain	793

SANDWICH - HALLOUMI & MUSHROOM

Peri Peri, Pitta, Extra Hot	719
Peri Peri, Pitta, Hot	678
Peri Peri, Pitta, Lemon & Herb	647
Peri Peri, Pitta, Mango & Lime	660
Peri Peri, Pitta, Medium	657
Pitta, Plain	637

SANDWICH - STEAK

Fillet, & Veg, Peri Peri, Extra Hot	496
Fillet, & Veg, Peri Peri, Hot	455
Fillet, & Veg, Peri Peri, Lemon & Herb	424
Fillet, & Veg, Peri Peri, Mango & Lime	437
Fillet, & Veg, Peri Peri, Medium	434
Fillet, & Veg, Plain	414

SANDWICH - SUPERGREEN

Peri Peri, Pitta, Extra Hot	526
Peri Peri, Pitta, Hot	485
Peri Peri, Pitta, Lemon & Herb	454
Peri Peri, Pitta, Mango & Lime	467
Peri Peri, Pitta, Medium	464
Pitta, Plain	444

SANDWICH - SWEET POTATO & BUTTERNUT

Peri Peri, Extra Hot, Pitta	552
Peri Peri, Hot, Pitta	511
Peri Peri, Lemon & Herb, Pitta	480
Peri Peri, Mango & Lime, Pitta	493
Peri Peri, Medium, Pitta	490
Plain, Pitta	470

SAUCE

Peri Peri Drizzle, Side	97
Perinaise, Condiments	159

TART

Custard, Naughty Natas	180

TEA

Infusions, All Flavours	0
Organic, Everyday	23

TOMATOES

Kids Menu	13

VEGETABLES

Roasted, Side	98

WRAP

Double, Peri Peri, Mango & Lime	721

WRAP - BEANIE

Peri Peri, Extra Hot	815
Peri Peri, Hot	774
Peri Peri, Lemon & Herb	743

NANDO'S

WRAP - BEANIE

Peri Peri, Mango & Lime	756
Peri Peri, Medium	753
Plain	733

WRAP - CHICKEN

Breast, Peri-Peri, Extra Hot	650
Breast, Peri-Peri, Hot	609
Breast, Peri-Peri, Lemon & Herb	578
Breast, Peri-Peri, Mango & Lime	591
Breast, Peri-Peri, Medium	588
Breast, Plain	568
Double, Peri Peri, Extra Hot	780
Double, Peri Peri, Hot	739
Double, Peri Peri, Lemon & Herb	708
Double, Peri Peri, Medium	718
Double, Plain	698

WRAP - HALLOUMI & MUSHROOM

Peri-Peri, Extra Hot	847
Peri-Peri, Hot	806
Peri-Peri, Lemon & Herb	775
Peri-Peri, Mango & Lime	788
Peri-Peri, Medium	785
Plain	765

WRAP - STEAK

Fillet, & Veg, Peri Peri, Extra Hot	600
Fillet, & Veg, Peri Peri, Hot	559
Fillet, & Veg, Peri Peri, Lemon & Herb	528
Fillet, & Veg, Peri Peri, Mango & Lime	541
Fillet, & Veg, Peri Peri, Medium	538
Fillet, & Veg, Plain	518

WRAP - SUPERGREEN

Peri Peri, Extra Hot	713
Peri Peri, Hot	672
Peri Peri, Lemon & Herb	641
Peri Peri, Mango & Lime	654
Peri Peri, Medium	651
Plain	631

WRAP - SWEET POTATO & BUTTERNUT

Peri Peri, Extra Hot	740
Peri Peri, Hot	699
Peri Peri, Lemon & Herb	668
Peri Peri, Mango & Lime	681
Peri Peri, Medium	678
Plain	658

PAPA JOHNS

BREAD

Bacon & Cheese, Sticks, Sides	118
Cinnamon, Knots	430
Garlic, Knots	100
Garlic & Cheese, Sticks, Sides	229
Garlic Pizza, Sticks, Sides	181

BROWNIES

Chocolate, Double	397

PAPA JOHNS

	KCAL
CAKE	
Chocolate, Lava	337
CHICKEN	
Poppers, Sides	436
Wings, BBQ, Sides	712
Wings, Buffalo, Sides	635
Wings, Plain, Sides	600
COOKIES	
Chocolate Chip	160
CORN	
Cobs	143
PEPPERS	
Jalapeno, Breaded, Bites, Sides	516
PIZZA - ALL THE MEATS	PER SLICE
Original Crust, Large	272
Original Crust, Medium	243
Original Crust, Small	220
Original Crust, XXL	312
Stuffed Crust, Large	320
Stuffed Crust, Medium	295
Stuffed Crust, XXL	356
Thin Crust, Large	237
Thin Crust, Medium	202
Thin Crust, XXL	266
PIZZA - AMERICAN HOT	PER SLICE
Original Crust, Large	216
Original Crust, Medium	195
Original Crust, Small	194
Original Crust, XXL	243
Stuffed Crust, Large	257
Stuffed Crust, Medium	242
Stuffed Crust, XXL	284
Thin Crust, Large	152
Thin Crust, Medium	153
Thin Crust, XXL	184
PIZZA - CHEESE & TOMATO	PER SLICE
Original Crust, Large	226
Original Crust, Medium	210
Original Crust, XXL	268
Stuffed Crust, Large	268
Stuffed Crust, Medium	262
Stuffed Crust, XXL	302
Thin Crust, Large	172
Thin Crust, Medium	160
Thin Crust, XXL	200
PIZZA - CHICKEN BBQ	PER SLICE
Original Crust, Large	253
Original Crust, Medium	230
Original Crust, Small	213
Original Crust, XXL	288
Stuffed Crust, Large	267
Stuffed Crust, Medium	275
Stuffed Crust, XXL	324

PAPA JOHNS

	KCAL
PIZZA - CHICKEN BBQ	PER SLICE
Thin Crust, Large	205
Thin Crust, Medium	178
Thin Crust, XXL	230
PIZZA - CHICKEN CLUB	PER SLICE
Original Crust, Large	236
Original Crust, Medium	216
Original Crust, Small	199
Original Crust, XXL	271
Stuffed Crust, Large	284
Stuffed Crust, Medium	268
Stuffed Crust, XXL	315
Thin Crust, Large	188
Thin Crust, Medium	164
Thin Crust, XXL	211
PIZZA - GARDEN PARTY	PER SLICE
Original Crust, Large	223
Original Crust, Medium	202
Original Crust, Small	193
Original Crust, XXL	257
Stuffed Crust, Large	270
Stuffed Crust, Medium	254
Stuffed Crust, XXL	301
Thin Crust, Large	177
Thin Crust, Medium	145
PIZZA - HAWAIIAN	PER SLICE
Original Crust, Large	207
PIZZA - HAWAIIAN, CHICKEN BBQ	PER SLICE
Original Crust, Large	231
Original Crust, Medium	205
Original Crust, Small	187
Original Crust, XXL	265
Stuffed Crust, Large	266
Stuffed Crust, Medium	251
Stuffed Crust, XXL	297
Thin Crust, Large	180
Thin Crust, Medium	158
Thin Crust, XXL	204
PIZZA - HAWAIIAN, PREMIUM	PER SLICE
Original Crust, Medium	187
Original Crust, Small	175
Original Crust, XXL	239
Stuffed Crust, Large	231
Stuffed Crust, Medium	234
Stuffed Crust, XXL	275
Thin Crust, Large	158
Thin Crust, Medium	136
Thin Crust, Medium	136
Thin Crust, XXL	179
PIZZA - HOT PEPPER PASSION	PER SLICE
Original Crust, Large	218
Original Crust, Medium	198
Original Crust, Small	191

PAPA JOHNS

PIZZA - HOT PEPPER PASSION	PER SLICE
Original Crust, XXL	257
Stuffed Crust, Large	258
Stuffed Crust, Medium	250
Thin Crust, Large	171
Thin Crust, Medium	141
Thin Crust, XXL	192

PIZZA - LAMB, ARABIAN PULLED	PER SLICE
Original Crust, Large	206
Original Crust, Medium	187
Original Crust, Small	173
Original Crust, XXL	238
Stuffed Crust, Large	243
Stuffed Crust, Medium	227
Stuffed Crust, XXL	273
Thin Crust, Large	157
Thin Crust, Medium	136
Thin Crust, XXL	178

PIZZA - MEATBALL PEPPERONI	PER SLICE
Original Crust, Large	262
Original Crust, Medium	241
Original Crust, Small	224
Original Crust, XXL	291
Stuffed Crust, Large	304
Stuffed Crust, Medium	288
Stuffed Crust, XXL	331
Thin Crust, Large	218
Thin Crust, Medium	196
Thin Crust, XXL	236

PIZZA - MEXICAN	PER SLICE
Original Crust, Large	237
Original Crust, Medium	214
Original Crust, Small	177
Original Crust, XXL	278
Stuffed Crust, Large	282
Stuffed Crust, Medium	220
Stuffed Crust, XXL	312
Thin Crust, Large	173
Thin Crust, Medium	159
Thin Crust, XXL	200

PIZZA - PEPPERONI DOUBLE	PER SLICE
Original Crust, Small	249
Original Crust, Large	279
Original Crust, Medium	261
Original Crust, XXL	311
Stuffed Crust, Large	340
Stuffed Crust, Medium	313
Stuffed Crust, XXL	355
Thin Crust, Large	234
Thin Crust, Medium	213
Thin Crust, XXL	256
Premium, Layered, Original Crust, Large	325
Premium, Layered, Original Crust, Medium	233

PAPA JOHNS

PIZZA - PEPPERONI DOUBLE	PER SLICE
Premium, Layered, Original Crust, Small	269
Premium, Layered, Original Crust, XXL	359
Premium, Layered, Stuffed Crust, Large	374
Premium, Layered, Stuffed Crust, Medium	349
Premium, Layered, Stuffed Crust, XXL	406
Premium, Layered, Thin Crust, Large	267
Premium, Layered, Thin Crust, Medium	235
Premium, Layered, Thin Crust, XXL	324

PIZZA - PIRI PIRI CHICKEN	PER SLICE
Original Crust, Large	234
Original Crust, Medium	213
Original Crust, Small	192
Original Crust, XXL	270
Stuffed Crust, Large	295
Stuffed Crust, Medium	265
Stuffed Crust, XXL	315
Thin Crust, Large	188
Thin Crust, Medium	163
Thin Crust, XXL	213

PIZZA - PULLED PORK, SPICY	PER SLICE
Original Crust, Large	245
Original Crust, Medium	224
Original Crust, Small	200
Original Crust, XXL	281
Stuffed Crust, Large	286
Stuffed Crust, Med	271
Stuffed Crust, Med	271
Stuffed Crust, XXL	321
Thin Crust, Large	196
Thin Crust, Medium	172
Thin Crust, XXL	221

PIZZA - SAUSAGE & PEPPERONI	PER SLICE
The Papa's Favourite, Original Crust, Large	295
The Papa's Favourite, Original Crust, Medium	275
The Papa's Favourite, Original Crust, Small	264
The Papa's Favourite, Original Crust, XXL	355
The Papa's Favourite, Stuffed Crust, Large	368
The Papa's Favourite, Stuffed Crust, Medium	340
The Papa's Favourite, Stuffed Crust, XXL	399
The Papa's Favourite, Thin Crust, Large	296
The Papa's Favourite, Thin Crust, Medium	245
The Papa's Favourite, Thin Crust, XXL	303

PIZZA - SPICY ITALIAN	PER SLICE
Original Crust, Large	273
Original Crust, Medium	245
Original Crust, Small	229
Original Crust, XXL	309
Stuffed Crust, Large	321
Stuffed Crust, Medium	298
Stuffed Crust, XXL	350
Thin Crust, Large	219
Thin Crust, Medium	189

PAPA JOHNS	KCAL
PIZZA - SPICY ITALIAN	PER SLICE
Thin Crust, XXL	242
PIZZA - TANDOORI SPICE	PER SLICE
Original Crust, Large	248
Original Crust, Medium	225
Original Crust, Small	205
Original Crust, XXL	283
Stuffed Crust, Large	295
Stuffed Crust, Medium	277
Stuffed Crust, XXL	327
Thin Crust, Large	193
Thin Crust, Medium	168
Thin Crust, XXL	216
PIZZA - THE GREEK	PER SLICE
Original Crust, Large	233
Original Crust, Medium	212
Original Crust, Small	193
Original Crust, XXL	268
Stuffed Crust, Large	281
Stuffed Crust, Medium	264
Stuffed Crust, XXL	312
Thin Crust, Large	179
Thin Crust, Medium	154
Thin Crust, XXL	202
PIZZA - THE WORKS	PER SLICE
Original Crust, Large	260
Original Crust, Medium	232
Original Crust, Small	212
Original Crust, XXL	298
Stuffed Crust, Large	322
Stuffed Crust, Medium	284
Stuffed Crust, XXL	342
Thin Crust, Medium	190
Thin Crust, XXL	251
POTATO WEDGES	
Sides	420
RIBS	
Memphis BBQ	658
PIZZA EXPRESS	
ANTIPASTO	
Classic, Italian, Intro	785
Classic, Italian, Sharing, Intro, ½ Plate	750
AUBERGINE	
Parmigiana, Melanzane, Main	607
BOLOGNESE	
Pasta, Piccolo	387
Pennette, Main	651
BREAD	
Garlic, Intro	258
Garlic, with Mozzarella, Intro	326
BROCCOLINI	
Side	167

PIZZA EXPRESS	KCAL
BROWNIES	
Chocolate, GF, Dolcetti, not including Coffee	215
Chocolate, GF	552
Piccolo	215
BRUSCHETTA	
Con Funghi, Intro	386
Originale, Intro	412
CAKE	
Chocolate, with Fresh Strawberry, Mini, Piccolo	251
Chocolate Fondant	668
Chocolate Fudge, Mini, Dolcetti	251
Chocolate Fudge	491
Chocolate Fudge, with Ice Cream	491
Sticky Toffee, Bundt, with Salted Caramel Gelato	638
CALZONE	
Calabrese, Main	1346
Classico, Main	1001
Salami E Salsiccia, Main	984
Verdure, Main	1280
CANNELLONI	
Main	766
CAVATAPPI	
Formaggi, Main	1093
CHEESECAKE	
Strawberry & Mint Fool	133
Vanilla	369
Vanilla, with Ice Cream	549
CHICKEN ARRABIATA	
Leggera, Pollo, Main	483
CHIPS	
Polenta, Side	558
COLESLAW	
Side	330
CRUMBLE	
Fruit, Winter, Mulled	333
DESSERT	
Caffe Reale, Dolcetti, not including Coffee	191
Chocolate Glory	687
Dough balls with Nutella	480
Dough Balls with Nutella Docetti	241
Honeycombe Cream Slice	575
Honeycombe Cream Slice & Ice Cream	687
Leggera, Limoncello, Tartufo	202
Lemon Posset Crunch, Dolcetti, not including Coffee	194
Semi Freddo Reale, Dolcetti	134
Summer Pudding	255
Toffee Fudge Glory	631
DIP	
Garlic Butter, ¼ Pot	67
DOUGH BALLS	
Doppio, Formaggi, Sharing, Intro, ½ Portion	441
Doppio, Sharing, Intro, ½ Portion	385
Formaggi, Intro	438

PIZZA EXPRESS

DOUGH BALLS

	KCAL
GF, Intro	382
Intro	361
Mini, Side	125

DOUGH BALLS - GARLIC BUTTER

& Side Salad, GF, Piccolo	238
& Side Salad, Piccolo	196

DOUGH BALLS - OLIVE OIL

& Balsamic Vinegar, & Side Salad, GF, Piccolo	225
& Balsamic Vinegar, & Side Salad, Piccolo	187

DRESSING

House, Tbsp	133
Light, 2 Tbsp	89

FRESELLA

Starter	630

ICE CREAM - CHOCOLATE

Chocolate, Coppa, Gelato	253

ICE CREAM - SALTED CARAMEL

Coppa, Gelato	288

ICE CREAM - STRAWBERRY

Coppa, Gelato	221

ICE CREAM - VANILLA

Coppa, Gelato	260
Gelato, Piccolo	113
Gelato, with Chocolate Sauce, Piccolo	146
with Cone, & Chocolate Sauce, Piccolo	154
Gelato, with Cone, Piccolo	120
Gelato, with Fresh Strawberry, Piccolo	120
Gelato, with Fruit Coulis, Cone, & Strawberry, Piccolo	134
Gelato, with Fruit Coulis, Piccolo	125
Chocolate Sauce, Cone, & Fudge, Gelato, Piccolo	194
Fruit Coulis, & Cone, Gelato, Piccolo	132
Fruit CoulisFresh Strawberry, Gelato, Piccolo	134
Fudge Cubes, Gelato, Piccolo	153
Toffee Sauce, Cone & Fudge Cubes, Gelato, Piccolo	190
Toffee Sauce, Gelato, Piccolo	143
Toffee Sauce & Cone, Gelato, Piccolo	150

ICE LOLLY

Ice Pop, Piccolo	17

LASAGNE

Classica, Main	752
Verde, Main	744
Verdi	744

MELANZANINE

Starter	223

NOCI

Harissa Mix	319

OLIVES

Marinate, Intro	122

PASTA

Bianca, Piccolo	389
Burro, Piccolo	311
Napoletana, Piccolo	316

PIZZA EXPRESS

PASTA

	KCAL
Pollo, Main	923
Pollo, Pesto, Main	1195

PIADINA

Bread	232
Caesar	426
Capresse	460
Chicken & Avocado	493
Italian Meat	532
PLT	432

PIE

Banoffee, & Ice Cream	524

PIZZA

	PER PIZZA
American, Classic, GF	1020
American, Classic, Main	844
American, Hot, HGP, Romanita, Lunch	493
American, Light Mozzarella, Piccolo, GF	408
American, Piccolo	395
American, Romanita, Lunch	490
American, Simple, Pepperoni	1102
American, with Light Mozarella, Piccolo	357
American Hot, Classic, Main	807
American Hot, Romana, Main	928
American Hot, Supermarket, 8 inch	586
American Hottest, Romana 65, Main	1261
Basilicata, Romana, Main	1436
Caprina Rossa, Romana, Main	901
Caronara, Romana, Main	1057
Da Morire, Romana, Main	940
Diavolo, Romana, Main	943
Etna, Romana, Main	1227
Fiorentina, Classic, GF	1045
Fiorentina, Classic, Main	910
Formaggi, Classic, Main	820
Four Seasons, Classic, GF	894
Four Seasons, Classic, Main	679
Giardiniera, Classic, GF	1115
Giardiniera, Classic, Main	909
Il Padrino, Romana, Main	1032
La Regina, Romana 65	993
La Reine, Classic, Main	777
La Reine, Light Mozzarella, Piccolo, GF	396
La Reine, Light Mozzarella, Piccolo	326
La Reine, Piccolo, GF	411
La Reine, Romanita, Lunch	405
Leggera, American, Hot, Main	396
Leggera, Padana, Main	488
Leggera, Pollo ad Astra, Main	486
Leggera, Sloppy Giuseppe, Main	450
Leggera Gustova (Approximate)	550
Margherita, Classic, GF	899
Margherita, Classic, Main	729
Margherita, Light Mozzarella, Piccolo	309

PIZZA EXPRESS

PIZZA	PER PIZZA
Margherita, Light Mozzarella, Piccolo, GF	359
Margherita, Piccolo, GF	388
Margherita, Piccolo	328
Margherita, Romana, Light Mozzarella, Piccolo	367
Margherita, Romana, Piccolo, GF	495
Margherita, Romana, Piccolo	426
Margherita, Romanita, Lunch	911
Margherita, Romano, Light Mozzarella, Piccolo, GF	437
Margherita, Romano, Light Mozzarella, Piccolo	367
Margherita Bufala, Romana 65, Main	935
Melanzane, Romana, Main	926
Mushroom, Light Mozzarella, Piccolo	312
Mushroom, Light Mozzarella, Piccolo, GF	363
Mushroom, Piccolo, GF	377
Mushroom, Piccolo	330
Nicoise, Romana, Main	1204
Padana, Romana, Main	888
Padana, Romanita, Lunch	546
Pianta, Classic, Main	860
Pianta Romana, Main	824
Pollo, Light Mozzarella, Piccolo, GF	382
Pollo, Light Mozzarella, Piccolo	312
Pollo, Piccolo, GF	396
Pollo, Piccolo	362
Pollo ad Astra, Romana, Main	925
Pollo Ad Astra, Romanita, Lunch	479
Pollo Forza	877
Pollo Forza, Romana, Main	1168
Polpette Bolognese, Romana, Main	1160
Pomodoro, Pesto, Leggera, Main	401
Pomodoro, Pesto, Romana, Main	1151
Porchetta	1207
Prosciutto Fichi	1014
Quattro Formaggi, Romana, Main	886
Romana, Melanzane	887
Rustichella, Romana, Main	1077
Sloppy Giuseppe, Classic, Main	842
Sloppy Giuseppe, Classic, GF	1167
Soho 65, Classic, Main	1063
Spinach & Mascarpone, Sienese	1405
Toscana Romana, Main	1169
Trifolata, Mushroom	914
Veneziana, Classic, Main	836
Veneziana, Romana, Main	796
Veneziana, Romanita, Lunch	440

PIZZA BASE

Main, GF	431
Main	448
Piccolo, Main, GF	199
Piccolo	224

POTATOES

Nocciola, Side	288

PIZZA EXPRESS

PROFITEROLES

Salted Caramel, Dolcetti, not including Coffee	242

RISOTTO

Arancini, Ragu, Rice	371
Fresco, Intro	443
Fresco, Main	867
Pollo Funghi, Starter	367
Prosciutto Piselli, Main	767
Prosciutto Piselli	383

SALAD

Bosco, Main	737
Bosco, Mini, Lunch	444
Bosco, with Chicken, Main	909
Caesar, Side	313
Chicken, Caesar, Grand, Main	698
Fichi Fresca	788
Leggera, Chicken, Superfood	633
Leggera, Salmon, Superfood	686
Mixed, Piccolo	18
Mixed Leaf, Side	134
Mozzarella, Buffalo, & Tomato, Intro	311
Nicoise, Main	604
Nicoise, Mini, Lunch	340
Pollo, Main	737
Pollo, Mini, Lunch	363
Pollo, Verdure	862
Pollo Pancetta, Main	784
Primavera	934
Superboost, Side	227
Superfood, Mini, Lunch	272
Vegetable, & Goats Cheese, Warm, Main	690

SORBET

Lemon Curd, Dolcetti	84
Lemon Curd, Main	167
Raspberry, Dolcetti, not including Coffee	86
Raspberry, Piccolo	61
Raspberry	147
Raspberry, with Cone, Piccolo	72
Raspberry, with Fruit Coulis, & Cone, Piccolo	79

SOUP

Butternut	529
Tomato	514

SQUID

Calamari, Intro	636

STEW

Contadino, Sausage & Lentil	483

TALEGGIO

Oven Baked, Sharing Starter, ½ Portion	377

TIRAMISU

Portion	242

TOMATOES

Roasted, Intro	67

	KCAL		KCAL
PIZZA EXPRESS		**PIZZA HUT**	
TORTA		**FLATBREAD**	
Double Chocolate Espresso, Dolcetti	374	BBQ Steak	540
Lemon, & Mascarpone	529	Chicken Delight	443
Lemon Meringue, Dolcetti	185	Shrimply Delicious	433
PIZZA HUT		Tuna Nicoise	513
APPLES		Virtuous Veg	378
Salad Station	10	**FRIES**	
BACON		Cheesy, Fried, Side	1069
Bits, Salad Station	104	Cheesy, Oven Baked, Side	680
BEETROOT		Fried, Side	888
Diced, Salad Station	5	Oven Baked, Side	498
BITES		Sweet Potato, Side	772
Cheese, & Onion, Fried	361	**ICE CREAM**	
Cheese, & Onion, Oven Baked	334	Chocolate	163
BREAD		Strawberry	174
Garlic	511	Vanilla, Extra	81
Garlic, with Cheese	689	**ICE CREAM FLOAT**	
BREADSTICKS		Cream Soda, Black Cherry	320
Salad Station	87	Cream Soda	320
CARROTS		Cream Soda	320
Shredded, Salad Station	10	**KETCHUP**	
CHEESECAKE		Pot	99
Chocolate, Chunk	438	**LASAGNE**	
CHICKEN		Beef	790
Bites, BBQ	441	Beef	790
Bites, Plain	381	**LETTUCE**	
Bites, Sweet Chilli	468	Mix, Salad Station	2
Wings	612	**MACARONI CHEESE**	
COLESLAW		Main	824
Salad Station	38	**MAYONNAISE**	
COOKIES		Garlic, Salad Station	97
Dough, Chocolate Chip, Hot	596	Light, Salad Station	74
Dough, S'mores, Hot	676	**MILK SHAKE**	
Dough, Salted Caramel, Hot	579	Chocolate, & Orange	680
COUS COUS		Chocolate	515
Tomato, & Basil, Salad Station	28	Oreo	804
CRISPS		Salted Caramel	530
with Cheese Sauce, & Onions, Fried	1730	Strawberry	482
with Cheese Sauce, & Onions, Microwaved	1687	**MUSTARD**	
CROUTONS		Creamy	261
Salad Station	85	**OIL**	
CUCUMBER		Garlic, & Chilli, Salad Station	166
Salad Station	2	**ONION RINGS**	
DIP		Fried, Side	520
Blue Cheese, Salad Station	68	Oven Baked, Side	338
DRESSING		**ONIONS**	
Caesar, Salad Station	48	Crispy, Salad Station	125
French, Low Fat, Salad Station	18	Red, Salad Station	7
Olive Oil, & Balsamic Vinegar, Salad Station	134	**PASTA**	
Thousand Island, Salad Station	45	BBQ, Salad Station	27
DRINK		Cheesy, Sweetcorn, Salad Station	37
Mango, Slush	206	**PEPPER**	
		Jalapeno, Poppers, Fried	438

PIZZA HUT
PEPPER

	KCAL
Jalapeno, Poppers, Oven Baked	312
Jalapeno, Salad Station	2

PEPPERS

Mixed, Salad Station	3

PIZZA

	PER SLICE
BBQ Americano, Cheesy Bites Crust	324
BBQ Americano, Deep Pan, Large	315
BBQ Americano, Deep Pan, Reg	202
BBQ Americano, GF	184
BBQ Americano, Stuffed Crust, Large	324
BBQ Americano, Stuffed Crust, Reg	233
BBQ Americano, Thin Crust, Large	231
BBQ Americano, Thin Crust, Reg	178
BBQ Mac n' Cheese, Stuffed Crust, Large	398
BBQ Mac n' Cheese, Stuffed Crust, Reg	277
Californian King Of the Coast, Cheesy Bites Crust	292
Californian King Of the Coast, Deep Pan, Large	283
Californian King Of the Coast, Deep Pan, Reg	184
Californian King Of the Coast, GF	166
Californian King Of the Coast, Stuffed Crust, Large	292
Californian King Of the Coast, Stuffed Crust, Reg	215
Californian King Of the Coast, Thin Crust, Large	199
Californian King Of the Coast, Thin Crust, Reg	170
Chicken Supreme, Cheesy Bites Crust	295
Chicken Supreme, Deep Pan, Big Sharer	265
Chicken Supreme, Deep Pan, Large	286
Chicken Supreme, Deep Pan, Reg	183
Chicken Supreme, GF	165
Chicken Supreme, Stuffed Crust, Large	295
Chicken Supreme, Stuffed Crust, Reg	214
Chicken Supreme, Thin Crust, Big Sharer	147
Chicken Supreme, Thin Crust, Large	202
Chicken Supreme, Thin Crust, Reg	159
Hawaiian, Cheesy Bites Crust	281
Hawaiian, Deep Pan, Big Sharer	263
Hawaiian, Deep Pan, Large	272
Hawaiian, Deep Pan, Reg	176
Hawaiian, GF	158
Hawaiian, Stuffed Crust, Large	281
Hawaiian, Stuffed Crust, Reg	207
Hawaiian, Thin Crust, Big Sharer	145
Hawaiian, Thin Crust, Large	188
Hawaiian, Thin Crust, Reg	135
Heavenly Veg, Cheesy Bites Crust	313
Heavenly Veg, Deep Pan, Large	304
Heavenly Veg, Deep Pan, Reg	196
Heavenly Veg, GF	177
Heavenly Veg, Stuffed Crust, Large	313
Heavenly Veg, Stuffed Crust, Reg	226
Heavenly Veg, Thin Crust, Large	220
Heavenly Veg, Thin Crust, Reg	171
Mac n' Cheese, Stuffed Crust, Large	399

PIZZA HUT
PIZZA

	PER SLICE
Mac n' Cheese, Stuffed Crust, Reg	278
Margherita, Cheesy Bites Crust	289
Margherita, Deep Pan, Big Sharer	272
Margherita, Deep Pan, Large	280
Margherita, Deep Pan, Reg	182
Margherita, GF	164
Margherita, Stuffed Crust, Large	289
Margherita, Stuffed Crust, Reg	213
Margherita, Thin Crust, Big Sharer	155
Margherita, Thin Crust, Large	196
Margherita, Thin Crust, Reg	158
Meat Feast, Cheesy Bites Crust	336
Meat Feast, Deep Pan, Big Sharer	303
Meat Feast, Deep Pan, Large	327
Meat Feast, Deep Pan, Reg	203
Meat Feast, GF	196
Meat Feast, Stuffed Crust, Large	336
Meat Feast, Stuffed Crust, Reg	233
Meat Feast, Thin Crust, Big Sharer	185
Meat Feast, Thin Crust, Large	242
Meat Feast, Thin Crust, Reg	178
New Orleans Chicken Sizzler, Cheesy Bites Crust	292
New Orleans Chicken Sizzler, Deep pan, Big Sharer	357
New Orleans Chicken Sizzler, Deep pan, Large	287
New Orleans Chicken Sizzler, Deep Pan, Reg	178
New Orleans Chicken Sizzler, GF	165
New Orleans Chicken Sizzler, Stuffed Crust, Large	292
New Orleans Chicken Sizzler, Stuffed Crust, Reg	206
New Orleans Chicken Sizzler, Thin Crust, Big Sharer	239
New Orleans Chicken Sizzler, Thin Crust, Large	199
New Orleans Chicken Sizzler, Thin Crust, Reg	159
Pepperoni, Cheesy Bites Crust	307
Pepperoni, Deep Pan, Large	298
Pepperoni, Deep Pan, Reg	194
Pepperoni, GF	175
Pepperoni, Stuffed Crust, Large	307
Pepperoni, Stuffed Crust, Reg	224
Pepperoni, Thin Crust, Large	216
Pepperoni, Thin Crust, Reg	169
Philly Cheese Steak, Cheesy Bites Crust	370
Philly Cheese Steak, Deep Pan, Large	365
Philly Cheese Steak, Deep Pan, Reg	241
Philly Cheese Steak, GF	223
Philly Cheese Steak, Stuffed Crust, Large	373
Philly Cheese Steak, Stuffed Crust, Reg	271
Philly Cheese Steak, Thin Crust, Large	280
Philly Cheese Steak, Thin Crust, Reg	217
Supreme, Cheesy Bites Crust	331
Supreme, Deep Pan, Large	322
Supreme, Deep Pan, Reg	205
Supreme, GF	188
Supreme, Stuffed Crust, Large	331

PIZZA HUT

PIZZA	PER SLICE
Supreme, Stuffed Crust, Reg	236
Supreme, Thin Crust, Large	238
Supreme, Thin Crust, Reg	181
Texas Meat Meltdown, Cheesy Bites Crust	358
Texas Meat Meltdown, Deep Pan, Large	349
Texas Meat Meltdown, Deep Pan, Reg	229
Texas Meat Meltdown, GF	173
Texas Meat Meltdown, Stuffed Crust, Large	358
Texas Meat Meltdown, Stuffed Crust, Reg	256
Texas Meat Meltdown, Thin Crust, Large	264
Texas Meat Meltdown, Thin Crust, Reg	201
Triple Pepperoni, Deep Pan, Big Sharer	339
Triple Pepperoni, Thin Crust, Big Sharer	224
Veggie, Cheesy Bites Crust	276
Veggie, Deep Pan, Big Sharer	273
Veggie, Deep Pan, Large	267
Veggie, Deep Pan, Reg	171
Veggie, GF	152
Veggie, Stuffed Crust, Large	276
Veggie, Stuffed Crust, Reg	201
Veggie, Thin Crust, Big Sharer	155
Veggie, Thin Crust, Large	183
Veggie, Thin Crust, Reg	146

POTATO SALAD

Salad Station	27

RIBS

BBQ	562
Rack, Meal, Fried	1473
Rack, Meal, Oven Baked	1182

SALSA

Salad Station	14

SAUCE

BBQ	119
Chocolate, Extra	71
Hot & Spicy	65
Hut House Seasoning	322
Mayonnaise, Garlic	243
Mayonnaise, Light	186
Salted Caramel, Extra	70
Sweet Chilli	175

SHRIMP

Popcorn	305

SORBET

Mango	179

SULTANAS

Salad Station	55

SWEETCORN

Salad Station	15

TOMATOES

Cherry, Salad Station	3

TORTILLA CHIPS

Salad Station	96

PIZZA HUT

WAFFLES

Chocolate	685

PRET A MANGER

APPLES

Chopped	86
Juice, Sparkling, Pure Pret	139
Spiced, Infusion	45

BAGUETTE

Artichoke, Olives, & Tapenade, Vegan	454
Avocado, Olives, & Tomato, with Rocket	532
Bacon, Posh, Airports Only	518
Bahn Mi, Crunchy, Veggie	418
Beetroot, Smashed, Pistachios, & Feta	531
Brie, Tomato, & Basil, White	432
Brie & Cranberry	579
Butternut Squash, Wensleydale, & Cranberry	542
Cheese, Prosciutto, Tomatoes, Mayo, & Basil, White	531
Cheese, Cheddar, & Pickle, Cheddar, Posh, White	620
Chicken, & Bacon, Caesar, White	598
Egg Mayo, & Bacon, Breakfast	337
Egg Mayo, & Roasted Tomatoes, Breakfast	309
Egg Mayo, Asparagus, Watercress, & Parmesan	528
Ham, & Greve Cheese, Mustard Mayo, White	588
Ham, & Egg, Mustard Mayo, Classic, White	560
Ham, & Pickles, Jambon Beurre, White	355
Ham Hock, Stuffing, & Apple	597
Italian Veggie	539
Mozzarella, Chipotle, Hot	468
Salmon, & Soft Cheese, Smoked, White	454
Salmon, Smoked, & Free Range Egg, Breakfast	325
Tuna, Nicoise	531
Tuna Mayo, & Cucumber, Pole & Line Caught, White	540

BANANA

Fresh	62

BARS

Chocolate Brownie	305
Dairy Free Chocolatey Coconut Bite	205
Love Bar	329
Orange, Cardamom, Milk Chocolate	134
Pret Bar	266
Raw, Fruit, Seed	202

BEANS

Baked, with Avocado, Power Pot	251

BEEF

Short Rib, Korean, in Brioche Roll	527

BERRIES

Wild, Infusion	25

BREAD

Baguette, Losange, for Soup	177
Baguette, Stone Baked, Mini	204

BREAKFAST

Acai, & Almond Butter, Bowl	380
Bacon Brioche	420

PRET A MANGER

BREAKFAST

Bacon & Egg Brioche	490
Egg Mayo, & Avocado	344
Ham & Egg Brioche	412
Poached Egg, Sausage & Beans, Power Pot	260
Sausage & Egg Brioche	546
Veggie Brioche	346

BREAKFAST CEREAL

Bircher, Dairy Free, Bowl	252
Bircher Muesli Bowl	308
Honey & Granola Pret Pot	281
Porridge, Coconut	198
Porridge, No Topping	242

BROWNIES

Chocolate, Salted Caramel Vegan	223

CAKE

Banana, Slice	224
Carrot, Slice	321
Choc Bar	355
Chocolate, Triple, Pioneer	598
Fruit Teacake, Pioneer	279
Lemon Drizzle, Slice, Pioneer	698
Mince Pie	315
Pecan Slice	436
Pistachio, & Mandarin	507
Sticky Toffee, & Pecan	558
Tiffin, Christmas	410
Victoria Sponge, Pioneer	641
Victoria Sponge, Pret a Manger*	503

CHEESECAKE

Lemon, Pot	406

CHOCOLATE

Dark with Sea Salt	136

CLEMENTINES

Fresh	63

COCONUT

Chips, Roasted	105
Water, Pret Pure	66

COFFEE

Americano, Black	1
Americano, White, Iced	36
Americano White, Semi Skimmed Milk	14
Cappuccino	92
Cappuccino, Soya	92
Cappucino, Oat Milk	96
Espresso	0
Filter Coffee	0
Filter Coffee, Semi Skimmed Milk	14
Flat White, Almond Milk	56
Flat White, Coconut	102
Flat White, Festive	135
Flat White, Oat Milk	81
Flat White	80

PRET A MANGER

COFFEE

Flat White, Pumpkin Spiced	104
Flat White, Soya	77
Frappe, Chocolate	439
Frappe, Classic	251
Latte, Coconut	150
Latte, Love Bar	145
Latte, Oat Milk	132
Latte, Skimmed Milk	118
Latte, Soya, Iced	114
Latte, Soya	113
Macchiato	5
Mocha, Coconut	216
Mocha, Mint	220
Mocha, Oat Milk	186
Mocha, Semi Skimmed Milk	185
Mocha, Soya	181

COOKIES

Chocolate Chunk	327
Chocolate Praline, Melt in the Middle	319
Double Chocolate Orange	389
Fruit, Oat & Spelt	339

CORN CAKES

Chocolate Covered	239

CRANBERRIES

in Coats, Yoghurt Coating	241

CRISPS

Croxton Manor Cheese & Red Onion	210
Kale	67
Maldon Sea Salt	203
Sea Salt & Organic Cider Vinegar Crisps	196
Smokey Chipotle	203

CROISSANT

Almond	366
Chocolate & Hazelnut	379
French, Butter	304
Ham, Cheese, Tomato & Bacon	298
Mozzarella & Tomato	329

DANISH PASTRY

Cinnamon	398

DRESSING

Dijon, Small	144
Green, Zingy	85
Teriyaki	36
Yoghurt, Lemon, & Mayo, Large	138

DRIED FRUIT & NUTS

Mango & Seeds	122

DRINK

Cucumber Seltzer	56

FLATBREAD

Artichokes, Olive Tapenade, Rocket, & Basil	422
Chicken, Lebanese	496
Chicken, Pesto, & Rocket	518

PRET A MANGER

FLATBREAD

	KCAL
Falafel	529
Greek, Green	402
Mediterranean Tuna	533
Mexican Avocado	508
Plain	211
Squash, with Feta & Mint	337
Super-Veg Rainbow	353
Sweet Potato Falafel, Coconut, & Cashew	455

FRUIT

	KCAL
British Berries	5
Five Berry Bowl	364
Five Berry Pot	158
Fruit Salad, Pret's	112
Mango & Lime	91
Seedless Grapes	109
Superfruit Salad, Pot, Pret a Manger*	107

FRUIT & NUT

	KCAL
Mix	175
Mix, with Chocolate Covered Raisins	177

FRUIT COMPOTE

	KCAL
Topping, Breakfast	26

GINGER BEER

	KCAL
Pure Pret	139

GINGERBREAD

	KCAL
Godfrey, Pret's Gingerbread Man	201
Melvin the Melting Snowman	257

HONEY

	KCAL
Breakfast Topping	107

HOT CHOCOLATE

	KCAL
Coconut	288
Oat Milk	256
Original	256
Soya	251

JUICE

	KCAL
Apple	125
Blood Orange	132
Carrot	50
Clementine	110
Daily Greens	92
Ginger & Apple, Shot	55
Green Goodness	176
Hot Shot	47
Orange, Lge	168
Pomegranate, & Hibiscus, Still, Pure Pret	108

JUICE DRINK

	KCAL
Beet Beautiful	188
Cranberry & Raspberry, Still	159
Ginseng & Echinacea, Sparkling, Yoga Bunny	135
Grape & Elderflower, Sparkling, Pure Pret	129
Mandarin & Lychee, Pure, Still	106
Mango & Passion Fruit, Still	209
Melon, & Basil	171

PRET A MANGER

JUICE DRINK

	KCAL
Orange, & Passion Fruit, Still	133
Super Greens	269

KOMBUCHA

	KCAL
Lemon, & Ginger, Organic	37

LEMON

	KCAL
& Ginger, Infusion	15

LEMONADE

	KCAL
& Ginger, Still	160
Sparkling	109

MACARONI CHEESE

	KCAL
& Greens, Vegan	558
Beef, Short Rib, & Cauliflower	709
Ham Hock & Sprout	631
Kale & Cauli	553
Prosciutto	590

MANGO

	KCAL
Fresh	116

MILK

	KCAL
Babyccino, with Chocolate Sprinkles	14
British Organic, Kids	94
Coconut	150
Oat	118

MOUSSE

	KCAL
Chocolate	453

MUFFIN

	KCAL
Breakfast	431
Double Berry	442
Prets Christmas	466

NUTS

	KCAL
Naked	259

PAIN AU RAISIN

	KCAL
Pain au Raisin	361

POPCORN

	KCAL
Bar	176
Rock Salt, Light	143
Sweet & Salt, Light	163

PRETZELS

	KCAL
Plain	304

SADA SEV

	KCAL
Smashed Beetroot, & Feta, Pot	176

SALAD

	KCAL
Asian Greens, Veggie Pot	170
Avocado, Super-Greens, Pot	171
Cauliflower, & Turmeric, Super-Veg	306
Chicken, Italian, Chef's	345
Chicken, Pesto, & Mozzarella, Buffalo	365
Crayfish, & Avocado, No Bread	215
Egg, & Avocado, Protein Pot	224
Egg, & Spinach, Protein Pot	104
Egg, Poached, & Avocado, Protein Pot	197
Falafel, Mezze	480
Greens, Grains & Chicken	258

PRET A MANGER

SALAD

Rainbow Veggie, Pot	186
Roast Beets, Squash, & Feta, Box	238
Super Beans, Brocolli, & Turmeric Cauli, no Dressing	209
Sweet Potato Falafel & Smashed Beets, Box	334
Teriyaki Salmon Sushi, without Dressing	316
Tuna, Nicoise	191

SANDWICH

Aubergine, & Halloumi, Brioche	492
Cheese, Kids	422
Chicken, & Cucumber, Granary Bread	390
Chicken Avocado	485
Chickpeas, Curried, & Mango Chutney	476
Chipotle Pulled Chicken, Brioche	398
Christmas Lunch	482
Christmas Lunch, Veggie	531
Classic Super Club	528
Crayfish, & Avocado	383
Egg Mayo, Coronation	520
Free Range Egg Mayo	367
Cracking Egg Salad	375
Falafel, Halloumi, & Pickles, Brioche	520
Falafel & Red Tapenade	540
Ham, & Cheese	547
Ham, Kids	300
Mature Cheddar & Pret Pickle	520
New Yorker, on Rye, Veggie	582
Scottish Smoked Salmon	378
Super Greens & Reds	449
Tuna, & Cucumber	448
Very Merry Christmas Lunch	525

SEEDS

Tamari Pumpkin	186

SHORTBREAD

Plain	396

SMOOTHIE

Acai Super Berry	255
Almond, Protein Power	450
Berry Blast	239
Blueberry, Protein Power	425
Coconut Crush	168
Green, Breakfast Bowl	311
Mango Smoothie	145
Rhubarb	185
Strawberry Smoothie	211
Vitamin Volcano Smoothie	163

SOUP

Broth, Dried Chilli, Extra	1
Butternut Squash, Spiced	240
Carrot, & Coriander, Lightly Spiced	181
Chicken, & Chorizo, Smoky	234
Chicken, & Vegetable, Red Thai	235
Chicken, Broccoli & Brown Rice	133

PRET A MANGER

SOUP

Chicken, Cream of, No Cream	141
Chicken, Curry, Coconut	222
Chilli, Vegan, Soup Of The Day	213
Kale, Lentil, & Roasted Spices	217
Miso, Veggie	44
Pea, & Mint	189
Pork, & Lentil, Ragu	218
Tomato, Souper	198
Vegetable, Tagine	187

SYRUP

Shot, Caramel	49
Shot, Hazelnut	47
Shot, Love Bar	46
Shot, Mince Pie	50
Shot, Mint	63
Shot, Pumpkin Spice	49
Shot, Vanilla	49

TART

Pret's Bakewell Tart	410

TEA

Black, Iced	0
Black, Iced, with Strawberry, Cucumber, & Mint	55
Ceylon, Breakfast	14
Chamomile	0
Earl Grey, Black	14
Fennel, & Mint	0
Green, & Peach	88
Green, Iced	0
Green, Iced, with Blood Orange, & Pomegranate	50
Green, White Matcha, Oolong	0
Latte, Chai, Iced	180
Latte, Chai	182
Latte, Golden Turmeric	111
Latte, Matcha	108
Peppermint	0
Rooibos Cacao	0
Tropical Green Tea	0
Turmeric Tonic	0

TOASTIE

Brie, Avocado & Tomato	562
Chicken, Basil, & Red Pepper	564
Egg, Cheddar, & Tomato	595
Egg Florentine	575
Halloumi & Red Pepper	556
Ham, Cheese & Mustard	570
Tuna Melt Toastie	552

TORTILLA

Avocado, Beans, Toasted	435
Avocado, Cheddar, & Chipotle, Toasted	578
Banana, Blueberry, & Almond Butter	387
Chicken, Chipotle, Toasted	497
Egg, Bacon, & Avocado, Toasted	555

PRET A MANGER

TORTILLA

Eggs Florentine, Toasted	527
Mushroom, Florentine, Toasted	432

VEG POT

Courgetti, Veggie	132

WATER

Spring, Sparkling	0

WRAP

Avocado, & Chipotle Chickpeas, Salad	444
Avocado, & Herb Salad	514
Butternut, & Pistachio, Spicy	313
Chakalaka, Beans, & Vegetables	340
Chana Chaat, Mint, & Mango Chutney	453
Chicken, Spicy, Hot	496
Falafel, & Halloumi, Hot	659
Hoisin Duck Wrap	457
Houmous, & Crunchy Vegetables, Vegan	386
Miso, Aubergine, & Edamame	365
Nicoise Salad, Veggie	500
Ragu, & Red Pepper, Vegan, Hot	421
Summer Salad	339
Swedish Meatball, Hot	666

YOGHURT

Coconut, Mango Chia Pot	190
Dark Chocolate, & Toasted Coconut, Pot	362
Mango, Chia, Pot	137

YOGHURT - DAIRY FREE

Chocolate, Coconut, Chia, Blueberries, Pomegranate	162

STARBUCKS

BARS

Fruit & Nut, Cranberry, Pumpkin seed & Blueberry	235

COFFEE - AMERICANO

Grande	17
Short	6
Tall	11
Venti	23

COFFEE - AMERICANO, ICED

Grande	17
Tall	11
Venti	23

COFFEE - CAPPUCCINO

Almond Milk, Grande	87
Almond Milk, Short	52
Almond Milk, Tall	77
Almond Milk, Venti	129
Coconut Milk, Grande	165
Coconut Milk, Short	85
Coconut Milk, Tall	118
Coconut Milk, Venti	202
Semi Skimmed Milk, Grande	115
Semi Skimmed Milk, Short	78
Semi Skimmed Milk, Tall	97
Semi Skimmed Milk, Venti	161

STARBUCKS

COFFEE - CAPPUCCINO

Skimmed Milk, Grande	82
Skimmed Milk, Short	55
Skimmed Milk, Tall	70
Skimmed Milk, Venti	115
Soy, Grande	92
Soy, Short	62
Soy, Tall	74
Soy, Venti	123
Whole Milk, Grande	136
Whole Milk, Short	92
Whole Milk, Tall	116
Whole Milk, Venti	192

COFFEE - CAPPUCCINO, ICED

Almond Milk, Grande	64
Almond Milk, Tall	48
Almond Milk, Venti	71
Coconut Milk, Grande	70
Coconut Milk, Tall	65
Coconut Milk, Venti	113
Semi Skimmed Milk, Grande	94
Semi Skimmed Milk, Tall	77
Semi Skimmed Milk, Venti	141
Skimmed Milk, Grande	68
Skimmed Milk, Tall	56
Skimmed Milk, Venti	101
Soy, Grande	71
Soy, Tall	64
Soy, Venti	116
Whole Milk, Grande	113
Whole Milk, Tall	100
Whole Milk, Venti	168

COFFEE - COLD BREW

Skimmed Milk, Solo	6
Festive Grande	33
Festive Tall	25
Festive Venti	41

COFFEE - CORTADO

Almond Milk	27
Coconut Milk	41
Semi Skimmed Milk	47
Skimmed Milk	36
Soy	40
Whole Milk	60

COFFEE - ESPRESSO

Con Panna, Doppio	36
Con Panna, Solo	31
Doppio	48
Solo	6

COFFEE - ESPRESSO, MACCHIATO

Almond Milk, Doppio	10
Almond Milk, Solo	6
Coconut Milk, Doppio	11

STARBUCKS

COFFEE - ESPRESSO, MACCHIATO

Coconut Milk, Solo	6
Semi Skimmed Milk, Doppio	11
Semi Skimmed Milk, Solo	7
Skimmed Milk, Doppio	11
Soy, Doppio	11
Soy, Solo	6
Whole Milk, Doppio	12
Whole Milk, Solo	7

COFFEE - FILTER

Grande	5
Short	3
Tall	4
Venti	6

COFFEE - FLAT WHITE

Whole Milk, Short	119

COFFEE - LATTE

Almond Milk, Grande	100
Almond Milk, Short	50
Almond Milk, Tall	75
Almond Milk, Venti	126
Coconut Milk, Venti	204
Coconut Milk, Grande	163
Coconut Milk, Short	81
Coconut Milk, Tall	121
Semi Skimmed Milk, Grande	188
Semi Skimmed Milk, Short	95
Semi Skimmed Milk, Tall	143
Semi Skimmed Milk, Venti	248
Skimmed Milk, Grande	131
Skimmed Milk, Short	67
Skimmed Milk, Tall	102
Skimmed Milk, Venti	174
Soy, Grande	148
Soy, Short	75
Soy, Tall	110
Soy, Venti	185
Whole Milk, Grande	223
Whole Milk, Short	113
Whole Milk, Tall	172
Whole Milk, Venti	299
Eggnog, Grande	344
Eggnog, Short	169
Eggnog, Tall	271
Gingerbread, Almond Milk, Grande	254
Gingerbread, Almond Milk, Short	144
Gingerbread, Almond Milk, Tall	198
Gingerbread, Coconut Milk, Grande	313
Gingerbread, Coconut Milk, Short	171
Gingerbread, Coconut Milk, Tall	238
Gingerbread, Semi Skimmed Milk, Grande	343
Gingerbread, Semi Skimmed Milk, Short	185
Gingerbread, Semi Skimmed Milk, Tall	258

STARBUCKS

COFFEE - LATTE

Gingerbread, Skimmed Milk, Grande	291
Gingerbread, Skimmed Milk, Short	161
Gingerbread, Skimmed Milk, Tall	223
Gingerbread, Soy, Grande	312
Gingerbread, Soy, Short	171
Gingerbread, Soy, Tall	237
Gingerbread, Whole Milk, Grande	392
Gingerbread, Whole Milk, Short	208
Gingerbread, Whole Milk, Tall	291
Toffee Nut, Almond Milk, Grande	260
Toffee Nut, Almond Milk, Short	150
Toffee Nut, Almond Milk, Tall	203
Toffee Nut, Coconut Milk, Grande	318
Toffee Nut, Coconut Milk, Short	177
Toffee Nut, Coconut Milk, Tall	243
Toffee Nut, Semi Skimmed Milk, Grande	348
Toffee Nut, Semi Skimmed Milk, Short	191
Toffee Nut, Semi Skimmed Milk, Tall	264
Toffee Nut, Skimmed Milk, Grande	296
Toffee Nut, Skimmed Milk, Short	166
Toffee Nut, Skimmed Milk, Tall	228
Toffee Nut, Soy, Grande	317
Toffee Nut, Soy, Short	176
Toffee Nut, Soy, Tall	242
Toffee Nut, Whole Milk, Grande	397
Toffee Nut, Whole Milk, Short	213
Toffee Nut, Whole Milk, Tall	297

COFFEE - LATTE, ICED

Almond Milk, Grande	73
Almond Milk, Tall	57
Almond Milk, Venti	90
Coconut Milk, Grande	78
Coconut Milk, Tall	65
Coconut Milk, Venti	102
Semi Skimmed Milk, Grande	87
Semi Skimmed Milk, Tall	77
Semi Skimmed Milk, Venti	126
Skimmed Milk, Grande	63
Skimmed Milk, Tall	56
Skimmed Milk, Venti	90
Soy, Tall	64
Soy, Venti	104
ISoy, Grande	71
Whole Milk, Grande	104
Whole Milk, Tall	100
Whole Milk, Venti	149

COFFEE - MACCHIATO

Caramel, Almond Milk, Grande	172
Caramel, Almond Milk, Short	86
Caramel, Almond Milk, Tall	123
Caramel, Soy, Grande	207
Caramel, Soy, Short	104

STARBUCKS

COFFEE - MACCHIATO

	KCAL
Caramel, Whole Milk, Short	137

COFFEE - MACCHIATO, CARAMEL, ICED

Almond Milk, Grande	162
Almond Milk, Tall	121
Almond Milk, Venti	188
Skimmed Milk, Tall	142

COFFEE - MACHIATO, CARAMEL

Almond Milk, Venti	211
Coconut Milk, Grande	250
Coconut Milk, Short	124
Coconut Milk, Tall	183
Coconut Milk, Venti	308
Semi Skimmed Milk, Grande	240
Semi Skimmed Milk, Short	122
Semi Skimmed Milk, Tall	209
Semi Skimmed Milk, Venti	329
Skimmed Milk, Grande	193
Skimmed Milk, Short	97
Skimmed Milk, Tall	165
Skimmed Milk, Venti	261
Soy, Tall	167
Soy, Venti	280
Whole Milk, Grande	269
Whole Milk, Tall	240
Whole Milk, Venti	376

COFFEE - MACHIATO, CARAMEL, ICED

Coconut Milk, Grande	207
Coconut Milk, Tall	154
Coconut Milk, Venti	236
Semi Skimmed Milk, Grande	230
Semi Skimmed Milk, Tall	171
Semi Skimmed Milk, Venti	261
Skimmed Milk, Venti	219
Soy, Grande	205
Soy, Tall	153
Soy, Venti	235
Whole Milk, Grande	271
Whole Milk, Tall	202
Whole Milk, Venti	306

COFFEE - MACHIATTO, CARAMEL, ICED

Skimmed Milk, Grande	191

COFFEE - MISTO

Almond Milk, Grande	59
Almond Milk, Short	30
Almond Milk, Tall	45
Almond Milk, Venti	75
Coconut Milk, Grande	95
Coconut Milk, Short	48
Coconut Milk, Tall	73
Coconut Milk, Venti	120
Semi Skimmed Milk, Grande	106
Semi Skimmed Milk, Short	54

STARBUCKS

COFFEE - MISTO

	KCAL
Semi Skimmed Milk, Tall	81
Semi Skimmed Milk, Venti	134
Skimmed Milk, Grande	73
Skimmed Milk, Short	37
Skimmed Milk, Tall	56
Skimmed Milk, Venti	92
Soy, Grande	82
Soy, Short	42
Soy, Tall	63
Soy, Venti	104
Whole Milk, Grande	126
Whole Milk, Short	65
Whole Milk, Tall	97

COFFEE - MOCHA

& Whip Cream, Coconut Milk, Tall	298
& Whipped Cream, Almond Milk, Grande	317
& Whipped Cream, Almond Milk, Short	180
& Whipped Cream, Almond Milk, Tall	253
& Whipped Cream, Coconut Milk, Grande	374
& Whipped Cream, Coconut Milk, Short	208
& Whipped Cream, Semi Skimmed Milk, Grande	403
& Whipped Cream, Semi Skimmed Milk, Short	222
& Whipped Cream, Semi Skimmed Milk, Tall	321
& Whipped Cream, Skimmed Milk, Grande	353
& Whipped Cream, Skimmed Milk, Short	198
& Whipped Cream, Skimmed Milk, Tall	282
& Whipped Cream, Soy, Grande	371
& Whipped Cream, Soy, Short	207
& Whipped Cream, Soy, Tall	297
& Whipped Cream, Whole Milk, Grande	456
& Whipped Cream, Whole Milk, Short	249
& Whipped Cream, Whole Milk, Tall	363

COFFEE - MOCHA, ICED

& Whipped Cream, Almond Milk, Grande	313
& Whipped Cream, Almond Milk, Tall	230
& Whipped Cream, Almond Milk, Venti	351
& Whipped Cream, Coconut Milk, Grande	341
& Whipped Cream, Coconut Milk, Tall	253
& Whipped Cream, Coconut Milk, Venti	382
& Whipped Cream, Semi Skimmed Milk, Grande	355
& Whipped Cream, Semi Skimmed Milk, Tall	265
& Whipped Cream, Semi Skimmed Milk, Venti	398
& Whipped Cream, Skimmed Milk, Grande	331
& Whipped Cream, Skimmed Milk, Tall	245
& Whipped Cream, Skimmed Milk, Venti	371
& Whipped Cream, Soy, Grande	340
& Whipped Cream, Soy, Tall	252
& Whipped Cream, Soy, Venti	381
& Whipped Cream, Whole Milk, Grande	381
& Whipped Cream, Whole Milk, Tall	286
& Whipped Cream, Whole Milk, Venti	426

STARBUCKS

COFFEE - MOCHA, WHITE CHOC

Whipped Cream, Almond Milk, Grande	371
Whipped Cream, Almond Milk, Short	203
Whipped Cream, Almond Milk, Tall	288
Whipped Cream, Coconut Milk, Grande	425
Whipped Cream, Coconut Milk, Short	230
Whipped Cream, Coconut Milk, Tall	326
Whipped Cream, Semi Skim Milk, Grande	453
Whipped Cream, Semi Skimmed Milk, Short	244
Whipped Cream, Semi Skimmed Milk, Tall	346
Whipped Cream, Skimmed Milk, Grande	406
Whipped Cream, Skimmed Milk, Short	221
Whipped Cream, Skimmed Milk, Tall	313
Whipped Cream, Soy, Grande	423
Whipped Cream, Soy, Short	229
Whipped Cream, Soy, Tall	325
Whipped Cream, Whole Milk, Grande	503
Whipped Cream, Whole Milk, Short	269
Whipped Cream, Whole Milk, Tall	383

FRAPPUCCINO - CARAMEL

with Whipped Cream, Almond Milk, Grande	380
with Whipped Cream, Almond Milk, Mini	218
with Whipped Cream, Almond Milk, Tall	274
with Whipped Cream, Coconut Milk, Grande	373
with Whipped Cream, Coconut Milk, Mini	251
with Whipped Cream, Coconut Milk, Tall	278
with Whipped Cream, Semi Skimmed Milk, Grande	374
with Whipped Cream, Semi Skimmed Milk, Mini	256
with Whipped Cream, Semi Skimmed Milk, Tall	275
with Whipped Cream, Skimmed Milk, Grande	358
with Whipped Cream, Skimmed Milk, Mini	247
with Whipped Cream, Skimmed Milk, Tall	262
with Whipped Cream, Soy, Grande	364
with Whipped Cream, Soy, Tall	267
with Whipped Cream, Soy Milk, Mini	250
with Whipped Cream, Whole Milk, Grande	379
with Whipped Cream, Whole Milk, Mini	266
with Whipped Cream, Whole Milk, Tall	280

FRAPPUCCINO - CARAMEL CREAM

with Whipped Cream, Almond Milk, Grande	300
with Whipped Cream, Almond Milk, Mini	164
with Whipped Cream, Almond Milk, Tall	224
with Whipped Cream, Coconut Milk, Grande	321
with Whipped Cream, Coconut Milk, Mini	175
with Whipped Cream, Coconut Milk, Tall	242
with Whipped Cream, Semi Skimmed Milk, Grande	332
with Whipped Cream, Semi Skimmed Milk, Mini	181
with Whipped Cream, Semi Skimmed Milk, Tall	251
with Whipped Cream, Skimmed Milk, Grande	314
with Whipped Cream, Skimmed Milk, Mini	171
with Whipped Cream, Skimmed Milk, Tall	236
with Whipped Cream, Soy, Grande	320
with Whipped Cream, Soy, Tall	241

STARBUCKS

FRAPPUCCINO - CARAMEL CREAM

with Whipped Cream, Soy Milk, Mini	175
with Whipped Cream, Whole Milk, Grande	353
with Whipped Cream, Whole Milk, Mini	192
with Whipped Cream, Whole Milk, Tall	267

FRAPPUCCINO - CARAMEL LIGHT

No Whip, Skimmed Milk, Grande	134
No Whip, Skimmed Milk, Mini	59
No Whip, Skimmed Milk, Tall	96

FRAPPUCCINO - CHAI TEA

with Whipped Cream, Almond Milk, Grande	293
with Whipped Cream, Almond Milk, Mini	156
with Whipped Cream, Almond Milk, Tall	211
with Whipped Cream, Coconut Milk, Grande	313
with Whipped Cream, Coconut Milk, Mini	167
with Whipped Cream, Coconut Milk, Tall	228
with Whipped Cream, Semi Skimmed Milk, Grande	324
with Whipped Cream, Semi Skimmed Milk, Mini	173
with Whipped Cream, Semi Skimmed Milk, Tall	236
with Whipped Cream, Skimmed Milk, Grande	306
with Whipped Cream, Skimmed Milk, Mini	163
with Whipped Cream, Skimmed Milk, Tall	222
with Whipped Cream, Soy, Grande	313
with Whipped Cream, Soy, Mini	167
with Whipped Cream, Soy, Tall	227
with Whipped Cream, Whole Milk, Grande	343
with Whipped Cream, Whole Milk, Mini	184
with Whipped Cream, Whole Milk, Tall	252

FRAPPUCCINO - CHOCOLATE CREAM

with Whipped Cream, Almond Milk, Grande	317
with Whipped Cream, Almond Milk, Mini	165
with Whipped Cream, Almond Milk, Tall	226
with Whipped Cream, Coconut Milk, Grande	325
with Whipped Cream, Coconut Milk, Mini	177
with Whipped Cream, Coconut Milk, Tall	235
with Whipped Cream, Semi Skimmed Milk, Grande	336
with Whipped Cream, Semi Skimmed Milk, Mini	183
with Whipped Cream, Semi Skimmed Milk, Tall	243
with Whipped Cream, Skimmed Milk, Grande	317
with Whipped Cream, Skimmed Milk, Mini	173
with Whipped Cream, Skimmed Milk, Tall	229
with Whipped Cream, Soy, Grande	324
with Whipped Cream, Soy, Mini	176
with Whipped Cream, Soy, Tall	234
with Whipped Cream, Whole Milk, Grande	339
with Whipped Cream, Whole Milk, Mini	193
with Whipped Cream, Whole Milk, Tall	247

FRAPPUCCINO - COFFEE

No Whip, Almond Milk, Grande	191
No Whip, Almond Milk, Mini	111
No Whip, Almond Milk, Tall	137
No Whipped Cream, Coconut Milk, Grande	207
No Whip, Coconut Milk, Mini	122

STARBUCKS
FRAPPUCCINO - COFFEE

No Whipped Cream, Coconut Milk, Tall	151
No Whipped Cream, Semi Skimmed Milk, Grande	215
No Whip, Semi Skimmed Milk, Mini	127
No Whipped Cream, Semi Skimmed Milk, Tall	157
No Whipped Cream, Skimmed Milk, Grande	201
No Whip, Skimmed Milk, Mini	118
No Whipped, Skimmed Milk, Tall	146
No Whipped Cream, Soy, Grande	206
No Whip, Soy, Mini	121
No Whipped Cream, Soy, Tall	150
No Whipped Cream, Whole Milk, Grande	230
No Whip, Whole Milk, Mini	137
No Whipped Cream, Whole Milk, Tall	170
Light, No Whipped Cream, Skimmed Milk, Grande	118
Light, No Whip, Skimmed Milk, Mini	59
Light, No Whipped Cream, Skimmed Milk, Tall	83

FRAPPUCCINO - DOUBLE CHOC CHIP CREAM

with Whipped Cream, Almond Milk, Grande	380
with Whipped Cream, Almond Milk, Mini	225
with Whipped Cream, Almond Milk, Tall	273
with Whipped Cream, Coconut Milk, Grande	391
with Whipped Cream, Coconut Milk, Mini	231
with Whipped Cream, Coconut Milk, Tall	288
with Whipped Cream, Semi Skimmed Milk, Grande	402
with Whipped Cream, Semi Skimmed Milk, Mini	238
with Whipped Cream, Semi Skimmed Milk, Tall	297
with Whipped Cream, Skimmed Milk, Grande	383
with Whipped Cream, Skimmed Milk, Mini	220
with Whipped Cream, Skimmed Milk, Tall	280
with Whipped Cream, Soy, Grande	390
with Whipped Cream, Soy, Mini	230
with Whipped Cream, Soy, Tall	287
with Whipped Cream, Whole Milk, Grande	421
with Whipped Cream, Whole Milk, Mini	250
with Whipped Cream, Whole Milk, Tall	313

FRAPPUCCINO - ESPRESSO

No Whip, Almond Milk, Grande	175
No Whip, Almond Milk, Mini	91
No Whip, Almond Milk, Tall	116
No Whipped Cream, Coconut Milk, Grande	186
No Whip, Coconut Milk, Mini	100
No Whipped Cream, Coconut Milk, Tall	124
No Whipped Cream, Semi Skimmed Milk, Grande	191
No Whip, Semi Skimmed Milk, Mini	104
No Whipped Cream, Semi Skimmed Milk, Tall	128
No Whipped Cream, Skimmed Milk, Grande	182
No Whip, Skimmed Milk, Mini	97
No Whipped Cream, Skimmed Milk, Tall	121
No Whipped Cream, Soy, Grande	185
No Whip, Soy, Mini	99
No Whipped Cream, Soy, Tall	124
No Whipped Cream, Whole Milk, Grande	201

STARBUCKS
FRAPPUCCINO - ESPRESSO

No Whip, Whole Milk, Mini	112
No Whipped Cream, Whole Milk, Tall	135

FRAPPUCCINO - ESPRESSO LIGHT

No Whip, Skimmed Milk, Grande	111
No Whip, Skimmed Milk, Mini	62
No Whip, Skimmed Milk, Tall	78

FRAPPUCCINO - GREEN TEA

with Whipped Cream, Almond Milk, Grande	286
with Whipped Cream, Almond Milk, Mini	183
with Whipped Cream, Almond Milk, Tall	200
with Whipped Cream, Coconut Milk, Grande	301
with Whipped Cream, Coconut Milk, Mini	192
with Whipped Cream, Coconut Milk, Tall	210
with Whipped Cream, Semi Skimmed Milk, Grande	310
with Whipped Cream, Semi Skimmed Milk, Mini	196
with Whipped Cream, Semi Skimmed Milk, Tall	216
with Whipped Cream, Skimmed Milk, Grande	296
with Whipped Cream, Skimmed Milk, Mini	189
with Whipped Cream, Skimmed Milk, Tall	207
with Whipped Cream, Soy, Grande	301
with Whipped Cream, Soy, Mini	192
with Whipped Cream, Soy, Tall	210
with Whipped Cream, Whole Milk, Grande	325
with Whipped Cream, Whole Milk, Mini	204
with Whipped Cream, Whole Milk, Tall	225

FRAPPUCCINO - JAVA CHIP

with Whipped Cream, Almond Milk, Grande	354
with Whipped Cream, Almond Milk, Mini	221
with Whipped Cream, Almond Milk, Tall	256
with Whipped Cream, Coconut Milk, Grande	435
with Whipped Cream, Coconut Milk, Mini	229
with Whipped Cream, Coconut Milk, Tall	314
with Whipped Cream, Semi Skimmed Milk, Grande	442
with Whipped Cream, Semi Skimmed Milk, Mini	234
with Whipped Cream, Semi Skimmed Milk, Tall	320
with Whipped Cream, Skimmed Milk, Grande	429
with Whipped Cream, Skimmed Milk, Mini	226
with Whipped Cream, Skimmed Milk, Tall	310
with Whipped Cream, Soy, Grande	434
with Whipped Cream, Soy, Mini	229
with Whipped Cream, Soy, Tall	314
with Whipped Cream, Whole Milk, Grande	457
with Whipped Cream, Whole Milk, Mini	242
with Whipped Cream, Whole Milk, Tall	332

FRAPPUCCINO - JAVA CHIP LIGHT

No Whip, Skimmed Milk, Grande	211
No Whip, Skimmed Milk, Mini	113
No Whip, Skimmed Milk, Tall	148

FRAPPUCCINO - MANGO PASSION

Tea, Grande	191
Tea, Mini	84
Tea, Tall	157

STARBUCKS
FRAPPUCCINO - MOCHA

with Whipped Cream, Almond Milk, Grande	361
with Whipped Cream, Almond Milk, Mini	208
with Whipped Cream, Almond Milk, Tall	258
with Whipped Cream, Coconut Milk, Grande	377
with Whipped Cream, Coconut Milk, Mini	219
with Whipped Cream, Coconut Milk, Tall	271
with Whipped Cream, Semi Skimmed Milk, Grande	385
with Whipped Cream, Semi Skimmed Milk, Mini	224
with Whipped Cream, Semi Skimmed Milk, Tall	278
with Whipped Cream, Skimmed Milk, Grande	371
with Whipped Cream, Skimmed Milk, Mini	215
with Whipped Cream, Skimmed Milk, Tall	267
with Whipped Cream, Soy, Grande	376
with Whipped Cream, Soy, Mini	218
with Whipped Cream, Soy, Tall	271
with Whipped Cream, Whole Milk, Grande	400
with Whipped Cream, Whole Milk, Mini	234
with Whipped Cream, Whole Milk, Tall	290
No Whip, Skimmed Milk, Grande	143
No Whip, Skimmed Milk, Mini	81
No Whip, Skimmed Milk, Tall	96

FRAPPUCCINO - MOCHA, WHITE CHOCOLATE

with Whipped Cream, Almond Milk, Grande	379
with Whipped Cream, Almond Milk, Mini	197
with Whipped Cream, Almond Milk, Tall	275
with Whipped Cream, Coconut Milk, Grande	394
with Whipped Cream, Coconut Milk, Mini	206
with Whipped Cream, Coconut Milk, Tall	288
with Whipped Cream, Semi Skimmed Milk, Grande	402
with Whipped Cream, Semi Skimmed Milk, Mini	211
with Whipped Cream, Semi Skimmed Milk, Tall	294
with Whipped Cream, Skimmed Milk, Grande	389
with Whipped Cream, Skimmed Milk, Mini	203
with Whipped Cream, Skimmed Milk, Tall	283
with Whipped Cream, Soy, Grande	393
with Whipped Cream, Soy, Mini	206
with Whipped Cream, Soy, Tall	287
with Whipped Cream, Whole Milk, Grande	416
with Whipped Cream, Whole Milk, Mini	219
with Whipped Cream, Whole Milk, Tall	306

FRAPPUCCINO - MOCHA, WHITE CHOCOLATE, LIGHT

No Whip, Skimmed Milk, Grande	155
No Whip, Skimmed Milk, Mini	78
No Whip, Skimmed Milk, Tall	98

FRAPPUCCINO - STRAWBERRIES & CREAM

with Whipped Cream, Almond Milk, Grande	321
with Whipped Cream, Almond Milk, Mini	217
with Whipped Cream, Almond Milk, Tall	235
with Whipped Cream, Coconut Milk, Grande	341
with Whipped Cream, Coconut Milk, Mini	234
with Whipped Cream, Coconut Milk, Tall	251
with Whipped Cream, Semi Skimmed Milk, Grande	351

STARBUCKS
FRAPPUCCINO - STRAWBERRIES & CREAM

with Whipped Cream, Semi Skimmed Milk, Mini	242
with Whipped Cream, Semi Skimmed Milk, Tall	259
with Whipped Cream, Skimmed Milk, Grande	334
with Whipped Cream, Skimmed Milk, Mini	228
with Whipped Cream, Skimmed Milk, Tall	245
with Whipped Cream, Soy, Grande	340
with Whipped Cream, Soy, Mini	233
with Whipped Cream, Soy, Tall	250
with Whipped Cream, Whole Milk, Grande	370
Strawith Whipped Cream, Whole Milk, Mini	257
with Whipped Cream, Whole Milk, Tall	275

FRAPPUCCINO - VANILLA CREAM

with Whipped Cream, Almond Milk, Grande	292
with Whipped Cream, Almond Milk, Mini	148
with Whipped Cream, Almond Milk, Tall	207
with Whipped Cream, Coconut Milk, Grande	296
with Whipped Cream, Coconut Milk, Mini	160
with Whipped Cream, Coconut Milk, Tall	221
with Whipped Cream, Semi Skimmed Milk, Grande	316
with Whipped Cream, Semi Skimmed Milk, Mini	165
with Whipped Cream, Semi Skimmed Milk, Tall	225
with Whipped Cream, Skimmed Milk , Tall	208
with Whipped Cream, Skimmed Milk, Grande	294
with Whipped Cream, Skimmed Milk, Mini	156
with Whipped Cream, Soy, Grande	302
with Whipped Cream, Soy, Mini	159
with Whipped Cream, Whole Milk, Grande	329
with Whipped Cream, Whole Milk, Mini	176
with Whipped Cream, Whole Milk, Tall	236

FRAPPUCCINO - WHITE CHOC CREAM

with Whipped Cream, Almond Milk, Grande	336
with Whipped Cream, Almond Milk, Mini	173
with Whipped Cream, Almond Milk, Tall	245
with Whipped Cream, Coconut Milk, Grande	358
with Whipped Cream, Coconut Milk, Mini	184
with Whipped Cream, Coconut Milk, Tall	262
with Whipped Cream, Semi Skimmed Milk, Grande	369
with Whipped Cream, Semi Skimmed Milk, Mini	190
with Whipped Cream, Semi Skimmed Milk, Tall	271
with Whipped Cream, Skimmed Milk, Grande	350
with Whipped Cream, Skimmed Milk, Mini	180
with Whipped Cream, Skimmed Milk, Tall	256
with Whipped Cream, Soy, Grande	357
with Whipped Cream, Soy, Mini	184
with Whipped Cream, Soy, Tall	262
with Whipped Cream, Whole Milk, Grande	389
with Whipped Cream, Whole Milk, Mini	201
with Whipped Cream, Whole Milk, Tall	287

FRAPPUCCINO - ZEN TEA

Raspberry, Blackcurrant, Grande	192
Raspberry, Blackcurrant, Mini	87
Raspberry, Blackcurrant, Tall	158

STARBUCKS

HOT CHOCOLATE - CLASSIC

Item	KCAL
with Whipped Cream, Almond Milk, Grande	286
with Whipped Cream, Almond Milk, Short	173
with Whipped Cream, Almond Milk, Tall	241
with Whipped Cream, Almond Milk, Venti	363
with Whipped Cream, Coconut Milk, Grande	343
with Whipped Cream, Coconut Milk, Short	201
with Whipped Cream, Coconut Milk, Tall	285
with Whipped Cream, Coconut Milk, Venti	435
with Whipped Cream, Semi Skimmed Milk, Grande	372
with Whipped Cream, Semi Skimmed Milk, Short	215
with Whipped Cream, Semi Skimmed Milk, Tall	307
with Whipped Cream, Semi Skimmed Milk, Venti	473
with Whipped Cream, Skimmed Milk, Grande	323
with Whipped Cream, Skimmed Milk, Short	191
with Whipped Cream, Skimmed Milk, Venti	410
with Whipped Cream, Soy, Grande	341
with Whipped Cream, Soy, Short	200
with Whipped Cream, Soy, Tall	283
with Whipped Cream, Whole Milk, Grande	426
with Whipped Cream, Whole Milk, Short	242
with Whipped Cream, Whole Milk, Tall	348
with Whipped Cream, Whole Milk, Venti	540
with Whippped Cream, Skimmed Milk, Tall	269

HOT CHOCOLATE - FUDGE

Item	KCAL
Grande	315
Short	198
Tall	257

HOT CHOCOLATE - KIDS

Item	KCAL
with Whipped Cream, Almond Milk	173
with Whipped Cream, Coconut Milk	201
with Whipped Cream, Semi Skimmed Milk	215
with Whipped Cream, Skimmed Milk	191
with Whipped Cream, Soy	200
with Whipped Cream, Whole Milk	242

HOT CHOCOLATE - SIGNATURE

Item	KCAL
with Whipped Cream, Almond Milk, Short	271
with Whipped Cream, Almond Milk, Tall	396
with Whipped Cream, Coconut Milk, Short	275
with Whipped Cream, Coconut Milk, Tall	399
with Whipped Cream, Semi Skimmed Milk, Short	283
with Whipped Cream, Semi Skimmed Milk, Tall	418
with Whipped Cream, Skimmed Milk, Short	267
with Whipped Cream, Skimmed Milk, Tall	393
with Whipped Cream, Soy, Short	272
with Whipped Cream, Soy, Tall	401
with Whipped Cream, Whole Milk, Short	293
with Whipped Cream, Whole Milk, Tall	433

MILK

Item	KCAL
Steamed, Almond Milk, Grande	89
Steamed, Almond Milk, Short	44
Steamed, Almond Milk, Tall	68
Steamed, Almond Milk, Venti	113

STARBUCKS

MILK

Item	KCAL
Steamed, Coconut, Venti	191
Steamed, Coconut Milk, Grande	151
Steamed, Coconut Milk, Short	74
Steamed, Coconut Milk, Tall	115
Steamed, Semi Skimmed Milk, Grande	182
Steamed, Semi Skimmed Milk, Short	89
Steamed, Semi Skimmed Milk, Tall	139
Steamed, Semi Skimmed Milk, Venti	531
Steamed, Skimmed Milk, Grande	129
Steamed, Skimmed Milk, Short	63
Steamed, Skimmed Milk, Tall	98
Steamed, Skimmed Milk, Venti	163
Steamed, Soy, Grande	148
Steamed, Soy, Short	73
Steamed, Soy, Tall	113
Steamed, Soy, Venti	188
Steamed, Whole Milk, Grande	240
Steamed, Whole Milk, Short	118
Steamed, Whole Milk, Tall	184
Steamed, Whole Milk, Venti	305

SYRUP

Item	KCAL
Bar Mocha, 1 Pump - ½ fl oz - 17 g	26
Bar Mocha, 2 Pumps - 1 fl oz - 34 g	53
Bar Mocha, 3 Pumps - 1½ fl oz - 51 g	79
Bar Mocha, 4 Pumps - 2 fl oz - 68 g	106
Bar Mocha, 5 Pumps - 2 ½ fl oz - 85 g	132
Flavoured, 1 Pump - ¼ fl oz 10g	20
Flavoured, 2 Pumps - ½ fl oz - 20 g	40
Flavoured, 3 Pumps - 3/4 fl oz - 30 g	60
Flavoured, 4 Pumps - 1 fl oz - 40 g	81
Sugar Free	0

TEA

Item	KCAL
Chai, Grande	0
Chai, Latte, Almond Milk, Grande	183
Chai, Latte, Almond Milk, Short	92
Chai, Latte, Almond Milk, Tall	139
Chai, Latte, Almond Milk, Venti	230
Chai, Latte, Coconut Milk, Grande	192
Chai, Latte, Coconut Milk, Short	96
Chai, Latte, Coconut Milk, Tall	143
Chai, Latte, Coconut Milk, Venti	239
Chai, Latte, Semi Skimmed Milk, Grande	236
Chai, Latte, Semi Skimmed Milk, Short	119
Chai, Latte, Semi Skimmed Milk, Tall	179
Chai, Latte, Semi Skimmed Milk, Venti	297
Chai, Latte, Skimmed Milk, Grande	204
Chai, Latte, Skimmed Milk, Short	103
Chai, Latte, Skimmed Milk, Tall	154
Chai, Latte, Skimmed Milk, Venti	256
Chai, Latte, Soy, Grande	213
Chai, Latte, Soy, Short	108
Chai, Latte, Soy, Tall	162

STARBUCKS

TEA

Chai, Latte, Soy, Venti	268
Chai, Latte, Whole Milk, Grande	255
Chai, Latte, Whole Milk, Short	129
Chai, Latte, Whole Milk, Tall	194
Chai, Latte, Whole Milk, Venti	322
Chai, Tall	0
Chai, Venti	0
Chamomile, Grande	0
Chamomile, Tall	0
Chamomile, Venti	0
Earl Grey, Grande	0
Earl Grey, Tall	0
Earl Grey, Venti	0
Emperor's Clouds & Mist, Grande	0
Emperor's Clouds & Mist, Tall	0
Emperor's Clouds & Mist, Venti	0
English Breakfast, Grande	0
English Breakfast, Tall	0
English Breakfast, Venti	0
Green, Latte, Almond Milk, Grande	154
Green, Latte, Almond Milk, Short	65
Green, Latte, Almond Milk, Tall	113
Green, Latte, Almond Milk, Venti	204
Green, Latte, Coconut Milk, Grande	210
Green, Latte, Coconut Milk, Short	93
Green, Latte, Coconut Milk, Tall	158
Green, Latte, Coconut Milk, Venti	277
Green, Latte, Semi Skimmed Milk, Grande	239
Green, Latte, Semi Skimmed Milk, Short	107
Green, Latte, Semi Skimmed Milk, Tall	181
Green, Latte, Semi Skimmed Milk, Venti	315
Green, Latte, Skimmed Milk, Grande	190
Green, Latte, Skimmed Milk, Short	83
Green, Latte, Skimmed Milk, Tall	142
Green, Latte, Skimmed Milk, Venti	251
Green, Latte, Soya Milk, Grande	208
Green, Latte, Soya Milk, Short	92
Green, Latte, Soya Milk, Tall	156
Green, Latte, Soya Milk, Venti	275
Green, Latte, Whole Milk, Grande	291
Green, Latte, Whole Milk, Short	133
Green, Latte, Whole Milk, Tall	223
Green, Latte, Whole Milk, Venti	384
Hibiscus, Grande	0
Hibiscus, Tall	0
Hibiscus, Venti	0
Iced, Black Tea, Shaken, Grande	0
Iced, Black Tea, Shaken, Tall	0
Iced, Black Tea, Shaken, Venti	0
Iced, Chai, Latte, Almond Milk, Grande	181
Iced, Chai, Latte, Almond Milk, Tall	136
Iced, Chai, Latte, Almond Milk, Venti	227

STARBUCKS

TEA

Iced, Chai, Latte, Coconut, Tall	164
Iced, Chai, Latte, Coconut, Venti	274
Iced, Chai, Latte, Coconut Milk, Grande	217
Iced, Chai, Latte, Semi Skimmed Milk, Grande	236
Iced, Chai, Latte, Semi Skimmed Milk, Tall	179
Iced, Chai, Latte, Semi Skimmed Milk, Venti	298
Iced, Chai, Latte, Skimmed Milk, Grande	204
Iced, Chai, Latte, Skimmed Milk, Tall	154
Iced, Chai, Latte, Skimmed Milk, Venti	257
Iced, Chai, Latte, Soy, Grande	216
Iced, Chai, Latte, Soy, Tall	163
Iced, Chai, Latte, Soy, Venti	272
Iced, Chai, Latte, Whole Milk, Grande	270
Iced, Chai, Latte, Whole Milk, Tall	205
Iced, Chai, Latte, Whole Milk, Venti	341
Iced, Green Tea, Shaken, Grande	0
Iced, Green Tea, Shaken, Tall	0
Iced, Green Tea, Shaken, Venti	0
Iced, Hibiscus, Shaken, Grande	0
Iced, Hibiscus, Shaken, Tall	0
Iced, Hibiscus, Shaken, Venti	0
Jasmine Pearls, Grande	0
Jasmine Pearls, Tall	0
Jasmine Pearls, Venti	0
Mango, Black, Tea Lemonade, Grande	127
Mango, Black, Tea Lemonade, Tall	96
Mango, Black, Tea Lemonade, Venti	158
Mint Blend, Grande	0
Mint Blend, Tall	0
Mint Blend, Venti	0
Mint Citrus, Green Tea, Grande	0
Mint Citrus, Green Tea, Tall	0
Mint Citrus, Green Tea, Venti	0
Peach, Green, Tea Lemonade, Grande	127
Peach, Green, Tea Lemonade, Tall	96
Peach, Green, Tea Lemonade, Venti	158
Youthberry, Grande	0
Youthberry, Tall	0
Youthberry, Venti	0

TOPPING

Whipped Cream, Cold, Grande, Beverage	114
Whipped Cream, Cold, Venti, Beverage	104
Caramel - 4 g	15
Chocolate - 4 g	6
Sprinkles - 1 g	4
Whipped Cream, Cold, Tall, Beverage	81
Whipped Cream, Hot, Grande/Venti Beverage	72
Whipped Cream, Hot, Short, Beverage	52
Whipped Cream, Hot, Tall, Beverage	62

SUBWAY

BACON

2 Strips	40

SUBWAY

BEEF
	KCAL
Patty, Big	142
Steak, Portion	94

BREAD
Flatbread	220
Rolls, Submarine, 9 Grain Honey Oat, 6"	218
Rolls, Submarine, 9 Grain Wheat, 6"	205
Rolls, Submarine, Hearty Italian, 6"	209
Rolls, Submarine, Italian Herb & Cheese, 6"	242
Rolls, Submarine, Italian White, 6"	198

CHEESE
Cheddar, Processed	40
Monterey Cheddar	57
Peppered	39

CHICKEN
Breast, Portion	35
Strips, Teriyaki Glazed, Portion	101
Tikka, Portion	89

COOKIES
Chocolate Chip Candy	211
Chocolate Chunk	216
Double Choc Chip	215
Oatmeal Raisin	195
Raspberry Cheesecake	207

DANISH PASTRY
Apricot Crown	419
Cinnamon Swirl	207
Vanilla Crown	329

DOUGHNUTS
Chocolate	351
Sugared	352

EGGS
Patty, Portion	55

FLATBREAD
Bacon, Egg, & Cheese, with Salad, Breakfast	352
Bacon, with Salad, Breakfast	345
Beef, Big Beef Melt, with Salad	418
Chicken, & Bacon, Ranch Melt, with Salad	518
Chicken, Breast, with Salad, Low Fat	321
Chicken, Teriyaki, with Salad, Low Fat	337
Chicken, Tikka, with Salad, Low Fat	325
Egg, & Cheese, wiith Salad, Breakfast	316
Ham, with Salad, Low Fat	305
Italian BMT, with Salad	427
Meatball Marinara, with Salad	454
Mega Melt, with Salad, Breakfast	529
Sausage, Egg, & Cheese, with Salad, Breakfast	492
Sausage, with Salad, Breakfast	396
Spicy Italian, with Salad	498
Steak, & Cheese, with Salad	370
Subway Melt, with Salad	388
Tuna, with Salad	371
Turkey, & Ham, with Salad, Low Fat	308

SUBWAY

FLATBREAD
	KCAL
Turkey, Breast, with Salad, Low Fat	292
Veggie Delite, with Salad, Low Fat	236
Veggie Patty, with Salad	396

HAM
Portion	69

MEATBALLS
Bowl	314
Marinara, Sub Portion	218

MUFFIN
Blueberry	394
Chocolate Chunk	243
Double Chocolate Chip	351
Raspberry, & White Chocolate	389

NACHOS
Cheese, Melted	403

PEPPERONI
Salami, & Cheese, Spicy Italian, Portion	262
Salami, & Ham, Italian BMT, Portion	192

SALAD
Beef, Big Beef Melt, without Dressing	234
Chicken, & Bacon, Ranch Melt, without Dressing	334
Chicken, Breast, without Dressing	137
Chicken, Pizziola, without Dressing	274
Chicken, Teriyaki, without Dressing	141
Chicken, Tikka, without Dressing	121
Ham, without Dressing	153
Italian BMT, without Dressing	244
Meatball, Marinara, without Dressing	270
Spicy Italian, without Dressing	314
Steak, & Cheese, without Dressing	186
Subway Melt, with Cheese, without Dressing	205
Tuna, without Dressing	187
Turkey, & Ham, without Dressing	124
Turkey, Breast, without Dressing	108
Veggie Delite, without Dressing	52
Veggie Patty, without Dressing	212

SAUCE
Barbecue	39
Chilli, Hot	48
Chilli, Sweet	46
Chipotle Southwest	90
Deli Mustard	48
Honey Mustard	32
Mayonnaise, Lite	50
Ranch	43
Sweet Onion	34

SAUSAGE
Portion	176

SUBS - BACON
9 Grain Honey Oat Bread, Breakfast, 6"	291
9 Grain Wheat Bread, Breakfast, 6"	278
Hearty Italian Bread, Breakfast, 6"	282

SUBWAY

SUBS - BACON
	KCAL
Italian Herb & Cheese Bread, Breakfast, 6"	315
Italian White Bread, Breakfast, 6"	271

SUBS - BACON, EGG, & CHEESE
	KCAL
9 Grain Honey Oat Bread, Breakfast, 6"	350
9 Grain Wheat Bread, 6"	337
Hearty Italian Bread, Breakfast, 6"	361
Italian Herb & Cheese Bread, Breakfast, 6"	374
Italian White Bread, Breakfast, 6"	330

SUBS - BIG BEEF MELT
	KCAL
with Salad, 9 Grain Honey Oat Bread, 6"	416
with Salad, 9 Grain Wheat Bread, 6"	403
with Salad, Hearty Italian Bread, 6"	407
with Salad, Italian Herb & Cheese Bread, 6"	440
with Salad, Italian White Bread, 6"	396

SUBS - CHICKEN & BACON RANCH MELT
	KCAL
with Salad, 9 Grain Honey Oat Bread, 6"	516

SUBS - CHICKEN & BACON RANCH MELT
	KCAL
with Salad, 9 Grain Wheat Bread, 6"	503

SUBS - CHICKEN & BACON RANCH MELT
	KCAL
with Salad, Hearty Italian Bread, 6"	507
with Salad, Italian Herb & Cheese Bread, 6"	540
with Salad, Italian White Bread, 6"	496

SUBS - CHICKEN BREAST
	KCAL
with Salad, 9 Grain Honey Oat Bread, Low Fat, 6"	319
with Salad, 9 Grain Wheat Bread, Low Fat, 6"	306
with Salad, Hearty Italian Bread, Low Fat, 6"	310
with Salad, Italian Herb & Cheese Bread, Low Fat, 6"	343
with Salad, Italian White Bread, Low Fat, 6"	299

SUBS - CHICKEN PIZZIOLA
	KCAL
with Salad, 9 Grain Honey Oat Bread, 6"	456
with Salad, 9 Grain Wheat Bread, 6"	443
with Salad, Hearty Italian Bread, 6"	447
with Salad, Italian Herb & Cheese Bread, 6"	480
with Salad, Italian White Bread, 6"	436

SUBS - CHICKEN TERIYAKI
	KCAL
with Salad, 9 Grain Honey Oat Bread, Low Fat, 6"	335
with Salad, 9 Grain Wheat Bread, Low Fat, 6"	322
with Salad, Hearty Italian Bread, Low Fat, 6"	326
with Salad, Italian Herb & Cheese Bread, Low Fat, 6"	359
with Salad, Italian White Bread, Low Fat, 6"	315

SUBS - CHICKEN TIKKA
	KCAL
with Salad, 9 Grain Honey Oat Bread, Low Fat, 6"	323
with Salad, 9 Grain Wheat Bread, Low Fat, 6"	310
with Salad, Hearty Italian Bread, Low Fat, 6"	314
with Salad, Italian Herb & Cheese Bread, Low Fat, 6"	347
with Salad, Italian White Bread, Low Fat, 6"	303

SUBS - EGG & CHEESE
	KCAL
9 Grain Honey Oat Bread, Breakfast, 6"	314
9 Grain Wheat Bread, Breakfast, 6"	301
Hearty Italian Bread, Breakfast, 6"	305
Italian Herb & Cheese Bread, Breakfast, 6"	338
Italian White Bread, Breakfast, 6"	294

SUBWAY

SUBS - HAM
	KCAL
with Salad, 9 Grain Honey Oat Bread, Low Fat, 6"	303
with Salad, 9 Grain Wheat Bread, Kids Pak, 4"	182
with Salad, Hearty Italian Bread, Low Fat, 6"	294
with Salad, Italian Herb & Cheese Bread, Low Fat, 6"	327
with Salad, Italian White Bread, Kids Pak, 4"	177

SUBS - ITALIAN BMT
	KCAL
with Salad, 9 Grain Honey Oat Bread, 6"	425
with Salad, 9 Grain Wheat Bread, 6"	412
with Salad, Hearty Italian Bread, 6"	416
with Salad, Italian Herb & Cheese Bread, 6"	449
with Salad, Italian White Bread, 6"	405

SUBS - MEATBALL MARINARA
	KCAL
with Salad, 9 Grain Honey Oat Bread, 6"	452
with Salad, 9 Grain Wheat Bread, 6"	439
with Salad, Hearty Italian Bread, 6"	443
with Salad, Italian Herb & Cheese Bread, 6"	476
with Salad, Italian White Bread, 6"	432

SUBS - MEGA MELT
	KCAL
9 Grain Honey Oat Bread, Breakfast, 6"	527
9 Grain Wheat Bread, Breakfast, 6"	514
Hearty Italian Bread, Breakfast, 6"	518
Italian Herb & Cheese Bread, Breakfast, 6"	551
Italian White Bread, Breakfast, 6"	507

SUBS - SAUSAGE
	KCAL
9 Grain Honey Oat Bread, Breakfast, 6"	394
9 Grain Wheat Bread, Breakfast, 6"	381
Hearty Italian Bread, Breakfast, 6"	385
Italian Herb & Cheese Bread, Breakfast, 6"	418
Italian White Bread, Breakfast, 6"	374

SUBS - SAUSAGE, EGG & CHEESE
	KCAL
9 Grain Honey Oat Bread, 6"	490
9 Grain Wheat Bread, 6"	477
Hearty Italian Bread, Breakfast, 6"	481
Italian Herb & Cheese Bread, Breakfast, 6"	514
Italian White Bread, Breakfast, 6"	470

SUBS - SPICY ITALIAN
	KCAL
with Salad, 9 Grain Honey Oat Bread, 6"	495
with Salad, 9 Grain Wheat Bread, 6"	482
with Salad, Hearty Italian Bread, 6"	486
with Salad, Italian Herb & Cheese Bread, 6"	519
with Salad, Italian White Bread, 6"	475

SUBS - STEAK & CHEESE
	KCAL
with Salad, 9 Grain Honey Oat Bread, 6"	368
with Salad, 9 Grain Wheat Bread, 6"	355
with Salad, Hearty Italian Bread, 6"	359
with Salad, Italian Herb & Cheese Bread, 6"	392
with Salad, Italian White Bread, 6"	348

SUBS - SUBWAY MELT
	KCAL
with Salad, 9 Grain Honey Oat Bread, 6"	386
with Salad, 9 Grain Wheat Bread, 6"	373
with Salad, Hearty Italian Bread, 6"	377
with Salad, Italian Herb & Cheese Bread, 6"	410

SUBWAY

SUBS - SUBWAY MELT
with Salad, Italian White Bread, 6"	366

SUBS - TUNA
with Salad, 9 Grain Honey Oat Bread, 6"	369
with Salad, 9 Grain Wheat Bread, 6"	356
with Salad, Hearty Italian Bread, 6"	360
with Salad, Italian Herb & Cheese Bread, 6"	393
with Salad, Italian White Bread, 6"	349

SUBS - TURKEY & HAM
with Salad, 9 Grain Honey Oat Bread, Low Fat, 6"	306
with Salad, 9 Grain Wheat Bread, Low Fat, 6"	293
with Salad, Hearty Italian Bread, Low Fat, 6"	297
with Salad, Italian Herb & Cheese Bread, Low Fat, 6"	330
with Salad, Italian White Bread, Low Fat, 6"	286

SUBS - TURKEY BREAST
with Salad, 9 Grain Honey Oat Bread, Low Fat, 6"	290
with Salad, 9 Grain Wheat Bread, Kids Pak, 4"	184
with Salad, Hearty Italian Bread, Low Fat, 6"	281
with Salad, Italian Herb & Cheese Bread, Low Fat, 6"	314
with Salad, Italian White Bread, Kids Pak, 4"	180

SUBS - VEGGIE DELITE
with Salad, 9 Grain Honey Oat Bread, Low Fat, 6"	234
with Salad, 9 Grain Wheat Bread, Kids Pak, 4"	147
with Salad, Hearty Italian Bread, Low Fat, 6"	258
with Salad, Italian Herb & Cheese Bread, Low Fat, 6"	258
with Salad, Italian White Bread, Kids Pak, 4"	142

SUBS - VEGGIE PATTY
with Salad, 9 Grain Honey Oat Bread, 6"	394
with Salad, 9 Grain Wheat Bread, 6"	381
with Salad, Hearty Italian Bread, 6"	385
with Salad, Italian Herb & Cheese Bread, 6"	418
with Salad, Italian White Bread, 6"	373

TOASTIE
Cheese	214
Pepperoni Pizza	254

TUNA
Portion	135

TURKEY
Breast, & Ham, Portion	72
Breast, Portion	56

VEGETARIAN
Veggie Patty, Portion	160

TABLE TABLE

BEANS
Baked, in Tomato Sauce, Side, Kids Menu	51

BEEF
Roast, Kids Menu	535
Steak, Rib-eye, 10oz	1081
Steak, Rump, 8oz	863
Steak, Sirloin, 8oz	895
Topside, Sunday Lunch	828

BREAD
Garlic, Bread	110

TABLE TABLE

BREAD
Garlic, Side, Kids Menu	106
Garlic, Side	327
Garlic, with Cheese, Side	473

BROWNIES
Chocolate	533

BURGERS
Beef, with Cheese, Classic	1007
Beef, with Chips, Kids Menu	697
Chicken, Coronation	1065
Chickpea, & Spinach	882
Cluck 'N' Ale, Summer Menu	1387
Steak, Black, & Blue, Stack, Double	1253
Steak, with Bacon, Stack, Double	1273

CAKE
Chocolate, Fudge, Sensation	876

CAULIFLOWER CHEESE
Side	281
Sunday Lunch	281

CHEESECAKE
Baked	657

CHICKEN
Breast, Bacon, & Cheese, with Chips	821
Breast, Bacon, & Cheese, with Jacket Potato	808
Forestiere	730
Goujons, Buttermilk, Summer Menu	719
Goujons, with BBQ Dip	413
Paprika	607
Poppin, with Chips, & Beans, Kids Menu	525
Skewers, Jerk, Summer Menu	274
Wings, BBQ, 12	1001
Wings, BBQ, 6	500
Wings, Buffalo, 12	1009
Wings, Buffalo, 6	505

CHILLI
Con Carne, Beef	761

CHIPS
Side, Kids Menu	312
Side	416

COD
Bites, Breaded, Kids Menu	363

COLESLAW
Side, Kids Menu	40

CORN
Cob, Side, Kids Menu	29

CRUMBLE
Apple, Toffee, Salted	670

CURRY
Chicken, Thai Red	784

DESSERT
Chocolate, Challenge, Mini, Kids Menu	353
Eton Mess	481
Pizza, Chocolate, Kids Menu	371

TABLE TABLE

FISH & CHIPS

Battered, with Mushy Peas	1313
Battered, with Peas	1275

FRIES

Skinny, Side	328

FROZEN YOGHURT

Strawberry	280

FRUIT SALAD

Kids Menu	49

GAMMON

Steak, & Chips, with Egg, & Pineapple	815
Steak, & Chips, with Egg	837
Steak, & Chips, with Pineapple	793
Steak, & Jacket Potato, with Egg, & Pineapple	801
Steak, & Jacket Potato, with Egg	823
Steak, & Jacket Potato, with Pineapple	779

HADDOCK

Beer Battered, & Chips, with Mushy Peas	1146
Beer Battered, & Chips, with Peas	1108

HAM

Egg, & Chips	815

ICE CREAM

Vanilla, with Caramel Sauce, Kids Menu	259
Vanilla, with Caramel Sauce	354
Vanilla, with Chocolate Fudge Sauce	353
Vanilla, with Chocolate Sauce, Kids Menu	257
Vanilla, with Raspberry Sauce, Kids Menu	256
Vanilla, with Raspberry Sauce	350

LAMB

Rump, with Malbec Sauce	920

LASAGNE

Beef, & Pork	614
Spinach, & Ricotta	670

LIVER & BACON

Main	604

MAKHANI

Chicken	836

MIXED GRILL

Flat Iron Steak, Sausage, Chicken Breast, Gammon	1362
Rump Steak, Sausage, Chicken Breast, Gammon	1416

MUSHROOMS

Garlic, & Herb, Breaded	353

NACHOS

Kids Menu	230

ONION RINGS

Battered, Side	368

PARCELS

Filo, Mixed Vegetable	375
Mixed Vegetable, Filo, Sunday Lunch	806

PASTA

Penne, Tomato Sauce, Kids Menu	344

PATE

Pork, with Red Onion Chutney	431

TABLE TABLE

PEAS

Side, Kids Menu	47

PIE

Apple, Caramel, with Cream	522
Apple, Caramel, with Custard	454
Apple, Caramel, with Ice Cream	446
Beef, & Merlot	1352
Gammon, Chicken, & Pea	1024

PLATTER

BBQ, Summer Menu	1700
Sharing	1710
Sharing, with Buffalo Wings	2036

PORK

Loin, Sunday Lunch	915
Loin, Sunday Lunch	915
Roast, Kids Menu	652

POTATOES

Dippers, with Cheese, & Bacon	411
Jacket, Chicken, & Bacon, Mayo	699
Jacket, Prawns, & Marie Rose Sauce	581
Jacket, with Cheese, & Beans	853

PRAWN COCKTAIL

Classic	379

PRAWNS

BBQ, Summer Menu	420

QUICHE

Cheese, Three, Summer Menu	710

RIBS

Half Rack, BBQ, & Smoky Paprika Chicken	1047
Whole Rack, & Smoky Paprika Chicken	1401

RISOTTO

Pea, Basil, & Mozzarella	1034

SALAD

Beef, Pulled, Smoked, Main, Summer Menu	536
Beef, Pulled, Smoked, Starter, Summer Menu	239
Caesar, Chicken, & Kale	489
Caesar, Chicken, & Kale, with Bacon	552
Chicken, Jerk, & Mango, Summer Menu	301
Halloumi, Summer Menu	164
Mixed, Side	86
Prawn, Ginger, & Sesame	243

SANDWICH

Chicken, & Bacon, Mayo, Brown Bread	495
Chicken, & Bacon, Mayo, White Bread	489
Prawn, & Marie Rose Sauce, Brown Bread	409
Prawn, & Marie Rose Sauce, White Bread	403

SAUCE

Bearnaise, Steak Sauces	184
Diane, Steak Sauce	73
Peppercorn, Steak Sauce	46

SAUSAGE & MASH

Bangers, Kids Menu	391
Lunch Club Menu	783

TABLE TABLE

SAUSAGE & MASH

	KCAL
Main	897
Vegetarian, Bangers, Kids Menu	364

SCAMPI

Breaded, & Chips, with Mushy Peas	838
Breaded, & Chips, with Peas	800

SEA BASS

Fillet, with Potatoes	663

SORBET

Strawberry, & Black Pepper, Summer Menu	185

SOUP

Carrot, & Coriander	282
Minestrone	281
Mushroom, Cream Of	296
Pea, & Mint	295
Tomato, Black Pepper, & Thyme	293

SPAGHETTI BOLOGNAISE

Kids Menu	320

SUNDAE

Caramel, Popcorn, Summer Menu	765
Funny Face, Kids Menu	260
Vanilla, Ice Cream, Chocolate, Brownie, Rocky Road	767
Vanilla, Ice Cream, Dairy Milk, Cadbury	667

SWEET POTATO

Fries, Side	390

TART

Cheese, Cheshire, & Bramley Apple	715
Treacle	731

TOASTIE

Ham, & Cheese, White Bread	500
Ham & Cheese, Brown Bread	506

TRIFLE

Lemon, Gin, & Tonic	626
Strawberry Pimms, Summer Menu	603

TURKEY

Roast, Kids Menu	515
Sunday Lunch	791

VEGETABLES

Mixed, Green, Side	112
Sticks, Kids Menu	49
Sticks, Side, Kids Menu	28

WELLINGTON

Pork, Pulled, Hog Roast	1236
Salmon, with Cheese, Spinach, & Caper Sauce	1121

WRAP

Chicken, Build Your Own, Kids Menu	491
Salmon, Build Your Own, Kids Menu	495
Sausage, Vegetarian, Build Your Own, Kids Menu	491

THE REAL GREEK FOOD COMPANY LTD

ASPARAGUS

Grilled, Hot Meze	140

CHEESE

Halloumi, Grilled, Hot Meze	151

THE REAL GREEK FOOD COMPANY LTD

CHEESE

	KCAL
Halloumi, Skewers, Hot Meze	118
Halloumi, Skewers, Kids Menu	118

CHICK PEAS

Revithia, Cold Meze	286

CHICKEN

Skewers, Hot Meze	177
Skewers, Kids Menu	88

CHIPS

Side	528

COD

Salt, Hot Meze	346

CRUDITES

Cold Meze	37

DESSERT

Watermelon, Sweet & Salty	124
Yoghurt, Greek with Raspberries	223

DIP

Aioli, Parsley	176
Dip, Selection	589
Mayonnaise, Lemon, Preserved	279
Melitzanasalata, Cold Meze	236
Relish, Chilli, Smoked	42
Relish, Sun-Dried Tomato & Roast Red Pepper	92

DOLMADES

Cold Meze	254

FLATBREAD

Greek, Cold Meze	615
Greek, with Olive & Dukkah, Nibbles	538

HOUMOUS

Cold Meze	298

LAMB

Cutlets, Hot Meze	881
Kefte, Hot Meze	344
Skewers, Hot Meze	255

NUTS

Mixed, Athenian, Nibbles	479

OCTOPUS

Grilled, Hot Meze	447

OLIVES

Nibbles	317

PARCELS

Tiropitakia, Filo Pastry, Hot Meze	416

PORK

Skewers, Hot Meze	281

POTATOES

New, in Olive Oil & Lemon Juice, Hot Meze	293

RICE

Saffron, Hot Meze	406

SALAD

Cos	42
Tabouleh, Cold Meze	117
Watermelon, Mint & Feta, Cold Meze	102

THE REAL GREEK FOOD COMPANY LTD

SARDINES

Grilled, Hot Meze	619

SOUVLAKI

Lamb, Kefte	730
Lamb	607
Pork	633
Souvlaki, Halloumi & Vegetable	451

SQUID

Kalamari, Grilled, Hot Meze	286

TARAMASALATA

Cold Meze	913

TZATZIKI

Cold Meze	163

TOBY CARVERY

ANGEL DELIGHT

Strawberry, Mini, Kids Menu	79
Strawberry, with Popping Candy, Kids Menu	73

BEANS

Green	17
Romano	17

BEEF

Roast, Kids Menu	229
Roast, King Size	609
Roast	458

BOLOGNESE

Spaghetti, with Veggie Sticks, Kids Menu	263

BROCCOLI

Side	20

BROWNIES - CHOCOLATE

Whipped Cream, White Chocolate, & Rasperries	889
Mini, Whipped Cream, Kids Menu	370

CABBAGE

Red, with Cranberry, & Orange	12
with Onions	8

CAKE

Chocolate, Fudge	669
Chocolate, Fudge, with Custard	759
Chocolate, Fudge, with Ice Cream	804
Chocolate, Fudge, with Whipped Cream	1039

CARROTS

Side	24

CAULIFLOWER CHEESE

Side	17

CHEESE

Dorset, Bites, Chilli Seasoning	265
Fondue, Blue, with Bread, & Crudites	526

CHEESECAKE

Blueberry, & Vanilla, Strawberry Compote, Baked	742

CHICKEN

Breast, Roast, & Giant Yorkshire Pudding, Kids Menu	196
Wings, Honey, & Mustard	274

CRUMBLE - APPLE

Mango, & Passion Fruit, Custard, Mini, Kids Menu	343

TOBY CARVERY

CRUMBLE - APPLE

Plum, & Damson, Mini, Kids Menu	301
Plum, & Damson, with Custard	454
with Custard, Mini, Kids Menu	314

DESSERT

Bananas, & Custard, Kids Menu	223
Eton Mess, Strawberry, & Passion Fruit	914

GAMMON

Cheddar, Salad, Chutney & Baguette	795
Pomegranate Glaze, King Size	422
Pomegranate Glaze	317
Roast, Kids Menu	158

GRATIN

Potato, Carrot, Garlic, Creamy	121

GRAVY

Beef, & Onion	21
Onion, Vegetarian	23
Poultry	21

ICE CREAM

Kids Menu	190

ICE LOLLY

Frozen Yoghurt, Strawberry, Greek Style, Kids Menu	55

JELLY

Orange, with Mandarins, Kids Menu	100

LEEKS

Side	8

MEATBALLS

Pork, & Beef, with Gravy	356

MUSHROOMS

Creamy, Cheddar Sauce, with Bread	346

MUSTARD

Original	29
Wholegrain	32

ONIONS

in Gravy	30

PARCELS

Broccoli, & Brie	492

PARSNIP

Side	134

PEAS

Side	46

PIE

Allotment, House Salad, & Steamed Potatoes	455
Shepherds, with Carrot & Swede Mash, Kids Menu	228

PORK

Riblets, Pomegranate glaze	210
Roast, Kids Menu	212
Roast, with Crackling, King Size	564
Roast, with Crackling	424

PORK CRACKLING

& Apple Sauce	1033
Homemade	670

TOBY CARVERY

POTATO MASH
	KCAL
Side	46

POTATOES
Roast, Roasties	375
Roast, Roasties, with Cheese	494
Roast, 3 Potatoes	258

PRAWN COCKTAIL
King, with Bread	528
King, with Wholemeal Bread, Mini, Kids Menu	291

PROFITEROLES
with Belgian Chocolate Sauce, & Whipped Cream	645

RICE PUDDING
Vanilla, with Raspberries	350

SALAD
Superfood, with French Dressing	158
Superfood, with Roast Chicken, & French Dressing	543
Superfood, with Salmon, & French Dressing	526

SALMON
En Pappillote	368

SANDWICH
Beef, & Horseradish, Crispy Baguette, Roast	989
Beef, & Horseradish, Homebaked Bap, Roast	931
Cheddar, Apple, & Chutney, Crispy Baguette	1097
Cheddar, Apple, & Chutney, Homebaked Bap	1039
Full Feast, Crispy Baguette	936
Full Feast, Homebaked Bap	878
Gammon, Lettuce, & Tomato, Crispy Baguette	936
Gammon, Lettuce, & Tomato, Homebaked Bap	878
Pork, Stuffing, & Apple Sauce, Crispy Baguette	986
Pork, Stuffing, & Apple Sauce, Homebaked Bap	928
Prawns, King, Seafood Sauce, Crispy Baguette	1175
Prawns, King, Seafood Sauce, Homebaked Bap	1117
Turkey, Stuffing, & Cranberry Sauce, Baguette	895
Turkey, Stuffing, & Cranberry Sauce, Bap	837

SAUCE
Apple	20
Bread	36
Cranberry	34
Horseradish	26
Mint	21

SAUSAGE
& Yorkshire Pudding, Kids Menu	274
Pigs, In Blankets	520

SAUSAGE & MASH
Bangers, with Gravy	1182

SOUP
Of The Day, with Bread	263
Tomato, with Wholemeal Bread, Kids Menu	232

SPONGE
Treacle	482
Treacle, with Custard	572
Treacle, with Ice Cream	617
Treacle, with Whipped Cream	852

TOBY CARVERY

SPROUTS
	KCAL
Side	26

STUFFING
Sage, & Onion	73

SUNDAE - CHOCOLATE BROWNIE
Kids Menu	353

SUNDAE - ICE CREAM
Munchies, Chocolate, & Caramel Sauce, Sharing	1020
Munchies, Chocolate, & Caramel Sauce	582

SUNDAE - ICE CREAM, CHOCOLATE BROWNIE
Sensation	675

SUNDAE - ICE CREAM, HONEYCOMB
Toffee, Fudge, & Chocolate Sauce	509

SUNDAE - ICE CREAM, PEACH MELBA
Raspberries, with Demarara Crumb, Sharing	742
Raspberries, with Demerara Crumb	535

SWEDE
Side	20

SWEETCORN
Side	61

TART
Lemon, Creamy, with Strawberries, Whipped Cream	596
Pepper, & Pomegranate	520
Portabello, Bulls-eye	522

TERRINE
Pork, Apple, & Cider	369

TOAD IN THE HOLE
Main	463

TURKEY
Roast, Kids Menu	126
Roast, King Size	337
Roast	253

VEGETABLES
Sticks, & Cheesy, BBQ, Dip, Kids Menu	103

WELLINGTON
Carrot, & Chickpea, Spiced	749

YORKSHIRE PUDDING
with Ice Cream, Kids Menu	425

URBAN EAT

APPLES
& Grapes	46

BAGEL
New York Deli Style Pastrami & Emmental Cheese	385

CROISSANT
Gammon Ham, Emmental Cheese & Tomato	369
Ham & Cheese	369
Tomato, Mozzarella Cheese & Baby Spinach	368

FRUIT
Classic Salad Pot	68
Grape Pot	96
Melon & Grape Pot	80
Pineapple Chunks Pot	69

URBAN EAT

HOUMOUS

& Crudites, Snack Pot	110

PANINI

All Day Breakfast Ciabatta	521
Bacon & Hash Brown	639
Brie & Caramelised Onion, Ultimate	483
Cheese & Tomato	471
Chicken Fajita	503
Chicken Fajita Ciabatta	498
Christmas Dinner	594
Ham & Cheese	448
Mozzarella & Slow Roast Tomato	439
Three Cheese & Slow Roasted Tomato Ciabatta	431
Tuna Melt	406
Tuna Melt Ciabatta	397

PASTY

Beef	704

ROLL

Bacon	411

SALAD

Chicken Caesar	332
Oriental Prawn Noodle with Mango, Ultimate	217
Pasta, Cheese & Tomato	612
Pasta, Chicken & Bacon	503
Pasta, Chicken with Tomato & Basil	202
Pasta, Tuna & Sweetcorn, Basic	378
Ultimate Tabbouleh & Roast Vegetable	414

SANDWICH - ALL DAY BREAKFAST

on White	508
on White	368

SANDWICH - BACON

Bap, Breakfast	413

SANDWICH - BEEF

& Horseradish, on White Bread	377
& Horseradish, Rare, Scottish	373

SANDWICH - BLT

on Malted Wheat	485
on Malted Wheatgrain	444

SANDWICH - CHEESE

Mature Cheddar, & Onion Salad, Bap	668
Cheddar, & Soft, & Red Onion Relish, GF Roll	485
Cheddar, Ploughman's, on Malted Wheatgrain	450
Brie, & Cranberry, on Softgrain	399
Cheddar, & Tomato, on White, Halal	332
Roll, Cheddar	351
Sub, Mature Cheddar, Spring Onion, & Tomato	710
Mozzarella, Tomato, & Pesto, on Malted Wheatgrain	404
Two Cheese, & Onion	456

SANDWICH - CHICKEN

& Mayo, with Salad, Bap	556
Bombay, on Malted Wheatgrain	417
& Bacon, Dijon Mustard Mayo, Malted Wheatgrain	398
Coronation, on Malted Wheatgrain	436

URBAN EAT

SANDWICH - CHICKEN

& Bacon, on Malted Wheatgrain	530
& Slow Roasted Tomato, in a GF Roll	498
& Stuffing, on White	497
& Sweetcorn, on Malted Wheatgrain	422
& Bacon, with Avocado, on Malted Wheatgrain	485
Mayo, on Malted Wheatgrain	466
with Tomato & Salad Leaf on Malted Wheatgrain	245
Tikka, Yoghurt & Mint Dressing, Malted Wheatgrain	372
Mayo, & Sweetcorn, on Malted Wheatgrain, Halal	431
Roll, Pesto, & Slow Roasted Tomato	331
& Salad, on Malted Wheatgrain	380
Roll, with Mayo	383
Sub, with Bacon, & Mayonnaise	667

SANDWICH - CRAYFISH

& Rocket, with Lemon Mayo, on Malted Wheatgrain	332

SANDWICH - EGG

& Spinach, on Wheatgrain, Vegetarian	374
& Cress, on Malted Wheatgrain	327

SANDWICH - EGG MAYONNAISE

on White Bread, No Fuss	306
& Bacon, on Malted Wheatgrain	276
& Bacon, on White	369
Roll	325

SANDWICH - FALAFEL

Falafel, with Lemon & Coriander Houmous	341

SANDWICH - GAMMON

with Cheddar Cheese, & Pickle, on Softgrain	384
& English Mustard Mayo	299
& English Mustard Mayonnaise, on White	319
& Tomato Salad, on Malted Wheatgrain	247
Sub, & Salad	438

SANDWICH - HAM

& Mustard Mayo, on White	299
Roll, Smoked	278

SANDWICH - HOUMOUS

& Roast Vegetables, on Malted Wheatgrain	289

SANDWICH - PASTRAMI

& Monterey Jack Cheese, New York Deli Style	398

SANDWICH - PRAWN MAYONNAISE

on Oatmeal	439

SANDWICH - SALMON

Smoked, Cucumber & Dill Mayo, Malted Wheatgrain	410
& Soft Cheese, Smoked, on Oatmeal	304

SANDWICH - SAUSAGE

Cumberland, Bap, Breakfast	420
& Red Onion Chutney, on Softgrain	416

SANDWICH - TUNA

& Salad, on Malted Wheatgrain	302

SANDWICH - TUNA MAYONNAISE

& Sweetcorn, on White, Halal	390
Roll	386
& Cucumber, on Softgrain	423

URBAN EAT

SANDWICH - TUNA MAYONNAISE
& Sweetcorn, on White	266

SANDWICH - TURKEY
Sub, Turkey Feast	698
Turkey Feast	448

SANDWICH - VEGETARIAN
Vegetarian, Triple Pack	678

SLICES
Chicken & Bacon	506
Spicy Chicken	502

TOASTIE
Irish Mature Cheddar & Tomato on White	333

WRAP
Brie, Festive	551
Chicken, with Caesar Mayonnaise	647
Chicken Fajita, with Tomato Salsa	423
Shredded Duck, with Hoisin Sauce	446
Spicy Bean, Hot	524
Egg, Ultimate Bombay, with Salsa, Wholemeal	534

YOGHURT
Granola & Blueberry Compote	218
Granola & Strawberry Compote	218

WAGAMAMA

BANANA
Katsu, & Caramel Ice Cream	312

BEANS
Edamame, with Chilli	280
Edamame, with Salt	280

BEEF
Tataki, Chilled	165
Teriyaki, & Rice, Donburi	973

BROCCOLI
& Bok Choi, Wok-Fried	181

BUNS
Beef, Korean BBQ, & Red Onion, Steamed, Hirata	354
Chicken, Crispy, & Tomato, Steamed, Hirata	464
Mushroom, & Panko Aubergine, Steamed, Hirata	385
Pork, Belly, & Panko Apple, Steamed, Hirata	550

CAKE
Chocolate, Layer, & Ice Cream	485

CAULIFLOWER
Bang Bang	480

CHEESECAKE
Coconut, & Fig	394
White Chocolate, & Ginger	455

CHICKEN
Crispy, with Sesame, & Soy Sauce, Tori Kara Age	440
Grilled, & Soba Noodles, Kids Menu	419
Katsu, Breaded, & Sticky Rice, Amai Sauce, Kids	496
Katsu, Breaded, & Sticky Rice, Curry Sauce, Kids	496
Katsu, Grilled, & Sticky Rice, Amai Sauce, Kids	445
Katsu, Grilled, & Sticky Rice, Curry Sauce, Kids	445
Rice, Egg, Stir Fry, Cha Han, Kids Menu	433

WAGAMAMA

CHICKEN
Teriyaki, & Rice, Donburi	784

CHILLI
Side	2

COD
Cubes, Breaded, & Sticky Rice, Amai Sauce, Kids	610
Cubes, Breaded, & Sticky Rice, Curry Sauce, Kids	610

CURRY
Chicken, & White Rice, Raisukaree	1371
Chicken, & White Rice, Samla	1135
Chicken, Firecracker, & Steamed Rice	1229
Chicken, Katsu, & Sticky Rice	1145
Prawn, & White Rice, Raisukaree	1282
Prawns, Firecracker, & Steamed Rice	1110
Tofu, & Mushrooms, Yasai Samla	1108
Vegetable, Katsu, & Sticky Rice	1174

DESSERT
Mango, Spiced, & Coconut, Parfait	299

DUCK
Grilled, Teriyaki, with Rice, Donburi	1133
Lettuce, Wraps	339
Wrap, with Cucumber, & Hoisin Sauce	451

DUMPLINGS
Chicken, Steamed, Gyoza	223
Duck, Fried, Gyoza	377
Pork, Pulled, Steamed, Gyoza	236
Prawn, Fried, Gyoza	232
Yasai, Steamed, Gyoza	210

EGGS
Tea Stained, Side	94

FISH
White, Grilled, with Soba Noodles, Kids Menu	353

ICE CREAM
Caramel, Salted	496
Chocolate, & Shichimi	393
Coconut, Passion Fruit Sauce, & Coconut Flakes	449
Coffee, Vietnamese	471
Vanilla, Pod, Kids Menu	137
Yuzu	251

ICE LOLLY
Fruit, & Berry, Kids Menu	83

JUICE
Blueberry, Spice	193
Carrot	72
Fruit	146
Green, Clean	174
Green, Super	128
Orange	110
Positive	159
Power	160
Raw	97
Repair	188
Tropical	167

WAGAMAMA

KIMCHI
Side	18

NOODLES
Plain, Side	323

NOODLES - BEEF
Short Rib, Bone In, Ramen	1097
Steak, Sirloin, Chilli, Ramen	665
Steak, Sirloin, Teriyaki, Soba, Teppanyaki	813
Steak, Bulgogi, Soba, Omakase	778

NOODLES - CHICKEN
& Prawn, Pad-Thai, Teppanyaki	741
& Prawn, Yaki Soba, Teppanyaki	715
& Prawn, Yaki Udon, Teppanyaki	744
Coconut & Lemongrass Soup, Itame	820
Ginger, Udon, Teppanyaki	767
GF, Ramen	513
Grilled, Chilli, Ramen	590
Grilled, Ramen, Kids Menu	368
Grilled, Ramen	476
Pork, Prawns, & Mussels, Wagamama, Ramen	686
Soba, Teppanyaki, Kids Menu	374

NOODLES - DUCK
Grilled, Ramen	990

NOODLES - LAMB
Teriyaki, Soba, Omakase	890

NOODLES - PORK
Belly, Shirodashi, Ramen	959

NOODLES - PRAWN
Coconut & Lemongrass Soup, Itame	718

NOODLES - SALMON
Grilled, Teriyaki, Soba, Teppanyaki	803

NOODLES - SEAFOOD
GF, Ramen	821
Ramen	821

NOODLES - TOFU
& Vegetable, Pad-Thai, Teppanyaki	831
& Vegetables, Soba, Teppanyaki, Kids Menu	396
Vegetable Broth, Kare Burosu	629
Vegetable, Coconut Lemongrass Soup, Yasai Itame	842
Yasai Pad-Thai	765

NOODLES - VEGETABLE
Yasai, Ramen, Kids Menu	324
Yasai Yaki Soba, Teppanyaki	696
Yasai Yaki Soba	564

OMELETTE
Shiitake Mushroom, & Broccoli, with Rice, Donburi	725

PICKLE
Japanese, Side	30

PORK BELLY
in Breadcrumbs, & Sticky Rice, Tonkatsu, Omakase	1033
Sticky, with Miso Aubergine, Omakase	1394

PRAWNS
in Breadcrumbs, Crispy, Chilli Sauce, Ebi Katsu	298

WAGAMAMA

PRAWNS
Skewers, Lollipop, Kushiyaki	142

RIBS
Pork, Korean BBQ	698

RICE
Brown, Side	543
Steamed, Side	543
Sticky, Side	543

SALAD
Beef, Sirloin, & Shiitake Mushrooms	434
Chicken, & Prawn, Pad-Thai	342
Chicken, Chilli, Warm	487
Raw	108
Tofu, Chili, Warm	502

SORBET
Lemongrass, & Lime	152
Lemongrass, & Lime	152
Pink Guava, & Passionfruit	162

SOUP
Miso, & Japanese Pickles, Side	66

SQUID
Chilli	534

TART
Yuzu, & Lemon	306

TOFU
Rice, Egg, Stir Fry, Cha Han, Kids Menu	454

TUNA
Steak, Seared, with Quinoa, Omakase	522

VEGETABLES
Katsu, Breaded, & Sticky Rice, Amai Sauce, Kids	468
Katsu, Breaded, & Sticky Rice, Curry Sauce, Kids	468

WASABI CO LTD

BEEF
Sukiyaki Don	758

CHICKEN
Karaage, Side Dish	156
Karaage	468
Spicy, Don	819
Sweet Chilli	1078
Sweet Chilli Don	991
with Spicy Sauce	402
Yakitori, Fried	544
Yakitori, Side Dish	65

CHICKEN KATSU
Curry, Bento	923
Curry, Katsu Don	1136
Curry	614
Fried	285
Original	113
Yakisoba Bento Box	629

CHICKEN TERIYAKI
Don	732
Original	343

WASABI CO LTD

CURRY

Chicken	632
Tofu	689

DUMPLINGS

Gyoza, Chicken, Fried	15
Gyoza, Chicken, Steamed, Side Dish	43
Gyoza, Chicken, Steamed	8

JAHANG

Chicken	801
Tofu	693

NOODLES

Chicken Gyoza, Soumen	550
Stir Fry, Chicken Katsu Yakisoba	710
Stir Fry, Chicken Yakisoba	829
Stir Fry, Tofu Yakisoba	723

PRAWNS

Fried, Don	666
Tempura, Fried	93
Tempura, Side Dish	38
Tempura, Tanmen	1430

RICE

Side	528

SALMON

Fried	617

SOUMEN

Salmon	700
Spicy Chicken	556
Veg	334

SOUP

Miso, Bonito Stock	51
Miso, Sachet	1
Miso, Vegetarian	51

SUSHI

Wasabi Classic, with Chicken Katsu, Set	654
Avocado Hosomaki	55
California Futomaki	51
California Hand Roll	173
Chicken Katsu Salad	671
Chicken Teriyaki Hand Roll	156
Chicken Teriyaki Onigiri	182
Chicken Teriyaki Roll	42
Chirashi Salad, Traditional	632
Chumaki Set	346
Crabmeat & Avocado, Hosomaki	66
Crabmeat Gunkan	66
Cucumber Hosomaki	52
Dragon Roll Set	633
Edamame	154
Fried Prawn Hand Roll	188
Fried Prawn Roll	64
Fuji Set	805
Golden Roll Set	453
Hana Set	782

WASABI CO LTD

SUSHI

Harmony Set	792
Hosomaki Set, Mini	437
Japanese Omelette Nigiri	50
Mini Chirashi Set	122
Mixed Maki Set	521
Nigiri Iroha Set	317
Prawn Mayo Gunkan	81
Pumpkin Croquette Salad Set	730
Rainbow Set	664
Salmon & Masago Roll	46
Salmon Hosomaki	71
Salmon Love Set	388
Salmon Nigiri	50
Salmon Nigiri Set	343
Salmon Onigiri	191
Salmon Sashimi Set	211
Sashimi Set	242
Seared Salmon, Nigiri Set	216
Seaweed Onigiri	147
Seaweed Salad Gunkan	47
Shrimp Nigiri	35
Snomono Salad	402
Spicy Chirashi Sushi	705
Spicy Mini Chirashi Set	382
Spicy Salmon Gunkan	96
Spicy Salmon Roll	51
Spicy Yakatori, Set	515
Sunomono Salad Set	402
Sunrise Set	725
Surimi Crabmeat & Cucumber Roll	46
Tofu Nigiri	56
Tofu Roll	43
Tuna & Mustard Onigiri	133
Tuna & Sweetcorn Roll	64
Tuna Hosomaki	50
Tuna Nigiri	42
Veg Set, Mini	392
Wakame Seaweed Salad	60
Wasabi Classic, with Surimi Crabmeat Salad	591
Wasabi Special Bento	669
Yasai Roll Set, Vegetarian	647

TANMEN

Spicy Chicken	473
Veg	997

WIMPY

BACON

Slice, Burger Extra	65

BREAKFAST

All Day	896
Country	347
Hashbrown	408
Sausage, Bacon, & Scrambled Egg, Kids	396

WIMPY

BREAKFAST

	KCAL
Sunrise	335
The Great Wimpy	717

BROWNIES

Chocolate	570

BUNS

Bacon, Brekkie Bites	341
Bacon & Egg, Brekkie Bites	430
Sausage, & Egg, Brekkie Bites	512

BURGERS

Bender, in a Bun	539
Bender, in a Bun, with Cheese	580
Bender, with Chips, Kids	514
Bender, with Salad, Kids	335
Cheese, & Egg, Brekkie Bites	517
Cheese Burger, Double	647
Cheese Burger	433
Cheeseburger, Junior, with Chips, Kids	612
Cheeseburger, Junior, with Salad, Kids	433
Chicken, Fillet, Firecracker Sauce	498
Chicken, Fillet, with Wimpy Mayo	527
Fish Finger	647
Halfpounder, BBQ	974
Halfpounder, Hawaiian	942
Halfpounder, Jalapeno	880
Halfpounder, Original	876
Halfpounder, with Cheese, & Bacon	884
Hamburger	392
Junior, with Chips, Kids	572
Junior, with Salad, Kids	392
Kingsize	821
Mega	873
Open, Chicken, Gourmet	542
Open, Jalapeno	627
Open, Smoky BBQ	725
Quarterpounder, BBQ Bacon	710
Quarterpounder, Club	735
Quarterpounder, Hawaiian	679
Quarterpounder, Jalapeno	616
Quarterpounder, Original	613
Quarterpounder, Patty	264
Quarterpounder, with Cheese, & Bacon, Original	621
Quarterpounder, with Cheese, Original	613

BURGERS VEGETARIAN

Bean, Spicy	542
Mushroom, Open	664
Quorn, Lemon & Pepper	554

CAKE

Chocolate Fudge	522

CHEESE

Grated, Burger Extra	51
Mozzarella, Melts, 4 Melts	260
Slice, Burger Extra	41

WIMPY

CHICKEN

	KCAL
Chunks 123, with Chips, Kids	422
Chunks, with Salad, Kids	243
Platter, Gourmet	531

CHICKEN WITH

Chips, Chunks	745

CHIPS

Reg	267

COFFEE

Americano, Large	12
Americano, Reg	6
Cappuccino, Large	134
Cappuccino, Reg	109
Esspresso	6
Latte, Large	194
Latte, Reg	160
Mocha, Large	303
Mocha, Reg	213

COLESLAW

Side	130

CREAM

Side	72

CUSTARD

Side	125

DOUGHNUTS - BROWN DERBY

with Ice Cream, Chocolate Sauce, & Chopped Nuts	426

DRESSING

Caesar	219
French	60
Wimpy Mayo	199

EGGS

Fried, Burger Extra	90
Fried, on Toast, Brekkie Bites	350
Scrambled, on Toast, Brekkie Bites	304
Scrambled, on Toast, Kids	226

FISH & CHIPS

Cod	783
Scampi	616

FISH FINGERS

with Chips, Kids	359
with Salad, Kids	180

GRILLS

All Day Breakfast	896
Bender Sausage	679
Breakfast Sausage	567
International	1077
Wimpy	856

HASH BROWNS

Extra	98

HOT CHOCOLATE

with Cream, Large	283
with Cream, Reg	202

WIMPY

ICE CREAM

	KCAL
Soft, Portion	159
with Chocolate Sauce, Kids	176
with Strawberry Sauce, Kids	175

ICE CREAM FLOAT

7 Up	182
Pepsi, Diet	96
Pepsi	181
Pepsi Max	96
Tango Orange	135

JELLY

Orange, Pot, Kids	3
Strawberry, Pot, Kids	5

MILK SHAKE

Banana, Ice Cream	236
Banana, Thick	296
Chocolate, Ice Cream	267
Chocolate, Thick	297
Strawberry, Ice Cream	257
Strawberry, Thick	295
Vanilla, Ice Cream	215
Vanilla, Thick	262

MUFFIN

British, Breakfast	404
Hashbrown	404
Sausage, & Hashbrown	502

MUSHROOMS

Burger Extra	133

ONION RINGS

Side, 6 Rings	238

PEAS

Kids	86

PEPPERS

Jalapeno, Burger Extras	2

PINEAPPLE

Extra	40

POTATO FILLING

Bacon	65
Beans, Baked, Heinz	93
Cheese, Grated	171
Coleslaw	148
Mushrooms, Grilldled	133

POTATOES

Jacket, with Butter, & Salad	523

SALAD

Chicken, Breaded	345
Chicken, Gourmet	303
Fish	463
Scampi	376
Side, Kids	8
Side	56

SAUCE

BBQ	40

WIMPY

SAUCE

	KCAL
Chocolate	81
Firecracker	29
Ketchup	30
Mango	29
Maple Flavoured	86
Special	114
Strawberry	80
Wimpy Mayo	100

SAUSAGES

with Chips, Kids	398
with Salad, Kids	219

SMOOTHIE

Mango	233

SPONGE PUDDING

Sticky Toffee, with Cream	589
Sticky Toffee, with Custard	642
Sticky Toffee, with Ice Cream	612
Syrup, with Cream	529
Syrup, with Custard	581
Syrup, with Ice Cream	551

SUNDAE

Brownie	717
Eton Mess	301
Fruit Nut	207
Knickerbocker Glory	374
Rocky Road	396

SYRUP

Caramel, for Coffee	26
Vanilla, for Coffee	27

TEA

Herbal	2
with Milk	23

TEACAKES

Toasted, with Butter	295

TOAST

with Butter, & Jam, 2 Slices	318
with Butter, & Marmalade, 2 Slices	318

TOASTIE

Cheese, & Ham, White	388
Cheese, & Red Onion, White	343
Cheese, & Tomato, White	338
Cheese, with Chips, Kids	474
Cheese, with Salad, Kids	298
Chicken, BBQ, White	475
Hawaiian, White	403

TOPPING

Flake, Crushed, for Drinks	44
Flake	44
Fruit	18
Marshmallows, Mini, for Drinks	32
Marshmallows, Mini	32
Nuts, Chopped	30

WIMPY

TOPPING

	KCAL
Oreo Minis	118
Strawberries	9

TORTE

	KCAL
Apple, with Cream	385
Apple, with Custard	438
Apple, with Ice Cream	408

VEGETABLES

	KCAL
Carrot & cucumber Pot, Kids	24

WAFFLES

	KCAL
Chocolate, with Cream, Kids	402
Chocolate, with Ice Cream, Kids	386
Eskimo, with Chocolate Sauce	746
Eskimo, with Maple Flavoured Syrup	757
Eskimo, with Strawberry Sauce	746

Useful Resources

Weight Loss
Weight Loss Resources is home to the UK's largest calorie and nutrition database along with diaries, tools and expert advice for weight loss and health.
Tel: 01733 345592 Email: helpteam@weightlossresources.co.uk
Website: www.weightlossresources.co.uk

Products to Help You Keep Track
From food diaries to weight graphs and calorie counted recipe books visit the wlr shop.
Tel: 01733 345592 Email: helpteam@weightlossresources.co.uk
Website: www.weightlossresources.co.uk/shop

Dietary Advice
The British Dietetic Association has helpful food fact leaflets and information on how to contact a registered dietitian.
Tel: 0121 200 8080 Email: info@bda.uk.com
Website: www.bda.uk.com

Healthy Eating
The British Nutrition Foundation has lots of in depth scientifically based nutritional information, knowledge and advice on healthy eating for all ages.
Tel: 0207 7557 7930 Email: postbox@nutrition.org.uk
Website: www.nutrition.org.uk

Healthy Heart
The British Heart Foundation provides advice and information for all on all heart aspects from being healthy, to living with heart conditions, research and fundraising.
Tel: 0207 554 000 Email: via their website
Website: www.bhf.org.uk

Cancer Research
Cancer Research UK is the leading UK charity dedicated to research, education and fundraising for all forms of cancer.
Tel: 0300 123 1022 Email: via their website
Website: www.cancerresearchuk.org

Diabetes Advice
Diabetes UK is the leading charity working for people with diabetes. Their mission is to improve the lives of people with diabetes and to work towards a future without diabetes
Tel : 0345 123 2399 Email: info@diabetes.org.uk
Website: www.diabetes.org.uk

Beating Bowel Cancer
Beating Bowel Cancer is a leading UK charity for bowel cancer patients, working to raise awareness of symptoms, promote early diagnosis and encourage open access to treatment choice for those affected by bowel cancer.Tel: 08450 719301   Email: nurse@beatingbowelcancer.org
Website: www.beatingbowelcancer.org

Safety and Standards
The Food Standards Agency is an independent watchdog, set up to protect the public's health and consumer interests in relation to food.
Tel: 0207 276 8829 Email: helpline@foodstandards.gsi.gov.uk
Website: www.food.gov.uk

Feedback

If you have any comments or suggestions about The Calorie, Carb & Fat Bible, or would like further information on Weight Loss Resources, please call, email, or write to us:

Tel:	01733 345592
Email:	helpteam@weightlossresources.co.uk
Address:	Rebecca Walton,
	Weight Loss Resources Ltd,
	2C Flag Business Exchange,
	Vicarage Farm Road,
	Peterborough,
	PE1 5TX.

Reviews for The Calorie Carb & Fat Bible

'What a brilliant book. I know I'll be sinking my teeth into it.'
GMTV Nutritionist Amanda Ursell, BSc RD

'To help you make low-cal choices everyday, invest in a copy.'
ZEST magazine

'There is no doubt that the food listings are extremely helpful
for anyone wishing to control their calorie intake in order to lose
pounds or maintain a healthy weight.'
Women's Fitness magazine

'Useful if you don't want to exclude any overall food groups.'
Easy Living magazine

'Quite simply an astonishing achievement by the authors.'
Evening Post, Nottingham

'The book gives you all the basic information so you can work out
your daily calorie needs.'
Woman magazine

'This is a welcome resource in view of the 'national epidemic of obesity.'

Bryony Philip, Bowel Cancer UK

'The authors seem to understand the problems of slimming.'

Dr John Campion

'Jam-packed with info on dieting, and full to bursting point with the calorie, carbohydrate and fat values of thousands of different foods, it's the perfect weight loss tool.'

Evening Express, Aberdeen

'Excellent resource tool - used by myself in my role as a Practice Nurse.'

Pam Boal, Sunderland

'I recently bought your book called the Calorie, Carb & Fat Bible and would love to tell you what a brilliant book it is. I have recently started a weight management programme and I honestly don't know where I'd be without your book. It has helped me a lot and given me some really good advice.'

Rachel Mitchell

About Weight Loss Resources

weightlossresources.co.uk

"What this does is put you in control with no guilt, no awful groups and no negativity! Fill in your food diary, get support on the boards and watch it fall off!"

LINDAB, Weight Loss Resources Member

How Does It Work?

Weight Loss Resources is home to the UK's biggest online calorie and nutrition database. You simply tap in your height, weight, age and basic activity level - set a weight loss goal, and the programme does all the necessary calculations.

What Does It Do?

The site enables you to keep a food diary which keeps running totals of calories, fat, fibre, carbs, proteins and portions of fruit and veg. You can also keep an exercise diary which adds the calories you use during exercise. At the end of a week, you update your weight and get reports and graphs on your progress.

How Will It Help?

You'll learn a great deal about how your eating and drinking habits affect your weight and how healthy they are. Using the diaries and other tools you'll be able to make changes that suit your tastes and your lifestyle. The result is weight loss totally tailored to your needs and preferences. A method you can stick with that will help you learn how to eat well for life!

Try It Free!

Go to **www.weightlossresources.co.uk** and take a completely free, no obligation, 24 hour trial. If you like what you see you can sign up for membership from £6.95 per month.